Dementia

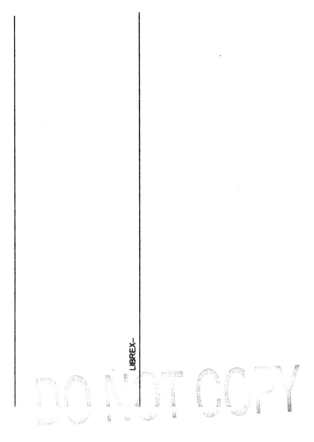

Dementia

Fourth edition

David Ames BA MD FRCPsych FRANZCP
Professor of Ageing and Health
National Ageing Research Institute
University of Melbourne, Parkville, Victoria, Australia

Alistair Burns MPhil MD FRCP FRCPsych
Professor of Old Age Psychiatry
University of Manchester, Manchester, UK

John O'Brien MA DM FRCPsych
Professor of Old Age Psychiatry
Institute for Ageing and Health, Newcastle University
Newcastle upon Tyne, UK

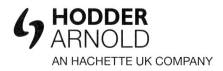
HODDER
ARNOLD
AN HACHETTE UK COMPANY

First published in Great Britain in 1994 by Chapman & Hall
Second edition published in 2000 by Arnold
Third edition published in 2005 by Hodder Arnold
This fourth edition published in 2010 by
Hodder Arnold, an member of Hodder Education, an Hachette UK Company,
338 Euston Road, London NW1 3BH

http://www.hodderarnold.com

Hachette UK's policy is to use papers that are natural, renewable and recyclable products and made from wood grown in sustainable forests. The logging and manufacturing processes are expected to conform to the environmental regulations of the country of origin.

Whilst the advice and information in this book are believed to be true and accurate at the date of going to press, neither the author[s] nor the publisher can accept any legal responsibility or liability for any errors or omissions that may be made. In particular (but without limiting the generality of the preceding disclaimer) every effort has been made to check drug dosages; however it is still possible that errors have been missed. Furthermore, dosage schedules are constantly being revised and new side-effects recognized. For these reasons the reader is strongly urged to consult the drug companies' printed instructions before administering any of the drugs recommended in this book.

British Library Cataloguing in Publication Data
A catalogue record for this book is available from the British Library

Library of Congress Cataloging-in-Publication Data
A catalog record for this book is available from the Library of Congress

ISBN-13   978 0 340 987 278

1 2 3 4 5 6 7 8 9 10

Publisher:	Caroline Makepeace
Project Editor:	Stephen Clausard
Production Controller:	Kate Harris
Cover Designer:	Lynda King
Indexer:	Laurence Errington

Cover image © Cathy Greenblat, www.cathygreenblat.com, from *Love, Loss and Laughter: Seeing Alzheimer's Differently*

Typeset in 9.5 Minion by Macmillan Publishing Solutions, Bangalore - 25
Printed and bound in the UK by MPG Books Ltd

What do you think about this book? Or any other Hodder Arnold title?
Please visit our website: www.hodderarnold.com

Contents

PART II MILD COGNITIVE IMPAIRMENT

PART III ALZHEIMER'S DISEASE

Contributors

Dag Aarsland MD PhD
Psychiatric Clinic, Stavanger University Hospital
Stavanger, Norway

George S Alexopoulos MD
Weill Cornell Medical College
White Plains, NY, USA

Osvaldo P Almeida MD PhD FRANZCP
Western Australian Centre for Health and Ageing, School of
Psychiatry and Clinical Neurosciences and Centre for Medical
Research, University of Western Australia; Department of
Psychiatry, Royal Perth Hospital
Perth, Australia

June Andrews
Iris Murdoch Building, University of Stirling
Stirling, UK

Sylvaine Artero PhD
INSERM U888, Nervous System Pathologies: Epidemiological and
Clinical Research, La Colombière Hospital
Montpellier, France

Clive Ballard MD MB ChB M MedSci MRCPsych
Consultant in Old Age Psychiatry
Wolfson Centre for Age Related Diseases, Guy's Campus
London, UK

Sube Banerjee MB BS MSc MD FRCPsych
Professor of Mental Health and Ageing
The Institute of Psychiatry, King's College London, PO26 Section of
Mental Health and Ageing, Health Service and Population Research
Department
London, UK

Carol Bannister BChB MRCPsych
Consultant in Old Age Psychiatry
The Fiennes Centre
Banbury, UK

Robert Barber FRCPsych MD
Consultant Psychiatrist
Centre for Health of the Elderly, Newcastle General Hospital
Newcastle upon Tyne, UK

Martin M Bednar
Executive Director
Neuroscience Research Unit, Pfizer Global Research and
Development
New London, USA

Alan Bensoussan BSc MSc PhD
Director
National Institute of Complementary Medicine University of
Western Sydney
New South Wales, Australia

German Berrios BA MA DPhilSci MD FRCPsych FBPsS FMedSci
Emeritus Chair of the Epistemology of Psychiatry
Emeritus Consultant and Head of Neuropsychiatry
Life Fellow, Robinson College
University of Cambridge
Cambridge, UK

Konrad Beyreuther
Director of Network Aging Research
University of Heidelberg
Heidelberg, Germany

Michael Bird BA MPsych PhD
Greater Southern Area Health Service
New South Wales, Australia; and
Australian National University
Canberra, Australia

Betty S Black PhD
Department of Psychiatry and Behavioral Sciences
Johns Hopkins University
Baltimore, USA

Stephen C Bowden PhD
Department of Psychology, University of Melbourne
Victoria, Australia

Patricia A Boyle PhD
Rush Alzheimer's Disease Center and Department of Behavioral
Science, Rush University Medical Center
Chicago, IL, USA

Henry Brodaty AO MB BS MD DSc FRACP FRANZCP
Professor, School of Psychiatry
University of New South Wales
Sydney, Australia

Kolbjørn Brønnick PhD
The Norwegian Centre for Movement Disorders, Stavanger
University Hospital
Stavanger, Norway

Richard Brown BSc MRCP MRCPsych
Specialist Registrar in Psychiatry
St Martin's Hospital
Canterbury, UK

Anna Burke MD
Geriatric Psychiatrist/ Dementia Specialist
Banner Alzheimer's Institute
Phoenix, Arizona, USA

E Jane Byrne MB ChB FRCPsych
Senior Lecturer in the Psychiatry of Old Age
School of Medicine, The University of Manchester
Manchester, UK

David Challis BA MSc PhD
Professor of Community Care Research and Director
PSSRU, University of Manchester
Manchester, UK

Dennis Chang MBBS MSc PhD
Centre for Complementary Medicine Research, College of Health
and Science, University of Western Sydney
New South Wales, Australia

Edmond Chiu AM MBBS DPM FRANZCP
Academic Unit for Psychiatry of Old Age, University of Melbourne
St George's Hospital
Melbourne, Australia

Phyllis Chua MB BS Mmed FRANZCP
Academic Unit for Psychiatry of Old Age
University of Melbourne, St George's Hospital
Melbourne, Australia

John Collinge MD FRCP FRCPath FmedSci
MRC Prion Unit and Department of Neurodegenerative Disease
UCL Institute of Neurology
London, UK; and
National Prion Clinic, National Hospital for Neurology and
Neurosurgery
London, UK

Claudia Cooper PhD MRCPsych
Senior lecturer in Psychiatry of Older People
Department of Mental Health Science, Centre for Ageing and
Mental Health Science, University College London
London, UK

Jody Corey-Bloom MD PhD
Department of Neurosciences, University of California San Diego
La Jolla, CA, USA

Sebastian J Crutch PhD CPsychol
Dementia Research Centre
University College London, Institute of Neurology
London, UK

Colm Cunningham
Iris Murdoch Building
Department of Applied Social Science
University of Stirling
Stirling, UK

Marika Donkin BA – Psychology (Hons) GradDipProfEthics
School of Psychiatry, University of New South Wales
Sydney, Australia

Vari Drennan MSc PhD RN RHV
Faculty of Health and Social Care Sciences
St. George's, University of London and Kingston University
London, UK

Rebecca Eastley MRCPsych
Consultant in Old Age Psychiatry
Avon and Wiltshire Mental Health Partnership NHS Trust
Southmead Hospital
Bristol, UK

Klaus P Ebmeier MD
Department of Psychiatry
Warneford Hospital
Oxford, UK

Antigoni Ekonomou PhD
Stem Cell Biology Laboratory/Translational Neuroscience Group
Wolfson Centre for Age-Related Diseases, King's College London
London, UK

Yonas Endale Geda MD MSc
Associate Professor of Neurology and Psychiatry, Alzheimer's
Disease Research Center, College of Medicine, Mayo Clinic
Rochester, MN, USA

Timo Erkinjuntti MD PhD FAAN FAHA
Professor of Neurology
Head of the University Department of Neurological Sciences
University of Helsinki, Head Physician, Department of Neurology
and Memory Resarch Unit, Helsinki University Central Hospital
Helsinki, Finland

Hans Förstl Prof Dr med
Direktor der Klinik und Poliklinik für Psychiatrie und
Psychotherapie, Klinikum rechts der Isar der TU München
München, Germany

Cleusa P Ferri PhD
Section of Epidemiology, HSPR, Institute of Psychiatry King's
College London, London, UK

Nicola Filippini DPhil
FMRIB Centre, University of Oxford, Department of Clinical
Neurology, John Radcliffe Hospital
Oxford, UK

Adam S Fleisher MD MAS
Department of Neurosciences, University of California San Diego
La Jolla, CA, USA; and
Banner Alzheimer's Institute
Phoenix, AZ, USA

Leon Flicker MBBS GDipEpid PhD FRACP
Director
Western Australian Centre for Health and Ageing, Centre for
Medical Research, Western Australian Institute for Medical
Research; and
Professor of Geriatric Medicine
School of Medicine and Pharmacology, University of Western
Australia

Paul T Francis PhD
Professor of Neurochemistry
Wolfson Centre for Age-Related Diseases, King's College London
London, UK

Serge Gauthier MD FRCPC
Director
Alzheimer Disease and Related Disorders Unit, McGill Centre for
Studies in Aging, Douglas Mental Health University Institute,
Professor, Departments of Neurology and Neurosurgery, Psychiatry
Medicine, McGill University
Montreal, Canada

Linda A Gerdner PhD RN FAAN
Consulting Assistant Professor
Stanford Geriatric Education Center, Center for Education in Family
and Community Medicine, Stanford University School of Medicine
Stanford
California, USA

Dilip Ghosh BSc PhD
Centre for Complementary Medicine Research, College of Health
and Science, University of Western Sydney
New South Wales, Australia

Glenda Halliday MD PhD
Neuroscience Research Australia
Randwick, Australia

Harald Hampel MD MSc
Department of Psychiatry, Psychosomatic Medicine and
Psychotherapy, Johann Wolfgang Goethe University
Frankfurt am Main, Germany; and
Chair of Psychiatry, Discipline of Psychiatry
School of Medicine, Trinity College, University of Dublin and Trinity
College Institute of Neuroscience (TCIN) and Trinity Centre for
Health Sciences, The Adelaide and Meath Hospital Incorporating
The National Children's Hospital (AMiNCH)

Tallaght, Dublin, Ireland; and
Department of Psychiatry and Psychotherapy
Ludwig-Maximilian University Munich
Alzheimer Memorial Center, Dementia Research Group
Munich, Germany

John Hodges FMedSci
Prince of Wales Medical Research Institute
Randwick NSW, Australia

John Holmes MA MD MRCP MRCPsych
Leeds Institute of Health Sciences
University of Leeds
Leeds, UK

Jane Hughes MSc BA (Econ) DSW CQSW
University of Manchester
Manchester, UK

Julian Hughes MA MB ChB PhD MRCPsych
Consultant in Old Age Psychiatry and Honorary Professor of
Philosophy of Ageing
Northumbria Healthcare NHS Foundation Trust and Institute for
Ageing and Health, Newcastle University
Newcastle upon Tyne, UK

Steve Iliffe FRCEP FRCP
Professor of Primary Care for Older People
Associate Director, DeNDRoN national co-ordinating centre
Department of Primary Care and Population Sciences, University
College London
London, UK

Paul Ince MD
Professor
Department of Neuroscience, Royal Hallamshire Hospital
Sheffield, UK

Linus Jönsson MD PhD
Vice President
I3 Innovus
Stockholm, Sweden

Jim Jackson MSc
Translational Medicine Programme, University of Edinburgh
Medical School
Edinburgh, UK

Robin Jacoby DM FRCP FRCPsych
Professor Emeritus of Old Age Psychiatry
The University of Oxford, The Warneford Hospital
Oxford, UK

Carmen Janvin Mpsych
Psychiatric Clinic, Stavanger University Hospital
Stavanger, Norway

Raj N Kalaria FRCPath
Professor
Institute for Ageing and Health, Wolfson Research Centre,
Newcastle University, Campus for Ageing and Vitality
Newcastle upon Tyne, UK

Robert E Kelly MD Jr
Weill Cornell Medical College
White Plains, NY, USA

Prof. Dr. Med Alexander F Kurz
Department of Psychiatry and Psychotherapy, Technische
Universität München
München, Germany

Nicola T Lautenschlager MD FRANZCP
Academic Unit for Psychiatry of Old Age
Department of Psychiatry, University of Melbourne, Melbourne
Victoria, Australia; and
School of Psychiatry and Clinical Neurosciences, University of
Western Australia
Perth, Western Australia, Australia

Iracema Leroi MD FRCPC MRCPSYCH
Consultant in Old Age Psychiatry
Lancashire Care NHS Trust, Blackburn, UK; Honorary Senior
Lecturer, Department of Psychiatry, University of Manchester
Manchester, UK

James Lindesay DM MRCPsych
Professor of Psychiatry for the Elderly
Department of Health Sciences, University of Leicester
Leicester, UK

Gill Livingston MD FRCPsych
Professor of Psychiatry of Older People
Department of Mental Health Science, Centre for Ageing and
Mental Health Science, University College London
London, UK

Constantine G Lyketsos MD MHS
Elizabeth Plank Althouse Professor of Psychiatry
School of Medicine and Bloomberg School of Public Health, Johns
Hopkins University; Director of Psychiatry, Johns Hopkins Bayview
Baltimore, MD, USA

Clare E Mackay PhD
Department of Psychiatry
Warneford Hospital
Oxford, UK

David MA Mann BSc PhD FRCPath
Professor of Neuropathology
University of Manchester, Salford Royal Hospital
Salford, UK

Jill Manthorpe MA
SCWRU
Kings College London
London, UK

Colin L Masters MD
Executive Director and Laureate Professor
Mental Health Research Institute
University of Melbourne, Parkville
Victoria, Australia

Maree Mastwyk RN RPN BN
Aged Psychiatry Service
Caulfield Hospital
Caulfield South, Victoria, Australia; National Ageing Research
Institute, Parkville, Victoria, Australia

Ian G McKeith MD BS FRC(Psych) FMed Sci (UK)
Professor of Old Age Psychiatry and Clinical Director
Wolfson Research Centre, Institute for Ageing and Health,
Newcastle University, Campus for Ageing and Vitality
Newcastle upon Tyne, UK

Catriona McLean
Head of Anatomical Pathology
Monash University
Alfred Hospital, Prahran
Victoria, Australia

Stephen L Minger PhD
Senior Lecturer in Stem Cell Biology
Wolfson Centre for Age-Related Diseases, King's College London
London, UK

Bronwyn Moorhouse BApp Sci PhD
Speech Pathologist
Royal Talbot Rehabilitation Centre
Kew, Australia

Emerson Moran
Palm Beach Gardens,
Florida, USA

David Neary MD FRCP
Department of Neurology, Greater Manchester Neuroscience
Centre, Salford Royal Foundation Trust
Salford, UK

Ian Nnatu MB BS MRCPsych Pg Dip(CBT)
Consultant Psychiatrist
West London Mental Health NHS Trust
London, UK

Shirley Nurock MSc
Former Carer; London Area Coordinator of the UK Alzhemer's
Society Quality Research in Dementia (QRD) Network;
Chair, CRAC Dementia (Council of Relatives to Assist
in the Care of Dementia)
London, UK

John O'Brien MA DM FRCPsych
Professor of Old Age Psychiatry
Wolfson Research Centre, Institute for Ageing and Health, Campus
for Ageing and Vitality
Newcastle, UK

Daniel W O'Connor MD FRANZCP
Professor of Old Age Psychiatry
Monash University, Kingston Centre
Cheltenham, Victoria, Australia

Desmond O'Neill MD FRCPI AGSF FRCP (Glasg)
Associate Professor in Medical Gerontology
Trinity College
Dublin, Ireland

Johannes Pantel MD
Department of Psychiatry, Psychosomatic Medicine and
Psychotherapy, Johann Wolfgang Goethe University
Frankfurt am Main, Germany

Ronald C Petersen PhD MD
Professor of Neurology, Cora Kanow Professor of Alzheimer's
Disease Research, Alzheimer's Disease Research Center
College of Medicine, Mayo Clinic
Rochester, MN, USA

Michael Philpot BSc MB BS FRCPsych
Consultant Psychiatrist
Maudsley Hospital
London, UK

Martin Prince MD
Section of Epidemiology, HSPR, Institute of Psychiatry King's
College London
London, UK

Nitin Purandare MBBS DPM MD DGM FRCPsych PhD
Senior Lecturer/ Honorary Consultant in Old Age Psychiatry
Psychiatry Research Group, School of Community Based Medicine,
University of Manchester
Manchester, UK

Peter V Rabins MD MPH
Department of Psychiatry and Behavioral Sciences, Johns Hopkins
Medical Institutions
Baltimore, USA

Ruth Remington PhD ANP GNP-BC
Associate Professor
University of Massachusetts Lowell, School of Health and
Environment, Department of Nursing
Lowell, USA

Craig Ritchie MBChB MRCPsych MSc DLSHTM
Senior Clinical Research Fellow Old Age Psychiatry
Division of Neurosciences and Mental Health, Imperial College
London
London, UK

Karen Ritchie MPsych PhD
INSERM U888, Nervous System Pathologies: Epidemiological and
Clinical Research, La Colombière Hospital
Montpellier, France

Jonathan D Rohrer MRCP
Dementia Research Centre, University College London
Institute of Neurology
London, UK

Gustavo C Román MD FACP FAAN FANA FRSM (Lond)
Medicine/Neurology, UTHSCSA
San Antonio, TX, USA

Martin N Rossor MA MD FRCP FmedSci
Dementia Research Centre, University College London
Institute of Neurology
London, UK

Christopher C Rowe MD FRACP
Department of Nuclear Medicine and Centre for PET, Austin Health
Victoria, Australia; and
Department of Medicine, Austin Health
Victoria, Australia

Greg Savage BSc (Hons) MSc PhD
Research Associate Professor and Clinical Neuropsychologist
Macquarie Centre for Cognitive Science (MACCS)
Macquarie University
Sydney, Australia

Ajit Shah MB ChB MRCPsych
Professor of Ageing
Ethnicity and Mental Health, University of Central Lancashire
Preston, UK; and Consultant Psychiatrist,
West London Mental Health NHS Trust
London, UK

Bindu Shanmugham MD MPH
Medical Director
Palo Alto Veterans Administration Health Care System
Livermore, CA, USA

Sarah Shizuko Morimoto PsyD
Weill Cornell Medical College
White Plains, NY, USA

Taryn C Silber
Summer Undergraduate Research Fellow
Alzheimer's Disease Research Center, College of Medicine
Mayo Clinic
Rochester, USA; and
University of Wisconsin-Madison
Madison, WI, USA

Margie Smith BSc Phd
Senior Scientist of Molecular Pathology
Royal Melbourne Hospital
Melbourne, Australia

Irene Smith Lassen BSc
Physiotherapist
Psychogeriatric Department, Aarhus University Hospital Risskov
Risskov, Denmark

Julie S Snowden PhD
Consultant Neuropsychologist and Honorary Professor of
Neuropsychology
Salford Royal Foundation Trust and University of Manchester
Manchester, UK

John Snowdon MD MPhil FRANZCP FRCPsych FRACP
Jara Unit
Concord Hospital
New South Wales, Australia

Robert Stewart MD MRCPsych
Institute of Psychiatry (King's College London)
London, UK

Elsdon Storey MBBS DPhil FRACP
Van Cleef Roet Centre for Nervous Diseases, Monash University
(Alfred Hospital Campus), Prahran
Victoria, Australia

Joe Stratford MBBS BSc MRCPsych
Consultant Psychiatrist for Older People
Stroud, Gloucestershire, UK

Caroline Sutcliffe BS MSc
University of Manchester
Manchester, UK

Pierre N Tariot MD
Banner Alzheimer's Institute, 901
East Willetta Street, , Phoenix, Arizona, USA

Jennifer Torr MBBS MMed(Psychiatry) FRANZCP
Director of Mental Health, Centre for Developmental Disability
Health Victoria, Monash University
Notting Hill, Victoria, Australia

Anne Unkenstein MA MAPS
Neuropsychologist
Cognitive, Dementia and Memory Service, Royal Park Campus
Royal Melbourne Hospital
Victoria, Australia

Anoop R Varma DM FRCP MD
Consultant Neurologist and Honorary Clinical Lecturer
Greater Manchester Neurosciences Centre, University of
Manchester, Salford Royal and North Manchester General
Hospitals
Salford, UK

Victor L Villemagne MD
Department of Nuclear Medicine and Centre for PET, Austin Health
Victoria, Australia; and
The Mental Health Research Institute of Victoria
Victoria, Australia; and
Department of Medicine, Austin Health
Victoria, Australia

James Warner
St Charles Hospital
London, UK

Jason D Warren PhD FRACP
Dementia Research Centre, University College London
Institute of Neurology
London, UK

Flavie Waters MSc MPsych PhD
Associate Professor
Centre for Clinical Research in Neuropsychiatry, School of
Psychiatry and Clinical Neurosciences, University of Western
Australia, and Older Adult Mental Health Research Unit, Perth
North Metropolitan Area Health Service
Perth, Australia

Alissa Westphal BAppSc Hons GradDipSc
Academic Unit for Psychiatry of Old Age
The University of Melbourne
Melbourne, Australia; Occupational Therapy
Royal Park Campus, Parkville,
Victoria, Australia

Gordon Wilcock DM FRCP (Hon) DSc
Professor of Clinical Geratology,
Nuffield Department of Medicine
University of Oxford
Oxford, UK

Beverley Williams RN RPN Credentialed MH Nurse
Aged Psychiatry Service
Caulfield Hospital, Caulfield South
Victoria, Australia

Robert S Wilson PhD
Rush Alzheimer's Disease Center, Department of Behavioral
Science and Department of Neurological Sciences, Rush University
Medical Center
Chicago, IL, USA

Anders Wimo MD PhD
Alzheimer's Disease Research Center, NCS, Department of
Neurobiology, Care Sciences and Society, Karolinska Institutet
Stockholm, Sweden

Bengt Winblad MD PhD
Alzheimer's Disease Research Center, NCS, Department of
Neurobiology, Care Sciences and Society, Karolinska Institutet
Stockholm, Sweden

Michael Woodward MB BS FRACP
Associate Professor
Aged and Residential Care Services, Heidelberg Repatriation
Hospital
Heidelberg West, Victoria, Australia

Foreword

THERE IS A BRIGHT LIGHT AT THE END OF THE DEMENTIA TUNNEL

The rapid passing of the five years since the publication of the 3rd edition of Dementia has seen many momentous, world changing events impacting on the environment, geo-politics, economy, technology and lifestyle. In this period, population ageing continued inexorably and with it the mounting incidence and prevalence of dementia, especially in low- and middle-income countries such as China and India. Scientific and clinical communities have laboured hard to respond to this challenge; a challenge that policy development and implementation have mostly not kept pace with, being weighed down as they are by ageism, political and bureaucratic inertia.

How then, can a busy clinician keep up with the continuous, voluminous and high quality productivity of our scientific and clinician researchers? David Ames, Alistair Burns and John O'Brien have again rose to this challenge in providing, through this 4th edition of Dementia, a masterful, comprehensive, succinct, relevant, balanced, scholarly and superbly clinician-friendly collection of up-to-date information in the field. They have guided their authors, who are the leaders in their respective fields, to achieve clinical relevance whilst keeping true to the scientific rigor of valid data; translating them to the real world of clinical care and practice. This laudably useful book is the result.

The editors have managed to distil this vast subject into a book of 80 chapters without sacrificing quality – a most remarkable feat of thorough planning and tight editorial management, as would be expected from two editors and one deputy editor of the two major influential Journals in this field!

This edition has at its beginning a carer's lived experience of her journey with her husband through the pathways of dementia – a valued addition to the updated experience of another carer who contributed to the 3rd edition – thus reflecting the humanity and values of the three editors, whose central aim in producing all four editions has been to bring light to the darkness of those affected by dementia. Therefore, the reader now finds many chapters describing the multi-disciplinary and multi-modal management practices and strategies which have emerged in recent times. The inclusion of an evidence-based chapter on vitamins and complementary medicines gives readers answers often asked by the public, and adds much to a holistic view of available treatment.

The very real and exciting scientific advances in genetics, imaging, biomarkers and pharmacological developments have been presented in a readily understandable and relevant manner. Readers will obtain deep and intellectually satisfying knowledge and understandings of these advances to help contribute to their daily tasks of helping people with dementia and their carers.

Whilst amyloid continues to dominate our attention, information about the "other protein", tau, has been placed within many chapters for added relevance and context. Chapters in stem cell therapy, vascular factors, fronto-temporal lobe degenerations and prion diseases add to broader thinking in this field, anticipating future directions in research and therapeutics.

Primary and social care, being the foundations of quality care, continue to have important positions in this edition. Discussions of ethical issues such as end-of-life decision making and relationships with the pharmaceutical industry remind all readers that science and clinical practice should always be firmly set on strong ethical foundations. Anything less diminishes ourselves and those we serve.

Those who may be less familiar with the protean acronyms and abbreviations occupying so much of scientific literature will find a very helpful list to assist them. Extensive references at the end of each chapter will direct those who wish to explore the topic in greater detail to related papers and books.

In reading this edition, readers will gain, if they have not already, a warm sense of optimism to replace the pessimistic gloom and doom of the past that occurred when the subject of dementia was raised in the clinical arena. Even if a cure is not anticipated in this text, it delivers a genuinely Hippocratic message that there is much we can do to help those with dementia and reduce the sufferings associated with it.

This 4th edition is a very worthwhile update on the 3rd edition, and I hope that David, Alistair and John will continue to work for the benefit of their colleagues and for people with dementia and their carers.

Edmond Chiu
Melbourne
August, 2010

Preface to the Fourth Edition

There is an old and probably apocryphal story about a performace of *Il Trovatore* in a provinicial Italian opera house. After a stentorian account of the big aria *di quella pira* had ended in a loudly forced top C, the tenor was generously applauded and encored the piece. After more applause he sang it yet again, but when elements of the audience called for a fourth rendition he put up his hands for silence. 'Friends', he said, 'I would love to sing the aria again for you, but if I do that I will have no more voice for the rest of the performance'. At this point the tones of one of the highly knowledgeable *loggionisti* rang out from the *seconda galleria* 'You will sing it until you get it right!'. After four goes at *Dementia* we are starting to hope that if it isn't yet right it is at least getting close!

When Hodder received our proposal of a fourth edition they commissioned a number of reviewer reports to assess whether there would indeed be any demand for a new edition and, if so, what form it should take. These reviewers and others who wrote about the third edition for various periodicals seemed to agree on a number of things. Some of them berated us for not including mention of Tom Kitwood and person centred care in the third edition (which was odd because if you look carefully he and it *are* indeed mentioned), there was a consensus that the numbering of subchapters in previous editions was a little confusing, and everyone seemed to think that the large section on dementia services in numerous countries had passed its use-by date and could now be retired. More than one reviewer felt that the third edition contained more about transgenic mice than some people wanted to know (i.e. anything!). We were very encouraged that another reviewer noted that the third edition had a notable lack of typographical errors and inaccurate references (clearly due to AB's obsessional checking of each line of text). While agreeing that a new edition would be timely, various reviewers encouraged us to include additional emphasis on the overlap of vascular and primary causes of dementia, prevention of dementia, a template for national service models, enhanced information about the management of behaviours of concern, care of those with dementia in acute hospitals, complementary therapies, music therapy and the relationship between health practitioners and the pharmaceutical industry. 'Go for it', said Hodder, 'and by the way could you please shave 100 pages off the length of the book'.

Most of the planning for this edition was then done over beer at a Chicago hotel during the 2008 International Conference on Alzheimer's Disease. Out went the national service chapters, the transgenic mice and some other esoteric topics. It was agreed that there would be no subchapters, but that each chapter would stand as a complete entity in its own right, though the sectional organization of the text would be retained after an overhaul. In came chapters on the lived experience of dementia, emerging techniques of molecular imaging, medical co-morbidity and hospital care, dementia and residential care, a detailed review of research on non-pharmacological management of disturbed behaviour, music therapy, the global challenge of dementia, an exemplary national service model, the relationship between the health professions and the drug industry and complementary therapies. The overlap between vascular and primary degenerative causes of dementia would be emphasized by having its own dedicated section. All but a classic and timeless handful of the remaining chapters have been completely rewritten, usually (but not always) by the authors who wrote them for the third edition. After a lot of discussion we decided not to include a chapter by a person with dementia, not because we don't think the views of people with dementia are important (we do), but because such a chapter would either end up being written largely by that person's carer or else the person's experience and expression of dementia would be highly atypical and hence not necessarily representative of the experience of most people with dementia. The chapter we did commission on the lived experience of dementia also has the advantage of giving a complete picture of one person's entire trajectory from beginning to end of the illness, which, by definition, no living person with dementia could yet offer.

Some people have commented on the rotating order of the editors' names on sequential editions of *Dementia*. This simply reflects the fact that we have taken it in turns to act as lead co-ordinating editor. On this occasion DA did the bulk of the editing while on three months sabbatical leave in London, based at the Imperial College Department of Psychiatry at Charing Cross Hospital, Fulham, in the last quarter of 2009, and while travelling in and around Northern Italy over Christmas/New Year 2009/2010. Thanks are due to Craig Ritchie for facilitating his attachment, to Sheila Mackenzie for clerical support there and to Sara Graham for the loan of her flat, where much of the work was done to the accompaniment of music broadcast by BBC Radio 3. The contribution of *Trenitalia* to the book's genesis should not be underemphasized either. Their complete inability to run a single service used by DA to an on-time schedule over 16 days gave numerous unforeseen extra opportunities for editing, and indeed one chapter was completely edited while an allegedly fast train to Milan was stuck in a tunnel north of Florence! Last we would like to thank our regular secretaries, Lynette Bon, Amanda Gaunt and Anne Maule for their patience and help, Stephen Clausard, Caroline Makepeace, Amy Mulick, Philip Shaw and all former and current staff of Hodder with whom we collaborated for their encouragement and assistance, our chapter authors for their marvellous contributions, and our wives and daughters for tolerating our distraction by the book when we could have been focusing on them.

David Ames, Alistair Burns, John O'Brien
Melbourne, Manchester, Newcastle-upon-Tyne
January 2010

Preface to the Third Edition

It is a pleasure to present the Third Edition of our textbook Dementia. We have found the success of the first and second edition very gratifying but were conscious of the need to justify the publication of a textbook of this size and scope in a field that is developing very rapidly. It is easy to imagine that such a potential dinosaur may quickly become outdated, will sit on shelves, be thought of affectionately but not be of much practical use to anyone.

However, we became convinced by a number of people, fuelled by our own determination, that we could not let a brand name die, and that a third edition was not only possible but might actually be appreciated by some people.

It is trite to say that the field has moved on since the last edition – of course it has. This is not just in the usual areas where one would expect it, i.e. basic science and treatment, but also, reassuringly, in areas such as service development and carer research.

We have kept the format as it was because it seems to work, but have introduced briefer overviews of services in areas throughout the world.

We owe a great thanks to the contributors who, in the main, have kept to time – we know and they know who they are! The publishers at Hodder Arnold, particularly Layla Vandenbergh, have been helpful and we are grateful to Ed Chiu for such a generous foreword. Most of all, our secretaries, Norma Welsh in Newcastle, Marilyn Kemp in Melbourne and particularly Barbara Dignan in Manchester, deserve the biggest thanks. Without their dedication the project would not have been completed.

AB
Manchester, UK
JO'B
Newcastle upon Tyne, UK
DA
Melbourne, Australia

Preface to the Second Edition

In the six years since the first edition of Dementia was published in 1994, advances in our knowledge and understanding of the disorder and its subtypes have proceeded at a truly breathtaking pace. Clearly we have a greater appreciation of the importance of genetic factors in dementia, whilst molecular biology has provided novel insights into possible pathogenic mechanisms. However, great advances have also been made in several other areas that, unfortunately, often receive less prominence than they deserve. For example, major progress has been made in the nosology, classification and diagnosis of the many subtypes of dementia and there are now several important sets of clinical and neuropathological diagnostic criteria published, many of which have already been the subject of prospective validation studies. Several subtypes of dementia that were of arguable significance when the first edition was published, such as dementia with Lewy bodies and frontotemporal dementia, have been recognized as important conditions with great clinical relevance. Concepts of vascular dementia have changed and the notion of multi-infarct dementia has now been replaced by more sophisticated models that recognize the fact that several different types of vascular pathology, not just cortical infarction, can cause dementia. In parallel with better understanding of the many conditions that cause dementia, there is also increasing recognition of the importance of heterogeneity and overlap at clinical, neurochemical and neuropathological levels between different disorders. This particularly applies to the overlap between vascular dementia and Alzheimer's disease. The advent in the last few years of cholinesterase inhibitors has for the first time allowed rational and, at least in some patients, moderately effective treatment of cognitive as well as non-cognitive features of Alzheimer's disease. These drugs may also prove helpful in treating some other subtypes of dementia. Services have improved considerably in many countries, allowing research advances to be directly applied to what must be the main goal, that of improving patient care.

However, we cannot at any level be complacent and clearly there is still a long way to go. Statistics regarding demographic changes abound, though it is a sobering thought that in Western society life expectancy has increased from 45 years in 1901 to 80 years in 2001. Such longevity, combined with the well-recognized increase in prevalence and incidence of dementia with age, will continue to lead to a huge increase in dementia cases over the next 30 years, especially in the developing world. Many problems remain.

We still lack sufficiently accurate *in vivo* diagnostic markers to replace the 'gold standard' of neuropathology. We still need to learn more about aetiological factors and the definitive neurobiological mechanisms that ultimately cause neuronal loss remain elusive. Current therapeutic approaches remain limited and effective disease-modifying and preventive strategies still have to be determined. Despite progress, services in many countries remain underdeveloped and too fragmented to cope with the increase in cases which lies ahead. The socioeconomic burden of dementia remains enormous and will continue to increase. Dementia is one of the major challenges facing all societies in the new millennium and will remain so for the foreseeable future.

This combination of exciting recent progress combined with continued challenges ahead was the major driving force for producing this second edition of Dementia, which has been radically restructured and updated. Several changes will be immediately apparent. First, the layout of the book reflects the richness and diversity of the different subtypes of dementia and, instead of a simple division between Alzheimer's disease and other dementias, there are now separate sections on each of the main causes of dementia. Second, a number of new chapters are included to provide comprehensive coverage of topics such as new diagnostic criteria, rating scales, investigations, neurobiological mechanisms, as well as all aspects of management including psychosocial and psychological approaches. There are too many new chapters to mention them all, but other important topics, such as moral, ethical and legal aspects of dementia, sexuality and current and new therapeutic options, are included. The section on services has been expanded to include more contributions from Europe as well as from China, South and Central America, the former Soviet Union and services for younger people with dementia. The inclusion of a chapter on Alzheimer's Disease Societies and Associations is a measure of the influence that these have had worldwide in supporting patients, carers and researchers. Dementia with Lewy bodies, increasingly recognized as the second main cause of degenerative dementia, is given prominent coverage with four new chapters. The section on focal dementias includes frontotemporal dementia, Pick's disease, semantic dementia and progressive aphasia and allows readers to observe the different approaches that can be used to define and understand such disorders. Overall, 17 new chapters are included whilst other chapters have been updated and, in most cases, entirely rewritten.

In choosing our authors, we have deliberately sought to try to achieve a balance between retaining sufficient authors from the first edition to provide some continuity whilst including some new contributors. We have also deliberately sought an authorship to reflect a mixture of those who are already internationally renowned experts and those whom we consider to be the rising stars of the future.

This second edition was commissioned by Chapman and Hall, who published the first edition, and has subsequently been published by Arnold, a member of the Hodder Headline Group. We are indebted to all who have been involved in the production of this book, including Peter Altman of Chapman and Hall, who was responsible for the first edition, Georgina Bentliff, Catherine Barnes and Sarah De Souza of Arnold and to our secretaries (Norma Welsh, Yvonne Liddicoat, Barbara Dignan) for their great efforts and help. We are also deeply grateful to Edmond Chiu for his generous Foreword and to Professor Elaine Murphy for providing the Epilogue. Most of all, we thank all our authors who found the time to produce such excellent chapters and upon whose efforts the success of this book will ultimately rely. Our aim was to produce fully comprehensive and up-to-date coverage of all aspects of dementia within a single text, which would prove accessible to clinicians, researchers and allied professional groups. As before, we leave you, our readers and reviewers, to judge the extent to which this aim has been achieved.

John O'Brien, David Ames, Alistair Burns
Newcastle upon Tyne, Melbourne,
Manchester, April 2000

Preface to the First Edition

It was with some trepidation that we decided to edit a large textbook on dementia. There are, and will continue to be, many texts on dementia and one has to consider critically the need for another. Dementia is one of the major challenges to face society in the twentieth century, numerically dwarfing other disorders which have caught the public's imagination. The attraction of being involved in this venture is that it attempts to encompass, in a single volume, all aspects of all types of dementia. However hard we have tried we could obviously not succeed in this and someone somewhere will complain we have omitted something important. In addition, this is a field which is expanding rapidly and we have tried therefore to concentrate on a solid core of information, which although requiring some updating in the future is likely to remain part of the mainstream view of the field.

We have divided the book into two parts, the first dealing with Alzheimer's disease and the second with other dementias. We recognize that this will be considered by many to be a false dichotomy and we accept that criticism. However, from an organizational point of view, some form of order was necessary and we hope this makes sense. Overlap between chapters is a difficult issue and while we have exercised the editorial Tippex to the best of our ability, some duplication remains. However, much of this is intentional and some chapters would have been denuded unnecessarily and could not have stood alone. Areas where we have unashamedly fostered such overlap include Chapters 7 and 8, Chapters 12 and 13 and Chapters 46 and 51. We feel this is a way of encouraging debate about contentious subjects as well as avoiding undue artistic tantrums.

We have been lucky in our choice of authors, the vast majority of whom have delivered their manuscripts on time and without much persuasion. To them, we give thanks, and to our recalcitrant contributors we heave a sigh of relief that we received their submissions at all. We are indebted to Annelisa Page and Peter Altman of Chapman & Hall for their tireless support and to our secretaries for their help. We also thank Professor Alwyn Lishman for his generous foreword.

We hope that our efforts have not been wasted and will leave you, the readers and reviewers, to judge.

AB
Manchester
RL
London

Acknowledgements and disclaimers

Christopher Rowe and Victor Villemagne, the authors of chapter 13, acknowledge that this work was supported in part by grant 509166 of the National Health and Medical Research Council of Australia, the Austin Hospital Medical Research Foundation, and Neurosciences Victoria.

Steve Illiffe, Jill Manthorpe and Vari Drennan, the authors of chapter 17, have received financial support from the Department of Health National Institute for Health Research (DH/NIHR) Programme Grants for Applied Research funding scheme for the EVIDEM (evidence-based interventions in dementia) programme 2007–2012. The views and opinions expressed in chapter 17 do not necessarily reflect those of the DH/NIHR.

Michael Bird (chapter 24) gratefully acknowledges, first, the support of the Australian Government Department of Health and Ageing, Office for Older Australians, who funded some of the research reported in this chapter. Second, profound thanks are due to all the people with dementia, their families and residential aged care nursing staff, who participated in the clinical interventions described and so generously assisted in providing research data. Third, he thanks Esme Moniz-Cook, who contributed some of the material here. Finally, thanks to Katrina Anderson, who assisted in preparation of this chapter.

An earlier version of chapter 35 was presented at the 4th International Colloquium of the International Association of Catholic Bioethicists in Cologne (2009). Julian Hughes is grateful to the organizers for permission to use the modified material. He is also grateful to Dr Stephen Louw for the stimulus he has given to the thoughts expressed in this chapter.

The authors of chapter 38 thank Dr Nori Graham for comments provided on a draft of the chapter.

The preparation of chapter 44 was supported by U01 AG06786, P50 AG016574, K01 MH068351, Robert H. and Clarice Smith and Abigail Van Buren Alzheimer's Disease Research Program & Harold Amos Medical Faculty Development Program (RWJ foundation).

Chapter 49 was originally written by Peter Lantos and Nigel Cairns and appeared as chapter 37 in the second edition of Dementia. It was updated by Colin Masters for the third edition and this fourth edition.

Johannes Pantel and Harald Hampel (chapter 53) wish to thank Ms Yvonne C Hoessler for valuable technical assistance with preparing the manuscript.

Sebastian Crutch (chapter 72) was supported by an Alzheimer's Research Trust Fellowship.

Flavie Waters, co-author of chapter 75, is supported by a National Health and Medical Research Council Australian Research Training Fellowship (404117), and a seeding grant from the Perth (Western Australia) North Metropolitan Area Health Service.

List of abbreviations used

2DE	2D electrophoresis	ANP	atrial natriuretic peptide
5-HT	5-hydroxytryptamine	AOS	apraxia of speech
6-CIT	six item cognitive impairment test	ApoE	apolipoprotein E
AAC	augmentative and alternative communication	APP	amyloid precursor protein
		AR	autosomal recessive
AACD	ageing-associated cognitive decline	ARB	angiotensin II receptor blockers
AAIQOL	Activity and Affect Indicators of Quality of Life	ARC	annual rate of change
		ARCD	age-related cognitive decline
AAMI	age-associated memory impairment	ART	antiretroviral drugs
AAN	American Academy of Neurology	ASHA	American Speech-Language-Hearing Association
ABCD	Arizona Battery for Communication Disorders of Dementia		
		ASL	arterial spin labelling
ABS	Agitated Behaviour Scale	AT1	angiotensin II type 1
ACA	amyloid (congophilic) angiopathy	ATA	atmospheres absolute
ACC	anterior cingulate cortex	Aβ	amyloid-β
ACE	angiotensin I-converting enzyme	BACE	β-secretase
ACE-I	angiotensin-converting enzyme inhibitors	BADS	Behavioural Assessment of the Dysexecutive Syndrome
ACE-R	Addenbrooke's Cognitive Examination – Revised	BASQID	Bath Assessment of Subjective Quality of Life
ACh	acetylcholine		
AChE	acetylcholinesterase	BAT	body awareness therapy
AChEI	acetylcholinesterase inhibitor	BBB	blood–brain barrier
AD	Alzheimer's disease	BChE	butyryl cholinesterase
ADAS	Alzheimer's Disease Assessment Scale	BD	Binswanger disease
ADAS-cog	Alzheimer's Disease Assessment Scale – cognitive subscale	BDNF	brain-derived neurotrophic factor
		BDS	Blessed Dementia Scale
ADC	AIDS dementia complex; apparent diffusion coefficient	BECCA	Befriending and Costs of Caring
		BEHAVE-AD	Behavioural Pathology in Alzheimer Disease Rating Scale
ADCS	Alzheimer's disease Cooperative Study		
ADCS-ADL	Alzheimer's Disease Cooperative Study Activities of Daily Living Scale	BIBD	basophilic inclusion body disease
		BIMCT	Blessed Information-Memory-Concentration Test
ADED	Association of Driver Rehabilitation Specialists		
		BLA	Barnes Language Assessment
ADFACS	AD Functional Assessment and Change Scale	BMT	behavioural management techniques
		BNT-2	Boston Naming Test – 2
ADI	Alzheimer's Disease International	BOLD	blood oxygen level dependent
ADL	activities of daily living	BP	blood pressure
ADM	adrenomedulline	BPRS	Brief Psychiatric Rating Scale
ADNI	AD Neuroimaging Initiative	BPSD	behavioural and psychological psychiatric symptoms of dementia
ADQOL	Alzheimer's disease-related Quality of Life		
AE	adverse events	BRSD	CERAD Behavioral Rating Scale for Dementia
AEP	auditory evoked potential		
AES	Apathy Evaluation Scale	BSB	bromostyrylbenzene
AF	atrial fibrillation	BSE	bovine spongiform encephalopathy
AHEAD	assessment of health economics in Alzheimer's disease	BSF	benign senescent forgetfulness
		bvFTD	behavioural variant of frontotemporal dementia
AL	assisted living		
ALD	adrenoleukodystrophy	BVMT-R	Brief Visuospatial Memory Test – Revised
aMCI	amnestic mild cognitive impairment	CA	conversational analysis; cost analysis
AMTS	Abbreviated Mental Test Score	CAA	cerebral amyloid angiopathy
ANI	asymptomatic neurocognitive impairment	CADL	community activities of daily living

CAM	complementary and alternative medicine
CAMCOG	Cambridge Cognitive Examination
CAMDEX	Cambridge Examination for Mental Disorders in the Elderly
cAMP	cyclic AMP
CANTAB	Cambridge Neuropsychological Test Automated Battery
CAS	Caregiver Activity Survey
CATIE-AD	Clinical Antipsychotic Trial of Intervention Effectiveness-AD
CATS	Caregiver Activities Time Survey
CBA	cost benefit analysis
CBD	corticobasal degeneration
CBF	cerebral blood flow
CBS	Cornell–Brown Scale
CBS	corticobasal syndrome
CCA	cost consequence analysis
CCB	calcium channel blockers
CCOHTA	Canadian Health Technology Assessment Guidelines for Pharmacoeconomics
CCSMA	Cache County Study of Memory in Aging
CD	Cost description
CDR	Clinical Dementia Rating
CDR-SB	Sum of Boxes of the Clinical Dementia Rating
CEA	cost effectiveness analysis
CERAD	Consortium to Establish a Registry for Dementia
CgA	chromogranin A
CGI	Clinical Global Impression
CGIC	Clinical Global Impression of Change
ChAT	choline acetyltransferase
ChEI	cholinesterase inhibitor
CHO	choline-containing compounds
CHS	Cardiovascular Health Study
CI	confidence interval
CIBIC	Clinician's Interview-Based Impression of Change
CIBIC-plus	Clinician's Interview-Based Impression of Change (plus caregiver input)
CILQ	Cognitively Impaired Life Quality Scale
CIND	Cognitive Impairment No Dementia
CJD	Creutzfeldt–Jakob disease
CLB	cortical Lewy bodies
CM	calming music
CMA	cost minimization analysis
CMAI	Cohen–Mansfield Agitation Inventory
CNS	central nervous system
CNV	contingent negative variation
COI	cost of illness
COME	catechol O-methyltransferase
COMFI	Communication Outcome Measure of Functional Independence
Cox	cyclooxygenase
CPA	cyproterone acetate
CQLI	caregiver quality of life index
CRE	creatine/phosphocreatine

CRP	C-reactive protein
CRV	cerebroretinal vasculopathy
CSDD	Cornell Scale for Depression in Dementia
CSF	cerebrospinal fluid
CSI-D	Community Screening Interview for Dementia
CST	cognitive stimulation therapy
CT	computed tomography
CTX	cerebrotendinous xanthomatosis
CUA	cost utility analysis
CVAE	cerebrovascular adverse events
CVD	cerebrovascular disease
CVLT-II	California Verbal Learning Test – Second edition
CYP	cytochrome P450
CysC	cystatin C
DAD	Disability Assessment in Dementia
DADL	domestic activities of daily living
DALY	disability adjusted life year
DASH	Dietary Approaches to Stop HT
DB	double blind
DCLB	dementia associated with cortical Lewy bodies
DCM	dementia care mapping
DD	depressive dementia
DDPAC	disinhibition–dementia–parkinsonism–amyotrophy complex
DES	diethylstilbestrol
DH	Department of Health
DHA	docosahexaenoic acid
DHEA	dehydroepiandrosterone
DHEAS	dehydroepiandrosterone sulphate
D-KEFS	Delis-Kaplan Executive Function System
DLB	dementia with Lewy bodies
DLBD	diffuse LB disease
DLDH	dementia lacking distinctive histology
DLPFC	dorsolateral prefrontal cortex
DMR	Dementia Questionnaire for Persons with Mental Retardation
DN	dystrophic neurites
DqoL	dementia quality of life instrument
DRS	Dementia Rating Scale
DS	Down syndrome
DTI	diffusion tensor imaging
DVLA	Driver and Vehicle Licencing Authority
DWI	diffusion-weighted imaging
DWMHI	deep white matter hyperintensities
EADC	European Alzheimer disease consortium
ED	erectile disorder
EEG	electroencephalogram
EFNS	European Federation of Neurological Societies
EM	electron microscopic
EMEA	European Medicines Agency
EMG	electromyography
EOAD	early-onset Alzheimer's disease

EOG	electro-oculography	HCTZ	hydrochlorothiazide
EP	evoked potential	HD	Huntington's disease
EPA	eicosapentaenoic acid	HDL	high density lipoprotein
EPI	Eysenck Personality Inventory	HE	Hashimoto's encephalopathy
EPS	extrapyramidal symptoms	HELP	heparin-mediated extracorporeal LDL/
ERG	electro-retinography; External Reference		fibrinogen precipitation
	Group	HERNS	hereditary endotheliopathy with
ERP	event-related potential		retinopathy, nephropathy and stroke
ERT	enzyme replacement therapies	HIC	high income countries
ESPS 2	Second European Stroke Prevention Study	HICP	Harmonized Indices of Consumer Prices
ESR	erythrocyte sedimentation rate	HIS	Hachinski Ischaemic Score
ET-1	endotheline	HM	hand massage
EVA	Evaluation of Vascular Care in AD	HMPAO	hexamethylpropyleneamine oxime
FA	fractional anisotropy	HOPE	Heart Outcomes Prevention Evaluation
FA	Friedreich's ataxia	HOT	hyperbaric oxygen treatment
FBD	familial British dementia	HPA	hypothalamic–pituitary–adrenal
FDA	Food and Drug Administration	HR	hazard ratio
FDG	fluoro-deoxy-glucose	HRQoL	health related quality of life
FDG-PET	2-[F]fluoro-2-deoxy-D-glucose positron	HRT	hormone replacement therapy
	emission tomography	HT	hypertension
FFI	fatal familial insomnia	HUI	Health Utilities Index
FIRDA	frontal intermittent rhythmic δ activity	HupA	Huperzine A
FLAIR	fluid attenuated inversion recovery	HVLT-R	Hopkins Verbal Learning test – Revised
FLCI	Functional Linguistic Communication	HVR	hereditary vascular retinopathy
	Inventory	HYE	healthy years equivalents
fMRI	functional magnetic resonance imaging	IADL	instrumental activities of daily living
FSH	follicle stimulating hormone	ICA	internal carotid artery
FTD	frontal lobe dementias	ICAM-1	intercellular adhesion molecule-1
FTE	full-time equivalent	ICD	International Classification of Diseases
FTLD	frontotemporal lobar degeneration	ICF	International Classification of Functioning,
FUS	fused in sarcoma		Disability and Health
FvFTD	frontal variant of FTD	ID	intellectual disabilities
GABA	gamma aminobutyric acid	IDE	insulin degrading enzyme
GAG	glycosaminoglycan	IF	intermediate filaments
GBD	Global Burden of Disease	IGF	insulin-like growth factor
GBS	Gottfries–Bråne-Steen	IHA	International Huntington Association
GCA	giant cell arteritis	IHD	ischaemic heart disease
GDNF	glial-derived neurotrophic factor	IL	interleukin
GDS	Global Deterioration Scale; Geriatric	IL-1	interleukin-1
	Depression Scale	IL-6	interleukin-6
GEM	Ginkgo Evaluation of Memory	IMCT	Information Memory Concentration Test
GMS	Geriatric Mental State Schedule	IMIA	individualized music intervention for
GNT	Graded Naming Test		agitation
GP	general practitioner	INS	implantable neurostimulator
GPCOG	general practitioner assessment of	IQ	intelligence quotient
	cognition	IQCODE	Informant Questionnaire for Cognitive
GSK3	glycogen synthase kinase 3		Decline in the Elderly
GSS	Gerstmann–Sträussler syndrome	ISS	Ischemic Stroke System
GWAS	genome-wide association studies	ITT	intent to treat
H_3	histamine-3	IVD	ischaemic vascular dementia
HAART	highly active antiretroviral therapy	KSS	Kearns–Sayre syndrome
HAAS	Honolulu Asia Aging Study	LB	Lewy body
HAD	HIV-associated dementia	LBD	Lewy body dementia
HAND	HIV-associated neurocognitive disorders	LBVAD	LB variant of Alzheimer's disease
HC	Huntington's chorea; healthy controls	LCTF	long-term care facilities
HCHWA-D	hereditary cerebral haemorrhage with	LD	Lafora body disease
	amyloidosis of the Dutch type	LDL	low-density lipoprotein

LE	limbic encephalitis		MSA	multisystem atrophy
LGG	late-onset GM2 gangliosidosis		MSQ	Mental Status Questionnaire
LH	luteinizing hormone		MSS	multisensory stimulation
LHRH	luteinizing hormone releasing hormone		MTA	medial temporal lobe atrophy
LLA	lipid lowering agent		MTHFR	methelenetetrahydrofolate reductase
LLF	late-life forgetfulness		MTI	magnetization transfer imaging
LLT	Location Learning Test		MTL	medial-temporal lobe
LMIC	low and middle income countries		NART	National Adult Reading Test
LOAD	late-onset Alzheimer's disease		NCI	neuronal cytoplasmic inclusion
LOCF	last observation carried forward		NCL	neuronal ceroid lipofuscinosis
LPA	logopenic/phonological aphasia		NFPA	nonfluent progressive aphasia
LRP1	low-density lipoprotein receptor-related protein 1		NFT	neurofibrillary tangle
			NGF	nerve growth factor
LSB	life story books		NGO	non-governmental organization
LTC	long-term care		NHS	National Health Service
LTCF	long-term care facilities		NIA-RI	National Institute on Aging and Reagan Institute
LTD	long-term depression			
LTP	long-term potentiation		NICE	National Institute for Clinical Excellence
mAb	monoclonal antibodies		NIFID	neuronal intermediate filament inclusion disease
MAC	macroangiopathic			
MADRS	Montgomery Åsberg Depression Rating Scale		NII	neuronal intranuclear inclusions
			NIMH	National Institutes of Mental Health
MALS	Maryland Assisted Living Study		NINDS	National Institutes of Neurological Disorders and Stroke
MBI	mild behavioural impairment			
MC	multicentre		NMDA	N-methyl-D-aspartate
MCA	Mental Capacity Act 2005		NMDAR	N-methyl-D-aspartate receptor
MCD	mild cognitive disorder		NMS	neuroleptic malignant syndrome
MCI	mild cognitive impairment		NOS	not otherwise specified
MDRS	Mattis Dementia Rating Scale		NOSGER	Nurses' Observation Scale for Geriatric Patients
MDS	minimum data set			
MEG	magnetoencephalography		NPD-C	Niemann–Pick disease type C
MELAS	mitochondrial encephalomyopathy with lactic acidosis and stroke-like episodes		NPH	normal pressure hydrocephalus
			NPI	Neuropsychiatric Inventory
MERRF	myoclonic epilepsy with ragged red fibres		NPI-NH	Neuropsychiatric Inventory – Nursing Home version
MIC	microangiopathic			
MID	multi-infarct dementia		NS	neuroleptic sensitivity
MLD	metachromatic leukodystrophy		NSAID	non-steroidal anti-inflammatory drug
MMN	mismatch negativity		NSC	neural stem cell
MMSE	Mini-Mental State Examination		NSE	neuronal specific enolase
MNCD	mild neurocognitive disorder		NSF	National Service Framework
MND	motor neurone disease; mild neurocognitive disorder		NSHS	National Sexual Health Strategy
			OAS	Overt Aggression Scale
MNGIE	mitochondrial myopathy, peripheral neuropathy, encephalopathy and gastrointestinal disease		OBRA-87	Omnibus Budget Reconciliation Act, 1987
			OBS	Organic Brain Scale
			OCD	obsessive compulsive disorder
MoCA	Montreal Cognitive Assessment		OOH	out-of-hours
MOSES	Multidimensional Observation Scale for Elderly Subjects		OR	odds ratio
			OT	occupational therapy; occupational therapist
MPA	medroxypreogesterone acetate			
MQ	memory quotient		PA	progressive nonfluent aphasia
MRC	Medical Research Council		PACNS	primary angiitis of the CNS
MRC CFAS	Medical Research Council Cognitive Function and Ageing Study		PADL	personal activities of daily living
			PAP	Psychomotor Activation Program
MRI	magnetic resonance imaging		PAR	population-attributable risk
MRS	magnetic resonance spectroscopy		PAS	periodic acid Schiff
MRT	magnetic resonance tomography		PASAT	Paced Serial Addition Test
MS	multiple sclerosis		PB	processing bodies

PBA-HD	Problem Behaviours Assessment for Huntington's Disease	QoLAD	quality of life-Alzheimer's disease
PC	placebo controlled	QoLAS	Quality of Life Assessment Schedule
PCA	posterior cortical atrophy; personal care attendant	QUALID	Quality of Life in Late Stage Dementia
		QWB	quality of wellbeing
PCD	personal communication dictionaries	QWBS	Quality of Well-being Scale
PCR	polymerase chain reaction	RAGE	receptor for advanced glycation endproducts
PD	Parkinson's disease; personal detractors		
PDD	Parkinson's disease dementia	R-ANOVA	repeated measure analysis of variance
PDE	phosphodiesterase	RBD	REM sleep behaviour disorder
PDE4	phosphodiesterase 4	rCBF	regional cerebral blood flow
PDS	Progressive Deterioration Scale	RCD	respiratory chain diseases
PEG	percutaneous endoscopic gastrostomy	RCFT	Rey Complex Figure Test
PEO	progressive external ophthalmoplegia	RCT	randomized controlled trial
PES-AD	Pleasant Events Schedule-Alzheimer's Disease	REACH	Resources for Enhancing Alzheimer's Carer Health
PET	positron emission tomography	REM	rapid eye movement
PiB	Pittsburgh Compound B	REMSD	REM sleep disorder
PiD	Pick's disease	RNP	ribonuclear protein particles
PKC	protein kinase C	ROI	region of interest
PL	plaques	RPD	rapidly progressive dementia
PLA	progressive logopenic aphasia	RR	relative risk
PNFA	progressive non-fluent aphasia	rs-fMRI	resting state functional magnetic resonance imaging
PoA	power of attorney		
PPA	primary progressive aphasia	RSN	resting state networks
PPAR-γ	perioxisome proliferator-activated receptor-γ	RT	reminiscence therapy
		RUD	Resource Utilization in Dementia
PPF	propentofylline	RUDAS	Rowland Universal Dementia Assessment Scale
PPIC	Profile of Pragmatic Impairment in Communication		
		RVCL	retinal vasculopathy with cerebral leukodystrophy
PPP	purchase power parities		
PPV	positive predictive value	SAH	subarachnoid haemorrhage
PRN	pro re nata	SAI	short latency afferent inhibition
PRoFESS	Prevention Regimen for Effectively Avoiding Second Strokes	SBO	specified bovine offal
		SCAG	Sandoz Clinical Assessment-Geriatric Scale
PROGRESS	Perindopril Protection Against Recurrent Stroke Study	SCE	spontaneous cerebral microemboli
		SCIE	Social Care Institute for Excellence
PrP	prion protein	sCJD	sporadic Creutzfeldt–Jakob disease
PS	presenilin	SCOPE	Study on Cognition and Prognosis in the Elderly
PSCI	post-stroke cognitive impairment		
PSD	post-stroke dementia	SCU	special care units
PSG	polysomnography	SD	semantic dementia
PSP	progressive supranuclear palsy	SDLT	senile dementia of LB type
PSP-P	PSP-parkinsonism	SEAC	Spongiform Encephalopathy Advisory Committee
PST	problem-solving therapy		
PSWC	periodic sharp wave complexes	SF-36	Short Form 36
PT	physiotherapy	SG	standard gamble; stress granules
p-tau	hyperphosphorylated tau protein	SIADH	syndrome of inappropriate antidiuretic hormone secretion
PUFA	polyunsaturated fatty acid		
PVH	periventricular hyperintensities	SIB	Severe Impairment Battery
PWB-CIP	Psychological Well-Being in Cognitively Impaired Persons	SIVD	subcortical ischaemic vascular dementia; small vessel ischaemic subcortical vascular disease and dementia
PWD	people with dementia		
PWI	perfusion-weighted imaging	SKT	Syndrom Kurz test
QALY	quality adjusted life years	SLE	systemic lupus erythematosus
qEEG	quantitive electroencephalography analysis	SLT	speech and language therapist
		SNP	single nucleotide polymorphism
QoL	quality of life	SP	spastic paraparesis; stratum pyramidale

spCJD	sporadic–Jakob disease		VantagE	Vascular Dementia trial studying Exelon
SPECT	single-photon emission computed tomography		VAS	visual analogue scale
			VBM	voxel-base morphometry
SPG	sphenopalatine ganglion		VCAM-1	vascular cell adhesion molecule-1
SPM	statistical parametric mapping		VCI	vascular cognitive impairment
SPMSQ	Short Portable Mental Status Questionnaire		VCI-ND	VCI-no dementia
SR	spaced retrieval		vCJD	Variant Creutzfeldt-Jakob disease
SSEP	somatosensory evoked potential		VE	vasogenic oedema
SSRI	selective serotonin reuptake inhibitor		VEP	visual evoked potentials
STMS	Short test of Mental Status		VGKC	voltage-gated potassium channel
SVD	small vessel disease		VGLUT	vesicular glutamate transporter
SVZ	subventricular zone		VL	viral load
TAR	transactive response		VLCFA	very long chain fatty acids
TAT	thrombin–antithrombin complex		VLDL	very low density lipoprotein
TBSS	tract-based spatial statistics		vMCI	vascular mild cognitive impairment
TD	tardive dyskinesia			
tHcy	total homocysteine		VT	validation therapy
TIA	transient ischaemic attack		WAIS-III	Wechsler Adult Intelligence Scale – Third edition
TIB	trouble indicating behaviour			
TICS	Telephone Interview for Cognitive Status		WCST	Wisconsin Card Sorting Test
TLS	translocation in liposarcoma		WD	Wilson's disease
TMS	transcranial magnetic stimulation		WFN	World Federation of Neurology
TMT	trail-making test		WhD	Whipple's disease
TNF	tumour necrosis factor		WHO	World Health Organization
TNF-α	tumour necrosis factor-α		WIB	well-being or ill-being
ToM	theory of mind		WKS	Wernicke–Korsakoff syndrome
TOMM40	translocase of mitochondrial membrane 40		WM	white matter
tPA	plasminogen activator		WMHI	white matter hyperintensities
TRH	thyrotropin-releasing hormone		WML	white matter lesion
t-tau	total tau protein		WMS-III	Wechsler Memory Scale – Third edition
TTO	time trade-off			
TYM	test your memory test		WTAR	Wechsler Test of Adult Reading
UPDRS	Unified Parkinson's Disease Rating Scale		YLD	years lived with disability
VaD	vascular dementia		YLL	years of life lost
V-ADAS-Cog	Vascular-Alzheimer's Disease Assessment Scale-cognitive subscale		ZRP	zone of reduced penetrance
			α2M	α2-macroglobulin

DEMENTIA: GENERAL ASPECTS

Dementia: historical overview

GERMAN BERRIOS

1.1 INTRODUCTION

All clinical categories, including those pertaining to the dementias, are the result of the coming together in the work of an author of selected behavioural markers, explanatory concepts and terms to refer to them. Complex social and economic variables will determine whether or not the ensuing 'convergence' will last. For reasons that have to do with the rhetoric of science, these social acts are sold to the throng as pure 'scientific acts'. For example, it would be naive to believe that the decision to consider a symptom-cluster such as, for example, 'dementia with Lewy bodies' as a 'new disease' is solely based on the 'discovery' of powerful, ineluctable and replicable correlations (Perry *et al.*, 1996). Given that not all correlations are privileged in this way, and that there is no clear theory linking all the symptoms to each other and to the Lewy bodies themselves, it is not difficult to surmise that such consideration is also driven by social variables. The current model of science as a pure pursuit of truth, however, leaves no space for broader explanations and hence all manner of social variables remain understudied.

This is not a new phenomenon, for the same complex mechanisms operated at the time when Kraepelin constructed the concept of Alzheimer's disease (AD) (Berrios, 1990b). The crucial issue here is that there is nothing wrong with the fact that social forces shape 'scientific facts' and hence contribute to the construction of psychiatric diseases. Indeed, understanding such mechanisms would render psychiatry more complete, the psychiatrist wiser and doctoring more useful to patients. Hopefully, the time will come when denying social processes may be considered as unethical and offensive to patients.

Knowledge of the history of dementia as a word, a concept and a behavioural syndrome is a precondition for scientific research. Successive historical convergences have shaped the current notion of dementia. A full study should map the changes in the history of 'dementia' at least since Roman times. For the purposes of this chapter, however, it should suffice to study a shorter period, stretching from the work of Boissier de Sauvages (1771), who still offered a static view of disease to Marie (1906) whose great treatise would read as very modern to anachronistic eyes. The former defined 'dementia' as a generic term; the latter saw in dementia a 'syndrome', which could be enacted by a variety of 'diseases' each with its recognizable phenomenology and putative neuropathology.

1.2 TERMS

Up to the 1700s, states of cognitive and behavioural deterioration of whatever origin ending up in psychosocial incompetence were called amentia, dementia, imbecility, morosis, *fatuitas*, anoea, foolishness, stupidity, simplicity, carus, idiocy, dotage and senility. In Roman times, the word 'dementia' was also used to mean 'being out of one's mind, insanity, madness, folly' (Lewis and Short, 1969). For example, in the first century BC, Cicero (1969) (*Tusculanan disputations*, Book 3, para 10) and Lucretius (1975) (*De Rerum Natura*, Book 1, line 704) used 'dementia' as a synonym of madness.

The term dementia first appears in the European vernaculars after the seventeenth century. In Blancard's (1726) English dictionary it is used as an equivalent of *anoea* or 'extinction of the imagination and judgment' (p. 21). By 1644, according to the *Oxford English Dictionary*, an adjectival form ('demented') entered the English language. In his Spanish–French dictionary Sobrino (1791) wrote: 'demencia = démence, folie, extravagance, égarement, alienation d'esprit' (p. 300). Rey (1995), in turn, states that *démence* appeared in French in 1381 to refer to 'madness, extravagancy' but that the adjective *dément* came into currency only from 1700. It would seem, therefore, that between the seventeenth and eighteenth centuries the Latin stem *demens* (without mind) had found a home in most European vernaculars. As we shall see, the full medicalization of 'dementia' started after the 1750s.

1.3   MEDICAL USAGE

Evidence for an early medical usage of the term dementia is found in the French Encyclopaedia (Diderot and d'Alembert, 1765):

> Dementia is a disease consisting in a paralysis of the spirit characterized by abolition of the reasoning faculty. It differs from *fatuitas*, morosis, *stultitia* and *stoliditas* in that in the latter there is a weakening of understanding and memory; and from delirium which is a temporary impairment in the exercise of the said functions. Some modern writers confuse dementia with mania, which is a delusional state accompanied by disturbed behaviour (*audace*); these symptoms are not present in subject[s] with dementia who exhibit foolish behaviour and cannot understand what they are told, cannot remember anything, have no judgment, are sluggish, and retarded … Physiology teaches that the vividness of our understanding depends on the intensity of external stimuli … in pathological states these may be excessive, distorted or abolished; dementia results from abolition of stimuli which may follow: 1. damage to the brain caused by excessive usage, congenital causes or old age, 2. failure of the spirit, 3. small volume of the brain, 4. violent blows to the head causing brain damage, 5. incurable diseases such as epilepsy, or exposure to venoms (Charles Bonnet reports of a girl who developed dementia after being bitten by a bat) or other substances such as opiates and mandragora.
>
> Dementia is difficult to cure as it is related to damage of brain fibres and nervous fluids; it becomes incurable in cases of congenital defect or old age … [otherwise] treatment must follow the cause …
>
> [The legal definition of dementia reads]: Those in a state of dementia are incapable of informed consent, cannot enter into contracts, sign wills, or be members of a jury. This is why they are declared incapable of managing their own affairs. Actions carried out before the declaration of incapacity are valid unless it is demonstrated that dementia predated the action.

> Ascertainment of dementia is based on examination of handwriting, interviews by magistrates and doctors, and testimony from informants. Declarations made by notaries that the individual was of sane mind whilst signing a will are not always valid as they may be deceived by appearances, or the subject might have been in a lucid period. In regards to matrimonial rights, démence is not a sufficient cause for separation, unless it is accompanied by aggression (*furour*). It is, however, sufficient for a separation of property, so that the wife is no longer under the guardianship of her husband. Those suffering from dementia cannot be appointed to public positions or receive privileges. If they became demented after any has been granted, a coadjutor should be appointed …

Although modern-sounding, this definition must be read with caution: its clinical description depends on contrasts and differences with delirium and a list of disorders which are no more; its legal meaning is based on the old Román accounts, and its mechanisms make use of the camera obscura metaphor and assume the passive definition of the mind that Condillac had borrowed from John Locke.

1.4   BEHAVIOURS REDOLENT OF CURRENT DEMENTIA DURING THIS PERIOD

In the literature of the seventeenth and eighteenth centuries (and indeed of earlier periods), it is possible to recognize behaviours that nowadays we may wish to refer as dementia being reported under different rubrics. For example, in relation to 'Stupidity or Foolishness', Thomas Willis (1684) wrote:

> although it chiefly belongs to the rational soul, and signifies a defect of the intellect and judgement, yet it is not improperly reckoned among the diseases of the head or brain; for as much as this eclipse of the superior soul proceeds from the imagination and the memory being hurt, and the failing of these depends upon the faults of the animal spirits, and the brain itself (p. 209).

Willis suggested that stupidity might be genetic ('original', as when 'fools beget fools') or caused by ageing ('Some at first crafty and ingenious, become by degrees dull, and at length foolish, by the mere declining of age, without any great errors in living') (p. 211), or other causes such as 'strokes or bruising upon the head', 'drunkenness and surfeiting', 'violent and sudden passions' and 'cruel diseases of the head' such as epilepsy.

The same is the case with Boissier de Sauvages (1771), one of the great classificators of the eighteenth century. Order 3rd (8th class) of his *Nosographie Methodique* encompasses delirium, paraphrosyne, imbecility, melancholia, demonomania and mania. Synonyms of 'Imbecility are *Bêtise* (stupidity, foolishness), *Niaiserie* (silliness), and *Démence*; in Greek *paranoia*, and in Latin *Dementia, Fatuitas, Vecordia*. The term is used to refer to patients who are fools (*fous*), imbeciles (*imbécilles*), mentally weak (*foibles d'esprit*), mad (*insensés*)' (p. 723). Boissier lists 12 subtypes of imbecility of which the first one is the imbecility of the elderly (*L'imbécillite de vieillard*), also known as puerile state, drivelling or senile madness, and which he explains thus: 'Because of the stiffness of their nervous fibres, old people are less sensitive to external impressions ...' (p. 724).

In the *Nosographie* (1818; first published 1798), Pinel dealt with cognitive impairment under amentia and morosis, which he explains as a failure in the association of ideas leading to disordered activity, extravagant behaviour, superficial emotions, memory loss, difficulty in the perception of objects, obliteration of judgement, aimless activity, automatic existence and forgetting of words or signs to convey ideas. He also referred to *démence senile* (para 116). Pinel did not emphasize the difference between congenital and acquired dementia (Pinel, 1806).

The above entries summarize well views on dementia before the nineteenth century. There was, first of all, a 'legal' meaning according to which dementia was a state of non-imputability. In France, this was enshrined in Article 10 of the Napoleonic Code: 'There is no crime when the accused is in a state of dementia at the time of the alleged act' (Code Napoléon, 1808). Second, there was a clinical meaning. This could be very general (i.e. a synonym of madness) or specific, i.e. a clinical condition that was differentiable from mania (which, at the time, described any state of acute excitement, be it schizophrenic, hypomanic or organic) and delirium (which referred, more or less, to what goes on nowadays under the same name). Although chronic, dementia could still be reversible, affect individuals of any age and be a final common pathway, i.e. the end deficit for many other mental disorders. This created a template for the alienists of the nineteenth century.

1.5 DEMENTIA DURING THE NINETEENTH CENTURY

There is a major difference between eighteenth-century views on dementia and what the historian finds a century later when dementia starts to refer more or less specifically to states of cognitive impairment mostly affecting the elderly, and almost always irreversible. The word 'amentia' was no longer used in this context and started to name a 'psychosis, with sudden onset following severe, often acute physical illness or trauma' (Meynert, 1890). The syndromatic view of the dementias was still in use but mainly in regards to the 'vesanic dementias', i.e. terminal states for all manner of mental disorders.

In his doctoral thesis, Esquirol (1805) used the word dementia to refer to loss of reason, as in *démence accidental*, *démence mélancolique*; then, he distinguished between acute, chronic and senile dementia. Acute dementia was short-lived, reversible, and followed fever, haemorrhage and metastasis; chronic dementia was irreversible and caused by masturbation, melancholia, mania, hypochondria, epilepsy, paralysis and apoplexy; lastly, senile dementia resulted from ageing,

and consisted in a loss of the faculties of the understanding (Esquirol, 1814). Esquirol's final thoughts on dementia were influenced by his controversy with Bayle (1822) who via his concept of *chronic arachnoiditis* propounded an anatomical ('organic') view of all the insanities and scorned Pinel's views that some vesanias might develop in a psychological space (Bayle, 1826).

Together with his student Georget, Esquirol supported a 'descriptivist' approach, at least in relation to some forms of mental disorder. He reported 15 dementia cases (seven males and eight females) with a mean age of 34 years (SD = 10.9), seven being, in fact, cases of general paralysis of the insane, showing grandiosity, disinhibition, motor symptoms, dysarthria and terminal cognitive failure. Also included was a 20-year-old girl who, in modern terms, suffered from a catatonic syndrome; and a 40-year-old woman with pica, cognitive impairment and space-occupying lesions in her left hemisphere and cerebellum (Esquirol, 1838). Although the mean age of these samples and the absence of cases of senile dementia may simply reflect a short life expectancy in Esquirol's day, or that at the Charenton Hospital some selection bias was in operation, it is more likely to reflect the view that age was not an important variable. Together with irreversibility, age became a defining criterion only by the second half of the nineteenth century.

Like his teacher Esquirol, aware of the importance of clinical description, Calmeil wrote: 'It is not easy to describe dementia, its varieties, and nuances; because its complications are numerous ... it is difficult to choose its distinctive symptoms' (p. 71). Dementia followed chronic insanity and brain disease, and was partial or general. Calmeil was less convinced than his co-student Georget that all dementias were associated with alterations in the brain.

In regard to senile dementia, Calmeil remarked: 'there is a constant involvement of the senses, elderly people can be deaf, and show disorders of taste, smell and touch; external stimuli are therefore less clear to them, they have little memory of recent events, live in the past, and repeat the same tale; their affect gradually wanes away ...' (p. 77). Although a keen neuropathologist, Calmeil concluded that there was no sufficient information on the nature and range of anomalies found in the skull or brain to decide on the cause of dementia (pp. 82–3) (Calmeil, 1835).

A Ghent alienist, thinking in Flemish and writing in French, Guislain believed that in dementia:

> All intellectual functions show a reduction in energy, external stimuli cause only minor impression on the intellect, imagination is weak and uncreative, memory absent, and reasoninq patholoqical. There are two varieties of dementia ... one affecting the elderly (senile dementia of Cullen) the other younger people. Although confused with dementia, idiocy must be considered as a separate group (p. 10). [In dementia,] 'the patient has no memory, or at least is unable to retain anything ... impressions evaporate from his mind. He may remember names of people but cannot say whether he has seen them before. He does not know what time or day of the week it is, cannot tell morning from evening, or say what 2 and 2 add to ... he has lost the instinct of

preservation, cannot avoid fire or water, and is unable to recognize dangers; has also lost spontaneity, is incontinent of urine and faeces, and does not ask for anything, he cannot even recognize his wife or children ... (p. 311) (Guislain, 1852).

Because in the past the mentally ill: 'had been categorized only in terms of a [putative] impairment of their mental faculties ...' (p. 2), Morel (1860) endeavoured to develop a taxonomy that distinguished between occasional and determinant causes of mental disorder (p. 251) and suggested six clinical groups: hereditary, toxic, associated with the neuroses, idiopathic, sympathetic and dementia. In regards to the latter, Morel (1860) believed that:

... if we examine dementia (amentia, progressive weakening of the faculties) we must accept that it constitutes a terminal state. There will, of course, be exceptional insane individuals who, until the end, preserve their intellectual faculties; the majority, however, are subject to the law of decline. This results from a loss of vitality in the brain ... Comparison of brain weights in the various forms of insanity shows that the heavier weights are found in cases of recent onset. Chronic cases show more often a general impairment of intelligence (dementia). Loss in brain weight – a constant feature of dementia – is also present in ageing, and is an expression of decadence in the human species. [There are] natural dementia and that dementia resulting from a pathological state of the brain ... some forms of insanity are more prone to end up in dementia (idiopathic) than others ... it could be argued that because dementia is a terminal state it should not be classified as a sixth form of mental illness ... I must confess I sympathize with this view, and it is one of the reasons why I have not described the dementias in any detail ... on the other hand from the legal and pathological viewpoints, dementia warrants separate treatment ... (pp. 837–8).

Morel's view is in keeping with his 'degenerationist' hypothesis, which he himself had developed three years earlier (Morel, 1857; Pick, 1989). One consequence of this view was that there were no specific brain alterations in dementia.

In spite of his early death, LF Marcé published a series of important articles on the neuropathology of senile dementia which challenged Morel's non-specificity hypothesis.

There is no space here to analyse with the same level of detail the evolution of the concept of dementia in other European countries, although it followed similar lines. Views in England, for example, were mainly derivative from French ones. In a popular textbook, and following Pinel, Esquirol and Calmeil, Prichard included a category which he called 'incoherence or dementia':

[it] is a very peculiar and well-marked form of mental disorder. The mind in this state is occupied, without ceasing, by unconnected thoughts and evanescent emotions; it is incapable of continued attention and reflection, and at length loses the faculty of distinct

perception or apprehension. Numerous examples of this disease, or decay of the mental powers are to be met within every receptacle containing a considerable assemblage of deranged persons ... incoherence is either a primary disease, arising immediately from the agency of exciting causes on a constitution previously health, or it is a secondary affection, the result of other disorders of the brain and nervous system which, by their long duration or severity, give rise to disease in the structure of those organs ... secondary incoherence or dementia follows long-protracted mania, attacks of apoplexy, epilepsy or paralysis, or fevers attended with severe delirium. This decay of the faculties has been termed fatuity or imbecility, and it has been confounded with idiotism, which in all its degrees and modifications is a very different state ... (pp. 83–5) (Prichard, 1835).

The same can be said of the views expressed by Bucknill and Tuke in their popular textbook:

Dementia may be either primary or consecutive; acute or chronic. It may also be simple or complicated; it is occasionally remittent but rarely intermittent. It is primary when it is the first stage of the mental disease of the patient; and when this occurs, it is, perhaps, one of the most painful forms of insanity; the patient often being acutely sensible of a gradual loss of memory, power of attention, and executive ability. At this period, the distinction is often well marked between the strictly intellectual and affective disorder ... dementia is much more frequently consecutive, that is the consequence of other diseases of the mind. Thus during 44 years, while 277 cases of mania and 215 of melancholia were admitted at the Retreat, only 48 of dementia were admitted during the same period; yet, at the end of that term, there were remaining in the institution, 20 patients in a state of dementia out of 91 inmates. Mania very often degenerates into dementia; as also do melancholia and monomania ... it should be observed, that the term dementia may be, and sometimes is, too indiscriminately employed. All writers of authority agree in representing impairment of the memory as one of the earliest symptoms of dementia; but we believe cases are occasionally classed under incipient dementia, in which close observation would show that the memory is unimpaired ... It is often rather a torpid condition of the mind, falling under the division 'apathetic insanity, which ought not to be confounded with dementia ...' (pp. 117–19) (Bucknill and Tuke, 1858).

The same concepts are found in German-speaking nations and the views of Heinroth, Feuchtersleben, Griesinger and Kahlbaum were influential until the beginning of the second half of the nineteenth century. Heinroth (1818/1975) used the term dementia in a very broad sense to refer to a state of mind that might accompany or follow other mental disorders, i.e. 'vesanic dementia', a term that late in the century was to become very popular, particularly in France. This concept, which is not related to age, is redolent of the later notion of secondary dementia, i.e. the state of psychosocial and cognitive incompetence that might follow a functional psychosis. Feuchtersleben's (1845/1847) usage is even more general. In his work he uses dementia as a synonym of madness and may refer to forms of acute madness with and without accompanying idiocy. There is only one form of dementia, which he refers to as *moria* and considered as more or less chronic and more or less cognitive. Although possibly ending up in a state of idiocy, the patient can show lucid intervals. Once again, age is of no relevance to moria and hence one must conclude that Feuchtersleben is referring to a form of vesanic dementia.

Griesinger's nosology is not altogether clear and has often been interpreted as being based on the belief that there is only one form of madness (*unitary psychoses concept*), which may go through at least three stages: depression (as in melancholia), exaltation (as in mania) and weakness (as in chronic madness and dementia). In the second edition of his great work, Griesinger (1861/1867) insists that the states of mental weakness 'do not constitute primary but consecutive forms of insanity' (p. 319). This suggests that he is also referring to a form of vesanic dementia, although he includes under this large class all the forms of mental handicap where no preliminary 'primary' forms of madness can be recognized. Under the heading 'dementia', Griesinger includes mental disorders fundamentally caused by a 'general weakness of the mental faculties' including loss of emotions. Age is not a factor in the development of dementia or apathetic dementia and hence it must also be concluded that Griesinger is referring to vesanic dementia.

The work of Kahlbaum, particularly his important book of 1863 on the definition and classification of mental disorders, marks the beginning of a new era in psychiatry. His incorporation of time as a variable in the analysis of madness (longitudinal definition) and his view that period of life is relevant to the form of the disease remain the pillars of psychiatric nosology today. The concept of 'Dementia' is dealt with in the third section of Kahlbaum's (1863) book under the name of *aphrenia*. This clinical category refers to states of mental impotence (*Zustand geistiger Impotenz*) (p. 153), which Kahlbaum equates to the old German notion of *Blödsinn*. After complaining that neither the Greeks nor Latin writers managed to specify a term for this condition, he insists that a word is needed to refer to states of cognitive and behavioural incompetence such as those seen in *dementia terminalis* (Berrios, 1996).

1.6   THE FRAGMENTATION OF DEMENTIA

During the second half of the nineteenth century, and based on the clinical observations and reconceptualization carried out by the French, German and English writers mentioned above, dementia starts to be considered as a syndrome and hence could be attached to a variety of disorders. The primary classification was to be between primary and secondary, the latter including all the vesanic dementias, i.e. states of defect that could follow any severe form of insanity. An increased use of light microscopy during the second half

of the century led to the view that primary forms of dementia could be caused by degenerations of cerebral parenchyma or by arteriosclerosis. By 1900, senile, arteriosclerotic, infectious and traumatic forms of dementia had been reported (Berrios and Freeman, 1991). 'Mixed forms', such as 'dementia praecox' were also suggested reflecting Kahlbaum's view that mental disorders appeared during specific biological transitions. The list of parenchymal forms became longer after the inclusion of states of degeneration from alcoholism, epilepsy, myxoedema and lead poisoning. The history of some of these forms will be discussed presently.

1.6.1   General paralysis of the insane

Bayle (1822) described cases, under the name *arachnitis chronique*, of what later was to be called 'general paralysis of the insane'. Whether this 'new phenomenon' resulted from 'a mutation in the syphilitic virus towards the end of the eighteenth century' is unclear (p. 623) (Hare, 1959). Equally dubious is the claim that its discovery reinforced the belief of alienists in the anatomoclinical view of mental disease (Zilboorg, 1941). In fact, it took more than 30 years for general paralysis to gain acceptance as a 'separate' disease. Bayle's 'discovery' was more important in another way, namely that it challenged the 'cross-sectional' view of disease; in the words of Bercherie (1980): 'for the first time in the history of psychiatry there was a morbid entity which presented itself as a sequential process unfolding itself into successive clinical syndromes' (p. 75).

By the 1850s, no agreement had yet been reached as to how symptoms were caused by the *periencephalite chronique diffuse* (as general paralysis was known at the time). Three clinical types were recognized: manic-ambitious, melancholic-hypochondriac and dementia; according to the 'unitary view', all three constituted stages of a single disease, the order of their appearance depending on the progress of the cerebral lesions. Baillarger (1883), however, sponsored a 'dualist' view: 'paralytic insanity and paralytic dementia are different conditions'. It is clear that the debate had less to do with the nature of the brain lesions than with how mental symptoms and their contents were produced in general: how could the 'typical' content of paralytic delusions (grandiosity) be explained? Since the same mental symptoms could be seen in all manner of conditions, Baillarger believed that chronic periencephalitis could account only for the motor signs – mental symptoms 'therefore, having a different origin' (p. 389). The absence of a link between lesion and symptom also explained why some patients recovered.

The view that general paralysis might be related to syphilis (put forward by Fournier, 1875) was resisted. Indeed, the term 'pseudogeneral paralysis' was coined to refer to cases of infections causing psychotic symptoms (Baillarger, 1889). In general, there is little evidence that alienists considered general paralysis as a 'paradigm-disease', i.e. a model for all other mental diseases. It can even be said that the new 'disease' created more problems than it solved (Berrios, 1985a).

1.6.2   The vesanic dementias

The term 'vesanic dementia' began to be used after the 1840s to refer to the clinical states of cognitive disorganization following insanity (Berrios, 1987); its meaning has changed with equal speed alongside psychiatric theory. According to the unitary insanity notion, vesanic dementia was a terminal stage (after mania and melancholia); according to degeneration theory, it was the final expression of a corrupted pedigree; and according to post-1880s' nosology, a final common pathway to some insanities. Vesanic dementias were reversible, and could occur at any age; risk factors such as old age, lack of education, low social class, bad nutrition, etc., accelerated the progression of the dementia or impeded recovery (p. 597) (Ball and Chambard, 1881).

The vesanic dementias included cases suffering from cognitive impairment associated with melancholia. Under the term *démence mélancolique*, Mairet (1883) reported a series of cases of depressed patients with cognitive impairment who on post-mortem showed changes in the temporal lobe; this led Mairet to hypothesize that the affected sites were related to feelings, and to suggest that nihilistic delusions appeared when the lesion spread to the cortex (Berrios, 1985a). Mairet's cases (some of which would now be called 'Cotard's syndrome') showed psychomotor retardation, refused food and died in stupor (Cotard, 1882; Berrios and Luque, 1995). Others, however, got better and these cases are redolent of what nowadays might be called 'depressive pseudodementia'.

Another contributor to the understanding of cognitive impairment in the affective disorders was George Dumas (1894), who suggested that it was 'mental fatigue that explained the psychological poverty and monotony of melancholic depressions' and that the problem was not 'an absence but a stagnation of ideas'; he was, therefore, the first to explain the disorder as a failure in performance.

The word 'pseudodementia', however, originated in a different clinical tradition. It was first used by Carl Wernicke to refer to 'a chronic hysterical state mimicking mental weakness' (Bulbena and Berrios, 1986). Not used until the 1950s, it was given a lease of life by writers such as Madden *et al.* (1952), Anderson *et al.* (1959) and Kiloh (1961). Current usage is ambiguous in that it relates to three clinical situations: a real (albeit reversible) cognitive impairment accompanying some psychoses, a parody of such impairment, and the cognitive deficit of delirium (Bulbena and Berrios, 1986).

1.6.3   Brain changes and ageing

Since the beginning of the nineteenth century, cases had been described of brain 'softening' followed by cognitive failure. Rostan (1823) reported 98 subjects thus affected, thought to be scorbutic in origin, and divided them into simple, abnormal and complicated (the latter two groups being accompanied by psychiatric changes). Mental symptoms might occur before, during and after the softening itself; thus, senile dementia and insanity might precede the brain changes. When it accompanied stroke, Rostan described cognitive failure and attacks of insanity suggesting that these symptoms were 'a general feature … not a positive sign of localisation'

(pp. 214–15). Durand-Fardel (1843) provided an account of the relationship between softening and insanity, warning that softening was used to refer both to a disease (stroke) and to a state of the brain. Psychiatric complications were acute and long term, the former including confusion, depression, irritability, acute insanity and loss of mental faculties (p. 139); the latter had gradual onset, and exhibited an impairment of memory, poverty of thinking, and a regression to infantile forms of behaviour, features which led to 'true dementia' (pp. 327–8).

Years later, Jackson (1875) reviewed the problem: 'softening … as a category for a rude clinical grouping was to be deprecated' (p. 335); he nonetheless followed Durand-Fardel's classification and suggested that, after stroke, mental symptoms might be immediate or occurring after a few hours or months; he recognized that major cognitive failure may ensue, and saw this as an instance of 'dissolution': emotional symptoms being release phenomena (for an analysis of this concept see Berrios, 1991). He believed that anxiety, stress and irritability might be harbingers of stroke.

1.6.4   The concept of arteriosclerotic dementia

Old age was considered an important factor in the development of arteriosclerosis (Berrios, 1994) and a risk factor in diseases such as melancholia (Berrios, 1991). By 1910, there was a trend to include all dementias under 'mental disorders of cerebral arteriosclerosis' (Barrett, 1913). Arteriosclerosis might be generalized or cerebral, inherited or acquired, and caused by syphilis, alcohol, nicotine, high blood pressure or ageing. In those genetically predisposed, cerebral arteries were considered as thinner and less elastic. Arteriosclerosis caused mental changes by narrowing of arteries and/or reactive inflammation. The view that arteriosclerotic dementia resulted from a gradual strangulation of blood supply to the brain was also formed during this period; consequently, emphasis was given to prodromal symptoms, and strokes were but the culmination of a process started years before.

Some opposed this view from the beginning. For example, Marie (1906) claimed that such explanation was a vicious circle, as alienists claimed that: 'ageing was caused by arteriosclerosis and the latter by ageing' (p. 358), and Walton (1912) expressed serious doubts from the histopathological point of view. The frequent presence in post-mortem of such changes also concerned pathologists who worried that they could not 'safely exclude cerebral arteriosclerosis of greater or lesser degree in any single case' of senile dementia (p. 677) (Southard, 1910). Based on a review of these arguments, Olah (1910) concluded that there was no such thing as 'arteriosclerotic psychoses'. However, the 'chronic global ischaemia' hypothesis won the day, and it was to continue well into the second half of the twentieth century. For some it became a general explanation; for example, North and Bostock (1925) reported a series of 568 general psychiatric cases in which around 40 per cent suffered from 'arterial disease', which – according to the authors – was even responsible for schizophrenia. The old idea of an apoplectic form of dementia, however, never disappeared.

1.6.5   Apoplectic dementia

'Apoplectic dementia' achieved its clearest enunciation in the work of Benjamin Ball (Ball and Chambard, 1881). 'Organic apoplexy' resulted from bleeding, softening or tumour and might be 'followed by a notable decline in cognition, and by a state of dementia which was progressive and incurable ... of the three, localised softening (*ramollissement en foyer*) caused the more severe states of cognitive impairment' (p. 581). Ball believed that prodromal lapses of cognition (episodes of somnolence and confusion with automatic behaviour, for which there was no memory after the event) and sensory symptoms were caused by atheromatous lesions. Visual hallucinations, occasionally pleasant, were also common. After the stroke, persistent cognitive impairment was frequent. Post-mortem studies showed in these cases softening of 'ideational' areas of cortex and white matter. Ball also suggested a laterality effect (p. 582) in that right hemisphere strokes led more often to dementia whereas left hemisphere ones caused perplexity, apathy, unresponsiveness and a tendency to talk to oneself (p. 583). Following Luys, he believed that some of these symptoms resulted from damage to corpus striatum, insular sulci and temporal lobe. During Ball's time, attention shifted from white to red softening. Charcot (1881) wrote on cerebral haemorrhage (the new name for red softening): 'having eliminated all these cases, we find ourselves in the presence of a homogeneous group corresponding to the commonest form of cerebral haemorrhage. This is, par excellence, sanguineous apoplexy ... as it attacks a great number of old people, I might call it senile haemorrhage' (p. 267).

1.6.6   Presbyophrenia and confabulation

The word 'presbyophrenia' was coined by Kahlbaum (1863) to name a subtype of the paraphrenias (insanities occurring during periods of biological change). Presbyophrenia was a form of paraphrenia senilis characterized by amnesia, disorientation, delusional misidentification and confabulation. Ignored for more than 30 years, the term reappeared in the work of Wernicke, Fischer and Kraepelin. Wernicke's classification of mental disorders was based on his theory of the three-partite relational structure consciousness (outside world, body and self) (Lanczik, 1988). Impairment of the link between consciousness and outside world led to presbyophrenia, delirium tremens, Korsakoff's psychosis and hallucinoses. Amongst the features of presbyophrenia, Wernicke included confabulations, disorientation, hyperactivity, euphoria and a fluctuating course; acute forms resolved without trace, chronic ones merged with senile dementia (Berrios, 1986).

In France, Rouby (1911) conceived of presbyophrenia as a final common pathway for cases suffering from Korsakoff's psychosis, senile dementia or acute confusion. Truelle and Bessière (1911) suggested, in turn, that it might result from a toxic state caused by liver or kidney failure. Kraepelin (1910) lumped presbyophrenia together with the senile and presenile insanities, and (as compared with Korsakoff's patients) believed presbyophrenic patients to be older, free from polyneuritis and history of alcoholism, and showing hyperactivity and elevated mood. Ziehen (1911) wrote that 'their marked memory impairment contrasts with the relative sparing of thinking'. Fischer (1912) suggested that disseminated cerebral lesions were the essential anatomical substratum of presbyophrenia.

During the 1930s, two new hypotheses emerged. Bostroem (1933) concluded on phenomenological grounds that presbyophrenia could be identified with mania, suggesting an interplay between cerebral arteriosclerosis and cyclothymic premorbid personality. Lafora (1935) emphasized the role of cerebrovascular pathology, and claimed that disinhibition and presbyophrenic behaviour were caused by a combination of senile and atherosclerotic changes. Burger-Prinz and Jacob (1938), however, questioned the view that cyclothymic features were a necessary precondition. Bessière (1948) claimed that presbyophrenia was a syndrome found in conditions such as senile dementia, brain tumours, traumatic psychoses and confusional states. More recently, it has been suggested that presbyophrenia may be a subform of AD characterized by a severe atrophy of locus caeruleus (Berrios, 1985b).

One of the features of presbyophrenia was confabulation. This complex symptom has not quite found a place in psychopathology (Berrios, 2000). Two phenomena are included under the name 'confabulation'. The first type concerns 'untrue' utterances of subjects with memory impairment; often provoked or elicited by the interviewer, these confabulations are accompanied by little conviction and are believed by most clinicians to be caused by the (conscious or unconscious) need to 'cover up' for some memory deficit. Researchers wanting to escape the 'intentionality' dilemma have made use of additional factors such as presence of frontal lobe pathology, dysexecutive syndrome, difficulty with the temporal dating of memories leading to an inability temporally to string out memory data etc.

The second type concerns confabulations with fantastic content and great conviction as seen in subjects with functional psychoses and little or no memory deficit. Less is said in the neuropsychological literature about this group, although (at least in the case of schizophrenia) it is correlated with a bad performance on frontal lobe tests. It is our belief that this group remains of crucial importance to psychiatrists. Little is known about the epidemiology of either type of confabulation.

In clinical practice, these two 'types' can be found in combination. It remains unclear why so many patients with Korsakoff's psychosis or frontal lobe disorder, in spite of the fact that they do meet the putative conditions for confabulation (amnesia, frontal lobe damage, difficulty with the dating of memories, etc.) do not confabulate. Furthermore, confabulations have also been reported in subjects with lesions in the non-dominant hemisphere and in the thalamus.

Under different disguises, the 'covering up' or 'gap filling' hypothesis is still going strong. Although superficially plausible, it poses a serious conceptual problem in regard to the issue of 'awareness of purpose': if full awareness is presumed, then it is difficult to differentiate confabulations from lying; if no awareness is presumed, then the semantics of the concept of 'purpose' is severely stretched and confabulations cannot be differentiated from delusions.

The received view of confabulations also neglects the clinical observation that confabulations (particularly provoked ones!) do occur in dialogical situations: for example, the way in which the patient is asked questions may increase the probability of producing a confabulation. This suggests that the view that confabulations are a disorder of a putative narrative function found in normal human subjects must be taken seriously. It is hypothesized here that this trait is normally distributed in the population. In the absence of adequate epidemiological information, research efforts should be directed at mapping the distribution of this narrative (or confabulatory) capacity in the community at large. Only then will it be possible to understand the significance of its disorders. In the long term, this approach will prove more heuristic than unwarranted speculation based on a few anecdotal cases.

Reported in relation to clinical conditions other than memory deficit, 'confabulation-like' behaviours can already be found in the clinical literature of the second half of the nineteenth century. Sully (1885) suggested that such behaviours might be related to a psychological function whose role was filling gaps in the flow of our lives and explained why 'our image of the past is essentially one of an unbroken series of conscious experiences'. Sully believed that this function also intervened when memory failed: 'just as the eye sees no gap in its field of vision corresponding to the "blind" spot of the retina, but carries the impression over this area, so memory sees no lacuna in the past, but carries its image of conscious life over each of the forgotten spaces' (p. 282).

Kraepelin (1886–1887) reported typical cases of confabulation associated with, among other things, general paralysis of the insane, melancholia and dementia; and later on suggested that 'pseudomemories' could be a symptom of paraphrenia (without cognitive impairment), and described a clinical variety called *paraphrenia confabulans* (Kraepelin, 1919). Under schizophrenic *akzessorischen Gedachtnisstörungen*, Bleuler (1911) discussed three related phenomena: *Gedächnisillusionen* (illusions or distortions of memory), *identifizierenden Erinnerungstäuschungen* (memory falsifications based on identification) and *Erinnerungshalluzinationen* (memory hallucinations). Of the former he wrote: 'memory illusions often constitute the main material for the construction of delusions in paranoids. The entire previous life of the patient may be changed in his memory in terms of this complex' (p. 115). On this definition, it is difficult, on the basis of their intrinsic features, to distinguish illusion of memory from confabulation. Indeed, symptom-naming is determined by whether schizophrenia or 'organic disorder' is the associated disease. Unsuccessfully, Bleuler (1911) tried to establish a differentiation on the basis of mechanism: 'until now, and in contrast to the views of some authors, I have not observed confabulation as it appears in organic cases; e.g. memory hallucinations which fill in memory gaps which at first

appear at a (usually external) given moment and mostly adapt themselves to such an occasion' (p. 117). Kleist (1960) described patients with 'progressive confabulosis' as 'cheerful, expansive, and with little in the way of thought or speech disorder' (p. 211); and Leonhard (1957) redescribed the condition as 'confabulatory euphoria'.

1.6.7   Alzheimer's disease

Alzheimer's disease has become the prototypical form of dementia. From this point of view, a study of its origins should throw light on the evolution of the concept of dementia. The writings of Alzheimer, Fischer, Fuller, Lafora, Bonfiglio, Perusini, Ziveri, Kraepelin and other protagonists are deceptively fresh, and this makes anachronistic reading inevitable. However, the psychiatry of the late nineteenth century is a remote country: concepts such as dementia, neurone, neurofibril and plaque were then still in process of construction and meant different things to different people. A discussion of these issues is beyond the scope of this chapter (see Berrios, 1990b).

1.6.7.1   THE NEUROPATHOLOGY OF DEMENTIA BEFORE ALZHEIMER

Enquiries into the brain changes accompanying dementia started during the 1830s but consisted in descriptions of external appearance (Wilks, 1865). The first important microscopic study was that of Marcé (1863) who described cortical atrophy, enlarged ventricles and 'softening'. The vascular origin of softening was soon ascertained (Parrot, 1873), but the distinction between vascular and parenchymal factors had to wait until the 1880s. From then on, microscopic studies concentrated on cellular death, plaques and neurofibrils.

1.6.7.2   ALZHEIMER AND HIS DISEASE

Alzheimer (1907) reported the case of a 51-year-old woman, with cognitive impairment, delusions, hallucinations, focal symptoms, and whose brain showed plaques, tangles and arteriosclerotic changes. The existence of neurofibrils had been known for some time (DeFelipe and Jones, 1988); for example, that in senile dementia 'the destruction of the neurofibrils appears to be more extensive than in the brain of a paralytic subject' (Bianchi 1906, p. 846). Fuller (1907) had remarked in June 1906 (i.e. five months before Alzheimer's report) on the presence of neurofibrillar bundles in senile dementia (p. 450). Likewise, the association of plaques with dementia was not a novelty: Beljahow (1889) had reported them in 1887, and so had Redlich and Leri a few years later (Simchowicz, 1924); in Prague, Fischer (1907) gave an important paper in June 1907 pointing out that miliary necrosis could be considered as a marker of senile dementia.

Nor was the syndrome described by Alzheimer new: states of persistent cognitive impairment affecting the elderly, accompanied by delusions and hallucinations were well known (Marcé, 1863; Krafft-Ebing, 1873; Crichton-Browne,

1874; Marie, 1906). As a leading neuropathologist Alzheimer was aware of this work. Did he then mean to describe a new disease? The answer is that it is most unlikely he did, his only intention having been to point out that such a syndrome could occur in younger people (Alzheimer, 1911). This is confirmed by commentaries from those who worked for him: Perusini (1909) wrote that for Alzheimer 'these morbid forms do not represent anything but atypical form of senile dementia' (p. 143).

1.6.7.3 THE NAMING OF THE DISEASE

Kraepelin (1910) coined the term in the eighth edition of his Handbook: at the end of the section on 'senile dementia' he wrote:

> the autopsy revels, according to Alzheimer's description, changes that represent the most serious form of senile dementia ... the *Drusen* were numerous and almost one third of the cortical cells had died off. In their place instead we found peculiar deeply stained fibrillary bundles that were closely packed to one another, and seemed to be remnants of degenerated cell bodies ... The clinical interpretation of this AD is still confused. Whilst the anatomical findings suggest that we are dealing with a particularly serious form of senile dementia, the fact that this disease sometimes starts already around the age of 40 does not allow this supposition. In such cases we should at least assume a 'senium praecox' if not perhaps a more or less age-independent unique disease process.

1.6.7.4 THE RECEPTION OF THE NEW DISEASE

Alzheimer (1911) showed surprise at Kraepelin's interpretation, and always referred to his 'disease' as *Erkrankungen* (in the medical language of the 1900s a term softer than *Krankheit*, the term used by Kraepelin). Others also expressed doubts. Fuller (1912), whose contribution to this field has been sadly neglected, asked 'why a special clinical designation – Alzheimer's disease – since, after all, they are but part of a general disorder' (p. 26). Hakkébousch and Geier (1913), in Russia, saw it as a variety of the involution psychosis. Simchowicz (1911) considered 'Alzheimer's disease' as only a severe form of senile dementia. Ziehen (1911) does not mention the disease in his major review of senile dementia. In a meeting of the New York Neurological Society, Ramsay Hunt (Lambert, 1916) asked Lambert, the presenter of a case of 'Alzheimer's disease' that 'he would like to understand clearly whether he made any distinction between the so-called Alzheimer's disease and senile dementia' other than ... in degree and point of age'. Lambert agreed suggesting that, as far as he was concerned, the underlying pathological mechanisms were the same (Lambert, 1916). Lugaro (1916) wrote: 'For a while it was believed that a certain agglutinative disorder of the neurofibril could be considered as the main "marker" (*contrassegno*) of a presenile form [of senile dementia], which was "hurriedly baptized" (*fretta battezzate*) as "Alzheimer's

disease"' (p. 378). He went on to say that this state is only a variety of senile dementia. Simchowicz (1924), who had worked with Alzheimer, wrote 'Alzheimer and Perusini did not know at the time that the plaques were typical of senile dementia [in general] and believed that they might have discovered a new disease' (p. 221). These views, from men who lived in Alzheimer's and Kraepelin's time, must be taken seriously (Berrios, 1990a).

Of late there has been an attempt to rewrite the history of AD. After having been lost for years, the case notes of Auguste D, the first patient with AD, were found in the late 1990s (Maurer and Maurer, 1998). As mentioned above the original report by Alzheimer (1907) clearly stated that Auguste suffered from severe confusion, delusions, hallucinations, focal symptoms and on post-mortem her brain showed plaques, tangles and, most importantly, *arteriosclerotic* changes. As if to confirm the ontology of AD, Graeber *et al.* (1998) reported that in tissue sections belonging to this case they confirmed the presence of neurofibrillar tangles and amyloid plaques. Most interestingly, and given that vascular changes are currently not supposed to be a diagnostic criterion, these authors have put Alzheimer right by stating that Auguste's brain showed no arteriosclerotic lesions. Furthermore, they report that the apolipoprotein E (ApoE) genotype of Auguste was ε3/ε3, 'indicating that mutational screening of the tissue is feasible'.

On the basis of these findings, can one say that back in 1910 Kraepelin was, after all, right in claiming that Alzheimer had 'discovered' a new disease? The answer has to be that one must judge his decision in terms of what Kraepelin knew at the time and of the academic pressure he was under. He knew what Alzheimer's report stated in 1907, what the latter might have verbally added, and upon Kraepelin's perusal of Auguste's case notes, which were requested by him from Frankfurt (indeed this is the reason why they were lost for such a long time). In clinical terms, Auguste was not a 'typical' case. At 51 she had delusions, hallucinations and Alzheimer's reported arteriosclerotic changes. None of these features is mentioned in Kraepelin's original claim. The question is, why?

It is also interesting that the so-called 'second case' of Alzheimer's (Graeber *et al.*, 1997), Johann F, reported in 1911, is now considered to have suffered a 'plaques-only' form of AD. The same authors suggest that knowledge of this case may have encouraged Kraepelin to report the discovery by Alzheimer of a new disease. Unfortunately, there is no evidence that Kraepelin knew of this case when he was writing the relevant section of the eighth edition of his *Lehrbuch*. More to the point is that he knew of Perusini's (1909) review as he himself had asked the young Italian assistant to collect four cases. In addition to Auguste D (which includes more information than that provided by Alzheimer in 1907), Perusini reviewed the cases of Mr RM, a 45-year-old basket maker who had epileptic seizures, of Mrs BA a 65-year-old who had marked clinical features of myxoedema, and Schl L, a 63-year-old who had suffered from syphilis since 1870, was Romberg-positive, had a pupillary syndrome and heard voices. Since these are likely to have been the cases on which Kraepelin based his decision to construct the new disease, it would be interesting if the neuropathology and neurogenetics of the other three cases (Auguste's has already been done) were to be investigated.

1.6.8 Pick's disease and the frontal dementias

Dementias believed to be related to frontal lobe pathology have once again become of interest, and authors often invoke the name of Arnold Pick (Niery *et al.*, 1988). However, when the great Prague neuropsychiatrist described the syndrome named after him, all he wanted was to draw attention to a form of localized (as opposed to diffuse) atrophy of the temporal lobe (Pick, 1892). This alteration was to give rise to a dysfunction of language and praxis, and be susceptible to diagnosis during life. Pick believed that lobar atrophies constituted a stage in the evolution of the senile dementias.

The story starts, as it should, before Pick. Louis Pierre Gratiolet (1854) was responsible for renaming the cerebral lobes after their overlying skull: thus 'anterior' became 'frontal' lobe. He made no assumption as to the function of the 'anterior extremity of the cerebral hemisphere'. 'Phrenologists', however, did and related reflective and perceptive functions (qualitatively defined) to the forehead (Anonymous, 1832) (for the science of phrenology see Combe, 1873; Lanteri-Laura, 1970). 'Modular' assumptions (i.e. a one-to-one correlation between mental function and brain site) involving the frontal lobes started only during the 1860s, following reports on dysfunction of language in lesions of the frontal lobes (Broca, 1861; Henderson, 1986). These claims ran parallel to those of Jackson's that the cerebral cortex was the general seat of personality and mind (Jackson, 1894). Meynert (1885) believed that 'the frontal lobes reach a high state of development in man' but still defined mental disorders as diseases of the 'fore-brain' (by which he meant 'prosencephalon' or human brain as a whole).

In his first report (the case of focal senile atrophy and aphasia in a man of 71) Pick (1892) did not inculpate the frontal lobes nor did he in his second case (Pick, 1901) (a woman of 59 with generalized cortical atrophy, particularly of the left hemisphere). The association with the frontal lobes appears only in his fourth case (Pick, 1906) (a 60-year-old man with 'bilateral frontal atrophy'). Which of these cases should, therefore, be considered as the first with Pick's disease? At the time, in fact, no one thought that Pick had described a new disease; Barrett (1913) considered the two first cases of Pick's as atypical forms of AD, and Ziehen (1911) did not see anything special in them.

During the same period, Liepmann, Stransky and Spielmeyer had described similar cases with aphasia and circumscribed cerebral atrophy (Mansvelt, 1954); so much so, that Urechia and Mihalescu felt tempted to name the syndrome 'Spielmeyer's disease' (Caron, 1934). This did not catch on, and in two classic papers on what he called 'Pick's disease', Carl (Schneider 1927; Schneider, 1929) constructed the new view of the condition by suggesting that it evolved in three stages – the first with a disturbance of judgement and behaviour, the second with localized symptoms and the third with generalized dementia. He recognized rapid and slow forms, the former with an akinetic and aphasic subtypes and

a malignant course, and the latter with a predominance of plaques (probably indistinguishable from AD).

1.7 THE AFTERMATH

The history of the word 'dementia' must not be confused with that of the concepts or behaviours involved. By 1800, two definitions of dementia were recognized and both had psychosocial incompetence as their central concept: in addition to cognitive impairment, the clinical definition included other symptoms such as delusions and hallucinations; irreversibility and old age were not features of the condition, and in general dementia was considered to be a terminal state to all sorts of mental, neurological and physical conditions. The adoption of the anatomoclinical model by nineteenth century alienists changed this. Questions were asked as to the neuropathological basis of dementia and this, in turn, led to readjustments in its clinical description. The history of dementia during the nineteenth century is, therefore, the history of its gradual attrition. Stuporous states (then called acute dementia), vesanic dementias and localized memory impairments, were gradually reclassified, and by 1900 the cognitive paradigm, i.e. the view that the essential feature of dementia was intellectual impairment, was established. From then on, efforts were made to explain other symptoms, such as hallucinations, delusions, and mood and behavioural disorders, as epiphenomena and as unrelated to whatever the central mechanism of dementia was. There has also been a fluctuating acceptance of the parenchymal and vascular hypotheses, the latter leading to the description of arteriosclerotic dementia. The separation of the vesanic dementias and of the amnestic syndromes led to the realization that age and ageing mechanisms were important, and by 1900 senile dementia became the prototype of the dementias; by 1970, AD had become the flagship of the new approach. During the last few years, the cognitive paradigm has become an obstacle, and a gradual re-expansion of the symptomatology of dementia is fortunately taking place (Berrios, 1989; Berrios, 1990a).

REFERENCES

Alzheimer A. (1907) Über eine eigenartige Erkrankung der Hirnrinde. *Allgemeine Zeitschrift für Psychiatrie und Psychisch-Gerichtlich Medizine* **64**: 146–8.

Alzheimer A. (1911) Über eigenartige Krankheitsfälle des späteren Alters. *Zeitschrift für die gesamte Neurologie und Psychiatrie* **4**: 356–85.

Anderson EW, Threthowan WH, Kenna JC. (1959) An experimental investigation of simulation and pseudodementia. *Acta Psychiatrica et Neurologica Scandinavica* **34** (Suppl. 132): 5–42.

Anonymous. (1832) An exposure of the unphilosophical and unchristian expedients adopted by antiphrenologists, for the purpose of obstructing the moral tendencies of phrenology. A review of John Wayte's book. *The Phrenological Journal and Miscellany* **7**: 615–22.

Baillarger J. (1883) Sur la théorie de la paralysie générale. *Annales Médico-Psychologiques* 35: 18–52; 191–218.

Baillarger J. (1889) Doit-on dans la classification des maladies mentales assigner une place á part aux pseudo-paralysies générales? *Annales Médico-Psychologiques* 41: 521–5.

Ball B, Chambard E. (1881) Démence. In: Dechambre A, Lereboullet L (eds). *Dictionnaire encyclopédique des sciences médicales*. Paris: Masson, 559–605.

Barrett AM. (1913) Presenile, arteriosclerotic and senile disorders of the brain and cord. In: White WA, Jelliffe SA (eds). *The modern treatment of nervous and mental diseases*. London: Kimpton, 675–709.

Bayle ALJ. (1822) *Recherches sur les maladies mentales*. Paris: Thése de Médecine.

Bayle ALJ. (1826) *Traité des maladies du cerveau*. Paris: Gabon et Compagnie.

Beljahow S. (1889) Pathological changes in the brain in dementia senilis. *Journal of Mental Science* 35: 261–2.

Bercherie P. (1980) *Les fondements de la clinique*. Paris: La Bibliothéque d'Ornicar.

Berrios GE. (1985a) 'Depressive pseudodementia' or 'melancholic dementia': a nineteenth century view. *Journal of Neurology, Neurosurgery, and Psychiatry* 48: 393–400.

Berrios GE. (1985b) Presbyophrenia: clinical aspects. *British Journal of Psychiatry* 147: 76–9.

Berrios GE. (1986) Presbyophrenia: the rise and fall of a concept. *Psychological Medicine* 16: 267–75.

Berrios GE. (1987) History of the functional psychoses. *British Medical Bulletin* 43: 484–98.

Berrios GE. (1989) Non-cognitive symptoms and the diagnosis of dementia historical and clinical aspects. *British Journal of Psychiatry* 154 (Suppl. 4): 11–16.

Berrios GE. (1990a) Memory and the cognitive paradigm of dementia during the nineteenth century: a conceptual history. In: Murray R, Turner T (eds). *Lectures on the history of psychiatry*. London: Gaskell, 194–211.

Berrios GE. (1990b) Alzheimer's disease: a conceptual history. *International Journal of Geriatric Psychiatry* 5: 355–65.

Berrios GE. (1991) Affective disorders in old age: a conceptual history. *International Journal of Geriatric Psychiatry* 6: 337–46.

Berrios GE. (1994) The psychiatry of old age: a conceptual history. In: Copeland J, Abou-Saleh M, Blazer D (eds). *The principles and practice of geriatric psychiatry*. Chichester: Wiley, 11–16.

Berrios GE. (1996) The classification of mental disorders: Part III. *History of psychiatry* 7: 167–82.

Berrios GE. (2000) Confabulations. In: Berrios GE, Hodges JR (eds). *Memory disorders in clinical practice*. Cambridge: Cambridge University Press, 348–68.

Berrios GE, Freeman H. (eds) (1991) *Alzheimer and the dementias*. London: Royal Society of Medicine.

Berrios GE, Luque R. (1995) Cotard's delusion or syndrome? A conceptual history. *Comprehensive Psychiatry* 36: 218–23.

Bessière R. (1948) La presbyophrénie. *L'Encéphale* 37: 313–42.

Bianchi L. (1906) *A textbook of psychiatry*. London: Baillière, Tindall and Cox.

Blancard S. (1726) *The physical dictionary wherein the terms of anatomy, the names and causes of diseases, chirurgical instruments, and their use, are accurately described*. London: John and Benjamin Sprint.

Bleuler E. (1911) *Dementia praecox*. Leipzig, Deuticke (English Translation: *Dementia praecox* (1950), New York: International Universities Press).

Boissier de Sauvages F. (1771) *Nosologie methodique, dans laquelle les maladies sont rangées par classes, suivant le systême de Sydenham, et l'Order des Botanistes*. Paris: Hérissant le Fils.

Bostroem A. (1933) Über Presbyophrenie. *Archiv für Psychiatrie und Nervenkrankenheiten* 99: 339–54.

Broca P. (1861) Perte de la parole, ramollissement chronique et destruction partielle du lobe anterieur gauche du cerveau. *Bulletin de la Société de Anthropologie Paris* 2: 235–8.

Bucknill JC, Tuke DH. (1858) *A manual of psychological medicine*. London: John Churchill.

Bulbena A, Berrios GE. (1986) Pseudodementia: facts and figures. *British Journal of Psychiatry* 148: 87–94.

Burger-Prinz H, Jacob H. (1938) Anatomische und klinische Studien zur senilen Demenz. *Zeitschrift für die gesamte Neurologie und Psychiatrie* 161: 538–43.

Calmeil LF. (1835) Démence. In: *Dictionnaire de médicine on repertoire general des sciences médicales*, 2nd edn. Paris: Bechet, 70–85.

Caron M. (1934) *Etude clinique de la maladie de pick*. Paris: Vigot Fréres.

Charcot JM. (1881) *Clinical lectures on senile and chronic diseases*. London: The New Sydenham Society.

Cicero. (1969) *Tusculanan disputations*. Translated by JE King. Vol XVIII. Cambridge: Loeb Classical Library.

Code Napoléon. (1808) *Edition originale et seule officielle*. Paris: l'Imprimerie Impériale.

Combe G. (1873) *Elements of phrenology*. Edinburgh: MacLachlan and Stewart.

Cotard J. (1882) Du délire des negations. *Archives de Neurologie* 4: 152–70; 282–96.

Crichton-Browne J. (1874) Senile dementia. *British Medical Journal* i: 601–3; 640–3.

DeFelipe J, Jones EG. (eds) (1988) *Cajal on the cerebral cortex. An annotated translation of the complete writings*. Oxford: Oxford University Press.

Diderot, d'Alembert. (eds) (1765) *Encyclopédie ou dictionnaire raisonné des sciences, des arts et des métieres, par une Societé de Gens de Lettres*. Vol 4, A. Paris: Briasson, David, Le Breton, Durand, 807–8

Dumas G. (1894) *Les états intellectuels dans la mélancolie*. Paris: Alcan.

Durand-Fardel M. (1843) *Traité du ramollissement du cerveau*. Paris: Baillière.

Esquirol E. (1805) *Des passions*. Paris: Didot Jeune.

Esquirol E. (1814) Démence. In: *Dictionaire des sciences médicales, par une Societé de Médicins et de Chirurgiens*. Paris: Panckouke, 280–93.

Esquirol E. (1838) *Des maladies mentales*. Paris: Baillière.

Feuchtersleben E. (first published in 1845, translated in 1847) *The principles of medical psychology*. Translated by HE Lloyds and BG Babington. London: Sydenham Society.

Fischer O. (1907) Miliare Nekrosen mit drusigen Wucherungen der Neurofibrillen, eine regelmaessege Verandaerung der Hirnrinde bei seniler Demenz. *Monatsschrift für Psychiatrie und Neurologie* **22**: 361–72.

Fischer O. (1912) Ein weiterer Beitrag zur Klinik und Pathologie der presbyophrenen Demenz. *Zeitschrift für die gesamte Neurologie und Psychiatrie* **12**: 99–135.

Fournier A. (1875) *Syphilis du cerveau*. Paris: Baillière.

Fuller SC. (1907) A study of the neurofibrils in dementia paralytica, dementia senilis, chronic alcoholism, cerebral lues and microcephalic idiocy. *American Journal of Insanity* **63**: 415–68.

Fuller SC. (1912) Alzheimer's disease (senium praecox): the report of a case and review of published cases. *Journal of Nervous and Mental Disease* **39**: 440–55; 536–57.

Graeber MB, Kosel S, Egensperger R *et al.* (1997) Rediscovery of the case described by Alois Alzheimer in 1911: historical, histological and molecular genetic analysis. *Neurogenetics* **1**: 73–80.

Graeber MB, Kosel S, Grasbon-Frodl E *et al.* (1998) Histopathology and APOE phenotype of the first Alzheimer's disease patient. *Neurogenetics* **1**: 223–38.

Gratiolet LP. (1854) *Mémoires sur les plis cérébraux de l'homme et des primates*. Paris: Bertrand.

Griesinger W. (first published in 1861, translated in 1867) Mental Pathology and Therapeutics. Translated by CL Robertson and J Rutherford. London: Sydenham Society.

Guislain J. (1852) *Leçons orales sur les phrénopathies*. Gand: L Hebbelynck.

Hakkébousch BM, Geier TA. (1913) De la maladie d'Alzheimer. *Annales Médico-Psychologiques* **71**: 358.

Hare E. (1959) The origin and spread of dementia paralytica. *Journal of Mental Science* **105**: 594–626.

Heinroth JC. (first published 1818, translated in 1975) *Textbook of disturbances of mental life*. Baltimore: Johns Hopkins University Press.

Henderson VH. (1986) Paul Broca's less heralded contributions to aphasia research. Historical perspective and contemporary relevance. *Archives of Neurology* **43**: 609–12.

Jackson JH. (1875) A lecture on softening of the brain. *Lancet* **ii**: 335–9.

Jackson JH. (1894) The factors of insanities. *Medical Press and Circular* **ii**: 615–25.

Kahlbaum KL. (1863) *Die Gruppierung der psychischen Krankheiten*. Danzig: AW Kafemann.

Kiloh LG. (1961) Pseudo-dementia. *Acta Psychiatrica Scandinavica* **37**: 336–51.

Kleist K. (1960) Schizophrenic symptoms and cerebral pathology. *Journal of Mental Science* **106**: 246–55.

Kraepelin E. (1886–1887) Über Erinnerungsfälschungen. *Archiv für Psychiatrie und Nervenkrankheiten* **17**: 830–43; **18**: 199–239, 395–436.

Kraepelin E. (1910) *Psychiatrie: Ein Lehrbuch für Studierende und Ärzte*. Leipzig: Johann Ambrosius Barth.

Kraepelin E. (1919) *Dementia praecox*. Translated by RM Barclay and GM Robertson. Edinburgh: Livingstone.

Krafft-Ebing R. (1873) De la démence sénile. *Annales Médico-Psychologiques* **34**: 306–7.

Lafora GR. (1935) Sobre la presbiofrenia sin confabulaciones. *Archivos de Neurobiologia* **15**: 179–211.

Lambert CI. (1916) The clinical and anatomical features of Alzheimer's disease. *Journal of Mental and Nervous Disease* **44**: 169–70.

Lanczik M. (1988) *Der Breslauer Psychiater Carl Wernicke*. Sigmaringen: Thorbecke.

Lanteri-Laura G. (1970) *Histoire de la phrenologie*. Paris: Presses Universitaires de France.

Leonhard K. (1957) *Aufteilung der endogenen Psychosen*. Berlin: Akademie-Verlag.

Lewis CT, Short C. (1969) *A Latin Dictionary*. Oxford: Clarendon Press (1st edition, 1879).

Lucretius. (1975) *De rerum natura*. Translation by WHD Rouse. Cambridge: Harvard University Press.

Lugaro E. (1916) La psichiatria tedesca nella storia e nell'attualita. *Rivista di Patologia Nervosa e Mentale* **21**: 337–86.

Madden JJ, Luhan JA, Kaplan LA *et al.* (1952) Non-dementing psychoses in older persons. *Journal of the American Medical Association* **150**: 1567–70.

Mairet A. (1883) *De la démence mélancolique*. Paris: Masson.

Mansvelt J. (1954) *Pick's disease*. Enchede: Van der Loeff.

Marcé LV. (1863) Recherches cliniques et anatomo-pathologiques sur la démence senile et sur les différences qui la separent de la paralysie générale. *Gazette Médicale de Paris* **34**: 433–5; 467–9; 497–502; 631–2; 761–4; 797–8; 831–3; 855–8.

Marie A. (1906) *La démence*. Paris: Doing.

Maurer K, Maurer U. (1998) *Alzheimer. Das Leben eines Arztes und die Karriere einer Krankheiten*. Munich: Piper.

Meynert T. (1885) *Psychiatry. A clinical treatise on diseases of the fore-brain*. Translated by B Sachs. New York: Putnam.

Meynert T. (1890) Amentia. In: *Klinische Vorlesungen über Psychiatrie auf Wissenschaftlichen Grundlagen, für Studierende und Ärzte, Juristen und Psychologen*. Vienna: Braumüller.

Morel BA. (1857) *Traité des dégénérescences physiques intellectuelles et morales de l'espèce humaine*. Paris: Baillière.

Morel BA. (1860) *Traité des maladies mentales*. Paris: Masson.

Niery D, Snowden JS, Northen B, Goulding P. (1988) Dementia of frontal lobe type. *Journal of Neurology, Neurosurgery, and Psychiatry* **51**: 353–61.

North HM, Bostock F. (1925) Arteriosclerosis and mental disease. *Journal of Mental Science* **71**: 600–1.

Olah G. (1910) Was kann man heute unter Arteriosklerotischen Psychosen verstehen. *Psychiatrie Neurologie Wochenschrift* **52**: 532–3.

Parrot J. Cerveau. (1873) VIII Ramollissement. In: Dechambre A, Lereboullet L (eds). *Dictionnaire encyclopédique des sciences médicales*, Vol 14. Paris: Mason and Asselin, 400–31.

Perry R, McKeith I, Perry E. (eds) (1996) *Dementia with Lewy bodies*. Cambridge: Cambridge University Press.

Perusini G. (1909) Über klinish und histologisch eigenartige psychische Erkrankungen des späteren Lebensalters. In: Nissl F, Alzheimer A (eds). *Histologische und histopatologische Arbeiten*, vol 3. Jena: Gustav Fischer, 297–351.

Perusini G. (1911) Sul valore nosografico di alcuni reperti istopatologici caratteristiche per la senilitá. *Rivista Italiana di Neuropatologia, Psichiatria ed Elettroterapia* **4**: 193–213.

Pick A. (1892) Über die Beziehungen der senilen Hirnatrophie zur Aphasie. *Prager Medicinische Wochenschrift* **17**: 165–7 (Translated by Berrios GE and Girling DM (1994) Introduction to and translation of 'On the relationship between senile cerebral atrophy and aphasia' by Arnold Pick. *History of Psychiatry*, 1994, 5: 539–49).

Pick A. (1901) Senile Hirnatrophie als Grundlage von Herderscheinungen. *Wiener Klinische Wochenschrift* **14**: 403–4.

Pick A. (1906) Über einen weiterer Symptomenkomplex im Rahmen der Dementia senilis, bedingt durch umschriebene sträkere Hirnatrophie (gemische Apraxie). *Monatschrift für Psychiatrie und Neurologie* **19**: 97–108.

Pick D. (1989) *Faces of degeneration.* Cambridge: Cambridge University Press.

Pinel Ph. (1806) *A treatise on insanity.* Translated by DD Davis. Sheffield: Cadell and Davies.

Pinel Ph. (1818) *Nosographic philosophique*, 6th edition. Paris: Brosson (first published: 1798).

Prichard JC. (1835) *A treatise on insanity.* London: Sherwood, Gilbert and Piper.

Rey A. (1995) *Dictionnaire historique de la langue Française*, 2 vols. Paris: Dictionnaire Le Robert.

Rostan L. (1823) *Recherches sur le ramollissement du cerveau*, 2nd edn. Paris: Bechet.

Rouby J. (1911) *Contribution á l'étude de la presbyophrénie.* Thèse de Médicine. Paris: E Nourris.

Schneider C. (1927) Über Picksche Krankheit. *Monatschrift für Psychiatrie und Neurologie* **65**: 230–75.

Schneider C. (1929) Weitere Beiträge zur Lehre von der Pickschen Krankheit. *Zeitschrift für the gesamte Neurologie und Psychiatrie* **120**: 340–84.

Simchowicz T. (1911) Histologische Studien über die Senile Demenz. *Histologische und histopathologischen Arbeiten über der Grosshirnrinde* **4**: 267–444.

Simchowicz T. (1924) Sur la signification des plaques séniles et sur la formule sénile de l'écorce cérébrale. *Revue Neurologique* **31**: 221–7.

Sobrino Aumentado o Nuevo Diccionario de las Lenguas Española, Francesa Y Latina. Leon de Francia, JB Delamollière, 1791.

Southard EE. (1910) Anatomical findings in 'senile dementia': a diagnostic study bearing especially on the group of cerebral atrophies. *American Journal of Insanity* **61**: 673–708.

Sully J. (1885) *Illusions. A psychological study*, 5th edn. London: Kegan Paul.

Truelle V, Bessière R. (1911) Recherches sur la presbyophrénie. *L'Encéphale* **6**: 505–20.

Walton GL. (1912) Arteriosclerosis probably not an important factor in the etiology and prognosis of involution psychoses. *Boston Medical and Surgical Journal* **167**: 834–6.

Wilks S. (1865) Clinical notes on atrophy of the brain. *Journal of Mental Science* **10**: 381–92.

Willis T. (1684) *Practice of physick.* Translated by S Pordage. London: T Dring, C Harper and J Leigh, 209–14.

Ziehen T. (1911) Les démences. In: Marie A (ed.) *Traité International de Psychologie Pathologique*, vol 2. Paris: Alcan, 281–381.

Zilboorg G. (1941) *A history of medical psychology.* New York: Norton.

2

The lived experience of dementia

SHIRLEY NUROCK

2.1 OUR STORY

'What do you mean, Alzheimer's disease? Surely he's too young!'

Apparently not. With these words (over the telephone) our lives were turned upside-down. My handsome, caring husband Leonard, a GP here in London, in his fifties, had been diagnosed with Alzheimer's disease (AD), our three children then in their early 'teens.

Yes, he had been more than usually forgetful over the last couple of years, infuriating me sometimes by mislaying keys or turning up at the wrong time or wrong place, but onset was insidious and I was preoccupied with my work, our hectic lifestyle, the children and their decisions about schools, universities and choice of subjects, and unthinkingly accepted his explanation of merely being stressed at work. This was the late 1980s and a new GP contract was coming into place that involved computerization and appointment of practice managers; not concepts he was familiar with.

The neurologist advised he stop work immediately, stop driving, just stay at home and keep as healthy as possible and don't move house, that would be the worst thing to do; 'Oh, and join the Alzheimer's Society'. That was it. He did. Or rather we did. Although aware that this was not good news, I was unfamiliar with the diagnosis and he seemed not to grasp its wider implications.

Given that his practice list was over 12 000, his assertion that only one or two of his patients may have AD seemed an underestimate. We lived in a five-storey narrow town house and the advice about not moving ultimately turned out to be one of the factors that led to earlier institutionalization than should have been the case.

I laid hands on as many books as I could (this was before the age of universal internet access) and slowly the full horror of the prognosis began to sink in; that this was a terminal illness, possibly I was going to be looking after him for years, our happy and charmed life with our loving family was not going to turn out as we had envisaged. I felt desperately sad for him and initially wondered if it could be a mistake, that he was being forgetful on purpose and would soon revert to his usual charming, distracted self. Denial soon turned to alarm as his memory deteriorated noticeably, then, selfishly, to anger. Never voiced, but I was angry with him for abandoning us in this way. What would become of us? What would become of me? In my forties, my life now on hold.

As we cried ourselves to sleep I embarked on that rollercoaster of emotions that was to last over 15 years. I think he felt humiliated and, aware that his mental faculties were failing, became increasingly frustrated and would mutter about throwing himself off the bridge. I genuinely believed he had a period of good quality life and love ahead and could always reassure him that he had much to live for and three affectionate children nearing adulthood. I had no choice but to give up my part-time work painting children's pictures, just at a time when numbers of commissions were soaring. Subsequently I recall panicking and frantically rushing round reorganizing our finances, signing new wills, powers of attorney and arguing with the pensions department about entitlement.

Imparting the news to friends and family was a relief, no more making excuses for Leonard's lapses of memory and increasing forgetfulness over names and faces. Most just looked bewildered and sadly many of our medical friends just vanished. Were they afraid it was contagious, sorry they couldn't make him better, or what? When effusive letters of condolence came from them some 15 years later I was not in forgiving mood. A brave few turned out to be true friends, visiting no matter how distressing they found our situation.

The children accepted what I told them and although always gentle with their father, I was aware that they retreated more into their own lives and friends. It was particularly hard for the two youngest, still at school and living at home. The youngest, our son, shy at the best of times, was consumed with embarrassment when I would turn up at school concerts or parents' evenings, husband-in-tow because there was nowhere else to leave him. If we were out as a family in public places our son had to help his father to the toilet. I appreciate how hard it was for him. Embarrassment became a feature of our lives and as one by one the children left home for pastures new and friends deserted us, loneliness became another. Even my husband noticed the latter and one day, not having spoken for weeks, clearly asked 'Where they all gone?' I knew but hadn't the heart to tell him.

Still active, he sought the outdoors and would spend hours pacing the nearby park. Within a year or two he was becoming a danger crossing roads so I would accompany him; in fact I have never walked so much in my life as those years. Often I would drive to the river and we would walk along the towpath to look at boats, seeking a tranquillity not possible in the city centre.

At home he invariably followed me round the house, sat next to me when I was speaking on the telephone and accompanied me to the bathroom, unwilling to let me out of his sight. Touching, and I understood why, but desperately lonely and starved of company and good conversation, I felt I was going crazy and remember on occasion pushing him away from my side.

He never saw a doctor, he was never ill in the way of having colds or 'flu. No one seemed to think I could be finding life hard, it was as if I didn't exist, I had no status. Even as a doctor's wife, I was unaware that there should be help available and that someone other than the none-too-helpful GP should know of our situation. That no expression of sympathy, concern or encouragement ever came from the medical profession was something I found hard to bear.

In desperation I tried to access drug trials, enquired at centres of research in the London area and followed up every relevant journal article, but to no avail. When eventually he was invited to an assessment, his Mini-Mental State Examination score was below the criteria for eligibility. Failed again, although of course that trial came to nothing. All those years ago an eminent neurologist assured me not to worry about the remote possibility of the children inheriting the condition since within 20 years there would be a cure. Where is it?

During the early years we took some holidays abroad. He loved the sun and I discovered that cruises were ideal; we had our own cabin, he couldn't get lost – well he could, we both did, but couldn't go far – he could pace the deck, visit new places, watch films. The motion of the ship and the wide sea proved almost hypnotic. I never knew what our fellow passengers made of us. I recall him asking the captain of the ship whether he was going to Leningrad too! These holidays were hard work mentally, but, on balance, worthwhile, a last attempt to lead as normal a life as possible.

A couple of years later agitation was added to the equation and I was forced on alert 24-hours a day. I still managed to lose him once and those 3 hours until he was found by the police were traumatic. For two years I slept on a mattress on the floor by his side of our bed so that when he got up to wander in the middle of the night he tripped and woke me. Thus I could prevent him walking out of the bedroom door and falling down the stairs. Locking doors, removing electric plugs, hiding basin plugs, turning off light switches, nightlights everywhere, flushing the toilet every time I went past, all became routine.

Eventually our GP, fed up with seeing me asking for more sleeping pills (for myself), said he would refer us to a private psychiatrist. Great, I thought, perhaps something could be done about my husband's agitation. It was only after two sessions that I realized I was the patient, that he thought I was depressed. I was furious. Yes, I probably was depressed but could not coping with my husband's illness be one reason why?

From the outset, being under 65 years of age, Leonard was not eligible to be seen by a geriatrician, but this psychiatrist did refer us to social services and an appointment was made for an assessment at the mental health day hospital and in turn this led to some helpful visits from an occupational therapist.

Antidepressants helped me, but I was aware he was depressed too. The psychiatrist's suggestion that I try him on my pills was a disaster – he became totally disoriented. I took matters into my own hands and in a convoluted way found a retired psychologist from the neuro-rehabilitation unit at The National Hospital and subsequently my husband attended regularly for over a year – again privately. When I collected him he was different, happier; it was worth anything to see him like that even if the effects lasted only a few hours. Helpfully I was given feedback on what he seemed unable to express to me, as in the time he knew I was going away for a week and had found a private respite home for him just outside London. Evidently he thought I would leave him there and never come back.

Local day centres were totally unsuitable. How could I leave him sitting in front of a TV with a rug over his knees in the company of 80-year-olds? It took months to track down a private centre run by a charity that had received a good review in an Alzheimer's Society magazine. When a place became available I was relieved to discover two other younger men attending. I had to convince my protesting husband that he was going there to help, he was a doctor after all. The three became good friends and although by this stage none could read, I am told some amusing conversations ensued on the subject of current affairs, but it didn't matter, it gave them a sense of companionship.

The downside was that it was on the other side of London, so Tuesdays and Thursdays I had a frantic rush to get him up and dressed for the hour's drive through the rush-hour traffic. I then ended up the opposite side of London with insufficient time to easily drive home and back to collect him.

By then I had decided I needed to know why I felt the way I did (dreadful) and enrolled on a part-time external Diploma in Psychology at London University. Lectures were in the evenings so I had to leave our son to give my husband supper and see him into bed. Subsequently I found a good public library near the day centre and would spend those days struggling with essays.

When he was in long-term care I went on to gain an MSc in gerontology. At the back of my mind was the thought that when all this was over I could have years ahead and would have to do something with my life. Sadly, going back to my former occupation was out of the question. During my years as a carer I have completely lost any creative ability and although I still paint as a hobby can no longer produce imaginative children's designs.

At first I didn't even realise I was a so-called 'carer'. I was using occasional sitters from a local private agency – in fact we went straight from hiring baby-sitters to husband-sitters, sometimes they were the same girls. Eventually, after much form-filling, social services allocated us home respite for 3 hours a week. This only worked well during a six-month 'pilot' when a carer with specific dementia training looked after him and I could go out with an easy mind. Usually it was a different carer each week and I spent the time away from home fretting and worrying.

In time a voluntary organization in the borough offered a 2-hour free sitting service once a week. The first afternoon a lovely Jamaican nurse arrived and I went off to the dentist. When I returned my husband was wandering about the house causing havoc and no sign of her. Evidently he had told her to go and, not being obliged to stay, she left. She had dreadlocks and beads in her hair and I think he was scared of her. When I tactfully tried to ask the office whether they had someone else, we were accused of being racist – no good telling them that my husband was not racist, that you cannot rationalize with someone with dementia and, if he was scared, no amount of talking would convince him otherwise. We went to the bottom of the waiting list.

Two years later we must have reached the top again and for a few blissful months a kindly lady would arrive at 8 pm on alternate Tuesdays and beg me to enjoy an evening out with friends. Night out, you're kidding! Friends! What friends? I would take a large glass of wine and a sleeping pill and shut myself in a bedroom until 8 o'clock next morning when she would knock on my door with my husband showered and dressed.

Those carers who say they find their role rewarding and spiritually uplifting fill me with disbelief. I could never see it like that, only as an appalling tragedy with catastrophic consequences for him and all who loved him and in the absence of any pastoral concern from within our community I turned away from religion altogether. Laughter was conspicuously absent; obviously my fault that unlike other carers I was unable to find amusing any of the incidents in our day-to-day life, it was just unremitting hard work laced with utter despair.

The agitation became worse and worse over the next couple of years. Eventually the unsympathetic geriatrician suggested something to calm him down. It was haloperidol. When we returned a month later I said he seemed worse, could barely talk or walk now and was showing signs of incontinence. The dose was doubled.

If only I had known then what I know now. In my ignorance I was unaware for whom haloperidol was meant or what the side effects were, and to this day I blame myself for his rapid descent into severe dementia. After only a few weeks he became a bent, drooling, shuffling shell of his former self, without facial expression and with involuntary foot jerking movements that were to stay with him for the rest of his days. I was distraught, no one seemed to listen to me and I felt powerless to help my poor husband. I had become a bystander watching horror after horror being heaped upon him as he hurtled down the dark tunnel of AD. It was heartbreaking, it was obscene, haloperidol yet another trigger to institutionalization.

As I collected Leonard from the day centre one day, the manager took me aside and said sorry they couldn't have him back if he carried on like this, he hadn't sat down all day, refused to eat, was falling and disrupting the others. When we arrived home I phoned the GP and for the first and only time asked for a home visit. A young locum doctor arrived, took one look at him shuffling round the living-room in tight circles, leaning sideways at an alarming angle and foaming at the mouth and said 'Take him to A & E'.

Midsummer's Eve and, if I had but known it, this was to be his Last Journey. He never came home again to live. The taxi driver surveyed us suspiciously as I spread a plastic sheet on the seat. It wasn't a heart attack or another fit as the locum suspected and after a few days on an acute medical ward he was transferred to the chaotic inpatient assessment ward at the Mental Health unit from where, despite my protests, it was eventually recommended he go into long-term care.

The last years of his life in first a home for the elderly mentally ill, where within a few weeks he broke a hip, and a few months later the other hip (no one saw these incidents happen), were a nightmare. I had been told I would feel only relief when he went into care. In fact it was harder. I was not in control of his life, how understanding staff were, how they handled him, what he was given to eat and I hated to see him wearing someone else's clothes. Alzheimer's disease had robbed him of his dignity and he had always been an immensely dignified man.

I spent hours with him each day trying to provide some quality of life and the sort of interaction never given in the Home. After breaking the second hip he never got back on his feet again so when he broke a femur – apparently due to staff's poor skills with the hoist – I refused to let him return there and he was eventually found a bed in continuing National Health Service care in a private nursing home not too far from where we lived.

I had to accept that nowhere would be perfect or provide the standard of care I wished for him, but I found it impossible to forgive the poor quality of his and the other residents' lives. To the Home manager's annoyance I employed some private carers; a strong man able to push the wheelchair up the hill to the park weather permitting; a delightful Irish lady to sit with him occasionally – and sing; a caring Russian girl to give him tea on Saturdays so that I could see my children outside the care home setting and visit my parents.

And my parents are still alive now, my father 98. They loved their son-in-law, their honorary doctor they called him, and couldn't accept what was happening to him, so out of turn. Neither could bear to visit him in the Home, so consequently saw little of me during those years as my time was spent beside Leonard.

I doubt being GP to a care home with so many frail elderly people is every doctor's dream, but the ability to diagnose concomitant illnesses of old age in non-verbal patients is key to their quality of life. On one occasion I had been insisting to the GP for over 2 weeks that something was very wrong, that it couldn't 'still be an allergy'. It was for me to telephone a dermatologist, a former colleague of my husband's, who that same day diagnosed bullous pemphigoid and started him on steroids. I had always believed nature should be allowed to take its course, but in another 24 hours, undiagnosed, he would have died the most appalling death as those massive blisters spread down his throat and other orifices.

How could I feel other than anger and helplessness? Interestingly, that year on steroids he reverted to something resembling his old self; smiles and occasional laughter not heard for years. When I suggested he stay on a low-dose given the feelings of well-being they promoted, I was told this wasn't ethical. What about all those ethical issues ill-prepared family carers are forced to confront at all stages of the disease? What is ethical about the way some care homes treat people with dementia?

Much as I disliked the Home and literally had to grit my teeth as I rang the entry bell each day, I always longed to see my husband, to touch him and prattle on with my usual monologue, my mental state so closely tied with how he was. If he was unwell, in pain, or looking distressed I would go home in the evening feeling distraught. If he was alert and calm I felt lighter and slept better. The wording on the birthday cake one year said Happy 88th Birthday; he was 68. Numbed and aghast in equal measure, I couldn't protest. Sadness was ever present, but now it was weariness, wondering what disaster would befall him next and an overriding sense of fear that engulfed me.

'What do you mean, MRSA? How?' The Home manager had no idea how or where, and gradually over the next few months with a series of chest infections, sores, and endless courses of antibiotics, Leonard went downhill. He looked so unhappy and anguished, painfully thin, just bones really, and had a greatly diminished quality of life. I had always worried how I would know when the end was approaching. Suddenly I knew. I had to force the nurse out of the room as I pleaded with the GP 'please no more antibiotics, just let him go in peace'. Ten days later he died, with myself, our son and son-in-law by his side. His journey through a living hell was over, a farewell that had lasted nearly 16 years. Watching him being wheeled out to the waiting ambulance on a cold drizzly February Friday was the bleakest day of my life.

Leonard, these you have missed: watching our children embarking on their paths to adulthood, through university, their careers, celebrating their successes. You were there, but not there. You saw both the girls on their wedding days wearing their beautiful white dresses because we stopped by the Home on our way to the ceremony, but I don't know if you recognized them or understood the momentousness of the day. You never had the pleasure of walking your daughters up the aisle or knowing your delightful sons-in-law and daughter-in-law. Our son grew up not knowing you for the brilliant, kind and caring man you had once been.

You would have adored the grandchildren, five of them now and, incredibly, twins on the way. You always doted on our children, how much more time you would have had in retirement to enjoy the next generation. I treasure the photograph of our first grandchild Sam on your lap just a few weeks before you died. You were staring wide-eyed at this little baby; I so hope you knew it was yours.

And our children… I still cannot fathom the extent to which their lives have been affected. The day after he graduated from Cambridge our son started his first job – in Scotland – as far away from home as possible. Now they are all married, all back in London and seem happy, although the spectre of AD, unspoken, must linger on occasion. Rightly or wrongly, I tried to shield them from the caring role, feeling that it should not be allowed to dominate their lives and I would never ever wish or expect them to look after me should I succumb in the future. I tried so hard to be a good wife and carer, mother and father, daughter and eventually grandmother, but in the end was so overwhelmed, so torn in a myriad directions, I am not sure I have succeeded as any of these.

Current research is trying to emphasize the positive aspects of caring. Few coping 24/7 with challenging behaviour, incontinence, social services and unhelpful carers are going to accept being told it is a positive and satisfactory experience. However, if carers survive the physical and emotional turmoil of a 'caring career' there is evidence that we emerge more confident, more empowered to deal with statutory authorities. Literally, we have fought a battle and come through it.

In my case the positive legacy includes teaching medical students, postgraduate clinical psychologists and nurses about the impact of dementia on families, active involvement on many major dementia research projects and the first carer to be awarded a research grant by the UK Alzheimer's Society. I continue my interest because our children are nearing middle age and, who knows, potentially at risk in the next decade or two.

The mental and physical costs are long-lasting: for me, anxiety, chronic insomnia and backache from all those years of 'lifting'. The year before he died I spent weeks in hospital and recuperating from *Legionella* and have never felt completely well since. Feeling totally knocked out, I remember sobbing by his side, convinced he would outlive me yet. The toll on family relationships; with my parents (who in some obscure way I think blame him for ruining their daughter's life); and wider family members who all had their own views on how I was looking after him and what I should, or should not, be doing for the best. The social legacy is immense in terms of work, lifestyle, relationships and, of course, finances.

However, life goes on: new friends, new hobbies, some amazing fellow carers, travel and a degree of contentment I never believed possible to achieve again. But tears are never far away and I would do anything to wind the clock back 25 years and be sharing happy memories with my beloved husband as we grow old together, rather than rushing around the country telling how it was.

2.2 POSTSCRIPT

My caring career started over 20 years ago. Awareness of dementia has increased exponentially with the predicted explosion of numbers likely to be affected in the future. Research inches forward and more is known about the benefits of psychological interventions. We already have evidence on what optimum care looks like and the special needs of younger people with dementia. We family carers believe there needs to be a change of attitude, more effort and the necessary funding to translate that evidence into delivering better quality care and training as the main route to improving life for those suffering now and until such time as a cure or effective symptom relief becomes available. The latter of course remains the ultimate goal.

Our turbulent journey, just one of millions being acted out across the globe, may serve as a caution to all those professionals involved in caring for this group.

3

Prevalence and incidence of dementia

DANIEL W O'CONNOR

3.1 SCOPE OF EPIDEMIOLOGY

Epidemiology is the study of the distribution and determinants of disease in human populations. It maps the frequency of disease and identifies people at higher or lower risk of contracting particular conditions. Once risk factors are confirmed, their impact can be reduced. Studies linking cigarette smoking with lung cancer, and hypertension with stroke, sparked successful campaigns to limit smoking and lower blood pressure. Ideally, epidemiological studies will identify reversible triggers to Alzheimer's disease (AD) and other dementias.

Links between life experience and disease are identified by means of observational, analytic and experimental approaches (Jablenksy, 2002). Observational studies entail large-scale surveys to measure the frequency of dementia and to note correlations with sociodemographic, biometric and lifestyle variables. Surveys, while costly and time-consuming, are essential in conditions like dementia that go mostly unrecognized by primary and specialist health services, even in developed countries. In one UK study, in a town with well-developed medical services, general practitioners recognized only half of all dementia cases (O'Connor et al., 1988).

Analytic studies contrast the backgrounds of people with dementia (drawn from community surveys or clinical practice) with those of matched controls to identify points of difference that might, on further study, prove to be risk factors. Case–control studies are economical but accurate matching is problematic and associations will emerge by chance if questions cover hundreds of items. To complicate matters, people with dementia cannot report accurately on exposure. Information must therefore be sought from relatives whose knowledge is imperfect and subject to bias.

Both types of study, observational and analytic, generate hypotheses to be tested in experimental trials, sometimes with unexpected results. The finding in some (but not all) case–control studies that hormone replacement therapy (HRT) conferred protection against dementia was not confirmed by a large controlled trial of HRT as a treatment of dementia, perhaps because women taking HRT were healthier and at lower risk (Almeida and Flicker, 2005). Apart from selection bias, reasons for discrepancies between analytic and experimental studies include confounding by pre-existing cognitive impairment, insufficient dosing and limited follow-up (Coley et al., 2008). Since dementia develops over many decades, interventions might need to be deployed decades earlier to be effective.

Particular risk factors for AD and vascular dementia (VaD) are addressed in Chapter 47, Risk factors for Alzheimer's disease and Chapter 61, What is vascular cognitive impairment?. This chapter focuses instead on the starting point of epidemiological knowledge, namely studies of the prevalence and incidence of dementia and its various subtypes. Wherever possible, information comes from community surveys rather than specialist settings.

3.2 METHODOLOGICAL ISSUES

The prevalence of dementia measures the proportion of people within a population who meet diagnostic specifications. Incidence measures the numbers of new cases of dementia within a defined period. Prevalence studies are simpler: people are divided into 'cases' of dementia and 'non-cases' at a single point in time. Some will have developed dementia recently: others have had it for many years. A community might therefore have a higher than usual prevalence because its residents with dementia survive longer. Incidence studies entail two surveys, a year or more apart, to determine the annual conversion of former 'non-cases' to 'cases'. They have greater scientific value since rates are not confounded by survival.

The first surveys of mental disorder date from the 1950s. Lin (1953), who supplemented brief evaluations of Taiwanese residents with information from relatives and hospitals, concluded that only 0.5 per cent of people aged over 60 years had 'senile dementia'. By contrast, Essen-Moller (1956) diagnosed 28 per cent of Swedes aged over 70 years with 'mild or severe dementia' based on detailed personal assessments by skilled clinicians. This 60-fold discrepancy might reflect genuine differences in dementia prevalence, but methodological factors were most likely to blame.

Even brief cognitive tests can distinguish correctly between healthy old people on the one hand and those with advanced dementia on the other. Discrepancies arise mostly at the cleavage point between 'normal ageing' on the one hand and 'early dementia' on the other. Since early dementia merges imperceptibly with age-related cognitive impairment, the dividing line is arbitrary.

Despite decades of research, there is no commonly-recognized protocol to screen, assess and diagnose dementia in community populations. **Table 3.1** summarizes the methods employed in large, well-documented reports from India (Chandra *et al.*, 1998), China (Zhang *et al.*, 2005) and

Spain (Gascón-Bayarri *et al.*, 2007). The studies vary in important details (participants' education, screening cut-points, special assessments and diagnostic criteria). These differences make it difficult to compare one study with another. Notwithstanding this, India looks to have a lower prevalence rate than China or Spain. How much this difference stems from the methods used to screen and diagnose dementia is unclear.

3.2.1   Screening

Population surveys are so expensive that most researchers use the Mini-Mental State Examination (MMSE; Folstein *et al.*, 1975) or other brief tests to select respondents for detailed evaluation. The 30-point MMSE, which takes only 10 minutes or so to administer and requires no specialist equipment, is well-suited to this task, at least in developed countries. In a meta-analysis of 21 community and primary studies, 83 per cent of people with dementia scored at or below the selected cut-point (usually 23 points) while 87 per cent of 'normals' scored above it (Mitchell, 2009). However, only a third of those 'failing' the MMSE met criteria for dementia so further investigation is mandatory.

Since the MMSE tests reading, writing and arithmetic, performance is shaped by education. In the UK, 11 per cent of 'normal' older people who left school before their fifteenth birthday scored 23 points or less compared with only 3 per cent of those with higher education. Conversely, the same cut-point missed 27 per cent of dementias in better educated people compared with only 12 per cent in those with limited education (O'Connor *et al.*, 1989a). Adjusting cut-points to reflect age- and education-specific norms seems not to

Table 3.1   Comparison of methods and results in three dementia prevalence studies.

	India	China	Spain
First author (year)	Chandra *et al.* (1998)	Zhang *et al.* (2005)	Gascón-Bayarri *et al.* (2007)
Respondents (N)	5126	34 927	1754
Sampling frame	Census	Census	Census
Sample, age	All aged over 55	Weighted sample aged over 55	Weighted sample aged over 70
Institutions	Not applicable	Included	Included
Education	73% illiterate	36% <1 year education	Not stated
Screening test	Modified MMSE+others	Modified MMSE	MMSE
Screen cut-point	≤10th percentile	≤10th percentile, by education	≤23 points
Diagnostic assessment	Clinical evaluation	Clinical evaluation	Clinical evaluation
Informant interviews	Yes	Some	Yes
Investigations	Neuropsychology, physical exam, lab tests, brain MRI	Neuropsychology, physical exam	Neuropsychology, physical exam, lab tests, brain CT
Diagnostic criteria	DSM-IV, NINCDS-ADRDA	NINCDS-ADRDA, NINCDS-AIREN	DSM-IV, NINCDS-ADRDA, NINCDS-AIREN
Dementia severity ratings	CDR		CDR
Dementia types[a]	AD	AD, VaD	AD, VaD, FTD, LBD
Research personnel	Trained interviewers, physician, neurologist	Medical students, neurologists, psychiatrists	Neurologist, neuropsychologist
Dementia prevalence, 75–84 years	1.7%	7.5%	8.7%

[a]Dementia types: Alzheimer (AD), frontotemporal (FTD), Lewy body (LBD), vascular (VaD).

improve validity in literate communities (Cullen *et al.*, 2005). A better strategy in two-phase studies is to evaluate all who score below the chosen cut-point together with a proportion of high scorers to limit the risk of missing early or atypical dementias.

The MMSE is not an appropriate screening tool in countries where older people are often illiterate and innumerate. The test has been modified, sometimes with great care to reflect local culture, relative difficulty and range of cognitive domains (e.g. Ganguli *et al.*, 1995). Other investigators combined test items less subject to educational bias (e.g. naming, praxis and recall) with reports from family members about cognitive and functional capacity. One such instrument, the Community Screening Instrument for Dementia (CSI-D), has high sensitivity and specificity in Native American, African American and Nigerian communities, particularly when scores are adjusted for years of education (Hall *et al.*, 2000). Further refinements emerged from a multi-national study of older people in India, China, Asia, Latin America and the Caribbean (Prince *et al.*, 2003).

In developed countries, up to half of all people with moderate and severe dementia will be missed if aged care facilities are ignored (O'Connor *et al.*, 1989b). With respect to geographic scope, some investigators approach all eligible residents of a suburb or town. Others employ complex strategies to select representative residents of entire cities, states or countries. A smaller locale promotes co-operation, reduces costs and makes follow-up easier. Larger scale studies ensure that findings can be generalized to the whole of a region or nation (Jablensky, 2002). The choice of approach is driven by study resources and objectives.

3.2.2   Diagnosis

Structured interviews administered by trained lay interviewers (e.g. the Geriatric Mental State; Copeland *et al.*, 1991) or clinicians (e.g. CAMDEX; Roth *et al.*, 1986) have been largely supplanted by assessments comprising a history, mental state examination, cognitive battery, informant interview, neurological examination, laboratory tests and neuroimaging with inputs from a physician, psychiatrist and neuropsychologist. Most recent European and North American surveys have adopted such a comprehensive approach (e.g. Fratiglioni *et al.*, 1999). Even in developing countries, the 10/66 Dementia Research Group, for example, deploys culturally appropriate cognitive tests, an informant interview, physical examination and laboratory tests (Prince *et al.*, 2007).

Informant interviews are essential. Since dementia impairs memory and insight, information must be sought from a relative or carer about the subject's personal details, cognition, functional status, medical and psychiatric history and medications. These details help to confirm the diagnosis of dementia, especially in its early stages, and to distinguish AD from other disorders. Informants' reports correlate highly with other markers of cognitive and functional capacity: underreporting and overreporting are remarkably uncommon (Jorm and Korten, 1988; O'Connor *et al.*, 1989c). Small numbers of respondents forbid contact with informants or have no surviving relatives. One stand-alone, structured

informant interview, IQ-CODE, has sound psychometric properties barely affected by education (Jorm, 2004).

If research findings are to carry weight, diagnostic criteria must be interpreted similarly in different centres (i.e. have high inter-rater reliability) and be accurate. In a study of five research centres in Australia, Europe and the United States, in which clinicians were asked to apply DSM-III-R and Clinical Dementia Rating (CDR) criteria to vignettes of older people identified in clinics and community surveys, between-centre agreement was generally high. It was lower at the border of 'normal ageing' and 'mild dementia' and for frail, deaf or depressed participants (O'Connor *et al.*, 1996).

The critical role of diagnostic glossaries was shown by Erkinjuntti *et al.* (1997) who used data from a multi-stage survey of 10 000 older Canadians to illustrate how criteria (and also assessment procedures) shape prevalence rates. Within the 19 per cent of respondents selected for further testing, 3 per cent met ICD-10 criteria for dementia compared with 29 per cent on DSM-III-R. Similar discrepancies emerged in a survey in rural India where prevalence rates ranged from 0.8 to 63 per cent, depending on the definitions applied (Jacob *et al.*, 2007).

Community diagnoses based on thorough clinical evaluations and informant histories have acceptable clinical validity. In a large British survey, only three of 56 people diagnosed with mild dementia by CAMDEX were passed as normal two years later (O'Connor *et al.*, 1991). Factors contributing to premature diagnoses included deafness, depression and unstable diabetes mellitus.

Validity is best confirmed by neuropathological examination but gathering post-mortem material in community populations is difficult. Holmes *et al.* (1999) obtained brain tissue from 80 aged people with dementia recruited from psychiatric, medical and social services in London, UK. Initial assessments comprising a structured diagnostic and informant interview (CAMDEX), physical examination and CT brain scan were followed by yearly re-examinations until death. Clinical and neuropathological diagnoses were based on detailed, standardized criteria and protocols. Of the 38 people judged in life to have probable AD, six had mixed pathologies and three had other conditions. Of the seven judged to have probable VaD, four had other conditions. In another longitudinal British community study, virtually all the 100 cases of dementia had significant neuropathology but most had mixed disease (Neuropathology Group of the MRCCFAS Study, 2001). Multiple pathologies are the norm in advanced old age and simple attributions to AD or VaD may not match reality.

Given all these issues, it is desirable to apply identical assessment and diagnostic procedures when comparing dementia rates in one community or country with another. This occurs very rarely. Only the Geriatric Mental State (Copeland *et al.*, 1991) and the 10/66 Dementia Research Group protocol (Prince *et al.*, 2007) have been deployed across multiple communities and countries.

There is little value in listing dozens of studies of the prevalence and incidence of dementia in general, and of specific dementing disorders, conducted using disparate methods. This chapter focuses instead on meta-analyses that pool the results of individual studies.

3.3   DEMENTIA

3.3.1   Prevalence

If dementia is truly more common in one part of the world, or in people from a particular background, knowledge of the responsible social or environmental triggers might lead to preventative or mitigating interventions.

In the first of several meta-analyses, Jorm *et al.* (1987) took findings from 22 reports to construct a mathematical model relating dementia prevalence to age and study characteristics. Rates varied widely but there was a consistent trend for prevalence to rise exponentially with age with a doubling in rates every 5.1 years (**Table 3.2**). This was confirmed by Hofman *et al.* (1991) who reanalysed data from 12 European studies conducted between 1977 and 1989 in which dementia was defined using DSM-III or equivalent criteria. No major differences emerged between countries. Broadly speaking, the prevalence of dementia as defined by DSM-III or its equivalent looks to be fairly uniform, at least in developed countries.

Two studies with strikingly high prevalence rates hint at an association between dementia and social deprivation. In the first, aged residents of three Arab Israeli villages were assessed using modified cognitive tests and informant interviews. A quarter met DSM-IV criteria for dementia, three times more than in comparable Jewish Israeli communities. Risk increased with age, female gender and illiteracy (Bowirrat *et al.*, 2001). In Australia, where many indigenous people have limited education and multiple medical co-morbidities, the prevalence of dementia above age 65 was reported as 27 per cent based on detailed, culturally appropriate assessments (Smith *et al.*, 2008). By contrast, rates were low in Cree Indian settlements in northern Canada where older people are actively engaged in fishing, trapping and crafts (Hendrie *et al.*, 1993).

3.3.2   Incidence

If it is true that prevalence increases exponentially with age, varying only in its time of onset, all of us will be affected at

some point in our lives. This hypothesis, which has major public health implications, was tested by Ritchie and Kildea (1995) who constructed a statistical model derived from 12 studies with data over age 80 and with adequate sampling procedures and diagnostic methods. This logistic model showed a flattening of growth at age 95, suggesting that dementia is not inevitable. Further evidence came from the Bronx Aging Study in which the risk of dementia grew steadily with age as expected. However, its rate of growth slowed from age 80 for both sexes (Hall *et al.*, 2005).

Few researchers have tracked incidence over time using identical methods to check if rates are falling, perhaps because of better health and well-being. Li *et al.* (2007), who applied similar screening, diagnostic and follow-up procedures in Beijing ten years apart, found a small, non-significant rise in incidence between 1989 and 1999. More such studies are required.

3.3.3   Survival

The number of new cases of dementia rises steeply with age. The longer new cases of dementia survive, the greater will be its prevalence. The best estimates of survival come from follow up of newly diagnosed cases since prevalence surveys capture only survivors. In the Leipzig Longitudinal Study which followed new cases of dementia for three years, 51 per cent died compared with 19 per cent of non-demented controls. Male sex, age, frailty and dementia severity increased risk further (Gühne *et al.*, 2006).

3.4   ALZHEIMER'S DISEASE

3.4.1   Prevalence

Table 3.3 presents findings from a meta-analysis of AD rates using data from 11 European studies conducted in the 1990s (Lobo *et al.*, 2000). Findings were close to those in an earlier,

Table 3.2   Prevalence rates (%) for dementia in four meta-analyses.

	Jorm *et al.* (1987)	Hofman *et al.* (1991)	Ritchie and Kildea (1995)	Fratiglioni *et al.* (1999)	
Number of studies	22	12	9	36	
Places	Europe, USA, Japan, Australasia	Europe	Europe, Canada, Japan	Europe, USA, Canada, Asia, Africa	
Age					**Mean**
65–69	1.4	1.4	1.5	1.5	1.5
70–74	2.8	4.1	3.5	3	3.5
75–79	5.6	5.7	6.8	6	6.3
80–84	10.5	13.0	13.6	12	13.1
85–89	20.8	21.6	22.3		22.1
90–94	38.6	32.2	31.5		31.7
95–99		34.7	44.5		41.2

overlapping meta-analysis by Rocca *et al.* (1991). As before, rates rise sharply with age.

Prevalence was lower overall in the 25 Chinese reports summarized by Dong *et al.* (2007), but females were at higher risk than men in both continents. In China, for instance, 3.8 per cent of men aged 80–84 years were diagnosed with AD compared with 11.0 per cent of women.

Corrada *et al.* (1995) applied logistic regression to identify methodological factors associated with variability in 15 published papers from Europe, the United States, Japan and China. After adjusting for age, higher rates were reported in studies that included mild cases and used laboratory tests to aid in diagnosis. Lower rates emerged from studies that used brain scans and cerebral ischaemia scores. This is not surprising. Studies that can afford laboratory tests are likely to be more thorough in other respects too and studies using brain scans might attribute cases, rightly or wrongly, to visible evidence of vascular pathology.

3.4.2   Incidence

Incidence studies, which entail a second sweep of a population to identify new cases, are better suited to identifying causative factors. **Table 3.4** summarizes findings from four meta-analyses. The incidence of AD rose with age in all four, just as expected. Rates were somewhat higher in two and lower in the others. It levelled off in extreme old age in one meta-analysis (Gao *et al.*, 1998) but not in another (Jorm and Jolley, 1998). Women were at increased risk in all three

studies that specified rates by gender. Possible explanations include women's lower levels of education and the premature onset of dementia in men due to head trauma, occupational toxicity and smoking (Andersen *et al.*, 1999; Fratiglioni *et al.*, 2000). Rates were a little lower in Asian countries than the United States and Europe, perhaps because of the lower prevalence of the ApoE ε4 allele in Japan and environmental and lifestyle differences (Jorm and Jolley, 1998).

In a refinement of an earlier meta-analysis, Ziegler-Graham *et al.* (2008) found that incidence rates doubled every 5.5 years quite consistently in 27 studies from Asia, Europe and the Americas. Base rates varied somewhat between regions but not to a statistically significant degree. Findings from three recent incidence surveys in the US (Miech *et al.*, 2002), Brazil (Nitrini *et al.*, 2004) and Canada (Tyas *et al.*, 2006) lay within the bounds identified in the meta-analyses.

3.4.3   Survival

Younger onset adds to the lethality of AD. In a follow-up study of 108 incident cases identified in the Baltimore Longitudinal Study of Aging, diagnosis was associated with a 39 per cent reduction in median life span for people aged 90 years compared with 67 per cent for those aged 65 years (Brookmeyer *et al.*, 2002).

3.5   VASCULAR DEMENTIA

3.5.1   Prevalence

Estimating the prevalence of VaD is difficult: definitions and assessment methods vary too widely to give confidence in study findings. In a review by Rocca and Kokmen (1999), for example, prevalence rates were higher in studies that combined 'mixed dementia' with VaD and based diagnoses on radiologists' reports of brain scans.

In a meta-analysis by Lobo *et al.* (2000), rates were lower than those for AD (**Table 3.5**). This fits with findings from community autopsy series in the UK and US showing a preponderance of AD pathology, though with high admixtures of

Table 3.3   Prevalence rates (%) of Alzheimer's disease in a meta-analysis of 11 European studies.

Age	Males	Females
65–69	0.6	0.7
70–74	1.5	2.3
75–79	1.8	4.3
80–84	6.3	8.4
85–89	8.8	14.2
90+	17.6	23.6

Data from Lobo *et al.* (2000).

Table 3.4   Incidence rates (cases per 1000 person years at risk) of Alzheimer's disease in four meta-analyses.

	Jorm and Jolley (1998)	Gao *et al.* (1998)	Fratiglioni *et al.* (2000)	Brookmeyer *et al.* (1998)
Number of studies	23	7	8	4
Places	Europe, USA, Asia	Europe, USA	Europe	USA
Age				
65–69	3.5	3.3	1.2	1.7
70–74	7.4	8.4	3.3	3.5
75–79	15.5	18.2	9.1	7.1
80–84	32.7	33.6	21.8	14.4
85–89	68.7	53.3	35.3	29.2
90–94	144.3	72.9		59.5
95+				121.0

Table 3.5 Prevalence rates (%) of vascular dementia in a meta-analysis of 11 European studies.

Age	Males	Females
65–69	0.5	0.1
70–74	0.8	0.6
75–79	1.9	0.9
80–84	2.4	2.3
85–89	2.4	3.5
90+	3.6	5.8

Data from Lobo *et al.* (2000).

vascular abnormalities (Lim *et al.*, 1999; Neuropathology Group of the MRCCFAS Study, 2001).

Rates of VaD look to be higher in Asia. When Fratiglioni *et al.* (1999) summarized findings from 25 European studies and five from Japan, Korea, India and China, the proportions of cases ascribed to VaD were 28 per cent in Europe and 38 per cent in Asia. It was diagnosed twice more often than AD in a series of Japanese studies, but exceptions exist. Ratios were similar, for example, in two studies conducted in China with US collaborators (Graves *et al.*, 1996).

Caucasian–Asian differences might be real, not artifactual. In one rigorous, seven-year Japanese study in which diagnoses were confirmed whenever possible by post-mortem examination, 61 per cent of dementias in men were attributed to vascular disease, a much higher rate than observed in equivalent studies in Europe and the United States (Yoshitake *et al.*, 1995). Lifestyle is possibly more influential than genes: rates of VaD in elderly Japanese-American men in the mainland US were similar to those of other North Americans (Graves *et al.*, 1996). By contrast, Japanese men in Hawaii, whose lifestyle is more authentically Asian, had VaD rates similar to those in Japan (White *et al.*, 1996).

3.5.1.1 INCIDENCE

Incidence rates vary widely from study to study for the reasons outlined above but are generally much lower than for AD. Males are possibly at higher risk than females in early old age but at lower risk later (Rocca and Kokmen, 1999; Fratiglioni *et al.*, 2000). Rates look to be higher in Asian populations than North American ones (Fratiglioni *et al.*, 2000), more in older studies than recent ones (Homma and Hasegawa, 2000).

3.6 OTHER DEMENTIAS

While most attention has been paid to AD and VaD, dementia due to other causes accounted for 11 per cent of cases in the 25 European prevalence surveys summarized by Fratiglioni *et al.* (1999).

In the six community surveys to have diagnosed Lewy body dementia using current criteria, prevalence rates ranged from 0 to 5 per cent with Lewy body cases accounting for between 0 and 30 per cent of all identified dementias. Rates were lower in studies led by neurologists in contrast to psychiatrists and

geriatricians (Zaccai *et al.*, 2005). Frontotemporal dementia arises mostly in younger age groups and is discussed below.

Dementias due to potentially reversible causes are rare. In a US medical records review of 560 new cases of dementia identified in the Rochester Epidemiology Project, non-degenerative causes were identified in 30 per cent of young onset patients but only 5 per cent in the older onset group. The most common causes were chronic mental illness, brain tumours, alcoholism and cerebral anoxia (Knopman *et al.*, 2006). No cases were identified of dementia due to normal pressure hydrocephalus, subdural haematoma, hypothyroidism, vitamin B_{12} deficiency or neurosyphilis.

3.6.1 Early-onset dementia

Dementia before 65 years of age is too rare to warrant a door-to-door survey. Instead, frequency estimates are derived from checks of memory clinics, hospital records and diagnostic registers. Given the gravity of these conditions for carers and service providers, most cases are likely to be captured in this way. In a London study in which 227 cases nominated by GPs, specialists and community services were reviewed in detail, diagnoses in age group 45–64 years were as follows: AD (35 per cent), VaD (18 per cent), frontotemporal dementia (15 percent), alcohol-related dementia (14 per cent) and other conditions (18 percent) including Lewy body dementia, Huntingdon's disease, multiple sclerosis, cortico-basal degeneration, Down's syndrome and unspecified conditions (Harvey *et al.*, 2003).

A different distribution emerged from a smaller records linkage study in Cambridgeshire, UK. Of 37 identified cases aged 45–64 years, most were labelled as either frontotemporal dementia (27 per cent) or Huntingdon's disease (22 per cent). Other conditions included equal numbers of AD, VaD and parkinsonian syndromes (Ratnavalli *et al.*, 2002).

Frontotemporal dementia appears to be more common than previously thought. In a sustained community-based search, Dutch neurologists and nursing home physicians identified 245 cases of whom 40 came to autopsy. The median age of onset was 58 years with a range of 33 to 80 years. The prevalence rose from 3.6 per 100 000 at age 50–59 to 9.4 at age 60–69 years and then fell to 3.8 at 70–79 years (Rosso *et al.*, 2003). Incidence rates have since been reported in the UK, with numbers similar to those for early-onset AD (Mercy *et al.*, 2008).

Irrespective of cause, early-onset dementia resulted in much increased mortality in a Dutch memory clinic cohort. Over a short follow-up period (mean two years), the risk of death was 43 times higher than for controls of the same age. For dementia with later onset, by contrast, the risk was only three times higher (Koedam *et al.*, 2008).

3.7 COMPARATIVE STUDIES

Putative socio-environmental risk factors will be identified more confidently if identical case-finding tools are applied to groups with vastly different social, educational, dietary, occupational and medical exposures. Studies of North American Whites, Blacks and Latinos generally show higher dementia rates in socially disadvantaged groups (Hendrie, 1999) but their backgrounds overlap too much to draw straightforward conclusions.

More revealing findings have emerged from a direct comparison of dementia in elderly Nigerian Africans and African Americans. This decade-long study applied identical screening tests and diagnostic evaluations comprising neuropsychology, informant interviews, personal evaluations and CT brain scans to residents of Ibadan, Nigeria and Indianapolis, USA (Hendrie et al., 1995). Contrary to expectation, the age-standardized prevalence rate of AD was lower in Nigerians aged over 65 years than African Americans (1.4 versus 6.2 per cent). Rates for dementia of all causes were lower too (2.3 versus 8.2 per cent). This disparity was not due to greater life expectancy in the United States. In a five-year follow-up, age-standardized annual incidence rates of AD were still lower in Ibadan, perhaps because of lower weight, blood pressure, glucose and cholesterol levels (Hendrie et al., 2001).

In a rural community in northern India, only 1 per cent of people aged over 65 met DSM-IV criteria for dementia despite low literacy levels when assessed in detail using tools modified from an earlier US survey. Gender and literacy made no difference (Chandra et al., 1998). In a two-year follow up, incidence rates were about a third those found in the US (Chandra et al., 2001) suggesting that northern Indian lifestyles are protective.

3.8 FUTURE TRENDS

According to burden of disease estimates, dementia contributes to more years lived with disability in later life than stroke, musculoskeletal disorders, cardiovascular disease and cancer (WHO, 2003). Given population ageing, the rapidly growing numbers of people with dementia will therefore impose great demands on families and social, residential and medical services throughout the world. To map this global impact, Brookmeyer et al. (2007) applied a complex mathematical model of incidence, progression and survival in AD to projected populations between 2006 and 2050. These very rough estimates suggest that the numbers of AD will quadruple from 27 to 106 million. Numbers in world areas might conceivably be as follows: Africa six million, North America nine million, Latin America 11 million, Europe 16 million and Asia 63 million. Modelling suggests that if interventions could delay both disease onset and progression by just one year, there would be nine million fewer cases overall. Prevention is therefore of paramount importance.

3.9 CONCLUSIONS

Surveys of dementia prevalence and incidence provide varying rates, most probably because of differences in study methodology. Future studies will be easier to interpret now that many investigators are using similar, and sometimes identical, approaches to assessment and diagnosis.

Alzheimer and vascular pathologies often coexist in advanced old age. Seemingly clear-cut diagnoses must therefore be interpreted cautiously.

Dementia might be more common in certain places and cultures. It is important to compare incidence (not prevalence) rates of AD, VaD, etc. in aged people from widely differing backgrounds. Observations of very low rates of dementia in Nigeria and northern India might prove to be of great significance.

REFERENCES

Almeida OP, Flicker L. (2005) Association between hormone replacement therapy and dementia: is it time to forget? *International Psychogeriatrics* **17**: 155–64.

Andersen K, Launer LJ, Dewey M et al. (1999) Gender differences in the incidence of AD and vascular dementia: the Eurodem studies. *Neurology* **53**: 1992–7.

Bowirrat A, Treves TA, Freidland RP, Korczyn AD. (2001) Prevalence of Alzheimer's disease in an elderly Arab population. *European Journal of Neurology* **8**: 119–23.

Brookmeyer R, Gray S, Kawas C. (1998) Projections of Alzheimer's disease in the United States and the public health impact of delaying disease onset. *American Journal of Public Health* **88**: 1337–42.

Brookmeyer R, Corrada MM, Curriero FC, Kawas C. (2002) Survival following a diagnosis of Alzheimer's disease. *Archives of Neurology* **59**: 1764–7.

Brookmeyer R, Johnson E, Ziegler-Graham K, Arrighi HM. (2007) Forecasting the global burden of Alzheimer's disease. *Alzheimer's and Dementia* **3**: 186–91.

Chandra V, Ganguli M, Pandav R et al. (1998) Prevalence of Alzheimer's disease and other dementias in rural India: the Indo-US study. *Neurology* **51**: 1000–8.

Chandra V, Pandav R, Dodge HH et al. (2001) Incidence of Alzheimer's disease in a rural community in India. *Neurology* **57**: 985–9.

Coley N, Andrieu S, Gardette V et al. (2008) Dementia prevention: methodological explanations for inconsistent results. *Epidemiologic Reviews* **30**: 35–66.

Copeland JRM, Dewey ME, Saunders P. (1991) The epidemiology of dementia: GMS-AGECAT studies of prevalence and incidence, including studies in progress. *European Archives of Psychiatry and Clinical Neuroscience* **240**: 212–17.

Corrada M, Brookmeyer R, Kawas C. (1995) Sources of variability in prevalence rates of Alzheimer's disease. *International Journal of Epidemiology* **24**: 1000–5.

Cullen B, Fahy S, Cunningham CJ et al. (2005) Screening for dementia in an Irish community sample using MMSE: a comparison of norm-adjusted versus fixed cut-points. *International Journal of Geriatric Psychiatry* **20**: 371–6.

Dong MJ, Peng B, Lin XT et al. (2007) The prevalence of dementia in the People's Republic of China: a systematic analysis of 1980–2004 studies. *Age and Ageing* **36**: 619–24.

Erkinjuntti T, Ostbye T, Steenhuis R, Hachinski V. (1997) The effect of different diagnostic criteria on the prevalence of dementia. *New England Journal of Medicine* **337**: 1667–74.

Essen-Moller E. (1956) Individual traits and morbidity in a Swedish rural population. *Acta Psychiatrica Scandinavica Supplementum* **100**: 1–160.

Folstein MF, Folstein SE, McHugh PR. (1975) Mini-Mental State: a practical method for grading the cognitive state of patients for clinicians. *Journal of Psychiatric Research* **12**: 189–98.

Fratiglioni L, De Ronchi D, Aguera-Torres H. (1999) Worldwide prevalence and incidence of dementia. *Drugs and Aging* **15**: 365–75.

Fratiglioni L, Launer LJ, Anderson K *et al.* (2000) Incidence of dementia and major sub-types in Europe: a collaborative study of population-based cohorts. *Neurology* **54** (Suppl. 5): S10–15.

Ganguli M, Ratcliff G, Chandra V *et al.* (1995) A Hindi version of the MMSE: the development of a cognitive screening instrument for a largely illiterate rural elderly population in India. *International Journal of Geriatric Psychiatry* **10**: 367–77.

Gao S, Hendrie HC, Hall KS, Hui S. (1998) The relationships between age, sex and the incidence of dementia and Alzheimer disease: a meta-analysis. *Archives of General Psychiatry* **55**: 809–15.

Gascón-Bayarri J, Reñé R, Del Barrio JL *et al.* (2007) Prevalence of dementia subtypes in El Prat de Llobregat, Catalonia, Spain: the PRATICON study. *Neuroepidemiology* **28**: 224–34.

Graves AB, Larson EB, Edland SD *et al.* (1996) Prevalence of dementia and its subtypes in the Japanese American population of King County, Washington State: the Kame project. *American Journal of Epidemiology* **144**: 760–71.

Gühne U, Matschinger H, Angermeyer MC, Riedel-Heller SG. (2006) Incident dementia cases and mortality: results of the Leipzig Longitudinal Study of the Aged. *Dementia and Geriatric Cognitive Disorders* **22**: 185–93.

Hall CB, Verghese J, Sliwinski M *et al.* (2005) Dementia incidence may increase more slowly after age 90: results from the Bronx Aging Study. *Neurology* **65**: 882–6.

Hall KS, Gao S, Emsley CL *et al.* (2000) Community screening for dementia (CSI 'D'): performance in five disparate study sites. *International Journal of Geriatric Psychiatry* **15**: 521–31.

Harvey RJ, Skelton-Robinson M, Rossor MN. (2003) The prevalence and causes of dementia in people under the age of 65 years. *Journal of Neurology, Neurosurgery and Psychiatry* **74**: 1206–9.

Hendrie HC. (1999) Alzheimer's disease: a review of cross-cultural studies. In: Mayeux R, Christen Y (eds). *Epidemiology of Alzheimer's: From gene to prevention.* Berlin: Springer-Verlag, 87–101.

Hendrie HC, Hall KS, Pillay N *et al.* (1993) Alzheimer's disease is rare in Cree. *International Psychogeriatrics* **5**: 5–14.

Hendrie HC, Osuntokun BO, Hall KS *et al.* (1995) Prevalence of Alzheimer's disease and dementia in two communities: Nigerian Africans and African Americans. *American Journal of Psychiatry* **152**: 1485–92.

Hendrie HC, Ogunniyi A, Hall KS *et al.* (2001) Incidence of dementia and Alzheimer disease in 2 communities: Yoruba residing in Ibadan, Nigeria and African Americans residing in Indianapolis, Indiana. *Journal of the American Medical Association* **285**: 739–47.

Hofman A, Rocca WA, Brayne C *et al.* (1991) The prevalence of dementia in Europe: a collaborative study of 1980-1990 findings. *International Journal of Epidemiology* **20**: 736–48.

Holmes C, Cairns N, Lantos P, Mann A. (1999) Validity of current clinical criteria for Alzheimer's disease, vascular dementia and dementia with Lewy bodies. *British Journal of Psychiatry* **174**: 45–50.

Homma A, Hasegawa K. (2000) Epidemiology of vascular dementia in Japan. In: Chiu E, Gustafson L, Ames D, Folstein MF (eds). *Cerebrovascular disease and dementia: Pathology, neuropsychiatry and management.* London: Martin Dunitz, 33–46.

Jablensky A. (2002) Research methods in psychiatric epidemiology: an overview. *Australian and New Zealand Journal of Psychiatry* **36**: 297–310.

Jacob KS, Kumar PS, Gayathri K *et al.* (2007) The diagnosis of dementia in the community. *International Psychogeriatrics* **19**: 669–78.

Jorm AF, Korten AE, Henderson AS. (1987) The prevalence of dementia: a quantitative integration of the literature. *Acta Psychiatrica Scandinavica* **76**: 465–79.

Jorm AF, Korten AE. (1988) Assessment of cognitive decline in the elderly by informant interview. *British Journal of Psychiatry* **152**: 209–13.

Jorm AF, Jolley D. (1998) The incidence of dementia: a meta-analysis. *Neurology* **51**: 728–33.

Jorm AF. (2004) The Informant Questionnaire on cognitive decline in the elderly (IQCODE): a review. *International Psychogeriatrics* **16**: 275–93.

Koedam EL, Pijnenburg YA, Deeg DJ *et al.* (2008) Early-onset dementia is associated with higher mortality. *Dementia and Geriatric Cognitive Disorders* **26**: 147–52.

Knopman DS, Petersen RC, Cha RH *et al.* (2006) Incidence and causes of nondegenerative nonvascular dementia: a population-based study. *Archives of Neurology* **63**: 218–21.

Li S, Yan F, Li G *et al.* (2007) Is the dementia rate increasing in Beijing? Prevalence and incidence of dementia 10 years later in an urban elderly population. *Acta Psychiatrica Scandinavica* **115**: 73–9.

Lim A, Tsuang D, Kukull W *et al.* (1999) Clinico-neuropathological correlation of Alzheimer's disease in a community-based case series. *Journal of the American Geriatrics Society* **47**: 564–9.

Lin TY. (1953) A study of the incidence of mental disorder in Chinese and other cultures. *Psychiatry* **16**: 313–36.

Lobo A, Launer LJ, Fratiglioni L *et al.* (2000) Prevalence of dementia and major sub-types in Europe: a collaborative study of population-based cohorts. *Neurology* **54** (Suppl. 5): S4–9.

Mercy L, Hodges JR, Dawson K *et al.* (2008) Incidence of early-onset dementias in Cambridgeshire, United Kingdom. *Neurology* **71**: 1496–9.

Miech RA, Breitner JCS, Zandi PP *et al.* (2002) Incidence of AD may decline in the early 90s for men, later for women. *Neurology* **58**: 209–18.

Mitchell AJ. (2009) A meta-analysis of the accuracy of the mini-mental state examination in the detection of dementia and mild cognitive impairment. *Journal of Psychiatric Research* **43**: 411–31.

Neuropathology Group of the Medical Research Council Cognitive Function and Ageing Study. (2001) Pathological correlates of late-onset dementia in a multi-centre, community based population in England and Wales. *Lancet* **357**: 169–75.

Nitrini R, Caramelli P, Herrera E *et al.* (2004) Incidence of dementia in a community-dwelling Brazilian population. *Alzheimer's Disease and Associated Disorders* **18**: 241–6.

O'Connor DW, Pollitt PA, Brook CPB, Reiss BB. (1989c) The validity of informant histories in a community study of dementia. *International Journal of Geriatric Psychiatry* 4: 203–8.

O'Connor DW, Pollitt PA, Hyde JB et al. (1988) Do general practitioners miss dementia in elderly patients? *British Medical Journal* 297: 1107–10.

O'Connor DW, Pollitt PA, Treasure FP et al. (1989a) The influence of education, social class and sex on Mini-Mental State scores. *Psychological Medicine* 19: 771–6.

O'Connor DW, Pollitt PA, Hyde JB et al. (1989b) The prevalence of dementia as measured by the Cambridge Mental Disorders of the Elderly Examination. *Acta Psychiatrica Scandinavica* 79: 190–8.

O'Connor DW, Pollitt PA, Jones BJ et al. (1991) Continued clinical validation of dementia diagnosed in the community using the Cambridge Mental Disorders of the Elderly Examination. *Acta Psychiatrica Scandinavica* 83: 41–5.

O'Connor DW, Blessed G, Cooper B et al. (1996) Cross-national interrater reliability of dementia diagnosis in the elderly and factors associated with disagreement. *Neurology* 47: 1194–9.

Prince M, Acosta D, Chiu H et al. (2003) Dementia diagnosis in developing countries: a cross-cultural validation study. *Lancet* 361: 909–17.

Prince M, Ferri CP, Acosta D et al. (2007) The protocols for the 10/66 dementia research group population-based research programme. *BMC Public Health* 7: 165.

Ratnavalli E, Brayne C, Dawson K, Hodges JR. (2002) The prevalence of frontotemporal dementia. *Neurology* 58: 1615–21.

Ritchie K, Kildea D. (1995) Is senile dementia "age-related" or "ageing-related"? – evidence from meta-analysis of dementia prevalence in the oldest old. *Lancet* 346: 931–4.

Rocca WA, Hofman A, Brayne C et al. (1991) Frequency and distribution of Alzheimer's disease in Europe: a collaborative study of 1980–1990 prevalence findings. *Annals of Neurology* 30: 381–90.

Rocca WA, Kokmen E. (1999) Frequency and distribution of vascular dementia. *Alzheimer Disease and Associated Disorders* 13 (Suppl. 3): S9–14.

Rosso SM, Kaat LD, Baks T et al. (2003) Frontotemporal dementia in the Netherlands: patient characteristics and prevalence estimates from a population-based study. *Brain* 126: 2016–22.

Roth M, Tym E, Mountjoy CQ et al. (1986) CAMDEX: a standardized instrument for the diagnosis of mental disorder in the elderly with special reference to the early detection of dementia. *British Journal of Psychiatry* 149: 648–709.

Smith K, Flicker L, Lautenschlager NT et al. (2008) High prevalence of dementia and cognitive impairment in indigenous Australians. *Neurology* 71: 1470–3.

Tyas SL, Tate RB, Wooldrage K et al. (2006) Estimating the incidence of dementia: the impact of adjusting for subject attrition using health care utilization data. *Annals of Epidemiology* 16: 477–84.

White L, Petrovich H, Ross W et al. (1996) Prevalence of dementia in older Japanese-American men in Hawaii: the Honolulu-Asia Aging Study. *Journal of the American Medical Association* 276: 955–60.

WHO. (2003) *World Health Report: Shaping the future*. Geneva: World Health Organization.

Yoshitake T, Kiyohara Y, Kato I et al. (1995) Incidence and risk factors of vascular dementia and Alzheimer's disease in a defined elderly Japanese population: the Hisayama study. *Neurology* 45: 1161–8.

Zaccai J, McCracken C, Brayne C. (2005) A systematic review of prevalence and incidence studies of dementia with Lewy bodies. *Age and Ageing* 34: 561–6.

Zhang ZX, Zahner GEP, Román GC et al. (2005) Dementia sub-types in China: prevalence in Beijing, Xian, Shangai and Chegdu. *Archives of Neurology* 62: 447–53.

Ziegler-Graham K, Brookmeyer R, Johnson E, Arrighi HM. (2008) Worldwide variation in the doubling time of Alzheimer's disease incidence rates. *Alzheimer's and Dementia* 4: 316–23.

Criteria for the diagnosis of dementia

CLIVE BALLARD AND CAROL BANNISTER

4.1 INTRODUCTION

There are two main diagnostic challenges within the dementia field: distinguishing patients with dementia from those without, and the accurate differential diagnosis of dementia subtypes (Kaye, 1998). The diagnosis of dementia has always had enormous prognostic implications, however, with the availability of licensed treatments for Alzheimer's disease (AD) (Rogers *et al.*, 1998; see Chapter 54, Established treatments for Alzheimer's disease: cholinesterase inhibitors and memantine) and vascular dementia (VaD) (see Chapter 63, Therapeutic strategies for vascular dementia and vascular cognitive disorders), and the likelihood of more effective treatments becoming available over the next decade, issues of differential diagnosis will become progressively more important.

This chapter reviews criteria and standardized approaches for the diagnosis of dementia, and then tackles the diagnosis of common specific dementia subtypes. There are few published studies validating some of the newer diagnostic criteria, which for this reason do not form the main focus of the chapter.

4.2 DIAGNOSIS OF DEMENTIA

The concept of dementia has evolved from the rather non-specific notion of an organic brain syndrome to a more specific operationalized concept (see Chapter 1, Dementia: historical overview). The ICD-10 criteria (World Health Organization, 1992) described dementia as 'a syndrome due to disease of the brain, usually of a chronic or progressive nature in which there is disturbance of multiple higher

cortical functions including memory, thinking, orientation, comprehension, calculation, learning capacity, language and judgement. Consciousness is not clouded. The impairments of cognitive function are commonly accompanied, and occasionally preceded by deterioration in emotional controls, social behaviour or motivation'. The DSM-IV (American Psychiatric Association, 1994) definition incorporates similar elements, emphasizing the necessity for deteriorating performance of activities of daily living (ADLs). A number of key elements exist across all diagnostic criteria, mainly that dementia is a brain disease, tends to be progressive and globally affects higher cognitive functions as well as emotional and social functioning. The DSM-IIIR criteria (American Psychiatric Association, 1987) (**Box 4.1**), attempted to operationalize these concepts and have been widely used as the basis for the diagnosis of dementia in research studies, with inter-rater reliability attaining scores of up to +0.7 (Baldereschi *et al.*, 1994). Although the key elements within these definitions are based on sound, common-sense principles, with which most clinicians would agree, there are a number of subtle difficulties. For example, the majority of definitions suggest that disturbances of consciousness or delirium should be absent. However, it is recognized that disturbances of consciousness are common in both VaD (Hachinski *et al.*, 1975) and dementia with Lewy bodies (DLB) (see Chapter 64, Dementia with Lewy bodies: a clinical and historical overview) and occur in a minority of AD patients (Robertson *et al.*, 1998).

There are also well-documented cases of patients with a variety of different dementia syndromes where the early manifestations were relatively focal, rather than global, cognitive impairment (Coen *et al.*, 1994). In addition, not all cases of dementia are progressive.

Box 4.1 DSM-IIIR criteria for dementia

1. Demonstrate evidence of impairment in short- and long-term memory. Impairment in short-term memory (inability to learn new information) may be indicated by inability to remember three objects after 5 minutes. Long-term memory impairment (inability to remember information that was known in the past) may be indicated by inability to remember past personal information (e.g. what happened yesterday, birthplace, occupation) or facts of common knowledge (e.g. past presidents, well-known dates).
2. At least one of the following:
   a. impairment in abstract thinking, as indicated by inability to find similarities and differences between related words, difficulty in defining words and concepts, and other similar tasks;
   b. impaired judgement, as indicated by inability to make reasonable plans to deal with interpersonal, family and job-related problems and issues;
   c. other disturbances of higher cortical function, such as aphasia (disorder of language), apraxia (inability to carry out motor activities despite intact comprehension and motor function), agnosia (failure to recognize or identify objects despite intact sensory function), and 'constructional difficulty' (e.g. inability to copy three-dimensional figures, assemble blocks or arrange sticks in specific designs);
   d. personality change, i.e. alteration or accentuation of premorbid traits.
3. The disturbance in 1 and 2 significantly interferes with work or usual social activities or relationships with others.
4. Not occurring exclusively during the course of delirium.
5. Either (a) or (b):
   a. There is evidence from the history, physical examination, or laboratory tests of a specific organic factor (or factors) judged to be aetiologically related to the disturbance.
   b. In the absence of such evidence, an aetiological organic factor can be presumed if the disturbance cannot be accounted for by any non-organic mental disorder, e.g. major depression accounting for cognitive impairment.

Despite these minor caveats, the majority of diagnostic criteria have good face validity, and are probably useful in clinical practice when applied flexibly. However, there are greater difficulties when applying these criteria in research studies. Much published dementia research has focused upon specific dementia subtypes, and has therefore avoided this issue. Within a research setting, the operationalized format of the DSM-IIIR criteria have advantages of established inter-rater reliability. Validity is not, however, a straightforward issue. Unlike specific disease processes such as AD or Pick's disease, dementia is ultimately a clinical diagnosis, and neuropathology cannot be used as a gold standard.

Semi-structured psychiatric interviews have been used as an alternative. The Cambridge Examination for Mental Disorders in the Elderly (CAMDEX; Roth et al., 1986) includes an informant history, physical examination and standardized cognitive assessment, to which operationalized criteria can be applied. The technique provides a standardized information base which can discriminate controls from patients with dementia with adequate reliability and validity, and is hence useful in either a clinical or research setting. The Geriatric Mental State Schedule (GMS; Copeland et al., 1976) is another semi-structured psychiatric interview which covers a range of psychiatric conditions and includes a brief cognitive screening section. It is applied directly as a patient interview and can be completed by medical or allied professionals with appropriate training. Diagnosis is based upon an algorithm (Copeland et al., 1986) which specifies degrees of certainty. The requirement for a computerized diagnostic system probably limits its value in clinical settings, although it has adequate reliability and validity in discriminating controls from dementia patients.

A technique utilized by many epidemiological studies has been to use a standardized cognitive screening instrument such as the Mini-Mental State Examination (MMSE) (Folstein et al., 1975), or a brief semi-structured interview, usually using a two-stage design with a more detailed evaluation of patients scoring below a set cut-off score (Boothby et al., 1994). Outside the context of a dual design, the cut-off score on a cognitive screening instrument is an unsatisfactory way of diagnosing dementia, given the great variability between individuals and the high level of impact that previous education, current psychiatric morbidity and motivation have upon test results.

The Clinical Dementia Rating Scale (CDR; Hughes et al., 1982) provides a mechanism for grading dementia severity in a relatively user-friendly manner. A description of typical performance for dementia patients with different severities of illness in a number of different domains are provided, with the rater required to make a judgement as to which category of severity most appropriately matches the impairments of an individual patient. More recently, a 'sum of boxes' method has been developed which increases the validity and reliability of the tool (O'Bryant et al., 2008). While this is not intended as a method to diagnose dementia per se, it provides an excellent method in tandem with a standardized definition to characterize the severity of impairments either in a clinical or research setting, and includes a category of 'questionable dementia' which is helpful in the global assessment of early cognitive impairments (Liu et al., 2007). Although the method was designed predominantly to improve the sensitivity of clinical staging in people with more severe dementia, the Functional Assessment Staging tool could be used in the same way.

Any of the standardized clinical definitions, particularly when used in conjunction with a severity rating, is likely to be very successful in the diagnosis of patients with moderate or severe dementia. The study populations utilized to investigate the reliability and validity of instruments, such as the CAMDEX and GMS, have been rather polarized. This has avoided the much more difficult issue of whether these criteria can distinguish between patients with no dementia and those with minimal or questionable dementia. Various terms have been utilized to describe older patients with early cognitive impairment who are clearly functioning below their pre-morbid level, but do not have dementia. Historically, labels such as benign senescent forgetfulness (Kral, 1978) and age-associated memory impairment (Crook et al., 1986) have been employed. Currently, the most widely used concept for early cognitive deficits is mild cognitive impairment (MCI; see Chapter 43, Mild cognitive impairment: a historical perspective and Chapter 44, Clinical characteristics of mild cognitive impairment). The original criteria focused very much upon amnestic deficits to identify 'pre-AD'. To meet the criteria for amnestic MCI, people have to perform 1.5 standard deviations below the mean of an age-matched group on a standardized memory task. The criteria therefore achieve a form of 'thresholding' which identifies a cluster of people at increased risk of AD together with a heterogeneous mix of people with mild memory deficits for a range of reasons. The concept has subsequently been broadened to include deficits in other or multiple cognitive domains, but further work is needed to clarify the utility of this approach for the identification of 'dementia' in general or non-AD dementias. Other frequently used concepts include Aging-Associated Cognitive Decline (AACD), which again relies upon thresholding but can also be applied to impairments in any cognitive domain; and Cognitive Impairment No Dementia (CIND) which relates to global cognitive performance in addition to operationalized clinical criteria. A detailed review of MCI and related concepts is beyond the remit of this chapter, although it would appear from numerous follow-up studies that between 4 and 12 per cent of people per year will develop dementia, depending upon the population sampled (higher in clinic settings, lower in the community (see Chapter 43, Mild cognitive impairment: a historical perspective and Chapter 44, Clinical characteristics of mild cognitive impairment). Research criteria for AD have been proposed, combining clinical and neuropsychological criteria with biomarkers (Dubois et al., 2007). Validation is awaited, but this is likely to be an important step forward for the 'pre-clinical' diagnosis of AD, but does not address the equally important challenge of the early identification of other dementias.

Concurrent psychiatric morbidity is a key confounding factor in the diagnosis of early cognitive impairments. Probably the most extreme example is so-called 'depressive pseudodementia' (Kiloh, 1961; Caine, 1981), where a patient experiences an apparently rapid onset of cognitive impairment in the context of a past history or family history of affective disorder and will probably exhibit concurrent depressive symptoms (Caine, 1981). The overlap between depression and cognitive impairment is, however, more complex (Feinberg and Goodman, 1984; see Chapter 74, Depression with

cognitive impairment). It is well established that depression affects both motivation and attention, therefore detrimentally influencing performance on ADLs and cognitive assessments. In addition, however, there is growing evidence of subtle neuropsychological deficits which may be specific to patients with late-onset depression, and which persist after treatment (Abas et al., 1990). This issue is further confounded by the fact the many psychotropic drugs detrimentally influence cognitive function, whilst some organic factors such as diffuse micro-vascular pathology may predispose to both cognitive impairment and depression (O'Brien et al., 1996). Other psychiatric conditions such as anxiety may also affect attention and performance on activities of daily living and formal cognitive assessments, whilst both depression and anxiety disorders are common in dementia sufferers, especially in the early stages of the illness. A proportion of patients with late-onset psychosis have a degree of cortical atrophy (Pearlson and Rabins, 1988), whilst a substantial minority of patients with early onset of psychotic disorders experience cognitive decline (Carpenter and Strauss, 1991). Again, except in patients with marked depressive pseudodementia who should be clinically diagnosed, it is unlikely that these factors will substantially affect misdiagnosis of patients with moderate or severe dementia, but they could have a substantial impact upon the diagnosis of minimal or mild dementia. Although well recognized by clinicians and described in a number of review articles, this is, however, an issue which has not received much research attention. In clinical practice a certain degree of pragmatism can be employed, whilst treating any concurrent psychiatric morbidity and evaluating the progress of any cognitive deficits over time. However, for research studies these diagnostic issues could be a confounding factor, which is why for example, patients with concurrent psychiatric symptoms are often excluded from pharmacological trials pertaining to dementia.

The inclusion of statements pertaining to disturbances of consciousness in the standardized diagnostic definitions of dementia is clearly designed to distinguish dementia from delirium. Some of the difficulties with this approach have been described, but in addition, although delirium is classically thought of as an acute condition, related to a treatable physical condition, a proportion of patients experience a sub-acute delirium, which can persist for months (Lipowski, 1989) and those most vulnerable to delirium are patients with pre-existing dementia. As a consequence, in practice it is not always straightforward to make the diagnosis, particularly in patients with chronic physical conditions predisposing to repeated delirium. Certainly within the CAMDEX and GMS validation studies, patients with delirium and dementia were distinguished with a good degree of inter-rater reliability and validity against expert clinical diagnosis and it is unlikely to apply to a large enough group of patients to make it a relevant issue in research studies. Within clinical services however, this issue will occasionally arise and is probably best dealt with by clinical judgement rather than standardized diagnostic criteria.

Most of the above discussion focuses on standardized methods of applying scales and diagnostic criteria. In clinical practice a number of different challenges exist over and above the value of the standardized instruments that are available. A recent systematic review suggests that dementia is under-diagnosed, with an estimated 50 per cent of primary care patients aged over 65 with dementia not diagnosed by their primary care physicians. This probably reflects a number of factors including case-complexity, pressure on time and the negative effects of reimbursement systems. Diagnosis is a step-wise process, which can be aided by cognitive assessments and simple diagnostic tools. It remains a key challenge to build a valid yet pragmatic and useable diagnostic approach which can be routinely and effectively used in everyday clinical practice.

In summary, standardized clinical definitions of dementia have good face validity and are probably useful in both clinical practice and research studies, particularly combined with a standardized rating of severity. There are however, specific groups of patients where diagnostic difficulties might exist, particularly patients with concurrent psychiatric morbidity, those with very mild degrees of cognitive impairment and patients with persistent delirium. For these groups, our understanding of the role of biomarkers in this process continues to progress. Developing simple and effective diagnostic protocols for clinical practice is probably the biggest current challenge.

4.3 DIFFERENTIAL DIAGNOSIS OF DEMENTIA SUBTYPES

4.3.1 Alzheimer's disease

More than 60 per cent of dementia patients have AD (Cummings and Benson, 1992). It is the most common dementia and is therefore the most important to diagnose accurately, particularly as licensed pharmacological treatments are available.

As with all types of dementia, a wide array of diagnostic criteria has been published, including various renditions of the DSM and ICD classifications. However, it was the introduction of the NINCDS-ADRDA criteria (McKhann et al., 1984) which represented a major landmark in dementia research, with the availability of reliable, valid operationalized criteria for AD. These criteria have been used far more widely than any others in research studies, and are also straightforward to utilize in a clinical setting. This section will therefore review the evidence pertaining to these criteria. The criteria themselves are shown in **Box 4.2**. Two degrees of certainty are described, probable AD, and possible AD. Section 1 is the most important and contains the operationalized element of the diagnosis. First it is necessary to establish that the person has dementia. Although the same caveats exist as were discussed in the previous section, the criteria make sensible recommendations that standardized assessments of cognitive function and ADLs are completed as well as a detailed clinical examination, in order to establish the presence of dementia. It also specifies that deficits are required in two or more areas of cognition, which should ensure that an individual is not suffering from a focal cognitive deficit. Progressive decline of memory and other cognitive functions is required. Disturbances of consciousness render patients unsuitable for a diagnosis of probable AD. Even though recent work does suggest that 20 per cent of AD patients do experience

disturbances of consciousness (Robertson et al., 1998), this is probably a sensible exclusion and a diagnosis of possible AD can still be made. An upper age limit of 90 is set, which is again sensible given the difficulties in determining the significance of cognitive impairment in patients within this age group. In the final part of section 1, it is stated that systemic disorders or other brain diseases that could account for the progressive cognitive deficits should be excluded. Although this is an appropriate recommendation, the lack of operationalization does permit variable interpretation.

Whilst application is clear cut when another significant brain disease is present, for example cerebrovascular disease, difficulties can arise in the presence of systemic disorders, such as hypothyroidism, which can result in cognitive deficits but are not necessarily the cause of cognitive impairment in a particular individual. In practice, the presence of a concurrent disorder which may contribute to the dementia does not preclude a diagnosis of possible AD, particularly if treatment has not resulted in an improvement of the dementia syndrome. Other typical clinical features and the results of investigations such as electroencephalogram (EEG) and computed tomography (CT) scans can be used in support of the diagnosis but are not a fundamental part of the operationalized criteria.

There are several advantages to applying these criteria in clinical practice. First, they require a standardized blood screen, detailed clinical evaluation and standardized cognitive assessment, but do not depend upon novel or expensive investigative techniques, which are unlikely to be available in many clinical centres. Second, they follow a logical diagnostic process similar to that adopted by most clinicians in the diagnosis of AD. Third, the criteria for probable AD would seem to be a suitably rigorous method for selecting patients with a clear-cut diagnosis in pharmacological interventions.

The NINCDS-ADRDA criteria have been widely evaluated in a large number of research studies, with excellent inter-rater reliability (Kukull et al., 1990; Baldereschi et al., 1994; Farrer et al., 1994). In addition, a number of clinico-pathological correlative studies have been completed demonstrating good agreement between clinical and neuropathological diagnosis (Martin et al., 1987; Morris et al. 1988; Tierney et al. 1988; Boller et al., 1989; Jellinger et al., 1989; Burns et al., 1990). Although 100 per cent diagnostic accuracy for probable AD has been reported in some studies, the overall specificity is approximately 80 per cent. Put into context, this is substantially better than can be achieved by utilizing a CT scan alone (Jacoby and Levy, 1980) and is better than has been achieved for the diagnosis of Parkinson's disease (PD) (Hughes et al., 1992).

Despite the good overall performance of these criteria, a number of caveats must be considered. First, the exact accuracy of clinical diagnostic criteria depends to some degree upon the neuropathological criteria (Nagy et al., 1998) chosen for diagnosis. Second, 5 per cent or more of patients with AD may have an atypical regional pattern of brain atrophy and a different clinical presentation. The best described example is posterior cortical atrophy (PCA), which typically presents with well-preserved memory and language but progressive, dramatic and relatively selective decline in vision and/or literacy skills such as spelling, writing and

Box 4.2 Criteria for clinical diagnosis of Alzheimer's disease

1. The criteria for the clinical diagnosis of PROBABLE Alzheimer's disease include:
   - dementia established by clinical examination and documented by the Mini-Mental test, Blessed Dementia Scale, or some similar examination, and confirmed by neuropsychological tests;
   - deficits in two or more areas of cognition;
   - progressive worsening memory and other cognitive functions;
   - no disturbance of consciousness;
   - onset between ages 40 and 90, most often after age 65; and absence of systemic disorders or other brain diseases that in and of themselves could account for the progressive deficits in memory and cognition.
2. The diagnosis of PROBABLE Alzheimer's disease is supported by:
   - progressive deterioration of specific cognitive functions such as language (aphasia), motor skills (apraxia) and perception (agnosia);
   - impaired activities of daily living and altered patterns of behaviour;
   - family history of similar disorders, particularly if confirmed neuropathologically; and
   - laboratory results of:
     - normal lumbar puncture as evaluated by standard techniques;
     - normal pattern or non-specific changes in EEG; such as increased slow-wave activity; and
     - evidence of cerebral atrophy on CT with progression documented by serial observation.
3. Other clinical features consistent with the diagnosis of PROBABLE Alzheimer's disease, after exclusion of causes of dementia other than Alzheimer's disease, include:
   - plateaus in the course of progression of the illness;
   - associated symptoms of depression, insomnia; incontinence, delusions, illusions, hallucinations, catastrophic verbal, emotional or physical outbursts, sexual disorders and weight loss;
   - other neurological abnormalities in some patients, especially with more advanced disease and including motor signs such as increased muscle tone, myoclonus or gait disorder;
   - seizures in advanced disease; and
   - CT normal for age.
4. Features that make the diagnosis of PROBABLE Alzheimer's disease uncertain or unlikely include:
   - sudden, apoplectic onset;
   - focal neurological findings such as hemiparesis, sensory loss, visual field deficits and incoordination early in the course of the illness; and
   - seizures or gait disturbances at the onset or very early in the course of the illness.
5. Clinical diagnosis of POSSIBLE Alzheimer's disease:
   - may be made on the basis of the dementia syndrome, in the absence of other neurological, psychiatric, or systemic disorder sufficient to cause dementia, and in the presence of variation in the onset, in the presentation, or in the clinical course;
   - may be made in the presence of a second systemic or brain disorder sufficient to produce dementia, which is not considered to be the cause of the dementia; and
   - should be used in research studies when a single, gradually progressive severe cognitive deficit is identified in the absence of other identifiable cause.
6. Criteria for diagnosis of DEFINITE Alzheimer's disease are:
   - the clinical criteria for probable Alzheimer's disease and histopathological evidence obtained from a biopsy or autopsy.
7. Classification of Alzheimer's disease for research purpose should specify features that may differentiate subtypes of the disorder, such as:
   - familial occurrence;
   - onset before age 65;
   - presence of trisomy-21; and
   - coexistence of other relevant conditions such as Parkinson's disease.

arithmetic. Third, the majority of studies have compared polarized groups of patients such as controls and those with moderate dementia, omitting many of the difficult to diagnose cases, and many of these studies were completed before there was wide clinical awareness of DLB as a major form of dementia. Most reports focusing on more diverse samples

including patients with DLB suggest that the criteria still perform well. For example, McKeith *et al.* (2000) reported a sensitivity and specificity of around 80 per cent for probable AD, whereas in an even more diverse sample, Litvan *et al.* (1998) reported a sensitivity of 95 per cent and specificity of 79 per cent for probable AD and, in a further study, Lopez *et al.* (1999) reported a sensitivity of 95 per cent and a specificity of 79 per cent for probable AD. Another difficulty is that many dementia patients have a combination of different disease pathologies, for example a substantial number of patients with AD pathology will have some degree of concurrent cerebrovascular disease and a small number of cortical Lewy bodies, which are often seen in the amygdale in people with otherwise clear-cut AD. Again, the exact degree of diagnostic accuracy will depend upon whether mixed cases are considered separately or as a subtype of AD, but in general the presence of mixed pathologies reduces the level of diagnostic accuracy (Holmes *et al.*, 1999). The issue of 'mixed pathology' is illustrated in a recent report from the Religious Order study (Schneider *et al.*, 2009). Although 88 per cent of the 179 people (average age, 86.9 years) with probable AD according to the NINCDS-ADRDA criteria had pathologically confirmed AD, 46 per cent had mixed pathologies, most commonly macroscopic infarcts ($n = 54$), neocortical Lewy body disease ($n = 19$) or both ($n = 8$).

What is referred to as AD within the NINCDS-ADRDA criteria represents a pathologically relatively advanced stage of the disease, and clinical criteria which enable clinical diagnosis of AD at an earlier stage of the disease process are an urgent objective. The concept of MCI has been useful in some regards, but the heterogeneity of people meeting criteria for MCI has been a limitation of the utility of the concept for clinical practice and as a basis for clinical trials. In the Religious Order study (Schneider *et al.*, 2009), only 54 per cent of the 134 people with MCI had pathologically diagnosed AD (59 per cent amnestic; 49 per cent non-amnestic), emphasizing the need to increase the specificity of diagnostic criteria for the identification of 'early' AD. Current thinking has moved forward to combine clinical, neuropsychological and biomarker information in an attempt to identify a more homogenous group of people with AD.

An expert consensus group has proposed research criteria for AD (Dubois *et al.*, 2007) in an attempt to improve identification of people in the earliest stages of the disease, but also to refine diagnostic accuracy across the full spectrum of the illness. Importantly, the research criteria are a bold attempt to incorporate increasing knowledge of biomarkers into clinical practice. For some time there has been convincing evidence indicating the utility of hippocampal and/or entorhinal atrophy on magnetic resonance imaging (MRI) and characteristic patterns of hypometabolism identified on positron emission tomography (PET) scanning in the early identification of AD. More recently there has been an increasing weight of evidence regarding the potential diagnostic value of quantifying disease-related proteins such as amyloid and tau. A longitudinal study from Gothenburg demonstrated that the combination of cerebrospinal fluid (CSF) T-tau and Aβ42 at baseline yielded a sensitivity of 95 per cent and a specificity of 83 per cent for detection of incipient AD in patients with MCI (Hansson *et al.*, 2006). Similarly, a prospective multi-centre study reported that increased retention of the PET ligand Pittsburgh compound B (11C-PIB), which binds to amyloid, identified 14 of the 17 (82 per cent) people who clinically converted to AD during follow up, whereas only one of the 14 PIB-negative MCI cases converted to AD (Okello *et al.*, 2009). For the first time

Dubois incorporates biomarkers as part of operationalized clinical criteria for AD.

These new criteria are centred on a clinical core of early and significant episodic memory impairment, operationally defined within the criteria (**Box 4.3**). They also stipulate that there must also be at least one or more abnormal biomarkers among structural neuroimaging with MRI, molecular neuroimaging with PET, and cerebrospinal fluid analysis of amyloid β or tau proteins (**Box 4.3**). This reflects the progress in our understanding of neuroimaging and CSF biomarkers but, given the current stage of knowledge, exact biomarker thresholds are not stipulated. The criteria represent a major step forward, but it is likely that refinement of the criteria, including more operationalized definitions of diagnostic thresholds for specific biomarkers will need to be incorporated as prospective validation studies progress.

4.3.2 Vascular dementia

Vascular dementia (VaD) is probably the second most common dementia, accounting for 10–20 per cent of dementia cases (Rocca *et al.*, 1991), either alone or in combination with neurodegenerative pathologies. There have been far fewer studies examining the diagnostic accuracy of criteria for VaD than for AD. The longest established criteria are based upon the Hachinski ischaemic score (Hachinski *et al.*, 1975; **Box 4.4**), originally derived on the basis of cerebral blood flow patterns in people with dementia. On the weighted scale, a score of 7 or more is taken to indicate VaD, whilst a score of 4 or less suggests that this is an unlikely diagnosis. Although the scale has been much criticized, either in its pure form, or in the modified form suggested by Rosen *et al.* (1980), sensitivities and specificities of approximately 80 per cent have been achieved for the diagnosis of 'pure' VaD cases (Loeb and Gandolfo, 1983; Small, 1985; Katzman *et al.*, 1988). However, the scale is far less successful in identifying mixed cases (Katzman *et al.*, 1988). Items within the scale such as abrupt onset, step-wise progression, fluctuation and focal neurological symptoms and signs, are geared much more to the identification of multiple infarctions than to other forms of vascular dementia (Chui, 1989), such as the insidious development of microvascular pathology, hypoxia or haemorrhage. In addition, individual symptoms within the scale are poorly operationalized and are therefore open to variable interpretation. Despite this, rather like the concept of hysteria, this scale has yet to be bettered and is likely to outlive its obituarists. More recently, two sets of operationalized criteria (**Box 4.5** and **Box 4.6**, pages 39 and 41) have been proposed, the California criteria (Chui *et al.*, 1992) and the NINCDS AIREN criteria (Román *et al.*, 1993). Diagnostic criteria for VaD are also included within ICD-10 (World Health Organization, 1992), DSM-IV (American Psychiatric Association, 1994) and the CAMDEX (Roth *et al.*, 1986). A preliminary study examining the ICD-10 research criteria was rather disappointing, suggesting that only 25 per cent of patients with clear vascular lesions on a CT scan fulfilled ICD-10 criteria for VaD (Wallin, 1994). Baldereschi *et al.* (1994) did, however, demonstrate a good inter-rater reliability of +0.66 for the diagnosis of VaD using these criteria.

Box 4.3 Research diagnostic criteria for Alzheimer's disease

Probable AD: A plus one or more supportive features B, C, D or E

Core diagnostic criteria

Presence of an early and significant episodic memory impairment that includes the following features:

1. Gradual and progressive change in memory function reported by patients or informants over more than six months
2. Objective evidence of significantly impaired episodic memory on testing: this generally consists of recall deficit that does not improve significantly or does not normalize with cueing or recognition testing and after effective encoding of information has been previously controlled
3. The episodic memory impairment can be isolated or associated with other cognitive changes at the onset of AD or as AD advances

Supportive features

Presence of medial temporal lobe atrophy

- Volume loss of hippocampus, entorhinal cortex, amygdala evidenced on MRI with qualitative ratings using visual scoring (referenced to well characterized population with age norms) or quantitative volumetry of regions of interest (referenced to well-characterized population with age norms)

Abnormal cerebrospinal fluid biomarker

- Low amyloid β_{1-42} concentrations, increased total tau concentrations, or increased phospho-tau concentrations, or combinations of the three
- Other well validated markers to be discovered in the future

Specific pattern on functional neuroimaging with PET

- Reduced glucose metabolism in bilateral temporal parietal regions
- Other well validated ligands, e.g. Pittsburg compound B or FDDNP

Proven AD autosomal dominant mutation within the immediate family

Exclusion criteria

History

- Sudden onset
- Early occurrence of the following symptoms: gait disturbances, seizures, behavioural changes

Clinical features

- Focal neurological features including hemiparesis, sensory loss, visual field deficits
- Early extra pyramidal signs

Other medical disorders severe enough to account for memory and related symptoms

- Non-AD dementia
- Major depression
- Cerebrovascular disease
- Toxic and metabolic abnormalities, all of which may require specific investigations
- MRI FLAIR or T2 signal abnormalities in the medial temporal lobe that are consistent with infectious or vascular insults

Chui *et al.* (2000) compared several different diagnostic criteria for VaD in 25 case vignettes, examining inter-rater reliability, as well as sensitivity and specificity against expert clinical judgement. The highest inter-rater reliability was achieved for the Hachinski scale, which performed better than the DSM-IV, the California criteria and the NINCDS AIREN criteria. Most of the criteria had poor sensitivity, but specificity was generally adequate. The DSM-IV criteria had the best sensitivity (50 per cent), and the best specificity was achieved by the NINCDS AIREN criteria (97 per cent). In a

Box 4.4 The Hachinski ischaemia score

Abrupt onset	2
Stepwise progression	1
Fluctuating course	2
Nocturnal confusion	1
Relative preservation of personality	1
Depression	1
Somatic complaints	1
Emotional incontinence	1
History of hypertension	1
History of strokes	2
Evidence of associated atherosclerosis	1
Focal neurological symptoms	2
Focal neurological signs	2

more extensive study, the same group (Chui *et al.*, 2000) examined the inter-rater reliability for the NINDS AIREN, ADDTC, DSM-IV, modified Hachinski score and ICD-10 criteria, identifying only moderate agreement (κ values 0.24–0.60) between the criteria, again the DSM-IV and the Hachinski score were the most liberal and the NINDS AIREN the most conservative. Gold *et al.* (1997) examined the diagnosis of VaD in a study of 113 autopsy-confirmed dementia cases. For a diagnosis of VaD, the Hachinski scale had the best specificity (0.88), with the NINCDS AIREN criteria achieving a specificity of 0.80. The California criteria had the best sensitivity (0.63). More recently, the validity of various operationalized clinical criteria for NaD (NINDS AIREN, DSM-IV, ADDTC, ICD10) against autopsy criteria has been examined. Eighty-nine patients (20 VaD, 23 mixed dementia, 46 AD) were included. Overall, the NINDS AIREN criteria for possible VaD (sensitivity 0.55, specificity specificity 0.84) and the possible ADDTC criteria (sensitivity 0.70, specificity 0.78) performed best. Consistent with previous studies, the NINDS AIREN criteria were the more conservative of the two. All of the criteria for probable VaD were too restrictive. A fuller breakdown is shown in **Table 4.1** (page 42). Across both of the Gold studies, none of the criteria performed well for mixed cases. There is a slight caveat in interpreting these results as the neuropathological criteria were strongly weighted towards infarcts, and would not have labelled people with extensive small vessel disease but no infarcts or lacunae as having VaD. In practice, this is likely to be a small proportion of individuals.

At present, NINDS AIREN and ADDTC criteria for possible VaD appear to be the most useful criteria, although an important caveat is that the neuroimaging component of the NINDS AIREN criteria discriminates poorly between people with and without dementia in the context of cerebrovascular disease (Ballard *et al.*, 2004). The Hachinski scale remains useful, particularly as a clinical instrument to help distinguish between VaD and other types of dementia in clinical practice.

The notoriously unreliable clinical diagnosis of 'mixed' AD and VaD, with no established clinical diagnostic criteria, is however a considerable concern, particularly as at least 40 per cent of dementia patients have an overlap of vascular and neurodegenerative pathologies. To give an indication of the scope of the problem, between 30 and 50 per cent of 'mixed dementia' cases are misclassified as VaD (Gold *et al.*, 1997). The potential overlap of pathologies is multifaceted and broadly classifying lesions as vascular or neurodegenerative may be inadequate; meaningful neuropathological classification of different types of vascular and neurodegenerative changes that reflect specific neurochemical and clinical symptom patterns that have prognostic value are required. Furthermore, these distinctions are arbitary unless they are clinically useful and guide the clinician with respect to treatment approaches.

There are three main substrates of dementia in patients with VaD: localized areas of infarction, microvascular disease, and more global neurodegeration associated with concurrent atrophy. Focusing on specific substrates of vascular dementia may help improve the diagnostic accuracy for both 'pure' and 'mixed' vascular dementia cases. The best example of this approach so far has been the development of criteria for subcortical ischaemic vascular dementia (SIVD) which describe VaD related to small vessel disease, combining the overlapping clinical syndromes of 'Binswanger's disease' (BD) and 'lacunar state'. Subcortical ischaemic vascular dementia is hypothesized to be caused by a loss of subcortical neurones or disconnection of cortical neurones from subcortical structures. The neuropsychological profile is described as characteristic of: i) a dysexecutive syndrome (difficulties in goal formulation, initiation, planning, organizing, sequencing, executing, set-shifting and abstracting); ii) slowed cognitive and motor processing speed; iii) other more general attentional impairments; and iv) memory deficits with impaired recall but relatively intact recognition. The concept appears useful, but has not yet been validated in a prospective clinicopathological study. Recent work highlighting neurochemical differences between SIVD, post-stroke dementia and mixed dementia (Perry *et al.*, 2005; Elliott *et al.*, 2009) emphasized the importance of further developing and validating criteria for specific VaD subtypes.

4.3.3 Dementia with Lewy bodies and Parkinson's disease dementia

A number of representative, hospital-based post-mortem series and studies based upon clinical cohorts have suggested that DLB is a common form of dementia, accounting for 10–20 per cent of cases in clinical settings (Lennox *et al.*, 1989; Hansen *et al.*, 1990; Kosaka, 1990; Perry *et al.*, 1990; Burns *et al.*, 1990). Diagnostic criteria were proposed by Byrne *et al.* (1991) and McKeith *et al.* (1992), and were superseded by international consensus criteria (McKeith *et al.* 1996). A number of validation studies of these criteria were reported (**Table 4.2**). Although probable DLB was diagnosed with a specificity of better than 80 per cent, sensitivity was an issue. Highlighted problems included the identification of fluctuating cognition, with two inter-rater reliability studies suggesting very poor agreement between different expert raters (Mega *et al.*, 1996; Litvan *et al.*, 1998) and the diagnosis of patients with a combination of cerebrovascular disease and cortical Lewy bodies (McKeith *et al.*, 2000). Importantly, diagnostic accuracy may also vary with dementia severity;

Box 4.5 Criteria for the diagnosis of ischaemic vascular dementia

Dementia

Dementia is a deterioration from a known or estimated prior level of intellectual function sufficient to interfere broadly with the conduct of the patient's customary affairs of life, which is not isolated to a single narrow category of intellectual performance, and which is independent of level of consciousness.

This deterioration should be supported by historical evidence and documented either by bedside mental status testing or ideally by more detailed neuropsychological examination, using tests that are quantifiable, reproducible, and for which normative data are available.

Probable ischaemic vascular dementia

The criteria for the clinical diagnosis of PROBABLE ischaemic vascular dementia (IVD) include ALL of the following:

- dementia;
- evidence of two or more ischaemic strokes by history, neurological signs and/or neuroimaging studies (CT or T1-weighted MRI); or occurrence of a single stroke with a clearly documented temporal relationship to the onset of dementia;
- evidence of at least one infarct outside the cerebellum by CT or T1-weighted MRI.
- The diagnosis of PROBABLE IVD is supported by:
- evidence of multiple infarcts in brain regions known to affect cognition;
- a history of multiple transient ischaemic attacks;
- history of vascular risk factors (e.g. hypertension, heart disease, diabetes mellitus);
- elevated Hachinski ischaemia scale (original or modified version).

Clinical features that are thought to be associated with IVD, but await further research include:

- relatively early appearance of gait disturbance and urinary incontinence;
- periventricular and deep white matter changes on T2-weighted MRI that are excessive for age;
- focal changes in electrophysiological studies (e.g. EEG, evoked potentials) or physiological neuroimaging studies (e.g. SPECT, PET, NMR spectroscopy).

Other clinical features that do not constitute strong evidence either for or against a diagnosis of PROBABLE IVD include:

- periods of slowly progressive symptoms;
- illusions, psychosis, hallucinations, delusions;
- seizures.

Clinical features that cast doubt on a diagnosis of PROBABLE IVD include:

- transcortical sensory aphasia in the absence of corresponding focal lesions on neuroimaging studies;
- absence of central neurological symptoms/signs, other than cognitive disturbance.

Possible ischaemic vascular dementiaa

A clinical diagnosis of POSSIBLE IVD may be made when there is dementia and one or more of the following:

- a history or evidence of a single stroke (but not multiple strokes) without a clearly documented temporal relationship to the onset of dementia; or
- Binswanger's syndrome (without multiple strokes) that includes all of the following:
  - early onset urinary incontinence not explained by urological disease, or gait disturbance (e.g. parkinsonian, magnetic, apraxic, or 'senile'gait) not explained by peripheral cause,
  - vascular risk factors, and
  - extensive white matter changes on neuroimaging.

Definite ischaemic vascular dementia

A diagnosis of DEFINITE IVD requires histopathological examination of the brain, as well as:

- clinical evidence of dementia;
- pathological confirmation of multiple infarcts, some outside of the cerebellum.

(Note: if there is evidence of Alzheimer's disease or some other pathological disorder that is to have contributed to the dementia, a diagnosis of MIXED dementia should be made).

Mixed dementia

A diagnosis of MIXED dementia should be made in the presence of one or more other systemic or brain disorders that are thought to be causally related to the dementia.

The degree of confidence in the diagnosis of IVD should be specified as possible, probable or definite, and the other disorders(s) contributing to the dementia should be listed. For example: mixed dementia due to probable IVD and possible Alzheimer's disease or mixed dementia due to definite IVD and hypothyroidism.

Research classification

Classification of IVD for RESEARCH purposes should specify features of the infarcts that may differentiate subtypes of the disorder, such as:

- location – cortical white matter, periventricular, basal ganglia, thalamus;
- size – volume;
- distribution – large, small or microvessel;
- severity – chronic ischaemia versus infarction;
- aetiology – atherosclerosis, embolism, arteriovenous, malformation, hypoperfusion.

Lopez et al. (2002) compared 180 patients with AD alone to 60 patients with AD and concurrent DLB. In patients with mild dementia, there was no specific clinical syndrome associated with concurrent Lewy bodies.

More recent studies have highlighted the frequent occurrence of rapid eye movement (REM) sleep behaviour disorder in DLB patients (Boeve et al., 2003; Boeve et al., 2004) and the potential value of investigational tools such as reduced uptake in the basal ganglia with dopamine transporters SPECT (DAT scan) (Walker et al., 2007; McKeith et al., 2007) and abnormal autonomic function on MIBG cardiac scintigraphy (Yoshita et al., 2001; Tateno et al., 2008). To address some of the issues raised from validation studies of the McKeith et al. (1996) criteria and to enable new developments to be incorporated, the consensus criteria have been updated (shown in **Box 4.7**). The core diagnostic criteria remain the same – fluctuating cognition, recurrent visual hallucinations and spontaneous motor features of Parkinson's disease, but the operationalization of these symptoms has been refined. In addition, although the presence of two of these features is still sufficient for a diagnosis of probable DLB, probable DLB can also now be diagnosed if one of these symptoms is present in combination with REM sleep behaviour disorder, severe neuroleptic sensitivity (Aarsland et al., 2005b) or low dopamine uptake in the basal ganglia (as indicated by dopamine transporters SPECT or PET scanning). Although carrying no direct diagnostic weighting, the list of features supporting a diagnosis of DLB has also been expanded and now includes MIBG cardiac scintigraphy. Based upon a hospital series, Aarsland et al. (2008) reported that 20 per cent of dementia patients met the revised criteria for probable DLB compared to 16 per cent meeting the McKeith et al. (1996) criteria for probable DLB. Whilst this does suggest that the new criteria improve case identification, more robust prospective validation is needed.

In the clinical diagnosis of DLB, considerable attention has also been paid to differentiation from AD. As the majority of DLB cases exhibit some pathological features of AD, the distinctions are in some ways arbitrary, although useful as they are associated with different clinical and neurochemical phenotypes. Seventy-five per cent of DLB patients have many of the neuropathological features of AD,

particularly senile plaques (Hansen et al., 1990). Although typically the density of neocortical plaques is similar to AD (Hansen et al., 1990), the burden of tangles is less than in 'pure' AD (Hansen et al., 1990). For example, when Lewy bodies occur in conjunction with Alzheimer pathology sufficient to meet CERAD criteria for probable or definite AD, neocortical neurofibrillary tangles are usually rare or absent, and tangles in the entorhinal cortex and hippocampus are intermediate between elderly controls and AD patients (Hansen et al., 1990). Fewer than 40 per cent of DLB patients meet criteria for a Braak stage IV or higher, although several recent studies indicate that these patients are less likely to present with a 'typical' DLB profile or to meet consensus criteria for probable DLB (Ballard et al., 2004).

The distinction between DLB and Parkinson's disease dementia (PDD) has also been controversial. There is a substantial overlap in symptoms between the two conditions, probably reflecting a common underlying cortical molecular pathology, with cortical Lewy bodies and more diffuse α synuclein pathology as common diagnostic features of both conditions at autopsy. Parkinson's disease dementia patients, however, have more severe loss of nigrostriatal dopaminergic neurons and greater cholinergic deficits (Ballard et al., 2006), but have less severe cortical Lewy body pathology and less severe concurrent AD pathology than DLB patients (Ballard et al., 2006). Diffuse cortical Lewy bodies appear to be the main substrate of dementia in PDD and the major cause of incident dementia in PD patients (Aarsland et al., 2005a). For research diagnosis within the consensus DLB criteria, the differential diagnosis of DLB and PDD is made on the basis of whether the parkinsonism is present for more than a year prior to the dementia. Building on the work of Litvan et al. (1998), new more specific criteria for the diagnosis of PDD have been proposed (Emre et al., 2007), requiring the presence of both dementia and PD, at least two out of four typical cognitive deficits such as executive dysfunction and visuospatial impairments and at least one neuropsychiatric symptom such as visual hallucinations, depression or apathy (**Box 4.8**). The criteria await validation.

Overall, the Mckeith et al. (1996) consensus criteria for DLB work reasonably well in clinical practice. The revised

Box 4.6 Criteria for clinical diagnosis of vascular dementia

The criteria for the clinical diagnosis of probable VaD include all of the following:

- Dementia defined by cognitive decline from a previously higher level of functioning and manifested by impairment of memory and of two or more cognitive domains (orientation, attention, language, visuospatial functions, executive functions, motor control and praxis), preferably established by clinical examination and documented by neuropsychological testing; deficits should be severe enough to interfere with activities of daily living not due to physical effects of stroke alone. Exclusion criteria: cases with disturbance of consciousness, delirium, psychosis, severe aphasia, or major sensorimotor impairment precluding neuropsychological testing. Also excluded are systemic disorders or other brain diseases (such as AD) that in and of themselves could account for deficits in memory and cognition.
- Cerebrovascular disease (CVD), defined by the presence of focal signs on neurological examination, such as hemiparesis, lower facial weakness, Babinski sign, sensory deficit, hemianopia and dysarthria consistent with stroke (with or without history of stroke) and evidence of relevant CVD by brain imaging (CT or MRI) including multiple large-vessel infarcts or a single strategically placed infarct (angular gyrus, thalamus, basal forebrain, or PCA or ACA territories), as well as multiple basal ganglia and white matter lacunes or extensive periventricular white matter lesions, or combinations thereof.
- A relationship between the above two disorders, manifested or inferred by the presence of one or more of the following:
  - onset of dementia within three months following a recognized stroke;
  - abrupt deterioration in cognitive functions; or fluctuating, stepwise progression of cognitive deficits.

Clinical features consistent with the diagnosis of probable VaD include the following:

- early presence of a gait disturbance (small-step gait or marche à petits pas, or magnetic apraxic-ataxic or parkinsonian gait);
- history of unsteadiness and frequent, unprovoked falls;
- early urinary frequency, urgency and other urinary symptoms not explained by urological disease;
- pseudobulbar palsy; and
- personality and mood changes, abulia, depression, emotional incontinence or other subcortical deficits including psychomotor retardation and abnormal executive function.

Features that make the diagnosis of vascular dementia uncertain or unlikely include:

- early onset of memory deficit and progressive worsening of memory and other cognitive functions such as language (transcortical sensory aphasis), motor skills (apraxia), and perception (agnosia), in the absence of corresponding focal lesions on brain imaging;
- absence of focal neurological signs, other than cognitive disturbance; and
- absence of cerebrovascular lesions on brain CT or MRI.

Clinical diagnosis of possible vascular dementia may be made:

- in the presence of dementia (Section 1) with focal neurological signs in patients in whom brain imaging studies to confirm definite CVD are missing; or
- in the absence of clear temporal relationship between dementia and stroke; or
- in patients with subtle onset and variable course (plateau or improvement) of cognitive deficits and evidence of relevant CVD.

Criteria for diagnosis of definite vascular dementia are:

- clinical criteria for probable vascular dementia;
- histopathological evidence of CVD obtained from biopsy or autopsy;
- absence of neurofibrillary tangles and neuritic plaques exceeding those expected for age; and
- absence of other clinical or pathological disorder capable of producing dementia.

Classification of vascular dementia for research purposes may be made on the basis of clinical, radiological and neuropathological features, for subcategories or defined conditions such as cortical vascular dementia, subcortical vascular dementia, Binswanger's disease and thalamic dementia.

The term 'AD with CVD' should be reserved to classify patients fulfilling the clinical criteria for possible AD and who also present clinical or brain imaging evidence of relevant CVD. Traditionally, these patients have been included with VaD in epidemiological studies. The term 'mixed dementia', used hitherto, should be avoided.

Table 4.1 Clinicopathological validation of the major criteria for vascular dementia (numbers extracted from Gold *et al.* (2002)).

n = 89 (20 VaD 23 mixed 46 AD)	Criteria	Sensitivity	Specificity
	DSMIV	0.5	0.84
	ICD 10	0.2	0.94
	Possible ADDTC	0.7	0.78
	Possible NINDS AIREN	0.55	0.84
	Probable ADDTC	0.2	0.91
	Probable NINDS AIREN	0.2	0.93

Table 4.2 Sensitivity, specificity, positive predictive value and negative predictive value of the consensus criteria for probable DLB: diagnostic validation studies.

	No. of cases	Diagnosis	Sensitivity	Specificity	PPV	NPV
Retrospective						
Mega *et al.* (1996)	24	AD, PD, PSP	0.4	1.0	1.0	0.93
Litvan *et al.* (1998)		DLB, PS, PSP, CBD, MSA, FTD, AD, CJD, VP	0.18	0.99	0.75	0.89
Luis *et al.* (1999)	56	DLB, AD, mixed DLB/AD	0.57	0.9	0.91	0.56
Lopez *et al.* (1999)	40	AD, PSP, FTD, DLB	0.34	0.94	/	/
Verghese *et al.* (1999)	18	DLB	0.61	0.84	0.48	0.96
Prospective						
Hohl *et al.* (2000)	10	AD, DLB, PSP	0.80	0.80	0.80	0.80
Holmes *et al.* (1999)	75	AD, VaD, DLB, mixed	0.22	1.0	1.0	0.91
McKeith *et al.* (2000)	50	DLB, AD, VaD	0.83	0.91	0.96	0.80
Lopez *et al.* (2002)	26	DLB, AD, mixed AD/VaD, PSP, CJD, FTD	38%	100%	/	/

AD, Alzheimer disease; CBD, cortico-basal degeneration; CJD, Creutzfeldt–Jakob disease; DLB, dementia with Lewy bodies; MSAK, multisystem atrophy; NPV, negative predictive value; PPV, positive predictive value; PSP, progressive supranuclear palsy; VaD, vascular dementia; VP, vascular parkinsonism.

criteria appear to be a step forward, with increased case identification. Dementia with Lewy bodies patients with concurrent vascular pathology or marked concurrent neurofibrillary tangle pathology are, however, more difficult to diagnose clinically. There are some useful clinical common sense steps that can be adopted to try and improve the accuracy in everyday practice. For example, visual hallucinations are much more indicative of DLB if they initially arise in the relatively early stages of the dementia, and become more frequent in AD patients during the moderate stages of the disease (Ballard *et al.*, 1999). Similarly parkinsonian symptoms are a less useful discriminator in the more severe stages of the disease where they become more frequent in the context of AD. In addition, better methods for evaluating fluctuating cognition may be useful, with three published standardized clinical rating methods (Ferman *et al.*, 2004). The proposed diagnostic criteria for PDD have good face validity, but require prospective validation.

4.3.4   Frontotemporal lobar degeneration

Frontotemporal dementia (FTD) results from frontotemporal lobar degeneration (FTLD). On gross pathology, there is circumscribed and often asymmetric lobar atrophy of the frontal lobes, adjacent anterior temporal regions, or both. Clinically, FTLDs reflect the initial distribution of neuropathology and present as several clinical syndromes depending on their predominant presenting symptoms, with a number of studies confirming the predominance of behavioural problems and language impairments (Lindau *et al.*, 1998; Chapter 68, Frontotemporal dementia, Chapter 69, Pick's disease: its relationship to progressive aphasia, semantic dementia and frontotemporal dementia, Chapter 70, The genetics and molecular pathology of frontotemporal lobar degeneration, Chapter 71, Semantic dementia and Chapter 72, Primary progressive aphasia and posterior cortical atrophy). In the development of consensus criteria, Neary *et al.* (1998) divided the clinical syndromes into 'FTD', 'progressive nonfluent aphasia', and 'semantic dementia'. All of the syndromes are important, but FTD, often referred to as behavioural variant, is the most frequent. Litvan *et al.* (1998) included several participants with FTD based upon the Manchester–Lund (1994) consensus statement in their clinicopathological study, reporting a sensitivity and specificity of 97 per cent for clinical diagnosis against autopsy confirmation. However, a further report has suggested that the inter-rater agreement between pathologists for the diagnosis of FTD is poor which makes interpretation of clinicopathological studies difficult. A recent validation study, based partly on detailed longitudinal assessment with partial autopsy conformation, indicated that the Neary consensus criteria for FTD identified 25/45 (56 per cent) of people at initial presentation and 33 (73 per cent) at some

---

Box 4.7 Revised criteria for the clinical diagnosis of dementia with Lewy bodies

1. *Central feature* (essential for a diagnosis of possible or probable DLB):

   dementia defined as progressive cognitive decline of sufficient magnitude to interfere with normal social or occupational function;

   prominent or persistent memory impairment may not necessarily occur in the early stages but is usually evident with progression;

   deficits on tests of attention, executive function and visuospatial ability may be especially prominent.

2. *Core* features (two core features are sufficient for a diagnosis of probable DLB, one for possible DLB):

   fluctuating cognition with pronounced variations in attention and alertness;

   recurrent visual hallucinations that are typically well formed and detailed;

   spontaneous features of parkinsonism.

3. *Suggestive features* (if one or more of these is present in the presence of one or more core features, a diagnosis of probable DLB can be made. In the absence of any core features, one or more suggestive features is sufficient for possible DLB. Probable DLB should not be diagnosed on the basis of suggestive features alone):

   REM sleep behavior disorder;

   severe neuroleptic sensitivity;

   low dopamine transporter uptake in basal ganglia demonstrated by SPECT or PET imaging.

4. *Supportive features* (commonly present but not proven to have diagnostic specificity):

   repeated falls and syncope;

   transient, unexplained loss of consciousness;

   severe autonomic dysfunction, e.g. orthostatic hypotension, urinary incontinence;

   hallucinations in other modalities;

   systematized delusions;

   depression;

   relative preservation of medial temporal lobe structures on CT/MRI scan;

   generalized low uptake on SPECT/PET perfusion scan with reduced occipital activity;

   abnormal (low uptake) MIBG myocardial scintigraphy;

   prominent slow wave activity on EEG with temporal lobe transient sharp waves.

5. A diagnosis of DLB is *less likely*:

   in the presence of cerebrovascular disease evident as focal neurologic signs or on brain imaging;

   in the presence of any other physical illness or brain disorder sufficient to account in part or in total for the clinical picture;

   if parkinsonism only appears for the first time at a stage of severe dementia.

6. Temporal sequence of symptoms:

   DLB should be diagnosed when dementia occurs before or concurrently with parkinsonism (if it is present). The term Parkinson disease dementia (PDD) should be used to describe dementia that occurs in the context of well-established Parkinson disease. In a practice setting the term that is most appropriate to the clinical situation should be used and generic terms such as Lewy body (LB) disease are often helpful. In research studies in which distinction needs to be made between DLB and PDD, the existing one-year rule between the onset of dementia and parkinsonism DLB continues to be recommended. Adoption of other time periods will simply confound data pooling or comparison between studies. In other research settings that may include clinicopathologic studies and clinical trials, both clinical phenotypes may be considered collectively under categories such as LB disease or alpha-synucleinopathy.

---

time over the course of the illness (Piguet *et al.*, 2009). Although the criteria provide a useful framework of the key symptoms, most expert commentators agreed that a revision is needed (Rascovsky *et al.*, 2007). Hypofrontality on SPECT scanning (Miller *et al.*, 1997), structural MRI (Rabinovici *et al.*, 2007) and neuropsychology are all useful in the diagnostis of individual patients, particularly for semantic dementia where typical MRI changes can be usefully identified with a rating scale (Davies *et al.*, 2009) and a typical pattern of deficits can be identified on standard and straightforward cognitive assessments (Davies *et al.*, 2008; Hodges *et al.*, 2008).

4.3.5 Other dementias

The ICD-10 criteria (World Health Organisation, 1992) include a description of dementia in Creutzfeldt–Jakob disease, dementia in Huntingdon's disease, dementia in human immunodeficiency virus disease and dementia in other specified diseases classified elsewhere (which incorporates a list including a variety of conditions such as epilepsy, hypothyroidism, intoxications, multiple sclerosis, neurosyphilis, nyacin deficiency, polyarthritis nodosa and vitamin B$_{12}$ deficiency). For specific systemic diseases, diagnosis can be more difficult than it first appears, as often the severity of cognitive

Box 4.8 Features of dementia associated with Parkinson's disease

Core features

1. Diagnosis of Parkinson's disease according to Queen Square Brain Bank criteria.
2. A dementia syndrome with insidious onset and slow progression, developing within the context of established Parkinson's disease and diagnosed by history, clinical and mental examination, defined as:
   - impairment in more than one cognitive domain;
   - representing a decline from premorbid level;
   - deficits severe enough to impair daily life (social, occupational or personal care), independent of the impairment ascribable to motor or autonomic symptoms.

Associated clinical features

1. Cognitive features:
   - attention: impaired. Impairment in spontaneous and focused attention, poor performance in attention tasks; performance may fluctuate during the day and from day to day;
   - executive functions: impaired. Impairment in tasks requiring initiation, planning, concept formation, rule finding, set shifting or set maintenance; impaired mental speed (bradyphrenia);
   - visuospatial functions: impaired. Impairment in tasks requiring visual-spatial orientation, perception, or construction;
   - memory: impaired. Impairment in free recall of recent events or in tasks requiring learning new material, memory usually improves with cueing, recognition is usually better than free recall;
   - language: core functions largely preserved. Word finding difficulties and impaired comprehension of complex sentences may be present.
2. Behavioural features:
   - apathy: decreased spontaneity; loss of motivation, interest, and effortful behaviour;
   - changes in personality and mood including depressive features and anxiety;
   - hallucinations: mostly visual, usually complex, formed visions of people, animals or objects;
   - delusions: usually paranoid, such as infidelity, or phantom boarder (unwelcome guests living in the home), delusions;
   - excessive daytime sleepiness.

Features which do not exclude PDD, but make the diagnosis uncertain

- Coexistence of any other abnormality which may by itself cause cognitive impairment, but judged not to be the cause of dementia, e.g. presence of relevant vascular disease in imaging.
- Time interval between the development of motor and cognitive symptoms not known.

Features suggesting other conditions or diseases as cause of mental impairment, which, when present make it impossible to reliably diagnose PDD

- Cognitive and behavioural symptoms appearing solely in the context of other conditions such as:
  - acute confusion due to:
    - systemic diseases or abnormalities;
    - drug intoxication;
  - major depression according to DSM IV.
- Features compatible with 'Probable Vascular dementia' criteria according to NINDS-AIREN (dementia in the context of cerebrovascular disease as indicated by focal signs in neurological exam such as hemiparesis, sensory deficits and evidence of relevant cerebrovascular disease by brain imaging AND a relationship between the two as indicated by the presence of one or more of the following: onset of dementia within three months after a recognized stroke, abrupt deterioration in cognitive functions, and fluctuating, stepwise progression of cognitive deficits).

impairments can be exacerbated without the underlying condition being the predominant cause of the dementia. For many of these conditions, where an underlying cause or specific gene can be identified, the validity of clinical criteria is obviously redundant as long as the clinical profile indicates the appropriate investigation. For prion diseases our understanding of biomarker profiles continues to develop (Bahl *et al.*, 2009).

4.4   CONCLUSION

In this chapter many potential difficulties in differential diagnosis have been highlighted. However, particularly for AD, the success of operationalized diagnostic criteria is considerable and they can be used with a degree of confidence for the diagnosis of most dementia patients. There are clearly a number of areas where further work is required, and for dementias other than AD further validation studies are needed to improve and establish accurate diagnostic methodology. The current chapter has not focused upon more detailed neuropsychological evaluation or biological markers, but it is likely in the future that more comprehensive research diagnostic criteria will include results from additional neuropsychological evaluation and more specialized investigation.

REFERENCES

Aarsland D, Perry R, Brown A et al. (2005a) Neuropathology of dementia in Parkinson's disease: a prospective, community-based study. Annals of Neurology 8: 773–6.

Aarsland D, Perry R, Larsen JP et al. (2005b) Neuroleptic sensitivity in Parkinson's disease and parkinsonian dementias. Journal of Clinical Psychiatry 66: 633–7.

Aarsland D, Rongve A, Nore SP et al. (2008) Frequency and case identification of dementia with Lewy bodies using the revised consensus criteria. Dementia and Geriatric Cognitive Disorders 26: 445–52.

Abas MA, Sahakian BJ, Levy R. (1990) Neuropsychological deficits and CT scan changes in elderly depressives. Psychological Medicine 20: 507–20.

American Psychiatric Association. (1987) Diagnostic and statistical manual of mental disorders, 3rd edn revised. Washington DC: American Psychiatric Association.

American Psychiatric Association. (1994) Diagnostic and statistical manual of mental disorders, 4th edn. Washington DC: American Psychiatric Association.

Bahl JM, Heegaard NH, Falkenhorst G et al. (2009) The diagnostic efficiency of biomarkers in sporadic Creutzfeldt–Jakob disease compared to Alzheimer's disease. Neurobiology of Aging 30: 1834–41.

Baldereschi M, Amato MP, Nencini P et al. (1994) Cross national inter-rater agreement on the clinical diagnostic criteria for dementia. Neurology 42: 239–42.

Ballard C, Ziabreva I, Perry R et al. (2006) Differences in neuropathology characteristics across the Lewy body dementia spectrum. Neurology 67: 1931–4.

Ballard CG, Burton EJ, Barber R et al. (2004) NINDS AIREN neuroimaging criteria do not distinguish stroke patients with and without dementia. Neurology 63: 983–8.

Ballard CG, Ayre G, O'Brien J et al. (1999) Simple standardised neuropsychological assessments aid in the differential diagnosis of dementia with Lewy bodies from Alzheimer's disease and vascular dementia. Dementia and Geriatric Cognitive Disorders 10: 104–8.

Boeve BF, Silber MH, Ferman TJ. (2004) REM sleep behaviour disorder in Parkinson's disease and dementia with Lewy bodies. Journal of Geriatric Psychiatry and Neurology 17: 146–57.

Boeve BF, Silber MH, Parisi JE et al. (2003) Synucleinopathy pathology and REM sleep behaviour disorder plus dementia or parkinsonism. Neurology 61: 40–5.

Boller F, Lopez O, Moossy J et al. (1989) Diagnosis of dementia: clinico pathologic correlations. Neurology 39: 76–9.

Boothby H, Blizard R, Livingston E et al. (1994) The Gospel Oak Study Stage III: The incidence of dementia. Psychological Medicine 24: 89–95.

Burns A, Luthert P, Levy R et al. (1990) Accuracy of clinical diagnosis of Alzheimer's disease. British Medical Journal 301: 1026.

Byrne EJ, Lennox G, Goodwin-Austin LB. (1991) Dementia associated with cortical Lewy bodies: proposed diagnostic criteria. Dementia 2: 283–4.

Caine ED. (1981) Pseudodementia. Archives of General Psychiatry 38: 1359–64.

Carpenter WT, Strauss JS. (1991) The prediction of outcome in schizophrenia IV: eleven year follow-up of the Washington IPSS cohort. Journal of Nervous and Mental Disease 179: 517–25.

Chui HC. (1989) Dementia: A review emphasising clinico-pathologic correlations and brain behaviour relationships. Archives of Neurology 46: 806–14.

Chui HC, Victoroff JI, Margolin D et al. (1992) Criteria for the diagnosis of ischaemic vascular dementia proposed by the state of California Alzheimer's Disease Diagnostic and Treatment Centres. Neurology 42: 473–80.

Chui HC, Mack W, Jackson E et al. (2000) Clinical criteria for the diagnosis of vascular dementia: a multicenter study of reliability and validity. Archives of Neurology 57: 191–6.

Coen RF, O'Mahoney D, Bruce I et al. (1994) Differential diagnosis of dementia: a prospective evaluation of the DAT inventory. Journal of the American Geriatric Society 42: 16–20.

Copeland JRM, Kelleher MJ, Kellet JM et al. (1976) A semi-structured clinical interview for the assessment and diagnosis of mental state in the elderly. Psychological Medicine 6: 439–49.

Copeland JRM, Dewey ME, Griffiths-Jones HM. (1986) Psychiatric case nomenclature and a computerised diagnostic system for elderly subjects: GMS and AGECAT. Psychological Medicine 16: 89–99.

Crook T, Bartus RT, Ferris SH et al. (1986) Age associated memory impairment: Proposed diagnostic criteria and measures of clinical change – report of a National Institute of Mental Health Workgroup. Developmental Neuropsychology 2: 261–76.

Cummings JL, Benson DF. (1992) Dementia: definition, prevalence, classification and approach to diagnosis. In: Cummings JL, Benson DF (eds). Dementia: A clinical approach. Boston: Butterworth-Heineman.

Davies RR, Scahill VL, Graham A et al. (2009) Development of an MRI rating scale for multiple brain regions: comparison with volumetric and with voxel-based morphometry. Neuroradiology 51: 491–503.

Davies RR, Dawson K, Mioshi E et al. (2008) Differentiation of semantic dementia and Alzheimer's disease using the Addenbrooke's Cognitive Examination (ACE). International Journal of Geriatric Psychiatry 23: 370–5.

Dubois B, Feldman HH, Jacova C et al. (2007) Research criteria for the diagnosis of Alzheimer's disease: Revising the NINCDS-ADRDA criteria. Lancet Neurology 6: 734–46.

Elliott MS, Ballard CG, Kalaria RN et al. (2009) Increased binding to 5-HT1A and 5-HT2A receptors is associated with large vessel infarction and relative preservation of cognition. Brain 132: 1858–65.

Emre M, Aarsland D, Brown R et al. (2007) Clinical diagnostic criteria for dementia associated with Parkinson's disease. Movement Disorders 22: 1689–707.

Farrer LA, Cupples LA, Blackburn S et al. (1994) Inter-rater agreement for the diagnosing of Alzheimer's disease: The MIRAGE Study. Neurology 44: 652–6.

Feinberg T, Goodman B. (1984) Affective illness, dementia and pseudodementia. Journal of Clinical Psychiatry 45: 99–103.

Ferman TJ, Smith GE, Boeve BF et al. (2004) DLB fluctuations: specific features that reliably differentiate DLB from AD and normal aging. Neurology 62: 181–7.

Folstein MF, Folstein SE, McHugh PR. (1975) Mini-mental state. A practical method for grading the cognitive state of patients for the clinician. Journal of Psychiatric Research 12: 189–98.

Gold G, Giannakopoulos P, Motes-Paicao C et al. (1997) Sensitivity and specificity of newly proposed clinical criteria for possible vascular dementia. Neurology 49: 690–4.

Hachinski VC, Ilief LD, Zilhka E et al. (1975) Cerebral blood flow in dementia. Archives of Neurology 32: 632–7.

Hansen L, Salmon D, Galasko D et al. (1990) The Lewy body variant of Alzheimer's disease: A clinical and pathological entity. Neurology 40: 1–8.

Hansson O, Zetterberg H, Buchhave P et al. (2006) Association between CSF biomarkers and incipient Alzheimer's disease in patients with mild cognitive impairment: a follow-up study. Lancet Neurology 5: 228–34.

Hodges JR, Martinos M, Woollams AM et al. (2008) Repeat and point: differentiating semantic dementia from progressive non-fluent aphasia. Cortex 44: 1265–70.

Hohl U, Tiraboschi P, Hansen LA et al. (2000) Diagnostic accuracy of dementia with Lewy bodies. Archives of Neurology 57: 347–51.

Holmes C, Cairns N, Lantos P, Mann A. (1999) Validity of current clinical criteria for Alzheimer's disease, vascular dementia and dementia with Lewy bodies. British Journal of Psychiatry 174: 45–51.

Hughes CP, Berg L, Danziger WL et al. (1982) A new clinical scale for the staging of dementia. British Journal of Psychiatry 140: 556–72.

Hughes AJ, Daniel SE, Kilford L et al. (1992) Accuracy of clinical diagnosis of idiopathic Parkinson's disease: A clinico-pathological study of 100 cases. Journal of Neurology, Neurosurgery and Psychiatry 55: 181–4.

Jacoby R, Levy R. (1980) Computerised tomography in the elderly 2. Senile dementia: diagnosis and functional impairment. British Journal of Psychiatry 136: 256–69.

Jellinger K, Danielczyk W, Fischer P et al. (1989) Diagnosis of dementia in the aged: clinico-pathological analysis. Clinico Neuropathology 8: 234–5.

Kaye JA. (1998) Diagnostic challenges in dementia. Neurology 51: 545–52.

Katzman R, Lacker B, Bernstein N. (1988) Advances in the diagnosis of dementia: accuracy of diagnosis and consequences of misdiagnosis of disorders causing dementia. In: Terry RD (ed.) Ageing and the brain. New York: Raven Press, 251–60.

Kiloh LG. (1961) Pseudodementia. Acta Psychiatrica Scandinavica 37: 336–51.

Kosaka K. (1990) Diffuse Lewy body disease in Japan. Neurology 237: 197–204.

Kral AA. (1978) Benign senescent forgetfulness. In: Katzman R, Terry RD, Black KL (eds). Alzheimer's disease: Senile dementia and related disorders. New York: Raven Press.

Kukull WA, Larson EB, Reifler BB et al. (1990) Inter-rater reliability of Alzheimer's disease diagnosis. Neurology 40: 257–60.

Lennox G, Lowe J, Morrell K et al. (1989) Antiubiquitin immunocytochemistry is more sensitive than conventional techniques in the detection of diffuse Lewy body disease. Journal of Neurology, Neurosurgery and Psychiatry 52: 67–71.

Lindau M, Almkvist D, Johanssen SE et al. (1998) Cognitive and behavioural differences of frontal lobe degeneration of the non-Alzheimer type and Alzheimer's disease. Dementia 9: 205–13.

Lipowski ZJ. (1989) Delirium in the elderly patient. New England Journal of Medicine 320: 578–82.

Litvan I, MacIntyre A, Goetz G et al. (1998) Accuracy of the clinical diagnoses of Lewy body disease, Parkinson's disease, and dementia with Lewy bodies. Archives of Neurology 55: 969–78.

Liu HC, Wang PN, Wang HC et al. (2007) Conversion to dementia from questionable dementia in an ethnic Chinese population. Journal of Geriatric Psychiatry and Neurology 20: 76–83.

Loeb C, Gandolfo C. (1983) Diagnostic evaluation of degenerative and vascular dementia. Stroke 14: 399–401.

Lopez OL, Litvan I, Catt KE et al. (1999) Accuracy of four clinical diagnostic criteria for the diagnosis of neurodegenerative dementias. Neurology 53: 1292–9.

Lopez OL, Becker JT, Kaufer DI et al. (2002) Research evaluation and prospective diagnosis of dementia with Lewy bodies. Archives of Neurology 59: 43–6.

Luis CA, Barker WW, Gajaraj K et al. (1999) Sensitivity and specificity of three clinical criteria for dementia with Lewy bodies in an autopsy-verified sample. International Journal of Geriatric Psychiatry 14: 526–33.

Lund and Manchester Groups. (1994) Clinical and neuropathological criteria for fronto-temporal dementia. Journal of Neurology, Neurosurgery and Psychiatry 57: 416–18.

McKhann G, Drachman D, Folstein M et al. (1984) Clinical diagnosis of Alzheimer's disease. Report of the NINCDS ADRDA work group under the auspices of the Department of Health and Human Service Task forces on Alzheimer's disease. Neurology 34: 939–44.

McKeith IG, Perry RH, Fairbairn AF et al. (1992) Operational criteria for senile dementia of Lewy body type. Psychological Medicine 22: 911–22.

McKeith IG, Galasko D, Kosaka K et al. (1996) Consensus guidelines for the clinical and pathologic diagnosis of dementia with Lewy bodies (DLB). Neurology 47: 1113–24.

McKeith IG, Ballard CG, Perry RH et al. (2000) Prospective validation of consensus criteria for the diagnosis of dementia with Lewy bodies – a prospective neuropathological validation study. Neurology 50: 181.

McKeith I, O'Brien J, Walker Z et al. (2007) Sensitivity and specificity of dopamine transporter imaging with 123I-FP-CIT SPECT in dementia with Lewy bodies: a phase III, multicentre study. Lancet Neurology 6: 305–13.

Martin E, Wilson R, Penn R *et al.* (1987) Cortical biopsy results in Alzheimer's disease: correlation with cognitive deficits. *Neurology* 37: 1201–4.

Mega M, Masterman DL, Benson F *et al.* (1996) Dementia with Lewy bodies: reliability of clinical and pathologic criteria. *Neurology* 47: 1403–9.

Miller BL, Ikonta C, Ponton M *et al.* (1997) A study of the Lund Manchester Criteria for fronto-temporal dementia: clinical and single photos emission computerised tomography correlations. *Neurology* 48: 937–42.

Morris J, McKeel D, Fulling K *et al.* (1988) Validation of clinical diagnostic criteria for Alzheimer's disease. *Annals of Neurology* 24: 17–22.

Nagy Z, Esiri M, Hindley N *et al.* (1998) Accuracy of clinical operational diagnostic criteria for Alzheimer's disease in relation to different pathological diagnostic protocols. *Dementia* 9: 219–38.

Neary D, Snowden JS, Gustafson L *et al.* (1998) Frontotemporal lobar degeneration: a consensus on clinical diagnostic criteria. *Neurology* 51: 1546–54.

O'Brien J, Ames D, Schwietzer I. (1996) White matter changes in depression and Alzheimer's disease: A review of magnetic resonance imaging studies. *International Journal of Geriatric Psychiatry* 11: 681–94.

O'Bryant SE, Waring SC, Cullum CM *et al.* (2008) Staging dementia using Clinical Dementia Rating Scale Sum of Boxes scores: a Texas Alzheimer's research consortium study. *Archives of Neurology* 65: 1091–5.

Okello A, Koivunen J, Edison P *et al.* (2009) Conversion of amyloid positive and negative MCI to AD over 3 years: an 11C-PIB PET study. *Neurology* 73: 754–60.

Pearlson G, Rabins P. (1988) The late onset psychoses – possible risk factors. In: Jeste DV, Zisook S (eds). *Psychiatric clinics of North America*, vol II, 1. Philadelphia: W Saunders, 15–22.

Perry RH, Irving D, Blessed G *et al.* (1990) A clinically and pathologically distinct form of Lewy body dementia in the elderly. *Journal of Neurological Sciences* 95: 119–39.

Perry E, Ziabreva I, Perry R *et al.* (2005) Absence of cholinergic deficits in "pure" vascular dementia. *Neurology* 64: 132–3.

Piguet O, Hornberger M, Shelley BP *et al.* (2009) Sensitivity of current criteria for the diagnosis of behavioral variant frontotemporal dementia. *Neurology* 72: 732–7.

Rabinovici GD, Seeley WW, Kim EJ *et al.* (2007) Distinct MRI atrophy patterns in autopsy-proven Alzheimer's disease and frontotemporal lobar degeneration. *American Journal of Alzheimer's Disease and Other Dementias* 22: 474–88.

Rascovsky K, Hodges JR, Kipps CM *et al.* (2007) Diagnostic criteria for the behavioral variant of frontotemporal dementia (bvFTD): current limitations and future directions. *Alzheimer Disease and Associated Disorders* 21: 14–18.

Rocca WA, Hofman A, Brayne C *et al.* (1991) The prevalence of vascular dementia in Europe: facts and fragments from 1980–90 studies. *EURODERM – Annals of Neurology* 30: 817–24.

Robertson B, Blennow K, Gottfries CG *et al.* (1998) Delirium in dementia. *International Journal of Geriatric Psychiatry* 13: 49–56.

Rogers SL, Farlow MR, Doody RS *et al.* (1998) A 24-week, double-blind, placebo-controlled trial of donepezil in patients with Alzheimer's disease. *Neurology* 50: 136–45.

Román GC, Tatemichi T, Erkinjuntti T *et al.* (1993) Vascular dementia: diagnostic criteria for research studies. Report of the NINCDS AIRENS International Workshop. *Neurology* 43: 250–60.

Rosen WG, Terry RD, Fuld PA *et al.* (1980) Pathological verification of ischaemic score in the differentiation of dementias. *Annals of Neurology* 7: 486–8.

Roth M, Tymm E, Mountjoy C *et al.* (1986) CAMDEX: A standardized instrument for the diagnosis of mental disorder in the elderly, with special reference to the early detection of dementia. *British Journal of Psychiatry* 149: 698–709.

Schneider JA, Arvanitakis Z, Leurgans SE *et al.* (2009) The neuropathology of probable Alzheimer disease and mild cognitive impairment. *Annals of Neurology* 66: 200–8.

Small GW. (1985) Revised ischaemic score for diagnosing multi-infarct dementia. *Journal of Clinical Psychiatry* 46: 514–17.

Tateno M, Kobayashi S, Shirasaka T *et al.* (2008) Comparison of the usefulness of brain perfusion SPECT and MIBG myocardial scintigraphy for the diagnosis of dementia with Lewy bodies. *Dementia and Geriatric Cognitive Disorders* 26: 453–7.

Tierney M, Fisher R, Lewis A *et al.* (1988) The NINCDS/ADRDA workgroup criteria for the clinical diagnosis of probable Alzheimer's disease: A clinico-pathologic study of 57 cases. *Neurology* 38: 359–64.

Verghese J, Crystal HA, Dickson DW, Lipton RB. (1999) Validity of clinical criteria for the diagnosis of dementia with Lewy bodies. *Neurology* 53: 1974–82.

Walker Z, Jaros E, Walker R *et al.* (2007) Dementia with Lewy bodies: a comparison of clinical diagnosis, FP-CIT single photon emission computed tomography imaging and autopsy. *Journal of Neurology, Neurosurgery and Psychiatry* 78: 1176–81.

Wallin A. (1994) The clinical diagnosis of vascular dementia. *Dementia* 5: 181–4.

World Health Organization. (1992) *International Classification of Diseases and Health Related Problems*, 10th revision. Geneva: World Health Organization.

Yoshita M, Taki J, Yamada M. (2001) A clinical role for I-123 MIBG myocardial scintigraphy in the distinction between dementia of the Alzheimer's-type and dementia with Lewy bodies. *Journal of Neurology, Neurosurgery and Psychiatry* 71: 583–8.

Assessment of the patient with apparent dementia

REBECCA EASTLEY AND GORDON WILCOCK

5.1 INTRODUCTION

All people presenting with apparent dementia should have a comprehensive assessment which identifies any potentially treatable physical or psychiatric causes, or co-morbid conditions, identifies psychosocial needs so support can be planned for the patient and carer, and establishes a diagnosis so symptomatic pharmacological treatments can be offered (Burns and Illiffe, 2009). Patients and carers often value a diagnosis even if no treatments are available as it can help with coping strategies for managing distressing and inexplicable symptoms. It also allows for a discussion about prognosis which enables plans to be made for anticipated future care needs. This chapter discusses the diagnostic assessment for a person presenting with apparent dementia.

5.2 DEMENTIA

Dementia is a clinical syndrome that results from acquired brain disease. It is usually a chronic and progressive condition although it can have a sudden onset in vascular dementia (VaD). There should be no impairment of consciousness. The clinical features of dementia can broadly be categorized into three groups: impairments in cognitive function; impairments in ability to perform activities of daily living; psychological or psychiatric features.

Cognitive deficits can include impairment in memory, executive function, language, orientation, calculation and learning. Memory impairment is a prominent feature of Alzheimer's disease (AD) and is a requisite symptom for the diagnosis of dementia in both the Diagnostic and Statistical Manual of Mental Disorders, third edition revised (DSM-IV; American Psychiatric Association, 1994) and the tenth edition of the International Classification of Diseases (ICD-10; World Health Organization, 1992). However, memory impairment is not a prominent feature of all dementias. Memory function is usually well preserved when people with frontotemporal dementias (FTD) first present, and the cognitive impairments in VaD will vary according to where the brain lesions are sited. A clinical diagnosis of dementia requires the presence of deficits in more than one cognitive domain.

The ability to perform activities of daily living is compromised in dementia. Initially, the person with dementia may have difficulty with complex tasks that depend on the interaction of several intact cognitive processes. They may have difficulty shopping, or managing paperwork. These changes are often insidious and compensated for by carers who gradually take over more of these roles in the household. As the dementia progresses, more basic tasks become difficult and help is required with dressing, washing and continence. At first the help may be by way of prompting but, as dyspraxia and agnosia develops, physical assistance may be required. Eventually the person with dementia may require help with the most basic tasks to sustain life, such as drinking and eating.

The third cluster of symptoms termed non-cognitive or neuropsychiatric symptoms are common in people with dementia (Peters *et al.*, 2006). In a population study, Lyketsos and colleagues (2000) reported that 61 per cent of people with dementia exhibited at least one neuropsychiatric symptom in the previous month, with apathy (27 per cent), depression (24 per cent) and agitation/aggression (24 per cent) being the most common symptoms. Psychotic symptoms occur in dementia, but in varying frequency in different subtypes. Delusions and hallucinations are more common in dementia with Lewy bodies (DLB) than AD (Ballard *et al.*, 1999) and are rare in FTD (Mendez *et al.*, 2008).

Post-mortem brain studies indicate that most people with dementia have mixed pathology, with AD and vascular pathology being the most common finding (MRC/CFAS, 2001). However, the most common single clinical diagnosis is AD and this diagnosis accounts for about 50 per cent of cases of dementia. Vascular dementia and mixed AD/VaD account for about 25 per cent of cases. Dementia with Lewy bodies accounts for 15–20 per cent of cases in hospital post-mortem series (Weiner, 1999) and is the second most common cause of neurodegenerative dementia after AD. Again, mixed pathological changes are the rule and cases of pure DLB without plaques, tangles or vascular changes are uncommon (Holmes *et al.*, 1999). Frontal lobe dementia is less common than AD, DLB or VaD overall, but it is the second most common form of primary neurodegenerative dementia in middle age, accounting for up to 20 per cent of presenile dementia cases (Snowden *et al.*, 2002).

5.3   MILD COGNITIVE IMPAIRMENT

Increasingly, clinicians are likely to see people who have subjective symptoms of cognitive impairment, particularly memory loss, but no significant impairment in their ability to perform day to day activities. Those people who have objective evidence of impairment on cognitive testing are termed to have mild cognitive impairment (MCI) (see Chapter 43, Mild cognitive impairment: a historical perspective and Chapter 44, Clinical characteristics of mild cognitive impairment). For many, MCI probably represents preclinical AD as eventually the dementia syndrome develops. However, there may be a period of stability over several years with no cognitive or functional deterioration. There is also an overlap between cognitive changes seen in MCI and that of normal ageing, suggesting a continuous rather than discrete pathological process (Small *et al.*, 2003). Although the ability to perform daily living tasks is not impaired, other non-cognitive symptoms have a high prevalence. In a population-based study including 320 people with MCI, 29 per cent of participants exhibited clinically significant neuropsychiatric symptoms in the previous month with depression, apathy and irritability being the most common (Lyketsos *et al.*, 2002). People presenting with MCI should have the same comprehensive assessment as those with more severe impairments.

5.4   DELIRIUM

Delirium should always be considered as a differential diagnosis as it is a common cause of cognitive impairment, especially in inpatient settings. Siddiqi and colleagues (2006)

systematic review, including 42 studies, reported delirium occurring in between 11 and 42 per cent of medical inpatients. Delirium is often superimposed on dementia as people with existing cognitive impairment are more at risk of developing delirium, and delirium is associated with an increased risk of developing dementia (Fick *et al.*, 2002). Some causes of delirium can lead to dementia if not recognized and treated. Core features of delirium are a recent onset of fluctuating consciousness with impaired awareness, and impaired cognitive function or perceptual abnormalities. The rapid onset, often within hours or days, coinciding with an identifiable medical or iatrogenic cause, usually makes the diagnosis. Fluctuation in cognitive functioning is a hallmark characteristic of DLB which can present similarly.

5.5   DEPRESSION

The traditional wisdom was that depressive pseudodementia should not be missed as it represented an important treatable cause of apparent dementia. We now understand that the relationship between depression and dementia is more complex (see Chapter 74, Depression with cognitive impairment). Elderly people with depression often show structural brain changes and deficits on standard cognitive tests which do not always resolve with treatment of the mood disorder (Abas *et al.*, 1990). Depression is also a common co-morbid condition in people with dementia. Patients with 'reversible dementia' presumed to be secondary to depression are at higher risk of subsequently developing dementia on follow up than those with depression alone (Alexopoulos *et al.*, 1993; Sáez-Fonseca *et al.*, 2007). Where depression is identified treatment should be initiated as both mood and cognitive symptoms can be improved, although in the case of the latter this improvement may not be sustained.

5.6   POTENTIALLY REVERSIBLE DEMENTIA

The incidence of 'reversible cases' of dementia appears to be declining. This could be due to an improvement in assessment in primary care leading to earlier interventions for potentially treatable causes (Weytingh *et al.*, 1995). It may also be a function of earlier studies including more inpatients with more recent studies being community based where reversibility is much less prevalent. Clarfield's (2003) meta-analysis involved 39 studies including 5620 patients with dementia. Potentially reversible causes were identified in 9 per cent of cases and were more likely to be found in younger patients, and those with a recent onset of cognitive impairment. However, only 0.28 per cent partially reversed and 0.31 per cent fully reversed with treatment. Metabolic disorders including hypothroidism and vitamin B_{12} deficiency were the most common potentially reversible causes but few cases of cure were identified (Clarnette and Patterson, 1994; Eastley *et al.*, 2000). Intracerebral causes of tumour, normal-pressure hydrocephalus and subdural haematoma made up only 2.2 per cent of cases.

5.7 THE ASSESSMENT

Whether the patient presents in an emergency room, in-patient unit or memory clinic, the principles of assessment remain the same. The assessment comprises eliciting a history from the subject and an informant, a mental state and physical examination, routine investigations including blood screening and neuroimaging, and further investigations as indicated by clinical findings.

5.7.1   History

Assessment begins with taking a history. Patients themselves may be aware of early cognitive problems and complain of mislaying items or having difficulty remembering names. Direct questioning may reveal evidence of problems with orientation, initiating, planning and carrying through activities, reading, or handling money. Special attention should be given to symptoms of language impairment, dyspraxia, agnosia and visuospatial impairment.

Non-cognitive symptoms, such as a change in personality, behavioural disturbance and psychiatric symptoms (see Chapter 8, Neuropsychiatric aspects of dementia and Chapter 9, Measurement of behaviour disturbance, non-cognitive symptoms and quality of life), are usually best elicited from an informant who knows the patient well. Crucially, an informant history allows the clinician to determine the patient's pre-morbid functioning (Galvin et al., 2005). Ideally, informants should be interviewed separately as they may feel unable to discuss embarrassing changes in their relative's behaviour, or their own stress as a carer.

Important diagnostic pointers can also be identified by the informant history of the clinical course of cognitive change (Young and Inouye, 2007). An insidious onset and gradual decline in cognitive function is the typical history of neurodegenerative conditions such as AD. Sudden acute changes in cognition or function may suggest a vascular cause. Onset associated in time with a physical illness may suggest delirium, but this may be superimposed on an existing dementia and careful enquiry should be made of any pre-existing symptoms. Sometimes apparent sudden changes are actually due to social changes which have put the patient in a new challenging position. Carer illness, moving house or even acquiring a new household appliance which the patient is unable to master may suddenly reveal difficulties to unsuspecting family members.

Many medical conditions can impact brain function. Hypertension, diabetes mellitus, hyperlipidaemia and smoking are risk factors for dementia and may be amenable to therapeutic intervention. A history of cardiac arrhythmia, anoxia and anaemia may be aetiologically relevant. Hypothyroidism can lead to cognitive impairment and should always be considered when there is a history of thyroid disease. Liver and renal disease may impact cognitive function but are rare causes of dementia.

Patients should be asked directly about any past psychiatric illness. A history of affective illness is a risk factor for depression which may be relevant to the current presentation. Details about the symptom profile of any past episodes of psychiatric disorder can be helpful, particularly if cognitive problems were prominent during a previous illness but resolved with treatment.

Alcohol dependence or abuse is more likely to be missed in elderly people than younger adults (Caracci and Miller, 1991). Alcohol is neurotoxic and alcohol dependence associated with thiamine deficiency may cause Wernicke's encephalopathy and Korsakoff's psychosis (see Chapter 77, Alcohol-related dementia and Wernicke–Korsakoff syndrome).

New medications or a change in dosage coinciding with the onset or exacerbation of cognitive problems should alert the clinician to the possibility of an iatrogenic cause, but long-standing medications may also be implicated. Tricyclic antidepressants, long-acting hypnotics, neuroleptics, the older anticonvulsants and any medication with anti-cholinergic activity may impact cognitive function. Ancelin et al. (2006) found that 80 per cent of their subjects taking drugs with high anticholinergic activity met the criteria for MCI. Most clinicians would be aware of the anticholinergic activity of older tricyclics or medications such as oxybutynin given for urinary incontinence, but more medications than generally appreciated, including digoxin and furosemide, may have clinically significant anticholinergic effects. Direct questioning sometimes reveals that patients are taking relative's medications or are regular users of over the counter medications.

Family histories can indicate that the person might be at increased risk of developing a particular condition, such as depression or AD, and more rarely may point to an otherwise unsuspected diagnosis.

5.7.2   Mental state examination

The mental state examination begins with the first contact with the patient, whether this is at home or in a clinic setting. Untidiness, inappropriate clothing or poor personal hygiene may indicate dyspraxia or self-neglect from severe depression. A mood disorder may be suggested by a downcast or anxious expression. Disinhibition may be demonstrated by an inappropriate greeting.

Language function is assessed during the interview and by formal testing. Abnormalities in the rate and form of speech may be indicative of an affective disorder or underlying neurological dysfunction. There may be a decreased rate or poverty of speech in depression or FTD. Patients who repeat answers, phrases or words from preceding questions are perseverating, a sign of frontal impairment. Dysarthria, the disorder of the articulation of speech, can be caused by lesions of the upper or lower motor neurons, extrapyramidal and cerebellar pathways. There may be paraphasias, fluent or non-fluent aphasia.

People with memory impairment may have difficulty recalling whether they have sustained mood symptoms and those who are more severely impaired may lack the ability to express their distress in cognitive terms. Special attention should be given to the presence of biological symptoms of depression, an informant history and a behavioural assessment. Suicide ideation should be assessed if there are any depressive symptoms whether the person has dementia or not. Lability of mood is classically seen in vascular dementia and cognitive impairment, and when extreme is termed emotional incontinence.

Psychotic symptoms may arise secondary to functional psychiatric illness, in which case they are usually mood congruent. In delirium, delusions are often paranoid in flavour and not well systematized. Some abnormal beliefs occurring in a person with dementia can often be understood in terms of the person trying to make sense of their experiences. Family members may be accused of stealing things, or neighbours of coming into the house and moving things. Systematized delusions and visual hallucinations are common in DLB.

5.7.3   Cognitive assessment

The cognitive examination should cover an assessment of attention and concentration, orientation, memory, language, executive function and praxis. Standardized cognitive tests should form part of the examination. The Mini-Mental State Examination is currently the most widely used cognitive assessment tool (Folstein et al., 1975). It is scored out of 30 with a score below 24 suggesting dementia. It takes around 10–15 minutes to administer but lacks sensitivity for mild cases of dementia. The clock-drawing test evaluates general executive functioning of the frontal lobes, as well as visuo-spatial abilities (Shulman, 2000). It is quick and often well tolerated by patients but its usefulness is limited by complicated scoring systems, and lack of sensitivity for mild impairment. Some tests, such as the General Practitioner Assessment of Cognition (GPCOG) (Brodaty et al., 2002) and the six-item cognitive impairment test (6-CIT) (Brooke and Bullock, 1999), were designed for use in primary care. A new assessment tool, the 'Test Your Memory Test' TYM (Brown et al., 2009) has been designed to be quick to administer and score and initial results suggest the TYM test has a higher sensitivity for detecting AD than the Mini-Mental State Examination. All test results should be interpreted cautiously, taking into account all relevant factors such as previous intellectual functioning, cultural and language issues, any sensory impairments and concurrent depressive symptoms (see Chapter 6, Screening and assessment instruments for the detection and measurement of cognitive impairment, for a more detailed discussion of short cognitive assessment instruments).

When there is diagnostic uncertainty, more detailed neuropsychological assessment may be required and is usually undertaken by a neuropsychologist (see Chapter 7, Neuropsychological assessment of dementia). Neuropsychological testing can lead to a change in initial diagnosis in up to 26 per cent of cases, being particularly helpful in cases where there is subtle cognitive impairment (Hentschel et al., 2005).

5.7.4   Physical examination

Like the mental state examination, the physical examination begins as soon as you meet the patient. Some conditions may be apparent from the patient's appearance alone.

There may be obvious discomfort when they get out of the chair in the waiting-room, or unsteadiness on standing. Shaking hands when introduced may reveal the forced grasping seen in frontal lobe lesions. The gait can be observed when walking to the consulting room or through the house. Is there evidence of ataxia, the broad-based gait of normal pressure hydrocephalus, or the parkinsonian shuffling steps? Does the patient get out of breath with minimal exertion? Abnormal movements such as resting tremors or chore-athetoid movements may be obvious before a neurological examination is performed.

Noting the skin colour takes seconds and may reveal the paleness of anaemia, jaundice, cyanosis, or the plethoric appearance of polycythaemia.

A vascular cause for the cognitive impairment may be indicated by the rate and rhythm of the pulse, the presence of hypertension, heart murmurs, carotid bruits, or poor peripheral circulation. A slow regular pulse may suggest heart block, overtreatment with some drugs, for example beta-blockers, or hypothyroidism. Sitting and standing blood pressure should be measured in case of orthostatic hypotension.

Chest examination may reveal evidence of infection, cardiac failure, or occasionally pleural effusion.

Any abnormal findings may be important, but liver disease stigmata, the presence of an aortic aneurysm, or discomfort on bladder palpation may be directly relevant to the aetiology. Faecal loading in the large bowel sometimes accounts for new behavioural problems. Constipation can be caused by medications with anticholinergic activity and also opiate derivatives, which themselves may exacerbate cognitive impairment.

Any abnormalities in posture, gait and movement may already have been noted but should also be formally assessed. Intention and static tremors are found when there is a cerebellar disorder, and the pill-rolling tremor is characteristic of parkinsonism. Action tremors may be exaggerated in thyrotoxicosis, uraemia and liver disease.

Of particular importance in the cranial nerve examination is any sign of facial weakness, abnormal eye movements, nystagmus and visual field defects. Ophthalmoscopy should be performed routinely as it may reveal signs of systemic disease, such as diabetic or hypertensive retinopathy, as well as papilloedema secondary to raised intracranial pressure.

Abnormalities in the pyramidal and the extra-pyramidal motor systems may help to confirm the diagnosis of VaD, DLB, Parkinson's disease and amyotrophic lateral sclerosis. Myoclonus may be associated with epilepsy, or Creutzfeldt–Jakob disease.

The grasp, sucking and snout reflexes are examples of primitive reflexes which are normal in infants. People with frontal dementias usually acquire primitive reflexes in the early stages of their illness, otherwise their occurrence is usually associated with advanced dementia. The grasp reflex, a flexion of the thumb and fingers, can be elicited by stroking the patient's palm between their thumb and index finger. The sucking reflex can be provoked by touching the lips with a wooden spatula or other instrument, and as the name implies involves contraction of the muscles used for sucking. A pout provoked by tapping the centre of closed lips is the snout reflex.

Sensation is particularly difficult to assess in a person with dementia and in addition an impairment of lower limb vibratory sense and proprioception is a common normal finding in many elderly people. However, sensory examination can still be useful and may reveal abnormalities suggestive of cerebrovascular lesions, peripheral neuropathy in diabetes or vitamin B_{12} deficiency and, more rarely these days, tabes dorsalis and subacute combined degeneration of the cord.

5.7.5   Initial investigations

Several guidelines and consensus statements recommend a battery of blood tests to exclude systemic conditions which may be causing the cognitive impairment (Knopman et al., 2001; National Institute for Health and Clinical Excellence, 2006). The earlier these possible causes are identified and treated the better the chances are that cognitive function can be improved, or at least further deterioration halted or slowed. Commonly recommended routine blood tests include full blood count, erythrocyte sedimentation rate (ESR) or C-reactive protein (CRP), renal function, thyroid function, calcium, glucose, vitamin B_{12}, serum folate and liver function tests.

Other tests including lipids, syphilis serology, HIV testing, mid-stream urine, chest x-ray and ECG are recommended if indicated by clinical findings, rather than forming part of an initial screen.

5.7.6   Structural neuroimaging

Structural neuroimaging, either computed tomography (CT) or magnetic resonance imaging (MRI) is now a standard recommendation in order to help establish the subtype of dementia, mainly to distinguish AD from VaD and FTD, and to exclude other cerebral pathology including tumours, subdural haematomas and normal pressure hydrocephalus (NICE, 2006; see Chapter 11, Structural brain imaging). Compared to CT, MRI is superior in terms of anatomical visualization of cerebral infarcts and white-matter changes, however it is more costly, may be less available, and excludes people with pacemakers and metal implants. Some people find the MRI scanning procedure frightening or uncomfortable and this may be an additional consideration to be taken into account. Structural neuroimaging may show medial temporal lobe atrophy in AD, and frontal lobe atrophy in FTD.

5.7.7   Functional neuroimaging

In addition to imaging techniques that look at brain structure, there are techniques that look at the function of brain tissue and can visualize brain activity *in vivo* (see Chapter 12, Functional brain imaging and connectivity in dementia). Functional imaging tends to be reserved as a second-line investigation to structural neuroimaging when the diagnosis is in doubt and can help differentiate between AD, VaD, FTD and DLB. Perfusion hexamethylpropyleneamine oxime (HMPAO) single-photon emission computed tomography

(SPECT) has higher specificity than clinical criteria for differentiating AD from other types of dementia, but is less sensitive than clinical criteria (Dougall et al., 2004). If HMPAO SPECT is unavailable, then 2-[F]fluoro-2-deoxy-D-glucose positron emission tomography (FDG PET) can be considered as an alternative option.

In DLB there is nigrostriatal degeneration with a significant reduction in striatal dopamine transporter (Piggott et al., 1999). The dopaminergic presynaptic ligand, ^{123}I-labelled 2β-carbomethoxy-3β-(4-iodophenyl)-N-(3-fluoropropyl) nortropane (^{123}I-FP-CIT) and SPECT have been shown to have high sensitivity and specificity for differentiating DLB from AD (McKeith et al., 2007), and may prove to be clinically useful in establishing the diagnosis in those with possible DLB (O'Brien et al., 2009).

5.7.8   Other investigations

5.7.8.1   CEREBROSPINAL FLUID EXAMINATION

Lumbar puncture is only indicated as an investigation if an infective or inflammatory cause is suspected. There has been a lot of interest in cerebrospinal fluid (CSF) markers (see Chapter 53, Blood and cerebrospinal fluid biological markers for Alzheimer's disease), but currently only the CSF 14-3-3 protein assay is clinically useful, having high sensitivity and specificity for Creutzfeldt–Jakob disease (Hsich et al., 1996).

Three other CSF markers, β-amyloid$_1$ total tau, and phospho-tau (p-tau) proteins, have been the focus of much research interest as predictive markers for the progression of MCI to AD. However, the availability of these investigations is limited to specialist centres.

5.7.8.2   ELECTROENCEPHALOGRAPHY

Electroencephalography is not a routine investigation but may be helpful where the presentation is atypical and a seizure disorder, delirium or Creutzfeldt–Jakob disease is suspected. In delirium, there is usually diffuse slowing in the background rhythm and periodic sharp wave complexes are seen in Creutzfeldt–Jakob disease.

5.7.8.3   BRAIN BIOPSY

Brain biopsy is a very rare investigation which should only be considered when potential benefits outweigh the risks of complications, which include bleeding and seizures. Brain biopsy might be indicated if an infective or inflammatory cause was suspected and could not be confirmed any other way.

5.8   SUMMARY

A diagnosis of dementia can often be made in primary care. Specialist services provide expertise for differentiating between subtypes of dementia and where there is diagnostic uncertainty for atypical and early presentations. At present, there is no definitive diagnostic test even for AD, the most common cause of dementia, so assessment remains a predominantly human process relying on the core clinical skills of the assessment team.

REFERENCES

Abas MA, Sahakian BJ, Levy R. (1990) Neuropsychological deficits and CT scan changes in elderly depressives. *Psychological Medicine* 20: 507–20.

Alexopoulos GS, Meyers BS, Young RC *et al.* (1993) The course of geriatric depression with 'reversible dementia': a controlled study. *American Journal of Psychiatry* 150: 1693–9.

American Psychiatric Association. (1994) *Diagnostic and statistical manual of mental disorders*, 4th edn. Text revision. Washington DC: The American Medical Association.

Ancelin LM, Artero S, Portet F *et al.* (2006) Non-degenerative mild cognitive impairment in elderly people and use of anticholinergic drugs: longitudinal cohort study. *British Medical Journal* 332: 455–9.

Ballard C, Holmes C, McKeith I *et al.* (1999) Psychiatric morbidity in dementia with Lewy bodies: a prospective clinical and neuropathological comparative study with Alzheimer's disease. *American Journal of Psychiatry* 156: 1039–45.

Brooke P, Bullock R. (1999) Validation of the 6 item cognitive impairment test. *International Journal of Geriatric Psychiatry* 14: 936–40.

Brodaty H, Pond D, Kemp NM *et al.* (2002) The primary care physician COG: a new screening test for dementia designed for general practice. *Journal of American Geriatric Society* 50: 530–4.

Brown J, Pengas G, Dawson K *et al.* (2009) Self administered cognitive screening test (TYM) for detection of Alzheimer's disease: cross sectional study. *British Medical Journal* 338: 1426–8.

Burns A, Illiffe S. (2009) Dementia. *British Medical Journal* 338: 405–9.

Clarfield AM. (2003) The decreasing prevalence of reversible dementias: an updated meta-analysis. *Archives of Internal Medicine* 163: 2219–29.

Clarnette RM, Patterson CJ. (1994) Hypothyroidism: does treatment cure dementia? *Journal of Geriatric Psychaitry and Neurology* 7: 23–7.

Dougall NJ, Bruggink S, Ebmeier KP. (2004) Systematic review of the diagnostic accuracy of 99mTc-HMPAO-SPECT in dementia. *American Journal of Geriatric Psychiatry* 12: 554–70.

Eastley R, Wilcock GK, Bucks R. (2000) Vitamin B12 deficiency in dementia and cognitive impairment: the effects of treatment on neuropsychological function. *International Journal of Geriatric Psychiatry* 15: 226–33.

Fick DM, Agostini JV, Innouye SK. (2002) Delirium superimposed on dementia: a systematic review. *Journal of American Geriatric Society* 50: 1723–32.

Folstein MF, Folstein SE, McHugh PR. (1975) Mini-mental state: a practical method for grading the cognitive state of patients for the clinician. *Journal Psychiatric Research* 12: 189–98.

Galvin JE, Roe CM, Powlishta KK *et al.* (2005) The AD8: A brief informant interview to detect dementia. *Neurology* 65: 559–64.

Hentschel F, Kreis M, Damian M *et al.* (2005) The clinical utility of structural neuroimaging with MRI for diagnosis and differential diagnosis of dementia: a memory clinic study. *International Journal of Geriatric Psychiatry* 20: 645–50.

Holmes C, Cairns N, Lantos P, Mann A. (1999) Validity of current clinical criteria for Alzheimer's disease, vascular dementia and dementia with Lewy bodies. *British Journal of Psychiatry* 174: 45–50.

Hsich G, Kenney K, Gibbs CJ *et al.* (1996) The 14-3-3 brain protein in cerebrospinal fluid as a marker for transmissible spongiform encephalopathies. *New England Journal of Medicine* 335: 924–30.

Knopman DS, DeKosky ST, Cummings JL *et al.* (2001) Practice parameter: Diagnosis of dementia (an evidence-based review) Report of the Quality Standards Subcommittee of the American Academy of Neurology. *Neurology* 56: 1143–53.

Lyketsos CG, Steinberg M, Tschanz JT *et al.* (2000) Mental and behavioral disturbances in dementia: findings from the Cache County Study on Memory in Aging. *American Journal of Psychiatry* 157: 708–14.

Lyketsos CG, Lopez O, Jones B *et al.* (2002) Prevalence of neuropsychiatric symptoms in dementia and mild cognitive impairment: results from the cardiovascular health study. *Journal of the American Medical Association* 288: 1475–83.

McKeith I, O'Brien J, Walker Z *et al.* (2007) Sensitivity and specificity of dopamine transporter imaging with ^{123}I-FP-CIT SPECT in dementia with Lewy-bodies: a phase III multicentre study. *The Lancet Neurology* 6: 305–13.

Mendez MF, Shapira JS, Woods RJ *et al.* (2008) Psychotic symptoms in frontotemporal dementia: prevalence and review. *Dementia and Geriatric Cognitive Disorders* 25: 206–11.

MRC/CFAS. Pathological correlates of late-onset dementia in a multicentre, community-based population in England and Wales. (2001) Neuropathology Group of the Medical Research Council Cognitive Function Ageing Study (MRC CFAS). *The Lancet* 357: 169–75.

National Institute for Health and Clinical Excellence. (2006) Dementia A NICE–SCIE Guideline on supporting people with dementia and their carers in health and social care. (National Clinical Practice Guideline Number 42.) London: The British Psychological Society and Gaskell.

O'Brien JT, McKeith IG, Walker Z *et al.* (2009) Diagnostic accuracy of ^{123}I-FP-CIT SPECT in possible dementia with Lewy bodies. *The British Journal of Psychiatry* 194: 34–9.

Peters KR, Rockwood K, Black SE *et al.* (2006) Characterizing neuropsychiatric symptoms in subjects referred to dementia clinics. *Neurology* 66: 523–8.

Piggott MA, Marshall EF, Thomas N *et al.* (1999) Striatal dopaminergic markers in dementia with Lewy bodies, Alzheimer's and Parkinson's diseases: rostrocaudal distribution. *Brain* 122: 1449–68.

Sáez-Fonseca JA, Lee L, Walker Z. (2007) Long-term outcome of depressive pseudodementia in the elderly. *Journal of Affective Disorders* 101: 123–9.

Shulman KI. (2000) Clock-drawing: Is it the ideal cognitive screening test? *International Journal of Geriatric Psychiatry* **15**: 548–61.

Siddiqi N, House AO, Holmes JD. (2006) Occurrence and outcome of delirium in medical in-patients: a systematic literature review. *Age and Ageing* **35**: 350–64.

Small BJ, Mobly JL, Laukka EJ et al. (2003) Cognitive deficits in preclinical Alzheimer's disease. *Acta Neurologica Scandinavica. Supplementum* **179**: 29–33.

Snowden JS, Neary D, Mann DMA. (2002) Frontotemporal dementia. *British Journal of Psychiatry* **180**: 140–3.

Weytingh MD, Bossuyt PM, van Crevel H. (1995) Reversible dementia: more than 10% or less than 1%? A quantitative review. *Journal of Neurology* **242**: 466–71.

Weiner MF. (1999) Dementia associated with Lewy bodies. *Archives of Neurology* **56**: 1441–2.

World Health Organization. (1992) *The ICD-10 Classification of Mental and Behavioural Disorders: Clinical Descriptions and Diagnostic Guidelines.* Geneva: WHO.

Young J, Inouye SK. (2007) Delirium in old people. *British Medical Journal* **334**: 842–6.

6

Screening and assessment instruments for the detection and measurement of cognitive impairment

LEON FLICKER

6.1 INTRODUCTION

A frequently used method in the ascertainment of dementia in older people is the performance of a short cognitive test to determine the need to perform further testing to establish the diagnosis. The case for detection of milder forms of cognitive impairment has not been established, and therapeutic strategies targeted for patients with conditions such as mild cognitive impairment (MCI) (Petersen *et al.*, 2001) have not been developed. Another use for these tests is to detect changes in cognitive impairments over time. Thus, the focus of this chapter remains on the use of short cognitive tests to aid in the detection of older people with dementia, and to monitor the progression of cognitive impairment in people with dementia. These short cognitive tests are commonly described as 'screening instruments', but this is in fact a misnomer. Screening has been defined as 'an organized attempt to detect, among apparently healthy people in the community, disorders or risk factors of which they are unaware' (Cadman *et al.*, 1984). The US Preventive Services Task Force (2003) has concluded that the evidence is insufficient to recommend for, or against, routine screening for dementia in older adults. In reality, these short cognitive tests are used as a means of case finding in certain clinical situations for which there is a high prior probability of finding individuals with cognitive impairment, usually associated with dementia or in those individuals who are medically unwell, delirium.

6.2 DESCRIPTION OF TESTS

The short cognitive tests have been used in case finding for over 50 years. A minor change that has occurred in the more recently developed tests is the use of lengthier delayed recall tasks, both cued, and non-cued. One of the earliest instruments was the Mental Status Questionnaire (MSQ) (Kahn *et al.*, 1960). In 1968, Blessed *et al.* (1968) described the Information Memory Concentration (IMCT), which was validated against the criterion of neuropathology. Hodkinson (1972) described a shortened version of the IMCT and called this the Abbreviated Mental Test Score (AMTS). In North America, Pfeiffer (1975) described the Short Portable Mental Status Questionnaire (SPMSQ) and Folstein *et al.* (1975) devised the Mini-Mental State Examination (MMSE) which has undergone standardization (Molloy *et al.*, 1991). Subsequently, additional questions were added to the MMSE and a modified scoring system was introduced to produce a test called the 3MS (Teng and Chui, 1987). Other short tests that have been developed include Kokmen's Short Test of Mental Status (STMS) (Kokmen *et al.*, 1991), and the General Practitioner Assessment of Cognition (GPCOG) (Brodaty *et al.*, 2002), both of which include the clock-drawing test. A short test has been developed which does not utilize orientation or other questions prone to cultural bias: the Rowland Universal Dementia Assessment Scale (RUDAS) (Storey *et al.*, 2004). All these instruments have in common their brevity, take 10 minutes or less to administer and require relatively little training.

One of the main problems with these cognitive tests is the fact that they exhibit both floor and ceiling effects. There have been attempts to develop tests that would be more suitable for testing impaired patients (Plutchik *et al.*, 1971; Albert and Cohen, 1992). Longer tests and word lists have the advantage that they are less prone to ceiling effects, although their use often requires some training. These include the 7-minute screen (Solomon *et al.*, 1998), which is a test that comprises a cued recall task, verbal fluency, an orientation test and a clock-drawing task. Similarly the Syndrom Kurz test (SKT) (Lehfeld and Erzigkeit, 1997), has nine subtests which include naming, memory, attention, cued recall and visuospatial functioning. A very short version of delayed free and cued recall tests has been developed called the Memory Impairment Screen (Buschke *et al.*, 1999), which consists of just four items.

Several other survey instruments have been developed which have incorporated both cognitive screening instruments and diagnostic schedules. These include the Cambridge Diagnostic Examination for the Elderly (Roth *et al.*, 1986), Consortium to Establish a Registry for Alzheimer's Disease (Morris *et al.*, 1989), Geriatric Mental State schedule (Copeland *et al.*, 1976) and a Structured Interview for the Diagnoses of Dementia of the Alzheimer's type Multi-infarct Dementia and Dementias of other Aetiology according to ICD-10 and DSM-IIIR (SIDAM) (Zaudig *et al.*, 1991). The cognitive components of the Cambridge Diagnostic Examination for the Elderly (Roth *et al.*, 1986), the Alzheimer's Disease Assessment Scale (ADAS-cog) (Rosen *et al.*, 1984) and the Mental Deterioration Battery (Carlesimo *et al.*, 1996) take longer to administer and are not usually performed as initial brief tests, although the Organic Brain Scale (OBS) from the Geriatric Mental State has been used as a stand-alone test (Ames *et al.*, 1992).

6.3 USES FOR THESE TESTS

The need for these 'screening; instruments has arisen because there is good evidence that clinicians will commonly miss cases of dementia in their routine practice without the assistance of formal cognitive assessment (Williamson *et al.*, 1964; Mant *et al.*, 1988; Valcour *et al.*, 2000). It remains a clearly defined guideline that for those individuals suspected of a cognitive disorder, an assessment with at least one of these tests should be undertaken.

Even before the arrival of specific treatments for the symptoms of Alzheimer's disease (AD), the presence or absence of significant cognitive impairment had major implications for the management of patients. In particular, older individuals with multiple medical problems requiring medications could not be managed appropriately without an assessment for the presence of cognitive impairment and some idea of its severity. Also, there is some evidence that the earlier identification of people with dementia and appropriate referral to support services and counselling can alleviate some of the stresses associated with caring for people with dementia and delay institutionalization (Green and Brodaty, 2002).

These short cognitive tests have limited domains of measurement. **Table 6.1** refers to the domains of measurement of the common assessment tools. Orientation figures prominently in most of these tools and is a reflection of recent memory acquisition. In a longitudinal study of cognitive function in people with Alzheimer's disease, it was demonstrated that dementia affects immediate and short-term memory as well as language function (Flicker *et al.*, 1993). Since memory impairment is a sine qua non in the categorization of dementia in both the DSM-IV and ICD-10 criteria, it is hardly surprising that most short cognitive tests focus on this domain. It is also clear that these tests are highly correlated with each other. For example Stuss *et al.* (1996) observed that the proportion of variance accounted for by a single common component was in excess of 0.80 for the Mattis Dementia Rating Scale, an abbreviated six-item version of the Orientation Memory Concentration Test adapted from Blessed *et al.* (1968), a Mental State Questionnaire and an Ottawa Mental State Examination. Also, in this study there was no added benefit from longer tests and the shorter cognitive tests performed as well as longer tests with multiple domains. In another study the correlation between the AMTS and MMSE was greater than 0.85 (Flicker *et al.*, 1997). Similarly, correlations between the MMSE and the ADAS-Cog

Table 6.1 Cognitive domains in commonly used short cognitive tests.

Test	Personal information	Orientation	Short-term memory	Remote memory	Attention	Naming	Visuospatial visuoconstruction	Other
MSQ	◆	◆		◆				
IMC	◆	◆	◆	◆	◆	◆		
AMT	◆	◆	◆	◆	◆	◆		
MMSE		◆	◆		◆	◆	◆	◆
3MS	◆	◆	◆		◆	◆	◆	◆
SPMSQ	◆	◆		◆	◆			
OBS	◆	◆	◆	◆				◆
STMS		◆	◆	◆	◆		◆	◆
GPCOG		◆	◆				◆	
TICS	◆	◆	◆	◆	◆	◆	◆	◆
RUDAS			◆				◆	◆

have been found to be strong (0.90; Burch and Andrews, 1987), although the correlation between the MMSE and the STMS was limited to 0.74 (Kokmen *et al.*, 1991). In a comparison of the MMSE and 3MS, both the modified scoring system and the additional questions of the 3MS increased its discriminatory ability, but at the expense of increased burden of administration time and training requirements (McDowell *et al.*, 1997).

These short cognitive scales appear robust in many settings. The IMCT has been validated by means of telephone interviews (Kawas *et al.*, 1995) as has the Telephone Cognitive Assessment Battery (Debanne *et al.*, 1997) and the Telephone Version of the MMSE (Roccaforte *et al.*, 1992). The Telephone Interview for Cognitive Status (TICS) (Brandt *et al.*, 1988) is also a widely used instrument because its word list component is capable of delineating subjects who may have a memory disorder that does not fulfil criteria for dementia but could satisfy other diagnostic criteria such as amnestic MCI. These instruments have been used across national boundaries and have wide applicability. For example, the OBS has been found to have good validity in three separate countries (Ames *et al.*, 1992). Some attempt has been made to develop self-administered tests, such as the EASI (Horn *et al.*, 1989). The use of self-administered tests has recently been comprehensively reviewed (Cherbuin *et al.*, 2008) with some promising results for the informant-based tests, but otherwise this method of administration cannot be recommended for widespread use in clinical practice. There is also evidence that the place of testing can cause significant changes in the test score, with testing in a patient's own residence being associated with a higher score (Ward *et al.*, 1990).

These short cognitive screens obviously have their limitations, the most obvious being that they test only limited domains of cognition. Besides the use of full neuropsychological assessment, attempts have been made to develop other short tests of specific functions. An example of this is the Executive Interview (Royall *et al.*, 1992), which attempts to assess executive cognitive function. Also, the ability to draw a clock has been extensively studied as a short test which examines other cognitive domains. It has been used by itself or in conjunction with other cognitive tests such as the SPMSQ or MMSE, or as part of the 7-minute screen, GPCOG or STMS. Clock-drawing may miss a quarter of cognitively impaired individuals, and it has been suggested that the test may be able to detect cognitive alterations not related to delirium or dementia (Gruber *et al.*, 1997). In addition, Clock-drawing may provide additional information to the MMSE, as suggested by Ferrucci *et al.* (1996), with its scores being associated with future cognitive decline in older people independently of MMSE scores.

Short cognitive tests are known to be sensitive to bias associated with education, but adjustment for this effect does not necessarily improve test performance (Belle *et al.*, 1996). For this reason the RUDAS (Storey *et al.*, 2004) was developed, which has attempted to be less culturally biased and uninfluenced by educational attainment.

Another consideration is that these tests may not be sensitive to all stages of the disease. Stern *et al.* (1994) demonstrated that there was a quadratic relationship with dementia severity, with ADAS-Cog and IMCT scores showing greater deterioration for patients with moderate dementia compared with mildly and severely demented patients. This may represent the relative insensitivity of the tests for patients with the least and greatest impairment, or may reveal true patterns of progressive cognitive decline at different parts of the disease process.

Attempts have also been made to shorten these tests even further – for example the ten-item Abbreviated Mental Test Score (AMTS) has been further shortened to four items (Swain and Nightingale, 1997), but this seems to lead to a loss of predictive efficiency. The potential problem of inadequate specificity of short cognitive tests for population screening has been revealed in a community study: the Canadian Study of Health in Aging (Graham *et al.*, 1996). In this study the 3MS was used as a community screen before a diagnostic battery. Cognitive impairment, not dementia, was found to be more common than dementing processes, with the prevalence of cognitive impairment not dementia found to be 16.8 per cent, whereas the prevalence of all types of dementia combined was 8 per cent (Graham *et al.*, 1997). The conditions identified within this category of cognitive impairment included delirium, alcohol use, drug intoxication, depression, psychiatric disorders, memory impairment associated with the ageing process and intellectual disability.

6.4   INFORMANT–BASED TESTS

Perhaps the most exciting development in the detection of cognitive impairment in older people in recent times has been the refinement and validation of structured tests administered to informants. Examples of this type of test include the DECO Test-Deterioration Cognitive Observée (Ritchie and Fuhrer, 1992) and the Informant Questionnaire for Cognitive Decline in the Elderly (IQCODE) (Jorm and Korten, 1988). Important advantages of these tests are that they correlate relatively poorly with pre-morbid function and are relatively insensitive to the effects of education.

The other consideration about informant questionnaires is that they have shown lower correlations with the cognitive tests: somewhere in the order of 0.6 (Flicker *et al.*, 1997). This is an important consideration in that their relatively low correlation with cognitive testing per se implies they provide additional independent information, which may assist in the discrimination of people with functionally important cognitive impairment. The work by Ritchie and Fuhrer (1992) would suggest that they seem to be better able to discriminate mild dementia from normality as opposed to cognitive screens such as the MMSE, although this was not replicated by others (Flicker *et al.*, 1997). This may represent a difference in the choice of informants as much of the sample described by Ritchie and Fuhrer (1992) were recruited through France Alzheimer and may have represented carers that were well attuned to the problems associated with dementia, while in the other study (Flicker *et al.*, 1997) informants were drawn from attendees at a memory clinic.

A meta-analysis (Jorm, 1997) suggests that informant tests may perform better than short cognitive tests, but it is important to emphasize that there was great heterogeneity within this meta-analysis and clearly the test results were dependent on the subject samples and the samples of informants. A subsequent meta-analysis confirmed relative independence of education and pre-morbid ability, but also that these type of tests may be biased by depression and anxiety in the informant and the quality of the relationship between the informant and the subject (Jorm, 2004). Harwood *et al.* (1997) also demonstrated comparable discriminatory ability of the AMT and the IQCODE in a sample of medical inpatients over the age of 65 admitted to a general medical unit. In that study, the 16-item version of the IQCODE was utilized with good effect. The IQCODE has been validated by longitudinal changes of cognitive tests (Jorm *et al.*, 1996) and also has been validated retrospectively against post-mortem diagnosis (Thomas *et al.*, 1994).

One of the important considerations for the use of combinations of tests or additional items is that the correlation between individual tests should not be too great. The importance of asymmetry of associations between tests to increase the positive predictive value of combinations of tests has been highlighted by others (Marshall, 1989). Hooijer *et al.* (1993) found some improvement in diagnosis in using pairs of short screening tests. This was not the case in work by Little *et al.* (1987) where a short AMT score was found to have better predictive value than longer combined tests.

To date, most work has focused on using either informant tests or short cognitive tests separately as a screen for further investigations and management, but clearly the tests can be combined. This was raised by Flicker *et al.* (1997) where the lower correlations and asymmetry of the test properties within different populations could be utilized so that the combined tests' sensitivity and specificity would be improved. This is quite different to the use of the alteration of cut-points, where a trade off occurs between sensitivity and specificity. The judicious use of the combination of informant and short cognitive tests may potentially result in an increase in both sensitivity and specificity. The tests can be applied so that for the combination to be positive both tests are required to be positive, which is called 'in series'. Alternatively, the combination of tests could be judged positive if either test is positive, which is called in 'parallel'.

Such an effect has been demonstrated by Gallo and Breitner (1995) by means of a telephone-administered cognitive test followed by an assessment with the informant. The informant test was falsely described as being more specific, but in fact it was the combination of using the two tests in series that resulted in the increased specificity needed for this two-stage screen. Another example of this approach being used in challenging population research is the work of Hall and colleagues (Hall *et al.*, 1993; Hall *et al.*, 1995). In these studies a combination of short cognitive tests and informant testing was used in cross-cultural studies of African American, Cree Indian and Nigerian populations, and the relative insensitivity of the informant tests to the effects of culture and education improved the performance of these combinations. The combination of the MMSE and IQCODE has now been evaluated extensively. In three separate studies (Mackinnon and Mulligan, 1998; Mackinnon *et al.*, 2003; Knafelc *et al.*, 2003) the total evidence suggested that the combination of tests performed better than either test alone,

and that the tests could be combined usefully by either a requirement for both or either test to be positive (in parallel) or calculating a new score using a weighted sum rule.

Besides the characteristics of the population being assessed, it is important to realize that the absolute prevalence of the condition will also cause a need for an adjustment in the cut-points in both the cognitive and informant tests. Very low prevalence will increase the need for specificity, otherwise there will be a large number of patients to further investigate. This is necessitated in both research and clinical practice. It is important to emphasize that the cut-points used in the combination of these tests in either series or parallel, may be quite different to the ones normally employed by the tests in isolation.

6.5   COSTS OF THE TESTS

Until recently these tests have been administered freely without charge. The major expense has been that of the clinicians' time, both in training and administration. With the increasing constraints by intellectual property laws, two commonly used instruments, the MMSE and TICS are now licensed for use by Psychological Assessment Resources (Inc). The MMSE may be administered free of charge by individual clinicians in the course of clinical practice, from memory or from an original paper (Folstein *et al.*, 1975), or with permission from Psychological Assessment Resources, otherwise there is a charge for using the score sheets obtained from Psychological Assessment Resources. Similar charges apply to the TICS. It would seem unfortunate if such proprietary interests inhibit the use of these short tests as often the major obstacle to the initial diagnosis of dementia is applying one of these short tests when there is clinical concern.

6.6   CONCLUSION

There is now available a plethora of short cognitive tests which appear useful in helping clinicians to determine whether individuals require further assessment for the presence of a cognitive disorder. The tests seem to perform in a similar fashion. The characteristics of the population in which the tests are used seem to be at least as important to performance as the test themselves. The addition of informant test information appears more valuable rather than increasing the length and complexity of the cognitive screen. It is difficult to predict the performance of these tests, either singly, or in combination with informant tests, from one population to the next. An improvement in the efficacy of cognitive assessments can be most easily achieved by combining informant and short cognitive tests to a single summative score, or using informant and cognitive tests with specific cut-points and rules of combination. The most important limiting factor in clinical practice is encouraging clinicians to use any one of these tests. If clinical suspicion remains, the combination of both a short cognitive test with an informant test is recommended.

REFERENCES

Albert M, Cohen C. (1992) The test for severe impairment: an instrument for the assessment of patients with severe cognitive dysfunction. *Journal of the American Geriatrics Society* **40**: 449–53.

Ames D, Ashby D, Flicker L *et al.* (1992) Jim Who? Recall of national leaders by elderly people in three countries. *International Journal of Geriatric Psychiatry* **7**: 437–42.

Belle SH, Seaberg EC, Ganguli M *et al.* (1996) Effect of education and gender adjustment on the sensitivity and specificity of a cognitive screening battery for dementia: results from the MoVIES project. *Neuroepidemiology* **15**: 321–9.

Blessed G, Tomlinson BE, Roth M. (1968) The association between quantative measures of dementia and of senile change in the cerebral grey matter of elderly subjects. *British Journal of Psychiatry* **114**: 797–811.

Brandt J, Spencer M, Folstein M. (1988) The telephone interview for cognitive status. *Neuropsychiatry, Neuropsychology, and Behavioral Neurology* **1**: 111–7.

Brodaty H, Pond D, Kemp NM *et al.* (2002) The GPCOG: a new screening test for dementia designed for general practice. *Journal of the American Geriatrics Society* **50**: 530–4.

Burch Jr EA, Andrews SR. (1987) Comparison of two cognitive rating scales in medically ill patients. *International Journal of Psychiatry in Medicine* **17**: 193–200.

Buschke H, Kuslansky G, Katz M *et al.* (1999) Screening for dementia with the Memory Impairment Screen. *Neurology* **52**: 224–7.

Cadman D, Chambers L, Feldman W, Sackett D. (1984) Assessing the effectiveness of community screening programs. *Journal of the American Medical Association* **251**: 1580–5.

Carlesimo A, Caltagirone C, Gainotti G *et al.* (1996) The mental deterioration battery: normative data, diagnostic reliability and qualitative analyses of cognitive impairment. *European Neurology* **36**: 378–84.

Cherbuin N, Anstey KJ, Lipnicki DM. (2008) Screening for dementia: a review of self- and informant-assessment instruments. *International Psychogeriatrics* **20**: 431–58.

Copeland JRM, Kelleher MJ, Kellett JM *et al.* (1976) A semi-structured interview for the assessment of diagnosis and mental state in the elderly. The Geriatric Mental State 1. Development and reliability. *Psychological Medicine* **6**: 439–49.

Debanne SM, Patterson MB, Dick R *et al.* (1997) Validation of a telephone cognitive assessment battery. *Journal of the American Geriatrics Society* **45**: 1352–9.

Ferrucci L, Cecchi F, Guralnik JM *et al.* (1996) Does the clock drawing test predict cognitive decline in older persons independent of the Mini-Mental State Examination? The FINE study group, Finland, Italy, The Netherlands Elderly. *Journal of the American Geriatrics Society* **44**: 1326–31.

Flicker C, Ferris SH, Reisberg B. (1993) A two year longitudinal study of cognitive function in normal ageing and Alzheimer's Disease. *Journal of Geriatric Psychiatry and Neurology* **6**: 84–96.

Flicker L, Logiudice D, Carlin JB, Ames D. (1997) The predictive value of dementia screening instruments in clinical populations. *International Journal of Geriatric Psychiatry* **12**: 203–9.

Folstein MF, Folstein SE, McHugh PR. (1975) Mini-mental state: a practical method for grading the cognitive state of patients for the clinician. *Journal of Psychiatric Research* **12**: 189–98.

Gallo JJ, Breitner JC. (1995) Alzheimer's disease in the NAS-NRC Registry of aging twin veterans, IV. Performance characteristics of a two-stage telephone screening procedure for Alzheimer's dementia. *Psychological Medicine* **25**: 1211–19.

Graham JE, Rockwood K, Beattie BL *et al.* (1996) Standardization of the diagnosis of dementia in the Canadian study of health and ageing. *Neuroepidemiology* **15**: 246–56.

Graham JE, Rockwood K, Beattie BL *et al.* (1997) Prevalence and severity of cognitive impairment with and without dementia in an elderly population. *Lancet* **349**: 1793–6.

Green A, Brodaty H. (2002) Care-giver interventions. In: Qizilbash N (ed.). *Evidence based dementia practice.* Oxford: Blackwell Science, 764–94.

Gruber NP, Varner RV, Chen YW, Lesser JM. (1997) A comparison of the clock drawing test and the Pfeiffer short portable mental status questionnaire in a Geropsychiatry clinic. *International Journal of Geriatric Psychiatry* **12**: 526–32.

Hall KS, Hugh C, Hendrie C *et al.* (1993) The development of a dementia screening interview in two distinct languages. *International Journal of Methods in Psychiatric Research* **3**: 1–28.

Hall KS, Ogunniyi AO, Hendrie HC *et al.* (1995) A cross-cultural community based study of dementias: methods and performance of the survey instrument Indianapolis, USA, and Ibadan, Nigeria. *International Journal of Methods in Psychiatric Research* **6**: 129–42.

Harwood DM, Hope T, Jacoby R. (1997) Cognitive impairment in medical inpatients. 1: Screening for dementia – is history better than mental state? *Age and Ageing* **26**: 31–5.

Hodkinson HM. (1972) Evaluation of a mental test score for the assessment of mental impairment in the elderly. *Age and Ageing* **1**: 233–8.

Hooijer C, Jonker C, Lindeboom J. (1993) Cases of mild dementia in the community: improving efficacy of case finding by concurrent use of pairs of screening tests. *International Journal of Geriatric Psychiatry* **8**: 561–4.

Horn L, Cohen CI, Teresi J. (1989) The EASI: a self-administered screening test for cognitive impairment in the elderly. *Journal of the American Geriatrics Society* **37**: 848–55.

Jorm AF. (1997) Methods of screening for dementia: a meta-analysis of studies comparing an informant questionnaire with a brief cognitive test. *Alzheimer's Disease and Associated Disorders* **11**: 158–62.

Jorm AF. (2004) The Informant Questionnaire on cognitive decline in the elderly (IQCODE): a review. *International Psychogeriatrics* **16**: 275–93.

Jorm AF, Korten AE. (1988) Assessment of cognitive decline in the elderly by informant interview. *British Journal of Psychiatry* **152**: 209–13.

Jorm AF, Christiansen H, Henderson AS *et al.* (1996) Informant ratings of cognitive decline of elderly people: relationship to longitudinal change on cognitive tests. *Age and Ageing* **25**: 125–9.

Kahn R, Goldfarb A, Pollack M, Peck A. (1960) Brief objective measures of mental status in the aged. *American Journal of Psychiatry* **117**: 326–8.

Kawas C, Karagiozis H, Resau L et al. (1995) Reliability of the Blessed telephone Information-Memory-Concentration Test. Journal of Geriatric Psychiatry and Neurology 8: 238–42.

Knafelc R, LoGiudice D, Harrigan S et al. (2003) The combination of cognitive testing and an informant questionnaire in screening for dementia. Age and Ageing 32: 541–7.

Kokmen E, Smith GE, Petersen RC et al. (1991) The short test of mental status. Correlations with standardized psychometric testing. Archives of Neurology 48: 725–8.

Lehfeld H, Erzigkeit H. (1997) The SKT – a short cognitive performance test for assessing deficits of memory and attention. International Psychogeriatrics 9 (Suppl. 1): 115–21.

Little A, Hemsley D, Bergmann K et al. (1987) Comparison of the sensitivity of three instruments for the detection of cognitive decline in elderly living at home. British Journal of Psychiatry 150: 808–14.

McDowell I, Kristjansson B, Hill GB, Hébert R. (1997) Community screening for dementia: the Mini Mental State Exam (MMSE) and Modified Mini-Mental State Exam (3MS) compared. Journal of Clinical Epidemiology 50: 377–83.

Mackinnon A, Mulligan R. (1998) Combining cognitive testing and informant report to increase accuracy in screening for dementia. American Journal of Psychiatry 155: 1529–35.

Mackinnon A, Khalilian A, Jorm AF et al. (2003) Improving screening accuracy for dementia in a community sample by augmenting cognitive testing with informant report. Journal of Clinical Epidemiology 56: 358–66.

Mant A, Eyland EA, Pond DC et al. (1988) Recognition of dementia in general practice: comparison of general practitioners' opinions with assessments using the Mini-Mental State Examination and the Blessed Dementia Rating Scale. Family Practice 5: 184–8.

Marshall RJ. (1989) The predictive value of simple rules for combining two diagnostic tests. Biometrics 45: 1213–22.

Molloy DW, Alemayehu E, Roberts R. (1991) Reliability of a standardised Mini-Mental State Examination compared with the traditional Mini-Mental State Examination. American Journal of Psychiatry 148: 102–5.

Morris JC, Heymann A, Mohs RC et al. (1989) The consortium to establish a registry for Alzheimer's disease (CERAD). Part 1. Clinical and neuropsychological assessment of Alzheimer's disease. Neurology 39: 1159–65.

Petersen RC, Doody R, Kurz A et al. (2001) Current concepts in mild cognitive impairment. Archives of Neurology 58: 1985–92.

Pfeiffer E. (1975) A short portable mental status questionnaire for the assessment of organic brain deficiency in elderly patients. Journal of the American Geriatrics Society 23: 433–41.

Plutchik R, Conte H, Lieberman M. (1971) Development of a scale (GIES) for assessment of cognitive and perceptual functioning in geriatric patients. Journal of the American Geriatrics Society 19: 614–23.

Ritchie K, Fuhrer R. (1992) A comparative study of the performance of screening tests for senile dementia using receiver operating characteristics analysis. Journal of Clinical Epidemiology 45: 627–37.

Roccaforte WH, Burke WJ, Bayer BL, Wengel SP. (1992) Validation of a telephone version of the Mini-Mental State Examination. Journal of the American Geriatrics Society 40: 697–702.

Rosen WG, Mohs RC, Davis KL. (1984) A new rating scale for Alzheimer's disease. American Journal of Psychiatry 141: 1356–64.

Roth M, Tym E, Mountjoy CQ et al. (1986) CAMDEX: a standardised instrument for the diagnosis of mental disorder in the elderly with special reference to the early detection of dementia. British Journal of Psychiatry 149: 698–709.

Royall DR, Mahurin RK, Gray KF. (1992) Bedside assessment of executive cognitive impairment: the executive interview. Journal of the American Geriatric Society 40: 1221–6.

Solomon PR, Hirschoff A, Kelly B et al. (1998) A 7 minute neurocognitive screening battery highly sensitive to Alzheimer's disease. Archives of Neurology 55: 349–55.

Stern RG, Mohs RC, Davidson M et al. (1994) A longitudinal study of Alzheimer's disease: measurement, rate and predictors of cognitive deterioration. American Journal of Psychiatry 151: 390–6.

Storey J, Rowland J, Basic D et al. (2004) The Rowland Universal Dementia Assessment Scale (RUDAS): A Multicultural Cognitive Assessment Scale. International Psychogeriatrics 16: 13–31.

Stuss DT, Meiran N, Guzman DA et al. (1996) Do long tests yield a more accurate diagnosis of dementia than short tests? A comparison of 5 neuropsychological tests. Archives of Neurology 53: 1033–9.

Swain DG, Nightingale PG. (1997) Evaluation of a shortened version of the abbreviated mental test in a series of elderly patients. Clinical Rehabilitation 11: 243–8.

Teng EL, Chui HC. (1987) The Modified Mini-Mental State (3MS) examination. Journal of Clinical Psychiatry 48: 314–18.

Thomas LD, Gonzales MF, Chamberlain A et al. (1994) Comparison of clinical state, retrospective informant interview and the neuropathologic diagnosis of Alzheimer's Disease. International Journal of Geriatric Psychiatry 9: 233–6.

US Preventive Services Task Force Agency for Healthcare Research and Quality, Rockville, MD (2003) Screening for Dementia, Topic Page. June 2003. Available from: www.ahrq.gov/clinic/uspstf/uspsdeme.htm.

Valcour VG, Masaki KH, Curb JD, Blanchette PL. (2000) The detection of dementia in the primary care setting. Archives of Internal Medicine 160: 2964–8.

Ward HW, Ramsdell JW, Jackson JE et al. (1990) Cognitive function testing in comprehensive geriatric assessment: a comparison of cognitive test performance in residential and clinic settings. Journal of the American Geriatrics Society 38: 1088–92.

Williamson J, Stokoe IH, Gray S et al. (1964) Old people at home: their unreported needs. Lancet 1: 1117–20.

Zaudig M, Mitelhammer J, Pauls A et al. (1991) SIDAM – A structured interview for the diagnoses of dementia of the Alzheimer's type, multi infarct dementia and dementias of other aetiology according to ICD-10 and DSM III R. Psychological Medicine 21: 225–36.

7

Neuropsychological assessment of dementia

GREG SAVAGE

7.1 INTRODUCTION

Dementia is a fundamentally neuropsychological concept, describing the cognitive and behavioural impact of a brain disorder which brings about an unravelling of the mind's workings: 'neuro' plus 'psychological'. Dementia can be the earliest manifestation of brain illness, and emerging signs of cognitive change often provide the first inkling that something is not quite right. A brief cognitive screening test is usually given by a geriatrician or neurologist and the result may be enlightening, but if the signs are subtle it may not. In any case, if the clinician suspects dementia is a possibility, a neuropsychological referral is often made to characterize any decline in cognition with comprehensive testing based on psychometric principles and with reference to robust normative data sets. The emergence of clinical neuropsychology as a mainstream specialty discipline in hospital outpatient clinics (e.g. so-called 'memory clinics') has allowed for the quantitative evaluation of cognitive decline with the kind of metric resolution which health-care professionals might reasonably expect of an empirical investigation.

This chapter outlines the role of neuropsychological assessment in helping to make a diagnosis of the underlying cause of dementia. It characterizes the neuropsychological domains affected in various kinds of dementia, the tests of those domains used to inform neuropsychological opinion, and the perspectives commonly taken by neuropsychologists in forming an opinion. Other chapters in this volume provide expert and comprehensive reviews of the clinical and cognitive features of conditions associated with dementia, and so this chapter will focus in a 'hands-on' manner on the process followed by the neuropsychologist in responding to referral questions. The chapter is intended to serve two audiences: neuropsychologists fielding dementia-related referrals, and other health professionals who make such referrals (and in particular, those who do not use neuropsychological services

routinely, but might do so given a better understanding of the assessment process).

The chapter adopts a broad definition of dementia, but one constrained by the overall perspective of this volume. As such, coverage focuses primarily on the essential dementia seen with Alzheimer's disease (AD), but extends significantly to other diseases and conditions associated with cognitive decline. Many of these present late in the life span and are prime contenders in the process of differential diagnosis of the underlying disease. Accordingly there is also discussion of typical test findings in cases of dementia with Lewy bodies (DLB), vascular dementia (VaD), the behavioural variant of frontotemporal dementia (bvFTD), the focal-onset semantic dementia (SD), and the cognitive impairment seen in depression, sometimes called depressive dementia (DD). Other conditions where dementia is not a primary feature will not feature here. Thus while dementia develops in neurodegenerative movement disorders such as Parkinson's disease and Huntington's disease, the early diagnosis and overriding clinical concerns relate to morbidity due to the primary movement disturbance. Dementia is also associated with infectious diseases, exposure to toxic substances, developmental intellectual disability and chronic and severe alcoholism. These kinds of dementia are less common and there are often prominent signs in the clinical history which serve to distinguish the diagnosis from the more common dementias, and to orient a neuropsychological referral to specialist services.

Dementia is usually defined in terms of deterioration in two areas: cognition, and activities of daily living (ADL). Moreover, the decline in cognition is usually required to involve memory in addition to at least one other domain (e.g. according to DSM-IV-TR; American Psychiatric Association, 2000). When there is measurable cognitive decline but the person is still coping adequately with daily activities, the term mild cognitive impairment (MCI) is typically used. This is a 'pending' nosological entity denoting a condition which is not normal, but dementia cannot be said to be present. Many people are referred to the neuropsychologist with this quasi-diagnosis, and these cases will be considered in the same manner as AD, as MCI tends to 'convert' to AD at an annual rate of around 10 per cent (Bruscoli and Lovestone, 2004); that is, many cases have preclinical AD at the time of referral.

7.2 PERSPECTIVES ON NEUROPSYCHOLOGICAL ASSESSMENT

Neuropsychological assessment of dementia cannot be purely psychometric: it is placed squarely in the context provided by a comprehensive interview with the patient, as well as an informant. This interview must leave the clinician with a clear understanding of the time-course of the emergence of signs/symptoms, and the patterning of what seem to be preserved versus declining abilities. A perspective on educational and vocational achievements will inform expectations about pre-morbid cognitive status, and the interview can provide important information about lifetime exposure to brain injuries or substances which could account for cognitive decline.

The assessment process outlined in this chapter is based on a cognitive neuropsychological approach to clinical testing (Mapou and Spector, 1995), which structures the testing session, and interprets test data, according to processing models developed in cognitive psychology. The process is flexible and hypothesis-driven in contrast with fixed-battery approaches, and conclusions about higher cognitive functions are parsimonious, taking into account the influences of 'foundation-level' abilities such as attention and speed of processing. Outcomes of the assessment are framed in cognitive terms (e.g. memory problems being amenable to cueing strategies or not) as opposed to performance-level terms (e.g. verbal memory being placed in the low average range), as these tend to be understandable by those making referrals, as well as those who care for the patient.

Neuropsychologists vary in terms of their utilization of psychometric properties of tests. Those taking a hypothesis-testing approach may administer subtests of larger batteries in an admix with more 'focused' tests, and might refer to a variety of normative databases without any formal statistical comparison. Aggregation of subtest scores into summary indexes can be seen as a confound, potentially obscuring clinically meaningful differences across subtests. In common with a fixed battery approach, the hypothesis-testing approach prescribes that tests should possess robust psychometric properties in terms of reliability and gracefully-graded sensitivity to variation in performance, even if the full potential for statistical analysis is not used. Both approaches judge cognitive performance relative to age-appropriate norms, and sometimes educational level is taken into account.

Measured levels of performance, as well as differences between performances for different domains, or over time, are characterized using a range of parameters. The flagship tests of the ubiquitous Wechsler suite are the Wechsler Adult Intelligence Scale – Third edition (WAIS-III; Wechsler, 1997a) and Wechsler Memory Scale – Third edition (WMS-III; Wechsler, 1997b); although fourth editions of both have

been published recently they are not yet in widespread use. Their IQ or Index scores have a normative mean (M) of 100 and a standard deviation (SD) of 15, and partitioning of the normal distribution of IQs/Indexes provides range descriptors such as Average (with IQs between 90 and 110), Low Average (80–90), High Average (110–120), and so on. These scores translate directly to Scaled Scores when subtests of the Wechsler tests are discussed ($M = 10$, SD = 3). Some tests provide percentile ranks, and others use T-scores ($M = 50$, SD = 10). Z scores (i.e. quantifying departure from average performance in SD units for a particular test) are frequently used as a common currency in comparing performances across a range of tests using different summary parameters.

7.2.1 Components of a battery for dementia assessment

A typical test battery used when dementia is suspected takes between 1 and 2 hours to administer and covers orientation, ability to attend and manipulate information in mind, speed of information processing (usually tested via psychomotor tasks), logical reasoning, constructional praxis, executive functioning, language and new learning and retention (usually for both verbal and non-verbal material). A context for interpreting performances in these domains is established by estimating pre-morbid intellectual level. Neuropsychologists often try to quantify current mood state, usually by administration of a formal self-report inventory.

The following section describes commonly used tests and their utility in differentiating between six potential diagnoses: AD, DLB, VaD, bvFTD, SD and DD. **Table 7.1** outlines likely patterns of preserved and impaired cognition in these disorders over the domains covered in this section.

7.2.1.1 TESTS OF ORIENTATION AND PERSONAL AND GENERAL INFORMATION

Neuropsychologists usually begin testing with non-confronting questions which are administered by most health professionals in some form; these are not psychometrically sophisticated, but answers here can provide significant insights into what to expect on later testing (e.g. mistaking current age by years, the year by a decade, the current local political leader by a number of past incumbents). Such strikingly aberrant responses are common in early AD; occasional incorrect responses may represent the 'patchy dysmnesia' often seen in depressive illness. The Information and Orientation subtest of the WMS-III has 14 items (a cut-off score for abnormality is available but seldom used); the first ten items of the Mini-Mental State Examination (MMSE; Folstein et al., 1975) or items from two sections of the Addenbrooke's Cognitive Examination Revised (ACE-R; Mioshi et al., 2006) may be used instead.

7.2.1.2 ESTIMATION OF PRE-MORBID INTELLECTUAL LEVEL

Inferences about cognitive decline are necessarily made with respect to expected levels of performance in the absence of

Table 7.1 Typical patterns of cognition for conditions associated with dementia.

Cognitive domain	Typical tests	Expected performance in various conditions					
		AD	DLB	VaD	bvFTD	SD	DD
Orientation	I/O MMSE ACE-R	Impaired	Intact	Impaired?	Intact	Intact	Variable
Attention/working memory	DSp(f) DSp(b) DS-C?	Intact early on	Impaired	Impaired?	Impaired	Intact	Impaired
Processing speed	DS-C SDMT	Intact	Intact?	Impaired?	Intact	Intact	Impaired
Reasoning	Sim PC	Intact early on	Intact?	Impaired?	Impaired	Impaired due to semantic loss?	Intact
Semantics	BNT GNT CF	Impaired	Intact	Impaired?	Intact	Impaired	Intact
Executive functioning	LF CF H&B Stroop	Mildly impaired?	Impaired	Impaired	Impaired	Intact early on	Impaired
Construction	RCFT BD	Mildly impaired	Impaired	Impaired?	Mildly impaired due to poor planning?	Intact	Mildly impaired due to poor planning?
Memory	LM VR RAVLT CVLT-II HVLT-R BVMT-R LLT	Impaired recall and recognition	Impaired recall, intact recognition?	Impaired recall and recognition?	Impaired recall, intact recognition?	Can be impaired due to semantic loss?	Impaired recall, intact recognition?

ACE-R, Addenbrooke's Cognitive Examination Revised; BD, Wechsler Adult Intelligence Scale – Third edition (WAIS-III) Block Design; BNT, Boston Naming Test; BVMT-R, Brief Visuospatial Memory Test – Revised; CF, Category fluency; CVLT-II, California Verbal Learning Test – Second edition; DS-C, WAIS-III Digit Symbol-Coding; DSp(b), WAIS-III Digit Span (backwards); DSp(f), WAIS-III Digit Span (forwards); GNT, Graded Naming Test; H&B, Hayling & Brixton Tests; HVLT-R, Hopkins Verbal Learning Test – Revised; I/O, Wechsler Memory Scale – Third edition (WMS-III) Information and orientation; LF, Letter fluency; LLT, Location Learning Test; LM, WMS-III Logical Memory; MMSE, Mini-Mental State Examination; PC, WAIS-III Picture Completion; RAVLT, Rey Auditory Verbal Learning Test; RCFT, Rey Complex Figure Test; SDMT, Symbol Digit Modalities Test; Sim, WAIS-III Similarities; VR, WMS-III Visual Reproduction.

brain illness. Typically there are no 'intact' baseline data available for the referred individual, and broadly placed estimates are made (e.g. average, high average, etc.). One method takes account of educational background, vocational achievements, and/or demographic variables (either informally or via input to normatively-derived regression equations). Another approach is to measure current ability in a domain which is usually resistant to even moderate dementia, such as word knowledge: correct reading aloud of so-called 'irregular' words whose pronunciations do not follow predictable spelling-sound rules suggests intact word knowledge, and tests incorporating graded difficulty afford a psychometric estimate of likely pre-morbid intellectual level. Typically used tests of word knowledge include the National Adult Reading Test (NART; Nelson, 1982). A recent variant, the Wechsler Test of Adult Reading (WTAR; Wechsler, 2001), was co-normed with the WAIS-III and WMS-III. Both these tests are well tolerated by most cases and produce a predicted IQ score which can be compared with current scores in a variety of cognitive domains. An important caveat holds in the assessment of possible dementia: word knowledge tests are invalid when deterioration of semantic knowledge forms part of the dementing syndrome, as in SD and AD. In SD, loss of verbal knowledge is a core feature, and reading of irregular words reveals 'surface dyslexia', whereby words are pronounced according to the usual rules. Thus in the NART or WTAR errors are made, underestimating pre-morbid intellect and reducing the chance of identifying actual decline in functioning. A generous interpretation of NART/WTAR-based pre-morbid IQ measures may be warranted when there is a suggestion of semantic decline.

A cognitively framed assessment then proceeds to assess foundation-level domains such as concentration and speed of thinking, as weaknesses here can undermine (and misrepresent) higher-level functioning.

7.2.1.3   TESTS OF CONCENTRATION AND WORKING MEMORY

The ability to engage in routine sequencing (concentration or focused attention) and to hold information in mind while working on a problem (so-called 'working memory') is assessed for two purposes. A general purpose serves to qualify interpretation of performances on more complex or focal cognitive abilities, and an efficient strategy on the part of the neuropsychologist is to establish how well the patient can attend quite early in the course of the assessment. Poor moment-to-moment concentration might 'recalibrate' expectations in the examiner, and suggest use of simplified versions of tests where floor-level performances are less likely. For example, if one can establish early on that a patient can hold only two or three digits in mind for immediate repetition, presentation of a 15-item word list is almost guaranteed not to yield useful information about learning ability, as the test will be overwhelming. Here, selection of a shorter variant is likely to be more useful, with the range of potential scores calibrated better to the patient's expected performance level.

A specific purpose for assessing concentration and working memory is to provide differential diagnostic information. Poor performance here can reflect dysfunction in frontal systems

and their connections to other brain regions. Patients with depressive and/or anxiety disorders, bvFTD, or DLB often perform poorly on tests such as the Digit Span and/or Letter-Number Sequencing subtests of the WAIS-III, and Mental Control from the WMS-III. Cases with mild AD do not tend to have prominent difficulty in this cognitive domain.

7.2.1.4   TESTS OF PROCESSING SPEED

Speed of mentation is hard to measure without introducing confounds related to the task employed. Some thinking speed tasks use motoric responses to visual stimuli, and care must be taken to ensure a putative speed measure is not overly reflecting the influence of other variables (e.g. difficulty seeing or fixating visual stimuli, or motoric difficulty/slowness). A widely used test of processing speed is the Digit Symbol-Coding subtest of the WAIS-III, which measures speed of transcription of symbols into a long series of numbered boxes, guided by a number–symbol matching key. The total number of symbols correctly transcribed within 2 minutes indicates speed of the translation from number to symbol. It can also index difficulty scanning the array in the key or motoric slowness, however, and comparison with performance on an ancillary subtest (Digit Symbol-Copy) is useful if these influences are suspected (symbols are simply copied into immediately adjacent boxes). A completely non-graphomotor speed measure can be inferred from performance on WMS-III Mental Control, which requires speeded production of well-known sequences in routine format (e.g. reciting the months in order) as well as non-routine format (e.g. months in reverse order). All these tests also tax working memory, and the long durations of the transcription tasks also test sustained attention.

Reduced speed of processing (and the confounded influence of working memory and sustained attention) is not usually compromised in mild or preclinical AD or in SD, but can be seen in bvFTD, DLB, VaD, DD and subcortical dementias.

Against a background established in terms of both likely pre-morbid capabilities and current foundation-level skills, testing of higher mental functions can proceed to be interpreted in a cognitive neuropsychological assessment framework.

7.2.1.5   TESTS OF REASONING

The ability to engage in abstract reasoning is an aspect of intellect which declines gracefully with the development of AD, and is impaired earlier and more prominently in conditions which involve early compromise to frontal systems functioning. The Similarities and Picture Completion subtests from the WAIS-III test reasoning based on verbal and pictorial materials respectively, and can elicit concrete and literal responses in dementias associated with hypofrontality such as bvFTD, DLB and often VaD.

7.2.1.6   TESTS OF LANGUAGE FUNCTIONING

A typical neuropsychological battery used in dementia-related referrals tends not to assess language comprehensively, but the ability to name objects is routinely assessed. Naming reflects semantic access (and/or representation) as well as phonological processing, and commonly used tests present line drawings of objects graded by frequency of encounter. The Boston Naming Test – 2 (BNT-2; Kaplan *et al.*, 2001) comprises 60 items, with a default entry point at item 30, and allows for phonological cueing if the patient cannot name the item spontaneously (assessing a so-called 'tip-of-the-tongue' state). It is often administered in either a 15- or 30-item short form. The Graded Naming Test (GNT; McKenna and Warrington, 1983) comprises 30 items but has a higher ceiling with the inclusion of quite obscure items. Care should be taken to recognize that certain items are culture-bound: for example, the UK-developed GNT considers a kangaroo to be an item of moderate difficulty, yet Australians consider this extremely easy; the BNT has a beaver as an easy item, but outside the United States a beaver might not be so easily named.

Dysnomia is a prominent sign in mild AD and focal dementias such as SD and progressive non-fluent aphasia (PNFA); degraded semantic knowledge is thought to be the problem in AD and SD, and a phonological account is proposed in PNFA. Integrity of semantic knowledge can also be assessed by testing vocabulary and general knowledge (e.g. using the Vocabulary and Information subtests of the WAIS-III). Syntactic aspects of language are usually preserved in all but severe cases of dementia, and formal testing is rarely undertaken.

7.2.1.7 TESTS OF CONSTRUCTION

Visuoconstructional ability is always tested in some form. The Rey Complex Figure Test (RCFT; Meyers and Meyers, 1995) affords good insights into constructional praxis, and evaluating the organizational approach taken in copying the figure informs an opinion about executive functioning. Dementia affecting posterior functions (e.g. in mild-moderate AD and in DLB) can produce distortion in reproduction of spatial relationships among elements of the figure, often culminating in a bizarrely misshapen copy. In contrast, copy of the Rey figure is seldom distorted in dementias with an anterior presentation (e.g. bvFTD, SD), although misalignment may occur due to a poorly planned approach. Matching of blocks to specified patterns is another frequently administered test (e.g. Corsi blocks, most often deployed in the Block Design subtest of the WAIS-III). This test can be failed at easy levels in mild AD, and while patients with bvFTD (and perhaps DLB) may have trouble, they can benefit from provision of structure: once the test is finished, many neuropsychologists revisit failed items using a transparent grid overlay which identifies the component blocks to aid initiation of a response.

7.2.1.8 TESTS OF EXECUTIVE FUNCTIONING

In an assessment tailored to be time efficient and minimally frustrating, many neuropsychologists avoid lengthy concept-formation tests such as the Wisconsin Card Sorting Test, and prefer brief tests of the same construct such as the Brixton

test (Burgess and Shallice, 1997). Here, the patient is required to anticipate the next location in a spatial sequence; the patient is warned at the outset that the sequential rule will change from time to time, and they will need to pick up on the new sequence. Ability to inhibit prepotent responses is often tested using a variant of the Stroop test: the Victoria version (Strauss *et al.*, 2006) is very quick to administer, measuring time taken to name the printed colours of 24 dots, then of 24 words and finally of 24 incongruent colour names (e.g. the word 'red' printed in blue ink). There is a natural tendency to read the word rather than state the ink colour used, and failure to inhibit this tendency indicates poor executive functioning. In a similar vein, the Hayling test (packaged with the Brixton) measures response latency and error rate in completing sentence fragments with intentionally nonsensical final words (e.g. London is a very busy: banana); executive failures lead to either frankly predictable completions (e.g. city), or marginally less predictable ones (e.g. location), or long latencies to produce an acceptable response.

Perhaps the most widely used test of executive functioning, included in most batteries, involves word generation under time pressure and compliance with a set of stated rules (e.g. Strauss *et al.*, 2006). Letter fluency (sometimes wrongly called phonemic fluency) requires production of as many words as possible which begin with a prescribed letter in a 1-minute period. There are three rules which patients must verify that they understand: no repeats, no proper nouns (explained in terms of 'words usually starting with a capital letter', with examples), and no variations on the same word (explained with examples). Trials are undertaken for three letters (usually F, A and S), and the total score indexes flexible thinking in a non-routine generation task requiring self-monitoring, rule observance, strategic exploitation of lexical 'free rides' (e.g. producing 'flip' might suggest 'flap' and 'flop' in quick succession), and adaptability in the face of 'blocking'. A variant which is more structured (and hence normally easier) simply requires generation of words on a given theme (with the only rule being no repeats). This category (or semantic) fluency test is sometimes only given once, but in the version used in the Delis-Kaplan Executive Function System (D-KEFS; Delis *et al.*, 2001), two trials are given with different topics, followed by a trial requiring alternation between two topics.

Fluency tests are very informative in dementia assessments, as the normal pattern of better performance on category fluency than letter fluency tends to be reversed in even mild or preclinical AD: letter fluency can be normal, but category fluency fails badly due to deteriorating semantic processing; this pattern may be seen in SD, but letter fluency can also be impaired. In depression, bvFTD, DLB and VaD letter fluency is typically impaired, with category fluency following suit or remaining largely intact.

7.2.1.9 TESTS OF MEMORY

Formal testing of learning and retention of new information assesses integrity of episodic memory functioning, and is intended to characterize the forgetfulness in everyday life which is such a frequent complaint – either by the patient or, more often, by significant others. Learning is sometimes tested with only one exposure to material, but preferably with repeated trials of exposure and testing, otherwise brief attentional lapses can confound interpretation. Testing of learning is performed immediately, but the most revealing data are usually provided after a delay of about 20–30 minutes. Testing might require free recall of information, cued recall, or recognition of the information when presented among potentially confusable information. This gradient between recall versus recognition failure maps onto cognitive constructs of retrieval versus encoding/consolidation problems, and this distinction is thought to have diagnostic value in discriminating among dementia types. In brief, retrieval problems are characterized by poor recall but near-normal recognition performances, due to failure of frontally mediated initiation of access to a stored memory trace; this pattern is typically observed in depression, DLB, VaD and bvFTD. In contrast, an encoding/consolidation problem is thought to represent temporal lobe dysfunction, as seen in AD, and perhaps in SD to the extent that the information source itself is degraded. In these conditions, an adequate memory trace is never formed and so patients perform poorly on both recall and recognition testing.

Assessment of unilateral memory disorders (e.g. in cases of stroke, tumour or epilepsy) has resulted in a tradition of testing memory using both verbal material (usually word lists, word pairings and/or prose passages) and non-verbal material (usually drawn diagrams, faces and/or object locations). Free recall of prose passages (e.g. WMS-III Logical Memory) is often tested, although performance here is not useful in distinguishing between a temporal lobe encoding/consolidation problem and a more frontally mediated retrieval-based impairment. In addition, large amounts of information are presented without multiple repeated trials, and attentional problems can confound interpretation. Performance on free recall word lists over repeated trials, combined with delayed recall and subsequent recognition testing addresses both these issues, and the Rey Auditory-Verbal Learning Test (Rey, 1958; Strauss et al., 2006) is widely used in dementia-related assessments. A similar test, the semantically clustered California Verbal Learning Test – Second edition (CVLT-II; Delis et al., 2000) is popular in the United States but inclusion of a few culturally bound items may confound its use in other English-speaking countries (e.g. where 'subway' is not an obvious member of the semantic cluster 'modes of transport'). These tests are particularly useful in the early detection of dementia, but the list length (15 and 16 items, respectively) may prove overwhelming in mild–moderate cases, resulting in floor effects which preclude measurement of deterioration over time. Easier semantically clustered versions such as the 12-item Hopkins Verbal Learning Test – Revised (HVLT-R; Benedict et al., 1998) or nine-item CVLT-II Short Form are extremely useful when screening of memory reveals strikingly impaired ability. Paired associate learning tests are very sensitive to temporal lobe damage, but verbal versions are usually administered in a cued recall format which allows for failure due to retrieval problems; development of associate-recognition modes of such tests

may improve specificity in detecting problems with encoding/consolidation.

In the non-verbal domain, memory for designs is frequently tested but relies on intact constructional ability. The Visual Reproduction subtest of the WMS-III measures recall for a series of designs with increasing complexity, each after a 10-second exposure; this immediate recall reflects working memory, but subsequent recall after 30 minutes reflects the more informative construct of retention. Incidental testing of recall for the Rey Complex Figure (i.e. without informing the patient ahead of time) indexes retention, but can only be interpreted validly when the initial copy was reasonably accurate and completed in an organized manner. The same caveats applied earlier to prose passages regarding attentional lapses and retrieval versus encoding/consolidation interpretations apply to these visually based free recall tests with only single exposure learning phases. The Brief Visuospatial Memory Test – Revised (BVMT-R; Benedict, 1997) is a non-verbal analogue to the HVLT-R, and uses repeated trials of free recall of six simple designs viewed at once for 10 seconds; subsequent recognition testing after delayed recall quantifies retrieval difficulty. The Faces subtest of the WMS-III tests immediate recognition memory for photographs of faces, avoiding the working memory confound of Visual Reproduction by testing at the end of a series of 24 items; delayed recognition tests retention. Finally, the Location Learning Test (LLT; Bucks et al., 2000) measures correct placement of drawings of ten common objects in a 5×5 grid over multiple trials. It has good metric properties which capture the degree of error in misremembering of location.

In all these tests, both verbal and non-verbal, patients with AD tend to have difficulty with both recall and recognition modes of testing, and patients with bvFTD, DLB, VaD and depression tend to have less difficulty on recognition testing.

7.3   COMMUNICATING A NEUROPSYCHOLOGICAL OPINION

The outcome of the assessment is usually conveyed in a formal report to the referrer. Neuropsychological reports are comprehensive documents which combine appraisal of the clinical history, qualitative aspects of behaviour on interview and throughout testing, and interpretation of test scores. Here, the operative word is interpretation: the score itself may be qualified by the manner in which it was achieved (e.g. normatively average repetition of digits might represent graceful arrival at a threshold of difficulty, or a chaotic pattern of early failures on easy items which persists through to extremely difficult items; the total score does not distinguish between these clinically quite different performances). Overall, the assessment process and the resulting opinion is fundamentally neuro**psychological**, not neuro**psychometric**. This should be reflected in the conclusions reached: an opinion should be conveyed in plain language with minimal recourse to statistics, and the logic underlying the interpretation of the findings should be transparent. If the referrer has primary responsibility for clinical care of the patient, they will usually discuss the findings and opinion in a review consultation, possibly in a synthesis with conclusions from other investigations. It is very useful to supplement this meeting with face-to-face feedback from the neuropsychologist to the patient, in the company of a carer; this provides the opportunity for clarification and for discussing potential management strategies (see Chapter 26, A predominantly psychosocial approach to behaviour problems in dementia: treating causality).

REFERENCES

American Psychiatric Association. (2000) *Diagnostic and Statistical Manual of Mental Disorders*, 4th edn, text revision. Washington DC: APA.

Benedict RHB. (1997) *Brief Visuospatial Memory Test – Revised*. Odessa, FL: Psychological Assessment Resources.

Benedict RHB, Schretlen D, Groninger L, Brandt J. (1998) Hopkins. Verbal Learning Test-Revised: Normative data and analysis of inter-form and test-retest reliability. *Clinical Neuropsychologist* 12: 43–55.

Bruscoli M, Lovestone S. (2004) Is MCI really just early dementia? A systematic review of conversion studies. *International Psychogeriatrics* 16: 129–40.

Bucks RS, Willison JR, Byrne LMT. (2000) *Location Learning Test: Manual*. Bury St Edmunds, UK: Thames Valley Test Company.

Burgess PW, Shallice T. (1997) *The Hayling and Brixton Tests*. Thurston, UK: Thames Valley Test Company.

Delis DC, Kaplan E, Kramer JH. (2001) *The Delis–Kaplan Executive Function System (D-KEFS)*. San Antonio, TX: The Psychological Corporation.

Delis DC, Kramer JH, Kaplan E, Ober BA. (2000) *California Verbal Learning Test*, 2nd edn, Adult Version. San Antonio, TX: The Psychological Corporation.

Folstein MF, Folstein SE, McHugh PR. (1975) "Mini-mental state": A practical method for grading the cognitive state of patients for the clinician. *Journal of Psychiatric Research* 12: 189–98.

Kaplan EF, Goodglass H, Weintraub S. (2001) *The Boston Naming Test*, 2nd edn. Philadelphia: Lippincott Williams & Wilkins.

McKenna P, Warrington E. (1983) *Graded Naming Test*. Windsor, UK: NFER-Nelson.

Mapou RL, Spector J. (1995) *Clinical neuropsychological assessment: A cognitive approach*. New York: Plenum Press.

Meyers JE, Meyers KR. (1995) *Rey Complex Figure Test and Recognition Trial*. Odessa, FL: Psychological Assessment Resources.

Mioshi E, Dawson K, Mitchell J *et al.* The Addenbrooke's Cognitive Examination Revised (ACE-R): A brief cognitive test battery for dementia screening. *International Journal of Geriatric Psychiatry* 21: 1078–85.

Nelson HE. (1982) *The National Adult Reading Test (NART)*. Windsor, UK: NFER-Nelson.

Rey A. (1958) *L'examen clinique en psychologie*. Paris: Presse Universitaire de France.

Strauss E, Sherman EMS, Spreen O. (2006) *A compendium of neuropsychological tests: Administration, norms, and commentary*, 3rd edn. New York: Oxford University Press.

Wechsler D. (1997a) *Wechsler Adult Intelligence Scale*, 3rd edn. San Antonio, TX: The Psychological Corporation.

Wechsler D. (1997b) *Wechsler Memory Scale*, 3rd edn. San Antonio, TX: The Psychological Corporation.

Wechsler D. (2001) *Wechsler Test of Adult Reading*. San Antonio, TX: The Psychological Corporation.

Neuropsychiatric aspects of dementia

IRACEMA LEROI AND CONSTANTINE G LYKETSOS

8.1 INTRODUCTION

The neuropsychiatric changes in dementia are nearly universal and may result in extremely challenging management problems. This is in spite of the definition of dementia being based on the cognitive and functional changes alone. The neuropsychiatric symptoms include personality changes, mood deterioration, perceptual abnormalities, psychomotor disturbances (such as agitation, aggression, wandering and purposeless behaviour) and neurovegetative changes, including changes in sleep and appetite. Collectively, these manifestations of dementia syndromes can be regarded under the rubric of 'behavioural and psychological symptoms of dementia (BPSD; Finkel *et al.*, 1996); however, they have been variously termed as 'neuropsychiatric symptoms', 'behavioural disturbances', 'non-cognitive changes' and 'challenging behaviours'. Here we will refer to them as the neuropsychiatric symptoms of dementia. The importance and ubiquity of these symptoms is highlighted by Alois Alzheimer's first clinical description of Alzheimer's disease (AD) in 1907. In this case study, he stated:

> The first noticeable symptoms of illness shown by this 51-year old woman was suspiciousness of her husband. Soon, a rapidly increasing memory impairment became evident; she could no longer orient herself in her own dwelling, dragged objects here and there and hid them, and at times, believing that people were out to murder her, started to scream loudly (Alzheimer, translated by Jarvik and Greenson, 1987).

Neuropsychiatric or 'behavioural' problems are considered second only to decline in activities of daily living as the most problematic symptoms for carers, with agitation, aggression and personality change each being rated as the most troublesome symptoms overall for 16 per cent of carers (Georges *et al.*, 2008). Furthermore, neuropsychiatric problems are a common first presentation of AD and often prompt referral for assessment. In some cases, changes in personality or behaviour in later life, namely a putative diagnosis of 'mild behavioural disturbance' may be a harbinger of later dementia, in an analogous way that a proportion of people with 'mild cognitive impairment' go on to develop later significant cognitive impairment warranting a diagnosis of dementia (Taragano *et al.*, 2009).

8.2 IMPACT OF NEUROPSYCHIATRIC SYMPTOMS

The impact of neuropsychiatric complications on patients, carers and the community is significant and according to the Alzheimer Europe Dementia Carers' survey, 50 per cent of carers report that such symptoms are the most problematic aspect of caring for someone with AD (Georges *et al.*, 2008). This impact is now being acknowledged as a focus around which national policy for dementia care should develop. For example, in the UK, a specific objective of the National Dementia Strategy (www.dh.gov.uk/en/SocialCare/

Deliveringadultsocialcare/Olderpeople/NationalDementia Strategy/DH_083362) (Department of Health, 2009) refers to the management of behavioural symptoms in care homes and was included in the policy in response to specific criticisms from various national bodies regarding the management of such problems in the care home setting. The cost of caring for those with neuropsychiatric symptoms in AD is significantly greater than for those without such symptoms, even after adjusting for the severity of the dementia and other co-morbidities (Murman et al., 2002).

Neuropsychiatric problems can lead to increased risk of injury to the dementia sufferer themselves and other patients with dementia in residential or nursing facilities, but also to carers, whether they be family or professional. Depression rates in the carers are significantly greater than in carers of those without neuropsychiatric problems (Gonzalez-Salvador et al., 2000). Injury and insult to care home staff resulting from neuropsychiatric complications can lead to high turn-overs of staff, which in turn can lead to a less positive work environment and can precipitate behavioural disturbances in residents. The risk of the patient being treated with restraints and antipsychotic medication also significantly increases with increasing severity of neuropsychiatric problems, which may in turn increase the risk of mortality, morbidity and dete-riorating cognition (Bianchetti et al., 1997).

The impact of neuropsychiatric symptoms on quality of life is far greater than the impact of functional limitations or cognitive decline (Banerjee et al., 2006). This finding has significance in that, whereas the cognitive and functional aspects of the dementia syndrome decline inexorably despite a relatively brief respite from decline enjoyed by some respon-ders to cognitive enhancers, the neuropsychiatric symptoms do not follow such a predictable course, and can arguably be largely eliminated through appropriate management. Elim-inating the symptoms could, in turn, impact significantly on improving quality of life for the dementia sufferer.

8.3 EPIDEMIOLOGY AND SPECTRUM OF NEUROPSYCHIATRIC SYMPTOMS OF DEMENTIA

Neuropsychiatric symptoms are extremely common in the dementias; however, a given symptom or syndrome may not reliably appear in any one dementia diagnosis. Unlike the predictable decline seen in cognitive and functional abilities of dementia sufferers, the neuropsychiatric symptoms fluc-tuate in their presence and intensity. The first presentation of neuropsychiatric symptoms, often in the form of depression with cognitive impairment, may precede the onset of a full dementia syndrome. For each episode of later-life depression over the age of 65 with accompanying cognitive symptoms, the risk of developing later AD increases (Wilson et al., 2002). Social withdrawal may occur almost three years prior to the onset of the full dementia syndrome, and anxiety and psy-chotic symptoms may also be harbingers of later cognitive decline (Taragano et al., 2009). These findings underscore the necessity for early detection of neuropsychiatric symptoms in the non-demented elderly population.

In mild cognitive impairment (MCI), which involves impairment in memory and possibly other areas of cognition in individuals whose day-to-day functioning is relatively preserved, neuropsychiatric symptoms affect 40–75 per cent of sufferers (Lyketsos et al., 2002; Hwang et al., 2004). In the Cardiovascular Health Study (CHS), of the 320 individuals who were identified as having MCI, 43 per cent exhibited neuropsychiatric symptoms, with depression, apathy and irritability being the most common (Lyketsos et al., 2002). Almost 30 per cent of those with neuropsychiatric symptoms were rated as 'clinically significant'. From the same study, for those with a diagnosis of dementia of any subtype, almost 75 per cent had at least one neuropsychiatric symptom.

Only a few population-based studies of neuropsychiatric disturbances in dementia have been undertaken, of which the Cache County Study of Memory in Aging (CCSMA) is a landmark (Breitner et al., 1999). Of the 5092 participants evaluated, which constituted 90 per cent of the elderly residential population of a particular county of the United States, 65 per cent ($n = 214$) had AD, 19 per cent ($n = 62$) had vascular dementia (VaD), and 16 per cent (53) had another DSM-IV dementia diagnosis. Based on items endorsed by caregivers on the Neuropsychiatric Inventory (NPI) (Cummings, 1997), 61 per cent ($n = 201$) of all the partici-pants with a diagnosis of dementia had one or more neuro-psychiatric symptoms in the month prior to interview, rates being much higher than the aged comparison group without dementia. Apathy, depression and agitiation/aggression were the most common (Lyketsos et al., 2000). Specifically, among those with a diagnosis of AD, 23 per cent ($n = 49$) had delusions and 13 per cent ($n = 28$) had hallucinations. In contrast, in those with a diagnosis of VaD, prevalences were 8 per cent ($n = 5$) and 13 per cent ($n = 8$) for these symptoms, respectively (Leroi et al., 2003). With regards to specific psychotic symptoms, misidentification phenomena and jealous delusions are more common in dementia than in schizophrenia, in which Schneiderian first-rank symptoms, such as auditory hallucinations of voices commenting, commanding or conversing, are more commonly seen. In AD specifically, the most common hallucinations are visual (80 per cent), far more common than auditory hallucinations (20 per cent) (Leroi et al., 2003).

The prevalence of neuropsychiatric symptoms in clinic-based populations of AD patients can be derived from the largest pooled dataset of AD patients, namely that created under the aegis of the European Alzheimer Disease Con-sortium. These cross-sectional data from 12 treatment centres included NPI scores of 2354 AD patients and revealed that, similarly to the population-based prevalence, apathy was the most common symptom, appearing in 55 per cent of patients, followed by anxiety and depression in about 37 per cent (Aalten et al., 2007). Delusions and hallucinations had a similar prevalence to the population-based findings as well.

Residential and nursing home prevalence figures differ slightly from the findings of population- or clinic-based cohorts of dementia sufferers, and this may in part be due to the more advanced stage of dementia sufferers no longer residing in a community setting. One of the first well-designed studies of neuropsychiatric symptoms in residents in nursing home facilities revealed that 91 per cent ($n = 73$) of the 80 residents evaluated had at least one psychiatric diagnosis and at least one behavioural problem, regardless of the presence of dementia (Tariot *et al.*, 1993).

The Maryland Assisted Living Study (MALS) examined a stratified random sample of assisted living (AL) residents in order to obtain a direct estimate of the prevalence of dementia and other psychiatric disorders in these facilities in central Maryland (Rosenblatt *et al.*, 2004). Based on NPI scores, 83 per cent of residents with dementia exhibited neuropsychiatric symptoms, of which 70 per cent had clinically significant symptoms as determined by an NPI domain score ≥4. The magnitude and frequency of neuropsychiatric symptoms was twice as great in small facilities (less than 15 beds) compared to larger facilities, suggesting that the characteristics of residential types need to be considered when determining the prevalence of neuropsychiatric symptoms in such settings (Leroi *et al.*, 2007).

The prevalence of neuropsychiatric symptoms may also depend on the specific dementia subtype, although AD and VaD cannot always be distinguished based on their profile of such symptoms (Leroi *et al.*, 2003). In contrast, the neuropsychiatric manifestations of frontal lobe dementias are embedded within the diagnostic criteria (McKhann *et al.*, 2001) and can be used to distinguish between subtypes: frontotemporal dementia (FTD), in which the core changes are characterized by an insidious onset and gradual decline in social functioning and regulation of personal conduct, accompanied by emotional blunting, loss of insight and behaviours that may be stereotypic, perseverative or stimulus bound; semantic dementia (SD), in which a predominance of left-sided temporal lobe pathology leads to compulsive behaviours; and progressive non-fluent aphasia (PNA), in which language dysfunction is the core presenting feature. Unlike SD, FTD tends to have a predominance of right-sided temporal dysfunction and tends to present with aberrant social behaviour, hyperorality, hypersexuality and changes in religious and ideological belief systems (Mychack *et al.*, 2001).

In the Lewy body diseases, such as dementia with Lewy bodies (DLB) and dementia associated with Parkinson's disease (PDD), visual hallucinations are particularly prominent with prevalences of up to 76 and 54 per cent in the two dementia types, respectively (Aarsland *et al.*, 2001). In Parkinson's disease (PD) without dementia, the same neuropsychiatric presentation is evident, but with a lower frequency, suggesting that a spectrum of similar but increasing pathology exists across the three disorders depending on the distribution of Lewy bodies and subsequent damage to cholinergic pathways (Tiraboschi *et al.*, 2000).

8.4   RISK FACTORS FOR THE DEVELOPMENT OF NEUROPSYCHIATRIC SYMPTOMS

In the UK, a large, population-based study of health in the elderly, the Medical Research Council Cognitive Function and Ageing Study (MRC CFAS), prospectively followed 13 004 individuals over the age of 64. Of the 587 individuals with dementia, neuropsychiatric symptoms were found to be associated with level of cognitive functioning (Savva *et al.*, 2009). Irritability was more common in those with less severe cognitive functioning as reflected by a Mini-Mental State Examination (MMSE) score of ≥22, whereas wandering, elation, apathy and psychosis was more common in those in the lower range of cognitive functioning (MMSE <17). Depression and anxiety tended to occur in younger people with dementia as well as those with vascular risk factors, such as a previous heart attack or a personal history of emotional problems. In contrast, vascular risk factors alone were associated with a lower rate of misidentification and confabulation. Genetic factors may play a role, including an association between the presence of the apolipoprotein E (ApoE) ε4 and the low-activity allele of the serotonin transporter gene, however, the evidence remains controversial (Lee and Lyketsos, 2003).

Finally, pre-morbid personality traits may predispose to the later development of neuropsychiatric symptoms in AD, particularly neurotic personality traits, or the tendency to experience negative emotions (Dawson *et al.*, 2000). However, this relationship is far from straightforward and pre-morbid. For example, neuroticism appears not to predict depression in dementia but rather, anxiety and total NPI scores. A pre-morbid personality of lower 'agreeableness' also appears to correlate with an 'agitation/apathy' syndrome derived by factor analysis of 208 AD patients (Archer *et al.*, 2007).

8.5   CLASSIFICATION OF SYMPTOMS

Various classification schemes have been proposed to capture the range of behavioural and psychiatric presentations in dementia. The current debate centres around whether to 'lump' or 'split' the symptoms into specific and definable syndromes or consider them as monosymptomatic phenomena. Historically, the monosymptomatic approach has underpinned landmark prevalence studies of the neuropsychiatric symptoms in AD, such as that of Burns *et al.* (1990). In this study, the prevalence of symptoms, derived from the Geriatric Mental State Schedule (GMS; Copeland *et al.*, 1976), considered each symptom as a separate entity and did not take the frequent co-occurrence of symptoms into consideration. This approach later gave way to the syndromal approach, which attempts to address several of the methodological liabilities of the monosymptomatic approach and is based on the observation of co-occurrence of several behavioural symptoms in individual patients.

Statistical methods have been employed to examine neuropsychiatric symptoms syndromally, as per the 'lumping' approach. These include factor and principal component analytic approaches, as well as cluster approaches including latent class analyses. Whereas several syndromes have emerged from these approaches, a summary of findings from the factor analytic approaches could be considered as encompassing the following syndromes: psychosis, depression, aggression, apathy and hyperactivity/agitation (McShane, 2000). One of the recent larger analyses was based on the European Alzheimer Disease Consortium's cross-sectional study of 2808 patients with dementia from 12 different centres (Aalten *et al.*, 2008). Using principal component analyses, four neuropsychiatric syndromes were identified across various dementia types and, similarly to those summarized by McShane (2000), included: 'hyperactivity' (agitation, aggression, euphoria, disinhibition, irritability, aberrant motor behaviour), 'psychosis' (hallucinations and delusions), 'affective symptoms' (depression and anxiety) and 'apathy' (apathy and eating behaviours). Demographic and clinical characteristics were taken into consideration and revealed that stage of disease and use of cholinesterase inhibitors influenced the symptom clusters.

In contrast to the factor analytic approaches, latent class analysis is a method which examines whether individuals tend to cluster into groups (classes) based on their individual clinical profile rather than examining the groupings of clinical characteristics across individuals, as in the former case. The latter method has revealed that three groups or classes of AD patients typically manifest: those with no neuropsychiatric symptoms (40 per cent) or with a monosymptomatic disturbance (19 per cent). A second class (28 per cent) has a predominantly affective syndrome, while a third class (13 per cent) presents with a psychotic syndrome (Lyketsos *et al.*, 2000). A similar pattern using latent class analysis emerged from the analysis by Moran *et al.* (2004), however, aggression, rather than psychosis, appeared more distinctly as a separate grouping.

The argument supporting a 'split' in symptoms is based on findings of distinct underlying neuropathology of different individual symptoms. For example, delusions in AD have been associated with the presence of neurofibrillary tangles, and may be associated with an 'affective syndrome', whereas hallucinations appear to be more closely associated with degeneration of cholinergic pathways (Perry *et al.*, 1990; Lyketsos *et al.*, 2000). Hence it may be misleading to 'lump' these different symptoms under the rubric of 'psychosis of AD'.

8.6   ASSESSMENT AND DIAGNOSIS OF THE NEUROPSYCHIATRIC SYMPTOMS OF DEMENTIA

The assessment of neuropsychiatric symptoms should be considered an essential part of a complete assessment of a patient with dementia. Several assessment tools and rating scales have been validated and can aid in the detection and diagnosis of the symptoms as well as their quantification (see Chapter 9, Measurement of behaviour disturbance, noncognitive symptoms and quality of life). Quantifying the frequency and severity of the symptoms can be important, particularly as they may be the key focus of therapy since quantification allows a clear determination of the outcome of the therapeutic intervention. The most commonly used and best-validated tools for assessing the full range of symptoms include the NPI (Cummings, 1997), which is considered the gold standard assessment tool and is often used as an efficacy outcome measure in clinical trials. A clinician-rated version available in several languages, the NPI-C, has recently been developed and is likely to be used widely in the future (Medeiros *et al.*, 2009).

Another commonly used full spectrum tool is the Behavioural Pathology in Alzheimer Disease Rating Scale (BEHAVE-AD) (Reisberg *et al.*, 1987). Other rating scales focus on specific behavioural syndromes such as the Cornell Scale for Depression in Dementia (CSDD) (Alexopoulos *et al.*, 1988), which is an informant-rated depression scale; the Cohen-Mansfield Agitation Inventory (Cohen-Mansfield, 1986) for assessment of agitation and aggression; and the Apathy Evaluation Scale (AES) (Marin *et al.*, 1991) for the assessment of apathy and loss of motivation.

Aside from the use of rating scales and tools, the clinical assessment of neuropsychiatric symptoms can be enhanced through the use of diagnostic criteria specific for particular syndromes. Such diagnostic criteria, although not widely used in the clinical setting, have come about due to attempts to operationalize the examination of separate behavioural phenomena. The symptoms have been classified into distinct sets of unique, validated criteria, similar to the approach to categorization of symptoms used by the American Psychiatric Association's Diagnostic and Statistical Manual of Mental Disorders. The approach so far has been restricted to the development of criteria for AD patients, which limits its utility. However, from a research perspective this approach fosters reliability and enables the development of a sound evidence-base for management strategies. Examples of such diagnostic criteria include: 'psychosis of AD' (Jeste and Finkel, 2000); 'depression of AD' (Olin *et al.*, 2002); and ' AD-associated affective disorder' or 'AD-associated psychotic disorder' (Lyketsos *et al.*, 2001).

8.7   PATHOPHYSIOLOGY OF NEUROPSYCHIATRIC SYMPTOMS OF DEMENTIA

Some of the most significant recent advances in our understanding of the neuropsychiatric symptoms of dementia have arisen from new findings of the underlying pathophysiology of these symptoms. A thorough understanding of such pathophysiological processes will aid validation of the clustering of the neuropsychiatric symptoms and syndromes and further clarify whether mechanisms distinct from those underlying cognitive symptoms exist.

Agitation, aggression and irritability can occur in up to 70 per cent of AD sufferers in their first year of diagnosis (Jost and Grossberg, 1996). A proportion of those with agitation will have underlying delusions, however, agitation may occur independently of psychotic symptoms and is most often associated with more advanced functional impairment (Levy *et al.*, 1996). Considered an 'enigmatic syndrome' in AD, the underlying neurobiology of agitation and aggression is unclear (Cummings, 2000). There is some evidence for a link between these symptoms and the glutamatergic system, which may be disrupted due to the formation of neurofibrillary tangles (NFT) in frontal and cingulate cortices (Tekin *et al.*, 2001). This pathology may result in an exaggerated response to triggers and other symptoms such as depression, anxiety and psychosis, through the lowering of the threshold that triggers aggressive behaviour (Senanarong *et al.*, 2004).

Psychosis is one of the most common presenting neuropsychiatric features in dementia, particularly in AD and DLB, where visual hallucinations may be the presenting symptoms. Delusions occur very frequently, particularly in the earlier stages of dementia and in those who are older (Leroi et al., 2003). Post-mortem neuropathological and neurochemical studies have generally considered hallucinations and delusions under the common rubric of 'psychosis' and suggest that those with psychosis and AD have more extensive degenerative changes in frontal and temporal areas, compared with those AD sufferers with no psychosis (Cummings, 2000). However, there is growing support for considering hallucinations and delusions separately when considering the pathophysiology of 'psychosis'. In particular, the association between lower levels of choline acetyltransferase levels in parietal and temporal lobes of dementia sufferers with hallucinations (Perry et al., 1990) and the relative efficacy of cholinesterase inhibitors in treating hallucinations in dementia suggests a cholinergic basis for hallucinations. In contrast, delusions are increasingly associated with the presence of NFTs in post-mortem samples and frontal hypometabolism on functional imaging (Cummings, 2000). Furthermore, it is unlikely that damage in a single brain area could account for the complexity of a set of symptoms that constitute 'psychosis'. It is more likely that disruption at any point along key networks, such as the medial and dorsolateral frontal cortices together with the limbic areas comprising the anterior cingulate to ventral striatum pathway, is responsible (Mega et al., 2000).

Depression in dementia is common, with 20 and 32 per cent of AD and dementia patients, respectively, experiencing depression in the month prior to assessment (Lyketsos et al., 2000; Lyketsos et al., 2002). Prevalence estimates of depression tend to vary in dementia due to several complicating factors such as the frequent co-morbidity with apathy, the overlap with other non-cognitive symptoms of dementia such as neurovegetative disturbances, the relative subtlety of presentation in later life, and finally, the inability of the depressed dementia patient to communicate their distress (Lee and Lyketsos, 2003). The predisposing factors and underlying pathophysiology of depression in dementia may differ in different groups of patients, despite the resulting clinical syndrome being relatively homogeneous. For example, a proportion of those developing depression after the onset of AD will have had a family history of mood disorder or have suffered depression in early or midlife and the subsequent presentation is a recurrence or emergence of predisposition. In contrast, for some, depression may represent an emotional reaction to cognitive deficits, cerebrovascular damage, or a direct consequence of the neurodegenerative process (Lee and Lyketsos, 2003). The latter process is most likely the same as that underlying 'late-life depression', which is commonly a harbinger of a dementia syndrome. In depression in AD, noradrenergic neuronal loss in the locus coeruleus and serotonergic neuronal loss in the dorsal raphe nucleus may in part drive the syndrome (Förstl et al., 1992) and this is further supported by findings that in AD, neuronal loss is more extensive in the locus coeruleus, known to be a key area in the pathology of depression, than in the nucleus basalis (Zarow et al., 2003).

Apathy, or loss of motivation, is considered the most common neuropsychiatric manifestation in dementia and in the European Alzheimer disease consortium (EADC) study was found to occur in almost 65 per cent of AD patients (Aalten et al., 2007). Apathy as a syndrome appears to be stable across several forms of dementia, including VaD, DLB and FTD (Aalten et al., 2008). As with depression, apathy may be a prodrome of a dementia syndrome and in MCI, co-morbidity with the 'lack of interest' component of the apathy syndrome predicted a higher rate of conversion to AD (Onyike et al., 2007; Robert et al., 2008). Apathy is very often under-recognized, yet it has significant consequences with greater levels of impairment in activities of daily living, more associated cognitive impairments and greater carer burden. The most likely pathophysiology underlying apathy syndromes is that which involves a lesion at any point along the distributed frontal-subcortical network. Depending on where the network might be lesioned may determine the particular manifestation of the apathy syndrome. For example, lesions involving the mesiofrontal circuit, of which the anterior cingulate gyrus forms a part and which mediates goal-directed and motivated behaviour, is likely to manifest in lack of drive or action. Lesions involving the dorsolateral frontal cortex are more likely to disrupt the cognitive and executive functioning abilities required to generate goal-directed behaviours (Landes et al., 2001). The importance of these regions to the apathy syndrome is supported by various studies, including the post-mortem findings of greater NFT burden in the anterior cingulate of those with AD and apathy (Tekin et al., 2001), and the neuroimaging findings suggesting that apathy is associated with decreased perfusion and metabolism of frontosubcortical brain areas and the anterior cingulate (Benoit et al., 2002).

8.8 CONCLUSIONS

The neuropsychiatric symptoms of the various dementia syndromes are common and nearly universal. It is now evident that certain neuropsychiatric phenoptypes are linked with particular underlying pathophysiological processes. These symptoms, which may appear even before the cognitive and functional decline has become apparent, have significant consequences for both the patient and their caregiver. On an optimistic note, while therapeutic approaches to the cognitive and functional decline remain limited, the neuropsychiatric symptoms remain the most treatment responsive aspects of dementia.

REFERENCES

Aalten P, Verhey F, Boziki M et al. (2007) Neuropsychiatric syndromes in dementia; results from the Eurpoean Alzheimer disease consortium. *Dementia and Geriatric Cognitive Disorders* 24: 457–63.

Aalten P, Verhey FRJ, Boziki M et al. (2008) Consistency of neuropsychiatric syndromes across dementias: Results from the

European Alzheimer disease consortium. *Dementia and Geriatric Cognitive Disorders* **25**: 1–8.

Aarsland D, Ballard C, Larsen JP, McKeith I. (2001) A comparative study of psychiatric symptoms in dementia with Lewy bodies and Parkinson's disease with and without dementia. *International Journal of Geriatric Psychiatry* **16**: 528–36.

Alexopoulos GS, Abrams RC, Young RC, Shamoian CA. (1988) Cornell Scale for depression in dementia. *Biological Psychiatry* **23**: 271–84.

Archer N, Brown RG, Reeves SJ *et al.* (2007) Premorbid personality and behavioural and psychological symptoms in probable Alzheimer disease. *The American Journal of Geriatric Psychiatry* **15**: 202–13.

Banerjee S, Smith SC, Lamping DL *et al.* (2006) Quality of life in dementia: more than just cognition. An analysis of associations with quality of life in dementia. *Journal of Neurology, Neurosurgery and Psychiatry* **77**: 146–8.

Benoit M, Koulibaly PM, Migneco O *et al.* (2002) Brain perfusion in Alzheimer's disease with and without apathy: a SPECT study with statistical parametric mapping analysis. *Psychiatric Research: Neuroimaging* **114**: 103–11.

Bianchetti A, Benvenuti P, Ghisla KM *et al.* (1997) An Italian model of dementia Special Care Units: results of a preliminary study. *Alzheimer Disease and Associated Disorders* **11**: 53–6.

Breitner JCS, Wyse BW, Anthony JC *et al.* (1999) APOE epsilon-4 count predicts age when prevalence of Alzheimer's disease increases then declines: the Cache County Study. *Neurology* **53**: 321–31.

Burns A, Jacoby R, Levy R. (1990) Psychiatric phenomena in Alzheimer disease. Parts I–III. *British Journal of Psychiatry* **157**: 3–6.

Cohen-Mansfield J. (1986) Agitated behaviors in the elderly. II. Preliminary results in the cognitively deteriorated. *Journal of the American Geriatric Society* **34**: 722–7.

Copeland J, Kelleher M, Kellett J *et al.* (1976) The Geriatric Mental State Schedule: 1 Development and reliability. *Psychological Medicine* **6**: 439–49.

Cummings JL. (1997) The Neuropsychiatric Inventory: Assessing psychopathology in dementia patients. *Neurology* **48** (Suppl. 6): S10–16.

Cummings JL. (2000) Cognitive and behavioral heterogeneity in Alzheimer's disease: seeking the neurobiological basis. *Neurobiology of Aging* **21**: 845–61.

Dawson DV, Welsh-Bohmer KA, Siegler IC. (2000) Premorbid personality predicts level of rated personality change in patients with Alzheimer Disease. *Alzheimer Disease and Associated Disorders* **14**: 11–19.

Department of Health. (2009). Living well with Dementia: A National Dementia. Available from: www.dh.gov.uk/en/Publicationsandstatistics/Publications/PublicationsPolicyAndGuidance/DH_094058 [Accessed 31 July, 2009].

Finkel SI, Costa e Silva J, Cohen G *et al.* (1996) Behavioral and psychological signs and symptoms of dementia: a consensus statement on current knowledge and implications for research and treatment. *International Psychogeriatrics* **8** (Suppl. 3): 497–500.

Förstl H, Burns A, Luthert P *et al.* (1992) Clinical and neuropathological correlates of depression in Alzheimer's disease. *Psychological Medicine* **22**: 877–84.

Georges J, Jansen S, Jackson J *et al.* (2008) Alzheimer's disease in real life – the dementia carer's survey. *International Journal of Geriatric Psychiatry* **23**: 546–51.

Gonzalez-Salvador T, Lyketsos CG, Barker A *et al.* (2000) Quality of life in dementia patients in long-term care. *International Journal of Geriatric Psychiatry* **15**: 181–9.

Hwang TJ, Masterman DL, Ortiz F *et al.* (2004) Mild cognitive impairment is associated with characteristic neuropsychiatric symptoms. *Alzheimer's Disease and Associated Disorders* **18**: 17–21.

Jarvik L, Greenson H. (1987) Translation of "About a peculiar disease of the cerebral cortex", 1907 by A. Alzheimer. *Alzheimer Diseases and Associated Disorders* **1**: 7–8.

Jeste V, Finkel SI. (2000) Psychosis of Alzheimer's disease and related dementias: diagnostic criteria for a distinct syndrome. *American Journal of Geriatric Psychiatry* **8**: 29–34.

Jost BC, Grossberg GT. (1996) The evolution of the psychiatric symptoms in Alzheimer's disease: a natural history study. *Journal of the American Geriatric Society* **44**: 1078–81.

Landes AM, Sperry SD, Strauss ME, Geldmacher DS. (2001) Apathy in Alzheimer's disease. *Journal of the American Geriatrics Society* **49**: 1700–07.

Lee HB, Lyketsos CG. (2003) Depression in Alzheimer's disease: Heterogeneity and related issues. *Biological Psychiatry* **54**: 353–62.

Leroi I, Voulgari A, Breitner JCS, Lyketsos CG. (2003) The epidemiology of psychosis in dementia. *American Journal of Geriatric Psychiatry* **11**: 83–91.

Leroi I, Samus QM, Rosenblatt A *et al.* (2007) A comparison of small and large assisted living facilities for the diagnosis and care of dementia: the Maryland Assisted Living Study. *International Journal of Geriatric Psychiatry* **22**: 224–32.

Levy ML, Cummings JL, Fairbanks LA *et al.* (1996) Longitudinal assessment of symptoms of depression, agitation, and psychosis in 181 patients with Alzheimer's disease. *American Journal of Psychiatry* **153**: 1438–43.

Lyketsos CG, Lopez O, Jones B *et al.* (2002) Prevalence of neuropsychiatric symptoms in dementia and mild cognitive impairment: results from the cardiovascular health study. *Journal of the American Medical Association* **288**: 1475–83.

Lyketsos CG, Steinberg M, Tschanz JT *et al.* (2000) Mental and behavioural disturbances in dementia: Findings from the Cache County study on memory aging. *American Journal of Psychiatry* **157**: 708–14.

Lyketsos CG, Breitner J, Rabins PV. (2001) An evidence-based proposal for the classification of neuropsychiatric disturbances in Alzheimer's disease. *The International Journal of Geriatric Psychiatry* **15**: 1037–42.

McKhann GM, Albert MS, Grossman M *et al.* (2001) Clinical and pathological diagnosis of frontotemporal dementia: report of the Work Group on Frontotemporal dementia and Pick's Disease. *Archives of Neurology* **58**: 1803–9.

McShane R. (2000) What are the syndromes of behavioural and psychological symptoms of dementia. *International Psychogeriatrics* 12: 147–53.

Marin RS, Biedrzycki RC, Firinciogullari S. (1991) Reliability and validity of the Apathy Evaluation Scale. *Psychiatry Research* 38: 143–62.

Medeiros K, Robert P, Gauthier S *et al.* (2009) The NPI-C: A clinician-rated assessment of neuropsychiatric symptoms in dementia. *International Psychogeriatrics* 21 (Suppl. 2): S92–3.

Mega MS, Lee L, Dinov ID *et al.* (2000) Cerebral correlates of psychotic symptoms in Alzheimer's disease. *Journal of Neurology, Neurosurgery and Psychiatry* 69: 167–71.

Moran M, Walsh C, Lynch A *et al.* (2004) Syndromes of behavioural and psychological symptoms in mild Alzheimer's disease. *International Journal of Geriatric Psychiatry* 19: 359–64.

Murman DL, Chen Q, Powell MC *et al.* (2002) The incremental direct cost associated with behavioral symptoms in AD. *Neurology* 59: 1721–9.

Mychack P, Kramer JH, Boone KB, Miller BL. (2001) The influence of right frontotemporal dysfunction on social behavior in frontotemporal dementia. *Neurology* 56 (Suppl. 4): S11–15.

Olin JT, Schneider LS, Katz IR *et al.* (2002) Provisional diagnostic criteria for depression of Alzheimer disease. *Americal Journal of Geriatric Psychiatry* 10: 125–8.

Onyike CU, Sheppard JM, Tschanz JT *et al.* (2007) Epidemiology of apathy in older adults: The Cache County Study. *American Journal of Geriatric Psychiatry* 15: 365–75.

Perry EK, Marshall E, Kerwin J *et al.* (1990) Evidence of a monoaminergic-cholinergic imbalance related to visual hallucinations in Lewy body dementia. *Journal of Neurochemistry* 55: 1454–6.

Reisberg B, Borenstein J, Salob SP *et al.* (1987) Behavioral symptoms in Alzheimer's disease: phenomenology and treatment. *Journal of Clinical Psychiatry* 48 (Suppl): 9–15.

Robert PH, Berr C, Volteau M *et al.* (2008) Importance of lack of interest in patients with mild cognitive impairment. *American Journal of Geriatric Psychiatry* 16: 770–6.

Rosenblatt A, Samus QM, Steele CD *et al.* (2004) The Maryland Assisted living Study: Prevalence, Recognition and Treatment of Dementia and other Psychiatric Disorders in the Assisted Living Population of Central Maryland. *Journal of the American Geriatrics Society* 52: 1618–25.

Savva GM, Zaccai J, Matthews FE *et al.* (2009) Prevalence, correlates and course of behavioural and psychological symptoms of dementia in the population. *The British Journal of Psychiatry* 194: 212–19.

Senanarong V, Cummings JL, Fairbanks L *et al.* (2004) Agitation in Alzheimer's disease is a manifestation of frontal lobe dysfunction. *Dementia and Geriatric Cognitive Disorders* 17: 14–20.

Taragano FE, Allegri RF, Krupitzki H *et al.* (2009) Mild behavioral impairment and risk of dementia. *Journal of Clinical Psychiatry* 70: 584–92.

Tariot PN, Podgorski CA, Blazina L, Leibovici A. (1993) Mental disorders in the nursing home: Another perspective. *American Journal of Psychiatry* 150: 1063–9.

Tekin S, Mega MS, Masterman DM *et al.* (2001) Orbitofrontal and anterior cingulate cortex neurofibrillary tangle burden is associated with agitation in Alzheimer disease. *Annals of Neurology* 49: 355–61.

Tiraboschi P, Hansen LA, Alford M *et al.* (2000) Cholinergic dysfunction in diseases with Lewy bodies. *Neurology* 54: 407–11.

Wilson RS, Barnes LL, Mendes de Leon CF *et al.* (2002) Depressive symptoms, cognitive decline, and risk of Alzheimer disease in older persons. *Neurology* 59: 364–70.

Zarow C, Lyness SA, Mortimer JA, Chui HC. (2003) Neuronal loss is greater in the locus coeruleus than nucleus basalis and substantia nigra in Alzheimer disease and Parkinson's disease. *Archives of Neurology* 60: 337–41.

Measurement of behaviour disturbance, non-cognitive symptoms and quality of life

AJIT SHAH AND IAN NNATU

9.1 BEHAVIOURAL AND PSYCHOLOGICAL SYMPTOMS OF DEMENTIA

9.1.2 Definition of behavioural and psychological symptoms of dementia

The behavioural and psychological symptoms of dementia (BPSD) have been defined as 'a heterogenous range of psychological reactions, psychiatric symptoms and behaviours occurring in people with dementia of any aetiology' (Finkel and Burns, 2000) and include: disorders of behaviour, mood, thought content and perception (Burns *et al.*, 1990a; Burns *et al.*, 1990b; Burns *et al.*, 1990c; Burns *et al.*, 1990d), and disorder of personality alteration (Shah *et al.*, 2005). The definition of any individual BPSD should be hierarchical and allow discrimination between the cognitive and BPSD domains, different BPSD domains, and individual symptoms within a given BPSD domain (Shah, 2000).

9.1.3 Disorders of behaviour

9.1.3.1 DEFINITION

A typical example of disturbed behaviour is aggression, but similar arguments can be rehearsed for other disorders of behaviour. Although varying definitions for aggression have been used (Shah, 1999a), a useful working definition is: 'Aggressive behaviour is an overt act, involving the delivery of noxious stimuli to (but not necessarily aimed) at another organism, object or self, which clearly is not accidental' (Patel and Hope, 1992a).

9.1.3.2 SAMPLES, SETTINGS, METHODS OF DATA COLLECTION AND MEASUREMENT INSTRUMENTS

Box 9.1 illustrates the samples studied and methods of data collection in several settings: community; outpatient clinics; residential and nursing homes; and, acute admission and continuing care geriatric and psychogeriatric wards (Shah, 1999a). Essential properties of instruments measuring BPSD are illustrated in **Box 9.2**. An important characteristic of some instruments measuring aggression is the spontaneous tendency for aggression to decline during a period of serial measurements as observed with the Staff Observation Aggression Scale (Palmstierna and Wistedt, 1987) on psychogeriatric wards (Nilsson *et al.*, 1988; Shah, 1999b).

9.1.3.3 COMMENT

Although many instruments measure aggression, not all the psychometric and other properties have been adequately evaluated. Individual instruments have been developed for use in specific settings, for specific diagnostic groups and by specific groups of raters, and their generalizability to other settings, diagnostic groups and categories of raters is unclear. For example, the RAGE scale, although developed for use by nursing staff to measure aggression in psychogeriatric in-patients with dementia (Patel and Hope, 1992b), has been used in nursing homes for all diagnostic groups (Shah *et al.*, 1997).

9.1.4 Disorders of personality alteration

9.1.4.1 DEFINITION

Personality changes in dementia include emergence of new features (Petry *et al.*, 1988; Dian *et al.*, 1990; Siegler *et al.*,

Box 9.1 Aggression: samples studied and methods of data collection

Samples:

Undifferentiated dementia	Haider and Shah, 2004; Shah *et al.*, 2004; Shah *et al.*, 2005; Onishi *et al.*, 2006; Hinton *et al.*, 2008; Koopmans *et al.*, 2009
Alzheimer's disease	Reisberg *et al.*, 1987; Burns *et al.*, 1990a; Burns *et al.*, 1990e; Burns *et al.*, 1990f; Devanand *et al.*, 1992a; Lyketsos *et al.*, 2001; Shah *et al.*, 2005; Suh and Kim, 2004; Senanarong *et al.*, 2005
Vascular dementia	Sultzer *et al.*, 1993; Shah *et al.*, 2005; Pinto and Seethalakshmi, 2006
Huntington's disease	Burns *et al.*, 1990f

Methods of data collection:

Case-notes	Reisberg *et al.*, 1987; Haider and Shah, 2004
Semi-structured telephone interview	Devanand *et al.*, 1992a
Postal questionnaire directed at staff	Lukovits and McDaniel, 1992
Postal questionnaire directed at informal carers	Lukovits and McDaniel, 1992
Staff completed incident forms	Shah, 1995
Informal staff reports	Hallberg *et al.*, 1993
Staff completed specially designed forms	Winger *et al.*, 1987
Staff completed formal rating scales	Koopmans *et al.*, 2009
Informal carers completed formal rating scales	Ryden, 1988
Informal carers completed informal forms	Onishi *et al.*, 2006
Semi-structured interviews	Devanand *et al.*, 1992b; Shah *et al.*, 2004; Suh and Kim, 2004; Senanarong *et al.*, 2005; Shah *et al.*, 2005; Pinto and Seethalakshmi, 2006; Hinton *et al.*, 2008
Direct observations	Hallberg *et al.*, 1993
Voice recordings	Hallberg *et al.*, 1990
Mechanical body movements	Rindlisbacher and Hopkins, 1992

Box 9.2 Psychometric and other properties of instruments measuring BPSD in dementia (data from Zaudig, 1996)

- Patient characteristics
- User characteristics
- Type of instruments
- Setting for administration
- Data source
- Output of the instrument
- Psychometric properties
  - Reliability
  - Test–retest
  - Inter-rater
  - Internal consistency
  - Validity
  - Face
  - Content
  - Concurrent
  - Construct
  - Predictive
  - Incremental
  - Sensitivity to change
  - Spontaneous tendency to decline over serial measurements
- Time frame for symptoms
- Training needs
- Methods of administration
- Qualification of users
- Acceptability to rates
- Costs

1991; Chatterjee *et al.*, 1992; Lautenschlager and Förstl, 2007) or exaggeration of existing features (Lautenschlager and Förstl, 2007).

9.1.4.2   SAMPLES, SETTINGS AND METHODS OF DATA COLLECTION

Box 9.3 illustrates the methods of data collection, samples and the settings in which personality alterations have been examined. Studies have included a comparison group of normal aged individuals (Rubins *et al.*, 1987a; Rubins *et al.*, 1987b; Petry *et al.*, 1988; Cummings *et al.*, 1990; Dian *et al.*, 1990; Jacoub and Jorm, 1996; Rankin *et al.*, 2005; Talassi *et al.*, 2007), vascular dementia (Sultzer *et al.*, 1993) and frontotemporal dementia (FTD) (Miller *et al.*, 1997; Rankin *et al.*, 2005), and compared Alzheimer's disease (AD) with norms for inpatients (Meins and Dammast, 2000). Comparison with pre-morbid personality and normal aged individuals allows identification of personality changes (Siegler *et al.*, 1991; Chatterjee *et al.*, 1992) and exclusion of personality changes as an artefact of ageing, respectively (Rubins *et al.*, 1987a; Rubins *et al.*, 1987b; Petry *et al.*, 1988; Cummings *et al.*, 1990; Dian *et al.*, 1990; Rankin *et al.*, 2005; Talassi *et al.*, 2007). Difficulties in measuring the type, nature

Box 9.3 Samples, settings and methods of data collection for personality alteration

Samples:

Undifferentiated dementias	Siegler *et al.*, 1991; Balsis *et al.*, 2005
Vascular dementia	Dian *et al.*, 1990; Sultzer *et al.*, 1993; O'Connor, 2000
Alzheimer's disease	Rubins *et al.*, 1987a; Rubins *et al.*, 1987b; Petry *et al.*, 1988; Petry *et al.*, 1989; Bozzola *et al.*, 1992; Chatterjee *et al.*, 1992; Sultzer *et al.*, 1993; Jacoub and Jorm, 1996; Meins and Dammast, 2000; Rankin *et al.*, 2005; Talassi *et al.*, 2007
Frontotemporal dementia	Miller *et al.*, 1997; Rankin *et al.*, 2005; Mendez *et al.*, 2006
Huntington's disease	Kirkwood *et al.*, 2002

Settings:

Community sample	Nilsson, 1983; Jacoub *et al.*, 1994; O'Connor, 2000
Dementia centre	Miller *et al.*, 1997
Memory clinic sample	Meins and Dammast, 2000
Mixed group of psycho-geriatric inpatients	Pearson, 1990; Pearson, 1992

Methods of data collection:

Specially designed personality questionnaires administered to relatives	Petry *et al.*, 1988, Chatterjee *et al.*, 1992; Petry *et al.*, 1989; Dian *et al.*, 1990; Siegler *et al.*, 1991; Bozzola *et al.*, 1992; Jacoub *et al.*, 1994; Jacoub and Jorm, 1996; Balsis *et al.*, 2005; Rankin *et al.*, 2005; Talassi *et al.*, 2007
As above and an open interview	Rubins *et al.*, 1987a, Rubins *et al.*, 1987b
Specially designed personality questionnaire administered to patients	Nilsson, 1983; Pearson, 1990, Pearson, 1992; Rankin *et al.*, 2005

and severity of personality change include: reduced insight; judgement and memory may preclude use of self-reports (Petry *et al.*, 1988; Meins and Dammast, 2000; Rankin *et al.*, 2005) and this may be particularly important in FTD (Rankin

et al., 2005); and account from relatives may be biased by their emotional feelings (Dian *et al.*, 1990; Jacoub *et al.*, 1994; Meins and Dammast, 2000) and personality (Meins, 2000).

9.1.4.3   MEASUREMENT INSTRUMENTS

The items irritability and disinhibition on the Neuropsychiatric Inventory (NPI) (Cummings *et al.*, 1994) coupled with case-note review examined socially disruptive and antisocial behaviour in AD and FTD (Miller *et al.*, 1997). The Brooks and McKinlay (1983) personality inventory, originally used in brain injury patients, has been administered to relatives of dementia sufferers (Petry *et al.*, 1988; Petry *et al.*, 1989; Cummings *et al.*, 1990; Talassi *et al.*, 2007). The 11 personality items on the Blessed Dementia Rating Scale (Blessed *et al.*, 1968) have been used alone (Bozzola *et al.*, 1992; Balsis *et al.*, 2005) and in combination with six open-ended questions (Rubins *et al.*, 1987a; Rubins *et al.*, 1987b). In psychiatric inpatients and day patients with organic disorders, impulsiveness correlated with extraversion but not psychoticism on the Eysenck Personality Inventory (EPI) (Pearson, 1990; Pearson, 1992). Subjects with mild–moderate dementia and neurotic disorders scored highly for neuroticism on the EPI in a community sample (Nilsson, 1983). The pre-morbid trait of neuroticism in AD was associated with 'troublesome behaviour' (Meins *et al.*, 1998).

9.1.4.4   CLINICAL FEATURES

Changes in personality features include: coarsening of affect, disinhibition, increase in passivity, apathy, sponteneity, irritability, belligerence, demanding attention, indifference, egocentricity, less conscientiousness, lower extraversion, higher neuroticism and higher openness (Seltzer and Sherwin, 1983; Ishii *et al.*, 1986; Petry *et al.*, 1988; Petry *et al.*, 1989; Cummings *et al.*, 1990; Siegler *et al.*, 1991; Bozzola *et al.*, 1992; Chatterjee *et al.*, 1992; Jacoub and Jorm, 1996; Meins and Dammast, 2000). Patients with AD, compared to normal elderly, had greater changes on 12 personality traits of being more out of touch, less self-reliant, less mature, less enthusiastic, less stable, more unreasonable, more lifeless, more unhappy, less affectionate, less kind, more irritable and less generous after the onset of dementia (Petry *et al.*, 1988); similar results were observed in vascular dementia (Dian *et al.*, 1990). A significant shift from positive to negative characteristics was observed after the onset of AD in 12 of the 18 adjectives forming the Brooks and McKinlay Personality Inventory (Talassi *et al.*, 2007). Acquired extroversion has been reported to be associated with FTD (Mendez *et al.*, 2006). Forensic behaviours like indecent exposure and shoplifting were more common in FTD than AD (Miller *et al.*, 1997). At three-year follow up, four patterns of personality alteration in AD emerged: change at onset with little change as the disease progressed; ongoing change as the disease progressed; no change at all; and, regression of previously altered personality characteristics (Petry *et al.*, 1989). Personality changes can precede a clinical diagnosis of AD (Balsis *et al.*, 2005) and Huntington's disease (Kirkwood *et al.*, 2002).

9.1.4.5   COMMENT

The relationship between personality changes and BPSD may be part of the same phenomena, aetiologically linked or discrete entities. Several personality change features listed above overlap with features of frontal lobe dysfunction (Dian et al., 1990) and depression (Sultzer et al., 1993). Paucity of data on psychometric and other properties of instruments measuring personality suggests the need for rigorous evaluation of existing instruments (Strauss and Pasupathi, 1994) and development of new instruments measuring personality features that are sensitive from the pre-morbid to illness state and allow for personality change as an artefact of ageing (Strauss et al., 1997).

9.1.5   Disorders of mood

9.1.5.1   DEFINITION

Patients with depression may have cognitive deficits and it may precede the onset of dementia, either as an early presentation of incipient dementia or as a risk factor (Verhey and Visser, 2000). Also, depressive symptoms and illness in dementia require careful definition due to overlap with features of personality changes and cognitive impairment, especially frontal lobe dysfunction (Weiner et al., 1997).

9.1.5.2   SAMPLES, SETTINGS AND METHODS OF DATA COLLECTION

Box 9.4 illustrates the diagnostic categories, settings and methods of data collection. Despite an absence of 'gold standard' diagnosis of depression in dementia (Verhey and Visser, 2000), instruments have been validated against definitions of depression according to DSM-III (Reifler et al., 1986; Cummings et al., 1987; MacKenzie et al., 1989), DSM-IIIR (Burns et al., 1990d; Skoog, 1993; Weiner et al., 1997), DSM-IV (Brodaty and Luscombe, 1996), Research Diagnostic Criteria (Alexopoulos et al., 1988) and ICD-10 (Burns et al., 1990b).

9.1.5.3   MEASUREMENT INSTRUMENTS

Box 9.4 illustrates the self-rated and interviewer-rated scales, but data on psychometric and other properties for most of these instruments are limited. They are generally less accurate as cognitive impairment increases and insight decreases (Ott and Fogel, 1992) because good attention, concentration, memory and judgement are required for their completion (Burke et al., 1989) and the discrepancy between depression reported by patients and carers increases in this context (Ott and Fogel, 1992). Thus, instruments using collateral sources of information (e.g. relatives or nurses) in addition to clinical examination have been developed: Depressive Signs Scale (Katona and Aldridge, 1985); the Cornell Scale (Alexopoulos et al., 1988); and the Depression in Dementia Mood Scale (Sunderland et al., 1988). The Cornell Scale has been most widely used (Shah et al., 2004; Shah et al., 2005; Aalten et al., 2006; Debruyne et al., 2009).

Box 9.4 Sample, settings and methods of data collection for disorders of mood

Sample:

Undifferentiated dementia	Skoog, 1993; Shah et al., 2004; Aalten et al., 2006
Vascular dementia	Cummings et al., 1987; Brodaty and Luscombe, 1996; Shah et al., 2005
Alzheimer's disease	Burns et al., 1990b; Lyketsos et al., 2001; Tran et al., 2003; Shah et al., 2005; Lam et al., 2006; Debruyne et al., 2009

Settings:

Community	Skoog, 1993; Lyketsos et al., 2001; Shah et al., 2004; Aalten et al., 2006; Shah et al., 2005
Outpatient clinic	Cummings et al., 1987; Brodaty and Luscombe, 1996
Nursing homes	Brodaty et al., 2001
Mixed settings	Alexopoulos et al., 1988; Burns et al., 1990b
Acute and continuing care psychogeriatric wards	Akoo and Shah, 1998; Ellanchenny and Shah, 2001

Methods of data collection:

Self-rating scales	Ott and Fogel, 1992; Tran et al., 2003; Debruyne et al., 2009
Interviewer-rated scales directed at patients	Cummings et al., 1987; Ott and Fogel, 1992; Brodaty and Luscombe, 1996
Interviewer-rated scales directed at carers	Brodaty and Luscombe, 1996; Shah et al., 2004; Shah et al., 2005; Aalten et al., 2006; Lam et al., 2006; Debruyne et al., 2009
Combination of interviewer and observer rating	Sunderland et al., 1988; Ott and Fogel, 1992
Combination of interview and collateral sources	Katona and Aldridge, 1985; Alexopoulos et al., 1988
Pure observer scales	Shah and Gray, 1997; Akoo and Shah, 1998; Ellanchenny and Shah, 2001

9.1.5.4   COMMENT

The prevalence of depressive symptoms and illness in AD was 0–87 per cent (median 41 per cent) and 0–86 per cent (median 19 per cent), respectively (Wragg and Jeste, 1989; Verhey and Visser, 2000). This variability may be due to: depression measuring instruments may be insensitive in severe dementia or those with severe dementia may not be able to experience complex emotions like depression (Burns *et al.*, 1990b); and depression in dementia may lack classical features of depression (Verhey and Visser, 2000), especially severe dementia (Burns *et al.*, 1990b).

9.1.6   Disorders of thought content and perception

9.1.6.1   DEFINITION AND CLASSIFICATION

The definitions of hallucinations and delusions in dementia are the same as for other psychiatric disorders (Cummings *et al.*, 1987). Presence for at least 7 days is an added requirement to exclude delirium. Auditory (Cummings *et al.*, 1987; Burns *et al.*, 1990d), visual (Cummings *et al.*, 1987; Reisberg *et al.*, 1987; Burns *et al.*, 1990d) and olfactory (Rubins and Kinscherf, 1989) hallucinations have been studied. Delusions were divided into four groups: simple persecutory; complex persecutory; grandiose; and those associated with specific neurological deficits (Cummings, 1985). Another classification for delusions was: delusions of theft, delusions of suspicion and systematized delusions (Burns *et al.*, 1990c). There are four types of misidentifications: people in the house; misidentification of mirror image; misidentification of television; and misidentification of people (Burns *et al.*, 1990d).

9.1.6.2   SAMPLES, SETTINGS, METHODS OF DATA COLLECTION AND MEASUREMENT INSTRUMENTS

Box 9.5 illustrates the samples, settings, methods of data collection and instruments used to measure psychotic symptoms. Several semi-structured interviews and specially designed forms measure psychotic symptoms along with several other BPSD, thus producing diluted data on pure psychotic features (Ballard *et al.*, 1995).

9.1.6.3   COMMENT

The prevalence of delusions (Cummings *et al.*, 1987; Reisberg *et al.*, 1987; Burns *et al.*, 1990c), hallucinations (Burns *et al.*, 1990d; Ballard *et al.*, 1995) in AD and vascular dementia range from 20 to 50, 17 to 36; 11 to 34 per cent, respectively. The boundaries between hallucinations, delusions and misidentification syndromes are often blurred (Whitehouse *et al.*, 1996) and delusions are difficult to differentiate from confabulations (Cummings *et al.*, 1987). The definitions and descriptions of the psychopathology require refinement and clarity (Trabucchi and Bianchetti, 1996). A systematized check list of 17 categories of psychotic symptoms is the only pure instrument designed to measure psychotic features, but it is poorly evaluated (Ballard *et al.*, 1995). Psychometric and other properties of instruments measuring psychotic symptoms have been poorly studied and require rigorous evaluation. Clinicians will generally only treat psychotic symptoms in dementia if the patient is distressed or if there is risk of harm to others or self, but none of the extant instruments measure these facets and such instruments require development.

9.1.7   A way forward

Research should be directed at comparing different instruments measuring the same BPSD domain with each other, generating data on all of their properties, refining these instruments to improve their properties, adapting them for use in different settings, different dementia diagnostics groups, different severities of cognitive impairment and by different types of raters to enable data collection in a comparable common currency, and developing guidelines and protocols for their use in research and clinical practice (Shah and Allen, 1999). This, in turn, would facilitate examination of the interrelationship between individual BPSD symptoms within and across different BPSD domains. This is beginning to happen with univariate analysis (Brodaty *et al.*, 2001), latent class analysis (Lyketsos *et al.*, 2001; Lam *et al.*, 2006) and factor analysis (Hope *et al.*, 1997; Dechamps *et al.*, 2008; Youn *et al.*, 2008; Savva *et al.*, 2009). Ultimately, such analysis will allow identification of the nosological validity of the empirically derived five BPSD domains by establishing symptom and syndromal clusters (Lyketsos *et al.*, 2001; Lam *et al.*, 2006) and, in turn, facilitate a greater understanding of the demographic, clinical, genetic, biochemical, neuro-physiological and neuroanatomical correlates of BPSD, and their longitudinal course and prognosis.

9.2   QUALITY OF LIFE

9.2.1   Definition of quality of life

There is no universally accepted definition of quality of life (QoL). Quality of life has been defined in several different ways and often it is not defined (Lawton, 1997). Perhaps the most comprehensive definition of QoL to date is that from the World Health Organization (WHO) which defined QoL as: 'individuals perception of their position in life in the context of the culture and value system in which they live, and in relation to their goals, expectations, standards and concerns' (WHOQoL, 1995).

Despite the lack of a universally accepted definition of QoL, it has been widely agreed that QoL is a multi-dimensional construct that includes the subjective experience of the patient in addition to objective criteria (Lawton, 1994; Ettema *et al.*, 2005). Lawton (1991) described QoL as a multi-dimensional construct that should include objective (observable) indices of well-being judged against socionormative criteria, in addition to the individual's own subjective perception of his or her own position in life. In recent years a much narrower concept health-related quality of life (HRQoL) has emerged. Health-related QoL has been defined

---

Box 9.5 Samples, settings, methods of data collection and instruments used to measure psychotic symptoms

Sample:

All nursing home residents	Brodaty *et al.*, 2001
Undifferentiated dementia	Haider and Shah, 2004; Shah *et al.*, 2004; De Vugt *et al.*, 2005; Aalten *et al.*, 2006; Onishi *et al.*, 2006; Dechamps *et al.*, 2008; Hinton *et al.*, 2008; Koopmans *et al.*, 2009
Vascular dementia	Cummings *et al.*, 1987; Shah *et al.*, 2005; Hsieh *et al.*, 2009
Lewy body dementia	Ballard *et al.*, 1995
Alzheimer's disease	Cummings *et al.*,1987; Burns *et al.*, 1990c; Burns *et al.*, 1990d; Lyketsos *et al.*, 2001; Tran *et al.*, 2003; Suh and Kim, 2004; Shah *et al.*, 2005; Lam *et al.*, 2006; Pinto and Seethalaksmi, 2006; Hancock and Lavner, 2008; Hsieh *et al.*, 2009
Huntington's disease	Dewhurst *et al.*, 1969
Frontotemporal dementia	Hancock and Lavner, 2008

Setting:

Community	Skoog, 1993; Lyketsos *et al.*, 2001; de Vugt *et al.*, 2005; Aalten *et al.*, 2006; Hinton *et al.*, 2008
Memory clinic	Ballard *et al.*, 1995; Tran *et al.*, 2003; Hancock and Lavner, 2008
Outpatient clinic	Cummings *et al.*,1987; Reisberg *et al.*, 1987; Lam *et al.*, 2006
Referrals to psychogeriatric service	Ballard *et al.*, 1995; Shah *et al.*, 2004; Shah *et al.*, 2005
Day hospital	Haider and Shah, 2004
Inpatients	Trabucchi and Bianchetti, 1996
Nursing homes	Brodaty *et al.*, 2001; Onishi *et al.*, 2006; Dechamps *et al.*, 2008; Hinton *et al.*, 2008; Koopmans *et al.*, 2009
Continuing care	Onishi *et al.*, 2006
Group homes	Onishi *et al.*, 2006
Mixed	Burns *et al.*, 1990c; Burns *et al.*, 1990d; Whitehouse *et al.*, 1996; Pinto and Seethalaksmi, 2006

Methods of data collection:

Patient interview	Cummings *et al.*, 1987; Skoog, 1993
Interview with caregiver	Shah *et al.*, 2004; Suh and Kim, 2004; Shah *et al.*, 2005; Aalten *et al.*, 2006; Lam *et al.*, 2006; Pinto and Seethalaksmi, 2006; Dechamps *et al.*, 2008; Hinton *et al.*, 2008; Koopmans *et al.*, 2009
Formal scales completed by caregivers	Tran *et al.*, 2003; Hancock and Lavner, 2008
Unvalidated scales completed by caregivers	Onishi *et al.*, 2006
Case-notes	Cummings *et al.*, 1987; Reisberg *et al.*, 1987; Haider and Shah, 2004

Instruments:

[a]BEHAVE-AD	Reisberg *et al.*, 1987
[a]MOUSEPAD	Allen *et al.*, 1996
Neuropsychiatric Inventory	Cummings *et al.*, 1994
Burns symptom checklist	Ballard *et al.*, 1995

[a]BEHAVE-AD, Behavioural Pathology in Alzheimer's Disease Rating Scale; MOUSEPAD, Manchester and Oxford Universities Scale for Psychopathological Assessment of Dementia.

---

as 'the individual's subjective perception of the impact of a health condition on life' (Banerjee *et al.*, 2002; Smith *et al.*, 2005).

9.2.2   Measurement of quality of life

The measurement of QoL in dementia poses unique challenges. Impairments in memory, language and judgement can interfere with the self-evaluation of dementia, particularly in the later, more advanced, stages of the disease. The lack of a universally accepted definition of QoL or a 'gold standard' measure of QoL raises important questions about the validity of available measures (Shah *et al.*, 2005). Concerns such as these have led to questions about whether instruments to measure QoL in dementia should be by self-rating, proxy rating or a combination of both (Banerjee *et al.*, 2002; Smith *et al.*, 2005). Proxy measures by informal or professional

---

Box 9.6 Quality of Life Scales in dementia (data from Black and Rabins, 2005)

Scale	Severity	Respondent
Alzheimer's disease-related quality of life (ADQRL) (Rabins *et al.*, 1999)	Mild to severe	Caregivers
Bath Assessment of Subjective Quality of Life (BASQID) (Trigg *et al.*, 2007)	Mild to moderate	Patients
Cornell-Brown Scale for Quality of Life in dementia (Ready *et al.*, 2002)	Mild to moderate	Clinician with carer and patient input
Cognitively Impaired Life Quality Scale (CILQ) (DeLetter *et al.*, 1995)	Severe	Nursing caregivers
Dementia care mapping (DCM) (Kitwood and Bredin, 1994)	Moderate to severe	Trained rater
Dementia quality of life instrument (DqoL) (Brod *et al.*, 1999)	Mild to moderate	Patients
DEMQOL (Smith *et al.*, 2007)	Mild to moderate	Proxy and patient
Pleasant Events Schedule-AD (PES-AD) (Logsdon and Teri, 1997)	Mild	Proxy and patient
Progressive Deterioration Scale (PDS) (De Jong *et al.*, 1989)	Mild to Severe	Proxy
Psychological Well-Being in Cognitively Impaired Persons (PWB-CIP) (Burgener and Twigg, 2002)	Severe	Proxy
Quality of life Assessment Schedule (QoLAS) (Selai *et al.*, 2001)	Mild to moderate	Patient and proxy
Quality of Life in Late Stage Dementia (QUALID) (Weiner *et al.*, 2007)	Severe	Proxy
Qualidem (Ettema *et al.*, 2007)	Mild to moderate	Professional care giver

carers may be necessary in severe dementia when patients have poor comprehension and communication skills (Smith *et al.*, 2005).

Generic and dementia-specific instruments are currently used to measure QoL in dementia. Generic measures allow for comparisons with other diseases, but some researchers have argued in favour of dementia-specific measures of QoL because the symptoms of dementia are very different to those of other disorders (Rabins and Kasper, 1997; Selai *et al.*, 2001).

9.2.3 Measurement instruments

Existing instruments for measuring QoL in dementia are illustrated in **Box 9.6**.

9.2.4 Comment

The measurement of QoL in dementia poses unique challenges. Impaired judgement, reduced insight, cognitive impairment, personality changes, affective and psychotic symptoms, physical morbidity and temporary fluctuations make the subjective assessment of QoL difficult. However, the measurement of QoL is beneficial in the screening and monitoring of psychosocial problems in individual patients, population surveys of perceived health problems, clinical audit, measuring outcome in health service and evaluation research, clinical trials and in cost utility analysis. Existing measures of QoL cannot yet be considered satisfactory in the absence of an agreed definition of QoL, operational criteria and a gold standard, lack of satisfactory data on psychometric and other properties and absence of normative data on the subjective perception of QoL. Future research efforts should focus on developing instruments that have robust psychometric data that are valid, reliable and sensitive to change.

REFERENCES

Aalten P, van Valen E, de Vugt ME *et al.* (2006) Awareness of behavioural problems in dementia patients: a prospective study. *International Psychogeriatrics* 18: 3–18.

Akoo S, Shah AK. (1998) Screening for depression by the nursing staff in an acute psychogeriatric unit. *Australasian Journal on Ageing* 17: 81–4.

Alexopoulos GS, Abrams RC, Young RC, Shamoian CA. (1988) Cornell Scale for depression in dementia. *Biological Psychiatry* 23: 271–84.

Allen NH, Gordon S, Hope T, Burns A. (1996) Manchester and Oxford Universities Scale for the Psychopathological Assessment of Dementia (MOUSEPAD). *British Journal of Psychiatry* 169: 293–307.

Ballard CG, Saad K, Patel A *et al.* (1995) The prevalence and phenomenology of psychotic symptoms in dementia sufferers. *International Journal of Geriatric Psychiatry* 10: 477–85.

Balsis S, Carpenter BD, Storandt M. (2005) Personality changes precedes clinical diagnosis of dementia of Alzheimer's type. *Journal of Gerontology Series B: Psychological Sciences and Social Sciences* 60: P98–101.

Banerjee S, Smith S, Murray J *et al.* (2002) DEMQOL: a new measure of health related quality of life in dementia. *Neurobiology of Ageing* 23 (Suppl. 1): S154.

Black BS, Rabins PV. (2005) Quality of life in dementia: conceptual and practical issues. In: O'Brien J, Ames D, Burns A (eds). *Dementia*. London: Hodder Arnold, 215–20.

Blessed G, Tomlinson BE, Roth M. (1968) The association between quantitative measures of dementia and of senile change in grey matter of elderly subjects. *British Journal of Psychiatry* 114: 797–811.

Bozzola FG, Gorelick PB, Freels S. (1992) Personality changes in Alzheimer's disease. *Archives of Neurology* 49: 297–300.

Brod M, Stewart AL, Sands L, Walton P. (1999) Conceptualization and measurement of quality of life in dementia: The dementia Quality of Life Instrument (DQoL). *The Gerontologist* 39: 25–35.

Brodaty H, Luscombe G. (1996) Studies on affective symptoms and disorders: depression in persons with dementia. *International Psychogeriatrics* **8**: 609–22.

Brodaty H, Draper B, Saab D *et al.* (2001) Psychosis and behaviour disturbance in Sydney nursing home residents: prevalence and predictors. *International Journal of Geriatric Psychiatry* **16**: 504–12.

Brooks DN, McKinlay W. (1983) Personality and behavioural change after severe blunt head injury: a relative's view. *Journal of Neurology, Neurosurgery and Psychiatry* **46**: 336–44.

Burgener S, Twigg P. (2002) Relationships among caregiver factors and quality of life in care recipients with irreversible dementia. *Alzheimer Disease and Associated Disorders* **16**: 88–102.

Burke WJ, Houston MJ, Boust SJ, Roccaforte WH. (1989) Use of Geriatric Depression Scale in dementia of Alzheimer's type. *Journal of the American Geriatric Society* **37**: 856–60.

Burns A, Jacoby R, Levy R. (1990a) Psychiatric phenomena in Alzheimer's disease IV: disorders of behaviour. *British Journal of Psychiatry* **157**: 86–94.

Burns A, Jacoby R, Levy R. (1990b) Psychiatric phenomena in Alzheimer's disease. III disorders of mood. *British Journal of Psychiatry* **157**: 81–86.

Burns A, Jacoby R, Levy R. (1990c) Psychiatric phenomena in Alzheimer's disease I: disorders of thought content. *British Journal of Psychiatry.* **157**: 72–76.

Burns A, Jacoby R, Levy R. (1990d) Psychiatric phenomena in Alzheimer's disease II: disorders of perception. *British Journal of Psychiatry.* **157**: 76–81.

Burns A, Jacoby R, Levy R. (1990e) Behavioural abnormalities and psychiatric symptoms in Alzheimer's disease: preliminary findings. *International Psychogeriatrics* **2**: 25–36.

Burns A, Folstein S, Brandt J, Folstein M. (1990f) Clinical assessment of irritability, aggression and apathy in Huntington and Alzheimer's disease. *Journal of Nervous and Mental Disease* **178**: 20–26.

Chatterjee A, Strauss ME, Smyth KA, Whitehouse PJ. (1992) Personality change in Alzheimer's disease. *Archives of Neurology* **49**: 486–91.

Cummings JL. (1985) Organic delusions: phenomenology, anatomical correlations and review. *British Journal of Psychiatry* **146**: 184–97.

Cummings JL, Miller B, Hill MA, Neshkes R. (1987) Neuropsychiatric aspects of multiinfarct dementia and dementia of Alzheimer's type. *Archives of Neurology* **44**: 389–93.

Cummings JL, Petry S, Dian L *et al.* (1990) Organic personality disorder in dementia syndromes: an inventory approach. *Journal of Neuropsychiatry* **2**: 261–7.

Cummings JL, Mega M, Gray K *et al.* (1994) The neuropsychiatric inventory: comprehensive assessment of psychopathology in dementia. *Neurology* **44**: 2308–14.

Debruyne H, Van Buggenhout M, Le Bastard N *et al.* (2009) Is the geriatric depression scale a reliable screening tool for depressive illness in elderly patients with cognitive impairment. *International Journal of Geriatric Psychiatry* **24**: 556–62.

Dechamps A, Jutand MA, Onifade C *et al.* (2008) Co-occurrence of neuropsychiatric syndromes in demented and psychotic institutionalised elderly. *International Journal of Geriatric Psychiatry* **23**: 1182–90.

De Jong R, Osterlund OW, Roy GW. (1989) Measurement of quality of life changes in patients with Alzheimer's disease. *Clinical Therapeutics* **11**: 545–54.

DeLetter MC, Tully CL, Wilson JF, Rich E. (1995) Nursing staff perceptions of quality of life of cognitively impaired elders: instrumental development. *Journal of Applied Gerontology* **14**: 426–43.

Devanand DP, Brockington CD, Moody BJ *et al.* (1992a) Behaviour syndromes in Alzheimer's disease. *International Psychogeriatrics* **4** (Suppl. 2): 161–84.

Devanand DP, Miller L, Richards M *et al.* (1992b) The Columbia University scale for psychopathology in Alzheimer's disease. *Archive of Neurology* **49**: 371–6.

De Vugt ME, Stevens F, Aalten P *et al.* (2005) A prospective study of the effects of behavioural symptoms on the institutionalisation of patients with dementia. *International Psychogeriatrics* **17**: 577–89.

Dewhurst K, Oliver J, Trick KL *et al.* (1969) Neuropsychiatric aspects of Huntington's disease. *Confinia Neurologica* **31**: 258–68.

Dian L, Cummings JL, Petry S, Hill MA. (1990) Personality alterations in multi-infarct dementia. *Psychosomatics* **31**: 415–19.

Ellanchenny N, Shah AK. (2001) Evaluation of three nurse-administered depression rating scales on acute and continuing care psychogeriatric wards. *International Journal of Methods in Psychiatric Research* **10**: 43–51.

Ettema TP, Droes R, de Lange J *et al.* (2005) The concept of quality of life in dementia in the different stages of the disease. *International Psychogeriatrics* **17**: 353–70.

Ettema TP, Droes R, de Lange J *et al.* (2007) QUALIDEM: development and evaluation of a dementia specific quality of life instrument – validation. *International Journal of Geriatric Psychiatry* **22**: 424–30.

Finkel SI, Burns A. (2000) Introduction to behavioural and psychological symptoms of dementia (BPSD). A clinical and research update. *International Psychogeriatrics* **12** (Suppl. 1): 9–12.

Haider I, Shah AK. (2004) A pilot study of behavioural and psychological signs and symptoms of dementia in patients of Indian sub-continent origin admitted to a dementia day hospital in the United Kingdom. *International Journal of Geriatric Psychiatry* **19**: 1195–204.

Hallberg IP, Norberg A, Ericckson A. (1990) Functional impairment and behaviour disturbances in vocally disruptive patients in psychogeriatric wards compared with controls. *International Journal of Geriatric Psychiatry* **5**: 53–61.

Hallberg IP, Edberg A, Normark A *et al.* (1993) Daytime vocal activity in institutionalised severely demented patients identified as vocally disruptive by nurses. *International Journal of Geriatric Psychiatry* **8**: 155–64.

Hancock P, Lavner AJ. (2008) Cambridge behavioural inventory for the diagnosis of dementia. *Progress in Neurology and Psychiatry* **12**: 23–5.

Hinton L, Tomaszewski Farias S, Wegelin J. (2008) Neuropsychiatric symptoms are associated with disability in cognitively impaired

Latino elderly with and without dementia: results from the Sacramento Area Latino study on aging. *International Journal of Geriatric Psychiatry* 23: 102–8.

Hope T, Keene J, Fairburn C *et al.* (1997) Behaviour changes in dementia. II: Are there behavioural syndromes? *International Journal of Geriatric Psychiatry* 12: 1074–8.

Hsieh CJ, Chang CC, Lin CC. (2009) Neuropsychiatric profiles of patients with Alzheimer's disease and vascular dementia in Taiwan. *International Journal of Geriatric Psychiatry* 24: 570–7.

Ishii N, Nishihara Y, Imamura T. (1986) Why do frontal lobe symptoms predominate in vascular dementia syndrome? *Neurology* 36: 340–5.

Jacoub P, Jorm A. (1996) Personality change in dementia of Alzheimer's type. *International Journal of Geriatric Psychiatry* 11: 201–7.

Jacoub P, Jorm A, Christensen H *et al.* (1994) Personality change in normal and cognitively impaired elderly: informant reports in a community sample. *International Journal of Geriatric Psychiatry* 9: 313–20.

Katona CLE, Aldridge CR. (1985) The dexamethazone test and depressive signs in dementia. *Journal of Affective Disorders* 8: 83–9.

Kitwood T, Bredin K. (1994) *Evaluating dementia care: The DCM method*, 6th edn. Bradford: University of Bradford, Bradford Dementia Research Group.

Kirkwood SC, Siemers E, Viken R *et al.* (2002) Longitudinal personality changes among presymptomatic Huntington disease gene carriers. *Neuropsychiatry, Neuropsychology and Behavioural Neurology* 15: 192–7.

Koopmans RT, van der Molen M, Raats M, Ettema TP. (2009) Neuropsychiatric symptoms and quality of life in patients in the final phase of dementia. *International Journal of Geriatric Psychiatry* 24: 25–32.

Lam LCW, Leung T, Lui VWC *et al.* (2006) Association between cognitive function, behavioural syndromes and two-year clinical outcome in Chinese subjects with late-onset Alzheimer's disease. *International Psychogeriatrics* 18: 517–26.

Lautenschlager NT, Förstl H. (2007) Personality change in old age. *Current Opinions in Psychiatry* 20: 62–6.

Lawton MP. (1991) A multi-dimensional view of quality of life in frail elders. In: Birren JE (ed). *The concept and measurement of quality of life in the frail elderly.* San Diego, CA: Academic Press, 3–27.

Lawton MP. (1994) Quality of Life in Alzheimer's disease. *Alzheimer Disease and Associated Disorders* 5: 21–32.

Lawton MP. (1997) Assessing quality of life in Alzheimer disease research. *Alzheimer Disease and Associated Disorders* 11 (Suppl. 6): 91–9.

Logsdon RG, Teri L. (1997) The Pleasant Events Schedule – AD: Psychometric properties and relationship to depression and cognition in Alzheimer's disease patients. *The Gerontologist* 37: 40–45.

Lukovits TG, McDaniel KD. (1992) Behavioural disturbance in severe Alzheimer's disease: a comparison of family member and nursing staff reporting. *Journal of the American Geriatric Society* 40: 891–5.

Lyketsos CG, Sheppard JME, Steinberg M *et al.* (2001) Neuropsychiatric disturbance in Alzheimer's disease clusters into three groups: the Cache county study. *International Journal of Geriatric Psychiatry* 16: 1043–53.

MacKenzie TB, Robiner WN, Knopman DS. (1989) Differences between patient and family assessments of depression in Alzheimer's disease. *American Journal of Psychiatry* 146: 1174–8.

Meins W, Frey A, Thiesemann R. (1998) Premorbid personality traits in Alzheimer's disease: do they predispose to non-cognitive behavioural symptoms? *International Psychogeriatrics* 10: 369–78.

Meins W. (2000) Impact of personality on behavioural and psychological symptoms of dementia. *International Psychogeriatrics* 12 (Suppl. 1): 107–9.

Meins W, Dammast J. (2000) Do personality traits predict the occurrence of Alzheimer's disease. *International Journal of Geriatric Psychiatry* 15: 120–4.

Mendez MF, Chen AK, Shapira JS *et al.* (2006) Acquired extroversion associated with bitemporal variant of frontotemporal dementia. *Journal of Neuropsychiatry and Clinical Neurosciences* 18: 100–7.

Miller BL, Darby A, Benson DF *et al.* (1997) Aggressive socially disruptive and antisocial behaviour associated with fronto-temporal dementia. *British Journal of Psychiatry* 170: 150–5.

Nilsson LV. (1983) Personality changes in the aged. A transectional and longitudinal study with Eysenk personality inventory. *Acta Psychiatrica Scandinavica* 68: 202–11.

Nilsson K, Palmsteirna B, Wistedt B. (1988) Aggressive behaviour in hospitalised psychogeriatric patients. *Acta Psychiatrica Scandinavica* 78: 172–5.

O'Connor DW. (2000) Epidemiology of behavioural and psychological symptoms of dementia. *International Psychogeriatrics* 12 (Suppl. 1): 41–5.

Onishi J, Suzuki Y, Umegaki H *et al.* (2006) Behavioural, psychological and physical symptoms in group homes for older adults with dementia. *International Psychogeriatrics* 18: 75–86.

Ott BR, Fogel BS. (1992) Measurement of depression in dementia: self v clinician rating. *International Journal of Geriatric Psychiatry* 7: 899–904.

Palmsteirna B, Wistedt B. (1987) Staff observation aggression scale: presentation and evaluation. *Acta Psychiatrica Scandinavica* 76: 657–63.

Patel V, Hope RA. (1992a) A rating scale for aggressive behaviour in the elderly – the RAGE. *Psychological Medicine* 22: 211–21.

Patel V, Hope RA. (1992b) Aggressive behaviour in elderly psychiatric inpatients. *Acta Psychiatrica Scandinavica* 85: 131–5.

Pearson PR. (1990) Impulsiveness and spiral maze performance in elderly psychiatry patients. *The Personality and Individual Differences* 11: 1309–10.

Pearson PR. (1992) The relationship of impulsiveness to psychoticism and extraversion in elderly psychiatric patients. *Journal of Psychology* 126: 443–4.

Petry S, Cummings J, Hill M, Shapira J. (1988) Personality alterations in dementia of Alzheimer's type. *Archives of Neurology* 45: 1187–90.

Petry S, Cummings J, Hill M, Shapira J. (1989) Personality alterations in dementia of Alzheimer's type: a three-year follow-up study. *Journal of Geriatric Psychiatry and Neurology* **2**: 203–7.

Pinto C, Seethalakshmi R. (2006) Behavioural and psychological symptoms of dementia in an Indian population: comparison between Alzheimer's disease and vascular dementia. *International Psychogeriatrics* **18**: 87–94.

Rabins PV, Kasper JD. (1997) Measuring quality of life in dementia: conceptual and practical issues. *Alzheimer Disease and Related Disorders* **11** (Suppl. 6): 100–4.

Rabins PV, Kasper JD, Kleinman L *et al.* (1999) Concepts and methods in the development of the ADQRL: an instrument for assessing health related quality of life in persons with Alzheimer's disease. *Journal of Mental Health and Aging* **5**: 33–48.

Rankin KP, Baldwin E, Pace-Savitsky C *et al.* (2005) Self awareness and personality change in dementia. *Journal of Neurology, Neurosurgery and Psychiatry* **76**: 632–9.

Ready RE, Ott BR, Grace J, Fernandez I. (2002) The Cornell–Brown Scale for Quality of Life in Dementia. *Alzheimer's Disease and Associated Disorders* **16**: 109–15.

Reifler B, Larson E, Teri I, Poulsen L. (1986) Dementia of Alzheimer's type and depression. *Journal of the American Geriatric Society* **34**: 855–9.

Reisberg B, Borensteen J, Sabb S *et al.* (1987) Behavioural symptoms in Alzheimer's disease: phenomenology and treatment. *Journal of Clinical Psychiatry* **48** (Suppl.): 9–15.

Rindlisbacher P, Hopkins RW. (1992) An investigation of the sundowning syndrome. *International Journal of Geriatric Psychiatry* **7**: 15–23.

Rubins EH, Kinscherf DA. (1989) Psychopathology of very mild dementia of Alzheimer's type. *American Journal of Psychiatry* **146**: 1017–21.

Rubins EH, Morris JC, Storandt M, Berg L. (1987a) Behavioural change in patients with mild senile dementia of Alzheimer's type. *Psychiatric Research* **21**: 55–62.

Rubins EH, Morris JC, Berg L. (1987b) The regression of personality change in senile dementia of Alzheimer's type. *Journal of the American Geriatric Society* **35**: 721–5.

Ryden M. (1988) Aggressive behaviour in persons with dementia who live in the community. *Alzheimer's Disease and Associated Disorders* **2**: 342–55.

Savva GM, Zaccai J, Matthews FE *et al.* on Behalf of the Medical Research Council Cognitive Function and Ageing Study. (2009) Prevalence, correlates and course of behavioural and psychological symptoms of dementia in the population. *British Journal of Psychiatry* **194**: 212–19.

Selai CE, Trimble MR, Rossor MN, Harvey RJ. (2001) Assessing quality of life in dementia: Preliminary psychometric testing of the Quality of Life Assessment Schedule (QoLAS). *Neuropsychological Rehabilitation* **11**: 219–43.

Seltzer B, Sherwin I. (1983) A comparison of clinical features in early onset and late onset primary degenerative dementia. *Archives of Neurology* **40**: 143–6.

Senanarong V, Poungvarin N, Jamjumras P *et al.* (2005) Neuropsychiatric symptoms, functional impairment and executive ability in Thai patients with Alzheimer's Disease. *International Psychogeriatrics* **17**: 81–90.

Shah AK. (1995) Violence among psychogeriatric inpatients with dementia. *International Journal of Geriatric Psychiatry* **10**: 887–91.

Shah AK. (1999a) Aggressive behaviour in the elderly. *International Journal of Psychiatry in Clinical Practice* **3**: 85–103.

Shah AK. (1999b) Some methodological issues in using aggression rating scales in institutions. *International Psychogeriatrics* **4**: 439–44.

Shah AK. (2000) What are the necessary characteristics of a behavioural and psychological symptoms in dementia rating scale? *International Psychogeriatrics* **12** (Suppl. 1): 205–9.

Shah AK, Allen H. (1999) Is improvement possible in the measurement of behaviour disturbance in dementia? *International Journal of Geriatric Psychiatry* **14**: 512–19.

Shah AK, Gray T. (1997) Screening for depression on continuing care psychogeriatric wards. *International Journal of Geriatric Psychiatry* **12**: 125–7.

Shah AK, Chui E, Ames D. (1997) The relationship between two aggression scales in nursing homes. *International Journal of Geriatric Psychiatry* **12**: 628–31.

Shah AK, Suh GK, Ellanchenny N. (2004) A cross-national comparative study of behavioural and psychological symptoms of dementia between UK and Korea. *International Psychogeriatrics* **16**: 219–36.

Shah AK, Foli S, Nnatu I. (2005) Measurement of behavioural disturbance, non-cognitive symptoms and quality of life. In: O'Brien J, Ames D, Burns A (eds). *Dementia*. London: Hodder Arnold, 72–80.

Shah AK, Suh GK, Ellanchenny N. (2005) A comparative study of behavioural and psychological symptoms of dementia in patients with Alzheimer's disease and vascular dementia referred to psychogeriatric services in Korea and the UK. *International Psychogeriatrics* **17**: 207–19.

Siegler IC, Welsh KA, Fillenbaum GG *et al.* (1991) Ratings of personality change in patients being evaluated for memory disorders. *Alzheimers Disease and Associated Disorders* **5**: 240–50.

Skoog I. (1993) The prevalence of psychotic, depressive and anxiety syndromes in demented and non-demented 85-year olds. *International Journal of Geriatric Psychiatry* **8**: 247–53.

Smith S, Lamping D, Banerjee S *et al.* (2005) Measurement of health related quality of life for people with dementia: development of a new instrument (DEMQOL) and an evaluation of current methodology. *Health Technology Assessment* **9**: 1–93.

Smith SC, Lamping DL, Banerjee S *et al.* (2007) Development of a new measure of health related quality of life for older people with dementia: DEMQOL. *Psychological Medicine* **37**: 737–46.

Strauss ME, Pasupathi M. (1994) Primary caregivers descriptions of Alzheimer patients' personality traits: temporal stability and sensitivity to change. *Alzheimers Disease and Related Disorders* **8**: 166–76.

Strauss ME, Lee MM, Di Filippo JM. (1997) Premorbid personality and behavioural symptoms in Alzheimer's disease. Some cautions. *Archives of Neurology* **54**: 257–9.

Suh GK, Kim SK. (2004) Behavioural and psychological signs and symptoms of dementia (BPSD) in antipsychotic-naive Alzheimer's disease patients. *International Psychogeriatrics* **16**: 337–50.

Sultzer DL, Levin HS, Mahler ME *et al.* (1993) A comparison of psychiatric symptoms in vascular dementia and Alzheimer's disease. *American Journal of Psychiatry* **150**: 1806–12.

Sunderland T, Alterman IS, Yount D *et al.* (1988) A new scale for the assessment of depressed mood in dementia patients. *American Journal of Psychiatry* **145**: 955–9.

Talassi E, Cipriani G, Bianchetti A, Trabucchi M. (2007) Personality change in Alzhiemer's disease. *Ageing and Mental Health* **11**: 526–31.

Trabucchi M, Bianchetti A. (1996) Clinical perspectives: what should we be studying? Delusions. *International Psychogeriatrics* **8** (Suppl. 3): 383–5.

Tran M, Bedard M, Molloy W *et al.* (2003) Associations between psychotic symptoms and dependence in activities of daily living among older adults with Alzheimer's disease. *International Psychogeriatrics* **15**: 171–80.

Trigg T, Skevington SM, Jones RW. (2007) How can we best assess the quality of life of people with dementia? The Bath Assessment of Subjective Quality of Life in Dementia (BASQID). *Gerontologist* **47**: 789–97.

Verhey FRJ, Visser PJ. (2000) Phenomenology of depression in dementia. *International Psychogeriatrics* **12** (Suppl. 1): 129–34.

Weiner MF, Svetlik D, Risser RC. (1997) What depressive symptoms are reported in Alzheimer's patients. *International Journal of Geriatric Psychiatry* **12**: 648–52.

Weiner MF, Martin-Cook K, Svetlik DA *et al.* (2007) The Quality of Life in late stage dementia (QUALID) Scale. *Journal of the American Medical Directors Association* **1**: 114–16.

Whitehouse P, Patterson MB, Strauss ME *et al.* (1996) Hallucinations. *International Psychogeriatrics* **8** (Suppl. 30): 387–92.

WHOQOL Group. (1995) The World Health Organization Quality of Life Assessment Position Paper from the WHO. *Social Science and Medicine* **41**: 1403–9.

Winger J, Schirm V, Stewart D. (1987) Aggressive behaviour in long term care. *Journal of Psychosocial Nursing and Mental Health* **25**: 28–33.

Wragg RE, Jeste D. (1989) Overview of depression and psychosis in Alzheimer's disease. *American Journal of Psychiatry* **146**: 577–87.

Youn JC, Lee DY, Lee JH *et al.* (2008) Development of a Korean version of the behaviour rating scale for dementia (BRSD-K). *International Journal of Geriatric Psychiatry* **23**: 677–84.

Zaudig M. (1996) Assessing behavioural symptoms of Alzheimer's type: categorical and quantitative approaches. *International Psychogeriatrics* **8** (Suppl. 2): 183–200.

10

Cross-cultural issues in the assessment of cognitive impairment

AJIT SHAH AND JAMES LINDESAY

10.1 INTRODUCTION

Cross-cultural studies comparing two or more ethnic groups in a single country, and those comparing populations across two or more countries, will be discussed with particular reference to methodology, measurement instruments, aetiology and protective and risk factors.

10.2 INTERNATIONAL DEMOGRAPHIC CHANGES AND THEIR IMPLICATIONS

The size of the elderly population is increasing worldwide because of increased life expectancy and falling birth rates (Shah and MacKenzie, 2007). Ninety million people have been estimated to live outside their country of birth (Bohning and Oishi, 1995).

The prevalence of dementia doubles every 5.1 years after the age of 60 years (Hofman et al., 1991). Thus, with the increase in the elderly population, the absolute number of dementia cases will also increase worldwide. In 2005, 24.3 million people worldwide were estimated to have dementia and 4.6 million new cases are predicted every year (Ferri et al., 2005).

10.3 DIAGNOSTIC ISSUES

Cognitive tests standardized in one cultural group may not be appropriate for another because they are influenced by culture, education, language, literacy, numeracy, sensory impairment, unfamiliarity with test situations and anxiety (Chandra et al., 1994; Lindesay et al., 1997; Lindesay, 1998; Prince et al., 2003; Stewart et al., 2003; Prince et al., 2004; Crane et al., 2006; Inzelberg et al., 2007; Jacob et al., 2007; Kalaria et al., 2008).

Education can influence performance on cognitive tests like the Mini-Mental State Examination (MMSE) (Folstein et al., 1975). The Chinese MMSE has developed different cut-off scores predicting dementia for different educational levels of respondents with good specificity and sensitivity (Katzman et al., 1988; Zhang et al., 1990; Sahadevan et al., 2000); this has also been suggested for other cultural groups (Murden et al., 1991; Gurland et al., 1992). Illiterate subjects may be unable to complete tests requiring reading, writing and drawing (Katzman et al., 1988; Chandra et al., 1994; Rajkumar and Kumar, 1996), and illiteracy may also reduce access to information related to orientation in time and general knowledge (Lindesay, 1998). Innumerate subjects may be unable to perform tests involving calculations (Chandra et al., 1994; Livingston and Sembhi, 2003). A study of ethnic minority elders in Liverpool, UK, reported a higher prevalence of dementia in those unable to speak English (McCrakken et al., 1997); this may have been an artefact of their inability to speak English. Subjects with lower levels of education may have difficulties in understanding the nature of the test and may feel that the questions are irrelevant and of little practical value (Chandra et al., 1994; Bhatnagar and Frank, 1997).

Tests identifying the discrepancy between age and date of birth (Bhatnagar and Frank, 1997; McCrakken *et al.*, 1997) may disadvantage those born in remote villages with poor birth registration facilities, and those who have altered age and date of birth to facilitate migration and entry into institutions (Rait *et al.*, 1997). Culture-specific questions (e.g. about monarchy or politicians) also disadvantage ethnic minority elders (Bhatnagar and Frank, 1997; McCrakken *et al.*, 1997), although these can be modified (e.g. date of independence of the country of origin) (Chandra *et al.*, 1994; Rait *et al.*, 1997). Cultural concepts of orientation in time and place (Ganguli *et al.*, 1995; Lindesay *et al.*, 1997) and pre-ferential use of Western or traditional calendars (Kua, 1992; Lindesay *et al.*, 1997; Rait *et al.*, 1997) can also influence performance. Orientation items work well within the dominant culture but less well in some ethnic minority groups (Rait *et al.*, 1997; Livingston and Sembhi, 2003); this was the case among Singapore Chinese (Kua, 1992), but not in Liverpool Chinese (McCrakken *et al.*, 1997).

10.4   MEASUREMENT INSTRUMENTS

Ideally, instruments that allow the subject to perform at their best without the influence of the extraneous factors listed above should be used. Several instruments measuring cognitive impairment have been developed by adapting existing instruments (mostly those developed in English) by either using a Delphi panel of experts from the culture of interest or more widespread consultation within the culture of interest, translation and back-translation by separate groups of bilingual translators and iterative field pretesting to ensure content, semantic, technical, criterion and conceptual equivalence with the parent version of the instrument for each item (Chandra *et al.*, 1994; Shah *et al.*, 2005a). The aim is to produce a culture-fair, education-free and analogous instrument. This should be followed by pilot testing to determine the distribution of the scores and the ability to discriminate between dementias of different severity (Chandra *et al.*, 1994). Clear validation against a gold standard diagnosis of dementia is also required, together with determination of various psychometric properties (Livingston and Sembhi, 2003; Shah *et al.*, 2005a). Ideally, the psychometric profile of the newly developed instrument should be similar to or better than in the parent version.

The MMSE has been developed in several languages including Arabic (Inzelberg *et al.*, 2007), Chinese (Serby *et al.*, 1987; Katzman *et al.*, 1988; Salmon *et al.*, 1989; Yu *et al.*, 1989; Xu *et al.*, 2003), Korean (Park and Kwon, 1990; Park *et al.*, 1991), Finnish (Salmon *et al.*, 1989), Italian (Rocca *et al.*, 1990), Yoruba (Hendrie, 1992), Spanish (Escobar *et al.*, 1986; Anzola-Perez *et al.*, 1996), Thai (Phanthumchinda *et al.*, 1991), Hindi (Ganguli *et al.*, 1995; Rait *et al.*, 2000a), Punjabi (Rait *et al.*, 2000a), Urdu (Rait *et al.*, 2000a), Bengali (Kabir and Herlitz, 2000; Rait *et al.*, 2000a), Malyalum (Shaji *et al.*, 1996), Gujarati (Lindesay *et al.*, 1997; Rait *et al.*, 2000a) and Sinhalese (de Silva and Gunatilake, 2002). Comparisons between these different versions are problematic because not all have been developed using rigorous procedures and/or a satisfactory psychometric evaluation.

The abbreviated Mental Test Score (Quereshi and Hod-kinson, 1974) has been developed in several south Asian languages and for use among African Caribbeans in the UK (Rait *et al.*, 1997; Rait *et al.*, 2000a; Rait *et al.*, 2000b). A Korean version of the Alzheimer's Disease Assessment Scale (Rosen *et al.*, 1984) has been developed (Youn *et al.*, 2002). The MMSE, selected items of the Consortium to Establish a Registry for Dementia (CERAD) neuropsychological test battery (Morris *et al.*, 1989) and the Cambridge Cognitive Examination (CAMCOG) component of the Cambridge Examination for Mental Disorders in the Elderly (CAMDEX) interview schedule (Roth *et al.*, 1986) have all been evaluated in older African Caribbean people in the UK (Richards and Brayne, 1996; Richards *et al.*, 2000). In this population, normative data are available for the orientation items of the MMSE, selected items of the CERAD neuropsychological test battery and the clock-drawing test (Stewart *et al.*, 2001a). The ten-word learning test from the CERAD battery has been shown to be successful in establishing a diagnosis of dementia in study populations in India, China, Southeast Asia, Latin America and the Caribbean (Prince *et al.*, 2003). The Alzheimer's Disease Questionnaire (Breitner and Folstein, 1984), which gathers information on history of cognitive impairment among first-degree relatives, has been translated into Chinese and Spanish, and has been administered by bilingual workers (Silverman *et al.*, 1992). The Informant Questionnaire on Cognitive Decline in the Elderly (IQCODE) (Jorm *et al.*, 1991) has been developed for use in illiterate Chinese populations (Fuh *et al.*, 1995). A dementia screening instrument, the Community Screening Interview for Dementia (CSI-D), a cognitive test for subjects and an informant interview, has been developed for use among Cree Indians in Canada (Hendrie *et al.*, 1993; Hall *et al.*, 2000), English-speaking Canadians (Hendrie *et al.*, 1993; Hall *et al.*, 2000) and Yoruba Nigerians in Ibadan (Hendrie *et al.*, 1995a; Hall *et al.*, 2000), Jamaicans (Hall *et al.*, 2000), African Americans in Indianapolis (Hall *et al.*, 2000), Koreans (Liu *et al.*, 2005), and in study populations in India, China, Southeast Asia, Latin America and the Caribbean (Prince *et al.*, 2003), with good psychometric properties. The Chula Mental Test, developed for use in Thailand by selecting and adapting items from several existing screening tests, has been found to reduce the influence of literacy on scores (Jitapunkul *et al.*, 1996). A Spanish (for use among Mexican Americans) (Royall *et al.*, 2003) and Brazilian Portuguese version (Fuzikawa *et al.*, 2003; Fuzikawa *et al.*, 2007) of the clock-drawing test have been evaluated; both these versions were reported to be education-free. A clock-reading test, developed in Germany, has been reported to be reliable and sensitive in detecting Alzheimer's disease (AD) and Lewy body dementia (LBD) (Schmidtke and Olbrich, 2007). A cognitive assessment instrument, the Kimberley Cognitive Assessment Tool, has been developed for indigenous Australians and has good psychometric properties, including good sensitivity and specificity in detecting dementia (LoGuidice *et al.*, 2006).

A unique approach involving the use of three instruments, the Geriatric Mental State Examination (GMS) (Copeland *et al.*, 1976), the CIS-D and the ten-word list-learning task from the CERAD battery appropriately translated into native languages, and an algorithm derived from these instruments, have been shown to have high sensitivity and specificity in the diagnosis of dementia in culturally diverse populations from India, China, Southeast Asia, Africa, Latin America and the Caribbean (Prince et al., 2003; Prince et al., 2008).

10.5   THE DIFFERENTIAL PREVALENCE AND INCIDENCE OF DEMENTIA SUBTYPES

Published studies of the prevalence of dementia in UK ethnic minority groups do not report on the relative prevalence of individual subtypes of dementia (Bhatnagar and Frank, 1997; Lindesay et al., 1997; McCrakken et al., 1997; Livingston et al., 2001). Anecdotally, it is believed that vascular dementia (VaD) may be more common than AD among Indian subcontinent elders (Bhatnagar and Frank, 1997) and African Caribbeans (Richards et al., 2000; Livingston et al., 2001; Stewart et al., 2001a; Livingston and Sembhi, 2003). In the UK, some risk factors for VaD are more prevalent in these ethnic groups than in the indigenous population, such as diabetes in Asians (Mather and Keen, 1985; Samanta et al., 1987), and hypertension and cardiovascular disease in Asians and African Caribbeans (Balarajan, 1996; Ritch et al., 1996). Native Americans with AD in the United States are reported to have a higher prevalence of cardiovascular risk factors including diabetes, hypertension and heart disease than white Americans (Weiner et al., 2003).

The prevalence of dementia in ethnic minority groups in other countries is also variable. A study of Chinese residents in nursing homes in the United States reported a prevalence of 95 per cent for dementia with the ratio of VaD to AD estimated as 4.4 to 1 (Serby et al., 1987), but there was no indigenous comparison group. Studies in the US have reported a higher prevalence of dementia in African Americans (Still et al., 1990; Heyman et al., 1991; Perkins et al., 1997) and Hispanics (Perkins et al., 1997) than in white Americans, although this was not found in a study of severe dementia in African Americans (Schoenberg et al., 1985). African Americans and Latinos had significantly higher prevalence and incidence of dementia than non-Latino white Americans (Gurland et al., 1995; Gurland et al., 1999), but these ethnic differences disappeared after controlling for age and educational attainment. Also, there was no difference between the three groups for individual subtypes of dementia. Another study reported a higher prevalence of VaD coupled with higher prevalence of strokes and hypertension in African Americans (Heyman et al., 1991; Perkins et al., 1997).

In a US post-mortem study, AD and dementia due to Parkinson's disease were more common in white Americans, and alcohol-related dementia and VaD were more common in African Americans (de la Monte et al., 1989). Another US study, using an informant risk questionnaire (Alzheimer's Disease Risk Questionnaire) administered to non-demented elderly day care centre attenders, reported a significantly increased risk of dementia in first-degree relatives of Jews and Italians compared with Chinese and Puerto Ricans (Silverman et al., 1992). This raises the issue of discrepant environmental exposure, as the first two groups had migrated to the US significantly earlier.

In a Canadian study, the prevalence of all dementias and AD was 4.2 and 0.5 per cent, respectively, in Cree Indians, and 4.2 and 3.5 per cent, respectively, in English-speaking Canadians (Hall et al., 1993). An Israeli study of presenile AD, using hospital discharge diagnosis as a proxy for incidence rates, reported age- and sex-adjusted incidence rates to be higher in European and American Jews than those from Asia or Africa (Treves et al., 1986), raising the possibility of both environmental and genetic risk factors. Pollitt (1997), quoting Zann (1994), reported that the prevalence of dementia in Aborigines in Northern Queensland was 20 per cent, with alcohol-related dementia accounting for the majority of cases.

A recent review of developing countries reported that the age-adjusted prevalence of dementia in those aged 65 years and older was consistently low in India and sub-Saharan Africa, although it was high in some Asian and Latin American countries (Kalaria et al., 2008). Although the rates are variable, the overall theme was of low prevalence in Asian and African countries. Similar findings were observed in the 10/66 Dementia Research Group studies when the DSM-IV diagnosis was used, but the prevalence rates were more consistent across countries when the 10/66 dementia algorithm and diagnosis were used (Llibre Rodriguez et al., 2008). Almost universally, the prevalence of dementia increases with ageing, and generally it is more common in women. A meta-analysis of the world literature reported that the incidence of VaD and AD exponentially increases with age (Jorm and Jolley, 1998). Eastern countries had a lower incidence of AD, but there was no difference in the incidence of VaD between European and eastern countries (Jorm and Jolley, 1998). The prevalence of AD is generally lower in Japan and China (Hasegawa et al., 1986; Shibayama et al., 1986; Li et al., 1989; Li et al., 1991) and that of VaD generally higher (Hasegawa et al., 1986; Shibayama et al., 1986; Li et al., 1989), although the ratio of the prevalence of AD to VaD is increasing in these countries (Fujishima and Kiyohara, 2002; Li et al., 2007).

The variable prevalence rates for dementia and its subtypes across different ethnic groups in a single country and across different countries may be due to methodological issues including: the sensitivity of screening instruments and case-finding methods (Osuntokun et al., 1992; Hall et al., 1993; Prince et al., 2003); diagnostic criteria (Osuntokun et al., 1992; Hall et al., 1993; Llibre Rodriguez et al., 2008); sampling frames and procedures (Osuntokun et al., 1992); screening personnel (Hall et al., 1993) and inter-rater reliability (Osuntokun et al., 1992); age and demographic characteristics of study populations (Osuntokun et al., 1992); educational attainment and literacy (Hall et al., 1993; Prince et al., 2003); and cultural factors (Shah et al., 2005a).

10.6   GENETIC AND ENVIRONMENTAL INFLUENCES

If the differences in the prevalence and incidence persist after the methodological issues are overcome, then cross-cultural studies have the potential to allow investigation of the underlying genetic and environmental risk and protective factors and the interaction between them (Amaducci *et al.*, 1991; Osuntokun *et al.*, 1992; Hall *et al.*, 1993). If the risk of dementia was solely due to genetic factors, then migrants would have the same incidence as in their country of origin (Graves *et al.*, 1994). Thus, comparison of the same ethnic group in different communities, at different stages of socio-economic development and differing environments, while maintaining genetic homogeneity, may allow identification of environmental risk factors (Graves *et al.*, 1994). To this end, cross-cultural incidence and prevalence studies designed to overcome the methodological difficulties, using screening and diagnostic instruments that are culture-fair, education-free and analogous with similar case-finding methods in age- and sex-stratified samples, are beginning to emerge (Prince *et al.*, 2003; Llibre Rodriguez *et al.*, 2008).

10.6.1   Environment

Despite comparable overall rates of dementia in Japan and the United States, the prevalence of VaD is highest in Japan, intermediate in Hawaii and lowest in the mainland US, with an opposite trend observed for AD (Graves *et al.*, 1994). The prevalence of AD among Japanese Americans in Washington (Graves *et al.*, 1996) and Honolulu (White *et al.*, 1996) is closer to white Americans than Japanese in Japan, suggesting an environmental aetiology. A prospective cohort study of Japanese Americans reported that those who led a traditional Japanese lifestyle had a slower decline in cognition over two years (Graves *et al.*, 1999), also suggesting the importance of environmental factors. Additionally, the lower prevalence of cardiovascular disease among Japanese Americans may also explain slower rates of cognitive decline (Graves *et al.*, 1999). Furthermore, increasing physical activity was associated with lower rates of dementia in the same Japanese American cohort (Taafe *et al.*, 2008). However, a study of first-generation Japanese migrants from Miyagi prefecture to Brazil (Meguro *et al.*, 2001a) reported a similar prevalence of dementia, VaD and AD to that in Miyagi prefecture in Japan (Ishii *et al.*, 1999), despite the migrants having a higher prevalence of diabetes mellitus and cerebrovascular disease (Meguro *et al.*, 2001b). The authors have posited that the prevalence of dementia was not affected by environmental factors because environmental effects may take considerable time to emerge, perhaps in subsequent generations.

The Indo-US cross-national study reported a prevalence of 0.84 per cent for all dementias among rural Indians near Delhi, a significantly lower figure than a community sample in Pennsylvania (Chandra *et al.*, 1998). An incidence study in the same geographical area reported one of the lowest incidences for AD in the world (Chandra *et al.*, 2001). A study of Singapore Malays and Chinese reported a higher prevalence of dementia among Malays than Chinese (Kua and Ko, 1995); the difference was mainly accounted for by a higher prevalence of multi-infarct dementia in Malay women compared to Malay men and Chinese women. A prevalence and incidence study comparing rates among Yoruba Nigerians in Ibadan and African Americans in Indianapolis reported lower prevalence and incidence rates for dementia and AD among the Nigerians (Hendrie *et al.*,

1995b; Hendrie *et al.*, 2001), again suggesting the importance of environmental aetiological factors.

10.6.2   Genetics

An early pilot population-based prevalence study reported a strong association between apolipoprotein E (ApoE) ε4 allele and AD in African Americans (Hendrie *et al.*, 1995a) suggesting that ApoE ε4 is a risk factor independent of ethnicity. However, this was not observed in Nigerians (Osuntokun *et al.*, 1995; Gureje *et al.*, 2006) and Kenyans (Chen *et al.*, 2010), despite a high prevalence of ε4 allele in the community in both countries. This discrepancy may be explained by differences in the expression of ApoE alleles or of ApoE receptors, interaction with unidentified modifier genes, or environmental factors interacting with genes. Furthermore, lower deposition of A4 β-amyloid has been found in post-mortem brains of Nigerian subjects without dementia compared to a similar series from Australia (Osuntokun *et al.*, 1994). Both these observations may help to explain a lower prevalence and incidence of AD in Nigeria.

A strong association between ApoE ε4 homozygous status and AD has been observed among Caucasians (non-Hispanic white Americans), African Americans and Hispanics in population-based prevalence studies in the US (Maestre *et al.*, 1995; Tang *et al.*, 1996; Sahota *et al.*, 1997); despite these associations, the relative risk of developing AD was found to be the highest in Caucasians compared with the other two groups, suggesting a gene–environment interaction. However, when considering heterozygous ApoE ε4 status, this relation was either weaker (Maestre *et al.*, 1995) or absent in African Americans (Tang *et al.*, 1996; Sahota *et al.*, 1997) in comparison with Caucasians and Hispanics. A similar weak association was found between ApoE ε4 status and cognitive impairment in African Caribbeans in the United Kingdom (Stewart *et al.*, 2001b). The presence of depressive symptoms and ApoE ε4 allele markedly increased the risk of dementia, including AD, in Japanese American men (Irie *et al.*, 2008).

A population-based incidence study, controlling for education, family history of AD and other risk factors like hypertension, demonstrated a strong association between combined homozygous and heterozygous ApoE ε4 status and AD in white Americans, African Americans and Hispanics in the United States (Tang *et al.*, 1998). Unfortunately, separate data for homozygous and heterozygous ApoE ε4 status were not available. Furthermore, in the presence of at least one ApoE ε4 allele, the cumulative risk of developing AD up to the age of 90 years was higher in the African American and Hispanic groups compared to the white American group; although, a Norwegian study reported that the effect of ApoE ε4 on AD becomes weaker with increasing age (Sando *et al.*, 2008a). These observations collectively suggest that the effect of ApoE ε4 on AD is weaker and 'dose dependent' in African Americans compared with white Americans and, to a lesser extent, Hispanics. It is possible that the presence of other environmental factors or modifier genes may reduce the ApoE ε4-associated risk of developing AD in African Americans (Sahota *et al.*, 1997; Tang *et al.*, 1998). These enviromental factors or modifier genes may be able to alter the risk of one dose of ApoE ε4 more easily than two doses (Maestre *et al.*, 1995).

Another explanation for these findings is that there may be differential linkage disequilibrium between unidentified AD susceptibility gene and ApoE ε4 alleles in different ethnic groups (Maestre *et al.*, 1995). A further explanation is the differential survival of those with ApoE ε4 alleles, although this observation is not supported by reports that ApoE ε4 in white subjects is unchanged with age (Maestre *et al.*, 1995; Tang *et al.*, 1996), and either unchanged (Tang *et al.*, 1996) or increased (Maestre *et al.*, 1995) with age in African Americans. Also, the frequency of ApoE ε4 in AD in white and African Americans is reported to decline (Maestre *et al.*, 1995) or remain unchanged (Tang *et al.*, 1996) with age. However, despite a decline in ApoE ε4 frequency in AD with age, other genetic and environmental factors may increase the risk of developing AD in African Americans and Hispanics in the absence of this allele (Tang *et al.*, 1998). A population-based incidence study of Japanese American men reported a significant association between ApoE ε4 and AD (Havlik *et al.*, 2000). Also, ApoE ε4 was found to be a risk factor for AD in women but not men in Venezuela, suggesting that gender may also be important (Molero *et al.*, 2001).

Chandra and Pandav (1998) have speculated that high serum cholesterol levels may interact with ApoE ε4 alleles to produce AD based on evidence of low serum cholesterol levels in rural Indians and a low prevalence of AD. Moreover, low serum levels of cholesterol were observed at least 15 years before the onset of dementia, particularly AD, and subsequently remained low in Japanese American men, and were suggested to be associated with early stages in the development of dementia (Stewart *et al.*, 2007). However, the Indian observations were not supported by the ApoE typing in the same population-based Indo-US prevalence study, where the frequency of ApoE ε4 was significantly lower in the Indian sample than in the US sample and the strength of association between ApoE ε4 and AD was the same in both samples (Ganguli *et al.*, 2000). Collectively, these findings may be one explanation for one of the lowest prevalence and incidence rates for AD in the world in the Indian sample (Chandra and Pandav, 1998; Chandra *et al.*, 2001). The authors concluded that the different prevalence in the two samples cannot be explained by differential risk or modifier risk pertaining to ApoE polymorphism, and they speculated that there may be additional risk or protective factors, survival effects or contributory environmental factors.

In a convenience sample of Cherokee Indians in Texas (US), the risk of developing AD declined with an increase in the genetic degree of Cherokee ancestry and this relationship was independent of ApoE ε4 allele (Rosenberg *et al.*, 1996). However, the protective effect of Cherokee ancestry declined with age. These findings suggest a complex interaction between genetic and environmental factors.

10.7 EDUCATION

The role of educational attainment as a risk factor for dementia is controversial, but its examination across different cultural groups may shed further light on the role of environmental factors or gene–environment interaction. Low levels of education were associated with very mild and mild dementia in Hong Kong (Lam *et al.*, 2008). Illiteracy was identified as a risk factor for incident cases of AD in a South Korean sample, and this link was more pronounced with increasing age (Lee *et al.*, 2008). Lower levels of education were associated with AD even when ApoE ε4 status was controlled for in a Norwegian sample (Sando *et al.*, 2008b). Levels of education were strongly correlated with the prevalence of dementia in Latinos, African Americans and non-Latino white Americans in the United States (Gurland *et al.*, 1995; Gurland *et al.*, 1999), but the differences in prevalence disappeared if age and education were controlled for, suggesting that education may be an important environmental risk factor independent of ethnicity. In a community study of African Caribbeans in London, hypertension and diabetes were specifically associated with cognitive impairment in those with low levels of education (Stewart *et al.*, 2001c). In a South Korean study, a similar association was found between cognitive impairment and systolic blood pressure, previous diagnosis of diabetes and random glucose levels in subjects with no formal education (Stewart *et al.*, 2003).

These findings may be explained by several hypotheses which require rigorous testing:

- Subjects with lower levels of education may have less well-controlled hypertension or diabetes (Gurland *et al.*, 1995; Gurland *et al.*, 1999; Stewart *et al.*, 2001c; Stewart *et al.*, 2003).
- Cognitive batteries may not be sufficiently sensitive to measure cognitive impairment in those with high levels of education (Stewart *et al.*, 2001c).
- Those with high levels of education may have developed sufficient cognitive reserve to be less vulnerable to the effects of hypertension and diabetes (Gurland *et al.*, 1995; Gurland *et al.*, 1999; Stewart *et al.*, 2001c; Stewart *et al.*, 2003).
- Cerebral damage due to hypertension or diabetes may be more severe in those with lower levels of education (Stewart *et al.*, 2003).

Paradoxically, in a study of subjects with familial Alzheimer's disease, high levels of education were associated with earlier onset of dementia (Mejia *et al.*, 2003). This was explained by earlier detection of symptoms in those with higher levels of education due to greater intellectual and environmental demands (Mejia *et al.*, 2003).

10.8 LIFE EXPECTANCY AND THE EPIDEMIOLOGICAL TRANSITION HYPOTHESIS

A theoretical model of the epidemiological transition in dementia has been developed using incidence and prevalence data from different countries (Suh and Shah, 2001). According to this model, all societies sequentially move through four hierarchical stages:

1. Low incidence–high mortality society
2. High incidence–high mortality society

3. High incidence–low mortality society
4. Low incidence–low mortality society

Within this model several factors contribute to the prevalence of dementia:

- The overall incidence (and thus the prevalence) will be low in societies where life expectancy is short because fewer subjects will reach the age of risk for dementia. The selective survival of those not at risk of dementia may further influence such a trend. It is possible that early mortality selects for genetic and/or constitutional factors that protect against neurodegenerative disorders.
- Mortality and survival after the onset of dementia also influence prevalence rates. In societies where survival after the onset of dementia is short, the prevalence may be low even if the incidence is not.
- The incidence itself is important because uneven distribution of protective or risk factors for dementia will vary the incidence.
- In socioeconomically less developed societies, infectious diseases associated with poor socioeconomic factors will reduce life expectancy with fewer individuals reaching the age of risk for dementia. Such a society had been described as a low incidence–high mortality society. With improvement in basic medical care the average life expectancy will increase and reach the threshold age of risk for dementia (Li et al., 2007; Lam et al., 2008). This will lead to a gradual transition from a low incidence–high mortality society to high incidence–high mortality society. The observed high prevalence of dementia in a socioeconomically deprived area of Brazil may represent this stage of epidemiological transition (Scazufca et al., 2008). Furthermore, in socioeconomically better developed societies the mortality associated with dementia may decline because of greater availability of medical care and technology. This will lead to a gradual transition from a high incidence–high mortality society to a high incidence–low mortality society. In socioeconomically very well-off societies, efforts to improve the control of risk factors for dementia (such as those for VD) may reduce the incidence of dementia, leading to a gradual transition to a low incidence–low mortality society. There is evidence that the ratio of AD to that of vascular disease is increasing in some Asian countries due to a reduction in the incidence of strokes (Fujishima and Kiyohara, 2002; Li et al., 2007).
- The transition from a low incidence–high mortality society to low incidence–low mortality society may unfold in several ways depending upon availability of medical services, advances in medical care and technology, public health policies and efforts undertaken to control risk factors for dementia and promote protective factors for dementia in a given society.

A similar epidemiological transition model has been developed for other mental disorders in old age (Shah, 2007). Another explanation for the low prevalence of dementia in an urban Indian area is selective migration, whereby people with dementia may return to their native rural areas (Vas et al., 2001).

10.9   FUTURE DIRECTIONS

The relationship between educational levels and dementia has been explained by several speculative hypotheses listed earlier. The role of education as an environmental factor in the development of dementia in the context of ApoE ε4 status and cardiovascular risk factors requires further study to test the various speculative explanatory models. This may have important implications for the prevention of dementia.

Cross-cultural studies of dementia have focused primarily on cognitive impairment. Behavioural and psychological symptoms of dementia (BPSD) have been less well studied in cross-cultural studies (Shah and Mukherjee, 2000; Shah et al., 2005b). Cross-cultural measures of BPSD that are culture-fair and analogous to those used in Western countries are emerging (Shah et al., 2004; Shah et al., 2005b; Shah et al., 2005c). Behavioural and psychological symptoms of dementia require close examination in cross-sectional and longitudinal studies of the prevalence and incidence of dementia in cross-cultural settings; these studies should be designed to examine genetic and environmental risk factors and the interaction between them for both cognitive impairment and BPSD.

Very few cross-cultural studies have examined neuro-chemical, neuroanatomical and neurohistological changes in dementia (Amaducci et al., 1991), and structural and functional imaging have hardly been used in cross-cultural studies. These techniques should be applied in rigorous population-based cross-cultural studies of both cognitive impairment and BPSD, using cross-culturally validated measures of cognitive impairment and BPSD. This approach would provide a powerful means of exploring environmental and genetic factors and the interaction between them. The clustering of less common dementias, such as Huntington's disease, prion dementias and Parkinson's dementia complex of Guam, in some cultural groups may also shed light on genetic and environmental interactions (Graham et al., 1998).

The epidemiological transition hypothesis for dementia also requires further study. This can initially be achieved using data from incidence and prevalence studies from individual countries, and data on socioeconomic status (e.g. gross national domestic product), life expectancy and proxy measures of the quality of medical services (e.g. infant mortality rates) – all available from the World Health Organization. One statistical model of the proposed epidemiological transition hypothesis is that of an inverted U-shaped curve following a quadratic equation $Y = A + BX - CX^2$ (where Y is the incidence of dementia, X is the socioeconomic status, and A, B and C are constants).

The development of these sophisticated international research programmes will require considerable development of specialist services for these groups worldwide if they are to be feasible (Shah, 2008; Shah et al., 2008).

REFERENCES

Amaducci L, Baldereschi M, Amato MP et al. (1991) The World Health Organisation cross-national research programme on age-associated dementias. Aging 3: 89–96.

Anzola-Perez E, Bangdiwala SI, De Llano GB et al. (1996) Towards community diagnosis of dementia: testing cognitive impairment in older persons in Argentina, Chile and Cuba. International Journal of Geriatric Psychiatry 11: 429–38.

Balarajan R. (1996) Ethnicity and variation in mortality from cardiovascular disease. Health Trends 28: 45–51.

Bhatnagar KS, Frank J. (1997) Psychiatric disorders in the elderly from the Indian subcontinent living in Bradford. International Journal of Geriatric Psychiatry 12: 907–12.

Bohning W, Oishi N. (1995) Is international migration spreading? Migration Review 29: 794–9.

Breitner JCS, Folstein M. (1984) Familial Alzheimer's dementia: a prevalent disorder with specific clinical features. American Journal of Psychiatry 14: 63–80.

Chandra V, Pandav R. (1998) Gene-environment interaction in Alzheimer's disease: a potential role for cholesterol. Neuroepidemiology 17: 225–32.

Chandra V, Ganguli M, Ratcliff G et al. (1994) Studies of the epidemiology of dementia: comparison between developed and developing countries. Ageing, Clinical and Experimental Research 6: 307–21.

Chandra V, Ganguli M, Pandav R et al. (1998) Prevalence of Alzheimer's and other dementias in rural India: the Indo-US study. Neurology 57: 985–9.

Chandra V, Pandav R, Dodge HH et al. (2001) Incidence of Alzheimer's disease in a rural community in the Indo-US study. Neurology 57: 985–9.

Chen CH, Mizuno T, Elston R et al. (2010) A comparative study to screen and APOE genotypes in an ageing East African population. Neurobiology of Ageing 31: 732–40.

Copeland JRM, Kelleher MJ, Kellett JM et al. (1976) A semi-structured interview for the assessment of diagnosis and mental state in the elderly. The Geriatric Mental State Schedule. 1. Development and reliability. Psychological Medicine 6: 439–49.

Crane PK, Gibbons LE, Jolley L et al. (2006) Differential item functioning related to education and age in an Italian version of the Mini-Mental State Examination. International Psychogeriatrics 18: 505–15.

De La Monte SM, Hutchins GM, Moore GW et al. (1989) Racial differences in the etiology of dementia and frequency of Alzheimer's lesions in the brain. Journal of the National Medical Association 81: 644–52.

De Silva HA, Gunatilake SB. (2002) Mini-Mental State Examination in Sinhalese: a sensitive test to screen for dementia in Sri Lanka. International Journal of Geriatric Psychiatry 7: 134–9.

Escobar JI, Burnham A, Karno M et al. (1986) Use of Mini-mental State Examination (MMSE) in a community population of mixed ethnicity. Journal of Nervous and Mental Diseases 174: 607–14.

Ferri CP, Prince M, Brayne C et al. (2005) Global prevalence of dementia: a Delphi consensus study. Lancet 366: 2112–17.

Folstein MF, Folstein SE, McHugh PR. (1975) 'Mini-mental State': a practical method for grading the cognitive state of patients for the clinician. Journal of Psychiatric Research 12: 189–98.

Fuh JL, Teng EL, Lin KN et al. (1995) The informant questionnaire on cognitive decline in the elderly (IQCODE) as a screening tool for dementia for a predominantly illiterate Chinese population. Neurology 45: 92–6.

Fujishima M, Kiyohara Y. (2002) Incidence and risk factors of dementia in a defined elderly Japanese population: the Hisayama study. Annals of New York Academy of Science 977: 1–8.

Fuzikawa C, Lima-Costa FM, Uchoa E et al. (2003) A population-based study of intra and inter-rater reliability of the clock drawing test in Brazil: the Bambui Health and Ageing Study. International Journal of Geriatric Psychiatry 18: 450–6.

Fuzikawa C, Lima-Costa FM, Uchoa E et al. (2007) Correlation and agreement between the Mini-Mental State Examination and the Clock Drawing test in older adults with low levels of schooling: the Bambui Health and Ageing Study (BHAS). International Psychogeriatrics 19: 657–68.

Ganguli M, Chandra V, Kamboh I et al. (2000) Apolipoprotein E polymorphism and Alzheimer's disease. Archives of Neurology 57: 824–30.

Ganguli M, Ratcliff G, Chandra V et al. (1995) A Hindi version of the MMSE: development of a cognitive screening instrument for a largely illiterate rural population in India. International Journal of Geriatric Psychiatry 10: 367–77.

Graham C, Howard R, Ya Y. (1998) Studies on dementia: dementia and ethnicity. International Psychogeriatrics 10: 183–91.

Graves AB, Larson EB, White LR et al. (1994) Opportunities and challenges in international collaborative epidemiological research of dementia and its subtypes. Studies between Japan and the US. International Psychogeriatrics 6: 209–23.

Graves AB, Larson EB, Edland SD et al. (1996) Prevalence of dementia and its subtype in the Japanese American in King County, Washington State. American Journal of Epidemiology 144: 760–71.

Graves AB, Rajaram L, Bowen JD et al. (1999) Cognitive decline and Japanese culture in a cohort of older Japanese Americans in King County. Journal of Gerontology Series B-Psychological Sciences and Social Sciences 54: S154–61.

Gureje O, Ogunniyi A, Baiyewu O et al. (2006) APOE epsilon4 is not associated with Alzheimer's disease in elderly Nigerians. Annals of Neurology 59: 182–5.

Gurland BJ, Wilder DE, Cross P et al. (1992) Screening scales for dementia: towards reconciliation of conflicting cross-cultural findings. International Journal of Geriatric Psychiatry 7: 105–13.

Gurland BJ, Wilder DE, Cross P et al. (1995) Relative rates of dementia by multiple definitions, over two prevalence periods in three sociocultural groups. American Journal of Geriatric Psychiatry 3: 6–20.

Gurland BJ, Wilder DE, Lantigua R et al. (1999) Rates of dementia in three ethnoracial groups. International Journal of Geriatric Psychiatry 14: 481–93.

Hall KS, Gao S, Emsley CL et al. (2000) Community screening interview for dementia (CIS-D): performance in five disparate study sites. *International Journal of Geriatric Psychiatry* **15**: 521–31.

Hall KS, Hendries HC, Brittain HM *et al.* (1993) The development of dementia screening interview in two distinct languages. *International Journal of Methods in Psychiatric Research* **3**: 1–28.

Hasegawa K, Homma A, Imai Y. (1986) An epidemiological study of age-related dementia in the community. *International Journal of Geriatric Psychiatry* **1**: 45–55.

Havlik RJ, Izmirlian G, Petrovitch H *et al.* (2000) ApoE ε4 predicts incident AD in Japanese American men: the Honolulu-Asia Aging Study. *Neurology* **54**: 1526–9.

Hendrie H. (1992) Indianapolis-Ibadan research project. In: Curb JD, Graves AB (eds). Multi-national studies of dementia. *The Gerontologist* 32 (Suppl. 2): 219.

Hendrie H, Hall KS, Pillay N *et al.* (1993) Alzheimer's disease is rare in Cree. *International Psychogeriatrics* **5**: 5–15.

Hendrie HC, Osuntokun BO, Hall KS *et al.* (1995a) Prevalence of Alzheimer's disease and dementia in two communities: Nigerian Africans and African Americans. *American Journal of Psychiatry* **152**: 1485–92.

Hendrie HC, Hall KS, Hui S *et al.* (1995b) Apolipoprotein E genotypes and Alzheimer's disease in a community study of elderly African Americans. *Annals of Neurology* **37**: 118–20.

Hendrie HC, Ogunniyi A, Hall KS *et al.* (2001) Incidence of dementia and Alzheimer's disease in 2 communities: Yoruba residing in Ibadan, Nigeria, and African Americans residing in Indianapolis, Indiana. *Journal of the American Geriatric Society* **285**: 739–47.

Heyman A, Fillenbaum G, Prosnitz B. (1991) Estimated prevalence of dementia among elderly black and white community residents. *Archives of Neurology* **48**: 594–8.

Hofman A, Rocca WA, Brayne C *et al.* (1991) The prevalence of dementia in Europe: a collaborative study of 1980-1990 findings. *International Journal of Epidemiology* **20**: 736–48.

Inzelberg R, Schechtman E, Abuful A *et al.* (2007) Education effects on cognitive function in a healthy aged Arab population. *International Psychogeriatrics* **19**: 593–606.

Irie F, Masaki KH, Petrovitch H *et al.* (2008) Apolipoprotein E epsilon 4 allele genotype and the effect of depressive symptoms on the risk of dementia in men: the Honolulu-Asia Aging Study. *Archives of General Psychiatry* **65**: 906–12.

Ishii H, Meguro K, Ishizaki J *et al.* (1999) Prevalence of senile dementia in a rural community in Japan: the Tajiri project. *Archives of Gerontology and Geriatrics* **29**: 249–65.

Jacob KS, Senthil Kumar P, Gayathri K *et al.* (2007) The diagnosis of dementia in the community. *International Psychogeriatrics* **19**: 669–78.

Jitapunkul S, Lailert C, Worakul P *et al.* (1996) Chula Mental Test: a screening test for elderly people in less developed countries. *International Journal of Geriatric Psychiatry* **11**: 715–20.

Jorm AF, Jolley D. (1998) The incidence of dementia: a meta-analysis. *Neurology* **51**: 728–33.

Jorm AF, Scott R, Cullen JS. (1991) Performance of Informant Questionnaire on Cognitive Decline in the Elderly (IQCODE) as a screening test for dementia. *Psychological Medicine* **21**: 785–90.

Kabir ZH, Herlitz A. (2000) The Bangla adaptation of mini-mental state examination (BMASE): an instrument to assess cognitive function in illiterate and literate individuals. *International Journal of Geriatric Psychiatry* **15**: 441–50.

Kalaria RN, Maestre GS, Arizaga R *et al.* (2008) Alzheimer's disease and vascular dementia in developing countries: prevalence, management and risk factors. *Lancet Neurology* **7**: 812–26.

Katzman R, Zhang M, Qu QY *et al.* (1988) A Chinese version of the Mini-mental State Examination: impact of illiteracy in a Shanghai dementia survey. *Journal of Clinical Epidemiology* **41**: 971–8.

Kua EH. (1992) A community study of mental disorders in elderly Singaporean Chinese using the GMS-AGECAT package. *Australia and New Zealand Journal of Psychiatry* **25**: 502–5.

Kua EH, Ko SM. (1995) Prevalence of dementia among elderly Chinese and Malay residents of Singapore. *International Psychogeriatrics* **7**: 439–46.

Lam LCW, Tam CWC, Lui VWC *et al.* (2008) Prevalence of very mild and mild dementia in community-dwelling older Chinese people in Hong Kong. *International Psychogeriatrics* **20**: 135–48.

Lee JY, Chang SM, Jang HK *et al.* (2008) Illiteracy and the incidence of Alzheimer's disease in the Yonchon County survey, Korea. *International Psychogeriatrics* **20**: 976–85.

Li G, Shen YC, Chen CH *et al.* (1989) An epidemiological survey of age-related dementia in an urban area of Beijing. *Acta Psychiatrica Scandinavica* **79**: 557–63.

Li G, Shen YC, Zhau YW *et al.* (1991) A three-year follow-up study of age-related dementia in an urban area of Beijing. *Acta Psychiatrica Scandinavica* **83**: 99–104.

Li S, Yan F, Chen C *et al.* (2007) Is the dementia rate increasing in Beijing? Prevalence and incidence of dementia 10 years later in an urban elderly population. *Acta Psychiatrica Scandinavica* **115**: 73–9.

Lindesay J. (1998) The diagnosis of mental illness in elderly people from ethnic minorities. *Advances in Psychiatric Treatment* **4**: 219–26.

Lindesay J, Jagger C, Mlynik-Szmid M. (1997) The mini-mental state examination (MMSE) in an elderly immigrant Gujarati population in the United Kingdom. *International Journal of Geriatric Psychiatry* **12**: 1155–67.

Liu SI, Prince M, Chiu MJ *et al.* (2005) Validity and reliability of a Taiwan Chinese version of the community screening instrument for dementia. *American Journal of Geriatric Psychiatry* **13**: 581–8.

Livingston G, Leavey G, Kitchen G *et al.* (2001) Mental Health of Migrants – the Islington Study. *British Journal of Psychiatry* **179**: 361–6.

Livingston G, Sembhi S. (2003) Mental Health of the ageing immigrant population. *Advances in Psychiatric Treatment* **9**: 31–7.

Llibre Rodriguez JJ, Ferri CP, Acosta D *et al.* (2008) Prevalence of dementia in Latin America, India and China: a population-based cross-sectional survey. *Lancet* **372**: 464–74.

LoGuidice D, Smith K, Thomas J *et al.* (2006) Kimberley Indigenous Cognitive Assessment Tool (KICA): development of a cognitive assessment tool for older indigenous Australians. *International Psychogeriatrics* **18**: 269–80.

McCrakken CFM, Boneham MA, Copeland JRM et al. (1997) Prevalence of dementia and depression among elderly people in black and ethnic groups. British Journal of Psychiatry 171: 269–73.

Maestre G, Ottman R, Stern Y et al. (1995) Apolipoprotein E and Alzheimer's disease: ethnic variation in genotypic risks. Annals of Neurology 37: 254–9.

Mather H, Keen M. (1985) The Southall diabetes survey: prevalence of known diabetes in Asians and Europeans. British Medical Journal 291: 1081–4.

Meguro K, Meguro M, Caramelli P et al. (2001a) Elderly Japanese emigrants to Brazil before World War II: II. Prevalence of dementia. International Journal of Geriatric Psychiatry 16: 775–9.

Meguro K, Meguro M, Caramelli P et al. (2001b) Elderly Japanese emigrants to Brazil before World War II: I. Clinical profiles based on specific historical background. International Journal of Geriatric Psychiatry 16: 768–74.

Mejia S, Giraldo M, Pineda D et al. (2003) Nongenetic factors as modifiers of the age of onset of familial Alzheimer's disease. International Psychogeriatrics 15: 337–49.

Molero AE, Pino-Ramirez G, Maestre GE. (2001) Modulation by age and gender of risk of Alzheimer's disease and vascular dementia associated with apolipoprotein E4 allele in Latin Americans: findings from the Maracaibo Ageing Study. Neuroscience Letters 307: 5–8.

Morris J, Heyman A, Mohs R et al. (1989) The consortium to establish a registry for Alzheimer's disease (CERAD). Part 1. Clinical and neuropsychological assessment of Alzheimer's disease. Neurology 39: 149–55.

Murden RA, McRae TD, Kaner S et al. (1991) Mini-mental state exam scores vary with education in blacks and whites. Journal of the American Geriatric Society 39: 149–55.

Osuntokun BO, Hendrie HC, Ogunniyi AO. (1992) Cross-cultural studies in Alzheimer's diesease. Ethnicity and Diseases 2: 352–7.

Osuntokun BO, Ogunniyi AO, Akang EEU et al. (1994) A4-amyloid in brains of non-demented Nigerians. Lancet 343: 56.

Osuntokun BO, Sahota A, Ogunniyi AO et al. (1995) Lack of association between apolipoprotein E ε4 allele and Alzheimer's disease in elderly Nigerians. Annals of Neurology 38: 463–5.

Park JH, Kwon YC. (1990) Modification of the Mini-mental State Examination for use in the elderly in a non-western society. Part I. Development of the Korean version of the Mini-Mental State Examination. International Journal of Geriatric Psychiatry 5: 381–7.

Park JH, Park YN, Ko HJ. (1991) Modification of the Mini-mental State Examination for use in the elderly in a non-western society. Part II: cut-off points and their diagnostic validities. International Journal of Geriatric Psychiatry 6: 875–82.

Perkins P, Annegers JF, Doody RS et al. (1997) Incidence and prevalence of dementia in a multiethnic cohort of municipal retirees. Neurology 49: 44–50.

Phanthumchinda K, Jitapunkul S, Sitthi-Amorn C et al. (1991) Prevalence of dementia in an urban slum population in Thailand: validity of screening methods. International Journal of Geriatric Psychiatry 6: 639–46.

Pollitt P. (1997) The problem of dementia in Australian Aboriginal and Torres Strait islander communities: an overview. International Journal of Geriatric Psychiatry 12: 155–63.

Prince M, Acosta D, Chiu H et al. (2003) Dementia diagnosis in developing countries: a cross-cultural validation study. Lancet 361: 909–17.

Prince M, Acosta D, Chiu H et al. (2004) Effects of education and culture on the validity of the Geriatric Mental State and its AGECAT algorithm. British Journal of Psychiatry 185: 429–36.

Prince MJ, de Rodriguez JL, Noriega L et al. (2008) The 10/66 Dementia Research Group's fully operational dementia computerised algorithm, comparison of 10/66 dementia algorithm a clinician diagnosis validation study. BMC Public Health. Doi:10.1186/1471-2458-8-219.

Quereshi KN, Hodkinson HM. (1974) Evaluation of a ten-question mental test in institutionalised elderly. Age and Ageing 3: 152–7.

Rait G, Burns A, Baldwin R et al. (2000a) Validating screening instruments for cognitive impairment in older south Asians in the United Kingdom. International Journal of Geriatric Psychiatry 15: 54–62.

Rait G, Morley M, Burns A et al. (2000b) Screening for cognitive impairment in older African-Caribbeans. Psychological Medicine 30: 957–63.

Rait G, Morley M, Lambat I, Burns A. (1997) Modification of brief cognitive assessments for use with elderly people from the South Asian sub-continent. Ageing and Mental Health 1: 356–63.

Rajkumar S, Kumar S. (1996) Prevalence of dementia in the community: a rural urban comparison from Madras, India. Australian Journal on Ageing 15: 9–13.

Richards M, Brayne C. (1996) Cross-cultural research into cognitive impairment and dementia: some practical experiences. International Journal of Geriatric Psychiatry 11: 383–7.

Richards M, Brayne C, Dening T et al. (2000) Cognitive function in UK community dwelling African Caribbean and white elders: a pilot study. International Journal of Geriatric Psychiatry 15: 621–30.

Ritch AES, Ehtisham M, Guthries S et al. (1996) Ethnic influence on health and dependency of elderly innercity residents. Journal of the Royal College of Physicians London 30: 215–20.

Rocca WA, Bonaiuto S, Lippi A et al. (1990) Prevalence of clinically diagnosed Alzheimer's disease and other dementing disorders. A door-to-door survey in Appigano, Macerata Province, Italy. Neurology 40: 626–31.

Rosen WG, Mohs RC, Davis KL. (1984) A new rating scale for Alzheimer's disease. American Journal of Psychiatry 141: 1356–64.

Rosenberg RN, Richter RW, Risser RC et al. (1996) Genetic factors for the development of Alzheimer's disease in Cherokee Indians. Archives of Neurology 53: 997–1000.

Roth M, Tym E, Mountjoy CQ et al. (1986) CAMDEX: A standardised instrument for diagnosis of mental disorder in the elderly with special references to early detection of dementia. British Journal of Psychiatry 149: 698–709.

Royall DR, Espino DV, Polk MJ et al. (2003) Validation of a Spanish translation of the CLOX for use in Hispanic samples: the

Hispanic EPESE study. *International Journal of Geriatric Psychiatry* 18: 135–41.

Sahadevan S, Lim PPJ, Tan NJL, Chan SP. (2000) Diagnostic performance of the mental status tests in older Chinese: influence of education and age on cut-off values. *International Journal of Geriatric Psychiatry* 15: 234–41.

Sahota A, Yang M, Gao S *et al.* (1997) Apolipoprotein E-associated risk of Alzheimer's disease in the African American population is genotype dependent. *Annals of Neurology* 42: 659–61.

Salmon DP, Reikkinen PJ, Katzman R *et al.* (1989) Cross-cultural studies of dementia – a comparison of the Mini-Mental state Examination performance in Finland and China. *Archives of Neurology* 46: 769–72.

Samanta DP, Burden AC, Fent B. (1987) Comparative prevalence of non-insulin-dependent diabetes mellitus in Asian and white Caucasian adults. *Diabetes Research and Clinical Practice* 4: 1–6.

Sando SB, Melquist S, Cannon A *et al.* (2008a) APOE epsilon 4 lowers the age of onset and is a high risk factor for Alzheimer's disease; a case control study from central Norway. *BMC Neurology* 8: 9. Available from: www.biomedcentral.com/1471-2377/8/9.

Sando SB, Melquist S, Cannon A *et al.* (2008b) Risk-reducing effect of education in Alzheimer's disease. *International Journal of Geriatric Psychiatry* 23: 1156–62.

Scazufca M, Menezes PR, Vallada HP *et al.* (2008) High prevalence of dementia among older adults from poor socioeconomic backgrounds in Sao Paulo, Brazil. *International Psychogeriatrics* 20: 394–405.

Schmidtke K, Olbrich S. (2007) The Clock Reading Test: validation of an instrument for the diagnosis of dementia and disorders of visuo-spatial cognition. *International Psychogeriatrics* 19: 307–22.

Schoenberg BS, Anderson DW, Haerer AF. (1985) Severe dementia: prevalence and clinical features in a biracial US population. *Archives of Neurology* 42: 740–3.

Serby M, Chou JC, Franssen EH. (1987) Dementia in an American Chinese nursing home population. *American Journal of Psychiatry* 144: 811–81.

Shah AK. (2007) The importance of socio-economic status of countries for mental disorders in old age: a development of an epidemiological transition model. *International Psychogeriatrics* 19: 785–7.

Shah AK. (2008) Do socio-economic factors, elderly population size and service development factors influence development of specialist mental health programme for older people. *International Psychogeriatrics* 20: 1238–44.

Shah AK, MacKenzie S. (2007) Disorders of ageing across cultures. In: Bhugra D, Bhui K (eds). *Textbook of cultural psychiatry.* Cambridge: Cambridge University Press, 323–44.

Shah AK, Mukherjee S. (2000) Cross-cultural issues in the measurement of behavioural and psychological signs and symptoms of dementia (BPSD). *Ageing and Mental Health* 4: 244–52.

Shah AK, Suh GK, Elanchenny N. (2004) A cross-national comparative study of behavioural and psychological symptoms of dementia between UK and Korea. *International Psychogeriatrics* 16: 219–36.

Shah AK, Lindesay J, Nnatu I. (2005a) Cross-cultural issues in the assessment of cognitive impairment. In: O'Brien J, Ames D, Burns A (eds). *Dementia.* London: Hodder Arnold, 147–64.

Shah AK, Dalvi M, Thompson T. (2005b) Behavioural and psychological signs and symptoms of dementia across cultures: current status and the future. *International Journal of Geriatric Psychiatry* 20: 1187–95.

Shah AK, Suh GK, Elanchenny N. (2005c) A comparative study of behavioural and psychological symptoms of dementia in patients with Alzheimer's disease and vascular dementia referred to psychogeriatric services in Korea and the UK. *International Psychogeriatrics* 17: 207–19.

Shah AK, Doe P, Deverill K. (2008) Ethnic minority elders: are they neglected in published geriatric psychiatry literature. *International Psychogeriatrics* 20: 1041–5.

Shaji S, Promodu K, Abraham I *et al.* (1996) An epidemiological study of dementia in a rural community in Kerala, India. *British Journal of Psychiatry* 168: 745–9.

Shibayama K, Kashara Y, Kobyashi H *et al.* (1986) Prevalence of dementias in a Japanese elderly population. *Acta Psychiatrica Scandinavica* 74: 144–51.

Silverman JM, Li G, Schear S *et al.* (1992) A cross-cultural family history study of primary progressive dementia in relatives of non-demented elderly Chinese, Italians, Jews and Peurto Ricans. *Acta Psychiatrica Scandinavica* 85: 211–17.

Stewart R, Richards M, Brayne C *et al.* (2001a) Cognitive function in UK community-dwelling /African Caribbean elders: normative data for a test battery. *International Journal of Geriatric Psychiatry* 16: 518–27.

Stewart R, Russ C, Richards M *et al.* (2001b) Apolipoprotein E genotype, vascular risk and early cognitive impairment in an African Caribbean population. *Dementia and Geriatric Cognitive Disorders* 12: 251–6.

Stewart R, Richards M, Brayne C, Mann A. (2001c) Vascular risk and cognitive impairment in an older British, African-Caribbean population. *Journal of the American Geriatric Society* 49: 263–9.

Stewart R, Kim J, Shin I *et al.* (2003) Education and the association between vascular risk factors and cognitive function: a cross-sectional study in older Koreans with cognitive impairment. *International Psychogeriatrics* 15: 27–36.

Stewart R, White LR, Xue QL *et al.* (2007) Twenty-six-year change in total cholesterol levels and incident dementia. *Archives of Neurology* 64: 103–7.

Still CN, Jackson KL, Brandes DA *et al.* (1990) Distribution of major dementias by race and sex in South Carolina. *Journal of South Carolina Medical Association* 86: 453–6.

Suh GK, Shah AK. (2001) A review of epidemiological transition in dementia: cross-national comparisons of the indices related to Alzheimer's disease and vascular dementia. *Acta Psychiatrica Scandinavica* 104: 4–11.

Taafe DR, Irie F, Masaki KH *et al.* (2008) Physical activity, physical function, and incident dementia in elderly men: the Honolulu-Asia Aging Study. *Journal of Gerontology Series A Biological Sciences and Medical Sciences* 63: 529–35.

Tang MX, Maestre G, Tsai WY *et al.* (1996) Relative risk of Alzheimer's disease and age-at-onset distributions based on ApoE genotypes among elderly African Americans, Caucasians and Hispanics in New York city. *American Journal of Human Genetics* **58**: 574–84.

Tang MX, Stern Y, Marder K *et al.* (1998) The ApoE ε4 allele and the risk of Alzheimer's disease among African Americans, whites and Hispanics. *Journal of the American Geriatric Society* **279**: 751–5.

Treves T, Korczyn AD, Zilber N *et al.* (1986) Presenile dementia in Israel. *Archives of Neurology* **43**: 26–9.

Vas CJ, Pinti C, Panikker D *et al.* (2001) Prevalence of dementia in an urban Indian population. *International Psychogeriatrics* **13**: 439–50.

Weiner MF, Rosenberg RN, Svetlik D *et al.* (2003) Comparison of Alzheimer's disease in native and white Americans. *International Psychogeriatrics* **15**: 367–75.

White L, Petrovitch H, Ross GW *et al.* (1996) Prevalence of dementia in older Japanese-American men in Hawaii. *Journal of the American Medical Association* **276**: 955–60.

Xu G, Meyer JS, Huang Y *et al.* (2003) Adapting Mini-mental State Examination for dementia screening among illiterate or minimally educated Chinese. *International Journal of Geriatric Psychiatry* **18**: 609–16.

Youn JC, Lee DY, Kim KW *et al.* (2002) Development of the Korean version of Alzheimer's Disease Assessment Scale (ADAS-K). *International Journal of Geriatric Psychiatry* **17**: 797–803.

Yu ESH, Liu WT, Levy P *et al.* (1989) Cognitive impairment among elderly adults in Shanghai, China. *Journal of Gerontology* **44**: S97–106.

Zann S. (1994) Identification of support, education and training needs of rural/remote health care service providers involved in dementia care. Rural Health, Support, Education and Training (RHSET). Project Progress Report. Queensland: Northern Regional Health Authority.

Zhang M, Katzman R, Salmon D *et al.* (1990) The prevalence of dementia and Alzheimer's disease in Shanghai, China: impact of age, gender and education. *Annals of Neurology* **27**: 428–37.

Structural brain imaging

ROBERT BARBER AND JOHN O'BRIEN

11.1 INTRODUCTION

This chapter focuses on the use of structural imaging, computed tomography (CT) and magnetic resonance imaging (MRI), in dementia.

The ability to visualize brain structure in life means MRI and CT have a central role in diagnosis. Traditionally, this role was limited to 'ruling out' pathologies that may be responsible for cognitive impairment, including so-called treatable or reversible causes. Increasingly imaging is used to assist in the diagnosis of dementia subtype. This function to 'rule in' causes has become possible because of advances in imaging methods which allow more subtle anatomical and pathological changes to be detected. It also reflects a conceptual shift towards diagnosing dementia subtypes using both exclusion and inclusion criteria, and recognition that imaging can enhance diagnostic accuracy. In addition, the result of a scan often has a pivotal role in helping individuals and their families understand and adjust to the diagnosis of dementia.

Imaging can also potentially identify biomarkers to aid presymptomatic diagnosis and provide new insights into the biology of dementia, and is increasingly being used as a surrogate outcome measure for clinical trials of putative disease modifying agents.

The significance of structural imaging to medical diagnostics was underlined when Sir Godfrey Hounsfield and Allan Cormack, who independently developed CT technology, were jointly awarded the Nobel Prize for Medicine in 1979. Two of the pioneers of MRI, Sir Peter Mansfield and Paul Lauterbur were also awarded Nobel Laureates in Medicine in 2003. There are now over 30 000 CT and 22 000 MRI scanners in operation worldwide, though availability varies considerably by country.

11.2 BACKGROUND TO COMPUTED TOMOGRAPHY AND MAGNETIC RESONANCE IMAGING

11.2.1 Computed tomography

The first human x-ray was taken in the 1890s and was a simple 'shadow' image of a hand on a photographic plate. The first patient brain scan was taken in 1972, taking several hours to acquire and process data for a single image or 'slice' ('tomography' is derived from the Greek *tomos* meaning 'slice'). Advances since have greatly improved patient experience and safety, resolution (spatial and temporal) and processing times, allowing the brain to be imaged in seconds. The recent development of multi-slice spiral CT has made three-dimensional (3D) reconstruction possible, so images are no longer limited to the axial plane. As with the very first x-ray, the CT image ultimately depends on electron density and the differential absorption of x-rays by body tissue, such that high-density structures like bone appear white, and low-density tissue, such as water and fat, appears black.

11.2.2 Magnetic resonance imaging

Magnetic resonance imaging is a non-invasive chemical probe capable of generating high-resolution 3D images of the body's internal structures. Water, composed of hydrogen nuclei or protons, constitutes about two-thirds of the human body and MRI utilizes the electromagnetic properties of the protons to construct a spatial representation of tissue. Under the controlled environment of the MRI scanner, protons are induced to act like microscopic radiotransmitters, and by detecting and processing their signal, macroscopic impressions of tissue structure can be obtained by 3D reconstruction. MRI scanners use powerful magnetic fields, up to 60 000 times greater than the Earth's magnetic field. Alterations in water (or in effect proton) content, and the local environment which affects proton properties, provides a basis for detecting pathological change and different types of body tissue. A difference in water content of less than 1 per cent is enough to distinguish normal and abnormal tissue.

One of the strengths of MRI is its versatility to visualize changes in both grey and white matter using different imaging sequences, as summarized in **Table 11.1** and illustrated in **Figure 11.1**. The potential benefit of combing some of the newer MRI sequences used in research settings are also summarized in **Table 11.1**. The potential benefit of combining different MRI sequences, and indeed structural and functional imaging, is currently an active area of research that ultimately aims to improve the clinical utility of neuroimaging.

11.2.3   Magnetic resonance imaging and computed tomography: indications and comparison

The different advantages and disadvantages of MRI and CT are summarized in **Table 11.2**. In addition to clinical factors, local service issues such as cost and availability will affect relative use of both imaging modalities.

Magnetic resonance imaging provides a sensitive method to study atrophy, cerebrovascular disease, white matter abnormalities and has advantages over CT in detecting certain diseases associated with cognitive impairment or seizures, such as multiple sclerosis (MS), Creutzfeldt–Jakob

Table 11.1   Main types of MRI sequences.

Conventional sequences:

T_1-*weighted*: commonly used clinical scan provides good definition of anatomy and grey/white matter contrast
T_2-*weighted*: provides high contrast and definition of soft tissue pathology (increased water content)
Proton density: provides good brain/CSF contrast

Newer sequences:

fluid attenuated inversion recovery (FLAIR): sensitive to changes in white matter (while suppressing the signal from the CSF)
magnetization transfer imaging (MTI): sensitive to changes in structural integrity of tissue
diffusion-weighted imaging (DWI): provides information about the microscopic diffusion of water molecules and integrity of axons.
    Diffusion tensor imaging (DTI) is a type of diffusion scan taken in multiple planes that can identify white matter tracts – so-called tractography. It gives an impression of the microstructure, coherence and connectivity of white matter tracks – see Chapter 12, Functional brain imaging and connectivity in dementia, for further details
perfusion-weighted imaging (PWI): provides information about the status of brain tissue perfusion

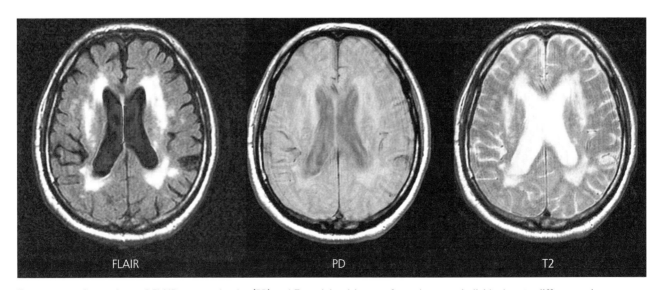

Figure 11.1   Comparison of FLAIR, proton density (PD) and T_2-weighted images from the same individual: note differences in appearance of white matter hyperintensities.

Table 11.2   Comparison between MRI and CT.

MRI	CT
Higher spatial and anatomical resolution	Shorter scan times
Superior soft tissue definition and contrast	Widely available
Image in multiple planes; therefore superior views of middle and posterior fossa, pituitary, brain stem and spinal cord	Lower cost
Uses non-ionizing radiation	Better tolerated
Wide application for quantitative analysis	Good for bone abnormalities
Greater sensitivity to detect white matter pathology and lesions causing epilepsy (such as inflammatory disease and hippocampal sclerosis)	Better for lesions with little or no water content (e.g. meningiomas) and detection of acute intracerebral haemorrhage

Table 11.3   Contraindications of MRI.

Claustrophobia/poorly tolerated (5–10 per cent): MRI scanners can be noisy and feel confined

Ferromagnetic implants, e.g. pacemakers, intracranial aneurysm clips, cochlear implants, neurostimulators: cardiac pacemakers can deprogramme and misfire so structural imaging with CT is the only option

Ferromagnetic objects in eyes

Orthopaedic implants are not contraindicated though may introduce local artefacts

disease (CJD), hippocampal sclerosis and inflammatory diseases. High spatial resolution (<1 mm) and superior soft tissue contrast also provides greater potential for early diagnosis. Moreover, brain structure can be examined in any plane and detailed volumetric quantification of regional and global morphology obtained, though multi-slice CT now offsets some of this advantage. Contraindications of MRI are summarized in **Table 11.3**.

As a general rule, CT is adequate for ruling out most intracerebral lesions, but has a more limited role than MRI for 'ruling in' degenerative disorders such as Alzheimer's disease (AD) and is less sensitive to vascular disease, especially when mild.

11.3   ASSESSMENT OF BRAIN ATROPHY

Early CT studies used simple linear measurements, such as the minimum width of the medial temporal lobe measured on temporal-lobe-oriented scans. These can be helpful in distinguishing patients with AD from healthy controls, but have less utility for distinguishing AD from other dementias (Jobst et al., 1992; O'Brien et al., 2000).

The majority of studies have used MRI to assess the extent and progression of atrophy and white matter pathology. These changes have been measured in different ways, ranging from simple and clinically applicable visual rating scales to sophisticated software programs only available in research centres. Few studies have compared the relative clinical utility of the different tools in different dementias, leaving uncertainty about which tool to best use in clinical practice. Nevertheless, in the case of AD, visual assessment of atrophy has a sensitivity and specificity for distinguishing AD from controls of between 70 and 90 per cent. Scales, such as the visual rating scale of medial temporal lobe atrophy (MTA)

(Scheltens et al., 1992), have the advantage of being simple and quick to use and provide information that correlates sufficiently well with quantitative in vivo analysis and neuropathological changes. Limitations include lack of detail and variable observer reliability.

In the research setting, MRI volumetric analysis is used for detailed quantification of even small amounts of atrophy. Historically, regions of interest were often manually traced, but this is time consuming and requires trained operators. More automated imaging software packages have been developed to provide a quicker and less operator-dependent way of assessing regional and global brain structures, both cross-sectionally and over time. Furthermore, unbiased techniques such as voxel-base morphometry (VBM) can examine changes in all parts of the brain, such as grey matter loss, rather than only predetermined regions. These automated techniques use different statistical modelling but cross-validation studies suggest they can produce comparable results, and they should become more applicable in clinical settings.

11.3.1   Cross-sectional and longitudinal studies

While cross-sectional studies compare atrophy in one disease group with either another, or normal age-related changes, longitudinal studies can measure the same structure in the same individual at two time points, thereby reducing the variance due to inter-subject differences. This technique is sufficiently sensitive to detect very small volume changes in the order of a few millilitres, which can be important during the presymptomatic or early stages of the disease when changes can be subtle (Scahill and Fox, 2007).

Regulatory authorities are keen for biomarkers to be used in clinical trials so the biological impact of new treatments can be appraised. Serial MRI has been used as surrogate end point in clinical trials in mild cognitive impairment (MCI) and AD. This can reduce the number of subjects required compared to clinical outcome measures.

Serial scanning has a number of methodological challenges: atrophy rates can vary considerably between subjects; serial scanning of patients with advancing dementia can be problematic; there are technical and cost implications; currently a gap of at least six months between scans is required before volume change can be consistently detected; and ultimately there is a need for post-mortem validation.

As we age, approximately 0.5 per cent of brain volume is lost every year, and as our brains become smaller our ventricles become larger, often at a faster rate. The pace of this change accelerates with age, particularly after 70 years, and appears to be associated with greater cognitive decline. The hippocampus appears to be particularly sensitive to the effects of ageing (as well as AD pathology) and atrophies at a faster rate than other structures. These age-related changes are common but not inevitable, and there is considerable variation between individuals. Atrophy is likely to be influenced by a number of factors, including genetic status (such as presence of apolipoprotein E (ApoE) ε4 alleles), health status (such as hypertension and diabetes), socioeconomic status and possibly dietary and hormonal factors. The impact of these variables may be evident by middle age.

Compared to age-matched controls, increased rates of brain atrophy and ventricular enlargement have been documented in most major forms of dementia, including AD, dementia with Lewy bodies (DLB), vascular dementia (VaD), frontotemporal dementia (FTD), corticobasal degeneration (CBD), progressive supranuclear palsy (PSP) and Huntington's disease (HD) (O'Brien et al., 2001; Whitwell et al., 2007a). However, serial measures of global atrophy are unlikely to distinguish patients with different dementia types, although measures of regional atrophy rates could. For example, in AD, the rate of hippocampal atrophy is greater than the global atrophy rate – approximately 3–8 per cent compared to 1–3 per cent depending on the study. Conversely, subjects with FTD have a greater rate of frontal lobe atrophy compared to those with AD (Krueger et al., 2010). Individuals developing MCI also have accelerated patterns of regional atrophy compared to cognitively normal individuals.

and bands, and DWMH into punctate foci, early confluent foci and large confluent areas (Fazekas et al., 1987). **Table 11.4** summarizes the radiological differences between DWMH and established infarcts (see also **Figure 11.3**). White matter lesions on conventional MRI sequences can be assessed using simple rating scales, semi-quantitative scales and volumetric analysis. As summarized in Chapter 12, Functional brain imaging and connectivity in dementia, diffusion tensor imaging (DTI) allows the integrity and connectivity of white matter tracts to be studied in normal ageing as well as disease states, revealing important insights.

It is important to recognize that WML are clinically and pathologically heterogeneous (see **Table 11.5**). They become more common with advancing age, and can be found in all major forms of dementias as well as a host of other conditions, including MS, hydrocephalus, various leukodystrophies, cerebral oedema, neurosarcoid and conditions such as late life depression. As such, the clinical significance of WML continues to be debated though in general as DWMH become more extensive the more likely they are to be clinically and pathologically significant, with underlying vascular mechanisms playing an important role. The location of DWMH could have an important bearing on the clinical phenotype, with the 'disconnection' of key cortical-subcortical circuits mediating their effect on brain function. Periventricular hyperintensities, on the other hand, may have a more limited impact on the clinical outcome and be less coupled to vascular mechanisms.

White matter lesions are common in late life with a prevalence of between 8 and 92 per cent depending on the study, and appear to progress over time, although not necessarily in a uniform way. Across a life span white matter is in a constant state of change, with processes of maturation continuing into middle age, followed by progressive loss of myelin integrity (Bartzokis et al., 2003). White matter changes are also influenced by various cardiovascular factors. Indeed, the emerging picture suggests WML and atrophy share similar risk factors, and there may well be an inter-relationship between these MRI variables; for example higher rates of cerebral atrophy and ventricular dilatation have been associated with more severe WML.

Importantly, WML could also be a target for treatment; treatment of hypertension was associated with reduced risk of WML progression in cognitively normal subjects (Firbank et al., 2007).

11.4   WHITE MATTER LESIONS

Magnetic resonance imaging has had a central role characterizing white matter abnormalities. The nature and significance of such changes, however, remains an area of uncertainty. white matter lesions (WML) that appear as areas of reduced attenuation or leukoaraiosis on CT scanning are hyperintense on proton density, T_2-weighted and FLAIR MR images.

WML can be divided into those immediately adjacent to the ventricles (periventricular hyperintensities; PVH) and those located in the deep white matter (deep white matter hyperintensities; DWMH). As shown in **Figure 11.2**, PVH can be further subdivided into caps (frontal and occipital)

11.5   ALZHEIMER'S DISEASE

11.5.1   Early and established Alzheimer's disease

Generalized brain atrophy and ventricular enlargement are common in AD and individuals with AD lose brain volume at approximately four times the rate of controls (2 versus 0.5 per cent) (O'Brien et al., 2001). However, these changes are relatively non-specific and, more characteristically, AD is associated with early and progressive atrophy of the medial temporal lobes. Individuals with AD have significantly

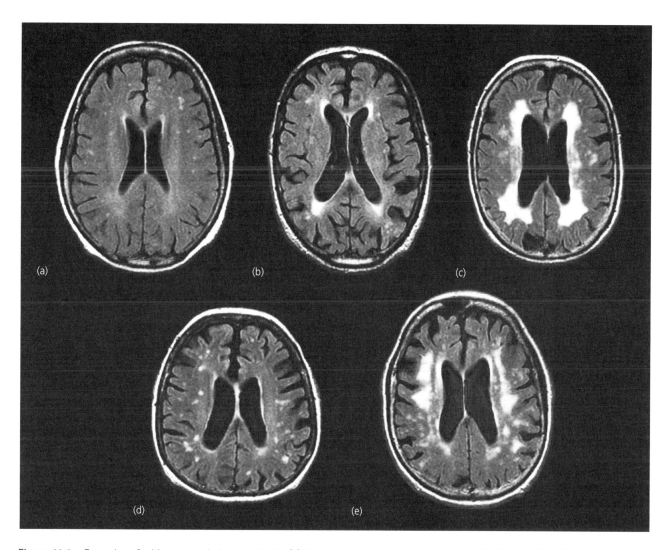

Figure 11.2   Examples of white matter lesions on FLAIR. (a) No periventricular hyperintensities (PVH); (b) mild PVH (frontal and occipital caps); (c) moderate to severe PVH (frontal and occipital caps); (d) punctate deep white matter hyperintensities (DWMH) (in frontal and parietal lobes); (e) large, early confluent DWMH.

Table 11.4   Differences between cerebral infarcts and deep white matter hyperintensities on MRI.

Infarcts	Deep white matter hyperintensities
Hypointense on T_1- and proton density weighted images	Hyperintense on T_2- and proton density weighted images
Hyperintense on T_2-weighted images	No change/invisible on T_1-weighted images
Well defined; wedge shape if peripheral	Range from punctuate to diffuse confluent lesions
Often single or low numbers	Often multiple
Often evidence of cortical extension	Restricted to white matter with no cortical extension
May be associated with focal enlargement of ventricles and sulci	Ventricles and sulci unchanged

smaller (by up to 40–50 per cent) hippocampi, para-hippocampi, which includes the entorhinal cortex, and amygdalae compared to normal controls. This is visualized as MTA on imaging as illustrated in **Figure 11.4** and **Figure 11.5**.

Medial temporal lobe atrophy occurs in 80–90 per cent of patients with AD compared to 5–10 per cent in control subjects. When measures of MTA are combined with other markers of reduced volume of the neocortex, differentiation

can be enhanced. For example, data from the AD Neuroimaging Initiative found combining measures of atrophy of the medial and lateral temporal lobe, cingulate and orbito-frontal areas gave a specificity of 93 per cent for discriminating healthy controls from those with AD (McEvoy *et al.*, 2009).

However, although MTA is a relatively sensitive marker of AD pathology, it is not specific to AD. Medial temporal lobe atrophy has been documented in a number of other

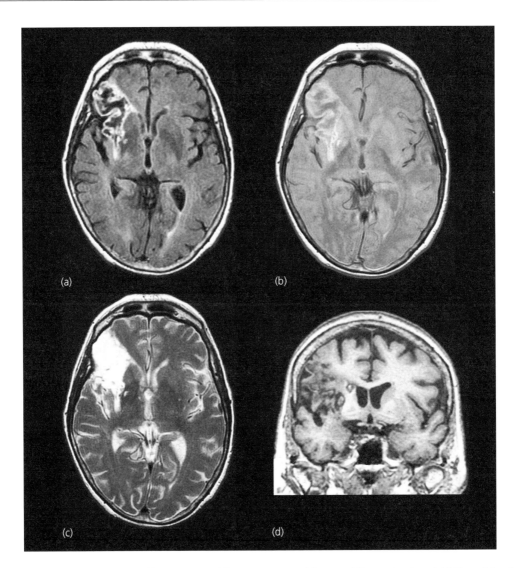

Figure 11.3 Example of frontal stroke on (a) axial FLAIR, (b) proton density, (c) coronal T$_1$-weighted, and (d) T$_2$-weighted.

Table 11.5 Histopathology associated with white matter lesions in dementias.

Lesion type	Pathology	Possible mechanisms
PVH	Less extensive PVH: loss of ependymal lining, increased interstitial fluid, gliosis, myelin pallor and dilatation of perivascular spaces	In part secondary to atrophy processes
	More extensive irregular PVH which extend into the deep white matter: likely to correspond to areas of reactive gliosis, lacunar infarction, loss of myelin, perivascular spaces and arteriolar thickening	Frontal caps extremely common in late life – could be considered 'normal' and secondary to age-related changes
		More extensive PVH probably linked to vascular risk factors
DWMH	Punctuate WMH: reduced myelination and perivenous damage	Punctate lesions are probably not associated with ischaemia/infarction
	Early confluent areas: show evidence of perivascular rarefaction of myelin, fibre loss and gliosis	Ischaemic damage implicated as lesions become larger and more confluent
	Confluent WMH: have a similar histopathology as irregular PVH, including microcystic infarcts	Other possible causes of white matter change include focal cerebral oedema, hypoxia, acidosis, chronic perfusion changes, Wallerian degeneration of axons secondary to neuronal loss in neocortex

DWMH, deep white matter hyperintensities; PVH, periventricular hyperintensities.

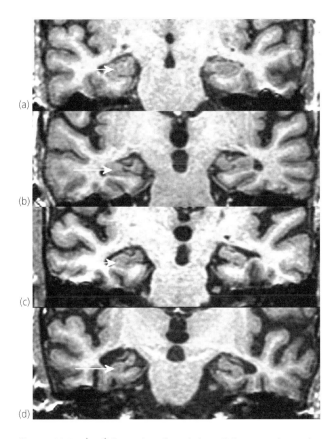

Figure 11.4 (a–d) Examples of graded medial temporal atrophy (MTA): arrows point to hippocampi.

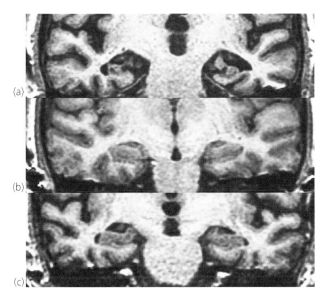

Figure 11.5 Comparison of medial temporal atrophy in (a) AD, (b) DLB and (c) normal controls.

conditions, such as VaD, DLB and FTD, though it may not always be as severe or common as in AD. Lesser degrees of MTA are also seen in Parkinson's disease, temporal lobe epilepsy, schizophrenia and depression. The lack of specificity of MTA may be because the atrophy reflects AD pathology, especially tau pathology (Burton *et al.*, 2009) that also occurs

in other dementias (O'Brien, 2007); MRI can provide secondary, not primary, evidence of AD (de Leon *et al.*, 2007).

Furthermore, there is an age-related atrophy of these structures that means the specificity of MTA as a biomarker for AD appears to decline with age, especially in the old (i.e. above 80 years). From a younger perspective, the pattern of atrophy in individuals who develop AD at a younger age (before 65 years) tend to have greater atrophy of the parietal (posterior cingulated and precuneus) and less medial temporal lobe atrophy (Frisoni *et al.*, 2007).

As AD progresses, atrophy occurs in nearly all limbic structures as well as the posterior cingulate cortex, possibly related to loss of afferent input from associated fibres. Overall, the distribution of atrophy is usually symmetrical and more prominent in medial and posterior brain structures than anterior structures, and develops in a way that is consistent with the Braak staging. By comparison, there is less atrophy in the frontal lobe, hypothalamus, thalamus, caudate and putamen, and relative sparing of the primary motor and sensory cortex, inferior occipitotemporal region and cerebellum (Baron *et al.*, 2001).

In terms of WML, most studies show that patients with AD have more extensive PVH and DWMH than controls. Loss of white matter integrity probably occurs for a number of reasons, including as a secondary downstream event to the primary cortical pathology, amyloid angiopathy and concurrent ischaemic damage.

In summary, MTA occurs early in the course of AD, and increases with increasing severity of dementia. As MTA is associated with the clinical diagnosis of AD, and associated with transition from MCI to AD, there have been recommendations to include estimates of MTA in revised criteria of the clinical diagnosis of early AD (Dubois *et al.*, 2007). Although MTA appears to be necessary for the development of AD, it is not sufficient to explain all symptomatic changes and, as Jack *et al.* (2002) speculate, MTA is a good marker for early AD, but as the disease progresses beyond the limbic areas, measures of neocortical atrophy may be better markers of advanced disease.

11.5.2 Prognostic significance of medial temporal lobe atrophy in individuals at risk of Alzheimer's disease and those with mild cognitive impairment

There is good evidence that MTA can occur before symptoms emerge and, by the time mild symptoms are apparent, hippocampal volume reductions may exceed 25 per cent.

The prognostic relevance of MTA in predicting cognitive decline and eventual dementia in individuals at risk of AD has been studied in two main groups: subjects with a familial, dominantly inherited form of AD and subjects with MCI. Findings to date suggest atrophy starts at least three years before clinical diagnosis of AD (Whitwell *et al.*, 2007a). This raises the prospect that there are changes that could be detected in due course to enable subjects 'at risk' to be identified. Indeed, this transitional phase from 'silent' pathology to emerging symptoms may be associated with the most aggressive phase of MTA. Similar techniques have been applied to identify presymptomatic structural changes in other genetic degenerative disorders, such as FTD and Huntington's disease (HD).

Individuals with MCI are at increased risk of developing dementia (see Chapter 44, Clinical characteristics of mild cognitive impairment). Detection of MCI is therefore important, and the role of neuroimaging in MCI has been extensively studied. Baseline temporal lobe atrophy correlates with future cognitive decline and conversion from MCI to AD (Hua *et al.*, 2008). As with presymptomatic studies, significant hippocampal (7–15 per cent) and entorhinal cortex volume (5–32 per cent) reductions are the most consistently described difference between subjects with MCI and cognitively unimpaired controls. Subjects who are moving along the trajectory from normal to MCI lose more of their hippocampal volume than those who remain stable. Overall, the results from visual rating of atrophy and cross-sectional and longitudinal volumetric studies have found the changes in MCI are intermediate between normal subjects and AD. The intermediate nature of these results is reflected in the relatively lower sensitivity (60 per cent) and specificity (80 per cent) of measures of MTA in discriminating MCI and controls compared to their discrimination of AD (Xu *et al.*, 2000). It is possible that composite MRI measures involving MTA plus other grey matter regions and white matter changes can improve the prediction of individual subjects with MCI who are at risk of developing AD (Misra *et al.*, 2009).

11.6   DEMENTIA WITH LEWY BODIES

Imaging changes in DLB are less well characterized than those of AD. Evidence indicates that DLB patients have greater preservation of medial temporal lobe structures than those with AD and VaD, as shown in **Figure 11.5** (Barber

et al., 2000; Barber *et al.*, 2001; Burton *et al.*, 2009). In addition, findings suggest there is atrophy of subcortical structures, including the putamen, substantia innominata and dorsal midbrain. Indeed, a pattern of relatively focused atrophy of the midbrain, hypothalamus and substantia innominata, with a relative sparing of the hippocampus and temporoparietal cortex is more likely to occur in DLB compared to AD (Whitwell *et al.*, 2007b). Post-mortem studies are generally consistent with these findings, and this may help explain differences in the profile of cognitive deficits between these disorders.

Although DLB is associated with visual hallucinations and occipital lobe changes in blood flow and metabolism on single photon emission computed tomography (SPECT), there are no gross structural changes in the occipital lobe on MRI (Middelkoop *et al.*, 2001).

Patients with DLB generally have greater whole brain atrophy compared to normal controls but less than those with AD. Annual rates of global atrophy in DLB are similar to those in AD and VaD, but greater than normal controls (O'Brien *et al.*, 2001).

Subjects with DLB probably share a similar distribution, prevalence and severity of WML to AD on MRI, intermediate in severity between normal controls and those with VaD (Barber *et al.*, 1999), though studies are not conclusive (Burton *et al.*, 2006). Preliminary data suggest WML in DLB are less likely to progress than those in AD and Parkinson's disease dementia (PDD).

11.7   FRONTOTEMPORAL DEMENTIA

Frontotemporal dementia is characterized by atrophy of the frontal and anterior temporal lobes. A normal MRI scan does not necessarily exclude the illness, especially early in the

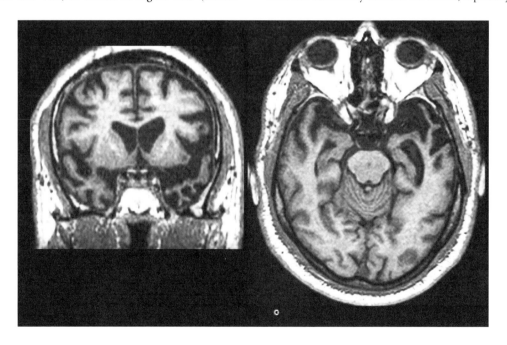

Figure 11.6   Patient with clinical diagnosis of semantic dementia showing bilateral anterior temporal lobe atrophy, left > right side: coronal and axial T$_1$-weighted images (courtesy of Prof T Griffiths).

illness, and in such instances functional imaging may assist in the diagnosis. If both structural and functional imaging are normal, however, the risk of making a false positive diagnosis of FTD may be increased (Kipps *et al.*, 2009). As subjects with FTD can have varying degrees of MTA, it is the pattern of prominent frontotemporal anterior atrophy that helps to differentiate it from other dementias, such as AD (especially with the anterior temporal pole more atrophied in FTD).

Table 11.6 MRI findings in other diseases associated with cognitive impairment.

Disorder	MRI findings
variant Creutzfeldt-Jakob disease (vCJD)	Symmetrical hyperintensity in the pulvinar (posterior) nuclei of the thalamus relative to the anterior thalamus (pulvinar sign). Other features are hyperintensity of the dorsomedial thalamic nuclei, caudate head and periaqueductal gray matter
sporadic CJD (sCJD)	High signal changes in the putamen, caudate and/or thalamus and cortical gyri (cortical ribboning). DWI has a high sensitivity and specificity for sCJD, (especially in detecting cortical changes c/w other MRI sequences)
Huntington's disease (HD)	Bilateral caudate atrophy – may also have reduced volume of other basal ganglia structures and frontal lobes
progressive supranuclear palsy (PSP)	Brain stem atrophy and non-specific mild atrophy
multisystem atrophy (MSA)	Olivopontocerebellar or basal ganglia atrophy depending on variant
normal pressure hydrocephalus (NPH)	Marked ventricular enlargement, with rounding of anterior horns of lateral ventricles. Ventricular enlargement is proportionate to sulcal widening – sulci normal, no significant white matter pathology

Table 11.7 Structural imaging requirements for current diagnostic systems for dementia.

Diagnosis	Specific diagnostic criteria	Comments
AD	NINCDS-ADRDA criteria (McKhann *et al.*, 1984): ↑ ventricles, gyri are narrowed, sulci are widened. General patterns may not be useful as diagnostic criteria in individual cases	All the major diagnostic criteria for AD focus on neuroimaging excluding competing causes of cognitive impairment and lack reference to possible neuroimaging inclusion criteria for AD, such as medial temporal lobe atrophy
DLB	Consensus criteria for DLB (McKeith *et al.*, 2005): Suggestive neuroimaging feature is low dopamine transporter uptake in the basal ganglia on functional neuroimaging. Additional supportive imaging features that commonly occur in DLB, but with lower specificity, include relative preservation of medial temporal lobe structures on structural neuroimaging, reduced occipital activity on functional neuroimaging, and low uptake myocardial scintigraph	Low dopamine transporter uptake in the basal ganglia on functional neuroimaging (notably (123)I-FP-CIT SPECT can be clinically useful in diagnostically uncertain cases, as an abnormal scan in a person with possible DLB is strongly suggestive of DLB
FTD	Consensus clinical criteria for frontotemporal dementia (Neary *et al.*, 1998): Abnormalities (structural and/or functional imaging) may be bilaterally symmetrical or asymmetric, affecting the left or right hemisphere disproportionally, though failure to demonstrate these prototypic appearances need not exclude diagnosis	In addition, two neuroimaging exclusion features are described: the presence of multifocal lesions and predominant post-central structural or functional deficits
VaD	California criteria for ischaemic vascular dementia (IVD) (Chui *et al.*, 1992): 'Probable' IVD – requires at least one infarct outside the cerebellum. 'Possible' IVD – does not require neuroimaging evidence of infarction The NINDS-AIREN criteria (Roman *et al.*, 1993): need to define the extent, topography and severity of vascular lesions 'Probable VaD' – multiple infarcts or strategic single infarcts or multiple subcortical or white matter lesions (at least 25 per cent of total white matter)	The NINDS-AIREN criteria have the most rigorous neuroimaging criteria. Specifically state that the absence of cerebrovascular lesions on brain CT or MRI makes the diagnosis of vascular dementia unlikely NINDS-AIREN versus California criteria: NINDS-AIREN criteria recognize that a single lesion may cause VaD and that radiological lesions regardless of location may be taken as evidence of cerebrovascular disease (excluding 'trivial' infarcts), require vascular change to fulfil criteria for both location and severity

AD, Alzheimer's disease; DLB, dementia with Lewy bodies; DSM, Diagnostic and Statistical Manual; FTD, frontotemporal dementia; ICD, International Classification of Diseases; VaD, vascular dementia.

Frontotemporal dementia consists of a number of clinical phenotypes with differing though overlapping MRI findings. The MRI findings in the behavioural variant of FTD is heterogeneous, with varying degrees of atrophy occurring along the frontal-to-temporal lobe axis, and in some instances including the parietal lobes (Whitwell *et al.*, 2009).

The other phenotypes of FTD include progressive non-fluent aphasia (PA) and semantic dementia (SD) with MRI changes largely confined to the temporal lobes. Progressive non-fluent aphasia is characterized by asymmetrical, left-sided perisylvian atrophy. As shown in **Figure 11.6**, temporal atrophy in SD tends to be more bilateral, though can be asymmetrical.

In common with most other dementias, annual rates of whole-brain atrophy are increased compared to controls. Provisional findings indicate WML are common, but as with AD and DLB, less severe than VaD. Their pathological basis, however, is likely to be different and reflect gliosis rather than ischaemic damage or amyloid angiopathy.

11.8   VASCULAR DEMENTIA

Clinically relevant ischaemic damage can be visualized on MRI as cortical infarcts, infarcts in strategic brain areas (such as the thalamus), multiple lacunar infarcts, extensive white matter change (usually defined as area > 25 per cent), or combinations thereof. There may also be evidence of both generalized and focal atrophy, either cortical or ventricular, corresponding to an area of infarction with subsequent local cell loss and atrophy. White matter changes in VaD are common and usually severe: large irregular PVH, confluent DWMH and basal ganglia hyperintensities are characteristic of VaD, reflecting a greater burden of ischaemia.

The relationship between cognitive impairment and vascular change remains an area of uncertainty and so interpreting the significance or otherwise of vascular changes on imaging can be difficult. For example, 'silent' lacunar infarcts as well as cerebral microbleeds are more common in non-cognitively impaired community-dwelling elderly people than previously recognized. Microbleeds are best visualized using gradient echo T_2 imaging, and are increased in normal ageing, dementias and VaD. Their pathogenesis is not yet fully determined, but may reflect microbleeding due to amlyoid angiopathy. Likewise, in clinical samples, small vessel disease on MRI is probably more commonly associated with VaD than large vessel disease, and subcortical ischaemic vascular disease is a significant risk factor for developing dementia (Jokinen *et al.*, 2009). Furthermore, the prevalence of mixed dementias is also more widely recognized, and postmortem studies have yet to show a clear link between lesion location and severity and clinical outcomes.

It is likely that 'non-vascular' variables influence whether cognitive deficits develop in the presence of vascular disease. For example, generalized changes such as cortical atrophy and MTA as well as variables such as age and level of education may play an important role in the development of post-stroke dementia and VaD attributed to small-vessel disease (Staekenborg *et al.*, 2008). Again, evidence from

Table 11.8   Examples of guidelines for imaging in dementia.

Selective criteria: example from guidelines	All-inclusive criteria: examples of statements from opinion leaders and guidelines
Canadian Consensus Conference on Dementia (Patterson *et al.*, 2001). Recommendations for neuroimaging	Knopman *et al.* (2001) Practice Parameters: Diagnosis of dementia (evidence-based guidelines) from the American Academy of Neurology. Recommend: structural neuroimaging with either a noncontrast CT or MRI scan in the routine initial evaluation of patients with dementia is appropriate
Cranial CT scan is recommended if one or more of the following criteria are present	
	Scheltens *et al.* (2002): neuroimaging, and MRI in particular, is increasingly regarded as an essential part of the investigation of a patient with dementia
A Age less than 60 years	
B Rapid, (e.g. over one to two months) unexplained decline in cognition or function	
C Short duration of dementia (less than two years)	
D Recent and significant head trauma	
E Unexplained neurological symptoms, e.g. new onset of severe headache or seizures	
F History of cancer (especially in sites and types that metastasize to the brain)	
G Use of anticoagulants or history of a bleeding disorder	
H History of urinary incontinence and gait disorder early in the course of dementia (as may be found in normopressure hydrocephalus)	
I Any new localizing sign (e.g. hemiparesis or Babinski reflex)	
J Unusual or atypical cognitive symptoms or presentation (e.g. progressive aphasia, gait disturbance)	

post-mortem studies suggest there is a synergistic relationship between vascular and degenerative pathologies, such that the presence of AD-type pathology can increase the clinical consequences of cerebrovascular disease, and vice versa. The recognition that vascular and degenerative disease share similar risk factors adds another level of complexity to their relationship.

11.9   OTHER DEMENTIAS

Other less common dementias with relatively distinct neuroradiological features on MRI are summarized in **Table 11.6**.

11.10   FINAL COMMENTS

Most guidelines take the view that all patients with dementia should have structural imaging performed at least once during their illness. Functional imaging is also likely to have an important role in enhancing diagnostic accuracy (see Chapter 12, Functional brain imaging and connectivity in dementia).

An important question is perhaps: 'If I need to make a diagnosis, what sort of imaging do I need to perform?' **Table 11.7** summarizes the different neuroimaging criteria for main diagnostic classifications of dementias. A CT will, for cost and practical reasons, usually be the imaging modality most often used, although an MRI, if accessible and feasible, would almost always be the superior imaging modality (**Table 11.8**). It is important to remember that information obtained from imaging needs to be interpreted in the context of other clinical findings, such as details from the history, mental and physical state as well as the most accurate other investigations to arrive at a clinical diagnosis.

REFERENCES

Barber R, Scheltens P, Gholkar A et al. (1999) White matter lesions on magnetic resonance imaging in dementia with Lewy bodies, Alzheimer's disease, vascular dementia, and normal aging. *Journal of Neurology, Neurosurgery and Psychiatry* 67: 66–72.

Barber R, Ballard C, McKeith IG et al. (2000) MRI volumetric study of dementia with Lewy bodies: A comparison with Alzheimer's disease and vascular dementia. *Neurology* 54: 1304–9.

Barber R, McKeith IG, Ballard C et al. (2001) A comparison of medial and lateral temporal lobe atrophy in dementia with Lewy bodies and Alzheimer's disease: MRI Volumetric Study. *Dementia and Geriatric Cognitive Disorders* 12: 198–205.

Baron JC, Chetelat G, Desgranges B et al. (2001) *In vivo* mapping of gray matter loss with voxel-based morphometry in mild Alzheimer's disease. *Neuroimage* 14: 298–309.

Bartzokis G, Cummings JL, Sultzer D et al. (2003) White matter structural integrity in healthy aging adults and patients with Alzheimer disease: a magnetic resonance imaging study. *Archives of Neurology* 60: 393–8.

Burton EJ, McKeith IG, Burn DJ et al. (2006) Progression of white matter hyperintensities in Alzheimer disease, dementia with lewy bodies, and Parkinson disease dementia: a comparison with normal aging. *American Journal of Geriatric Psychiatry* 14: 842–9.

Burton EJ, Barber R, Mukaetova-Ladinska EB et al. (2009) Medial temporal lobe atrophy on MRI differentiates Alzheimer's disease from dementia with Lewy bodies and vascular cognitive impairment: a prospective study with pathological verification of diagnosis. *Brain* 132 (Pt 1): 195–203.

Chui HC, Victoroff JI, Margolin D et al. (1992) Criteria for the diagnosis of ischaemic vascular dementia proposed by the State of California Alzheimer's Disease Diagnostic and Treatment Centres. *Neurology* 42: 473–80.

de Leon MJ, Mosconi L, Blennow K et al. (2007) Imaging and CSF studies in the preclinical diagnosis of Alzheimer's disease. *Annals of the New York Academy of Sciences* 1097: 114–45.

Dubois B, Feldman HH, Jacova C et al. (2007) Research criteria for the diagnosis of Alzheimer's disease: revising the NINCDS-ADRDA criteria. *Lancet Neurology* 6: 734–46.

Fazekas F, Chawluk JB, Alavi A et al. (1987) MR signal abnormalities at 1.5T in Alzheimer's disease and normal ageing. *American Journal of Roentgenology* 149: 351–6.

Firbank MJ, Wiseman RM, Burton EJ et al. (2007) Brain atrophy and white matter hyperintensity change in older adults and relationship with blood pressure. *Journal of Neurology* 254: 713–21.

Frisoni GB, Pievani M, Testa C et al. (2007) The topography of grey matter involvement in early and late onset Alzheimer's disease. *Brain* 130: 720–30.

Hua X, Leow AD, Lee S et al. (2008) 3D characterization of brain atrophy in Alzheimer's disease and mild cognitive impairment using tensor-based morphometry. *Neuroimage* 41: 19–34.

Jack Jr CR, Dickson DW, Parisi JE et al. (2002) Antemortem MRI findings correlate with hippocampal neuropathology in typical aging and dementia. *Neurology* 58: 750–7.

Jobst KA, Smith AD, Szatmari M et al. (1992) Detection in life of confirmed Alzheimer's disease using a simple measurement of medial temporal lobe atrophy by computed tomography. *Lancet* 340: 1179–83.

Jokinen H, Kalska H, Ylikoski R et al. (2009) Longitudinal cognitive decline in subcortical ischemic vascular disease – the LADIS Study. *Cerebrovascular Diseases* 27: 384–91.

Kipps CM, Hodges JR, Fryer TD et al. (2009) Combined magnetic resonance imaging and positron emission tomography brain imaging in behavioural variant frontotemporal degeneration: refining the clinical phenotype. *Brain* 132 (Pt 9): 2566–78.

Knopman DS, DeKosky ST, Cummings JL et al. (2001) Practice parameters: Diagnosis of dementia (an evidence-based review). Report of the Quality Standards Subcommittee of the American Academy of Neurology. *Neurology* 56: 1143–53.

Krueger CE, Dean DL, Rosen HJ et al. (2010) Longitudinal rates of lobar atrophy in frontotemporal dementia, semantic dementia, and Alzheimer's disease. *Alzheimer Diseases and Associated Disorders* 24: 43–8.

McEvoy LK, Fennema-Notestine C, Roddey JC. (2009) Alzheimer's disease: quantitative structural neuroimaging for detection and prediction of clinical and structural changes in mild cognitive impairment. *Radiology* **251**: 195–205.

McKeith IG, Dickson DW, Lowe J *et al.* (2005) Diagnosis and management of dementia with Lewy bodies: third report of the DLB Consortium. *Neurology* **65**: 1863–72.

McKhann G, Drachman D, Folstein M *et al.* (1984) Clinical diagnosis of Alzheimer's disease: report of the NINCDS-ADRDA Work Group under the auspices of Department of Health and Human Service Task Force on Alzheimer's disease. *Neurology* **34**: 939–44.

Middelkoop HA, van der Flier WM, Burton EJ *et al.* (2001) Dementia with Lewy bodies and AD are not associated with occipital lobe atrophy on MRI. *Neurology* **57**: 2117–20.

Misra C, Fan Y, Davatzikos C. (2009) Baseline and longitudinal patterns of brain atrophy in MCI patients, and their use in prediction of short-term conversion to AD: results from ADNI. *Neuroimage* **44**: 1415–22.

Neary D, Snowden JS, Gustafson L *et al.* (1998) Frontotemporal lobar degeneration: a consensus on clinical diagnostic criteria. *Neurology* **51**: 1546–54.

O'Brien JT. (2007) Role of imaging techniques in the diagnosis of dementia. *British Journal of Radiology* **80**: S71–7.

O'Brien JT, Metcalfe S, Swann A *et al.* (2000) Medial temporal lobe width on CT scanning in Alzheimer's disease: comparison with vascular dementia, depression and dementia with Lewy bodies. *Dementia and Geriatric Cognitive Disorders* **11**: 114–18.

O'Brien JT, Paling S, Barber R *et al.* (2001) Progressive brain atrophy on serial MRI in dementia with Lewy bodies, AD, and vascular dementia. *Neurology* **56**: 1386–8.

Patterson C, Gauthier S, Bergman H *et al.* (2001) The recognition, assessment and management of dementing disorders: conclusions from the Canadian Consensus Conference on Dementia. *Canadian Journal of Neurological Sciences* **28** (Suppl. 1): S3–16.

Román GC, Tatemichi T, Erkinjuntti T *et al.* (1993) Vascular dementia: diagnostic criteria for research studies. Report of the NINDS-AIRENS international workshop. *Neurology* **43**: 250–60.

Scahill RI, Fox NC. (2007) Longitudinal imaging in dementia. *British Journal of Radiology* **80**: 592–8.

Scheltens P, Leys D, Barkhof F *et al.* (1992) Atrophy of medial temporal lobes on MRI in "probable" Alzheimer's disease and normal ageing: diagnostic value and neuropsychological correlates. *Journal of Neurology, Neurosurgery and Psychiatry* **55**: 967–72.

Scheltens P, Fox N, Barkhof F, De Carli C. (2002) Structural magnetic resonance imaging in the practical assessment of dementia: beyond exclusion. *Lancet Neurology* **1**: 13–21.

Staekenborg SS, van Straaten EC, van der Flier WM *et al.* (2008) Small vessel versus large vessel vascular dementia: risk factors and MRI findings. *Journal of Neurology* **255**: 1644–51.

Whitwell JL, Jack CR Jr, Parisi JE *et al.* (2007a) Rates of cerebral atrophy differ in different degenerative pathologies. *Brain* **130**: 1148–58.

Whitwell JL, Weigand SD, Shiung MM *et al.* (2007b) Focal atrophy in dementia with Lewy bodies on MRI: a distinct pattern from Alzheimer's disease. *Brain* **130** (Pt 3): 708–19.

Whitwell JL, Przybelski SA, Weigand SD *et al.* (2009) Distinct anatomical subtypes of the behavioural variant of frontotemporal dementia: a cluster analysis study. *Brain* **132** (Pt 11): 2932–46.

Xu Y, Jack Jr CR, O'Brien PC *et al.* (2000) Usefulness of MRI measures of entorhinal cortex versus hippocampus in AD. *Neurology* **56**: 820–1.

Functional brain imaging and connectivity in dementia

KLAUS P EBMEIER, NICOLA FILIPPINI AND CLARE E MACKAY

12.1 INTRODUCTION

Neuroimaging offers a window into the living brain and thus provides unique access to understanding both normal and pathological processes associated with ageing. Structural imaging has diagnostic, and to some extent prognostic, value in dementia (see Chapter 11, Structural brain imaging). This chapter reviews the literature on functional imaging in dementia and also considers new methods for looking at both structural and functional connectivity in the brain. It explores whether these techniques, some of which are novel but some of which have been used for several decades, have added to our understanding of pathological ageing. In particular we will focus on whether any of the myriad of imaging acquisition and analysis techniques can be considered biomarkers, i.e. aid the clinician in diagnosis, prognosis or evaluating treatments.

Although several different technologies will be described, neuroimaging studies of brain function in dementia largely fall into two categories: (1) the study of resting blood flow and (2) measurement of brain changes due to a specific task. This chapter starts with a brief description of methodologies of emission tomography, functional magnetic resonance imaging and diffusion tensor imaging before describing applications in patients with dementia.

12.2 IMAGING METHODS

12.2.1 Single photon emission computed tomography

Single photon emission computed tomography (SPECT) uses γ emitting radioisotopes which are attached to biologically relevant molecules and injected intravenously to be distributed, among others, to the brain. The three-dimensional reconstruction of the tracer distribution in the brain gives a biologically meaningful map of, for example, blood flow, receptor binding capacity or similar measures. In order to focus the signal on the γ camera, collimators are used. These collimators only admit photons coming from a defined direction to the photosensitive crystal. By implication, this method of directional filtering only allows for a small proportion of emitted photons to be detected, which limits the sensitivity of SPECT. The attenuation of γ rays during their path through brain matter is usually modelled making assumptions of homogenous attenuation across the brain and head. Some common applications of SPECT are listed in **Table 12.1**. Gamma emitters with half-lives of 6–12 hours are usually employed, as the tracers tend to be produced some distance from the scanner. Because of this, limited numbers of exposures are possible. The γ emitting nuclei

Table 12.1   Some common applications of SPECT and PET.

Tracer	Isotope-mode	Physiology	Clinical use
HMPAO[a]	^{99m}T-SPECT	Perfusion	Yes
IMP[b]	^{123}I-SPECT	Perfusion	Yes
ECD[c]	^{99m}Tc-SPECT	Perfusion	Yes
Water	^{15}O-PET	Blood flow	Rare
Oxygen	^{15}O-PET	Oxygen uptake	No
FDG[d]	^{18}F-PET	Glucose uptake (aerobic + anaerobic)	Yes
Glucose	^{11}C-PET	Glucose uptake (aerobic)	No

[a] Hexamethylpropyleneamine oxime.
[b] N-isopropyl-(iodine-123)p-iodoamphetamine.
[c] Ethylene cysteinate dimer.
[d] Fluoro-deoxyglucose.

employed (^{123}I and ^{99m}Tc) are relatively large and tend to change the pharmacology of the substituted molecule. The extensive pharmacological development work necessary for such tracers may therefore be one of the explanations for the relatively limited number of γ (SPECT)-ligands available.

12.2.2   Positron emission tomography

Positron emission tomography (PET) uses positron emitters to label physiological brain processes. Positrons (positively charged electrons) are non-stable elementary particles; within millimetres travel they react with an electron to generate two photons with a defined energy moving at approximately 180° away from each other. The detection of such coincidence signals with a detector ring thus makes it possible to identify spatial as well as intensity information. Collimators are thus not necessary and signal detection is more sensitive. Positron emitting nuclei, particularly ^{11}C, are easily incorporated into biological molecules, without changing their chemical characteristics. Positron emission is relatively energetic – only short exposure to radiation is possible, the short decay half-lives require on-site radiochemistry to incorporate the nuclei into physiologically active compounds. In turn, short half-lives allow for repeated application of tracers. Usually transmission scans with a γ source in the detector rings are used to quantify the attenuation across the brain.

12.2.3   Functional magnetic resonance imaging

Magnetic resonance imaging (MRI) uses completely different physical principles from emission tomographies, both for the constitution and the spatial encoding of images (see Chapter 11, Structural brain imaging). The most frequently used technique for investigating function is blood oxygen level-dependent (BOLD) imaging. Oxy- and deoxyhaemoglobin have different ferromagnetic properties and therefore differentially affect a magnetic field. The relative concentration of oxyhaemoglobin increases in active brain areas, as blood flow increases more than oxygen extraction. The haemodynamic response function over time can be described in greater detail as a three-stage process. First, an initial small negative dip appears about 1 second after neuronal activation (Menon et al., 1993). This is believed to be due to the oxyhaemoglobin decrease that immediately follows neuronal activation. Second, the positive BOLD response peaks at about 5–7 seconds with a pronounced elevation of signal intensity due to increased blood flow coupled with a relatively smaller oxygen extraction resulting in an increased oxy-/deoxyhaemoglobin ratio. At the very beginning of the positive BOLD response an overshoot of the BOLD signal can often be noticed, presumably due to a slow cerebral blood volume adjustment in the face of a rapid increase in cerebral blood flow (Mandeville et al., 1999). Finally, the same principle explains the undershoot at the end of the activation that is followed by an abrupt below-threshold decrease of cerebral blood flow and by a persistently high cerebral blood volume which takes longer to return back to baseline values. A typical BOLD response based on a blocked design (or box car) experiment usually lasts between 20 and 30 seconds: 6–9 seconds are needed to reach peak activity, 8–20 seconds to return back to baseline. In spite of very fast MRI sequences used for functional magnetic resonance imaging (fMRI) (acquiring brain images every 50–100 ms), the vascular-haemodynamic response therefore represents an intrinsic limit to its temporal resolution. One advantage of fMRI compared with emission tomography lies in its higher spatial resolution of a few millimetres.

Blood oxygen level-dependent signal changes associated with neuronal activity are generally small, in the order of 2–5 per cent, and largely depend on the magnetic field strength of the scanner. Moreover, the strength of the detectable BOLD signal seems to vary across different brain regions (Birn et al., 2001), with visual areas having the strongest BOLD signal, whereas other brain areas, such as temporal and orbitofrontal are more difficult to study with traditional MRI sequences, due to signal loss and MRI field inhomogeneitiy artefacts.

Brain activations with well-defined BOLD signal have been obtained for functions, such as language, movement, hearing and memory. However, the BOLD signal as a measure of brain activity is still controversial. Indeed, signal changes may be generated more by synaptic than by neuronal body activity (Arthurs and Boniface, 2002). This implies that brain regions apparently active during fMRI experiments may be located at a distance from the true site of neuronal activity. Moreover, as synaptic activity can be either excitatory or inhibitory, the interpretation of fMRI results continues to be debated.

A significant advantage of fMRI over emission tomography-based techniques is that it is non-invasive, so repeated examinations are possible, and within each subject high signal to noise ratios can be achieved by repeating scans many times. On the other hand, fMRI is a loud procedure in a restricted environment and is problematic for anyone who suffers from claustrophobia. Brain lesions are likely sources of error for all functional imaging techniques, and head movement and susceptibility artefacts due to tissue–air boundaries are a particular problem for fMRI. For obvious reasons, such artefacts are more likely to occur in older age and in psychiatric patients. Functional MRI analyses continue to be developed in the research context, and are by no means standardized. The clinical use of fMRI in dementia is therefore an emerging field.

12.2.4   Blood flow magnetic resonance imaging (arterial spin labelling)

In a technique analogous to for example O-15 labelled H_2O-PET, MRI contrast media (e.g. gadolinium) can be injected and their brain concentration measured dynamically to obtain a quantitative measurement of cerebral blood flow (CBF). Studies have reported similar reductions in CBF in AD patients using this technique as have been established by PET and SPECT (Gonzalez et al., 1995). However, other MRI techniques, such as arterial spin labelling (ASL), have been recently developed for measuring quantitative CBF in a non-invasive way (Wong et al., 1997). Arterial spin labelling is based on the modification of blood magnetization in an artery (e.g. carotid) by magnetically labelling blood flowing into the brain. Arterial spin labelling thus uses a 'tracer', but instead of it being exogenous, as for PET, SPECT, XeCT or gadolinium MRI, the tracer is in this case magnetically labelled water in flowing blood. Blood flowing into the imaging slice exchanges with tissue water, thus also altering tissue magnetization (Detre et al., 1992). A perfusion-weighted image can be generated by subtracting an image in which inflowing water molecules have been spin labelled from an image without spin labelling. Although still very much in development, ASL can be used to obtain either a static measurement of resting blood flow, or can be measured dynamically to obtain a more quantitative fMRI signal. Compared with the BOLD signal, ASL offers certain advantages, such as improved sensitivity to slow changes in neural activity, reduced inter-subject variability and generally reduced sensitivity to susceptibility artefacts. Furthermore, ASL provides a quantitative measure of the CBF, which may be more closely related to neuronal activation than the BOLD signal (Miller et al., 2001). Arterial spin labelling can be useful for clinical studies as quantitative perfusion measurements provide information in studies where healthy and diseased participants are compared. Arterial spin labelling also allows for a more specific functional localization because

the blood flow signal can be better spatially localized to the site of neuronal activity, and the ASL signal reaches the activity peak earlier and has less variance in peak latency compared with the BOLD signal. Arterial spin labelling has been less extensively used than fMRI BOLD because of certain disadvantages. First, it is more difficult to implement, largely because it currently relies on non-proprietary sequences and therefore can only be run in laboratories with physics support. Second, it has less brain coverage and a poorer temporal resolution, mainly due to the pairwise acquisition of label and control images as well as the required delay time for the tagged blood to flow into imaging slices. Finally, it has a smaller signal change magnitude (typically less than 1 per cent) compared with BOLD, and for this reason it is unsuitable for tasks involving fast activity changes.

Using ASL, significantly reduced CBF in brain regions known to be affected by AD pathology, such as precuneus, posterior cingulate, parietal association cortex and inferior temporal lobe, have been consistently reported in AD patients relative to healthy controls (Johnson et al., 2005; Alsop et al., 2008). Alsop et al. (2008) reported significantly greater CBF values in AD patients relative to controls in the hippocampus, and more broadly the medial–temporal complex, after correcting for grey matter differences. This finding emphasizes the necessity to account for morphological differences when investigating functional or physiological differences in studies involving AD patients. Moreover, it suggests that potential compensatory or pathological mechanisms may modulate neural activity in brain regions where atrophy occurs.

Arterial spin labelling has also been tested in a more clinically oriented environment. Alzheimer's disease (AD) patients had reduced CBF values relative to frontal lobe dementia (FTD) patients in posterior brain regions, such as posterior cingulate and parietal lobes, whereas FTD patients had reduced CBF values in frontal regions relative to AD patients. The combined use of grey matter atrophy and perfusion values improved the discrimination between FTD patients and healthy controls, yielding a correct classification value of 74 per cent (71 per cent sensitivity, 76 per cent specificity). In addition, the combination of grey matter and CBF values improved the differential diagnosis between FTD and AD patients with 87 per cent correctly classified (90 per cent sensitivity, 83 per cent specificity) (Du et al., 2006). In another study comparing AD, MCI and healthy controls, the AD patients showed the lowest CBF values within the posterior cingulate, precuneus and parietal lobes relative to healthy controls and MCI, whereas the MCI patients had reduced CBF values in the right inferior parietal lobe compared with the healthy participants (Xu et al., 2007).

12.2.5   Diffusion tensor imaging

As described in Chapter 11, Structural brain imaging, most of the research into structural deficits associated with dementia primarily concerns grey matter. However, white matter pathology has also been reported in AD and is noted in many other neurodegenerative diseases. Diffusion tensor imaging (DTI) is a structural imaging technique that is used to investigate the integrity of white matter pathways in the brain. Diffusion-weighted images measure the movement of water molecules within tissue, and when acquired in multiple directions, are sensitized to diffusion in all directions in the brain. Two quantitative measurements can be obtained from DTI data. The first is a measurement of the total amount of diffusion in a voxel and is variously referred to as the apparent diffusion coefficient (ADC) or mean diffusivity (MD; to avoid confusion with major depression we will use the acronym ADC for this quantity). The second is a measurement of the extent to which diffusion is constrained in a particular direction and is usually called fractional anisotropy (FA). In white matter, for example, the orientation of the axons and myelin sheaths determine that diffusion will be easier along the tract (parallel) than across it (perpendicular), thus it is constrained and has a higher FA than grey matter (**See p1 of the plate section for Plate 1**). In contrast, grey and white matter has very similar values of ADC because the amount of water movement is approximately equal (**See p1 of the plate section for Plate 1**).

Alterations of ADC and FA have been reported in many diseases, but comparison between studies is often complicated by the wide range of analysis techniques available. The simplest technique is to define a region of interest (ROI) in which the mean ADC and/or FA can be calculated and compared between individuals. The advantage of this technique is its simplicity, but the disadvantage is that determining the ROI can be subjective and difficult to replicate, and information available in other areas of the brain may be missed. Voxelwise techniques allow comparisons to be made over the whole brain, but multi-subject registration is particularly problematic for FA data because of the variability of the white matter tracts. Tract-based spatial statistics (TBSS) is a voxelwise technique which attempts to reduce registration problems by only comparing FA and/or ADC in the centre of the tract (Smith *et al.*, 2006). The disadvantage here may be that interesting differences between groups may extend to, or be exclusive to, the edges of the white matter tracts, and may therefore be missed. Finally, by calculating the tensor of the diffusion direction (**See p1 of the plate section for Plate 1**), reconstructions of white matter tracts can be made (**See p1 of the plate section for Plate 1**). This 'tractography' method can be used to define individual tracts of interest for calculating mean FA or ADC.

12.3 BRAIN ACTIVITY PATTERNS USED IN CLINICAL PRACTICE

As the macroscopic anatomy and natural history of brain changes in the dementias are variable, it is not surprising that there are no strictly applicable 'rules' for diagnostic imaging. Alzheimer-like pathology can be found in a substantial proportion of the brains of non-demented patients (Ince 2001). In addition, the diagnoses of AD and vascular dementia (VaD) are not mutually exclusive so that mixed patterns are likely to occur in a significant proportion of patients. Finally, at an advanced stage all dementias tend to involve large portions of the brain, preferentially (and in all likelihood) association cortex, so any differential features will disappear.

Alzheimer's disease is said to initially present with posterior cingulate (Minoshima *et al.*, 1997) or medial temporal (Callen *et al.*, 2002) reductions in brain activity, but soon after bilateral posterior temporoparietal reductions in brain activity also appear (Holman *et al.*, 1992). In blood flow and glucose metabolism studies of patients with MCI, temporo-parietal association areas, posterior cingulate and hippocampus are associated with a higher risk of progressive cognitive decline (Wolf *et al.*, 2003). During later stages, reductions in prefrontal activity occur, so that some authors have suggested computing a ratio of association cortex activity over primary sensory-motor cortex activity as a diagnostic index for AD (Herholz *et al.*, 1999). Frontotemporal dementias, i.e. those that initially present with functional impairment of anterior parts of the brain, have a variety of underlying pathologies, from Pick's to AD. Vascular disease is likely to result in patchy lesions of brain perfusion, often asymmetrical in distribution, or localized in 'watershed' regions of the brain.

Experience in imaging clinical dementia with Lewy bodies (DLB) patients suggests little difference in perfusion patterns from AD, although occipitotemporal changes have been described (Ishii *et al.*, 1999; Minoshima *et al.*, 2001).

12.4 DIAGNOSTIC SENSITIVITY AND SPECIFICITY

As described in more detail in Chapter 60, Vascular factors and Alzheimer's disease, the clinical and pathological diagnoses of dementia are not always congruent. The question about the true 'gold standard' for the evaluation of imaging studies, therefore, arises: should functional imaging reflect the distribution and severity of brain cell loss, or should it be representative of patients' functional impairment or their symptoms and signs? Either association would be of interest, but the most important purpose of imaging is of course the facilitation of effective treatment. Often the predictive validity of imaging methods is not known, but it should be ascertainable using standard empirical methods. This is in contrast to studies trying to validate imaging data with post-mortem results. By the time the brain comes to histology, a large number of confounding factors will have had a role to play: the time interval and natural history intervening between scan and post-mortem examination; additional illness and treatment; the selection bias resulting from low uptake of post-mortem examinations.

12.5 DIAGNOSTIC ACCURACY OF FUNCTIONAL IMAGING CURRENTLY USED IN CLINICAL PRACTICE (PET AND SPECT)

12.5.1 Alzheimer's disease

Bilateral temporoparietal hypometabolism has been frequently reported for AD compared with normal volunteers (Alexander *et al.*, 2002; Herholz *et al.*, 2002a). Although a temporoparietal deficit pattern is indicative of AD, it cannot be regarded as specific, but it does discriminate between demented and non-demented individuals (Masterman *et al*,. 1997). A systematic review and meta-analysis of literature in SPECT and dementia (Dougall *et al*., 2003) found that using data pooled from 27 studies, SPECT successfully discriminated between healthy elderly controls and AD with a pooled sensitivity of 77 per cent against a pooled specificity of 89 per cent.

Additional significant abnormalities have been reported for AD in posterior cingulate (Minoshima *et al*.,1997) and hippocampus (Elgh *et al*., 2002). For very early AD, reductions in posterior cingulate tend to be greater than in parietotemporal and frontal association cortices (Minoshima *et al*., 1997). Functional imaging in AD increases diagnostic sensitivity at least compared with structural imaging, with blood flow and metabolism first reduced in posterior cingulate gyrus and precuneus, before advancing to medial temporal structures and parietotemporal association cortex.

Entorhinal cortex and hippocampal metabolic reductions have been successfully used as a classifier in the discrimination of cognitively normal controls from MCI (De Santi *et al*., 2001) with a diagnostic accuracy of 81 per cent, and from AD using the temporal neocortex with a diagnostic accuracy of 100 per cent (De Santi *et al*., 2001).

Neocortical metabolic reductions for AD are widely reported (De Santi *et al*., 2001). In a prospective longitudinal analysis using the ratio of deoxyglucose uptake in association cortex over primary sensory-motor cortex for classification, initial metabolic impairment was significantly associated with subsequent clinical deterioration, thus predicting for patients with mild cognitive deficits the progression to AD (Herholz *et al*., 1999).

In advanced AD, bilateral parietotemporal perfusion deficits are reported to be more frequent and severe (Nitrini *et al*., 2000) with a reported odds ratio (OR) of 17.0 (95 per cent CI 3.1–94.2) for severe AD (Mini-Mental State Examination (MMSE) <10) and an OR of 5.2 (95 per cent CI 1.1–24.4) for moderate AD (MMSE: 10–17).

Finally, in a study of 68 AD subjects, metabolism in the cerebellum of a severe AD group was found to be significantly reduced (Ishii *et al*., 1997) compared with 13 age-matched controls, which is of relevance as cerebellar activity is often taken as a 'normal' reference region (see below).

Initial studies using ASL and MRI to measure blood flow in Alzheimer's and FTD appear to confirm the established emission computed tomography results (Du *et al*., 2006).

12.5.1.1 PATHOLOGICALLY CONFIRMED STUDIES

A multi-centre study of PET in dementia with diagnostic verification by three-year clinical follow up (Silverman *et al*., 2001) concluded that regional brain metabolism was a sensitive indicator of AD. In the same study, a pathologically confirmed diagnosis of AD was predicted by PET with a sensitivity of 94 per cent (91 out of 97 subjects) against a specificity of 73 per cent (30 out of 41 subjects) against other patients presenting with symptoms of dementia. An overall diagnostic accuracy of 89 per cent was achieved for a subset of 55 patients who presented at the time of PET with questionable or mild dementia.

A PET study in a group considered 'diagnostically challenging or difficult to characterize by clinical criteria' (Hoffman *et al*., 2000) produced sensitivity and specificity values of PET against a histological diagnosis at autopsy of AD of 93 and 63 per cent, respectively. For comparison, clinical diagnosis of probable AD had sensitivity and specificity values of 63 and 100 per cent, respectively, concluding that the overall diagnostic accuracy of PET at 82 per cent was better than clinical diagnosis at 73 per cent. Two comparable SPECT studies with pathological verification of AD reported sensitivities of 86 and 63 per cent (43 dementia patients versus 11 healthy elderly controls) against specificities of 73 and 93 per cent (70 dementia patients versus 85 healthy elderly controls), respectively (Bonte *et al*., 1997; Jagust *et al*., 2001). In a perfusion SPECT study of 49 patients coming to autopsy, Bonte and colleagues found a specificity for a diagnosis of AD with and without Lewy bodies of 89.5 per cent, against a mixed group of patients with FTD, and a sensitivity of 86.7 per cent (Bonte *et al*., 2006).

12.5.2   Vascular dementia

Typical findings in VaD are multiple small areas of reduced perfusion and metabolism extending over cortical and subcortical structures and a high diagnostic accuracy has been reported for the discrimination of probable AD and VaD using this characteristic metabolic pattern (Mielke and Heiss, 1998). In addition, frontal lobes including cingulate and superior frontal gyri have been reported to be more affected in VaD than in AD (Lee *et al*., 2001). On the other hand, temporoparietal brain regions have been said best to discriminate AD from VaD with sensitivities reported as high as 90 and 82 per cent against 80 and 82 per cent specificity, respectively (Butler *et al*., 1995; deFigueiredo *et al*., 1995). SPECT has been reported to differentiate AD from multi-infarct dementia in a study with a 77 per cent correct classification rate, compared with structural MRI which correctly classified only 50 per cent in the same subject group (Butler *et al*., 1995).

12.5.3   Frontotemporal dementia

Highly significant metabolic abnormalities have been reported for PET in frontotemporoparietal association cortex, limbic area, basal ganglia and thalamus in FTD compared with normal volunteers. In particular, bilateral frontal hypoperfusion is a strong predictor of FTD versus AD in SPECT, with sensitivity and specificity estimated at 88 and 79 per cent, respectively (Sjögren *et al*., 2000). Medial temporal lobe reduction has been suggested as a marker to separate AD from FTD (Sjögren *et al*., 2000).

12.5.4   Dementia with Lewy bodies and differential diagnosis with depression

An autopsy-confirmed PET study of the differential diagnosis of DLB and AD subjects found occipital metabolic reductions as a potential ante-mortem marker to distinguish DLB from AD, with sensitivity and specificity values determined at 90 and 80 per cent, respectively (Minoshima *et al.*, 2001). SPECT studies have confirmed occipital reduction in perfusion as an indicator of DLB (Lobotesis *et al.*, 2001). Medial temporal and cingulate reductions in metabolism have been found to be significantly more pronounced in AD compared to DLB (Imamura *et al.*, 1997), while the occipital deficit in DLB appears irrespective of clinical severity (Okamura *et al.*, 2001).

SPECT has been reported to be a useful tool for the differential diagnosis of AD and depression, with perfusion deficits in depression lying between those of controls and AD and a reported sensitivity of 52 per cent (against 94 per cent with controls) using parieto-occipital perfusion as a marker (Stoppe *et al.*, 1995).

12.5.5   SPECT versus PET

A direct comparison (Herholz *et al.*, 2002b) of SPECT and PET produced an overall significant correlation of abnormal tracer uptake between PET and SPECT across the entire brain ($r = 0.43$) with better correspondence achieved in the temporoparietal and posterior cingulate association cortices. Using quantitative statistical parametric mapping (SPM), the same study reported that PET discriminated between healthy volunteers and AD with greater reliability than SPECT, since PET was less sensitive to statistical threshold effects. Clinical utility, e.g. predictive validity, of 2-[F]fluoro-2-deoxy-D-glucose positron emission tomography (FDG PET) appears to be higher than SPECT in small preliminary studies (Ishii and Minoshima, 2005), although opinions differ (Yuan *et al.*, 2009). In a small study directly comparing F-18-FDG PET and IMP-SPECT in patients with DLB, reductions of tracer uptake were found in posterior parietal and to a lesser extent in occipital cortex, with PET appearing to be more sensitive to changes (Ishii *et al.*, 2004).

12.5.6   Methodological issues for establishing diagnostic tools

PET and SPECT images can be analysed qualitatively using visual inspection methods or quantitatively using a variety of semi-automated methods.

For quantitative ROI analysis, the brain is divided into areas often approximating underlying structural anatomy. Mean values of functional activity are then averaged within these regions and compared with a dataset of controls (Defevre *et al.*, 1999). More objective methods have been developed recently, such as an automated multi-ROI programme 3DSRT (Kobayashi *et al.*, 2008), statistical parametric mapping (Friston *et al.*, 1995), discriminant function analysis (O'Brien *et al.*, 2001) and neural network analysis (Chan *et al.*, 1994). Three-dimensional stereotactic surface projection images improve the accuracy of visually detecting AD with PET (Burdette *et al.*, 1996). Finally, a combination of structural MRI or CT and functional imaging improves

the accuracy of diagnostic classification (O'Brien *et al.*, 2001).

12.6   THE CUTTING EDGE: BRAIN FUNCTION AND CONNECTIVITY IN DEMENTIA

Functional imaging has been able to add to the understanding of brain-behaviour correlates in dementia. Neuropsychological testing has shown that the first deficit in AD is episodic memory loss. The first reduction in rCBF has been shown to be in the area of the posterior cingulate gyrus and precuneus, which is known to be important in memory (Desgranges *et al.*, 1998). Supporting this correlation, a PET study revealed activation of the retrosplenial area of the cingulate cortex during an episodic memory encoding task which is also backed by the clinical picture subsequent to other lesions of the retrosplenial cingulate cortex, such as tumours, in this area.

The next area of functioning to show impairment is semantic memory and it is thought that this occurs when neurodegenerative changes extend to the adjacent temporal neocortex. It is possible that initial involvement of the transentorhinal region, as indicated by the first histological changes, then leads to disconnection of the hippocampus followed by the limbic structures and isocortical association areas. This disconnection hypothesis can also help to account for the variety and progression of symptoms in AD, as different areas become disconnected.

Short-term memory generally has been shown consistently to correlate with metabolism in the temporoparietal association cortex, with the left hemisphere for verbal and right for spatial memory, respectively (Trollor and Valenzuela, 2001). Asymmetries in hemisphere metabolism correlate with neuropsychological 'asymmetries' defined by the traditional verbal/non-verbal dichotomy (Haxby *et al.*, 1990). If there is 'asymmetrical' involvement, the left hemisphere is often the more affected side, though reasons for this are unknown. Bilateral parietotemporal hypoperfusion appears to be more frequent in male patients, those with early onset and patients with severe AD (Nitrini *et al.*, 2000).

Following memory, attention is the next domain to be affected in AD. The anterior cingulate is thought to be involved in attentional function and a particular correlation has been shown between divided attention and anterior cingulate activity (Matsuda, 2001). This is consistent with the clinical picture – it is thought that impairment of divided attention is responsible for problems in activities of daily living which occur in AD at a relatively early stage. With regard to psychiatric phenomena, functional imaging has shown that psychotic symptoms in AD correlate with reduced frontal and temporal metabolism (Mega *et al.*, 2000); negative symptoms have been linked to decreased perfusion in the frontal cortex (Galynker *et al.*, 2000); and apathy has been associated with significantly decreased blood flow in anterior temporal, orbitofrontal, anterior cingulate and dorsolateral prefrontal regions (Benoit *et al.*, 1999). With regard to depressive symptoms in AD, there is some evidence of correlation with reduced temporal lobe perfusion (Ebmeier *et al.*, 1998).

12.6.1 Cognitive activation studies in dementia

Recent functional activation studies have demonstrated that in mild to moderately severe AD, a cognitive or sensory challenge task can cause nearly normal levels of activation in areas that are hypometabolic or hypoperfused at rest. However, with increased disease severity the degree of activation declines (Devous, 2002). Furthermore, increased activation may be required in AD patients who perform a task, or indeed activation of additional brain areas which are not activated by healthy controls (Cardebat et al., 1998). It has been hypothesized that functional plasticity may be responsible for such a recruitment of new brain regions in patients.

Because the medial-temporal lobe (MTL) complex, and the hippocampus in particular, is the brain region to show earliest pathological signs in AD, and because of its involvement in memory processes, most fMRI studies of AD patients have used memory paradigms to investigate disease-related effects on brain activity. Functional MRI studies using encoding and retrieval memory tasks have consistently reported decreased activation in hippocampus and para-hippocampus compared with healthy volunteers (Rombouts et al., 2000). More controversial are reports for other neocortical brain regions, such as prefrontal cortex, where both decreased (Small et al., 1999) and increased (Sperling et al., 2003) activation have been observed in AD patients. Such increased activation in prefrontal cortex has been interpreted as compensatory reorganization (plasticity) or as a de-differentiation (mass activation) process (Prvulovic et al., 2005). Functional abnormalities have been observed in brain regions not directly affected by AD in the early stages of the disease, such as sensory-motor cortex (Buckner et al., 2000). However, because of the limited number of studies, further evidence is required.

More recently attention has been also focused on detecting AD-related BOLD signal changes in deactivation patterns. Interestingly, deactivation abnormalities associated with AD have been mainly found in a well-defined cluster of regions that is commonly called the 'default mode network'. This network includes prefrontal, anterior and posterior cingulate, lateral parietal, and inferior/middle temporal gyri, cerebellum and thalamic nuclei, and extends to MTL (Fox et al., 2005).

Other neurodegenerative diseases, such as FTD, DLB and VaD, have been less extensively studied. An fMRI activation study compared patients with early AD and FTD during a working memory task in order to try and differentiate between the groups. During performance of the task, there was reduced activation in the frontal, temporal and cingulate cortices in the FTD group compared with the AD group. There was, however, the opposite effect in the cerebellum, a region less consistently activated in functional working memory imaging studies. This cerebellar activation in FTD may reflect successful working memory specific compensation, since test performance of FTD patients were not different from the AD group (Rombouts et al., 2003). Activation studies may, therefore, be useful in helping to reveal subtle changes in brain functioning in the early stages of dementia, as well as improving our understanding of the neural circuits involved in the tasks.

12.6.2 Studies in mild cognitive impairment

Functional MRI has been advocated as a powerful technique to detect early functional brain changes in patients with MCI, where memory symptoms are still isolated, and before the structural atrophy observed in AD patients has become manifest.

Functional MRI studies in MCI subjects have focused on detecting brain functional abnormalities within the MTL complex using memory-based tasks. Results are less consistent than in AD studies, showing either increased (Dickerson et al., 2005) or decreased (Machulda et al., 2003) activation in MTL regions compared with healthy subjects.

It has been suggested that MCI subjects show increased MTL activation to compensate for incipient structural damage. In a study where MCI subjects were divided into two groups, those less impaired and those more impaired in an associative memory task, the less impaired group showed increased activation, whereas the more impaired group showed hippocampal decreased activation, compared with a group of healthy subjects (Celone et al., 2006).

A number of issues may explain the inconsistent results in fMRI studies of MCI and AD. First, differences in grey matter volume between the two groups may affect the results. Second, subjects recruited do not always have the same degree of impairment. This is particularly true for MCI studies, where variability of symptom severity, natural history, and in the range of years before converting to AD can be observed. Third, differences in the tasks used in different studies and in the task complexity may influence results, so that abnormalities in AD and MCI samples strongly depend on the type of task adopted. Last, progressive difficulties in understanding the task instructions with advancing disease may make comparisons between different samples difficult to interpret. To overcome this limitation, a new approach has been recently proposed to study brain functionality, called resting state functional magnetic resonance (rs-fMRI) (Fox and Raichle, 2007). During an rs-fMRI study participants lie in the scanner without any task or stimulation. The rs-fMRI approach is used to study 'networks' of regions that share a common time course of spontaneous fluctuations and appear to be functionally associated in their activity. Brain regions showing a strong covariance of activity over time are defined as 'resting state networks' (RSNs), and reflect intrinsic functional brain organization that changes in disease states. The use of rs-fMRI data has been proved to be of great value to investigate differences among healthy (Filippini et al., 2009) or diseased populations, particularly those suffering from or at risk of developing neurodegenerative disorders (Greicius et al., 2004).

12.6.3 Structural connectivity in Alzheimer's disease and mild cognitive impairment

As described in Section 12.2.5, Diffusion tensor imaging, DTI is a relatively new technique for investigating the integrity of white matter pathways in the brain. Increases in ADC and decreases in FA are regularly reported as a feature of normal ageing (Charlton et al., 2006), and histopathological studies show that this may be due to a loss of myelinated fibres (Tang *et al.*, 1997). Studies demonstrating a negative correlation between FA and performance on cognitive tasks lend support to the hypothesis that white matter deterioration underlies cognitive decline.

White matter hyperintensities are a common feature in patients with AD, but it remains unclear whether these are caused by vascular problems or neurodegeneration. Increased ADC and decreased FA have been reported throughout the temporal, frontal and parietal lobes in patients with AD (Chua *et al.*, 2008), and several authors have related white matter deficits to neuropsychological measures of cognitive decline (Bozzali *et al.*, 2002), indicating that these measurements have clinical relevance. Reduced FA has also been reported in patients with early AD (Choi *et al.*, 2005), MCI (Rose *et al.*, 2006) and even in healthy carriers of the apolipoprotein E ε4-allele, the best established risk factor for AD (Persson *et al.*, 2006). Although reductions in FA and increases in ADC are not specific to AD, these studies suggest that white matter degradation begins early in the disease process.

Although white matter abnormalities have been described in many areas of the brain in AD, there is some suggestion that the regional pattern of impairment can distinguish AD from other dementias. Zarei *et al.* (2009) used TBSS to distinguish AD from VaD. Relative to controls, patients with AD had reduced FA in the temporal lobe, whereas patients with VaD had more widespread reductions in FA in frontal and parietal areas. They identified a small region in the genu of the corpus callosum that was significantly more impaired in patients with VaD relative to those with AD. Zhang and co-workers (2009) reported that patients with FTD also have more widespread abnormalities of white matter than patients with AD. Like the patients with VaD in the previous study, patients with FTD had significantly lower FA and higher ADC in the genu of the corpus callosum (Zhang *et al.*, 2009). Taken together, these studies suggest that there are greater impairments of white matter integrity in patients with VaD and FTD relative to those with AD, and that the regional patterns of impairment may be useful for differential diagnosis.

12.6.4   Longitudinal studies

A number of functional imaging studies have investigated cognitive functioning over time. These have shown that patients with more severe perfusion or metabolic deficits in the temporoparietal cortex at initial evaluation show a more rapid cognitive decline over time (Devous, 2002). With regard to MCI, significant bilateral rCBF decreases are seen in the posterior cingulate, parietal and precuneus regions of those who later meet criteria for AD. Subsequently, at the stage of a clinical diagnosis of AD, additional rCBF abnormalities are seen in the hippocampus and parahippocampus (Minoshima *et al.*, 1997).

For individual patients, the particular neuropsychological pattern that develops during the progression of AD can be predicted by early metabolic asymmetries in the association cortices (Haxby *et al.*, 1990). This would indicate that there is a functional reserve in the brain, so that neuropsychological dysfunction is likely to follow rather than co-occur with rCBF changes.

More recently, longitudinal functional imaging studies have been proposed to assess the response to treatments for AD (Alexander *et al.*, 2002). Such activation studies are of particular interest, as they can help in identifying potentially reversible tissue damage.

12.7   CONCLUSIONS FOR THE CLINICIAN

One of the authors' central tenets is that the 'gold standard' of all imaging work has to be the patients' clinical state. By implication, 'predictive validity' is the concept of greatest interest: imaging results should predict patients' prognosis and in particular whether they are going to respond to a treatment. This does not contradict the basic notion that diagnosis has to be at the beginning of effective treatment, but it reflects the observation that brain pathological changes are not always specific to a particular illness; that there is a substantial overlap of pathological changes even with health, and that pathological illness 'entities' are likely to be caused by a varying admixture of genotype–environment interactions: AD is really a collective term for a number of conditions resulting in dementia, plaques and tangles. Histological diagnoses merely reflect recognizable final common pathways for a collection of pathological conditions and therefore do not necessarily predict treatment response or prognosis. In evaluating the usefulness of imaging methods, direct comparisons should be made with clinical outcome measures – histopathological follow-through studies are of interest, but will always be confounded by selection bias, intervening illness and other artefacts. The utility of any imaging biomarker depends on its specificity and sensitivity for differential diagnosis, their ability to detect disease early and/or their response to treatment. Although most imaging modalities described here have clinical relevance, it is likely that the individual measurements will be most useful in combination. One of the binds we encounter is that useful data on sensitivity and specificity, and more particularly positive and negative predictive value, require representative clinical cohorts. If the introduction of a new imaging method is to be evidence-based in a national health service and good evidence is only available after the establishment of a service, the creation of pilot services is necessary that are not technology driven, i.e. that are centred in a normal clinical setup that will generate results transferable to the service in general. The theoretical appeal of imaging methods, after all we believe that the dementias are brain diseases, holds out the promise of visualizing brain changes that are relevant to illness outcome and treatment response.

REFERENCES

Alexander GE, Chen K, Pietrini P *et al.* (2002) Longitudinal PET evaluation of cerebral metabolic decline in dementia: a potential outcome measure in Alzheimer's disease treatment studies. *American Journal of Psychiatry* **159**: 738–45.

Alsop DC, Casement M, de Bazelaire C *et al.* (2008) Hippocampal hyperperfusion in Alzheimer's disease. *Neuroimage* **42**: 1267–74.

Arthurs OJ, Boniface S. (2002) How well do we understand the neural origins of the fMRI BOLD signal? *Trends in Neuroscience* **25**: 27–31.

Benoit M, Dygai I, Migneco O *et al.* (1999) Behavioral and psychological symptoms in Alzheimer's disease. Relation between apathy and regional cerebral perfusion. *Dementia and Geriatric Cognitive Disorders* **10**: 511–17.

Birn RM, Saad ZS, Bandettini PA. (2001) Spatial heterogeneity of the nonlinear dynamics in the FMRI BOLD response. *Neuroimage* **14**: 817–26.

Bonte FJ, Weiner MF, Bigio EH, White CL. (1997) Brain blood flow in the dementias: SPECT with histopathologic correlation in 54 patients. *Radiology* **202**: 793–7.

Bonte FJ, Harris TS, Hynan LS *et al.* (2006) Tc-99m HMPAO SPECT in the differential diagnosis of the dementias with histopathologic confirmation. *Clinical Nuclear Medicine* **31**: 376–8.

Bozzali M, Falini A, Franceschi M *et al.* (2002) White matter damage in Alzheimer's disease assessed *in vivo* using diffusion tensor magnetic resonance imaging. *Journal of Neurology, Neurosurgery and Psychiatry* **72**: 742–6.

Buckner RL, Snyder AZ, Sanders AL *et al.* (2000) Functional brain imaging of young, nondemented, and demented older adults. *Journal of Cognitive Neuroscience* **12** (Suppl. 2): 24–34.

Burdette JH, Minoshima S, Vander Borght T *et al.* (1996) Alzheimer disease: improved visual interpretation of PET images by using three-dimensional stereotaxic surface projections. *Radiology* **198**: 837–43.

Butler RE, Costa DC, Greco A *et al.* (1995) Differentiation between Alzheimer's disease and multi-infarct dementia: SPECT vs MR imaging. *International Journal of Geriatric Psychiatry* **10**: 121–8.

Callen DJA, Black SE, Caldwell CB. (2002) Limbic system perfusion in Alzheimer's disease measured by MRI-coregistered HMPAO SPET. *European Journal of Nuclear Medicine and Molecular Imaging* **29**: 899–906.

Cardebat D, Demonet JF, Puel M *et al.* (1998) Brain correlates of memory processes in patients with dementia of Alzheimer's type: A SPECT activation study. *Journal of Cerebral Blood Flow and Metabolism* **18**: 457–62.

Celone KA, Calhoun VD, Dickerson BC *et al.* (2006) Alterations in memory networks in mild cognitive impairment and Alzheimer's disease: an independent component analysis. *Journal of Neuroscience* **26**: 10222–31.

Chan KH, Johnson KA, Becker JA *et al.* (1994) A neural network classifier for cerebral perfusion imaging. *Journal of Nuclear Medicine* **35**: 771–4.

Charlton RA, Barrick TR, McIntyre DJ *et al.* (2006) White matter damage on diffusion tensor imaging correlates with age-related cognitive decline. *Neurology* **66**: 217–22.

Choi SJ, Lim KO, Monteiro I, Reisberg B. (2005) Diffusion tensor imaging of frontal white matter microstructure in early

Alzheimer's disease: A preliminary study. *Journal of Geriatric Psychiatry and Neurology* **18**: 12–19.

Chua TC, Wen W, Slavin MJ, Sachdev PS. (2008) Diffusion tensor imaging in mild cognitive impairment and Alzheimer's disease: a review. *Current Opinion in Neurology* **21**: 83–92.

De Santi S, de Leon MJ, Rusinek H *et al.* (2001) Hippocampal formation glucose metabolism and volume losses in MCI and AD. *Neurobiology of Aging* **22**: 529–39.

Defevre LJ, Leduc V, Duhamel A *et al.* (1999) Technetium HMPAO SPECT study in dementia with Lewy bodies, Alzheimer's disease and idiopathic Parkinson's disease. *Journal of Nuclear Medicine* **40**: 956–62.

DeFigueiredo RJ, Shankle WR, Maccato A *et al.* (1995) Neural-network-based classification of cognitively normal, demented, Alzheimer disease and vascular dementia from single photon emission with computed tomography image data from brain. *Proceedings of the National Academy of Sciences of the United States of America* **92**: 5530–4.

Desgranges B, Baron JC, de la Sayette V *et al.* (1998) The neural substrates of memory systems impairment in Alzheimer's disease. A PET study of resting brain glucose utilization. *Brain* **121**: 611–31.

Detre JA, Leigh JS, Williams DS, Koretsky AP. (1992) Perfusion imaging. *Magnetic Resonance in Medicine* **23**: 37–45.

Devous MD. (2002) Functional brain imaging in the dementias: role in early detection, differential diagnosis, and longitudinal studies. *European Journal of Nuclear Medicine and Molecular Imaging* **29**: 1685–96.

Dickerson BC, Salat DH, Greve DN *et al.* (2005) Increased hippocampal activation in mild cognitive impairment compared to normal aging and AD. *Neurology* **65**: 404–11.

Dougall NJ, Bruggink S, Ebmeier KP. (2003) Clinical use of SPECT in dementia – a quantitative review. In: Ebmeier KP (ed.). *SPECT in dementia.* Basel: Karger Verlag, 4–37.

Du AT, Jahng GH, Hayasaka S *et al.* (2006) Hypoperfusion in frontotemporal dementia and Alzheimer disease by arterial spin labeling MRI. *Neurology* **67**: 1215–20.

Ebmeier KP, Glabus MF, Prentice N *et al.* (1998) A voxel-based analysis of cerebral perfusion in dementia and depression of old age. *Neuroimage* **7**: 199–208.

Elgh E, Sundstrom T, Nasman B *et al.* (2002) Memory functions and rCBF (99m)Tc-HMPAO SPET: developing diagnostics in Alzheimer's disease. *European Journal of Nuclear Medicine and Molecular Imaging* **29**: 1140–8.

Filippini N, Macintosh BJ, Hough MG *et al.* (2009) Distinct patterns of brain activity in young carriers of the APOE-ε4 allele. *Proceedings of the National Academy of Sciences of the United States of America* **106**: 7209–14.

Fox MD, Raichle ME. (2007) Spontaneous fluctuations in brain activity observed with functional magnetic resonance imaging. *Nature Reviews. Neuroscience* **8**: 700–11.

Fox MD, Snyder AZ, Vincent JL *et al.* (2005) The human brain is intrinsically organized into dynamic, anticorrelated functional networks. *Proceedings of the National Academy of Sciences of the United States of America* **102**: 9673–8.

Friston KJ, Holmes AP, Worsley KJ *et al.* (1995) Statistical parametric maps in functional imaging: a general linear approach. *Human Brain Mapping* **2**: 189–210.

Galynker II, Dutta E, Vilkas N et al. (2000) Hypofrontality and negative symptoms in patients with dementia of Alzheimer type. *Neuropsychiatry, Neuropsychology, and Behavioral Neurology* 13: 53–9.

Gonzalez RG, Fischman AJ, Guimaraes AR et al. (1995) Functional MR in the evaluation of dementia: correlation of abnormal dynamic cerebral blood volume measurements with changes in cerebral metabolism on positron emission tomography with fludeoxyglucose F 18. *American Journal of Neuroradiology* 16: 1763–70.

Greicius MD, Srivastava G, Reiss AL, Menon V. (2004) Default-mode network activity distinguishes Alzheimer's disease from healthy aging: evidence from functional MRI. *Proceedings of the National Academy of Sciences of the United States of America* 101: 4637–42.

Haxby JV, Grady CL, Koss E et al. (1990) Longitudinal study of cerebral metabolic asymmetries and associated neuropsychological patterns in early dementia of the Alzheimer type. *Archives of Neurology* 47: 753–60.

Herholz K, Nordberg A, Salmon E et al. (1999) Impairment of neocortical metabolism predicts progression in Alzheimer's disease. *Dementia and Geriatric Cognitive Disorders* 10: 494–504.

Herholz K, Salmon E, Perani D et al. (2002a) Discrimination between Alzheimer dementia and controls by automated analysis of multicenter FDG PET. *Neuroimage* 17: 302–16.

Herholz K, Schopphoff H, Schmidt M et al. (2002b) Direct comparison of spatially normalized PET and SPECT scans in Alzheimer's disease. *Journal of Nuclear Medicine* 43: 21–6.

Hoffman JM, Welsh-Bohmer KA, Hanson M et al. (2000) FDG PET imaging in patients with pathologically verified dementia. *Journal of Nuclear Medicine* 41: 1920–8.

Holman BL, Johnson KA, Gerada B et al. (1992) The scintigraphic appearance of Alzheimer's disease – a prospective study using technetium-99m-HMPAO SPECT. *Journal of Nuclear Medicine* 33: 181–5.

Imamura T, Ishii K, Sasaki M et al. (1997) Regional cerebral glucose metabolism in dementia with Lewy bodies and Alzheimer's disease: a comparative study using positron emission tomography. *Neuroscience Letters* 235: 49–52.

Ince PG. (2001) Pathological correlates of late-onset dementia in a multicentre, community-based population in England and Wales: Neuropathology Group of the Medical Research Council Cognitive Function and Ageing Study (MRC CFAS)1. *The Lancet* 357: 169–75.

Ishii K, Minoshima S. (2005) PET is better than perfusion SPECT for early diagnosis of Alzheimer's disease – for. *European Journal of Nuclear Medicine and Molecular Imaging* 32: 1463–5.

Ishii K, Sasaki M, Kitagaki H et al. (1997) Reduction of cerebellar glucose metabolism in advanced Alzheimer's disease. *Journal of Nuclear Medicine* 38: 925–8.

Ishii K, Yamaji S, Kitagaki H et al. (1999) Regional cerebral blood flow difference between dementia with Lewy bodies and AD. *Neurology* 53: 413–16.

Ishii K, Hosaka K, Mori T, Mori E. (2004) Comparison of FDG-PET and IMP-SPECT in patients with dementia with Lewy bodies. *Annals of Nuclear Medicine* 18: 447–51.

Jagust W, Thisted R, Devous MD et al. (2001) SPECT perfusion imaging in the diagnosis of Alzheimer's disease – A clinical-pathologic study. *Neurology* 56: 950–6.

Johnson NA, Jahng GH, Weiner MW et al. (2005) Pattern of cerebral hypoperfusion in Alzheimer disease and mild cognitive impairment measured with arterial spin-labeling MR imaging: initial experience. *Radiology* 234: 851–9.

Kobayashi S, Tateno M, Utsumi K et al. (2008) Quantitative analysis of brain perfusion SPECT in Alzheimer's disease using a fully automated regional cerebral blood flow quantification software, 3DSRT. *Journal of the Neurological Sciences* 264: 27–33.

Lee BF, Liu CK, Tai CT et al. (2001) Alzheimer's disease: scintigraphic appearance of Tc-99m HMPAO brain SPECT. *Kaohsiung Journal of Medical Sciences* 17: 394–400.

Lobotesis K, Fenwick JD, Phipps A et al. (2001) Occipital hypoperfusion on SPECT in dementia with Lewy bodies but not AD. *Neurology* 56: 643–9.

Machulda MM, Ward HA, Borowski B et al. (2003) Comparison of memory fMRI response among normal, MCI, and Alzheimer's patients. *Neurology* 61: 500–06.

Mandeville JB, Marota JJ, Ayata C et al. (1999) MRI measurement of the temporal evolution of relative $CMRO_2$ during rat forepaw stimulation. *Magnetic Resonance in Medicine* 42: 944–51.

Masterman DL, Mendez MF, Fairbanks LA, Cummings JL. (1997) Sensitivity, specificity, and positive predictive value of technetium 99-HMPAO SPECT in discriminating Alzheimer's disease from other dementias. *Journal of Geriatric Psychiatry and Neurology* 10: 15–21.

Matsuda H. (2001) Cerebral blood flow and metabolic abnormalities in Alzheimer's disease. *Annals of Nuclear Medicine* 15: 85–92.

Mega MS, Lee L, Dinov ID et al. (2000) Cerebral correlates of psychotic symptoms in Alzheimer's disease. *Journal of Neurology, Neurosurgery and Psychiatry* 69: 167–71.

Menon RS, Ogawa S, Tank DW, Ugurbil K. (1993) Tesla gradient recalled echo characteristics of photic stimulation-induced signal changes in the human primary visual cortex. *Magnetic Resonance in Medicine* 30: 380–6.

Mielke R, Heiss WD. (1998) Positron emission tomography for diagnosis of Alzheimer's disease and vascular dementia. *Journal of Neural Transmission* 53: 237–50.

Miller KL, Luh WM, Liu TT et al. (2001) Nonlinear temporal dynamics of the cerebral blood flow response. *Human Brain Mapping* 13: 1–12.

Minoshima S, Giordani B, Berent S et al. (1997) Metabolic reduction in the posterior cingulate cortex in very early Alzheimer's disease. *Annals of Neurology* 42: 85–94.

Minoshima S, Foster NL, Sima AAF et al. (2001) Alzheimer's disease versus dementia with Lewy bodies: Cerebral metabolic distinction with autopsy confirmation. *Annals of Neurology* 50: 358–65.

Nitrini R, Buchpiguel CA, Caramelli P et al. (2000) SPECT in Alzheimer's disease: features associated with bilateral parietotemporal hypoperfusion. *Acta Neurologica Scandinavica* 101: 172–6.

O'Brien JT, Ames D, Desmond P *et al.* (2001) Combined magnetic resonance imaging and single-photon emission tomography scanning in the discrimination of Alzheimer's disease from age-matched controls. *International Psychogeriatrics* **13**: 149–61.

Okamura N, Arai H, Higuchi M *et al.* (2001) [18F]FDG-PET study in dementia with Lewy bodies and Alzheimer's disease. *Progress in Neuropsychopharmacology and Biological Psychiatry* **25**: 447–56.

Persson J, Lind J, Larsson A *et al.* (2006) Altered brain white matter integrity in healthy carriers of the APOE epsilon 4 allele – A risk for AD? *Neurology* **66**: 1029–33.

Prvulovic D, Van de Ven V, Sack AT *et al.* (2005) Functional activation imaging in aging and dementia. *Psychiatry Research* **140**: 97–113.

Rombouts SA, Barkhof F, Veltman DJ *et al.* (2000) Functional MR imaging in Alzheimer's disease during memory encoding. *American Journal of Neuroradiology* **21**: 1869–75.

Rombouts SARB, van Swieten JC, Pijnenburg YAL *et al.* (2003) Loss of frontal fMRI activation in early frontotemporal dementia compared to early AD. *Neurology* **60**: 1904–8.

Rose SE, McMahon KL, Janke AL *et al.* (2006) Diffusion indices on magnetic resonance imaging and neuropsychological performance in amnestic mild cognitive impairment. *Journal of Neurology, Neurosurgery and Psychiatry* **77**: 1122–8.

Silverman DHS, Small GW, Chang CY *et al.* (2001) Positron emission tomography in evaluation of dementia: Regional brain metabolism and long-term outcome. *Journal of the American Medical Association* **286**: 2120–7.

Sjögren M, Gustafson L, Wikkelso C, Wallin A. (2000) Frontotemporal dementia can be distinguished from Alzheimer's disease and subcortical white matter dementia by an anterior-to-posterior rCBF-SPET ratio. *Dementia and Geriatric Cognitive Disorders* **11**: 275–85.

Small SA, Perera GM, DeLaPaz R *et al.* (1999) Differential regional dysfunction of the hippocampal formation among elderly with memory decline and Alzheimer's disease. *Annals of Neurology* **45**: 466–72.

Smith SM, Jenkinson M, Johansen-Berg H *et al.* (2006) Tract-based spatial statistics: Voxelwise analysis of multi-subject diffusion data. *Neuroimage* **31**: 1487–505.

Sperling RA, Bates JF, Chua EF *et al.* (2003) fMRI studies of associative encoding in young and elderly controls and mild Alzheimer's disease. *Journal of Neurology, Neurosurgery and Psychiatry* **74**: 44–50.

Stoppe G, Staedt J, Kogler A *et al.* (1995) 99mTc-HMPAO-SPECT in the diagnosis of senile dementia of Alzheimer's type – a study under clinical routine conditions. *Journal of Neural Transmission. General Section* **99**: 195–211.

Tang Y, Nyengaard JR, Pakkenberg B, Gundersen HJG. (1997) Age-induced white matter changes in the human brain: A stereological investigation. *Neurobiology of Aging* **18**: 609–15.

Trollor JN, Valenzuela MJ. (2001) Brain ageing in the new millennium. *The Australian and New Zealand Journal of Psychiatry* **35**: 788–805.

Wolf H, Jelic V, Gertz HJ *et al.* (2003) A critical discussion of the role of neuroimaging in mild cognitive impairment. *Acta Neurologica Scandinavica Supplement* **179**: 52–76.

Wong EC, Buxton RB, Frank LR. (1997) Implementation of quantitative perfusion imaging techniques for functional brain mapping using pulsed arterial spin labeling. *NMR in Biomedicine* **10**: 237–49.

Xu G, Antuono PG, Joneso J *et al.* (2007) Perfusion fMRI detects deficits in regional CBF during memory-encoding tasks in MCI subjects. *Neurology* **69**: 1650–6.

Yuan Y, Gu ZX, Wei WS. (2009) Fluorodeoxyglucose-positron-emission tomography, single-photon emission tomography, and structural MR imaging for prediction of rapid conversion to Alzheimer disease in patients with mild cognitive impairment: a meta-analysis. *American Journal of Psychiatry* **30**: 404–10.

Zarei M, Damoiseaux JS, Morgese C *et al.* (2009) Regional white matter integrity differentiates between vascular dementia and Alzheimer disease. *Stroke* **40**: 773–9.

Zhang Y, Schuff N, Du AT *et al.* (2009) White matter damage in frontotemporal dementia and Alzheimer's disease measured by diffusion MRI. *Brain* **132**: 2579–92.

Molecular brain imaging in dementia

VICTOR L VILLEMAGNE AND CHRISTOPHER C ROWE

13.1 MOLECULAR IMAGING IN DEMENTIA

Molecular neuroimaging techniques such as positron emission tomography (PET) have been used for the *in vivo* assessment of molecular processes at their sites of action, permitting detection of subtle pathophysiological changes in the brain at asymptomatic stages, when there is no evidence of anatomic changes on computed tomography (CT) or magnetic resonance imaging (MRI). The development of molecular imaging methods for non-invasively assessing disease-specific traits such as beta-amyloid (Aβ) burden in Alzheimer's disease (AD) is allowing early diagnosis at presymptomatic stages, more accurate differential diagnosis as well as, when available, the evaluation and monitoring of disease-modifying therapy (**Table 13.1**) (Mathis *et al.*, 2007; Villemagne *et al.*, 2008a).

Clinical imaging studies with amyloid radiotracers are providing quantitative information on Aβ burden *in vivo*, leading to new insights into Aβ deposition in the brain and facilitating research of neurodegenerative diseases where Aβ may play a role (Klunk *et al.*, 2004; Masters *et al.*, 2006; Mathis *et al.*, 2007; Rowe *et al.*, 2007). Most of the amyloid imaging studies worldwide had been conducted using ^{11}C-PiB, the most successful and widespread amyloid imaging agent to date.

On visual inspection, cortical retention of ^{11}C-PiB, regardless of disease severity, is markedly elevated in AD (Klunk *et al.*, 2004; Mintun *et al.*, 2006; Rowe *et al.*, 2007) while being generally lower and more variable in dementia with Lewy bodies (DLB), probably reflecting a larger spectrum of Aβ deposition (Rowe *et al.*, 2007; Maetzler *et al.*, 2009). In AD, ^{11}C-PiB retention is highest in frontal, cingulate, precuneus, striatum, parietal and lateral temporal cortex

(See p1 of the plate section for Plate 2). Occipital cortex, sensorimotor cortex and mesial temporal cortex are usually less affected (See p1 of the plate section for Plate 2). With the exception of ^{18}F-FDDNP that shows high retention in the mesial temporal cortex, a similar pattern of retention in AD is observed with most ^{11}C and [18]F β-amyloid ligands (**Figure 13.1**). ^{11}C-PiB binds reversibly, with fastest clearance from the cerebellar cortex and slowest from white matter (Rowe *et al.*, 2007). Absence of neuritic Aβ plaques in the cerebellar cortex of mild to moderate severity AD patients (Ikonomovic *et al.*, 2008) is reflected in the similar clearance of PiB from this region in normal and AD subjects (Rowe *et al.*, 2007), with the exception of familial AD cases (Klunk *et al.*, 2007; Villemagne *et al.*, 2009a; See p2 of the plate section for Plate 3) or prion diseases like Creutzfeldt–Jakob disease (CJD) (Boxer *et al.*, 2007; Villemagne *et al.*, 2009b; See p3 of the plate section for Plate 4). ^{11}C-PiB cortical retention was observed in the minority of Parkinson's disease (PD) patients, similar to findings in normal elderly subjects (Edison *et al.*, 2008; Johansson *et al.*, 2008; Maetzler *et al.*, 2009). ^{11}C-PiB-PET has facilitated differential diagnosis of dementia in patients with atypical onset or language onset (Rabinovici *et al.*, 2008).

Quantitative and visual assessment of PET images show a pattern of ^{11}C-PiB retention similar to the sequence of Aβ deposition derived from autopsy data (Braak and Braak, 1997; Thal *et al.*, 2002), with initial deposition in orbitofrontal cortex and gyrus rectus, followed by the cingulate gyrus and precuneus, the remaining prefrontal cortex and lateral temporal cortex, and finally the parietal cortex. The regional retention of ^{11}C-PiB reflects the regional density of Aβ plaques, as reported at autopsy (Bacskai *et al.*, 2007; Ikonomovic *et al.*, 2008), with a much higher plaque density in the frontal and other cortical areas than in hippocampus (Arnold *et al.*, 2000; Rowe *et al.*, 2007; Leinonen *et al.*, 2008).

[11]C-PiB retention is also elevated in subjects diagnosed with cerebral amyloid angiopathy (CAA; Johnson *et al.*, 2007), showing a slightly greater posterior to anterior brain distribution than AD cases. There is usually no cortical ^{11}C-PiB retention in patients with a clinical diagnosis of frontal temporal lobar degeneration (FTLD; Rowe *et al.*, 2007; Drzezga *et al.*, 2008; Rabinovici *et al.*, 2008; **See p3 of the plate section for Plate 4**) while analysis of ^{11}C-PiB binding in subjects diagnosed with mild cognitive impairment (MCI), a condition that progresses to AD at a rate of approximately 15 per cent per year (Petersen *et al.*, 1999; Morris *et al.*, 2001), has revealed two distinct ^{11}C-PiB retention patterns (**See p3 of the plate section for Plate 4**). About 60 per cent of MCI cases show cortical ^{11}C-PiB binding similar in distribution and sometimes in degree to AD, while the rest exhibit little or no cortical ^{11}C-PiB retention, similar to healthy controls (HC) (Kemppainen *et al.*, 2007; Pike *et al.*, 2007; Forsberg *et al.*, 2008; **See p3 of the plate section for Plate 4**).

About 25–35 per cent of asymptomatic age-matched HC present with cortical ^{11}C-PiB retention, predominantly in the prefrontal and posterior cingulate/precuneus regions (Mintun *et al.*, 2006; Rowe *et al.*, 2007; Villemagne *et al.*, 2008a;

Table 13.1 Potential roles for Aβ imaging.

Accurate diagnosis of AD

Prognosis of conversion to AD

Early diagnosis of Alzheimer's disease, allowing intervention when minimally impaired

Investigate the spatial and temporal pattern of Aβ deposition and its relation to disease progression, cognitive decline, and other disease biomarkers

Subject selection for anti-Aβ trials

Monitor the effectiveness of anti-Aβ therapy

Predict response to anti-Aβ therapy

Aizenstein *et al.*, 2008; **See p3 of the plate section for Plate 4**). These findings are in agreement with post-mortem reports that at least 30 per cent of non-demented older individuals over the age of 75 have amyloid plaques, with deposits occurring well before the onset of dementia (Morris and Price, 2001; Forman *et al.*, 2007). The retention of ^{11}C-PiB in HC correlates with subtle memory impairment and a greater risk of cognitive decline (Mintun *et al.*, 2006; Pike *et al.*, 2007; Villemagne *et al.*, 2008b), likely to represent what has been termed preclinical AD (Price and Morris, 1999).

13.2 AMYLOID LIGANDS

Aβ plaques and neurofibrillary tangles (NFT) are the hallmark brain lesions of AD. Selective tau imaging, for *in vivo* NFT quantification, is still in the early stages of development (Okamura *et al.*, 2005). Since Aβ is at the centre of AD pathogenesis, and given that several pharmacological agents aimed at reducing Aβ levels in the brain are being developed and tested, many efforts are focused on generating radiotracers or agents that allow Aβ imaging *in vivo* and are suited to widespread clinical application.

For a radiotracer to be useful as a neuroimaging Aβ probe, a number of key general properties are desirable: they should be lipophilic molecules that cross the blood–brain barrier (BBB), preferably not be metabolized, while reversibly binding to Aβ in a specific and selective fashion (Villemagne *et al.*, 2008a). Furthermore, low non-specific binding to white matter is desirable as Aβ deposition usually starts at layers III and IV of the cortex (Thal *et al.*, 2000), and spillover from high non-specific binding in white matter might mask or reduce the ability to detect this early deposition. Therapies, especially those targeting irreversible neurodegenerative processes, have a better chance of success if applied early. Therefore, early detection of the underlying pathological process is important.

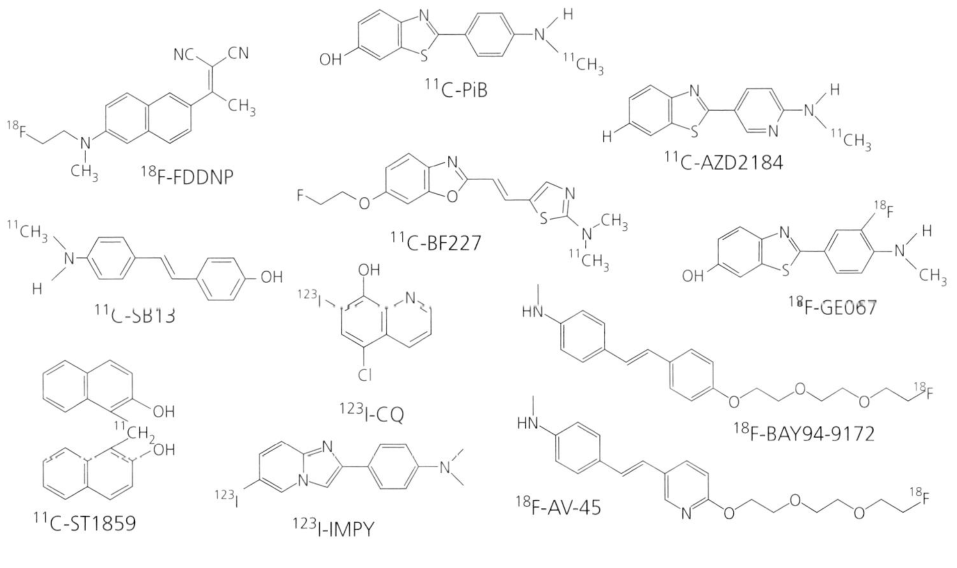

Figure 13.1 Amyloid ligands. Chemical structure of amyloid ligands that have been used in clinical studies.

Several compounds have been evaluated as potential Aβ probes. It has been known since the 1930s that Aβ plaques present in post-mortem AD brain tissue can be stained for histological examination with Congo red or Chrysamine-G. Klunk and Mathis and colleagues at the University of Pittsburgh developed numerous Congo red derivatives for potential use as *in vivo* Aβ probes, but these relatively large and acidic compounds' ability to cross the BBB was found to be marginal (Bacskai *et al.*, 2002). However, thioflavin T derivatives were found to have more favourable Aβ binding characteristics (Mathis *et al.*, 2003). In parallel, synthesis and initial characterization of ^{125}I bromostyrylbenzene (BSB) probes were described by Kung and colleagues from the University of Pennsylvania, Philadelphia (Kung *et al.*, 2001), and while they were found to strongly bind to Aβ amyloid plaques as assessed by fluorescent microscopy, they displayed low *in vivo* brain uptake (Kung *et al.*, 2002).

Anti-Aβ monoclonal antibodies that bind to specific epitopes within Aβ fibrils have been developed and used *in vitro* in human brain tissue (Majocha *et al.*, 1992). Because antibodies are poorly delivered into the central nervous system (CNS) when administered peripherally, they have failed as tracers for *in vivo* brain imaging studies.

Almost a decade after unsuccessful trials with anti-Aβ antibodies (Majocha *et al.*, 1992), amyloid imaging came to fruition with the first report of successful imaging in an AD patient with ^{18}F-FDDNP, a tracer characterized for binding both plaques and NFT (Shoghi-Jadid *et al.*, 2002). Since then, human amyloid imaging studies have been conducted in AD patients, normal controls and patients with other dementias using ^{11}C-PiB (Klunk *et al.*, 2004), ^{11}C-SB13 (Verhoeff *et al.*, 2004), ^{11}C-ST1859 (Bauer *et al.*, 2006), ^{11}C-BF227 (Kudo *et al.*, 2007), ^{11}C-AZD2138 (Nyberg *et al.*, 2009), ^{18}F-BAY94-91772 (Rowe *et al.*, 2008), ^{18}F-GE067 (Serdons *et al.*, 2009a) and ^{18}F-AV-45 (Sperling *et al.*, 2009a) with PET and with ^{123}I-IMPY (Newberg *et al.*, 2006) using single photon emission computed tomography (SPECT; **Figure 13.1**).

While all of the aforementioned tracers bind with varying degrees of success to Aβ fibrils and brain homogenates of AD patients, Congo red and thioflavin T – and some of their derivatives – have recently been shown to also bind to the soluble oligomeric forms of Aβ (Maezawa *et al.*, 2008). On the other hand, Aβ soluble species reportedly represent less than 1 per cent of the total brain Aβ (McLean *et al.*, 1999) and the reported affinity of PiB for these soluble oligomers seems to be significantly lower than for Aβ fibrils (Maezawa *et al.*, 2008). Concurring with these findings, is a recent report describing a patient with a novel APP mutation where Aβ does not fibrilize but remains in an oligomeric state, in whom PiB PET showed very mild cortical retention compared to that usually observed in sporadic AD (Tomiyama *et al.*, 2008). Until highly selective radiotracers are developed to bind the Aβ soluble species, the contribution of these oligomers to the amyloid imaging PET signal in sporadic AD from tracers such as ^{11}C-PiB is considered to be negligible (Mathis *et al.*, 2007).

Preliminary studies with SPECT Aβ radiotracers (**Figure 13.1**) showed limited utility for the evaluation of Aβ burden in AD (Newberg *et al.*, 2006). New SPECT radiotracers labelled with ^{123}I or those that could be potentially labelled with ^{99m}Tc are being evaluated (Lin *et al.*, 2009).

A marked progression in the development of amyloid-imaging tracers was the synthesis and characterization by Barrio and colleagues of a very lipophilic radiofluorinated 6-dialkylamino-2-naphthyethylidene derivative that has nanomolar affinity to Aβ fibrils (Agdeppa *et al.*, 2001). ^{18}F-FDDNP is reported to bind to both the extracellular Aβ plaques and the intracellular NFT in AD (Shoghi-Jadid *et al.*, 2002), while also binding to prion plaques from CJD (Bresjanac *et al.*, 2003). ^{18}F-FDDNP was used to obtain the first human PET images of Aβ in an 82-year-old woman with AD. Briefly, [^{18}F]FDDNP showed a differential clearance, being slower from areas of plaque deposition, such as the hippocampus, as pathologically confirmed later at post-mortem examination (Agdeppa *et al.*, 2001). In a follow-up study, AD patients again demonstrated higher accumulation and slower clearance of ^{18}F-FDDNP than controls in brain areas such as the hippocampus (Shoghi-Jadid *et al.*, 2002). Retention time of ^{18}F-FDDNP in these brain regions was correlated with lower memory performance scores in patients with AD (Small *et al.*, 2002). These findings were further confirmed in a larger series where AD and MCI participants were successfully differentiated from those with no cognitive impairment (Small *et al.*, 2006). However, the analysis required a 2-hour continuous scan and only demonstrated 9 per cent higher cortical uptake in AD. Direct comparison of ^{18}F-FDDNP with ^{11}C-PiB in monkeys (Noda *et al.*, 2008) and in human subjects showed very limited dynamic range of ^{18}F-FDDNP (Shin *et al.*, 2008; Tolboom *et al.*, 2009). ^{18}F-FDDNP still remains the only tracer showing retention in the medial temporal cortex of AD patients, suggesting higher binding affinity of FDDNP to NFT than to Aβ (Shin *et al.*, 2008). However, *in vitro* evaluation of FDDNP in concentrations similar to those achieved during a PET scan showed limited binding to both NFT and Aβ plaques (Thompson *et al.*, 2009).

^{11}C-PiB (**Figure 13.1**), the most successful and widely used of the currently available amyloid tracers has been shown to possess high affinity for fibrillar Aβ (Lockhart *et al.*, 2005). Recent studies have shown that PiB binds with high affinity to the N-terminally truncated and modified Aβ and Aβ N3-pyroglutamate species in senile plaques (Maeda *et al.*, 2007). *In vitro* assessment of ^{3}H-PiB binding to white matter homogenates failed to show any specific binding (Fodero-Tavoletti *et al.*, 2009). PiB is a derivative of thioflavin T, a fluorescent dye commonly used to assess fibrillization into β-sheet conformation (Levine, 1999), and as such PiB has been shown to bind to a range of additional Aβ containing lesions including diffuse plaques and CAA (Lockhart *et al.*, 2007), as well as to Aβ oligomers – albeit with lower affinity (Maezawa *et al.*, 2008), or other misfolded proteins with a similar β-sheet secondary structure such as α-synuclein (Fodero-Tavoletti *et al.*, 2007) and tau (Lockhart *et al.*, 2007; Ikonomovic *et al.*, 2008). Studies have shown that at the concentrations achieved during a PET examination, ^{11}C-PiB cortical retention in AD or DLB primarily reflects Aβ-related cerebral amyloidosis and not binding to Lewy bodies or NFT (Klunk *et al.*, 2003; Lockhart *et al.*, 2007; Fodero-Tavoletti *et al.*, 2007; Ikonomovic *et al.*, 2008).

Unfortunately, the 20-minute radioactive decay half-life of ^{11}C limits the use of ^{11}C-radiotracers to centres with an on-site cyclotron and ^{11}C radiochemistry expertise. Consequently, access to ^{11}C-labelled radiotracers is restricted and the high cost of studies is prohibitive for routine clinical use. To overcome these limitations, an Aβ imaging tracer labelled with ^{18}F was required. The 110-minute radioactive decay half-life of ^{18}F permits centralized production and regional distribution as currently practised worldwide in the supply of 18F-fluorodeoxyglucose (FDG) for clinical use. Several of the novel amyloid ligands are labelled with [18]F.

^{18}F-BAY94-9172 (a.k.a. Florbetaben) (**Figure 13.1**), developed by Kung and colleagues at the University of Pennsylvania, has been shown to bind avidly to neuritic and diffuse amyloid plaques and to CAA (Zhang *et al.*, 2005). BAY94-9172 was found to bind with high affinity to Aβ in brain homogenates and selectively labelled Aβ plaques in AD tissue sections (Zhang *et al.*, 2005). At tracer concentrations achieved during human PET studies, BAY94-9172 did not show binding to post-mortem cortex from subjects with FTLD. After injection into Tg2576 transgenic mice, *ex vivo* brain sections showed localization of ^{18}F-BAY94-9172 in regions with Aβ plaques as confirmed by thioflavin binding (Zhang *et al.*, 2005). In human studies, ^{18}F-BAY94-9172 neocortical retention was higher at 90 minutes post-injection in all AD subjects compared to age-matched controls and FTLD patients (**See p4 of the plate section for Plate 5**), with binding matching the reported post-mortem distribution of Aβ plaques (Rowe *et al.*, 2008). Multicentre clinical trials have confirmed these results.

Along with ^{18}F-BAY94-9172, Kung and colleagues at the University of Pennsylvania (Zhang *et al.*, 2005; **Figure 13.1**) developed other stilbene derivatives of which ^{18}F-AV-45 (Florpiramine) has proven suitable for human studies. The most salient feature of this tracer is its rapid reversible binding characteristics allowing scanning of subjects at 45–50 min after injection. A multicentre study in AD, MCI and HC has confirmed the ability of ^{18}F-AV-45 to discriminate between AD and age-matched controls (Sperling *et al.*, 2009a).

13.3   AMYLOID IMAGING AND OTHER MARKERS OF DISEASE

In vivo amyloid imaging is not only helping elucidate the relationship between Aβ deposition and cognition but is also allowing researchers to define and refine its relationship with cerebrospinal fluid (CSF) and genetic biomarkers, as well as to establish the relationships between Aβ deposition, neuropathology, brain atrophy and glucose metabolism.

[11]C-PiB PET studies have not only shown a robust difference in ^{11}C-PiB retention between AD patients and age-matched controls (Klunk *et al.*, 2004; Rowe *et al.*, 2007), but also inverse correlations with decreased CSF Aβ$_{42}$ (Fagan *et al.*, 2006; Koivunen *et al.*, 2008) and cerebral atrophy (Jack *et al.*, 2008; Mormino *et al.*, 2009). Amyloid imaging data concur both with post-mortem reports on the regional density and sequence of Aβ deposition (Braak and Braak, 1997; Arnold *et al.*, 2000; Thal *et al.*, 2002). They also agree with reports that these neuropathological changes precede

the clinical expression of AD by many years (Price and Morris, 1999; Bennett *et al.*, 2006), reflected in the large percentage of cognitively unimpaired individuals with significant ^{11}C-PiB retention in the brain (Mintun *et al.*, 2006; Pike *et al.*, 2007; Aizenstein *et al.*, 2008; Villemagne *et al.*, 2008b). Despite a strong inverse correlation between PiB and cerebral metabolism measured with FDG PET in temporal, parietal and posterior cingulate cortex, the correlation is not present in the frontal lobe or hippocampus (Klunk *et al.*, 2004; Edison *et al.*, 2007; Li *et al.*, 2008). Visual assessment of PET images by clinicians blinded to the diagnoses demonstrated that ^{11}C-PiB was more accurate than FDG to distinguish AD from HC (Ng *et al.*, 2007).

To date, the only consistent genetic marker for both the early (familial) and late-onset (non-familial) forms of AD is the polymorphism of the apolipoprotein E (ApoE) allele on chromosome 19 (Strittmatter *et al.*, 1993). ApoE ε4 is the primary genetic risk factor associated with sporadic AD, and its presence is thought to result in an earlier age of onset (Martins *et al.*, 2006). Examination of ApoE ε4 allele status revealed that, independent of clinical classification, ε4 carriers have significantly higher ^{11}C-PiB binding than non-ε4 carriers, further emphasizing the crucial role that ApoE plays in the metabolism of Aβ (Rowe *et al.*, 2007; Reiman *et al.*, 2009). In individuals with mutations within the APP or presenilin 1 genes associated with familial AD, there is very high PiB retention in the caudate nuclei in asymptomatic carriers, preceding symptoms and cortical PiB binding in the posterior cingulate/precuneus and, to a lesser degree, in prefrontal and temporal cortices, retention that seems to be independent of mutation type (Klunk *et al.*, 2007; Villemagne *et al.*, 2009a; **See p2 of the plate section for Plate 3**).

To date, the relationship between Aβ deposition and the development of clinical symptoms is not fully understood. Although Aβ burden as assessed by PiB-PET does not correlate with measures of memory impairment in AD, it does correlate with memory impairment in MCI (Pike *et al.*, 2007; Forsberg *et al.*, 2008; Mormino *et al.*, 2009) and healthy older subjects (Pike *et al.*, 2007; Villemagne *et al.*, 2008b). Interestingly, 60–80 per cent of the subjects classified as non-amnestic MCI do not show significant ^{11}C-PiB retention in the brain (Pike *et al.*, 2007; Wolk *et al.*, 2009). Conversely, 60–80 per cent of amnestic MCI subjects were shown to have significant ^{11}C-PiB retention in the brain (Pike *et al.*, 2007; Okello *et al.*, 2009; Wolk *et al.*, 2009). The observations that PiB retention in non-demented individuals relates to episodic memory impairment, one of the earliest clinical symptoms of AD, suggests that Aβ deposition is not part of normal ageing, and supports the hypothesis that Aβ deposition occurs well before the onset of symptoms and is likely to represent preclinical AD. The relation between the regional pattern of ^{11}C-PiB retention and its potential relation to cognition merits further comments. Multimodality studies in early AD have shown Aβ deposition in cortical regions that are associated with memory retrieval in young adults. This Aβ deposition pattern has been associated with the anatomy of the 'default network', a specific, anatomically defined brain system responsible for internal modes of cognition, such as self-reflection processes, conscious resting state, or episodic memory retrieval (Buckner *et al.*, 2005; Sperling *et al.*,

2009b). It has been proposed that deficits or disruption of the default activity in these cortical regions might predispose certain people to AD-related changes (Buckner *et al.*, 2005).

While one report of a two-year follow-up study in AD patients showed that despite some participants showing cognitive decline and worsening FDG hypometabolism, there was stable or even decreased ^{11}C-PiB binding (Engler *et al.*, 2006). However, another follow-up study with more subjects, including HC, MCI and AD, suggested a small increase in Aβ burden over one year but that cognitive decline was associated with measures of brain atrophy and not with Aβ deposition (Jack *et al.*, 2009). These findings, in addition to the evidence of Aβ deposition in a high percentage of MCI and asymptomatic HC, suggest that Aβ is an early and necessary, though not sufficient, cause for cognitive decline in AD (Villemagne *et al.*, 2008b). Perhaps specific *in vivo* tau imaging will help elucidate or bridge the gap between Aβ deposition and the persistent decline in cognitive function observed in AD. Ongoing large longitudinal studies including both structural and amyloid neuroimaging studies as well as genetic and biochemical biomarkers will permit a better understanding of the role and relevance of Aβ deposition in elderly controls and MCI subjects (Mueller *et al.*, 2005; Ellis *et al.*, 2009).

The observed dissociation between Aβ deposition and measures of cognition, synaptic activity and neurodegeneration in AD points towards other mechanisms, likely triggered by Aβ such as NFT formation, synaptic failure and eventually neuronal loss. The evidence points to the fact that Aβ toxicity in the form of oligomers and Aβ deposition in the form of aggregates precede by many years the appearance of clinical symptoms (Price and Morris, 1999; Hof *et al.*, 1996). These neurotoxic processes eventually lead to synaptic and neuronal loss, manifested as brain atrophy, glucose hypometabolism and cognitive impairment (Suo *et al.*, 2004; Jack *et al.*, 2009; Mormino *et al.*, 2009). Therefore, it is highly likely that PiB retention in non-demented individuals reflects preclinical AD (Mintun *et al.*, 2006; Rowe *et al.*, 2007; Villemagne *et al.*, 2008b). As previously suggested (Villemagne *et al.*, 2008a), this may be associated or attributed to a different susceptibility/vulnerability to Aβ, at both a cellular/regional level – frontal neurons seem to be more resistant to Aβ toxicity than hippocampal neurons (Capetillo-Zarate *et al.*, 2006; Resende *et al.*, 2007), as well as at an individual or personal level, either due to a particular cognitive reserve (Kemppainen *et al.*, 2008; Roe *et al.*, 2008), differences in Aβ conformation affecting toxicity and/or PiB binding (Lockhart *et al.*, 2005; Rosen *et al.*, 2009; Levine and Walker, 2010) or because an idiosyncratic threshold must be exceeded for synaptic failure and neuronal death to ensue (Suo *et al.*, 2004). These factors would help explain why some older individuals with a significant Aβ burden are cognitively unimpaired, while others with lower Aβ burden and no genetic predisposing factors have already developed the full clinical AD phenotype.

13.4 SUMMARY

The introduction of radiotracers for the non-invasive *in vivo* quantification of Aβ in the brain has revolutionized the approach to the evaluation of AD. Frank *et al.* (2003) proposed that an ideal biomarker for AD should be disease-specific, non-invasive, with sensitivity and specificity above 80 per cent. Amyloid imaging fulfils these criteria. Aβ burden as measured by PET matches histopathological reports of Aβ distribution in ageing and dementia, it appears more accurate than FDG for the diagnosis of AD, and is an excellent aid in the differential diagnosis of AD from FTLD. ApoE ε4 status is associated with higher Aβ burden. As new treatments in clinical trials are aimed at preventing or slowing AD progression, either by preventing Aβ generation or deposition, or increasing the clearance of Aβ, the role of imaging and quantifying Aβ burden *in vivo* is becoming increasingly crucial. Although these treatments are aimed at AD, the available data suggest that they may have value in other dementias such as DLB, where Aβ deposition is present.

Despite the development of promising new and reliable Aβ imaging ligands labelled with isotopes with longer radioactive half-lives (Rowe *et al.*, 2008; Serdons *et al.*, 2009b; Sperling *et al.*, 2009a; Sundgren-Andersson *et al.*, 2009), population screening is unlikely to involve neuroimaging approaches and, despite the unreliability of plasma assays to date (Zetterberg and Blennow, 2006), a simple blood test assessing central features of the disease, such as Aβ, as well as the use of near-infrared amyloid dyes (Raymond *et al.*, 2008) should soon be available to permit widespread screening of the at-risk population. On the other hand, molecular neuroimaging can provide highly accurate, reliable, and reproducible quantitative statements of Aβ burden, essential for therapeutic trial recruitment and for the evaluation of disease-specific treatments directed at removing Aβ.

REFERENCES

Agdeppa ED, Kepe V, Shoghi-Jadid K, Al E. (2001) *In vivo* and *in vitro* labeling of plaques and tangles in the brain of an Alzheimer's disease patient: a case study. *Journal of Nuclear Medicine* 42 (Suppl. 1): 65.

Aizenstein HJ, Nebes RD, Saxton JA *et al.* (2008) Frequent amyloid deposition without significant cognitive impairment among the elderly. *Archives of Neurology* 65: 1509–17.

Arnold SE, Han LY, Clark CM *et al.* (2000) Quantitative neurohistological features of frontotemporal degeneration. *Neurobiology of Aging* 21: 913–19.

Bacskai BJ, Klunk WE, Mathis CA, Hyman BT. (2002) Imaging amyloid-beta deposits in vivo. *Journal of Cerebral Blood Flow and Metabolism* 22: 1035–41.

Bacskai BJ, Frosch MP, Freeman SH *et al.* (2007) Molecular imaging with Pittsburgh Compound B confirmed at autopsy: a case report. *Archives of Neurology* 64: 431–4.

Bauer M, Langer O, Dal-Bianco P *et al.* (2006) A positron emission tomography microdosing study with a potential antiamyloid drug in healthy volunteers and patients with Alzheimer's disease. *Clinical Pharmacology and Therapeutics* 80: 216–27.

Bennett DA, Schneider JA, Arvanitakis Z *et al.* (2006) Neuropathology of older persons without cognitive impairment from two community-based studies. *Neurology* 66: 1837–44.

Boxer AL, Rabinovici GD, Kepe V et al. (2007) Amyloid imaging in distinguishing atypical prion disease from Alzheimer disease. Neurology 69: 283–90.

Braak H, Braak E. (1997) Frequency of stages of Alzheimer-related lesions in different age categories. Neurobiology of Aging 18: 351–7.

Bresjanac M, Smid LM, Vovko TD et al. (2003) Molecular-imaging probe 2-(1-[6-[(2-fluoroethyl)(methyl) amino]-2-naphthyl]ethylidene) malononitrile labels prion plaques in vitro. Journal of Neuroscience 23: 8029–33.

Buckner RL, Snyder AZ, Shannon BJ et al. (2005) Molecular, structural, and functional characterization of Alzheimer's disease: evidence for a relationship between default activity, amyloid, and memory. Journal of Neuroscience 25: 7709–17.

Capetillo-Zarate E, Staufenbiel M, Abramowski D et al. (2006) Selective vulnerability of different types of commissural neurons for amyloid beta-protein-induced neurodegeneration in APP23 mice correlates with dendritic tree morphology. Brain 129: 2992–3005.

Drzezga A, Grimmer T, Henriksen G et al. (2008) Imaging of amyloid plaques and cerebral glucose metabolism in semantic dementia and Alzheimer's disease. Neuroimage 39: 619–33.

Edison P, Archer HA, Hinz R et al. (2007) Amyloid, hypometabolism, and cognition in Alzheimer disease: an [11C]PIB and [18F]FDG PET study. Neurology 68: 501–8.

Edison P, Rowe CC, Rinne JO et al. (2008) Amyloid load in Parkinson's disease dementia and Lewy body dementia measured with [11C]PIB positron emission tomography. Journal of Neurology, Neurosurgery, and Psychiatry 79: 1331–8.

Ellis KA, Bush AI, Darby D et al. (2009) The Australian Imaging, Biomarkers and Lifestyle (AIBL) study of aging: methodology and baseline characteristics of 1112 individuals recruited for a longitudinal study of Alzheimer's disease. International Psychogeriatrics 21: 672–87.

Engler H, Forsberg A, Almkvist O et al. (2006) Two-year follow-up of amyloid deposition in patients with Alzheimer's disease. Brain 129: 2856–66.

Fagan AM, Mintun MA, Mach RH et al. (2006) Inverse relation between in vivo amyloid imaging load and cerebrospinal fluid Abeta(42) in humans. Annals of Neurology 59: 512–19.

Fodero-Tavoletti MT, Smith DP, McLean CA et al. (2007) In vitro characterization of Pittsburgh compound-B binding to Lewy bodies. Journal of Neuroscience 27: 10365–71.

Fodero-Tavoletti MT, Rowe CC, McLean CA et al. (2009) Characterization of PiB binding to white matter in Alzheimer disease and other dementias. Journal of Nuclear Medicine 50: 198–204.

Forman MS, Mufson EJ, Leurgans S et al. (2007) Cortical biochemistry in MCI and Alzheimer disease: lack of correlation with clinical diagnosis. Neurology 68: 757–63.

Forsberg A, Engler H, Almkvist O et al. (2008) PET imaging of amyloid deposition in patients with mild cognitive impairment. Neurobiology of Aging 29: 1456–65.

Frank RA, Galasko D, Hampel H et al. (2003) Biological markers for therapeutic trials in Alzheimer's disease. Proceedings of the biological markers working group; NIA initiative on

neuroimaging in Alzheimer's disease. Neurobiology of Aging 24: 521–36.

Hof PR, Glannakopoulos P, Bouras C. (1996) The neuropathological changes associated with normal brain aging. Histology and Histopathology 11: 1075–88.

Ikonomovic MD, Klunk WE, Abrahamson EE et al. (2008) Post-mortem correlates of in vivo PiB-PET amyloid imaging in a typical case of Alzheimer's disease. Brain 131: 1630–45.

Jack Jr CR, Lowe VJ, Senjem ML et al. (2008) 11C PiB and structural MRI provide complementary information in imaging of Alzheimer's disease and amnestic mild cognitive impairment. Brain 131: 665–80.

Jack Jr CR, Lowe VJ, Weigand SD et al. (2009) Serial PIB and MRI in normal, mild cognitive impairment and Alzheimer's disease: implications for sequence of pathological events in Alzheimer's disease. Brain 132: 1355–65.

Johansson A, Savitcheva I, Forsberg A et al. (2008) [(11)C]-PIB imaging in patients with Parkinson's disease: preliminary results. Parkinsonism and Related Disorders 14: 345–7.

Johnson KA, Gregas M, Becker JA et al. (2007) Imaging of amyloid burden and distribution in cerebral amyloid angiopathy. Annals of Neurology 62: 229–34.

Kemppainen NM, Aalto S, Wilson IA et al. (2007) PET amyloid ligand [11C]PIB uptake is increased in mild cognitive impairment. Neurology 68: 1603–6.

Kemppainen NM, Aalto S, Karrasch M et al. (2008) Cognitive reserve hypothesis: Pittsburgh Compound B and fluorodeoxyglucose positron emission tomography in relation to education in mild Alzheimer's disease. Annals of Neurology 63: 112–18.

Klunk WE, Wang Y, Huang GF et al. (2003) The binding of 2-(4'-methylaminophenyl)benzothiazole to postmortem brain homogenates is dominated by the amyloid component. Journal of Neuroscience 23: 2086–92.

Klunk WE, Engler H, Nordberg A et al. (2004) Imaging brain amyloid in Alzheimer's disease with Pittsburgh Compound-B. Annals of Neurology 55: 306–19.

Klunk WE, Price JC, Mathis CA et al. (2007) Amyloid deposition begins in the striatum of presenilin-1 mutation carriers from two unrelated pedigrees. Journal of Neuroscience 27: 6174–84.

Koivunen J, Pirttila T, Kemppainen N et al. (2008) PET amyloid ligand [C]PIB uptake and cerebrospinal fluid beta-amyloid in mild cognitive impairment. Dementia and Geriatric Cognitive Disorders 26: 378–83.

Kudo Y, Okamura N, Furumoto S et al. (2007) 2-(2-[2-Dimethylaminothiazol-5-yl]Ethenyl)-6-(2-[Fluoro]Ethoxy)Benzoxazole: a novel PET agent for in vivo detection of dense amyloid plaques in Alzheimer's disease patients. Journal of Nuclear Medicine 48: 553–61.

Kung HF, Lee CW, Zhuang ZP et al. (2001) Novel stilbenes as probes for amyloid plaques. Journal of the American Chemical Society 123: 12740–1.

Kung MP, Hou C, Zhuang ZP et al. (2002) Radioiodinated styrylbenzene derivatives as potential SPECT imaging agents for amyloid plaque detection in Alzheimer's disease. Journal of Molecular Neuroscience 19: 7–10.

Leinonen V, Alafuzoff I, Aalto S et al. (2008) Assessment of beta-amyloid in a frontal cortical brain biopsy specimen and by positron emission tomography with carbon 11-labeled Pittsburgh Compound B. *Archives of Neurology* **65**: 1304–9.

Levine 3rd H. (1999) Quantification of beta-sheet amyloid fibril structures with thioflavin T. *Methods in Enzymology* **309**: 274–84.

Levine 3rd H, Walker LC. (2010) Molecular polymorphism of Abeta in Alzheimer's disease. *Neurobiology of Aging* **31**: 542–8.

Li Y, Rinne JO, Mosconi L *et al.* (2008) Regional analysis of FDG and PIB-PET images in normal aging, mild cognitive impairment, and Alzheimer's disease. *European Journal of Nuclear Medicine and Molecular Imaging* **35**: 2169–81.

Lin KS, Debnath ML, Mathis CA, Klunk WE. (2009) Synthesis and beta-amyloid binding properties of rhenium 2-phenylbenzothiazoles. *Bioorganic and Medicinal Chemistry Letters* **19**: 2258–62.

Lockhart A, Ye L, Judd DB *et al.* (2005) Evidence for the presence of three distinct binding sites for the thioflavin T class of Alzheimer's disease PET imaging agents on beta-amyloid peptide fibrils. *Journal of Biological Chemistry* **280**: 7677–84.

Lockhart A, Lamb JR, Osredkar T *et al.* (2007) PIB is a non-specific imaging marker of amyloid-beta (Abeta) peptide-related cerebral amyloidosis. *Brain* **130**: 2607–15.

Maeda J, Ji B, Irie T *et al.* (2007) Longitudinal, quantitative assessment of amyloid, neuroinflammation, and anti-amyloid treatment in a living mouse model of Alzheimer's disease enabled by positron emission tomography. *Journal of Neuroscience* **27**: 10957–68.

Maetzler W, Liepelt I, Reimold M *et al.* (2009) Cortical PIB binding in Lewy body disease is associated with Alzheimer-like characteristics. *Neurobiology of Disease* **34**: 107–12.

Maezawa I, Hong HS, Liu R *et al.* (2008) Congo red and thioflavin-T analogs detect Abeta oligomers. *Journal of Neurochemistry* **104**: 457–68.

Majocha RE, Reno JM, Friedland RP *et al.* (1992) Development of a monoclonal antibody specific for ß/A4 amyloid in Alzheimer's disease brain for application to *in vivo* imaging of amyloid angiopathy. *Journal of Nuclear Medicine* **33**: 2184–9.

Martins IJ, Hone E, Foster JK *et al.* (2006) Apolipoprotein E, cholesterol metabolism, diabetes, and the convergence of risk factors for Alzheimer's disease and cardiovascular disease. *Molecular Psychiatry* **11**: 721–36.

Masters CL, Cappai R, Barnham KJ, Villemagne VL. (2006) Molecular mechanisms for Alzheimer's disease: implications for neuroimaging and therapeutics. *Journal of Neurochemistry* **97**: 1700–25.

Mathis CA, Wang Y, Holt DP *et al.* (2003) Synthesis and evaluation of 11C-labeled 6-substituted 2-arylbenzothiazoles as amyloid imaging agents. *Journal of Medicinal Chemistry* **46**: 2740–54.

Mathis CA, Lopresti BJ, Klunk WE. (2007) Impact of amyloid imaging on drug development in Alzheimer's disease. *Nuclear Medicine and Biology* **34**: 809–22.

McLean CA, Cherny RA, Fraser FW *et al.* (1999) Soluble pool of Aß amyloid as a determinant of severity of neurodegeneration in Alzheimer's disease. *Annals of Neurology* **46**: 860–6.

Mintun MA, Larossa GN, Sheline YI *et al.* (2006) [11C]PIB in a nondemented population: potential antecedent marker of Alzheimer disease. *Neurology* **67**: 446–52.

Mormino EC, Kluth JT, Madison CM *et al.* (2009) Episodic memory loss is related to hippocampal-mediated beta-amyloid deposition in elderly subjects. *Brain* **132**: 1310–23.

Morris JC, Price AL. (2001) Pathologic correlates of nondemented aging, mild cognitive impairment, and early-stage Alzheimer's disease. *Journal of Molecular Neuroscience* **17**: 101–18.

Morris JC, Storandt M, Miller JP *et al.* (2001) Mild cognitive impairment represents early-stage Alzheimer disease. *Archives of Neurology* **58**: 397–405.

Mueller SG, Weiner MW, Thal LJ *et al.* (2005) The Alzheimer's disease neuroimaging initiative. *Neuroimaging Clinics of North America* **15**: 869–77, xi–xii.

Newberg AB, Wintering NA, Plossl K *et al.* (2006) Safety, biodistribution, and dosimetry of 123I-IMPY: a novel amyloid plaque-imaging agent for the diagnosis of Alzheimer's disease. *Journal of Nuclear Medicine* **47**: 748–54.

Ng S, Villemagne VL, Berlangieri S *et al.* (2007) Visual assessment versus quantitative assessment of 11C-PIB PET and 18F-FDG PET for detection of Alzheimer's disease. *Journal of Nuclear Medicine* **48**: 547–52.

Noda A, Murakami Y, Nishiyama S *et al.* (2008) Amyloid imaging in aged and young macaques with [11C]PIB and [18F]FDDNP. *Synapse* **62**: 472–5.

Nyberg S, Jonhagen ME, Cselenyi Z *et al.* (2009) Detection of amyloid in Alzheimer's disease with positron emission tomography using [11C]AZD2184. *European Journal of Nuclear Medicine and Molecular Imaging* **36**: 1859–63.

Okamura N, Suemoto T, Furumoto S *et al.* (2005) Quinoline and benzimidazole derivatives: candidate probes for *in vivo* imaging of tau pathology in Alzheimer's disease. *Journal of Neuroscience* **25**: 10857–62.

Okello A, Koivunen J, Edison P *et al.* (2009) Conversion of amyloid positive and negative MCI to AD over 3 years: an 11C-PIB PET study. *Neurology* **73**: 754–60.

Petersen RC, Smith GE, Waring SC *et al.* (1999) Mild cognitive impairment: clinical characterization and outcome. *Archives of Neurology* **56**: 303–8.

Pike KE, Savage G, Villemagne VL *et al.* (2007) Beta-amyloid imaging and memory in non-demented individuals: evidence for preclinical Alzheimer's disease. *Brain* **130**: 2837–44.

Price JL, Morris JC. (1999) Tangles and plaques in nondemented aging and "preclinical" Alzheimer's disease. *Annals of Neurology* **45**: 358–68.

Rabinovici GD, Jagust WJ, Furst AJ *et al.* (2008) Abeta amyloid and glucose metabolism in three variants of primary progressive aphasia. *Annals of Neurology* **64**: 388–401.

Raymond SB, Skoch J, Hills ID *et al.* (2008) Smart optical probes for near-infrared fluorescence imaging of Alzheimer's disease pathology. *European Journal of Nuclear Medicine and Molecular Imaging* **35** (Suppl 1): S93–8.

Reiman EM, Chen K, Liu X *et al.* (2009) Fibrillar amyloid-beta burden in cognitively normal people at 3 levels of genetic risk for Alzheimer's disease. *Proceedings of the National Academy of Sciences of the United States of America* **106**: 6820–5.

Resende R, Pereira C, Agostinho P *et al.* (2007) Susceptibility of hippocampal neurons to Abeta peptide toxicity is associated with perturbation of Ca^{2+} homeostasis. *Brain Research* **1143**: 11–21.

Roe CM, Mintun MA, D'Angelo G *et al.* (2008) Alzheimer disease and cognitive reserve: variation of education effect with carbon 11-labeled Pittsburgh Compound B uptake. *Archives of Neurology* **65**: 1467–71.

Rosen RF, Walker LC, Levine 3rd H. (2009) PIB binding in aged primate brain: Enrichment of high-affinity sites in humans with Alzheimer's disease. *Neurobiology of Aging* March 27. [Epub ahead of print] (doi:10.1016/j.neurobiolaging.2009.02.011).

Rowe CC, Ng S, Ackermann U *et al.* (2007) Imaging beta-amyloid burden in aging and dementia. *Neurology* **68**: 1718–25.

Rowe CC, Ackerman U, Browne W *et al.* (2008) Imaging of amyloid beta in Alzheimer's disease with (18)F-BAY94-9172, a novel PET tracer: proof of mechanism. *Lancet Neurology* **7**: 129–35.

Serdons K, Terwinghe C, Vermaelen P *et al.* (2009a) Synthesis and evaluation of (18)F labeled 2-phenylbenzothiazoles as positron emission tomography imaging agents for amyloid plaques in Alzheimer's disease. *Journal of Medicinal Chemistry* **52**: 7090–102.

Serdons K, Verduyckt T, Vanderghinste D *et al.* (2009b) Synthesis of 18F-labelled 2-(4′-fluorophenyl)-1,3-benzothiazole and evaluation as amyloid imaging agent in comparison with [11C]PIB. *Bioorganic and Medicinal Chemical Letters* **19**: 602–5.

Shin J, Lee SY, Kim SH *et al.* (2008) Multitracer PET imaging of amyloid plaques and neurofibrillary tangles in Alzheimer's disease. *Neuroimage* **43**: 236–44.

Shoghi-Jadid K, Small GW, Agdeppa ED *et al.* (2002) Localization of neurofibrillary tangles and beta-amyloid plaques in the brains of living patients with Alzheimer disease. *American Journal of Geriatric Psychiatry* **10**: 24–35.

Small GW, Agdeppa ED, Kepe V *et al.* (2002) *In vivo* brain imaging of tangle burden in humans. *Journal of Molecular Neuroscience* **19**: 323–7.

Small GW, Kepe V, Ercoli LM *et al.* (2006) PET of brain amyloid and tau in mild cognitive impairment. *New England Journal of Medicine* **355**: 2652–63.

Sperling R, Johnson K, Pontecorvo MJ *et al.* (2009a) PET imaging of Beta-amyloid with florpiramine F18 (18F-AV-45): Preliminary results from a phase II study of cognitively normal elderly subjects, individuals with mild cognitive impairment, and patients with a clinical diagnosis of Alzheimer's disease. *Alzheimer's and Dementia* **5**: P197 [abstract].

Sperling RA, Laviolette PS, O'Keefe K *et al.* (2009b) Amyloid deposition is associated with impaired default network function in older persons without dementia. *Neuron* **63**: 178–88.

Strittmatter WJ, Saunders AM, Schmechel D *et al.* (1993) Apolipoprotein E: high-avidity binding to beta-amyloid and increased frequency of type 4 allele in late-onset familial Alzheimer disease. *Proceedings of the National Academy of Sciences of the United States of America* **90**: 1977–81.

Sundgren-Andersson AK, Svensson SPS, Swahn BM *et al.* (2009) AZD4694: Fluorinated Positron Emission Tomography (PET) radioligand for detection of beta-amyloid deposits. *Alzheimer's and Dementia* **5**: P267–8 [abstract].

Suo Z, Wu M, Citron BA *et al.* (2004) Abnormality of G-protein-coupled receptor kinases at prodromal and early stages of Alzheimer's disease: an association with early beta-amyloid accumulation. *Journal of Neuroscience* **24**: 3444–52.

Thal DR, Rub U, Schultz C *et al.* (2000) Sequence of Abeta-protein deposition in the human medial temporal lobe. *Journal of Neuropathology and Experimental Neurology* **59**: 733–48.

Thal DR, Rub U, Orantes M, Braak H. (2002) Phases of A beta-deposition in the human brain and its relevance for the development of AD. *Neurology* **58**: 1791–800.

Thompson PW, Ye L, Morgenstern JL *et al.* (2009) Interaction of the amyloid imaging tracer FDDNP with hallmark Alzheimer's disease pathologies. *Journal of Neurochemistry* **109**: 623–30.

Tolboom N, Yaqub M, van der Flier WM *et al.* (2009) Detection of Alzheimer pathology in vivo using both 11C-PIB and 18F-FDDNP PET. *Journal of Nuclear Medicine* **50**: 191–7.

Tomiyama T, Nagata T, Shimada H *et al.* (2008) A new amyloid beta variant favoring oligomerization in Alzheimer's-type dementia. *Annals of Neurology* **63**: 377–87.

Verhoeff NP, Wilson AA, Takeshita S *et al.* (2004) *In-vivo* imaging of Alzheimer disease beta-amyloid with [11C]SB-13 PET. *American Journal of Geriatric Psychiatry* **12**: 584–95.

Villemagne VL, Fodero-Tavoletti MT, Pike KE *et al.* (2008a) The ART of Loss: abeta imaging in the evaluation of Alzheimer's disease and other dementias. *Molecular Neurobiology* **38**: 1–15.

Villemagne VL, Pike KE, Darby D *et al.* (2008b) Abeta deposits in older non-demented individuals with cognitive decline are indicative of preclinical Alzheimer's disease. *Neuropsychologia* **46**: 1688–97.

Villemagne VL, Ataka S, Mizuno T *et al.* (2009a) High striatal amyloid beta-peptide deposition across different autosomal Alzheimer disease mutation types. *Archives of Neurology* **66**: 1537–44.

Villemagne VL, McLean CA, Reardon K *et al.* (2009b) 11C-PiB PET studies in typical sporadic Creutzfeldt-Jakob disease. *Journal of Neurology, Neurosurgery, and Psychiatry* **80**: 998–1001.

Wolk DA, Price JC, Saxton JA *et al.* (2009) Amyloid imaging in mild cognitive impairment subtypes. *Annals of Neurology* **65**: 557–68.

Zetterberg H, Blennow K. (2006) Plasma Abeta in Alzheimer's disease – up or down? *Lancet Neurology* **5**: 638–9.

Zhang W, Oya S, Kung MP *et al.* (2005) F-18 Polyethyleneglycol stilbenes as PET imaging agents targeting Abeta aggregates in the brain. *Nuclear Medicine and Biology* **32**: 799–809.

The neurophysiology of dementia

MICHAEL PHILPOT AND RICHARD BROWN

14.1 INTRODUCTION

The last century saw great progress in electrophysiological techniques. Conventional electroencephalography was effectively founded in the 1920s when it became possible to record such activity from the scalp. Evoked potentials and event-related potentials were first developed in the 1950s and 1960s, respectively. Quantitative analysis of the electroencephalogram (qEEG) became possible in the 1970s and recording of electromagnetic activity of the brain in the 1980s. Since then, methods of data acquisition and analysis have become ever more sophisticated.

This chapter deals with the application of neurophysiological techniques to the clinical management of the dementias and mild cognitive impairment (MCI). It will also review developments in neurophysiological research including the interest in identifying biomarkers for Alzheimer's disease (AD) and other neurodegenerative disorders. Technical details are beyond the scope of this review and the interested reader is referred to a specialist text such as Niedermeyer and Lopes da Silva (2005).

14.2 THE ELECTROENCEPHALOGRAM

14.2.1 Methods of EEG analysis

The traditional method of examining electroencephalogram (EEG) recordings is by visual assessment, looking for characteristic patterns of waveform, rhythm or spatial distribution. This is usually adequate for clinical purposes and in early clinical studies was augmented by scoring systems.

The use of EEG in research was revolutionized in the 1980s by statistical methods, such as fast Fourier transformation, that allowed complex waveforms to be converted into numerical or graphical information. Variables include absolute or relative power (the overall amplitude of a whole trace or within a waveband), mean frequency and graphical representation of the whole brain or in discrete regions of interest. Consequently qEEG – and indeed evoked and event-related potentials – can be analysed in terms of spectral data (frequency/amplitude), time (from an event or activation) or topographical location. Recording can be made while the subject is awake, at rest, asleep or during task performance. Recent techniques combining these methods enable measures of brain coherence (the degree to which similar responses occur in each hemisphere), connectivity (between hemispheres, posterior versus anterior brain or within neural networks), and the response to anticipated events. Lastly, the discovery that some dementias are associated with sleep abnormalities has led to a renewed interest in sleep EEG and polysomnography (PSG). The latter combines sleep EEG recording with electrooculography (EOG) to determine when rapid eye movement (REM) sleep is occurring, electromyography (EMG) using electrodes placed on the chin and legs to measure skeletal muscle tension, pulse oximetry, measures of respiration and often video.

14.2.2 EEG and ageing

The prevalence of EEG abnormalities increases with age with an emphasis in the temporal regions. There is a progressive slowing of the mean frequency, a reduction in α wave activity, an increase in the frequency and percentage of β activity and an increase in θ and δ activity (Dustman *et al.*, 1999). Most studies have been cross-sectional, comparing results in different age groups, but the few longitudinal studies carried out have found conflicting results. Förstl *et al.* (1996) found that waveband activity remains relatively stable over four years whereas Elmståhl and Rosén (1997) found an increase in α and θ power over a five-year period.

14.2.3   Mild cognitive impairment

The status of MCI as a possible prodrome to AD has prompted a number of EEG studies attempting to distinguish between MCI and normal ageing. Cognitive impairment developing in healthy older people has been predicted by baseline reductions in β power (Elmståhl and Rosén, 1997), and reduced α reactivity and increased θ power (Van der Hiele *et al.*, 2008). Hippocampal volume is a marker of memory impairment and in MCI correlations with θ activity (Grunwald *et al.*, 2001), reduced α power and mean frequency (Luckhaus *et al.*, 2008) and slow α activity (8–10.5 Hz) in temporoparietal regions (Babiloni *et al.*, 2009) have been found. These abnormalities correlated with the extent of white matter vascular lesions (Babiloni *et al.*, 2008). Several research groups have compared individuals with stable and progressive forms of MCI. Jelic *et al.* (2000) found that those who later developed obvious dementia had reduced EEG coherence, α and θ power. Luckhaus *et al.* (2008) found that reduced baseline α power in posterior regions best predicted cognitive decline at one-year follow up.

14.2.4   Alzheimer's disease

14.2.4.1   EEG FEATURES AND ASSOCIATIONS

EEG changes in AD can be thought of as an accentuation of normal age-related changes and lack specificity. The EEG may be visually normal in the early stages but as the disease progresses there is a general slowing with a symmetrical predominance of slow waves over the temporal and parietal regions (Binnie and Prior, 1994).

The following changes to qEEG are observed: a slowing of the α frequency, amplitude and relative power with a shift towards the anterior frontal regions; a decrease in relative and absolute β power; and, an increasing predominance of diffuse and symmetrical θ and δ waves in posterior regions, reflected by an increase in δ and θ power (Förstl *et al.*, 1996). Recent interest has focused on functional connectivity (or coherence) and many studies have now reported a reduction or disruption of neural networks in AD (Stam *et al.*, 2009; Dauwels *et al.*, 2010). Quantitative analysis of the EEG abnormalities correlate with the severity of cognitive impairment (Stam *et al.*, 2003), reduced cerebral blood flow (Ihl *et al.*, 1989) and hippocampal volume (Babiloni *et al.*, 2009), but the relationships are complex and inconsistent. The presence of qEEG abnormalities at diagnosis is associated with a more rapid progression of the disorder (van der Hiele *et al.*, 2008) and earlier death (Claus *et al.*, 1998).

Genetic risk factors may also influence EEG activity. Jelic *et al.* (1997) compared EEG coherence in AD patients homozygous for the apolipoprotein E (ApoE) ε4 allele with patients carrying either one or no ε4 allele. Coherence was reduced in the temporoparietal regions of the homozygotes. However, Kramer *et al.* (2008) found that alpha band synchronization was higher in ApoE ε4 carriers and AD patients, compared to non-carriers in both clinical groups.

14.2.4.2   DIAGNOSTIC USE OF EEG IN ALZHEIMER'S DISEASE

Methods of scoring the visual appearance of the EEG have modest success in differentiating AD from healthy elderly (e.g. Claus *et al.*, 1999) and AD and dementia with Lewy bodies (DLB; Roks *et al.*, 2008). qEEG is not routinely available in clinical practice but there have been many studies advocating its use as a diagnostic investigation, as well as a marker of prodromal or early cognitive impairment and disease progression (Adamis *et al.*, 2005). Although the simplest discrimination would be between AD patients and healthy elderly subjects, there has been little overall agreement about the optimal variables to use. Jelic and Kowalski (2009) reviewed qEEG studies between 1980 and 2008 and identified 46 that fulfilled eligibility criteria. There was a wide variety of diagnostic markers used, and indeed there was no consistency in the markers identified. There was a wide range in sensitivity and specificity and diagnostic odds ratios varied from 7 to 219. In general, the diagnostic performance of all markers was reduced in early or mild cases. Novel methods of analysis of EEG may enable further insights into frequency versus spatial distribution, connectivity between interacting brain regions, and diagnostic reliability (e.g. Dauwels *et al.*, 2010).

14.2.4.3   EEG AND CHOLINERGIC DRUGS

EEG abnormalities, including reduction in the mean frequency and an increase in slow wave activity, are associated with markers of the cholinergic system (Soininen *et al.*, 1992). A number of studies have used qEEG to assess the effects of cholinergic drugs. In general, published studies have shown a normalization of the EEG, i.e. a reduction in slow wave activity and an increase in fast activity. Effects have been found in patients taking drugs for several weeks, usually during clinical trials. Modest reductions in δ and θ power and an increase in fast activity were found following the long-term use of donepezil (Rodriguez *et al.*, 2004) and rivastigmine (Gianotti *et al.*, 2008). Beneficial effects in terms of increased EEG cortical activity occur in the frontal, temporal and parietal regions. Single-dose administration of cholinergic drugs has the same, although temporary, effect (Adler and Brassen, 2001) suggesting qEEG might be a useful marker of positive response to cholinesterase inhibitors.

14.2.5   Vascular dementias

Mild cerebrovascular disease is associated with appearance of slow and sharp waves in the temporal region. The EEG of multi-infarct dementia (MID) is similar to that of AD but focal and paroxysmal abnormalities are more prominent and there is greater asymmetry of activity although it may be normal in the early stages (d'Onofrio *et al.*, 1996).

Leuchter *et al.* (1994) found that patients with periventricular white matter hyperintensities had lower EEG coherence in the pre- and post-Rolandic areas. This effect was present in areas connected by fibres crossing the periventricular region but not in those connected by long cortico-cortical tracts, suggesting that vascular lesions might bring about difference types of neurophysiological disconnection depending on their distribution. Schreiter Gasser *et al.* (2008) compared patients with AD and mixed AD/vascular dementia (VaD). The mixed diagnosis group had increased power in the δ band and there was reduced power in the high frequency bands in AD. Topographical distribution was unaltered for slow frequency bands but showed decreased fast activity in the posterior regions.

14.2.6   Parkinson's disease dementia and dementia with Lewy bodies: a clinical aqnd historical overview

It is now thought that dementia in Parkinson's disease dementia (PDD) and DLB are part of a spectrum of disorders that share similar underlying pathology – the alpha-synucleinopathies (McKeith *et al.*, 2005; see Chapter 64, Dementia with Lewy bodies: a clinical and historical overview and Chapter 67, Cognitive impairment and dementia in Parkinson's disease). In cognitively intact patients with Parkinson's disease (PD), the EEG is essentially normal but diffuse slowing may be present (Serizawa *et al.*, 2008). In PD patients with dementia there is a further slowing, particularly in the posterior regions (Bonanni *et al.*, 2008). There is increased slow wave activity with transient temporal sharp waves (McKeith *et al.*, 2005). Bilateral frontal intermittent rhythmic δ activity (FIRDA; Roks *et al.*, 2008) may also be a useful diagnostic marker for DLB. Fluctuations in attention are another key feature of DLB and these might be reflected in greater variability and reduced coherence in alpha wave activity (Andersson *et al.*, 2008; Bonanni *et al.*, 2008).

14.2.7   Sporadic Creutzfeldt–Jakob disease and other spongiform encephalopathies

The characteristic EEG changes of sporadic Creutzfeldt–Jakob disease (sCJD) are bi-phasic or tri-phasic periodic sharp wave complexes (PSWC) occurring after the first three months of the condition and often preceded by FIRDA (Wieser *et al.*, 2006). The timing of the EEG can therefore be crucial and a study involving serial EEG recordings suggested that PSWC appear in conjunction with the motor symptoms of Creutzfeldt–Jakob disease (CJD). The positive predictive value of this marker is about 95 per cent (Steinhoff *et al.*, 2004). The typical EEG appearance becomes more likely the older the age of onset, and with a disease duration of greater than 12 months, and is seen most often in patients with the MM1 subtype (Collins *et al.*, 2006). These findings are not usually seen in the other spongiform encephalopathies and act as a discriminator for new variant CJD.

14.2.8   Other dementias

Although the EEG is usually normal in Pick's disease and frontotemporal dementia (Neary *et al.*, 1998), there is some disagreement about the prevalence of EEG abnormalities in frontotemporal lobar degeneration (FTLD) as a whole. Abnormalities have been reported in approximately 60 per cent of patients in one study (Chan *et al.*, 2004), but neither visual appearance of the EEG or qEEG were abnormal in another study (Pijnenburg *et al.*, 2008). In Huntington's disease there is a general poverty of rhythmic activity but an irregular low-voltage slow waveform emerges which correlates with the severity of cognitive impairment (Binnie and Prior, 1994).

14.2.9   Delirium

Delirium is often difficult to distinguish from dementia or even non-organic causes of mental dysfunction. An abnormal EEG, with generalized slowing, loss of the posterior dominant rhythm and loss of reactivity to eye opening and closing, generally indicates an organic cause but the abnormalities identifiable by visual inspection can depend on the underlying cause of the delirium (Jacobson and Jerrier, 2000). Thomas *et al.* (2008) found that a simple activation task (3 minutes of eye opening) improved the ability of qEEG to differentiate between patients with dementia and delirium, patients with dementia alone and cognitively unimpaired medical patients with 83 per cent accuracy.

14.2.10   Seizures associated with dementia

Epileptic seizures and focal EEG abnormalities occur in 10–20 per cent of AD patients, usually as a late complication of the disease although the incidence is relatively low (Scarmeas *et al.*, 2009). Predictors of seizures in AD include early onset, severity of dementia and the presence of focal epileptiform features on EEG. Seizure type is usually partial complex. Epilepsy may rarely masquerade as dementia. Høgh *et al.* (2002) described three patients with epilepsy presenting with a clinical picture of AD who subsequently responded to anticonvulsants.

14.2.11   Polysomnography

14.2.11.1   AGEING AND DEMENTIA

Complaints of difficulty sleeping increase with age. Throughout adult life there is a gradual reduction in total night-time sleep, sleep efficiency, percentages of slow wave, REM sleep and REM latency, sleep spindles and K-complexes. Sleep latency, percentages of stage 1 and 2 sleep and periods of wakefulness all increase (Ohayon *et al.*, 2004). The changes

Table 14.1 EEG features as a part of international diagnostic criteria in dementia.

Diagnosis	Diagnostic criteria	EEG features
Alzheimer's disease	NINCDS–ADRDA	
	1. McKhann *et al.*, 1984	1. Normal pattern/non-specific changes are supportive
	2. Dubois *et al.*, 2007	2. Do not feature in revised criteria
Vascular dementia	NINCDS–AIREN	Do not feature in diagnostic criteria
	Román *et al.*, 1993	
Dementia with Lewy bodies	DLB Consortium	Prominent slow wave activity with temporal lobe transient sharp waves are **supportive** features
	McKeith *et al.*, 2005	REM sleep behaviour disorder is a **suggestive** feature
Parkinson's disease dementia	Consensus Conference	Do not feature in diagnostic criteria
	Emre *et al.*, 2007	
Sporadic Creutzfeldt–Jakob disease	Consensus Conference	Generalized triphasic periodic sharp wave complexes (PSWC) at approximately one per second are one of the core features for a **probable** case
	Zerr *et al.*, 2009	
Frontotemporal lobar degeneration	Consensus Conference	EEG normal despite obvious dementia is supportive
	Neary *et al.*, 1998	

associated with ageing are more pronounced in dementia. There is a reduction in the period spent in deep sleep (stage 4 is often absent), very little REM sleep and frequent awakenings. Sleep spindles and K-complexes are poorly formed and often absent (Montplaisir *et al.*, 1998).

14.2.11.2 DEMENTIA AND DEPRESSION

Depression is characterized by a marked reduction in REM latency. This marker has been used to discriminate between depression and dementia (Reynolds *et al.*, 1988; Dykierek *et al.*, 1998). Reynolds *et al.* (1988) did include a comparison of patients with depressive 'pseudodementia' and those with progressive dementia complicated by depressive features. A combination of four sleep EEG measures had a diagnostic accuracy of 64 per cent. It is doubtful, however, whether the sleep EEG has much to offer in clinical practice. Co-morbid depression and dementia would not rule out a good response to antidepressants.

14.2.11.3 REM SLEEP BEHAVIOUR DISORDER

REM sleep behaviour disorder (RBD) is characterized by prominent motor behaviours, vivid and often frightening dreams during REM sleep, and is defined as the presence of REM sleep without atonia and a history of sleep-related injury or injurious behaviour. Sleep disorders are more common in DLB than AD and respond to treatment with rivastigmine (Grace *et al.*, 2000). The combination of PD and RBD is strongly associated with cognitive impairment (Gagnon *et al.*, 2009).

14.2.12 EEG in diagnostic criteria and clinical guidelines

The use of the EEG in the routine investigation of brain disorders other than epilepsy has largely been superseded by structural or functional neuroimaging. In the past, clinicians have been criticized for their injudicious requests for EEGs in the assessment of dementia and the low yield of results which effect the patient's management is well known (Binnie and Prior, 1994). Also, the wide range of diagnostic accuracy in studies of AD and MCI suggest that methods are still not optimal (Jelic and Kowalski, 2009). This is reflected by the absence of EEG and qEEG in most national and international guidelines for the assessment of AD. The most relevant neuropsychiatric settings indicating the use of EEG are acute presentations, suggesting encephalopathy, epilepsy or CJD, rather than other dementias. **Table 14.1** summarizes current criteria for a range of dementias in terms of the EEG evidence.

14.3 EVOKED POTENTIALS

An evoked potential (EP) is the sequence of EEG changes following a sensory stimulus. If the stimulus is repeated, the specific EEG pattern related to it can be discerned by averaging the responses and removing the effects of spontaneous background activity. EPs are made up of a number of wave forms or components representing electrical activity at different levels in the central nervous system usually occurring within 300 ms of the stimulus. They are numbered by convention or by reference to their latency and polarity. EPs are essentially passive responses, requiring no special effort on the part of the subject. This distinguishes them from event-related potentials, discussed under 14.4 Event-related potentials.

14.3.1 Visual evoked potentials

Visual potentials are evoked either by flashes of light or pattern reversal, as in chequerboard shifts or multifocal stimulation. These techniques are used to assess the integrity of the visual pathway and associated cortex. Potential latency and amplitude may be altered by a great number of factors including age, gender, head size, systemic disease, visual acuity, accommodation and attention (Celesia and Peachey, 2005).

A number of studies report the increased latency of components of FVEPs in AD, particularly the P2 wave which arises in the visual association cortex (Coburn et al., 2003). The latency delay of the P2 correlates with dementia severity. The early positive peak of the PRVEP (the P1/P100) which arises in the visual cortex is usually within normal limits (Philpot et al., 1990). A significant P2-P100 latency difference was initially thought to be a specific marker for AD (Harding et al., 1985) but was later shown to be non-specific (Sloan and Fenton, 1992). The diagnostic accuracy of the P2-P100 measure in studies of AD patients compared to healthy subjects is between 60 and 80 per cent (Coburn et al., 2003). Using traditional methods, inconsistent results have been reported in patients with MCI (Irimijiri et al., 2007). More recent studies using variations in visual stimulation techniques have produced encouraging results in comparisons between AD, MCI and healthy older people (Fernandez et al., 2007). The peripheral visual pathway, which can be assessed using electroretinography (ERG), is also affected in moderately severe AD (Celesia and Peachey, 2005).

Visual evoked potentials (VEP) and ERG abnormalities in PD can be reversed by dopamine agonists and also reflect dysfunction of peripheral and central pathways (Bodis-Wollner, 1997).

14.3.2   Auditory and somatosensory evoked potentials (AEP/SSEPs)

Repeated clicks or tones are used as the stimulus in auditory evoked potentials (AEPs) and the major waveforms are generated in the auditory brain stem and the auditory association areas. AEPs are also used in the assessment of demyelinating diseases, acoustic neuroma and coma. Delays in major peaks in dementia were first described by Hendrickson et al. (1979) but are non-specific and occur in a variety of conditions.

Somatosensory evoked potentials (SSEPs) are used in the functional assessment of peripheral nerves and in assessing brain function in unconscious patients. SSEP delay in dementia was first demonstrated by Levy et al. (1971) using ulnar nerve stimulation and later confirmed using the median nerve (Huisman et al., 1985). However, these changes are non-specific and have not received much research attention since. Abnormalities of EPs in response to stimulation of the cutaneous branch of the vagus nerve have recently been reported in AD and show some promise as a diagnostic marker (Polak et al., 2009).

14.4   EVENT-RELATED POTENTIALS

Event-related potentials (ERPs) require active cognitive participation from the subject and demonstrate the integrity of information processing pathways. The most commonly investigated waveform component is the positive peak occurring at around 300 ms after the stimulus or task, the P3/P300. In the oddball paradigm the subject has to differentiate between two stimuli; for example a frequently presented low tone and an infrequently presented high tone. The order of stimuli is semi-randomized to increase the unpredictability of the high or target tone. To ensure attention, subjects have to register their awareness of the target by pressing a button so that reaction time can also be measured.

The task attention demand can be a problem in older, cognitively impaired or unmotivated individuals. Mismatch negativity (MMN) forms part of the negative N2 peak arising at around 200 ms after stimulus offset and is elicited whether or not the subject makes a choice response. The 'mismatch' occurs between the sensory memory trace of the frequent stimulus and the target. contingent negative variation (CNV) describes the negative shift of the baseline following a warning stimulus given in expectation of a second stimulus. The change occurs between 200 and 500 ms and is terminated by the second stimulus.

14.4.1   Auditory ERPs

In cross-sectional studies of different age groups P3 (or P300) latency increases with age and amplitude reduces (Golob et al., 2007; Schiff et al., 2008). These changes are maximal in the temporoparietal region and the frontal region. However, latency, amplitude and distribution are all affected by the nature of task involved, the type of auditory stimulus employed and whether effort is required in processing (Polich and Corey-Bloom, 2005). MMN amplitudes are reduced in older adults (Schiff et al., 2008).

Many studies have reported the P3 latency delay and reduced amplitude in AD patients (Jackson and Snyder, 2008). P3 abnormalities correlate with the degree of cognitive impairment and worsen along with intellectual deterioration. MMN is reduced in patients with mild AD. Golob et al. (2007) found increased P50 amplitude and reduced P300 amplitude and delayed latency in patients with MCI. Subsequent follow up over five years showed that the P50 abnormality predicted those patients converting to mild AD. The same group have recently shown that all the later waveform latencies are delayed in the non-demented carriers of familial AD mutations and so may be a trait marker of AD (Golob et al., 2009).

Goodin (1990) reviewed 12 studies published up until 1988 and found that the average sensitivity of the P3/300 latency as a marker of dementia was just 51 per cent, ranging from 7 to 83 per cent. Results of more recent studies, which have included comparisons with depressed patients (Swanwick et al., 1996; Juckel et al., 2008) report sensitivities ranging from 81 to 100 per cent but the positive predictive value of an abnormal result is still relatively modest. Unfortunately, these measures are non-specific and occur in a variety of neurological and psychiatric disorders.

14.4.2   Visual ERPs

The oddball paradigm can be adapted to the visual modality. Here, a frequently presented pattern, letter or word is displayed with an infrequently presented one, or words may be paired with pictures. The visual modality has been used less than the auditory one to investigate AD but two recent studies have demonstrated potentially useful techniques to differentiate AD patients from healthy subjects (Chapman *et al.*, 2007) and AD and MCI patients from healthy subjects (Tales *et al.*, 2008). Using a variation of this method, Missionier *et al.* (2005) showed that an ERP measure reflecting working memory was absent in patients with progressive MCI compared to those with stable MCI. Similar results using another variation of this method were found for MCI patients with abnormalities of the N400 and P600 components. Those with latency delays had an 87 per cent chance of developing dementia within three years (Olichney *et al.*, 2008).

14.5 OTHER TECHNOLOGIES

14.5.1 Magnetoencephalography

Whole-head magnetoencephalography (MEG) can capture magnetic field information from up to 150 locations on the scalp enabling the mapping of the sources of abnormal fields or waveform frequencies and amplitudes. The technique has a higher temporal resolution than EEG, despite the tiny fields generated, that may be improved by combination with other imaging methods such as magnetic source imaging or functional magnetic resonance. Studies of AD patients have confirmed the decrease in fast wave activity, with increased slow wave activity and reduced coherence found using conventional EEG techniques (Criado *et al.*, 2006). Similar but less extreme changes have been found in MCI (Gómez *et al.*, 2009) and PD (Bosboom *et al.*, 2009). Recent work using graph theory to examine functional connectivity has confirmed disruption of neural networks in AD, particularly in lower α and β activity bands (Stam *et al.*, 2009).

14.5.2 Transcranial magnetic stimulation

Transcranial magnetic stimulation (TMS) employs powerful, rapidly alternating magnetic fields and allows a non-invasive method of electrically stimulating the brain. It has many applications in the investigation of neurological disorders and has been used in the treatment of depression (Chen *et al.*, 2008). In AD, interest has centred on the use of TMS to determine cortical excitability. There is increased motor cortex excitability that appears independent of inhibitory activity. Reduced intracortical inhibition has been demonstrated in corticobasal degeneration but not in AD or other forms of frontotemporal dementia (Alberici *et al.*, 2008). One specific technique – short latency afferent inhibition (SAI) – is thought to be a marker of cholinergic activity. Electrical stimulation of the median nerve can abolish the effects of TMS applied to the contralateral motor cortex. This effect only lasts about 10 ms but itself can be abolished by muscarinic antagonists (Chen *et al.*, 2008). SAI is reduced in AD and DLB, is normal in frontotemporal and VaD and can be normalized using rivastigmine (Di Lazzaro *et al.*, 2008).

Given the invasive nature of the technique it is unlikely to become a routine diagnostic procedure.

14.6 CONCLUSIONS

Before the advent of brain imaging, the EEG had a prominent role in clinical practice and probably still does in centres where neuroimaging is not readily available. The conventional resting EEG remains the most reliable and cost-effective method of neurophysiological investigation. Its main clinical uses remain the differentiation of organic disorders (including delirium) from non-organic disorders and to support the diagnosis of epilepsy. Nearly all the studies referred to in this chapter have compared well-characterized groups of subjects with each other, rather than including cases in which there have been real uncertainties about the diagnosis. Very few have confirmed diagnosis at post mortem. Perhaps as a result, techniques such as evoked and event-related potentials, MEG and TMS, do not yet have a place in routine clinical practice and, because of their lack of specificity, do not present a short cut to diagnosis. However, newly developed variations of old methods and more sophisticated means of analysing data give encouragement for future research.

REFERENCES

Adamis D, Sahu S, Treloar A. (2005) The utility of EEG in dementia: a clinical perspective. *International Journal of Geriatric Psychiatry* **20**: 1038–45.

Adler G, Brassen S. (2001) Short-term rivastigmine treatment reduces EEG slow-wave power in Alzheimer's patients. *Neuropsychobiology* **43**: 273–6.

Alberici A, Bonatao C, Calabria M *et al.* (2008) The contribution of TMS to frontotemporal dementia variants. *Acta Neurologica Scandinavica* **118**: 275–80.

Andersson M, Hansson O, Minthon L *et al.* (2008) Electroencephalogram variability in dementia with Lewy bodies, Alzheimer's disease and controls. *Dementia and Geriatric Cognitive Disorders* **26**: 284–90.

Babiloni C, Frisoni GB, Pievani M *et al.* (2008) White matter vascular lesions are related to parietal-to-frontal coupling of EEG rhythms in mild cognitive impairment. *Human Brain Mapping* **29**: 1355–67.

Babiloni C, Frisoni GB, Pievani M *et al.* (2009) Hippocampal volume and cortical sources of EEG alpha rhythms in mild cognitive impairment and Alzheimer disease. *Neuroimage* **44**: 123–35.

Binnie CD, Prior PF. (1994) Electroencephalography. *Journal of Neurology, Neurosurgery and Psychiatry* **57**: 1308–19.

Bodis-Wollner I. (1997) Visual electrophysiology in Parkinson's disease: PERG, VEP and visual P300. *Clinical Electroencephalography* **28**: 143–7.

Bonanni L, Thomas A, Tiraboschi P *et al.* (2008) EEG comparisons in early Alzheimer's disease, dementia with Lewy bodies and Parkinson's disease with dementia patients with a 2-year follow-up. *Brain* **131**: 690–705.

Bosboom JL, Stoffers D, Wolters ECh et al. (2009) MEG resting state functional connectivity in Parkinson's disease related dementia. *Journal of Neural Transmission* 116: 193–202.

Celesia GC, Peachey NS. (2005) Visual evoked potentials and electroretinograms. In: Niedermeyer E, Da Silva FL (eds). *Electroencephalography. Basic principles, clinical applications, and related fields*, 5th edn. Philadelphia: Lippincott Williams and Wilkins, 1017–43.

Chan D, Walters RJ, Sampson EL et al. (2004) EEG abnormalities in frontotemporal lobar degeneration. *Neurology* 62: 1628–30.

Chapman RM, Nowlis GH, McCrary JW et al. (2007) Brain event-related potentials: diagnosing early-stage Alzheimer's disease. *Neurobiology of Aging* 28: 194–201.

Chen R, Cros D, Curra A et al. (2008) The clinical diagnostic utility of transcranial magnetic stimulation: Report of an IFCN committee. *Clinical Neurophysiology* 119: 504–32.

Claus JJ, Ongerboer de Visser BW, Walstra GJ et al. (1998) Quantitative spectral electro-encephalography in predicting survival in patients with early Alzheimer's disease. *Archives of Neurology* 55: 1105–11.

Claus JJ, Strijers RLM, Jonkman EJ et al. (1999) The diagnostic value of electroencephalography in mild senile Alzheimer's disease. *Clinical Neurophysiology* 110: 825–32.

Coburn KL, Arruda JE, Estes KM, Amoss RT. (2003) Diagnostic utility of visual evoked potential changes in Alzheimer's disease. *Journal of Neuropsychiatry and Clinical Neurosciences* 15: 175–9.

Collins SJ, Sanchez-Juan P, Masters CL et al. (2006) Determinants of diagnostic investigation sensitivities across the clinical spectrum of sporadic Creutzfeldt–Jakob disease. *Brain* 129: 2278–87.

Criado JR, Amo C, Quint P et al. (2006) Using magnetoencephalography to study patterns of brain magnetic activity in Alzheimer's disease. *American Journal of Alzheimer's Disease and Other Dementias* 21: 416–23.

Dauwels J, Vialette F, Musha T, Cichocki A. (2010) A comparative study of synchrony measures for the early diagnosis of Alzheimer's disease based on EEG. *Neuroimage* 49: 668–93.

Di Lazzaro V, Pilato F, Dileone M et al. (2008) *In vivo* functional evaluation of central cholinergic circuits in vascular dementia. *Clinical Neurophysiology* 119: 2494–500.

d'Onofrio F, Salvia S, Petretta V et al. (1996) Quantified-EEG in normal aging and dementias. *Acta Neurologica Scandinavica* 93: 336–45.

Dubois B, Feldman HH, Jacova C et al. (2007) Research criteria for the diagnosis of Alzheimer's disease: revising the NINCDS-ADRDA criteria. *Lancet Neurology* 6: 734–46.

Dustman RE, Shearer DE, Emmerson RY. (1999) Life-span changes in EEG spectral amplitude, amplitude variability and mean frequency. *Clinical Neurophysiology* 110: 1399–409.

Dykierek P, Stadmuller G, Schramm P et al. (1998) The value of REM sleep parameters in differentiating Alzheimer's disease from old-age depression and normal aging. *Journal of Psychiatric Research* 32: 1–9.

Elmståhl S, Rosén I. (1997) Postural hypotension and EEG variables predict cognitive decline: results from a 5-year follow-up of healthy elderly women. *Dementia and Geriatric Cognitive Disorders* 8: 180–7.

Emre M, Aarsland D, Brown R et al. (2007) Clinical diagnostic criteria for dementia associated with Parkinson's disease. *Movement Disorders* 22: 1689–707.

Fernandez R, Kavcic V, Duffy CJ. (2007) Neurophysiologic analyses of low- and high-level visual processing in Alzheimer's disease. *Neurology* 68: 2066–78.

Förstl H, Sattel H, Besthorn C et al. (1996) Longitudinal cognitive, electroencephalographic and morphological brain changes in ageing and Alzheimer's disease. *British Journal of Psychiatry* 168: 280–6.

Gagnon JF, Vendette M, Postuma RB et al. (2009) Mild cognitive impairment in rapid eye movement sleep behaviour disorder and Parkinson's disease. *Annals of Neurology* 66: 39–47.

Gianotti LR, Kunig G, Faber PL et al. (2008) Rivastigmine effects on EEG spectra and three-dimensional LORETA functional imaging in Alzheimer's disease. *Psychopharmacology (Berlin)* 183: 323–32.

Golob EJ, Irimijiri R, Starr A. (2007) Auditory cortical activity in amnestic mild cognitive impairment: relationship to subtype and conversion to dementia. *Brain* 130: 740–52.

Golob EJ, Ringman JM, Irimijiri R et al. (2009) Cortical event-related potentials in preclinical familial Alzheimer's disease. *Neurology* 73: 1649–55.

Gómez C, Stam CJ, Hornero R et al. (2009) Disturbed beta band functional connectivity in patients with mild cognitive impairment: an MEG study. *Institute of Electronics and Electrical Engineers Transactions on Biomed Engineering* 56: 1683–90.

Goodin DS. (1990) Clinical utility of long latency 'cognitive' event-related potentials (P3): the pros. *Electroencephalography and Clinical Neurophysiology* 76: 2–5.

Grace JB, Walker MP, McKeith IG. (2000) A comparison of sleep profiles in patients with dementia with Lewy bodies and Alzheimer's disease. *International Journal of Geriatric Psychiatry* 15: 1028–33.

Grunwald M, Busse F, Hensel A et al. (2001) Correlation between cortical theta activity and hippocampal volumes in health, mild cognitive impairment and mild dementia. *Journal of Clinical Neurophysiology* 18: 178–84.

Harding GFA, Wright CE, Orwin A. (1985) Primary presenile dementia: the use of the visual evoked potential as a diagnostic indicator. *British Journal of Psychiatry* 147: 532–9.

Hendrickson E, Levy R, Post F. (1979) Averaged evoked responses in relation to cognitive and affective state of elderly psychiatric patients. *British Journal of Psychiatry* 134: 494–501.

Høgh P, Smith SJ, Scahill RI et al. (2002) Epilepsy presenting as AD: neuroimaging, electroclinical features, and response to treatment. *Neurology* 58: 298–301.

Huisman UW, Postuma J, Hooijer V et al. (1985) Somatosensory evoked potentials in healthy volunteers and patients with dementia. *Clinical Neurology and Neurosurgery* 87: 11–16.

Ihl R, Eilles C, Frolich F et al. (1989) Electrical brain activity and cerebral blood flow in dementia of the Alzheimer type. *Psychiatry Research* 29: 449–52.

Irimijiri R, Michalewski HJ, Golob EJ, Starr A. (2007) Cholinesterase inhibitors affect brain potentials in amnestic mild cognitive impairment. *Brain Research* 1145: 108–16.

Jackson CE, Snyder PJ. (2008) Electroencephalography and event-related potentials as biomarkers of mild cognitive impairment and mild Alzheimer's disease. *Alzheimer's and Dementia* 4 (Suppl. 1): S137–43.

Jacobson S, Jerrier H. (2000) EEG in delirium. *Seminars in Clinical Neuropsychiatry* 5: 86–92.

Jelic V, Julin P, Shigeta M *et al.* (1997) Apolipoprotein E ε4 allele decreases functional connectivity in Alzheimer's disease as measured by EEG coherence. *Journal of Neurology, Neurosurgery and Psychiatry* 63: 59–65.

Jelic V, Johansson SE, Almkvist O *et al.* (2000) Quantitative electroencephalography in mild cognitive impairment: longitudinal changes and possible prediction of Alzheimer's disease. *Neurobiology of Aging* 21: 533–40.

Jelic V, Kowalski J. (2009) Evidence-based evaluation of diagnostic accuracy of resting EEG in dementia and mild cognitive impairment. *Clinical EEG and Neuroscience* 40: 129–42.

Juckel G, Clotz F, Frodl T *et al.* (2008) Diagnostic usefulness of cognitive auditory event-related P300 subcomponents in patients with Alzheimer's disease. *Journal of Clinical Neurophysiology* 25: 147–52.

Kramer G, van der Flier WM, de Langen C *et al.* (2008) EEG functional connectivity and ApoE genotype in Alzheimer's disease and controls. *Clinical Neurophysiology* 119: 2727–32.

Leuchter AF, Dunjun JJ, Kufkin RB *et al.* (1994) Effect of white matter disease on functional connections in the aging brain. *Journal of Neurology, Neurosurgery and Psychiatry* 57: 1347–54.

Levy R, Isaacs A, Behrman J. (1971) Neurophysiological correlates of senile dementia. II. The somatosensory evoked response. *Psychological Medicine* 1: 159–65.

Luckhaus C, Grass-Kapanke B, Blaeser I *et al.* (2008) Quantitative EEG in progressing vs. stable mild cognitive impairment (MCI): results of a 1-year follow-up study. *International Journal of Geriatric Psychiatry* 23: 1148–55.

McKeith IG, Dickson DW, Lowe J *et al.* (2005) Diagnosis and management of dementia with Lewy bodies. 3rd report of the DLB consortium. *Neurology* 65: 1863–72.

McKhann G, Drachman DA, Folstein M *et al.* (1984) Clinical diagnosis of Alzheimer's disease – report of the NINCDS-ADRDA work group under the auspices of Department of Health and Human Services Task Force on Alzheimer's disease. *Neurology* 34: 939–44.

Missionier P, Gold G, Fazio-Costa L *et al.* (2005) Early event-related potential changes during working memory activation predict rapid decline in mild cognitive impairment. *Journal of Gerontology: Medical Sciences* 60A: 660–6.

Montplaisir J, Petit D, Gauthier S *et al.* (1998) Sleep disturbances and EEG slowing in Alzheimer's disease. *Sleep Research Online* 1: 147–51.

Neary D, Snowden JS, Gustafson L *et al.* (1998) Frontotemporal lobar degeneration. A consensus on clinical diagnostic criteria. *Neurology* 51: 1546–54.

Niedermeyer E, Lopes da Silva FL. (eds) (2005) *Electroencephalography. Basic principles, clinical applications and related fields*, 5th edn. Philadelphia: Lippincott Williams and Williams.

Ohayon MM, Carskadon MA, Guilleminault C, Vitiello MV. (2004) Meta-analysis of quantitative sleep parameters from childhood to old age in healthy individual: developing normative sleep values across the human lifespan. *Sleep* 27: 1255–73.

Olichney JM, Taylor JR, Gatherwright J *et al.* (2008) Patients with MCI and N400 or P600 abnormalities are at very high risk for conversion to dementia. *Neurology* 70: 1763–70.

Philpot MP, Amin D, Levy R. (1990) Visual evoked potentials in Alzheimer's disease: correlations with age and severity. *Electroencephalography and Clinical Neurophysiology* 77: 323–9.

Pijnenburg YA, Strijers RL, Made YV *et al.* (2008) Investigation of resting-state EEG functional connectivity in frontotemporal lobar degeneration. *Clinical Neurophysiology* 119: 1732–8.

Polak T, Markulin F, Ehils AC *et al.* (2009) Auricular vagus somatosensory evoked potentials in vascular dementia. *Journal of Neural Transmission* 116: 473–7.

Polich J, Corey-Bloom J. (2005) Alzheimer's disease and P300: review and evaluation of task and modality. *Current Alzheimer's Research* 2: 515–25.

Reynolds CF, Kupfer DJ, Houck PR *et al.* (1988) Reliable discrimination of elderly depressed and demented patients by electroencephalographic sleep data. *Archives of General Psychiatry* 45: 258–64.

Rodriguez G, Vitali P, Canfora M *et al.* (2004) Quantitative EEG and perfusional single photon emission computed tomography correlation during long-term donepezil therapy in Alzheimer's disease. *Clinical Neurophysiology* 115: 39–49.

Roks G, Korf ES, van der Flier WM *et al.* (2008) The use of EEG in the diagnosis of dementia with Lewy bodies. *Journal of Neurology, Neurosurgery and Psychiatry* 79: 377–80.

Román GC, Tatemichi TK, Erkinjuntti T *et al.* (1993) Vascular dementia. Diagnostic criteria for research studies: Report of the NINDS-AIREN International Workshop. *Neurology* 43: 250–60.

Scarmeas N, Honig LS, Choi H *et al.* (2009) Seizures in Alzheimer's disease: who, when, and how common? *Archives of Neurology* 66: 992–7.

Schiff S, Valenti P, Pellegrini A *et al.* (2008) The effect of aging on auditory components of event-related brain potentials. *Clinical Neurophysiology* 119: 1795–802.

Schreiter Gasser U, Rousson V, Hentschel F *et al.* (2008) Alzheimer's disease versus mixed dementias: an EEG perspective. *Clinical Neurophysiology* 119: 2255–9.

Serizawa K, Kamei S, Morita A *et al.* (2008) Comparison of quantitative EEGs between Parkinson disease and age-adjusted normal controls. *Journal of Clinical Neurophysiology* 25: 361–6.

Sloan EP, Fenton GW. (1992) Serial visual evoked potential recordings in geriatric psychiatry. *Electroencephalography and Clinical Neurophysiology* 84: 325–31.

Soininen H, Reinikainen K, Partanen J *et al.* (1992) Slowing of electroencephalogram and choline acetyl-transferase activity in definitive Alzheimer's disease. *Neuroscience* 49: 529–35.

Stam CJ, van der Made Y, Pijnenburg YA, Scheltens P. (2003) EEG synchronization in mild cognitive impairment and Alzheimer's disease. *Acta Neurologica Scandinavica* 108: 90–96.

Stam CJ, de Haan W, Daffertshofer A *et al.* (2009) Graph theoretical analysis of magneto-encephalographic functional connectivity in Alzheimer's disease. *Brain* 132: 213–24.

Steinhoff BJ, Zerr I, Glatting M *et al.* (2004) Diagnostic value of periodic complexes in Creutzfeldt-Jakob disease. *Annals of Neurology* **56**: 702–8.

Swanwick GRJ, Rowan M, Coen RF *et al.* (1996) Clinical application of electrophysiological markers in the differential diagnosis of depression and very mild Alzheimer's disease. *Journal of Neurology, Neurosurgery and Psychiatry* **60**: 82–6.

Tales A, Haworth J, Wilcock G *et al.* (2008) Visual mismatch negativity highlights abnormal pre-attentive visual processing in mild cognitive impairment and Alzheimer's disease. *Neuropsychologia* **46**: 1224–32.

Thomas C, Hestermann U, Walther S *et al.* (2008) Prolonged activation EEG differentiates dementia with and without delirium in frail elderly patients. *Journal of Neurology, Neurosurgery and Psychiatry* **79**: 119–25.

Van der Hiele K, Bollen EL, Vein AA *et al.* (2008) EEG markers of future cognitive performance in the elderly. *Journal of Clinical Neurophysiology* **25**: 83–9.

Wieser HG, Schindler K, Zumsteg D. (2006) EEG in Creutzfeldt-Jakob disease. *Clinical Neurophysiology* **117**: 935–51.

Zerr I, Kallenberg K, Summers DM *et al.* (2009) Updated clinical diagnostic criteria for sporadic Creutzfeldt-Jakob disease. *Brain* **132**: 2659–68.

Family carers of people with dementia

HENRY BRODATY AND MARIKA DONKIN

15.1   WHO ARE INFORMAL CARERS?

Alzheimer's Disease International (ADI) estimates that there are 30 million people with dementia worldwide (ADI, 2008). For approximately 75–80 per cent of persons with dementia (PWD) who live in the community, care is provided informally by unpaid carers (Schulz and Martire, 2004), typically family members, but also friends and neighbours. In 2007 there were at least 10 million people in the United States caring for a friend or family member with Alzheimer's disease (AD) or another dementia (Alzheimer's Association, 2007) and in the UK carers looked after approximately 700 000 PWD (Personal Social Services Research Unit London School of Economics, 2007).

Family carers, also called caregivers, are the 'cornerstone of support for people with dementia' (Ferri et al., 2005). Without carers, PWD would have a poorer quality of life and would need institutional care more quickly, and national economies would be inundated by the advancing demographic tidal wave.

In the US, most carers are helping relatives (87 per cent) (Alzheimer's Association and National Alliance for Caregiving, 2004). Approximately 60 per cent of dementia carers are female, and the majority are spouses, with daughters the next most prevalent type of carer (Schulz and Martire, 2004; Alzheimer's Association, 2008a). Males, primarily husbands and sons, comprise 40 per cent of carers (Alzheimer's Association, 2008a). This represents a doubling in the proportion of male carers of PWD from 1996 to 2008 (Alzheimer's Association, 2008b). In the UK, men aged 75 years and older are more likely than women to be caring for their spouse (Office for National Statistics, 2005).

More than 60 per cent of PWD live in the developing world (Alzheimer's Association, 2008a). Forecasts of the prevalence of dementia to the year 2040 are three times higher in developing than in the developed world (Kurz et al., 2008). The 10/66 Dementia Research Group assessed the care arrangements of 706 PWD in South East Asia, China, India, Latin America and the Caribbean and Nigeria. In all areas the majority of the carers were female, and typically in larger proportions than in the US and UK (ranging from 59 per cent in China and South East Asia to 95 per cent in Nigeria). As in the developed world, wives were most often the primary carers (21 per cent in China and South East Asia to 45 per cent in Nigeria), followed by daughters (15 per cent in India to 40 per cent in Nigeria). Daughters-in-law also featured prominently, comprising a mean of 11 per cent of all carers (with a range from 3 per cent in Latin America and the Caribbean to 24 per cent in India and South Asia). In India and South Asia daughters-in-law were the second largest group of carers after wives. PWD in the developing world tend to live in much larger extended family households than those in countries such as the US and UK (Prince, The 10/66 Dementia Research Group, 2004).

15.2   WHY DO FAMILY CARERS CARE?

Informal carers are motivated to provide care for several reasons, some of which are positive and beneficial and some of which are not. Positive reasons include a sense of love or reciprocity, spiritual fulfilment and feelings of mastery and accomplishment (Eisdorfer, 1991; Sanders, 2005). Carers who identify these reasons experience less burden, better health, relationships and social support (Cohen *et al.*, 2002). Less positive reasons include a sense of duty or cultural and social norms and pressures, guilt and greed (Eisdorfer, 1991). Carers thus motivated are more likely to suffer psychological distress and burden (Pyke and Bengston, 1996). While the negative aspects of caregiving receive more attention in the literature, Sanders (2005) reported that between 55 and 90 per cent of carers identified positive motivations for caregiving, including spiritual and personal growth, increased faith, accomplishment and mastery (Sanders, 2005).

A number of variables influence the way that carers view their role. Feeling more positively towards caregiving has been associated with lower educational level, greater social resources, satisfaction with social participation, better physical health status, being non-Caucasian and being older (Haley *et al.*, 1996; Kramer, 1997; Rapp and Chao, 2000). Dilworth-Anderson *et al.* (2005) found that African Americans identified more traditional, collectivist reasons for providing care than white Americans. In an earlier study, both strong and very weak cultural justifications for caregiving were associated with poorer self-rated health for African American carers (Dilworth-Anderson *et al.*, 2004; Dilworth-Anderson *et al.*, 2005). With the increasing prevalence of male carers, gender differences may be of particular interest, but research to date are lacking (Baker and Robertson, 2008).

15.3   HOW DO FAMILY CARERS CARE?

Care providers, who provide the day-to-day hands-on care, can be differentiated from care managers, who assist to arrange for others to provide care, for instance a nurse or personal care assistant (Archbold, 1981).

Providing care for a PWD is very demanding. Primary carers typically spend large proportions of their day assisting and supervising care recipients with activities of daily living (ADLs) and instrumental activities of daily living (IADLs). It is difficult to provide precise estimates as studies are limited by access to and willingness of carers to participate, impacting on the size and representativeness of samples. In a study of 1181 UK and European carers (a random sample from Alzheimer Europe's member organizations fairly evenly distributed between Germany, Poland, Spain, France and Scotland), 44 per cent reported spending at least 10 hours a day assisting the PWD (Georges *et al.*, 2008). A US survey of 227 dementia carers found that nearly one-quarter provided 40 hours of care or more per week, compared to 16 per cent for non-dementia carers. Thirty-two percent of these carers had sustained the commitment for five years or longer (Alzheimer's Association, 2007). The usefulness of this study is limited by its sample size. The Australian Survey of Disability, Ageing and Carers identified that 65 per cent of approximately 12 000 primary carers of PWD spent 40 hours or more per week in their caregiving role (Australian Institute of Health and Welfare, 2007).

Variables that influence the amount of time spent caring for a person with dementia (based on the most common caregiving relationship, wife to husband) include time since onset, the patient's level of disability and the amount of instrumental support available to the carer (Taylor *et al.*, 2008).

Estimates of informal care time typically only take account of time spent by the primary carer. Neubauer and colleagues (2008) found that including time spent by other carers increases the total estimate by more than 10 per cent. This figure may be an underestimate as it was based on interviews with the primary carer who responded on behalf of other carers, and the majority of the sample had only mild dementia (65 per cent).

The demands of caregiving are at least as high in the developing world. Interviews with 706 informal carers in developing countries indicated that they spend a median of between three (India, China, South and South East Asia) and nine (Nigeria) hours a day assisting people with dementia with ADLs (Prince, The 10/66 Dementia Research Group, 2004). One of the main differences between caregiving in these countries and the developed world is that people commonly live in three-generation households (Prince, The 10/66 Dementia Research Group, 2004). This does not appear to decrease carer burden. While there may be a number of care managers involved, there typically tends to be only one care provider performing most of the 'hands-on' care. Additionally, when the primary carer is not co-resident with the care recipient, having more people involved appears to create tension and conflict (Prince, The 10/66 Dementia Research Group, 2004). There is also a weakening of traditional kinship and support systems in some developing (particularly African) countries. Economic hardship, migration from rural areas and shifting values and priorities have meant that families are less able or willing to provide care in traditional ways for older people (Aboderin, 2004; Okojie, 2004).

15.4   EFFECTS OF DEMENTIA ON CARERS

The care that informal carers provide often comes at a considerable cost to their own health and well-being. For every PWD, there are several close family members deeply affected by the emotional, physical, social and financial costs associated with caregiving (Serrano-Aguilar *et al.*, 2006). Caregiving in general is associated with increased stress and burden, and contributes to psychological morbidity, particularly depression and anxiety, and poorer physical health (Brodaty and Hadzi-Pavlovic, 1990; Pearlin *et al.*, 1990; Schulz *et al.*, 1995; Clare *et al.*, 2002; Schulz and Martire, 2004). Dementia carers fare even worse than carers of people with other illnesses and disabilities (Schulz *et al.*, 1990; Mohide *et al.*, 1998; Ory *et al.*, 1999).

The relationship between caregiving and health outcomes is complex and many factors exacerbate or ameliorate how carers react to their role. Two models of factors leading to carer stress are useful. The modified Poulshock and Deimling model (**Figure 15.1**), shows that dementia leads to a burden

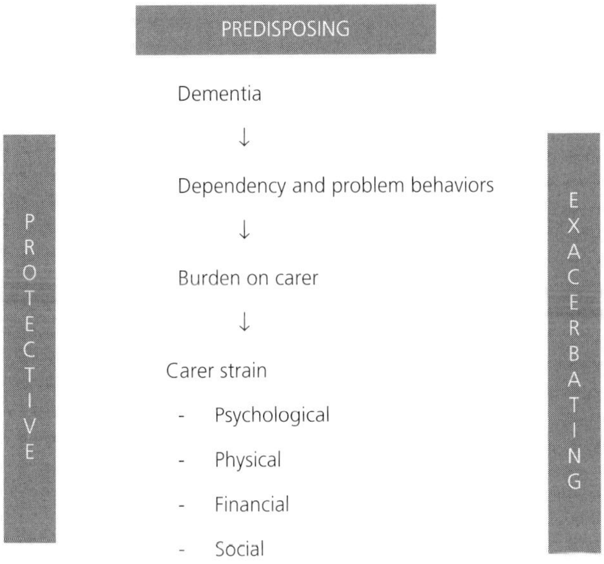

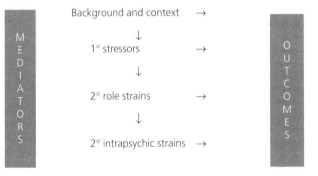

Figure 15.1 Poulshock and Deimling (1984) model of carer strain (modified).

Figure 15.2 Pearlin *et al.* (1990) model of carer strain.

of care which can manifest as strain in a number of ways (Poulshock and Deimling, 1984). Burden plays an important role between the impairment of the person with dementia and the impact that caregiving has on the carer and family. These can be exacerbated by factors such as behavioural disturbance in the PWD and physical or psychological ill-health in the carer, or ameliorated by social support and mature coping mechanisms (Poulshock and Deimling, 1984).

Pearlin and colleagues' (1990) model (**Figure 15.2**) outlines four main areas that contribute to carer stress: (1) background and context of the stress process, which includes carer and family characteristics, support and the impact of other life events. All other steps in the process are influenced by these key characteristics of the carer and caring context. (2) Primary or first degree stressors relate directly to the illness. Indicators of primary stressors are the cognitive status of the persons with dementia, their problematic behaviours and precautions and supervision required to deal with them, and the extent of their dependency on the carer for ADLs and IADLs. (3) Secondary role strains include family dynamics and conflict, and stress from the carer's life outside the caregiving role (including their employment and recreational

pursuits). These are not secondary in the sense that they are less potent, but because conditions surrounding the primary stressors are productive of secondary stressors (Pearlin *et al.*, 1990). (4) Intrapsychic strains are the carer's self-concept and psychological state. The relevant elements are self-esteem, mastery, role captivity, loss of self, competence and gain (Pearlin *et al.*, 1990; Campbell *et al.*, 2008). Factors which may mediate the relationship between stressors and outcome include coping style and availability and satisfaction with social support (Pearlin *et al.*, 1990).

Campbell and colleagues (2008) reviewed this model and found that the strongest predictors of carer burden were sense of 'role captivity' (carer feelings of being 'trapped' in their role), carer overload, adverse life events and quality of the relationship between carer and care receiver.

The following concepts are useful to understand the impact of dementia on the carer.

15.4.1 Objective burden

Objective burden reflects the dependency of the dementia patient. It is evidenced by loss of independence in ADLs and IADLs, reduced cognition, other abilities, companionship and communication, and behavioural and psychological symptoms of dementia (BPSD).

15.4.2 Subjective strain

Subjective strain is the appraisal of burden by the carer, including evaluation of their psychological state and resources (Gonyea *et al.*, 2005). There is considerable evidence that dementia carers around the world experience significant strain (Schulz *et al.*, 1995; Schulz and Williamson, 1997; Shaji *et al.*, 2003; Sanders, 2005; Connor *et al.*, 2008; Hirakawa *et al.*, 2008). Objective burden and subjective strain are surprisingly only loosely correlated (Campbell *et al.*, 2008), as it is not only the objective dementia-related load that determines carer burden levels, but the carer's subjective interpretation (Schulz *et al.*, 1995; Campbell *et al.*, 2008).

15.4.3 Psychological morbidity

The strain of caregiving can manifest as psychological morbidity, particularly depression and anxiety (Cooper *et al.*, 2006; Campbell *et al.*, 2008; Gaugler *et al.*, 2008). In developed countries, rates of depression among dementia carers range from 23 to 85 per cent (Prince, Adkins, 1999; Clare *et al.*, 2002) and rates of anxiety between 16 and 45 per cent (Schulz *et al.*, 1995; Livingston *et al.*, 2005; Cooper *et al.*, 2006; Cooper *et al.*, 2007). In developing countries, rates of psychiatric morbidity range from 40 to 75 per cent (Prince, The 10/66 Dementia Research Group, 2004).

Compared to other carers, dementia carers experience higher levels of psychological distress and lower levels of self-efficacy and subjective well-being. These differences are even larger when compared to non-carers (Pinquart and Sörensen, 2003). Campbell and colleagues (2008) indicated that depression results from feelings of resentment towards the PWD that comes from carers feeling 'trapped' and overwhelmed in their roles. Depression impairs carers' ability to manage new challenges, thereby making them more susceptible to experiencing negative life events (or at least perceiving events negatively) (Gonyea et al., 2005). Anxiety results from carers' fears about the future (Cooper et al., 2007) and in some studies is more prevalent than depression (Brodaty and Hadzi-Pavlovic, 1990).

Carer characteristics determine their psychological morbidity more than those of the care recipient (Cooper et al., 2006). Factors related to depression and anxiety include female gender, being a spousal carer, additional stressful life events, physical ill health, family history of mental illness, low quality of relationship between carer and care receiver, less life satisfaction, low levels of self-esteem and mastery, high neuroticism and levels of BPSD (Brodaty and Hadzi-Pavlovic, 1990; Schulz et al., 1995; Campbell et al., 2008).

15.4.4   Physical morbidity

Carers report more health problems and worse overall health compared to controls (Schulz et al., 1990; Baumgarten et al., 1992). Dementia caregiving has been associated with a higher risk of physical health problems, including cardiovascular disease, slower wound healing, higher metabolic risk, higher levels of chronic conditions (such as diabetes, arthritis, ulcers and anaemia), greater use of medications and health services, lower immunity and poorer immune response to vaccines (Haley et al., 1987; Pruchno and Potashnik, 1989; Baumgarten et al., 1992; Schulz and Williamson, 1997; Vedhara et al., 1999; Vedhara et al., 2003; Vitaliano et al., 2003; Schulz and Martire, 2004; Alzheimer's Association, 2007; Segerstrom et al., 2008). Segerstrom and colleagues (2008) found that negative repetitive thoughts predicted higher levels of depression in carers and lower antibody titres, whereas neutral repetitive thoughts predicted less depression and higher antibody titres, but also higher levels of the inflammatory cytokine IL-6 post-vaccination (Segerstrom et al., 2008).

Carers are also less likely to engage in preventative health behaviours such as exercise, and are more likely to smoke, drink alcohol and have poor sleep patterns, placing themselves at risk of further health problems (Schulz and Williamson, 1997).

15.4.5   Social isolation

Carers are often socially isolated as they tend to sacrifice their leisure pursuits and hobbies, restrict time with friends and family and to give up or reduce employment (Brodaty and Hadzi-Pavlovic, 1990; LoGiudice et al., 1999; Leong et al., 2001). Distance from family and friends can compound carer isolation. In one study, half the carers had contact with someone outside their household once per week or less and 13 per cent had no personal contacts outside the home in the previous 2 weeks (Brodaty and Hadzi-Pavlovic, 1990).

Social support and contact are associated with better psychological health for carers. Carers who were more satisfied with their social interactions showed fewer negative psychological symptoms (Serrano-Aguilar et al., 2006). Intervention may assist: an intervention that enhanced counselling and social support significantly increased the number of support persons for carers, their satisfaction with their support network, and the assistance they received with caregiving, compared to controls (Roth et al., 2005). The increased satisfaction with the social support network mediated a significant proportion of the intervention's impact on caregiver depression.

15.4.6   Financial

The worldwide direct costs of dementia were estimated in 2005 to be $US210 billion (Wimo et al., 2007). Formal care services for people with AD and other dementias cost the US at least $US60 billion (Wimo et al., 2007), and Europe at least $US80 billion (Wimo et al., 2007). Comparative figures for Australia and New Zealand were approximately $US3 billion (Wimo et al., 2007). Direct costs include medical consultations, investigations, pharmaceuticals, provision of personal and nursing care and residential care in the later stages.

These figures do not capture the total costs. Substantial indirect costs, usually omitted from estimates, are borne by carers. They include hours of informal care, loss of earnings as carers reduce their hours of paid work or move out of the workforce, and mortality burden (Access Economics, 2003; Brodaty et al., 2005). Total costs worldwide including indirect costs were $US315 billion in 2005, much higher than the direct cost estimate (Wimo et al., 2007). Almost 60 per cent of US family carers of PWD are also employed, of whom two-thirds reported that they missed work and 8 per cent that they turned down promotion opportunities. Up to 31 per cent had given up work to attend to caregiving responsibilities (Alzheimer's Association and National Alliance for Caregiving, 2004; Alzheimer's Association, 2007).

In the developing world, the costs of dementia in comparative terms represent a greater burden than in the developed world, and the economic disadvantage associated with caregiving is significant (Prince, The 10/66 Dementia Research Group, 2004). Wimo and colleagues (2007) estimated that direct costs of dementia in emerging market and developing countries totalled $US52 billion, with total costs reaching at least $US88 billion in 2005. In the countries surveyed, 32 per cent of carers on average (including 84 per cent in Nigeria) cut back on paid work to care for a family member with dementia and very few were able to access compensatory financial support such as government pensions. While health-care services are cheaper in absolute dollars than in developed countries, in relative terms these families spend a greater proportion of their income on health care for the PWD. Paradoxically, despite economic disadvantage, carers from poorer countries tend to use the more expensive services of private doctors as public services are unsatisfactory (Prince, The 10/66 Dementia Research Group, 2004).

15.5 PREDICTORS OF AND PROTECTORS FROM CARER DISTRESS

15.5.1 Demographic variables

Demographic variables associated with higher rates of psychological morbidity are female gender, being a spousal carer, particularly of a patient with early-onset dementia, cohabiting with the care receiver and having a lower income or being financially unstable (Robinson, 1989; Brodaty and Hadzi-Pavlovic, 1990; Morrissey et al., 1990; Dura et al., 1991; Schulz and Williamson, 1991; Baumgarten et al., 1992; Semple, 1992; Gallicchio et al., 2002; Livingston et al., 2005; Schulz et al., 2008). These are general trends and are not undisputed. Schulz et al. (1995) found inconclusive evidence about the relationship between age, gender and psychological morbidity. Brodaty and Hadzi-Pavlovic (1990) found that the higher levels of distress in female carers was mediated by the increased likelihood of behavioural disturbances in men and the high likelihood of them being supported by their wives.

Conversely, carer factors found to protect against strain and distress were male gender, being a non-spousal carer, living separately and being in a better financial position (Brodaty and Hadzi-Pavlovic, 1990; Schulz and Williamson, 1991; Baumgarten et al., 1992; Semple, 1992; Zarit and Whitlatch, 1992). Sons, as well as being the least likely group to be in a caregiving role, experienced the lowest levels of strain (Sanders, 2005; Hong and Kim, 2008).

15.5.2 Dementia variables

15.5.2.1 TYPE

Carers of people with AD, vascular dementia and dementia with Lewy bodies experience similar levels of stress (Draper et al., 1992; Lowery et al., 2000). Riedijk and colleagues (2006) found that carers of people with frontotemporal dementia (FTD) experienced significantly higher levels of burden than AD carers. The FTD care recipients demonstrated more neuropsychiatric and behavioural disturbances, which are associated with increased depression and burden (Schulz et al., 1995; Georges et al., 2008; Schulz and Sherwood, 2008). While Riedijk and colleagues found no differences between FTD and AD carers in terms of the amount of distress they experienced in response to the various disturbances, the increased frequency of these among people with FTD may explain the difference in burden. Other group differences worthy of note were the younger age of FTD patients and their longer duration of dementia.

15.5.2.2 DURATION

Carer strain has been associated with both shorter (Johnson and Catalano, 1983; Rabins et al., 1990; Reidijk et al., 2006) and longer (Zarit et al., 1986; Townsend et al., 1989) duration of dementia. Three theories attempt to explain this discrepancy. Supporting the relationship between shorter duration and strain, the adaptation hypothesis posits that over time carers adapt to the demands of their role (Johnson and Catalano, 1983; Rabins et al., 1990). Alternatively, the 'wear and tear' hypothesis proposes that the longer a carer remains in their role the more likely negative outcomes are to occur (Zarit et al., 1986; Townsend et al., 1989). The sequestration theory proposes that carers experiencing greater stress are more likely to admit their relative with dementia to a nursing home, thus removing these individuals from cross-sectional research correlating carer morbidity and dementia duration (Brodaty et al., 2005). Given these competing explanations, it is not surprising that other studies have reported no relationship between duration of caring and carer distress (Cooper et al., 2007).

Longitudinal studies indicate that length of caregiving interacts with education, social roles, amount of care provided and behavioural disturbances to account for psychosocial outcomes over time (Gaugler et al., 2005). Moen and colleagues (1995) found that the following variables moderated the relationship between duration of care and female carers' well-being: education (with better outcomes for more highly educated caregivers), life satisfaction prior to the caregiving role (with better outcomes when women were more satisfied with their earlier life), number of other roles (with better outcomes when women had fewer other roles), level of religious involvement (with better outcomes for those involved in religious pursuits), and paid employment (with better outcomes for those who worked). Walker and colleagues (1996) found that increased amount of care provided over time, particularly with ADLs, predicted reduced satisfaction and increased burden for caregivers, rather than duration itself. Early care experiences impact on the level of distress a carer demonstrates over time. Difficult transitions into the role (with a rapid onset, behaviourally disturbed individual, or where the carer is 'forced' into the role) are more likely to cause distress or the carer to discontinue and place the individual in a nursing home (Lawton et al., 2000). Carers who manage more problem behaviours, particularly early on when they are unprepared to deal with them, are more likely to experience negative outcomes (Gaugler et al., 2005).

15.5.2.3 SEVERITY

Most studies find no significant relationship between cognitive decline and carer psychological health (Draper et al., 1992; Schulz et al., 1995; Brodaty et al., 2005; Hirakawa et al., 2008). Many have found no relationship between degree of functional impairment and carer distress (Schulz et al., 1995), although in the developing world and when financial and social resources are lacking, functional decline can be an important source of carer strain (Shaji et al., 2003; Hong and Kim, 2008).

There is a strong relationship between neuropsychiatric and behavioural disturbance and carer distress, with symptoms such as apathy, aggression, delusions and wandering being associated with a decrease in carers' psychological well-being (Markowitz et al., 2003; Pinquart and Sörensen, 2003; de Vugt et al., 2005; Livingston et al., 2005; Hurt et al., 2008).

15.5.2.4   SUFFERING

Schulz and colleagues (2008) found that perceived suffering by persons with dementia was an independent contributor to the well-being of their carers, being positively associated with depression and medication use. They differentiated between emotional suffering (as measured by responses to three items: has the care recipient appeared anxious or worried, sad or depressed, or been crying and tearful in the last week) and existential suffering (as measured by responses to six items: has the care recipient threatened to hurt him/herself, been expressing feelings of hopelessness about the future, been commenting about the death of him/herself or others, been talking about feeling lonely, made comments about feeling worthless or being a burden to others, or made comments about feeling like a failure or about not having any worthwhile accomplishments in life), both of which were significantly and positively associated with depressive symptoms. Only existential suffering was associated with anti-depressant use, perhaps reflecting concerns of physicians responding to thoughts of self-harm. The analyses controlled for patient and illness characteristics, age, race and education, however they were based on the carer's perceptions of care recipients' suffering rather than direct measures.

15.5.3   Relationship factors

The type and quality of the relationship between carer and care receiver can predict the amount of carer distress. Spouses, particularly wives, tend to experience greater levels of distress than other carers in both Western (Brodaty and Hadzi-Pavlovic, 1990; Schulz and Sherwood, 2008) and non-Western cultures (Hong and Kim, 2008). Daughter-in-law carers also experience high levels of distress in countries (e.g. India, Korea, Nigeria) where filial obligation dictates that they perform the caregiving role (Hong and Kim, 2008). Primary carers or care providers experience higher levels of burden than care managers (Archbold, 1981; , 1984).

Low levels of past and current intimacy between the carer and the care recipient have been associated with higher levels of negative expressed emotion (hostility and criticism) directed at the person with dementia, lower levels of positive expressed emotion (warmth) (Fearon et al., 1998) and higher levels of carer distress (Brodaty and Hadzi-Pavlovic, 1990; Livingston et al., 2005). Cultural differences may mediate these associations. Carers in developing (particularly Asian) countries (due to factors associated with their language and family structures), tend to have lower levels of expressed emotion (Kurihara et al., 2000; Nomura et al., 2005).

Protective factors against distress are being a child or friend of the care receiver, and having a good previous and current interpersonal relationship, with high intimacy levels.

15.5.4   Carer variables

15.5.4.1   PERSONALITY

Carers who experience high levels of neuroticism, low optimism and negative expressed emotion, and who have insecure attachment styles, experience the most distress (Schulz et al., 1995; Nomura et al., 2005; Campbell et al., 2008; Cooper et al., 2008). Higher self-esteem and a secure attachment style are protective against distress and burden (Cooper et al., 2008; Lopez and Crespo, 2008).

15.5.4.2   PERCEPTION AND EXPERIENCE OF CAREGIVING ROLE

A lack of mastery or a sense of confidence in one's ability in the caregiving role is associated with increased strain and burden for carers (Campbell et al., 2008). The corollary holds too: a sense of mastery and competence as a carer and high self-esteem predict positive outcomes for carers (Schulz et al., 1995; Otswald et al., 1999; Connor et al., 2008).

Role captivity (feeling 'trapped' in one's role as a carer) also predicts burden levels and psychological ill health as it erodes the carer's sense of self and subsequently causes feelings of resentment towards the patient (Pearlin et al., 1990; Campbell et al., 2008).

15.5.4.3   COPING STRATEGIES

Dysfunctional and immature coping strategies (largely emotion-based strategies such as escape avoidance) are associated with increased anxiety and greater distress levels for carers (Cooper et al., 2006; Cooper et al., 2007). Problem-focused coping strategies (largely cognitively based such as positive reframing) can mitigate carer distress (Lazarus and Folkman, 1984; Pruchno and Resch, 1989; Cooper et al., 2007).

Surprisingly, in their review Cooper and colleagues (2007) also found that some cognitive coping styles, such as cognitive confronting (a confrontative and emotion focused approach) were associated with higher anxiety, and others, such as planful problem solving and cognitive confronting showed inconsistent results.

15.5.4.4   KNOWLEDGE AND INFORMATION

Lack of knowledge about dementia has been associated with poorer psychological health for formal paid carers (Pekkarinen et al., 2004). An international group of carers at the 2000 World Alzheimer Congress indicated that lack of information was an exacerbating factor for strain, and that increased understanding of dementia would be empowering (Brodaty and Green, 2002b), however interventions that have successfully improved carers' knowledge have not led to corresponding improvements in well-being or burden (Brodaty and Green, 2002a).

15.6   SUPPORT

Carer support can be formal or informal and can take the form of instrumental, emotional or informational support. Instrumental support includes help with daily living needs and housework, emotional support provides a 'shoulder to cry on' and informational support includes information and knowledge from both health professionals and other carers who have experienced similar situations. Formal support is provided by organizations such as aged care facilities or hospitals and informal support is provided by family and friends. Receiving support has generally been associated with better psychological health for carers (Brodaty and Hadzi-Pavlovic, 1990; Cohen, 2004) as it provides a buffer against burden and stress for them by increasing the perception that resources are available to handle stress (Cohen, 2004). However, not all support is beneficial; inappropriate or unwelcome support can be more stressful than helpful (Edwards and Cooper, 1988). Satisfaction with social support requires the perception by the carer that the right type of support is available at the desired level (Drentea et al., 2006).

Important moderators of the relationship between support and positive effects of psychological health include age, gender, trait neuroticism, culture and carer ideology. Older carers tend to value emotional support most highly and male carers prefer formal to informal support (Drentea et al., 2006). African American carers and those with low levels of neuroticism are more likely to rate perceived support positively than those with high levels of neuroticism and white Americans (Shurgot and Knight, 2005). People who hold 'non-traditional' caregiving ideologies (the idea that caregiving conflicts with their expectations and is unrewarding) are less likely to perceive that there is support available to them than people with more traditional approaches to caregiving (Lawrence et al., 2008).

15.7   NURSING HOME ADMISSION AND CARERS

Carers may choose to place their care recipient in a nursing home as the illness progresses, usually when the caregiving demands become overwhelming. While institutionalization reduces the direct obligations on the carer and can provide relief and reduced stress (Brodaty and Hadzi-Pavlovic, 1990; Aneshensel et al., 1995), it does not necessarily remove distress. Following nursing home admission, carers may experience increased guilt, anger, anxiety, depression, loss of self and financial difficulties (Tornatore and Grant, 2002; Schulz et al., 2004). These can persist for up to several years following institutionalization (Gaugler et al., 2007). The hypothesis that distress would be lessened for carers if care recipients were placed in group homes that had smaller numbers, more informal daily routines and more decision-making involvement of residents and informal carers, compared with traditional nursing homes, was not confirmed (te Boekhorst et al., 2008). There were no significant differences between carers of 67 care recipients in group homes and 97 in nursing homes on measures of competence, psychopathology and burden (te Boekhorst et al., 2008).

Demographic and psychosocial factors predict nursing home admission. Being employed and balancing too many demands, or being unemployed and financially unstable are associated with institutionalization, as are feeling burdened by the carer role, difficulty dealing with behavioural

manifestations of dementia, poorer relationship and poorer physical and psychological health (Brodaty et al., 1993; Tun et al., 2007; te Boekhorst et al., 2008).

15.8   CARER INTERVENTIONS

A wide range of interventions has been devised to buffer family carers from the negative effects that caring for a PWD has on them (Zarit and Femia, 2008). Interventions can be categorized into psychological, educational/information, support and multicomponent. Psychological interventions include psychoeducational and psychotherapeutic (skills training, provision of structured information, behavioural techniques and counselling), educational/information interventions involve information provision and dementia education only, support interventions include support groups, home visits and social support, and multicomponent involve both psychological and support components (Parker et al., 2008; Zarit and Femia, 2008).

Carer interventions have proved effective at increasing carer knowledge, reducing carer distress and depression and delaying nursing home placement for their care recipients, although some studies have shown modest or no effects (Brodaty et al., 2003; Pinquart and Sörensen, 2006; Selwood et al., 2007). The most successful intervention programmes are those that are tailored to the needs of the individual, are flexible, address issues to do with the subjective experience of burden, involve training in addition to education, include both the carer and care receiver, and focus on the medium to long term (Brodaty et al., 2003; Pinquart and Sörensen, 2006; Selwood et al., 2007; Zarit and Femia, 2008). The evidence for the effect of interventions on subjective burden is inconclusive, with the best effects found for individualized, comprehensive, multifaceted intervention programmes (Brodaty et al., 2003; Schulz and Martire, 2004; Gonyea et al., 2005; Pinquart and Sörensen, 2006).

Problems with the design and methodology of past carer intervention studies contributed to the modest effects obtained (Zarit and Femia, 2008). Some recent studies have addressed these shortcomings by giving consideration to the following: clarifying carers' needs, ensuring treatment is relevant to carers' needs, ensuring methodology meets the treatment goal and catering for the heterogeneity of carers (Zarit and Femia, 2008).

The Seattle Protocols are a systematic and structured, yet individualized approach to training family carers to reduce BPSD in people with AD. The protocols teach carers to monitor problems, identify possible events that trigger disturbances and develop effective responses (Teri et al., 2005). They have been effective at improving carer quality of life, reducing reactive responses to problem behaviours, improving burden levels (Teri et al., 2005) and depression, agitation and sleep disturbance (Teri et al., 1997; Teri et al., 2000; McCurry et al., 2005). The Resources for Enhancing Alzheimer's Carer Health (REACH) multi-site, multicomponent project using a variety of interventions is a six-year study conducted over six locations in the United States (Belle et al., 2006). Eisdorfer and colleagues (2003) reported the outcomes of a REACH comparative study involving a group receiving family therapy alone, a group receiving family therapy and a computer telephone support system and a minimal support control group. The group receiving therapy and telephone support showed a significant reduction in depressive symptoms for carers, while the therapy only group showed no significant effects. A follow-up study, REACH II, considered one of the most efficacious interventions to date (Stevens et al., 2009), was conducted over five sites with 692 Latino, Caucasian and African American carers divided into intervention and control groups. The intervention group received a comprehensive programme including provision of information, didactic instruction, role playing, problem solving, skills training, stress management and telephone support (Belle et al., 2006). Compared to controls, significant improvements in depression, burden, care recipient problem behaviours, self-care and social support were found for Caucasian and Hispanic carers, but not for African Americans (Belle et al., 2006).

A modified REACH programme, coined REACH OUT (designed to be more practical, feasible, and able to be successfully adopted in community settings) found positive pre-post effects on caregiver subjective burden, social support, caregiver frustration, depression and caregiver health (Burgio et al., 2009). Care recipient behaviour problems and mood disturbances pertaining to each dyad were also reduced. Furthermore, two of four care recipient risk behaviours improved, specifically caregivers reported that the care recipients were less likely to be left unsupervised and were less likely to wander following the intervention. Caucasian caregivers experienced a greater reduction of subjective burden than African American caregivers, African American caregivers showed greater improvement in positive aspects of caregiving than Caucasian caregivers and the intervention was more effective at reducing subjective burden for non-spousal caregivers than for spousal caregivers. Interventions were more successful for those from urban than from rural households.

Education alone appears to have little or limited benefit (Brodaty, 1994; Brodaty et al., 1994; Marriott et al., 2000). The education only community-based seminar series developed by the George G Glenner Alzheimer's Family Centre (Devor and Renvall, 2008), involving 20 courses of 6-hour seminars, with a total attendance of 300 carers, showed no significant influence on attendees' overload, stress or burden. At six-month follow up participants' self-perceived competence levels were higher (although there was no control group for comparative purposes). Those with the lowest baseline scores showed the most improvement in burden, overload and stress (Devor and Renvall, 2008). Support by itself also appears to confer little benefit. The Befriending and Costs of Caring (BECCA) long-term randomized controlled trial of befriending 236 carers by volunteers in England had no effect on carers' quality of life, anxiety, loneliness, perceived support or positive affect at 6-, 15- or 24-month follow ups (Charlesworth et al., 2008).

Multidimensional, flexible carer interventions that involve follow up and an ongoing relationship between helper and carer can delay nursing home placement (Brodaty et al., 2003). A 10-day structured carer intervention programme

delayed institutionalization of care recipients over seven years without sacrificing the psychological health of carers or increasing usage of health services and dementia drugs, and with significant cost savings over the first three years (Brodaty and Gresham, 1989; Brodaty and Peters, 1991; Brodaty et al., 1997). In a 17-year longitudinal study of 406 spousal carers, an intervention programme involving individual and family counselling, encouragement of support group participation and availability of ad hoc telephone counselling delayed time to nursing home placement significantly by a median of 1.5 years (Mittelman et al., 2006). The intervention was also successful at improving carer well-being, as demonstrated by fewer symptoms of depression, improved reaction to memory and behaviour problems and greater satisfaction with support networks (Mittelman et al., 2006). Other studies have demonstrated up to nine months' delay in institutionalization (Riordan and Bennett, 1998; Eloniemi-Sulkava et al., 1999). A randomized controlled trial (RCT) of five sessions of family counselling conducted in Manchester, New York and Sydney did not delay time to nursing home placement across the whole sample compared to usual care, but did so at the Australian site. Possible reasons were differences in aged care systems and financial disincentives to institutionalization and differences in the amount of counselling provided (more ad hoc counselling was provided in Sydney; Brodaty et al., 2009).

Several interventions led by occupational therapists have proved helpful in randomized controlled trials. In Holland, when patients were trained to use aids to compensate for cognitive decline and caregivers were instructed in coping behaviours and supervision, patients' and caregivers' quality of life, mood and health status improved as did caregivers' sense of control over life (Graff et al., 2006; Graff et al., 2007). The intervention was cost-effective (Graff et al., 2008). A US study that focused on environmental modification – five 90-minute home visits over three months by OTs who provided education and physical and social environmental modifications – resulted in patients having less decline in instrumental activities of daily living and self-care and fewer behavioural problems and spouse caregivers having less upset and for women greater self-efficacy in managing behaviours and functional dependency (Gitlin et al., 2001). The same group, using a more intense version of this intervention over six months and including more severely affected persons with dementia, essentially replicated their findings and demonstrated that benefits were maintained six months later through a maintenance programme of one home visit and three telephone calls (Gitlin et al., 2003; Gitlin et al., 2005). In a third study, a Tailored Activity Programme resulted in fewer problem behaviours and greater activity engagement as well as benefits for caregivers. The programme, which targeted enhancing three activities which were identified after careful assessments of patients, was conducted over four months during which therapists made six 90-minute home visits and two 15-minute telephone calls (Gitlin et al., 2008).

Incorporating technology into interventions can support the quality of life for carers and receivers, assist independent living and enhance safety and autonomy (Eisdorfer et al., 2003; Topo, 2009). Technological approaches include conference calling among family members of dementia patients;

telephone support systems with automated messages; stress monitoring and advice; respite calls for care recipients; online discussion groups; electronic reminder services; computer-based forums and question and answer sessions (internet and non-internet-based networks); email; electronic encyclopaedias and libraries; and computer-based decision support modules (Cassie and Sanders, 2008; Powell *et al.*, 2008). Eisdorfer and colleagues (2003) found that having access to technology-based interventions resulted in a decrease in depression at six and 18 months for both white and Cuban Americans compared to more traditional interventions. Beauchamp and colleagues (2005) assessed a multimedia workplace intervention for employed carers. The intervention, which could be tailored to fit the demographic features and needs of the carer, involved text materials and videos that model positive caregiving behaviour. Knowledge and education, coping strategies and cognitive and behavioural skills were covered. Exposure to the tool significantly improved carers' negative appraisals, improved symptoms of anxiety, depression and strain, and improved perception of gain. Its success was attributed to its accessibility on an as-needs basis, individual tailoring and multiple components. In a review of 15 papers describing five technology-based interventions for dementia carers, despite inconsistent outcomes and small studies, there were moderate improvements in carer stress and depression (Powell *et al.*, 2008). The obvious benefit of such interventions is that they can usually be accessed at all times of the day and night, at the carer's convenience. Further research in this area would be useful.

Developing countries rely primarily on families to provide support to people with dementia as health services are often ill-equipped to meet their needs (Dias *et al.*, 2008). Family carers in the developing world face additional challenges as awareness and understanding about dementia are lacking; symptoms may be perceived to be part of normal ageing, or denied because of the stigma attached to the illness (Patel and Prince, 2001; Senanarong *et al.*, 2004; Dias *et al.*, 2008). Effective interventions addressing issues and needs relevant to these carers are required. An RCT evaluated a home-based intervention in Goa, India consisting of basic education about dementia and common behaviour problems, strategies for managing problem behaviours, support to carers in ADLs, referral to psychiatrists or other medical professionals for assistance with BPSD, networking to assist the carers to form support groups and advice on government provisions for the elderly (Dias *et al.*, 2008). The intervention led to significant improvements in carer mental health and perceived burden for the 41 carers in the treatment group (compared to 40 controls). There were also reductions in the behavioural disturbances and improvements in the functional abilities of the dementia care recipients, but these were non-significant (Dias *et al.*, 2008). The programme used local health and human resources, making it affordable and easily accessible.

A six-month group counselling intervention was trialled with 50 carers (half assigned to the treatment and half to the control group) in Thailand (Senanarong *et al.*, 2004). Counselling, support, education and strategies for managing problem behaviours formed part of the intervention. At six months, the neuropsychiatric symptoms of the dementia care recipients had significantly declined. Carer distress associated

with these symptoms declined over time and compared with the control group, but not significantly. For both the Indian and Thai studies, small sample sizes were a limitation and possibly explained the lack of significance in some of the results. Additionally, the six month follow-up period may have been too short to demonstrate an effect, or to show whether the intervention had a long-term impact on carer and care receiver well-being.

An RCT in Moscow, Russia, involving a 5-week course covering basic education about dementia and specific training on managing problem behaviours, resulted in statistically significant reductions in carer burden and increases in quality of life that were close to significant (Gavrilova *et al.*, 2008). The effect sizes for these were in the moderate to high range (0.64 and 0.52, respectively), and larger than those typically seen in interventions undertaken in high income countries (Brodaty *et al.*, 2003; Gavrilova *et al.*, 2008). This supported the authors' hypothesis that an intervention focusing on education and training would have a greater impact in a setting where community awareness of dementia and appropriate formal care services are lacking. A number of the variables of interest were not significantly improved as a result of the intervention (including carer psychological morbidity and the severity of and distress caused by BPSD) possibly because of the small sample size ($n = 60$), lack of statistical power, and the use of a waiting list rather than active control group (Gavrilova *et al.*, 2008).

Alzheimer associations are another important form of intervention. Support organizations for people with dementia and their carers exist in over 70 countries worldwide (www.alz.co.uk). Referral of families to Alzheimer Associations is part of the clinician's therapeutic armamentarium (see Chapter 38, Alzheimer associations and societies). Respite care and community services also offer support to carers (see Chapter 17, Dementia care in the community: challenges for primary health and social care; Chapter 30, Residential care for people with dementia; Chapter 40, The global challenge of dementia: what can be done; and Chapter 41, Development of a national strategy for dementia: dementia and policy in the UK.

15.9   SPECIAL CATEGORIES OF CARERS

There are certain groups of carers who may experience additional challenges beyond those directly related to caregiving. Homosexual partners of people with dementia may feel that existing interventions and support services do not meet their needs and that the issues they face (for instance next of kin rights) are not well understood or addressed. One gay partner of a recently diagnosed dementia patient described his experience:

> there seemed to be an assumption that the disease only affected married couples or those with supportive families. The focus seemed to be on heroic husbands or wives, married for scores of years, who were now entering a supremely challenging phase in their relationship; or it was on devoted families who now

needed to consider how they could meet the needs of parents suffering from this most dreadful disease (Newman, 2005).

Moore (2002) found that homosexual carers in the United States experience prejudice and insensitivity in their interactions with health services, lack social and emotional support due to efforts to maintain privacy in their 'non-traditional' relationship, were unable to use employee benefits to assist their partner with dementia, face opposition from employers when attempting to take compassionate leave, and face legal difficulties with estate planning (Moore, 2002).

People from ethnic minorities, including indigenous groups, are less likely to have access to, and to use mental health services (Pollitt, 1997; LaFontaine *et al.*, 2007; Lawrence *et al.*, 2008). Contributing factors include a lack of understanding about dementia among these groups, language barriers or other communication barriers, lack of general practitioner (GP) knowledge of cultural differences in expression of mental illness and distress, distrust of Western medicine, ethnocentric attitudes and incorrect assumptions (for instance that certain ethnic groups will look after their relatives and do not require services) (Cortis, 2004; Mahoney *et al.*, 2005).

People with younger onset dementia and their carers face additional problems as they are more likely to be working and have dependent children. Carers are often unprepared for the task and have fewer appropriate services available to them (Chaston *et al.*, 2004; Arai *et al.*, 2007). Formal services (such as respite) are usually designed for older people and are inappropriate for people with dementia under 65 years of age. Informal supports may be fewer as family and friends are likely to be working and have dependants themselves, and are unable to empathize with the carer's experience. As a result, carers of people with younger onset dementia experience even higher levels of burden than carers of people with late-onset dementia (Luscombe *et al.*, 1998; Freyne *et al.*, 1999). Sometimes, the carers are the affected person's parents; their challenges are poignant.

Increasingly, people with Down syndrome and other intellectual disabilities are living to an age where they become susceptible to dementia (see Chapter 76, Dementia in intellectual disabilities). Often their parents, who have been their main carers, are facing age-related diseases themselves and anxieties arise about who will care for their dependants if these parents become disabled or die.

When a care recipient is in a second (or later) marriage, particularly when there are children from a previous marriage, it is more likely that disputes will arise about legal and guardianship issues. When people marry close to the time that one begins to dement, further issues can arise regarding capacity to marry, the partner's motivation (Peisah and Bridger, 2008), and possible issues to do with less well-developed feelings of reciprocity and obligation.

15.10   LEGAL ASPECTS

Legal guardianship and financial power of attorney are two relevant concepts with which carers should be familiar (see

Chapter 32, Legal issues and dementia). A guardian can make decisions about the person's services, place of residence and treatment (Raivio *et al.*, 2008). Financial power of attorney allows persons with dementia to nominate someone to make decisions about finances and property on their behalf (Alzheimer's Association, 2005). In some jurisdictions prior power of attorney becomes invalid when the appointer becomes incompetent. This can be circumvented, if the person with dementia declares that these proxy powers should endure after he or she loses competency. The person's right to self-determination and to have his or her wishes respected should be protected, and the sooner after a dementia diagnosis guardianship issues are considered the better (Alzheimer's Association, 2005; Raivio *et al.*, 2008). In England, the Mental Capacity Act 2005 provides a legal framework for people who lack capacity or who want to make provisions for a time when they no longer have capacity (Raivio *et al.*, 2008). There is considerable variation in laws between countries and even between jurisdictions within countries (Stoppe, 2009; Peisah *et al.*, 2009).

From the few available studies it appears that legal guardianship and financial power of attorney are not widely used by PWD, and are poorly understood by their carers. In one Italian study of 100 community-dwelling dementia patients, only 10–11 per cent of persons with moderate or severe AD had appointed a guardian and none of those with mild AD had done so (Ruggieri and Piccoli, 2003). The researchers attributed this to a lack of understanding about medicolegal issues among carers, and highlighted a need for guidelines on guardianship. Such guidelines do exist in the US and UK (Overman and Stoudemire, 1988; Lord Chancellor's Department, 2003), but their effectiveness is unclear (Raivio *et al.*, 2008).

Raivio and colleagues (2008) surveyed 1943 spousal carers of people with AD in Finland to examine the prevalence of legal guardians, financial powers of attorney and the need for further information about such issues. They found that only 4 per cent of the sample had appointed legal guardians, and 38 per cent had financial powers of attorney. Adoption of these legal measures was predicted by the severity of the condition, behavioural problems and carer strain (not demographic factors). Ten per cent of the carers had discussed legal issues with their doctors and approximately 50 per cent wanted to do so. It was clear that there was a strong need for information to assist carers handle economic and legal affairs for their relative with dementia.

Carers also have an important legal role in assisting care recipients to make decisions about treatment and participation in research. Informed consent is required before prescribing medication, which requires the patient to understand what the medication is for, the likely benefits, possible adverse events and any alternatives (Brodaty and Green, 2002b). If the PWD lacks capacity the carer may be asked to give proxy consent for pharmacotherapy, or to participate in a drug trial or other relevant research. Jurisdictions vary regarding the legislation and requirements for proxy consent. In some jurisdictions people with dementia can provide an advance directive or enduring guardianship order that comes into effect when they lose capacity. It is a complex issue and policy discussions regarding proxy consent have been continuing for at least three decades. In some jurisdictions in the United States, the uncertainty has led to institutions disallowing proxy consent for research (Kim *et al.*, 2009), despite broad public support for a policy of proxy (or surrogate) consent for AD research. A 2006 survey of 1515 Americans (aged 51 and older) showed majority support, between 68 and 83 per cent, depending on the scenario (Kim *et al.*, 2009).

Whether or not the person can give consent, it is likely that the carer will need to understand the purpose and limitations of treatment, ensure compliance, supervise medication and monitor any adverse events (Brodaty and Green, 2002b). The carer has responsibility to be informed about what is being prescribed, be realistic about what is likely to be achieved from undergoing treatment or a drug trial, inform the medical practitioner about adverse events, stop treatment when it is harmful and decide whether to discontinue medication that has ceased to be beneficial (Brodaty and Green, 2002b).

15.11   CONCLUSION

Dementia seldom afflicts just one person. Carers are an integral part of the journey from symptom onset through diagnosis and management to death. Carers, the 'second patient', deserve attention in their own right. They are an integral part of the dementia management equation. Those vulnerable to stress can be identified and interventions can reduce carers' distress and improve their quality of life. This in turn will lead to a better quality of life for the person with dementia and potentially increase their length of time living in the community.

REFERENCES

Aboderin I. (2004) Decline in material family support for older people in urban Ghana, Africa: understanding processes and causes of change. *Journals of Gerontology Series B-Psychological Sciences and Social Sciences* 59: S128–37.

Access Economics. (2003) *The dementia epidemic: Economic impact and positive solutions for Australia.* Canberra: Alzheimer's Australia.

Adkins VK. (1999) Treatment of depressive disorders of spousal caregivers of persons with Alzheimer's disease: A review. *American Journal of Alzheimer's Disease* 14: 289–93.

Alzheimer's Association. (2005) *Legal plans: assisting the person with dementia in planning for the future.* Alzheimer's Association.

Alzheimer's Association. (2007) *Alzheimer's Disease Facts and Figures.* Alzhemier's Association.

Alzheimer's Association. (2008a) 2008 Alzheimer's disease facts and figures. *Alzheimer's and Dementia* 4: 110–33.

Alzheimer's Association. (2008b) More men take the lead role in caring for elderly parents. Retrieved December 17, 2008. Available from: www.alz.org/news_and_events_in_the_news.asp.

Alzheimer's Association and National Alliance for Caregiving. (2004) *Families care: Alzheimer's caregiving in the United States.* Alzheimer's Association and National Alliance for Caregiving.

Alzheimer's Disease International. (2009) *World Alzheimer Report.* London: Alzheimer's Disease International.

Aneshensel C, Pearlin LI, Mullan JT et al. (1995) *Profiles in caregiving: The unexpected career.* San Diego, CA: Academic Press.

Arai A, Matsumoto T, Ikeda M, Arai Y. (2007) Do family caregivers perceive more difficulty when they look after patients with early onset dementia compared to those with late onset dementia. *International Journal of Geriatric Psychiatry* 22: 1255–61.

Archbold PG. (1981) Impact of parent caring on women. XII International Congress of Gerontology. Hamburg: West Germany.

Australian Institute of Health and Welfare. (2007) *Dementia in Australia: National data analysis and development.* Canberra: Australian Institute of Health and Welfare.

Baker KL, Robertson N. (2008) Coping with caring for someone with dementia: reviewing the literature about men. *Aging and Mental Health* 12: 413–22.

Baumgarten M, Battista RN, Infante-Rivard C et al. (1992) The psychological and physical health of family members caring for an elderly person with dementia. *Journal of Clinical Epidemiology* 45: 61–70.

Beauchamp N, Irvine AB, Seeley J, Johnson B. (2005) Worksite-based Internet multimedia program for family caregivers of persons with dementia. *The Gerontologist* 45: 793–801.

Belle S, Burgio L, Burns R et al. (2006) Enhancing the quality of life of dementia caregivers from different ethnic or racial groups. *Annals of Internal Medicine* 145: 727–38.

Brodaty H. (1994) Dementia and the family. In: Bloch S, Hafner J, Harari E, Szmukler GI (eds). *The family in clinical psychiatry.* Oxford: Oxford University Press, 224–46.

Brodaty H, Green A. (2002a) Who cares for the carer? The often forgotten patient. *Australian Family Physician* 31: 833–6.

Brodaty H, Green A. (2002b) Defining the role of the caregiver in Alzheimer's disease treatment. *Drugs and Aging* 19: 891–8.

Brodaty H, Gresham M. (1989) Effects of a training programme to reduce stress in carers of patients with dementia. *British Medical Journal* 299: 1375–9.

Brodaty H, Hadzi-Pavlovic D. (1990) Psychosocial effects on carers of living with persons with dementia. *Australian and New Zealand Journal of Psychiatry* 24: 351–61.

Brodaty H, Peters K. (1991) Cost effectiveness of a training program for dementia carers. *International Psychogeriatrics* 3: 11–22.

Brodaty H, McGilchrist C, Harris L, Peters KE. (1993) Time until institutionalization and death in patients with dementia: role of caregiver training and risk factors. *Archives of Neurology* 50: 643–50.

Brodaty H, Roberts K, Peters K. (1994) Quasi-experimental evaluation of an educational model for dementia caregivers. *International Journal of Geriatric Psychiatry* 9: 195–204.

Brodaty H, Gresham M, Luscombe G. (1997) The Prince Henry Hospital dementia caregivers' training programme. *International Journal of Geriatric Psychiatry* 12: 183–92.

Brodaty H, Green A, Koschera A. (2003) Meta-analysis of psychosocial interventions for caregivers of people with dementia. *Journal of the American Geriatric Society* 51: 657–64.

Brodaty H, Green A, Low L-F. (2005) Family carers for people with dementia In: Burns A, O'Brien J, Ames D (eds). *Dementia.* London: Hodder Arnold, 117–35.

Brodaty H, Mittelman M, Gibson L *et al.* (2009) The effects of counseling spouse caregivers of people with Alzheimer's disease taking donepezil and of country of residence on rates of admission to nursing homes and mortality. *American Journal of Geriatric Psychiatry* 17: 734–43.

Burgio LD, Collins IB, Schmid B *et al.* (2009) Translating the REACH caregiver intervention for use by area agency on aging personnel: the REACH OUT program. *Gerontologist* 49: 103–16.

Campbell P, Wright J, Oyebode J *et al.* (2008) Determinants of burden in those who care for someone with dementia. *International Journal of Geriatric Psychiatry* 23: 1078–85.

Cassie KMC, Sanders S. (2008) Familial caregivers of older adults. In: Cummings SM, Kropf NP (eds). *Handbook of psychosocial interventions with older adults: Evidence-based approach.* New York: Haworth Press, 293–320.

Charlesworth G, Shepstone L, Wilson E *et al.* (2008) Befriending carers of people with dementia: randomised controlled trial [see comment]. *British Medical Journal* 336: 1295–7.

Chaston D, Pollard N, Jubb D. (2004) Young onset dementia: a case for real empowerment. *Journal of Dementia Care* 12: 24–6.

Clare L, Wilson BA, Carter G *et al.* (2002) Depression and anxiety in memory clinic attenders and their carers: implications for evaluating the effectiveness of cognitive rehabilitation interventions. *International Journal of Geriatric Psychiatry* 17: 962–7.

Cohen CA, Colantonio A, Vernich L. (2002) Positive aspects of caregiving: rounding out the caregiving experience. *International Journal of Geriatric Psychiatry* 12: 331–6.

Cohen S. (2004) Social relationships and health. *American Psychologist* 59: 676–84.

Connor KI, McNeese-Smith DK, Vickrey BG *et al.* (2008) Determining care management activities associated with mastery and relationship strain for dementia caregivers. *Journal of the American Geriatrics Society* 56: 891–7.

Cooper C, Katona C, Orrell M, Livingston G. (2006) Coping strategies and anxiety in caregivers of people with Alzheimer's disease: the LASER-AD study. *Journal of Affective Disorders* 90: 15–20.

Cooper C, Balamurali TBS, Livingston G. (2007) A systematic review of the prevalence and covariates of anxiety in caregivers of people with dementia. *International Psychogeriatrics* 19: 175–95.

Cooper C, Owens C, Katona C, Livingston G. (2008) Attachment style and anxiety in carers of people with Alzheimer's disease: results from the LASER-AD study. *International Psychogeriatrics* 20: 494–507.

Cortis J. (2004) Meeting the needs of minority ethnic patients. *Journal of Advanced Nursing* 48: 51–8.

de Vugt ME, Stevens F, Aalten P *et al.* (2005) A prospective study of the effects of behavioral symptoms on the institutionalization

of patients with dementia. *International Psychogeriatrics* 17: 577–89.

Devor M, Renvall M. (2008) An educational intervention to support caregivers of elders with dementia. *American Journal of Alzheimer's Disease and Other Dementias* 23: 233–41.

Dias A, Dewey ME, D'Soua J *et al.* (2008) The effectiveness of a home care program for supporting caregivers of persons with dementia in developing countries: a randomised controlled trial from Goa, India. *Plos One* 3: 1–7.

Dilworth-Anderson P, Goodwin PY, Williams SW. (2004) Can culture help explain the physical health effects of caregiving over time among African American caregivers? *Journal of Gerontology: Social Sciences* 59B: S138–45.

Dilworth-Anderson P, Brummett BH, Goodwin P *et al.* (2005) Effect of race on cultural justifications for caregiving. *Journal of Gerontology* 60B: S257–62.

Draper BM, Poulos CJ, Cole AM *et al.* (1992) A comparison of caregivers for elderly stroke and dementia victims. *Journal of the American Geriatric Society* 40: 896–901.

Drentea P, Clay OJ, Roth DI, Mittelman MS. (2006) Predictors of improvement in social support: Five-year effects of a structured intervention for caregivers of spouses with Alzheimer's disease. *Social Science and Medicine* 63: 957–67.

Dura JR, Stukenberg KW, Kiecolt-Glaser JK. (1991) Anxiety and depressive disorders in adult children caring for demented parents. *Psychology and Aging* 6: 467–73.

Edwards J, Cooper C. (1988) Research in stress, coping and health: theoretical and methodological issues. *Psychological Medicine* 18: 15–20.

Eisdorfer C. (1991) Caregiving: an emerging risk factor for emotional and physical pathology. *Bulletin of the Menninger Clinic* 55: 238–47.

Eisdorfer C, Czaja S, Loewenstein DA *et al.* (2003) The effect of a family therapy and technology-based intervention on caregiver depression. *The Gerontologist* 43: 521–31.

Eloniemi-Sulkava U, Sivenius J, Sulkava R. (1999) Support program for demented patients and their carers: the role of dementia family care coordinator is crucial. In: Iqbal K, Swaab D, Winblad B, Wisinewski H (eds). *Alzheimer's disease and related disorders.* Chichester: John Wiley and Sons, 795–802.

Fearon M, Donaldson C, Burns A, Tarrier N. (1998) Intimacy as a determinant of expressed emotion in carers of people with Alzheimer's disease. *Psychological Medicine* 28: 1085–90.

Ferri CP, Prince M, Brayne C *et al.* (2005) Global prevalence of dementia: a Delphi consensus study. *Lancet* 366: 2112–7.

Freyne A, Kidd N, Coen R, Lawlor BA. (1999) Burden in carers of dementia patients: higher levels in carers of younger sufferers. *International Journal of Geriatric Psychiatry* 14: 784–8.

Gallicchio L, Siddiqi N, Langenberg P, Baumgarten M. (2002) Gender differences in burden and depression among informal caregivers of demented elders in the community. *International Journal of Geriatric Psychiatry* 18: 154–63.

Gaugler JE, Kane RL, Kane RA *et al.* (2005) The effects of duration of caregiving on institutionalization. *The Gerontologist* 45: 78–89.

Gaugler JE, Pot AM, Zarit SH. (2007) Long-term adaptation to institutionalization in dementia caregivers. *The Gerontologist* 47: 730–40.

Gaugler JE, Roth DL, Haley WE, Mittelman MS. (2008) Can counseling and support reduce burden and depressive symptoms in caregivers of people with Alzheimer's disease during the transition to institutionalization? Results from the New York University caregiver intervention study. *Journal of the American Geriatrics Society* **56**: 421–8.

Gavrilova SI, Ferri CP, Mikhaylova N *et al.* (2008) Helping carers to care: The 10/66 Dementia Research Group's randomized control trial of a caregiver intervention in Russia. *International Journal of Geriatric Psychiatry* **24**: 347–54.

Georges J, Jansen S, Jackson L *et al.* (2008) Alzheimer's disease in real life – the dementia carer's survey. *International Journal of Geriatric Psychiatry* **23**: 546–51.

Gilleard CJ. (1984) Problems posed for supporting relatives of geriatric and psychogeriatric day patients. *Acta Psychiatrica Scandinavica* **70**: 198–208.

Gitlin LN, Corcoran M, Winter L *et al.* (2001) A randomized, controlled trial of a home environmental intervention: effect on efficacy and upset in caregivers and on daily function of persons with dementia. *The Gerontologist* **41**: 4–14.

Gitlin LN, Winter L, Corcoran M *et al.* (2003) Effects of the home environmental skill-building program on the caregiver-care recipient dyad: 6-month outcomes from the Philadelphia REACH initiative. *The Gerontologist* **43**: 532–46.

Gitlin LN, Hauck WW, Dennis MP, Winter L. (2005) Maintenance of effects of the home environmental skill-building program for family caregivers and individuals with Alzheimer's disease and related disorders. *Journal of Gerontology: Medical Sciences* **60A**: 368–74.

Gitlin LN, Winter L, Burke J *et al.* (2008) Tailored activities to manage neuropsychiatric behaviors in persons with dementia and reduce caregiver burden: a randomized pilot study. *American Journal of Geriatric Psychiatry* **16**: 229–39.

Gonyea JG, O'Connor M, Carruth A, Boyle PA. (2005) Subjective appraisal of Alzheimer's disease caregiving: the role of self-efficacy and depressive symptoms in the experience of burden. *American Journal of Alzheimer's Disease and Other Dementias* **20**: 273–80.

Graff MJL, Vernooij-Dassen MJM, Thijssen M *et al.* (2006) Community based occupational therapy for patients with dementia and their caregivers: randomised controlled trial. *British Medical Journal* **333**: 1196–2001.

Graff MJL, Vernooij-Dassen MJM, Thijssen M *et al.* (2007) Effects of community occupational therapy on quality of life, mood, and health status in dementia patients and their caregivers: a randomized controlled trial. *Journal of Gerontology: Biological Science and Medical Sciences* **62**: 1002–9.

Graff MJ, Adang EMM, Vernooij-Dassen MJM *et al.* (2008) Community occupational therapy for older patients with dementia and their care givers: cost effectiveness study. *British Medical Journal* **336**: 134–8.

Haley WE, Levine EG, Brown SL, Bartolucci AA. (1987) Stress, appraisal, coping and social support as predictors of adaptational outcome among dementia caregivers. *Psychological Ageing* **2**: 223–30.

Haley WE, Roth DL, Coleton MI *et al.* (1996) Appraisal, coping and social support as mediators of well-being in black and white Alzheimer's family caregivers. *Journal of Consulting and Clinical Psychology* **64**: 121–9.

Hirakawa Y, Kuzuya M, Enoki H *et al.* (2008) Caregiver burden among Japanese informal caregivers of cognitively impaired elderly in community settings. *Archives of Gerontology and Geriatrics* **46**: 367–74.

Hong GR, Kim H. (2008) Family caregiver burden by relationship to care recipient with dementia in Korea. *Geriatric Nursing* **29**: 267–74.

Hurt C, Bhattacharyya S, Burns A *et al.* (2008) Patient and caregiver perspectives of quality of life in dementia. An investigation of the relationship to behavioural and psychological symptoms in dementia. *Dementia and Geriatric Cognitive Disorders* **26**: 138–46.

Johnson CL, Catalano DJ. (1983) A longtitudinal study of family supports to impaired elderly. *Gerontologist* **23**: 612–8.

Kim SY, Kim HM, Langa KM *et al.* (2009) Surrogate consent for dementia research: a national survey of older Americans. *Neurology* **72**: 149–55.

Kramer BJ. (1997) Gain in the caregiving experience: Where are we? What next? *The Gerontologist* **2**: 218–32.

Kurihara T, Kato M, Tsukahara T *et al.* (2000) The low prevalence of high levels of expressed emotion in Bali. *Psychiatry Research* **94**: 229–38.

Kurz A, Schulz M, Reed P *et al.* (2008) Personal perspectives of persons with Alzheimer's disease and their carers: A global survey. *Alzheimer's and Dementia* **4**: 345–52.

LaFontaine J, Ahuja J, Bradbury NM *et al.* (2007) Understanding dementia amongst people in minority ethnic and cultural groups. *Journal of Advanced Nursing* **60**: 605–14.

Lawrence V, Murray J, Samsi K, Banerjee S. (2008) Attitudes and support needs of Black Caribbean, south Asian, and White British carers of people with dementia in the UK. *The British Journal of Psychiatry* **193**: 240–6.

Lawton MP, Moss M, Hoffman C, Perkinson M. (2000) Two transitions in the daughter's caregiving careers. *The Gerontologist* **40**: 437–48.

Lazarus RS, Folkman S. (1984) *Stress, appraisal and coping.* New York: Springer.

Leong J, Madjar I, Fiveash B. (2001) Needs of family carers of elderly people with dementia living in the community. *Australasian Journal on Ageing* **20**: 133–8.

Livingston G, Mahoney R, Regan C, Katona C. (2005) The caregivers for Alzheimer's disease Problems Scale (CAPS): development of a new scale within the LASER-AD study. *Age and Ageing* **34**: 287–90.

LoGiudice D, Waltrowicz W, Brown K *et al.* (1999) Do memory clinics improve the quality of life of carers? A randomized pilot trial. *International Journal of Geriatric Psychiatry* **14**: 626–32.

Lopez J, Crespo M. (2008) Analysis of the efficacy of a psychotherapeutic program to improve the emotional status of caregivers of elderly dependent relatives. *Aging and Mental Health* **12**: 451–61.

Lord Chancellor's Department. (2003) *Making decisions-helping people who have difficulty deciding for themselves. A guide for healthcare professionals. L. C. s. Department.* London: Lord Chancellor's Department, 1–31.

Lowery K, Mynt P, Aisbett J *et al.* (2000) Depression in the carers of dementia sufferers: a comparison of the carers of patients suffering from dementia with Lewy Bodies and the carers of patients with Alzheimer's disease. *Journal of Affective Disorders* **59**: 61–5.

Luscombe G, Brodaty H, Freeth S. (1998) Younger people with dementia: diagnostic issues, effects on carers and use of services. *International Journal of Geriatric Psychiatry* **13**: 323–30.

McCurry S, Gibbons L, Logsdon RG *et al.* (2005) Nighttime insomnia treatment and education for Alzheimer's disease: a randomized controlled trial. *Journal of the American Geriatric Society* **53**: 793–802.

Mahoney DF, Cloutterbuck J, Neary S, Zhan L. (2005) African American, Chinese, and Latino family caregivers' impressions of the onset and diagnosis of dementia: cross-cultural similarities and differences. *The Gerontologist* **45**: 783–92.

Markowitz JS, Gotterman EM, Sadik K, Papadopoulos G. (2003) Health-related quality of life for caregivers of patients with Alzheimer's disease. *Alzheimer's Disease and Associated Disorders* **17**: 209–14.

Marriott A, Donaldson C, Tarrier N, Burns A. (2000) Effectiveness of cognitive-behavioural family intervention in reducing the burden of care in carers of patients with Alzheimer's disease. *British Journal of Psychiatry* **176**: 557–62.

Mittelman MS, Haley WE, Clay OJ, Roth DL. (2006) Improving caregiver well-being delays nursing home placement of patients with Alzheimer disease. *Neurology* **67**: 1592–9.

Moen P, Robison J, Dempster-McClain D. (1995) Caregiving and women's well-being: a life course approach. *Journal of Health and Social Behavior* **36**: 259–73.

Mohide EA, Torrance GW, Streiner DL *et al.* (1998) Measuring the wellbeing of family caregivers using the time trade-off technique. *Journal of Clinical Epidemiology* **41**: 475–82.

Moore W. (2002) Lesbian and gay elders: connecting care providers through a telephone support group. *Journal of Gay and Lesbian Social Services* **14**: 23–41.

Morrissey E, Becker J, Rupert MP. (1990) Coping resources and depression in the caregiving spouses of Alzheimer patients. *British Journal of Medical Psychology* **63**: 161–71.

Neubauer S, Holle R, Menn P *et al.* (2008) Measurement of informal care time in a study of patients with dementia. *International Psychogeriatrics* **20**: 1160–76.

Newman R. (2005) Partners in care: being equally different lesbian and gay carers. *Psychiatric Bulletin* **29**: 266–7.

Nomura H, Inoue S, Kamimura N *et al.* (2005) A cross-cultural study on expressed emotion in carers of people with dementia and schizophrenia: Japan and England. *Social Psychiatry and Psychiatric Epidemiology* **40**: 564–70.

Office for National Statistics. (2005) *Focus on older people.* Newport, UK: Office for National Statistics.

Okojie FA. (2004) Ageing in sub-Saharan Africa: toward a redefinition of needs, research, and policy directions. *Journal of Cross Cultural Gerontology* **3**: 3–19.

Ory MG, Hoffman RR, Yee JL *et al.* (1999) Prevalence and impact of caregiving: a detailed comparison between dementia and nondementia caregivers. *The Gerontologist* **39**: 177–85.

Otswald S, Hepburn K, Caron W *et al.* (1999) Reducing caregiver burden: a randomized psychoeducational intervention for caregivers of persons with dementia. *Gerontologist* **39**: 299–309.

Overman Jr W, Stoudemire A. (1988) Guidelines for legal and financial counseling of Alzheimer's disease patients and their families. *American Journal of Psychiatry* **145**: 1495–500.

Parker D, Mills S, Abbey J. (2008) Effectiveness of interventions that assist caregivers to support people with dementia living in the community: A systematic review. *International Journal of Evidence-Based Healthcare* **6**: 137–72.

Patel V, Prince M. (2001) Ageing and mental health in a developing country: who cares? Qualitative studies from Goa, India. *Psychological Medicine* **31**: 29–38.

Pearlin LI, Mullan JT, Semple SJ, Skaff MM. (1990) Caregiving and the stress process: An overview of concepts and their measures. *The Gerontologist* **30**: 583–94.

Peisah C, Bridger M. (2008) Abuse by marriage: the exploitation of mentally ill older people. *International Journal of Geriatric Psychiatry* **23**: 883–8.

Peisah C, Forlenza O, Chiu E. (2009) Ethics, capacity, and decision making in the practice of old age psychiatry: an emerging dialogue. *Current Opinion in Psychiatry* **22**: 519–21.

Pekkarinen L, Sinervo T, Perala ML, Elovainio M. (2004) Work stressors and the quality of life in long-term care units. *Gerontologist* **44**: 633–43.

Personal Social Services Research Unit London School of Economics. (2007) *Dementia UK: The full report.* Alzheimer's Society. London, Institute of Psychiatry, King's College London.

Pinquart M, Sörensen S. (2003) Differences between caregivers and noncaregivers in psychological health and physical health: a meta-analysis. *Psychology and Aging* **18**: 250–67.

Pinquart M, Sörensen S. (2006) Helping caregivers of persons with dementia: which interventions work and how large are their effects? *International Psychogeriatrics* **18**: 577–95.

Pollitt P. (1997) The problem of dementia in Australian Aboriginal and Torres Strait Islander communities: an overview. *International Journal of Geriatric Psychiatry* **12**: 155–63.

Poulshock S, Deimling G. (1984) Families caring for elders in residence: issues in the measurement of burden. *Journal of Gerontology* **39**: 230–9.

Powell J, Chiu T, Eysenbach G. (2008) A systematic review of networked technologies supporting carers of people with dementia. *Journal of Telemedicine and Telecare* **14**: 154–6.

Prince M. The 10/66 Dementia Research Group. (2004) Care arrangements for people with dementia in developing countries. *International Journal of Geriatric Psychiatry* **19**: 170–7.

Pruchno RA, Resch NL. (1989) Aberrant behaviors and Alzheimer's disease: Mental health effects on spouse caregivers. *Journal of Gerontology: Social Sciences* **44**: S177–82.

Pruchno RA, Potashnik SL. (1989) Caregiving spouses: Physical and mental health in perspective. *Journal of the American Geriatrics Society* **37**: 697–705.

Pyke KD, Bengston VL. (1996) Caring more or less: individualistic and collectivist systems of family eldercare. *Journal of Marriage and the Family* **58**: 379–92.

Rabins PV, Fitting MD, Eastham J, Zabora J. (1990) Emotional adaptation over time in care-givers for chronically ill elderly people. *Age and Ageing* 19: 185–90.

Raivio MM, Maki-Petaja-Leinonen AP, Laakkonen ML *et al.* (2008) The use of legal guardians and financial powers of attorney among home-dwellers with Alzheimer's disease living with their spousal caregivers. *Law, Ethics and Medicine* 34: 882–6.

Rapp SR, Chao D. (2000) Appraisals of strain and of gain: Effects on psychological wellbeing of caregivers of dementia patients. *Aging and Mental Health* 4: 142–8.

Reidijk SR, De Vugt ME, Duivenvoorden HJ *et al.* (2006) Caregiver burden, health-related quality of life and coping in dementia caregivers: a comparison of Frontotemporal Dementia and Alzheimer's Disease. *Dementia and Geriatric Cognitive Disorders* 22: 405–12.

Riordan J, Bennett A. (1998) An evaluation of an augmented domiciliary service to older people with dementia and their carers. *Aging and Mental Health* 2: 137–43.

Robinson KM. (1989) Predictors of depression among wife caregivers. *Nursing Research* 38: 359–63.

Roth DL, Mittelman MS, Clay OJ *et al.* (2005) Changes in social support as mediators of the impact of a psychosocial intervention for spouse caregivers of persons with Alzheimer's Disease. *Psychology and Aging* 20: 634–44.

Ruggieri RM, Piccoli F. (2003) Legal and assistance aspects of Alzheimer's disease: analysis of 100 cases. *Neurological Science* 24: 125–9.

Sanders S. (2005) Is the glass half empty or half full? Reflections on strain and gain in caregivers of individuals with Alzheimer's Disease. *Social Work in Health Care* 40: 57–73.

Schulz R, Martire LM. (2004) Family caregiving of persons with dementia: prevalence, health effects, and support strategies. *American Journal of Geriatric Psychiatry* 12: 240–9.

Schulz R, Sherwood PR. (2008) Physical and mental health effects of family caregiving. *American Journal of Nursing* 108 (9 Suppl): 23–7; quiz 27.

Schulz R, Williamson GM. (1991) A 2-year longitudinal study of depression among Alzheimer's caregivers. *Psychology and Aging* 6: 569–78.

Schulz R, Williamson GM. (1997) The measurement of caregiver outcomes in Alzheimer disease research. *Alzheimer Disease and Associated Disorders* 11: 117–24.

Schulz R, Vistainer P, Williamson GM. (1990) Psychiatric and physical morbidity effects of caregiving. *Journal of Gerontology: Psychological Sciences* 45: P181–91.

Schulz R, O'Brien AT, Bookwala J, Fleissner K. (1995) Psychiatric and physical morbidity effects of dementia caregiving: prevalence, correlates, and causes. *The Gerontologist* 35: 771–91.

Schulz R, Belle S, Czaja SJ *et al.* (2004) Long-term care placement of dementia patients and caregiver health and well-being. *Journal of the American Medical Asssociation* 292: 961–7.

Schulz R, McGinnis KA, Zhang S *et al.* (2008) Dementia patient suffering and caregiver depression. *Alzheimer Disease and Associated Disorders* 22: 170–6.

Segerstrom SC, Schipper LJ, Greenberg RN. (2008) Caregiving, repetitive thought, and immune response to vaccination in older adults. *Brain, Behavior and Immunity* 22: 744–52.

Selwood A, Johnston K, Katona C *et al.* (2007) A systematic review of the effect of psychological interventions on family caregivers of people with dementia. *Journal of Affective Disorders* 101: 75–89.

Semple SJ. (1992) Conflict in Alzheimer's caregiving families: Its dimensions and consequences. *The Gerontologist* 32: 648–55.

Senanarong V, Jamjumras P, Harmphadungkit K *et al.* (2004) A counseling intervention for caregivers: effect on neuropsychiatric symptoms. *International Journal of Geriatric Psychiatry* 19: 781–8.

Serrano-Aguilar PG, Lopez-Bastida J, Yanes-Lopez V. (2006) Impact on health-related quality of life and perceived burden of informal caregivers of individuals with Alzheimer's Disease. *Neuroepidemiology* 27: 136–42.

Shaji KS, Smitha K, Lal KP, Prince MJ. (2003) Caregivers of people with Alzheimer's disease: a qualitative study from the Indian 10/66 Dementia Research Network. *International Journal of Geriatric Psychiatry* 18: 1–6.

Shurgot G, Knight B. (2005) Influence of neuroticism, ethnicity, familism, and social support on perceived burden in dementia caregivers: pilot test of the Transactional Stress and Social Support Model. *Journal of Gerontology: Psychological Sciences* 60B: S331–4.

Stevens AR, Lancer K, Smith ER *et al.* (2009) Engaging communities in evidence-based interventions for dementia caregivers. *Family and Community Health* 32 (Suppl. 1): S83–92.

Stoppe G. Competence assessment in dementia. Retrieved 5 August, 2009. Available from: edcon-dementia.net/en/consensus.php?id = 4.

Taylor Jr DH, Kuchibhatla M, Ostbye T. (2008) Trajectories of caregiving time provided by wives to their husbands with dementia. *Alzheimer Disease and Associated Disorders* 22: 131–6.

te Boekhorst S, Pot AM, Depla M *et al.* (2008) Group living homes for older people with dementia: the effects on psychological distress of informal caregivers. *Aging and Mental Health* 12: 761–8.

Teri L, Logsdon RG, Uomoto J, McCurry SM. (1997) Behavioral treatment of depression in dementia patients: A controlled clinical trial. *Journal of Gerontology: Psychological Sciences* 52B: P159–66.

Teri L, Logsdon RG, Peskind E *et al.* (2000) Treatment of agitation in Alzheimer's disease: a randomized placebo controlled clinical trial. *Neurology* 55: 1271–8.

Teri L, McCurry SM, Logsdon R, Gibbons LE. (2005) Training community consultants to help family members improve dementia care: A randomized controlled trial. *The Gerontologist* 45: 802–11.

The 10/66 Dementia Research Group. (2004) Care arrangements for people with dementia in developing countries. *International Journal of Geriatric Psychiatry* 19: 170–7.

Topo P. (2009) Technology studies to meet the needs of people with dementia and their caregivers: A literature review. *Journal of Applied Gerontology* 28: 5–37.

Tornatore J, Grant L. (2002) Burden among family caregivers of persons with Alzheimer's disease in nursing homes. *The Gerontologist* 42: 497–506.

Townsend A, Noelker L, Deimling G, Bass D. (1989) Longtitudinal impact of interhousehold caregiving on adult children's mental health. *Psychological Aging* 4: 393–401.

Tun S, Murman D, Long HL *et al.* (2007) Predictive validity of neuropsychiatric subgroups on nursing home placement and survival in Alzheimer's disease patients. *American Journal of Geriatric Psychiatry* 15: 314–27.

Vedhara K, Cox NKM, Wilcock GK *et al.* (1999) Chronic stress in elderly carers of dementia patients and antibody response to influenza vaccination. *Lancet* 3531: 627–31.

Vedhara K, Bennett PD, Clark S *et al.* (2003) Enhancement of antibody responses to influenza vaccination in the elderly following a cognitive-behavioural stress management intervention. *Psychotherapy and Psychosomatics* 72: 245–52.

Vitaliano PP, Zhang J, Scanlan JM. (2003) Is caregiving hazardous to one's physical health? A meta-analysis. *Psychological Bulletin* 129: 946–72.

Walker AJ, Acock AC, Bowman SR, Li F. (1996) Amount of care given and caregiving satisfaction: a latent growth curve analysis. *Journal of Gerontology: Psychological Sciences* 51B: P130–42.

Wimo A, Winblad B, Jonsson L. (2007) An estimate of the total worldwide societal costs of dementia in 2005. *Alzheimer's and Dementia* 3: 81–91.

Zarit S, Femia E. (2008) Behavioral and psychosocial interventions for family caregivers. *American Journal of Nursing* 108 (9 Suppl.): 47–53; quiz 53.

Zarit SH, Whitlatch CJ. (1992) Institutional placement: Phases of the transition. *The Gerontologist* 32: 665–72.

Zarit SH, Todd PA, Zarit JM. (1986) Subjective burden of husbands and wives as caregivers: A longitudinal study. *The Gerontologist* 26: 260–6.

16

One caregiver's view

EMERSON MORAN

*Emerson Moran is a writer in Florida. Pat, his wife, was diagnosed with early onset Alzheimer's disease in 1999. Previously, Mr Moran was a communications executive with the American Medical Association. This article is adapted from his remarks at an AMA scientific news briefing in New York City in January 2004. (**See p4 of the plate section for Plate 6**.)*

The first time Pat didn't know who I was felt like we'd each been kidnapped.

Her early onset Alzheimer's had been at the centre of our life for several years, but I never expected our connection to fracture so soon. After all, I'd just quit a 10-year job to better manage our living with the disease by moving from Washington, DC, to South Florida, where Pat loved the warmth, water, bright flowers and the exotic birds.

That evening, after supper, we'd gone to the ocean to visit Pat's pelicans – when they fly low, she waves and calls them to come 'over here, over here'. At sunset, we headed home, about 15 minutes away. I remember the big thunderheads ahead of us, out over the Everglades, the wind shearing off their tops like anvils. It was like a Frederic Edward Church painting.

Halfway home, Pat was distressed and frightened. She asked who I was, what was I doing to her, where was I taking her. She tried to open the car door to escape. I was scared. Shortness of breath, dry mouth, jumbled thoughts. It was hard to look calm, talk and drive calmly at the same time.

At home, we looked at photos of our Philadelphia Quaker wedding, of trips to Tuscany and Cape May Point, of family and friends. She couldn't recognize the facts of our history, but she cried over our emotional memories. She didn't know my name, but knew we'd loved each other a long time. That was good enough for me then, and still is.

When I first saw Pat 20 years ago it was like in those movies when they freeze the frame. My frame froze. I've been with her in that frame ever since. What I didn't know for years and years was that Alzheimer's was in our frame, too.

Pat's Alzheimer's was diagnosed five years ago, but had already been controlling our life for a long time. We just didn't deal with it. Denial is a powerful force.

We had a very tough time at first. After all, a diagnosis of Alzheimer's is a death sentence, isn't it? And that's the first thing I felt: death, despair, deep depression, grief and fear – gripping, chilling, stunning fear. When CS Lewis lost his wife – she was the love of his life, too – he wrote that no one ever told him how much grief feels like fear. Well, yes it does.

We got through that, and, gradually and gratefully, and with a lot of help, we found ways to cope. We also discovered that our ability to deal with Alzheimer's progressed right along with the disease's progression. What we never expected was how far we'd end up going, geographically and spiritually, to manage our living with Alzheimer's before Alzheimer's totally managed us.

We tried to perpetuate our old way of life for a long time, and then reached a point where it made no sense, where our old 'normal' didn't work anymore. In the landscape of our life, normal had moved. We had to move with it, by creating a new landscape and a new normal, and by building a new life frame, with Alzheimer's now the biggest figure in our picture.

We began our new way of life Labor Day weekend 2002 when we moved 985 miles from Washington to Florida, leaving behind old job, old home, old normal. It felt like jumping off a cliff. The 2-day drive was easier than I thought it would be. We could never do it today. But, back then, Pat could still handle herself alone in a strange bathroom; eat without help in a crowded, noisy restaurant; feel safe in an unfamiliar motel room. She was happy in the car. She munched M&Ms, and sang along to the Beatles and Sarah Brightman. We stopped in St Augustine – the oldest permanent European settlement in North America – and took the horse and carriage ride to the Fountain of Youth, of all places.

A week later, she didn't know who I was. I'd read the Alzheimer's books, like *The 36 Hour Day*, and knew intellectually that this moment was certain to arrive. But, Lord, I thought, not this day! Please, not this day!

Later, I had one of those dreams where I'm trying to get some place. This time I was struggling to get to the airport in some desolate, desert-like place. I had to climb up a steep incline, crawl down a deep depression, and back up over rocks and through dust. The airline check-in desk was up above me, to the right, on the edge of a cliff. Out of nowhere, a pickup truck blocked my way, machine gun in the back, like those 'technicals' the Somalian war lords drove in *Black Hawk Down*. There was shooting, confusion. Then I woke up, full of dread and apprehension.

Yes, changing our life was like jumping off a cliff. But we had to jump. It was the only way to break away from our old way of life. I took a family leave from the job I'd had for 10 years. That, plus accumulated vacation, bought four months to sort things out, and to just be together. We decided that I'd quit my job. We'd move to Florida, where we had family and friends. Cost of living was going to be much lower, and we figured I could earn enough freelancing to get by. What we hoped to do was carve out a way of living that would:

- keep us together as many hours in each day as possible;
- embrace Pat with care and comfort and laughter;
- allow me to work from home;
- prop me up with enough emotional and physical support to keep us going.

Looking back, I can see how we actually changed the equation of what had been a pretty conventional career-driven middle-class American existence. In our old formula, work was cemented solidly at the centre, with everything else in orbit, around the edges. In our new formula, we put Pat and Alzheimer's in the centre, with work kicked out into an orbit of its own, not quite on the edge, but not in the centre, either.

This is pretty easy to articulate after the fact. But at the time it felt like radical, uprooting, life-altering, mind-boggling, heart-thumping, cliff-jumping change. Some simple things have helped a lot. Here are six that seem real clear to me from where we sit today:

1. Family: **there is a higher power in a loving family** – we feel it and it fuels us every day. When we met, Pat was a widow, I was divorced. She never had the chance to have her own kids. Then along came my crowd. Now it's up to three married sons (one, a Marine Corp F-18 fighter pilot, serving twice in Iraq), six grandchildren, plus three step-grandchildren, my sister, brother, nieces, nephews, cousins and their kids, my own ancient parents – we now live 2 minutes away – and they all love Pat. Even my first wife loves Pat!

2. Early on, in those darkest weeks after 'The Diagnosis', a colleague told me: '**This is not the end of the world.** You still have years ahead of quality and value and love together'. That stuck like glue. It's my creed.

3. A friend reminded me: 'This is that rainy day they tell you about. **The future is now**'. Whatever you have now, use it for what you need to do now.

4. To best care for Pat I had to **take care of myself** – physically, mentally and emotionally. Early on, I was mad as hell and didn't even know it until I exploded in front of a co-worker and kicked a door so hard that they tell me it's still dented. By 3.00 pm the next day I was sitting in front of a psychologist with a lot of experience dealing with Alzheimer's families. We made a deal. I'd stick with Dr Jacobek's counselling, and she would help me stay as 'whole' as possible, no matter what happened, all the way to the end, and beyond. That was almost five years ago, and we're still at it, 1200 miles apart, over the phone,

every 10 days. **Therapy is my gut check**, my outlet of last resort. I'm not sure how Pat and I could carry on without it.

Working out – physical exercise – is therapeutic, too. I'm not a jock, but today, working out is actually a refuge for me. Neighbourhood power walks; the gym's monthly 'geezer discount'; free weights in the garage. The cadence, the repetitions, the breathing are meditative. The endorphins fight depression.

5. **Get Pat all the help we can find**. We've been blessed with skilled, attentive doctors, and we learned that it's a good idea to have the same internist. He treats us as individuals and as a couple. Pat can't be left alone while I work. Handling this defines how we function. A sign on Dixie Highway in our new hometown led us to a local day programme for Alzheimer's. It was a big factor in deciding where to live.

The programme is 10 minutes from home, in a church, next to our local high school. Pat's there from 8.00 am to 4:00 pm Monday through Friday. The morning roundtrip is my commute to work and Pat's time there gives me a chance to get my own job done.

The programme's home is a 40-year-old Lutheran church hall, across a vacant lot from our local high school ('Home of the Gators'). More therapeutic than just day care, it's staffed by professionals, small enough for lots of gentle attention, and full of fun.

At Christmas, one registered nurse brought her kids' pet goat, wearing reindeer antlers. Pat still remembers the 'rein-goat,' a remarkable memory for a woman whose only moment of meaning usually is the one she is in.

One patient, a former golf pro, taught Pat how to putt. Some days, I wouldn't mind being there myself. Then there's Stacia, a crusty, no-nonsense, loving 70-something Polish angel who couldn't stand retirement and seems to find great satisfaction helping people just like us. Stacia brings Pat home in the afternoon, helps around the house, takes Pat to get her hair and nails done, and stays with her when my work takes me away. Stacia's parting words usually are, 'I'll take care of Pat. You take care of yourself'.

6. **Medication to manage and modify Pat's behaviour** is the final factor that holds the whole thing together. Pat has exploded with all the agitation, rage and aggression that can accompany Alzheimer's. It's terrifying when it erupts. I learned the hard way to keep a table between us for protection.

A wise geriatric psychiatrist prescribed a strong antipsychotic that many people with schizophrenia use to help keep their lives in order. This little pill calms the rage, quiets the aggression and takes away the agitation, without taking away anything else. I don't know how we would get through the day, much less live at home together, without it.

With or without medication, though, Rule Number One is this: You will never win an argument with someone with Alzheimer's. Never. Don't even try.

Rule Number Two is old and golden: Do unto Pat as I would have Pat do unto me. Pat can't bathe herself, choose between red or blue blouse, put on earrings, shave her legs, read the paper, chew steak or pizza, pour herself a cup of coffee, or find our bathroom on her own and in time. She can, however, always find the chocolate chip cookies. We joke about putting the cookies in the bathroom. Thankfully, 'Depends' have taken the crises out of incontinence.

The Pat I fell in love with had a wonderful artistic talent (sketches and watercolours mostly), but the Alzheimer's blocked the path to her creativity years ago. Passion for her art once consumed her. Today she won't even pick up a crayon. We still have her rough drawings and pencilled story line for a children's book on meerkats in the Kalahari Desert, a cherished, unfinished work, frozen in time by her disease, an artefact of Alzheimer's.

Her brain blocks other forms of communications. Most times, she can't find the words to ask for what she wants, tell me about her day, or name who's talking to her on the phone. She says 'Thank me', instead of 'Thank you' – then giggles at the odd sound of it.

What she can do is whistle, as she never did before. It's the first sound she makes in the morning and the last at night. I tell her she's in 'full pucker'. Old movie tunes from the 1940s are favourites. Over Christmas, she was stuck on 'Easter Parade'. Sometimes I whistle with her; it's one of the few things we can still do in harmony; intimacy, redefined.

We've always loved movies, and our own critique afterwards. But now Pat can't follow a movie or TV shows with complex story lines. However, she really likes 'Sponge Bob', and belly-laughs at 'Seinfeld'. We joke a lot. I tell her that, with Alzheimer's, there's no such thing as TV reruns.

Except for 9/11. We lived in DC, on Connecticut Avenue, close enough to hear sirens and see smoke from the Pentagon. Pat experienced 9/11 on TV over and over, each time the first time, each time brand new, on September 11 and September 12: right up to today. She still gets scared when she sees the images. But then, so do I. I'm pretty sure that my own post-9/11 priorities propelled how and when we changed our life so profoundly.

What we are doing has a high cost. Nearly 45 per cent of our income goes for health insurance, medications, the day programme, Stacia helping at home. Just like hundreds of thousands of other American families, we do this on our own.

Much has changed. The kids up North have to pay their own airfare when they come down to see us. We've ended our week-long family vacations at Cape May Point. But then, where we live now sure removes the urge for a mid-winter get-away in the sun. There's no more eating out several nights a week, but my home cooking is improving. I roasted the Thanksgiving turkey over charcoal, with cornbread stuffing and a maple syrup glaze. A pot of chilli is on the stove as I write this.

Shopping is more Sears than Bloomingdales, eBay and web discounts. I clip coupons. I've discovered warehouse shopping – toilet paper in 35-roll bundles, 300-ounce Tide. Plus, a perk of paradise, $19 orchids in full bloom.

Our favourite time of the day is bedtime, which is earlier and earlier. Pat starts shutting down when the sun starts going down. She seems to settle into her own private peace in bed, curled up, eyes closed, covers pulled into a tight cocoon. She'll lay awake for 2 or 3 hours while I read, watch TV, talk to my family on the phone. We listen to music; New Age Celtic tunes strike her Irish chords. I ask, but she can't tell me, what goes on behind her closed eyes, except to say, 'I'm working on things'.

She doesn't pay much attention to the TV, unless it's the Chicago Cubs baseball team. When we lived in Chicago in the 1990s, Pat loved taking the elevated train to Wrigley Field. One night, the broadcasters cut from the playing field to the cheering fans. Pat seemed sound asleep. It was loud, it was late, I turned off the TV. In the darkness Pat said, 'Put it back. It's fun'.

Pat and I are the lucky ones. Somehow, so far, we are pulling this off, a day at a time and we do have fun. We laugh a lot, and we play a lot.

The great irony is that they tell us that Alzheimer's is a catastrophic disease but, on any given day, we don't feel like we're in the middle of a catastrophe. In many ways, we are happier now than ever before. We talk about it. We agree that surrender, acceptance and loving each other no matter what are big reasons why.

I've been to the support groups and I've seen that not all Alzheimer's families are as fortunate. There's terrible pain and fierce anger out there. It hurts just to be near it.

I read a terrible news story maybe four years ago, from Washington. Just up 16th Street from the White House, in front of the Capital Hilton, a woman driving a Ford Taurus stopped at the light. Her father was sitting beside her. The paper said he had Alzheimer's, that she took care of him. Before the light could turn green, she pulled a gun, killed him and turned it on herself. The light changed to green, the traffic moved around them, and there they sat, at the bloody end of their own sad road.

I worry how close many other families have gotten to that point. I bet more than we'd like to think, not the point of violence, certainly, but maybe, secretly, wishing the end would come sooner rather than later.

This disease really is different, you know. There is no real treatment yet. Drugs can briefly slow down the clock, but there will be no remission, no cure, not for Pat and not, yet, for the 4 or 5 million others in the USA just like her.

We hope our 'together' lasts a long time, but, like many Alzheimer's patients, Pat's body has not been kind to her. Doctors call it 'co-morbidity' – coronary artery disease, breast cancer, diverticulitis, fibromyalgia, depression – and she's only in her mid-60s. In a medical crisis, do we treat or not treat? What's moral, what's ethical? Do we risk the distress of heart surgery, colostomy, chemotherapy? Or do we let nature take its course? Where's the right and wrong?

Nothing prepared us for issues like these. Pat can't decide for herself. It's up to me. Some nights, when answers don't come, the loneliness of Alzheimer's can be worse than the certainty of how it's all going to end, no matter what we do.

Alzheimer's is a medical Mount Everest that no one has figured out how to conquer. When they do, when they break through to the summit, it'll be too late for us, but not for many of the others. I guess that's the best hope there is with Alzheimer's: that money, hard work, luck and genius will pry loose the mystery of this disease that is so slowly being unlocked from inside this human genome of ours.

Pat and I work hard every day to just live life on life's terms. One melody Pat whistles is an old Irving Berlin tune called 'Always'. I have no idea where she gets it from. I 'Googled' the lyrics. They're up on our refrigerator door, held there by a tacky magnet from the boardwalk at the New Jersey seashore. This is the refrain:

> The days may not be fair – always.
> That's when I'll be there – always.
> Not for just an hour,
> Not for just a day,
> Not for just a year – but always.

I can't bear to think of the silence in my life when the whistling stops.

Pat sometimes looks at me, startled, and asks, 'Where's Emerson?' I tell her, 'I don't know, but if you see him, tell him I'm looking for him, too'. And we laugh. Always.

16.1   POSTSCRIPT

Pat's nursing home – it's four years now – is a short walk from home, through a neighbourhood park, past a gazebo, across a soccer field. What I missed most the first night alone was her snoring. Odd how reassuring that rough rattle in the dark. On good-weather days I bike, her laundry in a backpack; folding her clothes helps me feel normal.

The dementia unit, bright and airy, is called Chelsea Meadows. Walls washed with South Beach pastels are spotted with pictures of laughing children, sailboats, beach scenes, a three-foot-tall banana split. A wide hardwood walkway for the wanderers rings the space.

The hands-on staff are caring and committed. The food, even puréed, is good. But neither food nor fanciful name can hide the horrible reality that Pat's disease has done just about everything it will do to her. Except kill her. That will happen here, in an artificial village bereft of healing or hope, a homey mausoleum tilted outward on the perfect edge of nothing. The hospice calls it 'dying in place'.

One afternoon I find Pat in a wheelchair, head slumped forward, her blue Irish eyes closed. Celtic Woman's 'Last Rose of Summer' is playing. She could be dozing — or knocked out by meds that dull her physical and psychic pains. (**See p5 of the plate section for Plate 7.**)

I approach, singing 'Let Me Call You Sweetheart', off key. Not a move or a flutter. I caress one freckled cheek, plant a kiss on the other. I press my forehead to hers. 'Pretty nice, huh?' Eyelids do not flicker, no soft smile, nothing.

Her lips part. Then one word: 'Beautiful'. My skin prickles, my breath catches. It is a clear, finely formed 'beautiful', the 't' a taut 'tuh', the first multi-syllable word in months, a word that falls perfectly on the moment. Then it is gone. The flash of synaptic lightning passes.

She hasn't spoken since, her 'being' at a silent distance, removed to an inner deep space, close, perhaps, to the infinite. Makes sense. After all, Pat's 'beautiful' sounded just like the voice of God herself.

(Adapted from *In a Place of Dying*, by Emerson Moran. *New York Times*, September 16, 2008.)

17

Dementia care in the community: challenges for primary health and social care

STEVE ILIFFE, JILL MANTHORPE AND VARI DRENNAN

17.1 INTRODUCTION

Dementia is one of the main causes of disability in later life. In terms of the global burden of disease, it contributes 11.2 per cent of all years lived with disability; higher than stroke (9.5 per cent), musculoskeletal disorders (8.9 per cent), heart disease (5 per cent) and cancer (2.4 per cent) (World Health Organization, 2003). Nevertheless, in comparison to other areas of long-term disease management, dementia care currently constitutes only a small proportion of a primary care family doctor's workload, with only one or two new cases a year per primary care doctor in a demographically average population. While family doctors may have few cases, their engagement with those patients and their families is likely to be over years, as the median length of time from diagnosis to death is 10 years for those under 65 at diagnosis and four years for those over 80 years (Xie et al., 2008). As populations rapidly age, this situation will change. Health care systems in many countries are anticipating the need to develop new services and reconfigure existing ones to respond to the increasing prevalence of dementia.

In England, both the National Institute for Clinical Excellence (NICE) and Social Care Institute for Excellence (SCIE) dementia guidelines (NICE, 2006) and the National Dementia Strategy (Department of Health, 2009) propose a systematic approach to the continuing care of people with dementia in the community, to correct the evident deficits in care identified, over a period of many years, by a range of bodies from the Alzheimer's Disease Society (1995), founded in 1979, to the National Audit Office (2007). The same phenomenon of unintegrated services is found throughout Europe (Waldemar et al., 2007).

Service development for people with dementia must cross boundaries between health and social care agencies, between secondary and primary care sectors, and between the disciplines of medicine, nursing and social care. The purpose of this chapter is to identify effective ways to create such cross-boundary working in the sector where most people with dementia will receive most services and support; in primary care. Different health-care systems and funding streams make a prescriptive approach unhelpful, but nevertheless we believe there are key ideas, approaches and techniques that can cross cultures and systems. To help this process of learning from others' experiences we have adopted a polyglot terminology. 'Caregiver' is used to mean family members, neighbours or friends who provide practical and emotional support to people with dementia, and who would be called 'carers' or informal carers in the UK. 'Family doctors' are primary care physicians in some parts of the world and general practitioners (GPs) in others. 'Primary care nurses' include those nurses who work alongside family doctors and more specialist nurses working in the community (like the UK's District or Community Nurses), particularly those working with older people. Social workers do different things in different countries, but they all seem able to recognize each other and have a common practice base (Manthorpe and Moriarty, 2007). Social care and support, on the other hand, may be provided by commercial, local government or community, voluntary and religious organizations.

Underpinning our argument is the knowledge that proposals for skill acquisition or service development rest on a weak evidence base, particularly for psychosocial interventions. The systematic reviews that we cite make it clear that the paucity of evidence arises from the quality of studies rather than the number. Only with the cholinesterase inhibitor drugs can we be confident that the evidence of effectiveness is grounded in large trials with realistic time frames.

Dementia syndromes are progressive neurodegenerative diseases which follow a variable but inexorable trajectory. We have organized this chapter to follow that trajectory, starting with early symptoms, moving to diagnosis and early support, then mid-stage dementia and behavioural and psychological symptoms in dementia (BPSD). The chapter ends with a discussion of higher intensity care at home and in care homes, including end-of-life care. In each section we attempt to answer four questions: what is known about this subject? what do primary care practitioners need to learn? how will they know they are effective? and what service developments are needed?

17.2   EARLY RECOGNITION OF DEMENTIA IN PRIMARY CARE

17.2.1   What is known about this subject?

The benefits of reaching a diagnosis include ending uncertainty about the cause of symptoms and behaviour change, with greater understanding among family members of the problems experienced by the person with dementia. The aim is to increase access to helpful support resources, to promote positive coping strategies, and to facilitate planning and fulfilment of short-term goals (Bamford et al., 2004). Using cholinesterase inhibitor medication to modify symptoms in a worthwhile way for a minority of people with dementia who have Alzheimer's disease is a further advantage (NICE, 2006).

Dementia is probably under-diagnosed and under-treated with an estimated half of primary care patients with dementia not diagnosed by their primary care physicians (Boustani et al., 2003). Wide variation in family doctors' abilities and confidence in diagnosing and managing dementia has been consistently reported across different countries (Pucci et al., 2004). There is also ample evidence that diagnosis is often delayed, with misattribution of early symptoms to normal ageing by both people with dementia and their families, and professionals. This delay occurs despite evidence that early cognitive impairment is associated with increased frequency of consultations in primary care, and gait disturbances and cognitive complaints are the most common presenting symptoms (Ramakers et al., 2007).

In addition to memory problems, presenting problems may be communication difficulties, disturbance of spatial awareness and loss of the ability to perform activities of daily living independently. Missed appointments and problems around taking medication are also common (Bamford et al., 2007). Community nurses and social care practitioners may be some of the first professionals to see that these changes are affecting an older person (Manthorpe and Iliffe, 2007) if they

live on their own. Changes in personality and/or mood may lead family members to ask family doctors to identify what is wrong. Some may make an initial, potentially inaccurate diagnosis of depression, although depression may coexist alongside dementia.

Early recognition of dementia syndrome is an area of practice where there is considerable potential for uncertainty and confusion, including the difficulty in distinguishing between the (adverse) consequences of receiving the diagnosis of dementia and the problems that occur while living with dementia.

17.2.2   What do practitioners need to learn?

Although lack of insight may be an early feature of dementia syndrome, people with dementia may be more aware of their diagnosis than is suspected (Pearce et al., 2002; Clare, 2004) because older people and the general public are now much informed about dementia and its symptoms. Many primary care nurses and social care staff will be asked if they think an older person is getting dementia. Some primary care nurses will lack confidence in responding to these questions (Bryans et al., 2003). They need to be both knowledgeable about early symptoms of dementia syndromes but also familiar with the locally agreed first points of contact for people with such anxieties if they are to answer such questions with confidence.

Professional development among family doctors should aim to enrich the 'illness scripts' that practitioners use to recognize dementia, emphasizing the functional symptoms that can occur early in the disease process and reducing the reliance on subjective memory loss as a cardinal symptom. Concerns about causing harm by overzealous pursuit of early diagnosis can be offset by reframing the task as one of making 'timely diagnoses', in which changes in cognition or behaviour that worry the individual or those around them are taken seriously, investigated and clarified. This is essentially a clinical judgement rather than one that can be made (in primary care) by use of cognitive function tests, although such tests are useful adjuncts to clinical reasoning.

17.2.3   How will they know they are effective?

Enhanced skills in earlier recognition of dementia will minimize misattribution and reduce the length of time from symptom onset to diagnostic assessment, so that specialist services will see a change in their case mix, with fewer late presentations during crises and more early ones. Clinical records will contain more entries about risks being discussed and diagnostic hazards managed. These will need to be shared with primary care nurses and social care practitioners to ensure that mixed messages are not given.

17.2.4   What service developments are needed?

Professional development across community-based disciplines is the first priority, with development of 'memory clinics' a secondary task. In addition, at a local level mechanisms are required for developing and disseminating agreed service access routes, or care pathways for people with symptoms or concerns across agencies. Without such 'maps', the potential for conflict, omissions and delay increases (Waldorff et al., 2001).

However, there is a role for prevention of dementia that is largely underdeveloped. Service commissioners and providers should strengthen public health initiatives that have the potential to reduce dementia prevalence by modifying vascular risk. Cognitive function changes are measurable in people with cardiovascular risk factors in middle age, making targeted primary prevention of both heart and brain disease imperative. There is the real possibility that vigorous control of cardiovascular risks at community level could postpone the onset of dementia syndromes, and there is already some evidence of this happening in the US (Langa et al., 2008). No similar pattern is obvious yet in the UK (Langa et al., 2009), but this may be a time-lag effect, and we may see the incidence of dementia fall. Public health initiatives may be situated in health services but they are as likely to take place in sport, culture, environmental and transport services, where opportunities for exercise and social participation can be tuned to localities and populations. If older people feel that facilities such as local public leisure centres and swimming pools are not for them, for example, then this needs to be addressed by providers and commissioners.

17.3   DIAGNOSIS AND EARLY SUPPORT

17.3.1   What is known about this subject?

The problem of under-diagnosis of dementia is probably not due to lack of diagnostic skills, but rather to the interaction of case-complexity, pressure on time and the negative effects of reimbursement systems (Stoppe et al., 2007; Hinton et al., 2007). Primary care physicians appear to adopt a 'watchful waiting' stance with people with potential dementia symptoms (Bamford et al., 2007). This is due to a number of factors, including the tendency to assume such cognitive changes are merely due to 'old age' (Vernooij-Dassen et al., 2005), limited access to specialist mental health services and restrictions on the prescribing of cholinesterase inhibitors in the early stages of the illness, in some countries.

Diagnosis is not an act but a stepwise process which requires a supportive framework. De Lepeliere and colleagues (2008) explored the variety of techniques used for detection of dementia throughout Europe and concluded that a systematic, stepwise strategy could be employed to improve timely detection of dementia, that referral pathways could be more effective than specific guidelines, and that a strong, multidisciplinary service infrastructure enables the diagnostic process. In other words, diagnosis may depend on the availability of 'treatment' – in the case of dementia this includes psychosocial support for patients and their social networks as well as medication.

Telling people their diagnosis does seem to be what some people with dementia want to have (Jha et al., 2001), and

younger professionals want to provide (Sullivan and O'Conor, 2001). The fear of triggering individual distress, denial and withdrawal from contact with services is one factor that inhibits practitioners from discussing dementia as a diagnosis (Iliffe and Wilcock, 2005), and there appears to be a lack of clinical skill in managing this diagnostic transition. Disclosure of the suspected or certain diagnosis is rated by primary care physicians as one of the most difficult areas in dementia management, who are more likely than psychiatrists to use euphemisms (Bamford et al., 2004). The use of such euphemisms complicates relationships with other primary care practitioners who may be uncertain what the patient has been told and confused about whether to put the patient in touch with a support group such as the Alzheimer's Society or what to record in their own notes.

Members of social networks need support from the beginning. Counselling and support may preserve their self-rated health if they are already engaged in emotional or practical care work (Mittelman et al., 2007). Psychosocial interventions that include group activity can reduce caregiver feelings of 'burden' and increase their satisfaction (Andren and Elmståhl, 2008). The characteristics of effective psychosocial interventions are: psychoeducation (which addresses barriers to change); a family systems perspective; being multifaceted in solving problems and being applied flexibly to meet different needs in different families. Dementia services that take a family-based approach also include community nursing services that have an explicit and long-term focus on caregivers' support, such as Admiral Nurses in England who aspire to a 'predominantly supportive and educational function as opposed to [having] a case-management role' (Burton and Hope, 2005).

17.3.2   What do practitioners need to learn?

A person-centred approach can help alleviate four key problems: fears associated with other people 'finding out' the diagnosis; rapid deterioration in abilities; socially embarrassing behaviour; and a loss of involvement in care planning (Husband, 1999). The techniques available to all practitioners in primary care include combinations of reality orientation, memory strategies and reframing. Reality orientation, for example, focuses on the likely slow progression in early dementia and offsets catastrophic fears that may be triggered by mild memory lapses. Memory enhancement strategies include shorter term goal setting, and maintaining social and family roles that reinforce memory. Reframing dementia as a disability that can be accommodated shifts the emphasis from preoccupations with the diagnosis and not being perceived as a fool, and fosters understanding of the anger or frustrations associated with inabilities to perform daily tasks.

Reluctance to make use of services or support is not uncommon, and practitioners need to remember that take up is a result of a complex decision-making process often unrelated to objective circumstances. Conflict theory provides useful insights into such decision-making, particularly service avoidance (Markle-Reid and Browne, 2001), though a number of services may be inappropriate for people with parts of the developed world where individual or personal budgets can provide much better support by responding to people's needs at the time and supporting rather than undermining family and other assistance (Carr and Robbins, 2009). In some countries the effectiveness of community care policies is meaning that people who do eventually enter care homes are often very ill or very frail. High intensity care may be akin to palliative care.

The move to a care home is determined by the severity of cognitive impairment and functional loss, the presence of depression in the person with dementia, and (in some but not all studies) incontinence (Hope *et al.*, 1998, Thomas *et al.*, 2004). Case management can delay moves to care home among targeted subgroups (Challis *et al.*, 2002).

In the UK, the majority of people with dementia live and die at home or in a care home.

There are three ways in which people with dementia can die (Cox and Cook, 2002). First, there are people who have a diagnosis of dementia, but their death is caused by another medical condition (e.g. cancer or heart disease). Second, people may die with interplay of another illness and dementia, where the dementia has not impacted greatly on their functioning. Third, there are people who are described as having end-stage dementia, where the associated consequences of the dementia impact upon all domains of their life and they ultimately die of the complications of this condition. Each of these different ways will directly influence the place and experience of death for an individual and their family members. There is therefore not a single experience and patients and carers live with dementia for years often with different trajectories of functional decline and needs (Mularski *et al.*, 2007).

Professional and policy guidance on care for people with dementia nearing the end of life emphasizes the benefits of advance care planning, co-ordinated working between health and social care, and the adaptation and use of palliative care frameworks and clinical tools for people with long-term conditions (Alzheimer Europe, 2006; Alzheimer Europe, 2008). However, policy guidance and end-of-life initiatives, though laudable, have outstripped the available evidence on end-of-life care for people with dementia and their caregivers that live at home and in care homes (Goodman *et al.*, 2010).

17.5.2   What do practitioners need to learn?

Understanding the caregiver's strengths and their relationship with the person with dementia may be an important guide to how support is offered and given. Offering support early should become part of routine practice, but only if the professional knows where to signpost the patient or caregiver. Local service maps are important so that patients and carers do not face the frustrations of being passed from pillar to post. Professionals need to know the best sources of information about their locality and how to report unmet needs to those responsible for locality planning and service development.

Compared to those with other conditions, people with dementia are more likely to experience symptoms, including persistent pain, and are more likely to be untreated in the last six months of life (McCarthy *et al.*, 1997). The focus of attention may be on other issues, like nutrition and hydration, with pain being relatively neglected (Goodman *et al.*, 2010). This is a complex problem because of the communication difficulties that are a feature of advanced dementia, and should therefore be the focus of professional development for all practitioners who contribute to end-of-life care.

17.5.3   How will they know they are effective?

Good care homes and good home care services can reduce fewer inappropriate hospital admissions and transfers, and out of hours contacts. Good care homes will meet regulatory demands but there will also be confidence among local communities and perhaps a sense of pride that a local care home is part of the community. Care homes that work with volunteers and are supportive of residents' families will become well known. Local professionals often know which homes they would want to enter or where they might wish a relative to live if the need arose. We will know care homes are effective if they have limited staff turnover and if there are waiting lists for their services. The same applies to home care services. Staff may be able to support each other if this culture is fostered. They will be then more able to offer support for families and other residents who are bereaved. Fewer admissions to hospital and greater confidence that people's statements of wishes and any advance decisions will be respected can be indicators that end-of-life care is being well managed.

17.5.4   What service developments are needed?

The salience of flexibility, autonomy and responsiveness in home care teams is an important lesson for other service providers, which may be able to learn lessons from home care management styles. End-of-life guidelines should be reviewed and monitored to make sure that they are realistic and do not add to a 'tick box culture'. Staff may need time to develop skills in this area and to pass these to new staff and to family members. The support services for staff in large organizations, such as counselling or access to in-house employment support services, should be thought about in small or medium care enterprises. Time for supervision and reflection should be built into contracts for care.

17.6   CONCLUSION

Kodner's (2006) analysis of a successful model of integrated care for frail older adults from US evidence argues that provider networks which join together through standardized referral procedures, service agreements, joint training, shared information systems, and even common ownership of resources, enhance access to services, provide seamless care and maintain quality. In this chapter we have drawn on this and other evidence to suggest ways to create such cross-boundary working in the sector where most people with dementia will receive most services and support; in primary care.

REFERENCES

Alzheimer Europe. (2006) *The use of advance directives by people with dementia.* Luxembourg: Alzheimer Europe Luxembourg.

Alzheimer Europe. (2008) *Position and recommendations on end-of-life care.* Luxembourg: Alzheimer Europe.

Alzheimer's Disease Society. (1995) *Dementia in the community: management strategies for general practice.* London: Alzheimer's Disease Society.

Andren S, Elmståhl S. (2008) Psychosocial interventions for family caregivers of people with dementia reduces caregiver's burden: development and effect after 6 and 12 months. *Scandinavian Journal of Caring Sciences* 22: 98–109.

Balestreri L, Grossberg A, Grossberg GT. (2000) Behavioural and psychological symptoms of dementia as a risk factor for nursing home placement. *International Psychogeriatrics* 12: 59–62.

Ballard C, Fossey J, Chithramohan R *et al.* (2001) Quality of care in private sector and NHS facilities for people with dementia: cross sectional survey. *British Medical Journal* 323: 426–7.

Bamford C, Lamont S, Eccles M *et al.* (2004) Disclosing a diagnosis of dementia: a systematic review. *International Journal of Geriatric Psychiatry* 19: 151–69.

Bamford C, Eccles M, Steen N, Robinson L. (2007) Can primary care record review facilitate earlier diagnosis of dementia? *Family Practice* 24: 108–16.

Boustani M, Peterson B, Hanson L *et al.* (2003) Screening for dementia in primary care: a summary of the evidence for the US preventive services task force. *Annals of Internal Medicine* 138: 927–37.

Bowman C, Whistler J, Ellerby M. (2004) A national census of care home residents. *Age and Ageing* 33: 561–6.

Brauner DJ, Muir JC, Sachs GA. (2000) Treating nondementia illnesses in patients with dementia. *Journal of the American Medical Association* 283: 3230–5.

Brodaty H, Thomson C, Thompson C, Fine M. (2005) Why caregivers of people with dementia and memory loss don't use services. *International Journal of Geriartric Psychiatry* 20: 537–46.

Bryans M, Keady J, Turner S *et al.* (2003) An exploratory survey into primary care nurses and dementia care. *British Journal of Nursing* 12: 1029–37.

Bullock R, Passmore P, Iliffe S. (2007) Can we afford not to have integrated dementia services? *Age and Ageing* 36: 357–8.

Burton J, Hope KW. (2005) An exploration of the decision-making processes at the point of referral to an Admiral Nurse team. *Journal of Psychiatric and Mental Health Nursing* 12: 359–64.

Carr S, Robbins D. (2009) *The implementation of individual budget schemes in adult social care.* London: SCIE.

Challis D, von Abendorff R, Brown P *et al.* (2002) Care management, dementia care and specialist mental health services: an evaluation. *International Journal of Geriartric Psychiatry* 17: 315–25.

Cheston R, Jones K, Gilliard J. (2003a) Group psychotherapy and people with dementia. *Aging and Mental Health* 7: 452–61.

Cheston R, Jones K, Gilliard J. (2003b) Remembering and forgetting: group with people who have dementia. In: Adams T, Manthorpe J (eds). *Dementia care.* London: Arnold.

Clare L. (2004) Awareness in early stage Alzheimer's disease: A review of methods and evidence. *British Journal of Clinical Psychology* 43: 177–96.

Cox S, Cook A. (2002) Caring for people with dementia at the end of life. In: Hockley J, Clark D (eds). *Palliative care for older people in care homes.* Buckingham: Open University Press, 86–103.

De Lepeliere J, Wind A, Iliffe S *et al.* (2008) The primary care diagnosis of dementia in Europe: An analysis using multi-disciplinary, multi-national expert groups. *Aging and Mental Health* 12: 568–76.

Department of Health. (2009) *The National Dementia Strategy.* London: Department of Health.

Drennan V, Cole L. (2009) Promoting continence and managing incontinence with people with dementia living at home: one more challenge for integration. *Journal of Integrated Care* 17: 15–28.

Doraiswamy PM, Leon J, Cummings JL *et al.* (2002) Prevalence and impact of medical comorbidity in Alzheimer's disease. *Journals of Gerontology. Series A. Biological Sciences and Medical Sciences* 57: M173–7.

Georges J, Jansen S, Jackson J *et al.* (2008) Alzheimer's disease in real life-the dementia carer's survey. *International Journal of Geriatric Psychiatry* 23: 546–51.

Goodman C, Evans C, Wilcock J *et al.* (2010) End of life care for community dwelling older people with dementia: an integrated review. *International Journal of Geriatric Psychiatry* 25: 329–37.

Harari D, Igbedioh C. (2009) Restoring continence in frail older people living in the community: what factors influence successful treatment outcomes? *Age and Ageing* 38: 228–33.

Hope T, Keene J, Gedling K. (1998) Predictors of institutionalization for people with dementia living at home with a carer. *International Journal of Geriatric Psychiatry* 13: 682–90.

Hinton L, Franz C, Reddy G *et al.* (2007) Practice constraints, behavioural problems and dementia care: primary care physicians perspectives. *Journal of General Internal Medicine* 22: 1625–7.

Husband HJ. (1999) The psychological consequences of learning a diagnosis of dementia: three case examples. *Aging and Mental Health* 3: 179–83.

Iliffe S, Wilcock J. (2005) The identification of barriers to the recognition of and response to dementia in primary care using a modified focus group method. *Dementia* 4: 12–23.

Iliffe S, Jain P, Wong G *et al.* (2009) Dementia diagnosis in primary care: looking outside the educational box. *Aging Health* 5: 51–9.

Jha A, Tabet N, Orrell M. (2001) To tell or not to tell – comparison of older patients' reaction to their diagnosis of dementia and depression. *International Journal of Geriatric Psychiatry* 16: 879–85.

Kodner D. (2006) Whole-system approaches to health and social care partnerships for the frail elderly: an exploration of North

Managing medical co-morbidities and general hospital admission for people with dementia

JOHN HOLMES

18.1 INTRODUCTION

General hospitals can be dangerous places for people with dementia. Over the past few years the ways that general hospitals manage people with dementia (PWD) has come under increased scrutiny, with a growing realization that PWD are frequently found in many departments across the general hospital, and often experience poor care for both their dementia and the physical problem for which they were admitted. Staff may lack training, skills and experience in dealing with PWD, and impersonal care pathways designed for those who are cognitively intact often do not work well for PWD; both of these factors contribute to the fact that PWD in general hospitals often experience poorer outcomes. Ward environments are confusing, and the multiple ward changes found in many care pathways in general hospitals only contribute to this confusion. Added to this is the close relationship between dementia and delirium, conditions with different aetiologies but many shared clinical features, and we can see that dementia is an important problem that general hospitals must address if they are to deliver good care to all who use their services. This chapter will set out the scale and nature of the problem, before examining some potential solutions that could bring better outcomes for all stakeholders.

People aged 65 years or older occupy about two-thirds of beds in the UK National Health Services (Department of Health, 2001). A small proportion of these beds are in mental health units, but the vast majority are in general hospitals. Admissions of older people are spread throughout almost all hospital departments, with care of the elderly and general medicine having the greatest number, but few of the medical or surgical specialities being exempt, dealing as they do in the main with problems associated with increasing age – osteoporotic hip fracture, coronary artery disease, peripheral vascular disease, etc., and where we find older people, we find older people with dementia; admitted with a concurrent physical problem (or more often multiple problems), where coexisting pathologies are made more difficult to unravel by the presence of cognitive impairment. So, is dementia a problem for general hospitals? The epidemiology in this setting would suggest so, but first there are some important matters to consider.

18.2 RECOGNITION OF DEMENTIA IN THE GENERAL HOSPITAL

To begin to manage people with dementia in the general hospital setting, first we must recognize the presence of dementia. This is not as straightforward as it seems, both for researchers and for clinicians. The assessment of mental state, and particularly cognitive function, may be difficult in a very sick patient. The differentiation between dementia and delirium, and the added challenge of delirium superimposed on dementia, require information that the patient themselves often cannot provide due to memory impairment, yet if this information is not obtained then it is easy to see how both delirium and an underlying infection can go unrecognized and how dementia is not diagnosed. Many researchers have taken the easy option of measuring cognitive impairment using tools such as the Mini-Mental State Examination (Folstein *et al.*, 1975), but have not separated out dementia from delirium, an approach which is not helpful. In research studies, diagnosis of dementia requires at least a standardized assessment of cognitive function, together with a structured informant history that provides some information on the temporal nature and severity of cognitive and other symptoms, and a categorization that recognizes three different states – dementia, delirium and delirium superimposed on dementia. Few have taken this approach; one systematic review of the prevalence of mental health problems in general hospitals (Royal College of Psychiatrists, 2005) reveals 33 studies using blunt measures of cognitive function, 17 studies using adequate detection methods for dementia, 31 studies using adequate detection methods for delirium and none using a method for detecting coexisting dementia and delirium. The studies examining dementia reveal ranges in prevalence from 5 to 45 per cent across a range of hospital departments, with a pooled prevalence of 31 per cent. The range of prevalences seen reflects not just different methodologies used, but also underlying differences in the true prevalence between hospital specialities. Even if we accept that some of these cases will have a superimposed delirium, it seems that dementia is pandemic in our hospitals. This is further confirmed by a recent study in older people in a general medical setting where the research team carefully separated out cases of delirium and found rates of dementia of 42 per cent, with only half having a previous diagnosis (Sampson *et al.*, 2009). This suggests that general hospitals are a good place to set up screening programmes for previously undiagnosed dementia. We also need to bear in mind that the prevalences quoted will soon be out of date; an ageing population means increased prevalences of dementia in all settings; dementia in the general hospital cannot be ignored.

Where researchers struggle, so do clinicians. Dementia and delirium are closely intertwined; delirium is common in the acutely unwell patient with multiple pathologies (Siddiqi *et al.*, 2006), and dementia is the largest single risk factor for the development of delirium (Schor *et al.*, 1992). If a delirium is present there are likely to be several provoking factors, all of which may need addressing for successful resolution of the delirium. Where there are other sources of information about previous cognitive function this should be sought; in the absence of information to the contrary it seems best, when confronted with an acutely unwell confused patient, to assume prevalent delirium or a risk of incident delirium and treat as such using multicomponent approaches that ensure good, holistic care (Inouye *et al.*, 1999; Marcantonio *et al.*, 2001), while investigating and addressing potential causes of delirium and seeking further information about the temporal onset of symptoms.

18.3   OUTCOMES IN PEOPLE WITH DEMENTIA IN THE GENERAL HOSPITAL

Prevalence studies reveal dementia as a significant problem for general hospital providers, and the scale of the problem is

magnified when outcomes for this population are examined. Increased mortality, increased length of stay, increased institutionalization and decreased independence on discharge are all reported (Royal College of Psychiatrists, 2005), and these outcomes are important for a wide range of stakeholders. Patients and carers may be most interested in survival, whereas general hospital providers are interested in length of stay and social care providers pay attention to the care packages required to help people return home or the cost of institutional care. This broad impact demonstrates the cross-cutting nature of dementia across health and social care, and serve as a reminder that dementia is of interest not just to mental health services, but to the whole health and social care economy. This cross-cutting importance is not reflected in the commissioning or inspection of health and social care in England, although attempts by the English Department of Health to form partnerships across these agencies through its Partnerships for Older People Programme have had some success. Improvements in outcomes in one sector may well benefit other sectors too. However, it may be possible to improve outcomes only when we understand why outcomes are so poor in people with dementia, and this will be explored next.

One obvious reason for poor outcomes for PWD in the general hospital is the presence of dementia itself. The cognitive and motivational problems that dementia bring mean that rehabilitation instructions may not be followed or medication is not taken as prescribed. Basic necessities such as food and drink may not be to hand or may be taken away untouched; 60 per cent of older people in UK general hospitals are malnourished and dementia must be a contributor to this (Age Concern, 2006). These and other facts seem to reveal a deep-seated ambivalence about the ownership of dementia; it is perceived by many general hospital staff as being a mental health problem and so nothing to do with them (Holmes *et al.*, 2002). This is perpetuated by the lack of pre- and post-qualification training in dementia care that exists for health-care professionals in general hospitals (Department of Health, 2009b). In turn, mental health staff see the physical illness causing the general hospital presentation, and expect general hospital colleagues to be able to cope. It is therefore not surprising that general hospital staff who, day-to-day, are expected to care for people with dementia, feel they lack the knowledge and skills to do so successfully (Atkin *et al.*, 2005). The same research revealed that some staff recognized their shortcomings, wanting training to improve their skills, but others continued to perceive it as someone else's problem in the vain hope that it would simply disappear, a hope that will rapidly dissipate when population projections are examined.

A lack of familiarity with dementia and its care, combined with misinformation based on folklore and prejudice, and a culture of risk-avoidance, can work against people with dementia in the general hospital. An inability to make a cup of tea safely in the ward's assessment kitchen is branded a failure and rewarded with entry into institutional care, an easier outcome to arrange than the design of a complex care package to sustain someone at home. A suggestion that an assessment is carried out at home, in familiar surroundings, prompts the response 'What if they refuse to come back?'.

A person who walks around a ward seeking stimulation rather than sitting meekly by their bed is termed a 'wanderer'; and an assumption that this behaviour will be replicated at home, leading to unacceptable risk, results in unnecessary institutionalization. Urinating in a waste-bin is viewed as anti-social behaviour, although the toilets lack signage that is visible from bed areas. The capacity to make a decision to return home and the capability to manage at home are confused, so that the capable but incapacitous are institutionalized in what is perceived to be in their best interests. Add to this the pressure from concerned but misguided relatives who equate dementia with care homes, and think that institutional care magically removes all risk, and it is easy to understand why PWD can face a struggle to get home.

This reflects the situation at the coal face of general hospital care, but the same is also apparent at strategic and managerial levels too. Care pathways exist for most of the common chronic and acute physical conditions, addressing community care, admission into hospital, care during the admission and discharge home or to an intermediate care facility. Although these may work well for uncomplicated cases, the presence of dementia makes many of these pathways break down. Pathway design seems to have a blind spot, not recognizing that many people the pathway should help are not able to benefit, either because the pathway assumes full cognition (e.g. a chronic obstructive pulmonary disease pathway requiring full adherence to bronchodilator and steroid treatments) or because they are specifically excluded from certain parts of the pathway. The latter is common (though not universal) in the discharge-facilitating intermediate care services that are common in the UK (Department of Health, 2009b), where a diagnosis of dementia can be enough to shut off access to pathways out of hospital, resulting in increased length of stay. The assumption that PWD cannot benefit from rehabilitation is at best spurious; one study showed that people with mild and moderately severe dementia were able to be successfully rehabilitated after hip fracture, with only those who had severe dementia getting no benefit (Huusko et al., 2000). A further problem with pathways is that people with dementia are often old, and their multiple co-morbidities would fit several pathways at once; there may be a trade-off between, for example, specialist cardiac care for an acute coronary syndrome and best care of a concurrent chest infection and hypothyroidism. The treatment of such physical illness in people with dementia should take account of their dementia, meaning not just a history and examination focusing upon chest pain and its sequelae, but an all-encompassing assessment of the whole person. Some parts of our healthcare system have become extremely focused on single bodily systems, and that does not work for PWD.

Another feature of general hospital care that does not help PWD is that of multiple bed moves, within and between wards and sometimes between hospitals. The hospital is entered via the Accident and Emergency Department, followed by a spell of a short-stay assessment ward, then a period on an acute ward with maybe a transfer to a rehabilitation bed. Acquisition of a hospital-acquired infection may bring a further move, to a side-room or isolation ward, and once clear of infection the patient is unlikely to return to their original ward, going instead wherever a bed is available at the time. This results in a breakdown in continuity of care; with each move there is a new set of faces to get to know, a new set of strangers to ask probing questions, to get to know food likes and dislikes, to deliver personal care of the most intimate nature. Each move is an opportunity to lose essential equipment such as spectacles, dentures and hearing aids. What chance is there of orientation with these multiple moves, which bring increased risk of delirium (McCusker et al., 2001)? Some of the orientation questions used in cognitive testing become almost meaningless after a series of moves, the name or floor of the building becoming unobtainable. A recent assessment was requested of a man with dementia who had become aggressive and punched a hospital porter; it transpired that it had been decided to move him to another ward at 2.30am, and his response to being asked to vacate his bed in the middle of the night by a group of strangers did not, in that context, seem as extreme as it first appeared.

There are many barriers to rehabilitation and discharge for PWD in general hospitals, but they all have a common effect, that of leading to increased length of stay. On the face of it this seems bad for the health-care provider, since increased time in hospital leads to increased cost. There are also costs to the individual too, however. More time in hospital being helped is less time doing things independently, and even basic activities of daily living skills can be rapidly lost if people have things done for them rather than being allowed to care for themselves, if necessary with prompting. Such an approach may take more time, but the result is greater independence. More time in hospital means more exposure to the risks of being in hospital, with falls and the resulting fractures bringing an orthopaedic transfer, or exposure to pathogens bringing hospital-acquired infections; neither these nor other unnecessary complications help to hasten the return home.

18.4   IMPROVEMENTS IN CARE

The picture of dementia care in general hospitals painted above seems rather bleak, but for many it is sadly true. However, there are several ways to improve care and bring better outcomes. These range from changes in ward design and layout through to pathway redesign and staff training. Of these, probably the most important is staff training. Colleagues in general hospitals need to understand that dementia is part of their core business, rather than a condition dealt with elsewhere. We should not expect all to become dementia experts, but we should expect a basic knowledge of dementia, its presentation and diagnosis, common behaviours and their management, how to communicate with PWD, the legal framework for capacity and consent, and how to deliver physical care in an appropriate way that does not appear threatening. The English National Dementia Strategy (Department of Health, 2009b) highlights the training issue, calling for training in dementia care for general hospital staff and for a stronger presence for dementia in curricula for undergraduate health-care professionals. This training has to be supported by managers, with time made available to attend training sessions. Training may be provided by knowledgeable general hospital colleagues, but may be better provided by mental health staff working as part of a liaison mental health team, bridging the gap between physical and mental health care.

The basic knowledge and skills required of general hospital colleagues will need back-up from more experienced mental health professionals. As well as providing training, members of a liaison mental health team can provide specialist advice in more complex cases. Such mental health teams are far from universal (Holmes *et al.*, 2003), but where they exist they are able to provide prompt expert assessment and have the potential to improve outcomes (Royal College of Psychiatrists, 2005). These teams may be the first point of contact with mental health services, and they have a vital role in signposting people with dementia to services such as memory clinics where cognitive function can be monitored and appropriate support offered. Liaison staff can work with general hospital colleagues in drawing up care plans that address both physical and mental health-care needs, promoting person-centred care and independence and providing input into discharge planning and care package design that will enable successful discharge back to independent living.

Care for PWD in the general hospital can be improved by the development of services outside hospital too. One example is that of rapid-access home care. Someone with dementia may wait several days or weeks for a care package to be provided, but prompt availability of home care may bring more rapid discharge.

Environmental changes can make a difference. Ideally, ward layouts should be designed with dementia in mind, but in the absence of this some simple changes can help. These include appropriate use of colour so that particular ward areas share the same colour scheme. Clear signage that is visible from bed areas will help patients to identify toilets better, and orientation to time can be helped by ensuring clocks are visible and show the correct time; use of calendars may also help. Heavily patterned materials for curtains etc. should be avoided to reduce the risk of visual illusions, and noise should be kept to a minimum to avoid misinterpretation.

PWD may forget to eat what is put in front of them, but they are more likely to eat simple finger foods than meals requiring cutlery. The social aspect of eating can be enhanced by eating with others round a table rather than sat alone by a hospital bed; someone with dementia may be able to take a lead from others who are eating at the same time. Some hospitals recognize patients at nutritional risk through specially coloured food trays, highlighting that assistance with eating is required, and ensuring that food is not taken away by housekeeping staff uneaten. Attention to medication is also important; someone with dementia may need prompting and supervision to ensure that medication is taken at the right time and not left untouched.

One problem already mentioned is a lack of pathways out of hospital for people with dementia. Recent guidance from the English Department of Health (Department of Health, 2009a) makes it clear that intermediate care services should not exclude PWD, and training in dementia care for staff in these services may also be necessary. Care pathways for common conditions should be able to work for PWD; designing pathways with people with dementia in mind will not adversely affect the cognitively intact and will offer greater chance of rehabilitation and a return to independent living. Inclusion of dementia in care pathways requires sign-up from all stakeholders at the beginning of pathway development rather than it being added on as an afterthought.

18.5   CONCLUSION

This chapter has touched on some of the important issues in delivering better general hospital care for PWD. Although it is not exhaustive, it is apparent that many potential solutions are not particularly expensive or high-tech. When commissioners and providers of general hospital care understand the key importance of dementia across the whole health and social care economy we will see better care provision for PWD in this setting, and admission to hospital will no longer be fraught with danger.

REFERENCES

Age Concern. (2006) *Hungry to be heard: the scandal of malnourished older people in hospital.* London: Age Concern England.

Atkin K, Holmes J, Martin C. (2005) Provision of care for older people with co-morbid mental illness in general hospitals: general nurses' perceptions of their training needs. *International Journal of Geriatric Psychiatry* 20: 1081–3.

Department of Health. (2001) *National service framework for older people.* London: Department of Health.

Department of Health. (2009a) *Intermediate care: Halfway home.* London: Department of Health.

Department of Health. (2009b) *Living well with dementia: A National Dementia Strategy.* London: Department of Health.

Folstein MF, Folstein SE, Mchugh PR. (1975) "Mini-mental state". A practical method for grading the cognitive state of patients for the clinician. *Journal of Psychiatric Research* 12: 189–98.

Holmes J, Bentley K, Cameron I. (2002) *Between two stools: Psychiatric services for older people in general hospitals.* Leeds: University of Leeds.

Holmes J, Bentley K, Cameron I. (2003) A UK survey of psychiatric services for older people in general hospitals. *International Journal of Geriatric Psychiatry* 18: 716–21.

Huusko TM, Karppi P, Avikainen V et al. (2000) Randomised, clinically controlled trial of intensive geriatric rehabilitation in patients with hip fracture: subgroup analysis of patients with dementia. *British Medical Journal* 321: 1107–11.

Inouye SK, Bogardus Jr ST, Charpentier PA et al. (1999) A multicomponent intervention to prevent delirium in hospitalized older patients. *New England Journal of Medicine* 340: 669–76.

Marcantonio ER, Flacker JM, Wright RJ, Resnick NM. (2001) Reducing delirium after hip fracture: a randomized trial. *Journal of the American Geriatrics Society* 49: 516–22.

McCusker J, Cole M, Abrahamowicz M *et al.* (2001) Environmental risk factors for delirium in hospitalized older people. *Journal of the American Geriatrics Society* **49**: 1327–34.

Royal College of Psychiatrists. (2005) *Who cares wins: Improving the outcome for older people admitted to the general hospital.* Leeds: Royal College of Psychiatrists.

Sampson EL, Blanchard MR, Jones L *et al.* (2009) Dementia in the acute hospital: prospective cohort study of prevalence and mortality. *British Journal of Psychiatry* **195**: 61–6.

Schor JD, Levkoff SE, Lipsitz LA *et al.* (1992) Risk factors for delirium in hospitalized elderly. *Journal of the American Medical Association* **267**: 827–31.

Siddiqi N, House AO, Holmes JD. (2006) Occurrence and outcome of delirium in medical in-patients: a systematic literature review. *Age and Ageing* **35**: 350–64.

19

The role of nursing in the management of dementia

MAREE MASTWYK AND BEVERLEY WILLIAMS

Dementia care is not the care of the dying: it is about meaningful life for the living (Wylie, 2003).

19.1   INTRODUCTION

Jokes about dementia abound – 'with Alzheimer's disease (AD) you get to meet someone new every day'. When it comes to caring for someone with dementia, this is no longer a joke. The patient may not remember you from yesterday and if they do, it may be that all they remember is the emotion that seeing you engenders – happiness or irritability. Every day you need to introduce yourself to the patient and explain the task to be undertaken. He or she is in an unfamiliar environment, surrounded by strangers and may be frightened. A fundamental tenet of nursing is to provide a safe, secure environment, so we need to ameliorate that fear.

Dementia care is a nursing specialty just like paediatrics or coronary care. It is important that the nurse has an interest in or, better, a passion for this area and recognizes that the journey through dementia is unique for each individual (**Box 19.1**). Put simply, it is of crucial importance to make the journey as comfortable as possible. To achieve this, perform a nursing assessment that includes consultation with the patient; learn their history, background, abilities and shortfalls, likes and dislikes. Keep in mind the basic human needs: nutrition, hydration, exercise, sleep, hygiene, safety and comfort and be aware that if these needs are not being met, the patient may exhibit 'challenging' behaviours in order to be heard.

19.2   PATIENT AUTONOMY – ANY STAGE OF THE ILLNESS IN ANY SETTING

A patient newly diagnosed with dementia may still be working, caring for dependent children, retired, a committee member of the local golf club, or minding grandchildren during the week. People with dementia retain the ability to think, reason and function, although they may show signs of

---

Box 19.1

The nurse needs:

- Understanding, patience, resilience, sense of humour
- Interest/passion in caring for the person with dementia
- Education, guidance and support in the role

difficulty in these areas, and still make a contribution to the community. They are capable of making decisions, having opinions and planning for the future. Self-awareness is present for a considerable time, though those in contact with them, both personally and professionally, often fail to notice (Bossen *et al.*, 2009). Patients want to be heard, to give and receive information, to promote health and safety and to gain both emotional and cognitive support (Bossen *et al.*, 2009).

The emphasis today is on person-centred care (Kitwood, 1993) to maintain autonomy and dignity. This can only be accomplished if the opinions of the patient are sought and respected (Pringle-Specht *et al.*, 2009). The patient with dementia needs a partner to compensate for cognitive losses and promote more efficient use of remaining functional abilities (Pringle-Specht *et al.*, 2009), not one who takes control. Nurses need to foster the patient's independence for as long as possible. Not only cognitive/functional deficits need to be considered when drafting a care plan, but the patient's abilities, interests and culture too. Self-esteem has an impact on the way we feel about ourselves, interact with other people, handle problems, our level of relaxation and safety (ReachOut Australia, 2009). It does for the patient as well.

People with dementia can share their knowledge, experience and needs and are now included in focus groups with other stakeholders, for example driving cessation (Perkinson *et al.*, 2005). Alzheimer's Association 'fact sheets' include suggestions from people with dementia (Communication, 2009). Pringle-Specht and Bossen consulted Taylor, a person with probable AD for their paper 'Partnering for care: the evidence and the expert,' in March, 2009. People with dementia are able to guide us in designing strategies for care.

In later stages the family can be a valuable resource of information about the patient. However, until the patient is unable to communicate, he or she can be consulted directly about future plans, needs and wants. Alzheimer's Australia (Fact sheet – 'About you …. Early planning,' 2005) recommend planning with the patient early in the diagnosis of dementia to enable them to express their desires, wants and needs for consideration at the time when they are no longer able to express themselves, including medical, financial and legal concerns. This planning should include end of life decisions as well (see Chapter 35, Ethical issues and dementia, Chapter 36, End-of-life decisions and dementia

and Chapter 37, Care and management of the patient with advanced dementia).

Planning by the family on behalf of the patient can be distressing to the family as well. If important decisions are made in consultation with the patient early, this can remove a potential source of stress from the family as the patient's life nears its end.

Person-centred care requires person-centred staff and management to promote and provide a supportive environment (**Box 19.2**). Residents in a nursing home will still have some self-awareness and some ability to participate in decisions. Allowing them to make small simple choices for themselves can help maintain their self-esteem.

19.3   HOSPITAL NURSING CARE

Caring for a patient with dementia in a hospital requires patience and a calm approach as care is provided. Most patients will recall aspects of a hospital admission, despite their dementia. Even if the patient has severe dementia, unpleasant feelings and emotions from previous admissions may still be remembered, so nurses need to approach the patient in a friendly, non-threatening manner. Remember, the patient is in a strange, noisy environment and surrounded by strangers.

19.3.1   Care of a patient in a general ward

- Provide a single room if possible to minimize noise and confusion; preferably one with an en suite so that the toilet can be found easily.
- Greet the patient by name.
- Introduce yourself, ask if the patient remembers you when you go into the room on later occasions and introduce yourself again if necessary.
- Explain every procedure, even if it happens every day during the patient's admission, and even if you are only in the patient's room to replace a filled urine bottle. You may need to remind the patient frequently why they are in hospital. This may be frustrating for you but is more frustrating and confusing for the patient if there is no understanding.
- Focus the patient's attention. If two nurses are required for a procedure, only one should instruct the patient if the patient is required to do something to participate.
- If you need a distraction, chat about the patient's past life – job, family, hobbies. Remember that these early memories will be the last to go.
- Ask permission before helping yourself to the patient's locker or wardrobe. We see these cupboards as an extension of our working environment – the patient may interpret you helping yourself to soap, toothpaste, etc. as theft.
- The patient may not be able to report pain – look for non-verbal cues: grimacing, restlessness, agitation.
- Use caution when giving pro re nata (PRN) medication for agitation – pain may be the cause.

Box 19.2

Role of nursing:

- Promote independence
- Provide a safe, secure environment for patients and staff
- Advocate on the patient's behalf, when needed
- Educate patient, family, other nurses and staff
- Promote health, prevent illness/injury

- Extend visiting hours for next-of-kin, other family members and friends – hospitals are extremely noisy environments and some noises can be frightening. If a trusted visitor is with the patient, they can help explain what is going on and keep the patient calm.
- Place an orientation board in the line of sight of the patient with the day, date, location and why the patient is there.
- Facilitate watching favourite programmes on television.
- Ask the family to bring familiar objects and photos into the room and the patient's favourite music to play in the room.

19.3.2 Accident and Emergency Department

Try to find a quiet corner for the patient or, the least noisy corner. Try to minimize the stimulus from hospital equipment/hustle and bustle as much as possible. Every time you approach the patient, introduce yourself. As the number of people with dementia increases, James and Hodnett (2009) recommend the creation of a designated area for dementia patients, away from the noise of phones, pagers and alarms. The trolley should face a window, away from the busy activity and potentially frightening equipment of the Accident and Emergency Department (James and Hodnett, 2009). Position photos of the local area at a low enough level to see from the trolley and perhaps stimulate reminiscence (James and Hodnett, 2009). Provide calming music to reduce the impact of the unit's noise, tactile items, such as balls, for distraction, anaesthetic gel before venepuncture, clear toilet signage – perhaps a visual prompt – and adequate pain relief (**Box 19.3**; James and Hodnett, 2009). Increased stress and pain can cause changes in behaviour – 'exiting behaviour' trying to 'walk away' from the cause of pain, change in facial expressions (James and Hodnett, 2009). Hospital volunteers can be of benefit to the patient, staff and carers by remaining with the patient and explaining procedures to the patient and family where appropriate (James and Hodnett, 2009). Providing training in dementia care for staff will improve patient outcomes by reducing stress for both patient and staff (James and Hodnett, 2009).

19.4 PAIN AND MEDICATION

Experiencing pain is different for everybody. People have different pain thresholds which can be lowered by fatigue and depression. For those who are cognitively intact the presence of pain is more easily articulated. Thus preferred, effective medications and other methods of pain relief are more easily provided.

Cognitive impairment is a substantial barrier to the assessment and management of pain. It is common for older patients to experience pain associated with arthritis, spinal canal stenosis, diabetic neuropathy, painful legs, etc. A patient with dementia may be incapable of reporting pain verbally. The nurse needs to know the patient's past and current medical history both to identify possible causes and to facilitate appropriate management.

If the patient is unable to communicate adequately, our observations and knowledge of the patient need to be relied upon. Gait, facial expressions (frown, grimace), skin colour, behaviour, placing cold or hot things on a body part can all be observable indicators of pain. Vital signs (heart rate, blood pressure, temperature) can provide important information especially in the assessment of non-verbal elderly dementia patients. Observe, gather information from all team members, consult with the doctor, commence an analgesic regimen and continue to observe, evaluate and document.

Medications, when used well, can assist in pain management. However, consideration must be given to the fact that older people have an increased sensitivity to some drugs, especially opiates. If an increased sedative effect is present, this may lead to falls and fractures, loss of muscle strength, immobility and decreased cognition (see Chapter 18, Managing medical co-morbidities and general hospital admission for people with dementia).

Depending on the cause of the pain, regular paracetamol is a safer option than anti-inflammatories, which may have gastrointestinal or other side effects.

An effective approach to pain relief is to combine medication with a non-drug approach: massage, heat, exercise – all to increase circulation – or distraction. As tiredness can increase pain, consider the patient's sleep pattern too.

Medications prescribed earlier may now be unnecessary or causing side effects. Regular medication reviews are required to avoid unnecessary polypharmacy. Used wisely, medications can help with symptoms of pain, agitation and anxiety. They can improve sleep at night to increase daytime participation in activities.

19.5 RESIDENTIAL CARE

19.5.1 Assessment

Dementia care today is based on 'person-centred care', founded on a holistic model designed and developed by the

---

Box 19.3

Key points when caring for a person with dementia in any environment are:

- Remember: the patient is in a strange environment, surrounded by strangers
- INTRODUCE yourself and the task to prevent fear in the patient
- Allow autonomy, enhance self-esteem (allow choices, maintain abilities)
- One stimulus/voice at a time to focus the patient's attention
- Treat patient with dignity
- Maintain routine
- Do not 'infantilize' the patient
- The patient will remember EMOTION

late Tom Kitwood and Kathleen Bredin in the late 1980s (Kitwood, 1993). The basic tenets of this work are:

- uniqueness – everyone is different;
- complexity – we all see things differently and are influenced by the changes and events that occur during our lifetimes (Alzheimer's Australia W.A. Ltd., 2009).

Most facilities will have their own patient assessment tool. Whichever tool is used, the assessment needs to be person-centred and keep to the patient's at home routine as much as possible. For example, if they showered at home in the evening, can this be maintained? Information gathering should involve the patient, include the family and close friends, list abilities, needs, and details of the person's life story so that new staff can quickly gain an insight into the person they may be caring for on that day. Of course, assessment of falls risk, compliance with special diets, etc. also need to be included, but the emphasis needs to be on the patient – their life, culture, loves, hates, usual routine. Moving into a care facility will cause confusion and the patient will need support. Talking to the patient helps them feel welcome and use of knowledge obtained will assist in maintaining the patient's self-esteem and feelings of safety, thus reducing anxiety, and contributing to a settled environment for all. A brief, 'dot-point' biography of the patient in the front of the notes would be helpful. Two patients with the same diagnosis may be very different!

Once the assessment is complete, it is important to establish a routine and to utilize the care plan in the daily care of the patient. If the patient is capable of dressing 'with supervision' it would be an insult to dignity, autonomy and self-esteem to dress them yourself for expediency. It is important to work to the pace of the patient. Information gathered during the assessment can also be used to distract the patient at times of potential distress/anxiety and used in reminiscence and validation therapy. The assessment needs to be reviewed and amended regularly as needs change over time.

19.5.2   A note on culture

Some residential facilities are culture specific and have carers from the same cultural background. The patient's culture needs to be considered if this is not the case. Despite cognitive deficits, participating in religious practices can still bring comfort. Perhaps family or friends can help provide this. Immigrant patients may have spoken the local language fluently prior to diagnosis, but with the progression of dementia, may revert back to their native tongue. Patients approached with dignity and respect are more likely to respond positively than negatively. Non-verbal communication – facial expression, tone of voice, gentle directing – can be powerful.

19.6   ENVIRONMENT – PHYSICAL

Patients with dementia may have perceptual difficulties. Even in the absence of difficulties due to dementia, an older person may have impaired sight, deafness or a gait disturbance. They need a simple, uncluttered, well-lit environment that is safe to navigate. Family can assist by personalizing the patient's living space to make it identifiable by the patient. Colour and material choices are also important. Even in an old building, appropriate changes can be made at times of building maintenance. An ideal environment needs:

- to be calm and welcoming, and not too busy. Advise all staff to avoid unnecessary noise (e.g. not to drop a large bundle of cutlery into a sink).
- contrasting colours between walls, floors and doors. Toilet doors particularly need to be a different colour to other doors, so that the patient can identify and find the toilet when needed. In bathrooms, if the walls, floor, tiles, toilet, basin are all white, a patient with visuo-spatial difficulties may be unable to find the toilet and may become agitated, incontinent or use the black lined rubbish bin instead.
- to avoid surfaces/paints that reflect light. Sun glare may give the appearance of spills on the floor.
- floor coverings that are easy to clean, not slippery and that absorb noise. The floor surface should be level. Particular care needs to be taken if bedroom areas are carpeted and day rooms are surfaced with linoleum. Surface changes may produce a falls risk.
- hand rails on all walls.
- adequate lighting. No dark corners or shadows which may distort shapes to produce something frightening.
- appropriate signage – at eye level, perhaps use the accepted universal symbols for the toilet as well as the word 'toilet'; pictorial dinner plate with knife and fork on either side for the dining room etc.
- an outside area to walk in, sit in or, perhaps, garden in.
- background music – patient choice, or relaxing, non-stimulating music.
- to provide a patient's individual bedroom area – personalized with familiar furniture and recognizable belongings, family photograph on the door, pictures/photographs on the walls. Asking the family to help with this will help them feel they are still contributing to the care of the patient.

19.7   ENVIRONMENT – SOCIAL

Everyone requires daily mental stimulation. A patient who cannot walk, talk or participate actively in group activities can still be a passive observer. Previous leisure activities can still be enjoyed with a little creative modification. Most people enjoy dancing. Patients who cannot dance will still benefit from being present in the room while others dance – they can enjoy the movement, music and rhythm. Sports fans can still enjoy watching sports on television. Appropriate diversion therapies can be provided by occupational or diversional therapists (see Chapter 21, Occupational therapy in dementia care).

Multi-sensory stimulation has come from a Dutch initiative, the snoezelen room, which is useful with agitated dementia patients. As its objective is to stimulate the patient's senses – sight, sound, smell, touch and taste – the room may contain: comfortable seating, a solar projector, bubble column, a revolving mirror ball, soft gentle music (i.e. sounds of nature, aromatherapy oils/candles and many other innovative ideas). Such rooms promote relaxation through sensory stimulation and can be calming for agitated patients, though monitoring is needed because everyone's experience is different and some patients may become distressed or more agitated (Wylie, 2003).

Any sensory stimulation can be therapeutic. This might include sitting in the fresh air, enjoying the warmth of the sun, the sounds of leaves in the breeze and birds chirping, or smelling the aromas of cooking when one is unable to cook.

Photo albums of family and friends, annotated with names of people and places or a communication/visitors' book can be provided for the patient to read. Family and friends can contribute to this book continually and can see who and when others have visited, and it can be used to provide conversation/reminiscence prompts.

Music can be an entertainment, used as a therapy to promote memories in reminiscence therapy or to calm agitated patients (Alzheimer's Australia, 2009; see Chapter 29, Sexuality and dementia). The choice of music should be the patient's, not what the staff or family choose. It is the patient's home, everybody else is a guest.

19.8   TIME, PLACE, PERSON

19.8.1   Orientation

The patient's peace of mind is more important than their knowledge of time and place. If a 93-year-old woman thinks that her aunt still lives down a certain street 'near here', there is no point in causing distress by telling her that she is 93, the year is 2010 and that her aunt could not possibly still be alive. It would be better to comment on the fond memories she must have and encourage her to talk about those.

When orientation of the patient is important, such as meal or shower times, the patient should be greeted appropriately in a non-threatening way, to alleviate any fear felt at being approached by a stranger, and to gain co-operation. A little thought is required to provide the information needed for the task without putting the patient under pressure. For example, 'Hello Julia, I'm Nancy, one of the nursing staff. It's 12 o'clock and lunch will be served very soon. Let me walk with you to the dining room'. In this instance, orientation to person, time of day and purpose for activity are explained and the patient does not need to make a decision.

When dementia patients do not recognize family members, it is often distressing to the family but not necessarily to the patient. The patient may still remember the emotion associated with that family member and smile and say 'hello' when they enter the room. It is important to point out to the family that even though the patient cannot say their name they are still happy to see them.

19.8.2   Perception

Other factors to consider are disturbances of perception and misinterpretation of stimuli. The patient's reality is different to ours. They may tell their family that they want to go home. If the family take the patient home for a visit, the patient may say that he or she still wants to go home. Perhaps 'home' means a place of calm and safety, where they feel comfortable and at peace. While in a state of anxiety, a patient may become agitated and become a challenge for staff attempting to provide care.

19.8.2.1   PERCEPTUAL IMPAIRMENT

Due to confusion, the patient with dementia could find themselves living in a state of fright. A black jumper on furniture may look like an animal; a patient with Balint's syndrome (difficulties with visual perception) may not be able to see what is directly in front of them causing feelings of insecurity, making them prone to falls or unable to see food on a plate. Dementia may affect visuospatial awareness: glaring light on pale floors may look like water and the patient may try to step over it, risking a fall.

The nurse needs to be alert to the patient's sensory impairments in order to provide assistance when required. This may include helping with meals, moving clothing from furniture or directing the patient away from potentially dangerous or anxiety provoking situations. This may be as simple as standing in a patch of light on the floor.

19.9   COMMUNICATION THERAPIES

Deficits in the ability to communicate are often an early symptom of dementia: word finding difficulties, partial comprehension of conversation, problems with reading and writing. Communication is made up of three parts: 55 per cent body language (facial expression, posture, gestures); 38 per cent tone and pitch of voice; only 7 per cent is speech (Alzheimer's Australia, 2009). It is dependent on the listener listening and patiently giving the speaker time to speak. Give the patient the respect of waiting for their response rather than second guessing or speaking for them.

19.9.1   Therapies for moderate–severe dementia

19.9.1.1   REMINISCENCE THERAPY

Reminiscence therapy (RT) involves discussion of past events and can be a positive activity even if the patient cannot participate actively (Alzheimer's Australia, 2009). Groups are often led by nurses. Photographs, pictures, music, TV shows, books, can be used to trigger memories. It is important to know your patient before involving them in RT, as some memories may be distressing. RT does not always need to be conducted as a structured group therapy. It can also be used as a device for distraction at any time – in the Accident and Emergency Department or anywhere that the patient is becoming agitated.

19.9.1.2   VALIDATION THERAPY

The patient's reality is different to ours. By entering their reality, we can establish feelings of trust and security in the patient, and alleviate distress and anxiety (Alzheimer's Australia, 2009). Validation therapy (VT) consists of exploring an issue raised by the patient, even if it obviously has no bearing on the present. It is useful when the patient's short-term memory has deteriorated to the point that understanding of the present is cognitively beyond them and they have reverted to memories from their past (Alzheimer's Australia, 2009). The person attending the patient can promote discussion about their memories and the emotions they felt in that time. It does not matter that the details do not correlate with reality. The patient's peace of mind is the goal. VT can be used to engage the patient in conversation and promote mental stimulation or to distract or redirect them from doing something inappropriate without causing distress.

A 'This Is Your Life' book compiled by a family member or friend can be an excellent communication tool. Such a book can include photographs, letters, personal details, such as: immediate family tree, details of birth, anecdotes from family folklore, qualification certificates. Keep one idea to each page to avoid overwhelming the patient and place labels on photos rather than testing the patient (Alzheimer's Australia, 2009, Fact Sheet Communication).

19.10   EXERCISE/ACTIVITIES

Exercise has a beneficial effect on both physical and mental health. In a literature review, Leone *et al.* (2008) found that exercise, particularly, can have a positive effect on depressive symptoms, chronic diseases, and on the behavioural and psychological symptoms of dementia (BPSD). Exercise may lessen the risk of the onset of dementia and can stimulate cognition and the performance of activities of daily living in people with dementia (Alzheimer's Australia, 2008). The risk of falls can be reduced through balance and strength training (Alzheimer's Australia, 2008).

Benefits of exercise include:

- improved general well-being;
- improved blood flow;
- strengthened immune and hormone systems;
- increased lean muscle mass;
- increased metabolism;
- improved balance and coordination;
- positive effect on BPSD;
- enjoyment.

Types of exercise:

- aerobic (walking, dancing, any exercise which requires movement);
- progressive strength training (resistance and weight bearing);
- flexibility and balance training (tai chi, bending/ stretching).

All activities need to be tailored to the needs and capabilities of the individual (Alzheimer's Australia, 2008).

19.11   THE NEED FOR SLEEP

Consideration must be given to sleep hygiene. Lack of sleep impacts negatively on the patient's behaviour and ability to participate/function in activities in a meaningful way. An appropriate sleeping environment must be provided and other basic needs met: absence of pain, hunger, empty bowel/ bladder. Staff should be mindful of daytime rest periods – catnaps are acceptable, lengthy periods of sleep are not. Patients need to be involved in daytime activities/exercise both indoors and out in order to feel tired at night. The sleep/wake cycle can be reversed in dementia and daytime activities can assist normal diurnal awareness. Night sedation should be a last resort after all other strategies have been attempted.

19.12   NUTRITION

Nutrition for people with dementia can be assisted by the environment in which food is served. A noisy environment can be distracting and frightening. A lack of sensory cues (smell, sight, touch, taste and sound) will not encourage a person with dementia to eat (Marshall, 2003). Patients who have come from a small home unit into a multi-bed facility may find meal times confusing and overwhelming. A calm environment, background music and the opportunity to help with cooking and serving all may stimulate appetite (Marshall, 2003).

Food should be presented attractively. Smaller, more frequent meals or nutritious finger foods may benefit small eaters. Fluids should be offered frequently and in small quantities to be taken more easily. Some patients may require assistance to eat because of a perceptual difficulty or severe dementia. Some may need a trigger or cue, such as a guiding hand over theirs, to remind them of the action of eating. A staff member eating with the patients may be of benefit. Adequate time to eat must be provided and plates not removed hastily because kitchen staff need to go to lunch. Care is provided to benefit the patient not the staff.

19.13   BEHAVIOURAL AND PSYCHOLOGICAL SYMPTOMS OF DEMENTIA

Not all dementia patients exhibit BPSD. Nursing education requires knowledge of the different types of dementia, associated symptoms and expected progression of each disease. Basic understanding of the functional parts of the brain must underpin any understanding of the behaviours exhibited. Two people with the same diagnosis and same degree of atrophy may not necessarily display the same problem behaviours. Symptoms and responses to treatment change during the course of the illness.

Challenging behaviours are not deliberate and staff should not take behaviours personally. It is a waste of time arguing with a patient who does not have the capacity to understand. A person with dementia may not be able to process your words, however, if delivered with a smile, warmth, a soft tone of voice and gentle touch the person may respond in a more appropriate manner. Communication is both verbal and non-verbal. The message conveyed in a non-verbal manner may be more powerful than spoken words.

BPSD (see also Chapter 8, Neuropsychiatric aspects of dementia and Chapter 9, Measurement of behaviour disturbance, non-cognitive symptoms and quality of life) may include: aggression, agitation, resistance to personal care, wandering, intrusiveness, pacing, sleep disturbance, verbal outbursts or obscene abusive language, stealing, hiding, hoarding, inappropriate toileting, inappropriate sexual behaviour, repetitive acts, suspicion and accusations, anxiety, delusions, hallucinations, depression, depressed mood, apathy.

When are these behaviours most likely to occur?

- Attending personal care/bathing
- Dressing
- Meal times
- Late afternoon (sundowner syndrome occurs due to failing light)
- Night time
- Any time

Those behaviours that are disruptive to others need to be addressed. However, some, such as pacing and repetitive acts, need not necessarily disrupt anyone. Patients can rummage in a box or drawer provided for the purpose, or wander if it is safe in the ward area. Sundowner syndrome may be alleviated by turning on lights, closing curtains and removing shadows from the room. A behaviour only requires intervention if it is distressing to the patient or others. The nursing aim is to minimize the occurrence of any negative behaviour.

Bathing often triggers BPSD. This is perhaps due to fear, embarrassment and/or physical discomfort. An alternative to routine showering or bathing, such as a traditional bed/sponge bath using warmed cloths steeped in non-rinse cleanser, may help (O'Connor et al., 2009).

Multi-sensory activities and exercise can reduce BPSD. Depression in AD can be moderated by behaviour therapy administered by a trained carer, aggression by psychomotor therapy, apathy by use of snoezelen room/multi-sensory stimulation (Herrmann, 2005). Mental stimulation and exercise are basic human needs and unmet needs can create problems.

Other stimulating strategies to moderate or prevent BPSD are addressed in Chapter 23, The role of physiotherapy in the management of dementia and Chapter 24, Therapeutic effects of music in people with dementia. Most require human contact, so the personal interaction between the patient and person providing the care may be the key (O'Connor et al., 2009).

Sudden behavioural changes may be due to an infection, dehydration, electrolyte imbalance, constipation or nutritional deficiency. These are all treatable, reversible conditions. In addition, everyone, patients and staff can have good and bad days.

19.13.1   Distractions – 'quick–fix' solutions

Another technique to deal with BPSD is to recognize the precipitant and redirect or distract the patient to try to prevent the behaviour. The fundamental requirement for a quick-fix solution is to know your patient. If the patient is becoming testy, agitated or frustrated, greeting them by name with warmth and an outstretched hand may be all that is needed, or asking the patient about life pre-retirement, their tennis game – anything to distract the patient and focus their attention on something else.

There are many reasons why a patient with dementia may exhibit a problem behaviour; most probably precipitated by an unmet need. The solution does not always need to be pharmacological. In managing a challenging behaviour, a holistic problem-solving approach can be adopted to formulate strategies to modify/eliminate/better manage the behaviour.

A simple problem-solving model consists of:

Gathering information: What is the behaviour of concern? When does it happen? What are the triggers? How long does it persist? Who/what is it directed towards? Is it due to boredom? Is it stimulated by a memory of the past? Can the family shed any light? Is there an organic basis: urinary tract infection, pain, sensory loss, constipation?

Assessment: By team – pooling of information from all sources.

Planning: All members of the team contribute to developing a strategy to change the behaviour. A review date is set.

Implementation: ALL members of the team follow the plan on a daily basis; no saboteurs.

Evaluation: By team members of success or failure of the strategy. Accurate documentation and communication between team members is imperative.

Reiteration: Modification of management strategies based on the known successes/failures of those strategies already tried.

19.14   CARE OF THE FAMILY

... loved ones are not lost to us although they may have dementia (Young-Mason, 2009).

Family members grieve and fear for the patient from the moment of diagnosis. At different times they will feel lost, angry and frustrated. There are carer support services available to which the nurse can refer carers while providing care at home and during the transition from home care to a residential facility. Alzheimer's associations conduct sessions for carers to learn effective ways of dealing with problem behaviours (see Chapter 15, Family carers of people with dementia and Chapter 38, Alzheimer associations and societies).

The issues facing carers after institutionalization of the patient are under-researched. Some carers visit rarely while others stay most days. Some carers feel redundant, guilty or isolated. All carers will require support from the nurse as well, especially when the patient is newly admitted. It helps to involve them with the patient's care – with the assessment, decorating the patient's room, providing stimulation through reminiscence, taking the patient for walks, etc. They will require explanations if the patient's behaviour is problematic or if health is compromised. A family member with Enduring Power of Attorney may need guidance regarding choice of appropriate treatment at times if an advanced care plan is not in place.

19.15   CARE OF THE NURSE

Qualified nurses working exclusively with patients with dementia will largely be working in administration, management or in the community. Most care in dementia-specific nursing homes is provided by personal care attendants (PCAs), supervised by a registered nurse. In this situation, the nurse's job is to educate, support and lead by example.

19.15.1   Staff education

In any medical facility there are a host of different workers who come in contact with patients – from medical staff to cleaners. All staff in a facility that regularly caters for patients with dementia require some degree of training. In a facility in Suffolk, England, non-clinical staff doubted the necessity of dementia training to their jobs, but post-training reviews demonstrated that training was valuable to all departments, including laundry staff (Moden, 2009).

If most patient care is given by PCAs, trained nurses will be required to share their knowledge and provide education for the benefit of patients and untrained staff. Educational resources for ancillary staff are available from Alzheimer's associations.

Staff turnover in nursing homes is high. Recent research indicates that effective leadership, education and support contribute to the retention of carers in nursing homes (Chenoweth et al., 2010). The provision of education and clinical supervision alleviates stress and positively affects job satisfaction (Brodaty et al., 2003). It needs to be acknowledged that the work can be unpleasant and seemingly unrewarding but education and support can mitigate the negativity. To implement such an approach, the facility's management needs to be supportive.

Strategies to provide a forum for nurses to receive education and support in the workplace do not need to be expensive. They could include:

* regular support sessions;
* regular education sessions;
* debriefing sessions or extraordinary meetings to discuss specific issues that occur between regular meeting times, such as the death of a long-term resident, a challenging patient behaviour or a difficult family member;
* remunerate night staff for attendance and keep a register to ensure that every staff member has the opportunity to attend regularly.

In addition, challenging behaviours need to be dealt with actively and appropriately.

The people providing the care need to have a voice. A forum in which these voices can be heard should provide a safe, secure environment for the nurses, as some people feel shy about sharing their views in groups. Individual supervision may be necessary in some circumstances. Supportive facility managers acknowledge the need for regular staff forums and budget for them. Perhaps, by providing a structured, safe environment for the patients in a supportive environment for the nursing staff, an effective milieu for both may be created.

19.16   CONCLUSION

This chapter is written from a practical perspective. When all else fails, it is important to remember that common sense is a great tool when dealing with the complexity and diversity we face with people. Patients with dementia, in some cases, amplify the requirement that we think clearly and make well judged and informed decisions. The victims of dementia are not limited to the patient alone. This chapter aims to provide ideas to stimulate discussion that result in better support for the care of the unfortunate people who endure these degenerative and devastating illnesses. Our patients need to be treated with respect and kindness.

People are whole people until the moment of their death.
(Pringle-Specht et al., 2009)

REFERENCES

Alzheimer's Australia WA Ltd 'Person Centred Care.' 2004. Accessed 12 September, 2009. Available from: www.alzheimers.asn.au.

Alzheimer's Australia Fact Sheet 'Keep on moving: Physical Exercise and dementia.' July, 2008. Accessed 30 September, 2009. Available from: www.alzheimers.org.au.

Alzheimer's Australia Fact Sheet 'Communication.' April, 2009. Accessed 30 September, 2009. Available from: www.alzheimers.org.au.

Alzheimer's Australia Fact Sheet 'About you ... early planning' July, 2005. Accessed 23 August, 2009. Available from: www.alzheimers.org.au.

Bossen AL, Pringle-Specht JK, McKenzie SE. (2009) Needs of people with early-stage Alzheimer's disease: reviewing the evidence. *Journal of Gerontological Nursing* **25**: 8–15.

Brodaty H, Draper B, Low LF. (2003) Nursing home staff attitudes towards residents with dementia: strain and satisfaction with work. *Journal of Advanced Nursing* **44**: 583–90.

Chenoweth L, Jeon Y-H, Merlyn T, Brodaty H. (2010) A systematic review of what factors attract and retain nurses in aged and dementia care. *Journal of Clinical Nursing* **19**: 156–67.

Herrmann N. (2005) Some psychosocial therapies may reduce depression, aggression or apathy in people with dementia. *Evidence-based Mental Health* **8**: 104.

James J, Hodnett C. (2009) Taking the anxiety out of dementia. *Emergency Nurse* **16**: 10–13.

Kitwood T. (1993) The person and process in dementia. *International Journal of Geriatric Psychiatry* **8**: 541–5.

Leone E, Deudon A, Robert P. (2008) Physical activity, dementia and BPSD. *Journal of Nutrition and Aging* **12**: 457–60.

Marshall M. (2003) Nutrition. In: Hudson R (ed.). *Dementia nursing, a guide to practice*. Melbourne, Australia: Ausmed Publications Pty Ltd.

Moden L. (2009) Passionate about dementia care training. *Nursing Older People* **21**: 15.

O'Connor DW, Ames D, Gardner B, King M. (2009) Psychosocial treatments of behaviour symptoms in dementia: a systematic review of reports meeting quality standards. *International Psychogeriatrics* **21**: 225–40.

Perkinson MA, Berg-Weber ML, Carr D *et al.* (2005) Driving and dementia of the Alzheimer type: Beliefs and cessation strategies among stakeholders. *The Gerontologist* **45**: 676–85.

Pringle-Specht JK, Taylor R, Bossen AL. (2009) Partnering for care: The evidence and the expert. *Journal of Gerontological Nursing* **35**: 16–22.

ReachOut Australia Fact sheet *'Feeling OK about who you are.'* 25 Jun 2009. Accessed August 19, 2009. Available from: www.reachout.com.

Wylie K. (2003) Enriching the environment. In: Hudson R (ed.). *Dementia nursing, a guide to practice*. Melbourne, Australia: Ausmed Publications Pty Ltd.

Young-Mason J. (2009) Family and friends create hope and understanding for those with dementia. *Nursing and the Arts* **23**: 43–4.

Social work and care/case management in dementia

DAVID CHALLIS, JANE HUGHES AND CAROLINE SUTCLIFFE

20.1 INTRODUCTION

Social work, like any professional or occupational group, is inseparable from the organizational and legislative context in which it takes place since this defines the parameters of practice. Prior to the introduction of care/case management, descriptions of social work in services for adults, including older people, tended to focus on profession-specific activities, to the neglect of outputs such as the function of linking the individual to networks of care. Moreover, social work with older people, including those with dementia, was typically short term (Hunter *et al.*, 1990). Assessments were often undertaken in a relatively narrow and service-oriented fashion, followed by an allocation of service prior to closure (Challis, 2003). Continuing management of long-term problems for people living in the community was neglected. The advent of care/case management has required a useful redefinition of social work in relation to long-term care of older people. It can be most simply defined as a strategy for organizing and co-ordinating care services at the level of the individual. Care/case management therefore involves mobilizing and influencing various agencies and services to achieve clearly formulated goals, rather than each provider pursuing separate and perhaps diverse goals (Challis, 1993). It is helpfully understood in terms of six criteria: the performance of core tasks; effective coordination; explicit goals; a specific target population; a long-term care focus; and an impact on service development as well as individual cases. This is summarized in **Box 20.1**.

Specialist care/case management for older people with dementia is an area of practice in which there is much scope for innovation and development (Challis *et al.*, 2009). Moreover there is evidence of its effectiveness within this group provided that it is appropriately targeted. In many

developed countries, care/case management services have, it has long been argued, been intended for those people at risk of admission to long-term care reflecting a policy of 'downward substitution' by the provision of more cost-effective community-based alternatives (Challis, 2003). Two examples demonstrate the international applicability of care/case management as a means to provide effective community-based care for older people with dementia. Early research in the United States revealed that this target group experienced a

---

Box 20.1 Key characteristics of care management

- **Core tasks**: case finding and screening; assessment; care planning; monitoring and review
- **Functions**: co-ordination and linkage of care services
- **Goals**: providing continuity and integrated care; increased opportunity for home-based care; make better use of resources; promote well-being of older person
- **Target population**: long-term care needs; multiple service requirements; risk of institutional placement
- **Differentiating features of long-term care**: intensity of involvement; breadth of services spanned; lengthy duration of involvement with older person
- **Multilevel response**: linking practice-level activities with broader resource and agency level activities

greater reduction in their use of health care and had lower costs within an approach where care/case managers had small caseloads; undertook frequent home visits; with appropriate use and knowledge of local resources (Eggert *et al.*, 1990). In England, an exemplar care/case management site also demonstrated its capacity to support those with dementia in their own homes. Key characteristics of the service were: trained and experienced staff; small caseloads targeted on the most vulnerable older people; long-term support; financial management arrangements in which unit costs were explicit, care packages costed and, within limits, budgets devolved to front line staff; and systematic records for assessment and monitoring (Challis *et al.*, 2002a).

20.2   CURRENT PATTERNS OF PRACTICE

Increasingly, countries are developing strategies for the care of people with dementia which include enhanced care at home, thereby demonstrating the important contribution of social work and care/case management to such service development. This is, for example, detailed in Dutch, English, French and Irish strategic plans for people with dementia with care/case management identified as the means to co-ordinate the necessarily multiple service inputs as an alternative to admission to long-stay establishment (O'Shea and O'Reilly, 1999; Ministry of Health Welfare and Sports, 2008; Republique Francaise, 2008; Department of Health, 2009). In Australia, the strategic vision for the development of services suggests a not dissimilar role for social workers, that of helping people with dementia and their families 'navigate' the community care system with provision located within mainstream services (AHMC, 2006). By contrast, within the Norwegian strategy for people with dementia there is an emphasis on care planning, the development of home care services, and the development of a competent workforce (Norwegian Ministry of Health and Care Services, 2007).

The core tasks of long-term care embodied in care/case management, detailed in **Figure 20.1**, offer an approach suitable for the community-based care of vulnerable people with long-term conditions. Since older people with dementia typically have complex health and social care needs, it is important that agencies have in place procedures and protocols within care/case management arrangements which facilitate an appropriate level of response, a feature more likely to be associated with a differentiated approach to care/case management. This is an approach in which a distinction is made between older people with complex needs often requiring a multi-service response and those with less complex needs which are often met by a single service response provided by one agency (Hughes *et al.*, 2005). However, it is not always available. In England for example, little progress was made in the development of a differentiated approach to care/case management immediately after the introduction of the community care reforms. Rather, care/case management services were, in the main, provided for the majority rather than for a selected group of older service users. It was also apparent that intensive care/case management, an important component of a differentiated approach, was rare within older people's services (Weiner *et al.*, 2002). The purpose of intensive care/case management is to permit more flexible responses through improved co-ordination and appropriateness of care by use of a designated care manager, and is a prerequisite for the provision of complex packages of care to enable older people with dementia to continue living in their own homes (Applebaum and Austin, 1990; Challis, 1994; Challis *et al.*, 2001).

A model of care/case management that can successfully support older people with dementia at home has been proposed using eight standards of good practice that include intensive care/case management. Four of these relate to the framework within which care/case management is undertaken: provision by specialist multidisciplinary teams; integrated arrangements for commissioning domiciliary and respite services; joint financial arrangements facilitating health and social care provision; and organizational arrangements promoting a differentiated approach to ensure an appropriate level of response. The remaining four are associated with the process of care/case management: a continuing targeting process to ensure a level of response suitable to a person's needs; a multidisciplinary assessment process appropriate in

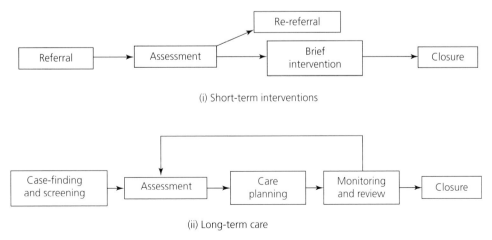

(i) Short-term interventions

(ii) Long-term care

Figure 20.1   A model of care. Source: Challis D, Chessum R, Chesterman J *et al.* (1990) *Case management in social and health care: The Gateshead Community Care Scheme.* PSSRU, University of Kent, Canterbury.

terms of content and timing; care planning which supports and enhances quality of life; and sufficient monitoring and review to ensure adjustments to care plans occur when required (Hughes *et al.*, 2005; Abell *et al.*, 2010).

20.3   INTENSIVE CARE/CASE MANAGEMENT

The Lewisham Case Management Scheme offered a practical demonstration of care management providing community support to older people with dementia living at home (Challis *et al.*, 2009). It was cited in the government's national dementia strategy as an examplar of intensive care/case management preventing inappropriate care home admissions and was one of a family of similar studies (Challis and Davies, 1986; Challis *et al.*, 1995; Challis *et al.*, 2002a; Department of Health, 2009). Specifically, it was established within a multi-disciplinary setting for a target population of individuals with a diagnosis of dementia, identified as having unmet needs and at risk of entry to institutional care, despite input from statutory services. The aim of the scheme was to provide effective integrated community-based long-term care spanning the health and social service interface. The service was provided by social services care/case managers based in a community mental health team for older people. Most importantly, care/case managers were able to purchase care in response to identified need within defined parameters. This enabled the development of a specialist paid helper service which was available to those in the experimental group, receiving care/case management input. The service setting and roles are summarized in **Figure 20.2**. Evaluation of the scheme used a quasi-experimental approach, where individuals in one community mental health team for older people receiving care/case management, the experimental group, were compared to those in a similar community mental health setting without a care/case management service, the control group. A range of indicators were used covering aspects of needs, quality of care, and quality of life, encompassing the perspectives of the older person, carers (including family, friends and paid carers), and the assessing researcher.

Box 20.2 details the process of assessment and care/case management within the scheme. With regard to implementing

Shorter-term care

| Community mental health team for older people
Doctors, Nurses, Psychologist,
Occupational Therapists, Social workers
Key workers |

+

Longer-term care

| Case managers
Social workers with budget
Service to patients with dementia
Care management |

Figure 20.2   Lewisham Case Management Scheme: setting and roles. Source: Challis *et al.* (2009).

Box 20.2 Practice interventions and strategies

Case finding and screening

- targeting of appropriate cases

Assessment

- structured approach
- severity of need assessed

Implementing the care plan

- goal defined
- strategies of intervention and resources identified

Monitoring, review and case closure

- achievement of goals reassessed
- problems reviewed
- outcome by domain of assessed need evaluated

---

the care plan, the goals of intervention in care/case management were identified by retrospective analysis of 80 care plans. These were analysed under seven categories: supportive, therapeutic, practical, preventive, social, destinational and organizational. The most frequently reported were supportive (68 per cent), therapeutic (66 per cent) and practical (56 per cent). Supportive goals were almost exclusively intended for the benefit of informal carers, the most frequently reported categories were to relieve carer burden, provide respite and assist carers. Therapeutic interventions were most often directed at devising strategies to reduce problem behaviours associated with the individual's deteriorating state. Practical goals were most frequently focused on assistance with personal care, health care and domestic care of the older person. These demonstrate that the prime objectives of the scheme were to support, sustain and enhance the quality of life of the older person in his/her own home, and thereby to assist the carers.

In the second year of the Lewisham Case Management Scheme its effects began to show in a lower rate of admission to care homes for older people with dementia in the experimental group, than under standard arrangements for those in the control group, resulting in lower associated costs for residential care. Although the community tenure effect in this study appeared more muted than in other care/case management studies (Challis *et al.*, 1995; Challis *et al.*, 2002a) at six months, older people in the experimental group were more satisfied with their lifestyle at home, and there was evidence of a reduction in their needs specifically associated with activities of daily living. No differences were found between the groups in levels of depression, and there was no impact on levels of problem behaviours. Furthermore, at 12 months there was a significant reduction in the amount of care input by and distress experienced for carers of the older people in the experimental group.

It was, however, apparent that older people in both groups were receiving support from a relatively resource-rich community-based old age psychiatry service, untypical of most of England. Social care provider costs were higher for those receiving care/case management, since care/case manager visits and the paid helper service were not available to those receiving standard services. On the other hand, for carers of those in receipt of care/case management there was a positive gain, since financial and other costs were lower for this group compared to the carers of those receiving standard services. Moreover, when all costs to society were accounted for, including informal care, the weekly cost of supporting older people with dementia and their carers was not significantly higher for those receiving intensive care/case management, although that of the main component, statutory services, was greater.

As demonstrated above, this specialist scheme was successful in providing care to older people with dementia to enable them to remain at home rather than enter long-term care and provided effective support to their carers. This approach is consistent with other UK and international evidence relating to the provision of specialist care for this group of older people (Chu et al., 2000; Eloniemi-Sulkava et al., 2001; Minkman et al., 2009). Moriarty and Webb (2000) noted factors that could optimize care for people with dementia and their carers. These included responsive care management systems, effective monitoring systems, and home care and day care services sensitive to changes in an individual's care needs and which provide practical support to carers. The latter is particularly important since the centrality of support for carers remains a constant theme (Moriarty, 1999; Brodaty et al., 2005; Gaugler et al., 2005; HM Government, 2008), and national and international policy has endorsed this service model (AHMC, 2006; Republique Francaise, 2008; Department of Health, 2009).

20.4   CONCLUSIONS

The emergence of dementia-specific services may lead to further inter-professional role blurring which, if managed correctly, could be the basis of improved care for people with dementia and their carers. Within this, social work and care/case management have a distinct role in relation to the provision of long-term community-based care. Developments in England over the last 20 years provide evidence of a change in the role, focus and setting for social workers and other professions working with people with dementia with an increasing emphasis on care/case management as a means of co-ordinating complex packages of care as an alternative to care home placement (SSI/SWSG, 1991; Department of Health, 2001; Department of Health, 2009). A changed role for social workers has been suggested with the introduction of personal budgets for social care services (cash for care), permitting older people and their carers to organize and manage their own care, although it is likely that social workers will still be required to perform this care co-ordination for the most frail elders. Indeed, there is evidence that greater flexibilities and personalized care can be provided

by care/case managers with budgets (Challis and Davies, 1986; Challis et al., 1995; Challis et al., 2002a; Glendinning et al., 2008). Concurrently there has been both an increase in community-based multidisciplinary teams for older people with mental health problems similar to those operating in adult mental health and learning disability services, and an increase in those with social workers as core members (Challis et al., 2002b; Tucker et al., 2009). Within this setting it is essential that arrangements are in place to facilitate the multidisciplinary assessment of people with dementia and particularly to ensure that specialist clinicians contribute to this process. A number of UK studies suggest potential gains from greater integration of secondary health care with the decisions made in the context of care/case management (Brocklehurst et al., 1978; Peet et al., 1994; Sharma et al., 1994; Challis et al., 2004). The experience of Australia, which has the community care reforms most analogous to those in England, gives credence to this type of arrangement (Challis et al., 1995; Howe and Kung, 2003). It is anticipated that the effective care of people with dementia will benefit from these new service configurations which pay less attention to traditional boundaries whether professional or organizational than hitherto.

For social work there are two challenges consequent on these changes which have an international resonance. First, the profession-specific contribution to the care of older people with dementia and their carers has changed to primarily that of responsibility for the care for people living at home and, by virtue of changes to long-term care funding, gate-keepers for admission to residential or nursing home care. Second, and in antithesis to this clarity, the social work role in respect of the care of people with dementia has become less profession specific. Within multidisciplinary teams there are more opportunities for the sharing of tasks offering informal small-scale opportunities for service substitution. Research conducted within a specialist mental health team for older people has found that the process of assessment can be undertaken by any of the members within it (Lindesay et al., 1996), and more recently, there is increasing evidence of community nurses working within teams for older people (Weiner et al., 2003). There is thus a tendency for there to be less specificity of role for staff as services become more community based. This leads unsurprisingly to a degree of insecurity among professional groups, because each derives their unique quality from a training and occupational function. Roles come to be negotiated rather than simply professionally defined within groups to a greater extent in community-based services and therefore may be seen as less clearly delineated by professional origin. This process may well occur to a greater exent as the process of closer integration between health and social care develops.

REFERENCES

Abell J, Hughes J, Reilly S et al. (2010) Case management for long-term conditions: developing targeting processes. *Case Management Journals* 11: 11–8.

Applebaum R, Austin C. (1990) *Long term care case management, design and evaluation.* New York: Springer.

Australian Health Ministers Conference (AHMC) (2006) *National Framework for Action on Dementia: 2006–2010*, Department of Health, Sydney. Available from: http://152.91.25.226/internet/main/publishing.nsf/Content/D64BD892C6FDD167CA2572180007E717/$File/nfad.pdf.

Brocklehurst J, Carty M, Leeming J, Robinson J. (1978) Care of the elderly: medical screening of old people accepted for residential care. *Lancet* **2**: 141–2.

Brodaty H, Thomson C, Thompson C, Fine M. (2005) Why caregivers of people with dementia and memory loss don't use services. *International Journal of Geriatric Psychiatry* **20**: 537–46.

Challis D. (1993) Alternatives to institutional care. In: Levy R, Howard R, Burns A (eds). *Treatment and care in old age psychiatry.* Petersfield: Wrightson.

Challis D. (1994) *Implementing caring for people: Care management. Factors influencing its development in the implementation of community care.* London: Department of Health.

Challis D. (2003) Achieving co-ordinated and integrated care among long term care services: the role of care management. In: Brodsky J, Habib J, Hirschfeld M (eds). *Key policy issues in long term care.* Geneva: World Health Organisation.

Challis D, Davies B. (1986) *Case management in community care.* Aldershot: Gower.

Challis D, Darton R, Johnson L *et al.* (1995) *Care management and health care of older people: The Darlington Community Care Project.* Aldershot: Arena.

Challis D, Darton R, Hughes J *et al.* (2001) Intensive care-management at home: an alternative to institutional care. *Age and Ageing* **30**: 409–13.

Challis D, Chesterman J, Luckett R *et al.* (2002a) *Care management in social and primary health care. The Gateshead Community Care Scheme.* Aldershot: Ashgate.

Challis D, Reilly S, Hughes J *et al.* (2002b) Policy, organisation and practice of specialist old age psychiatry in England. *International Journal of Geriatric Psychiatry* **17**: 1018–26.

Challis D, Clarkson P, Williamson J *et al.* (2004) The value of specialist clinical assessment of older people prior to entry to care homes. *Age and Ageing* **33**: 25–34.

Challis D, Sutcliffe C, Hughes J *et al.* (2009) *Supporting people with dementia at home. Challenges and opportunities for the 21st century.* Aldershot: Ashgate.

Chu P, Edwards J, Levin R, Thomson J. (2000) The use of clinical case management for early stage Alzheimer' patients and their families. *American Journal of Alzheimer's Disease and Other Dementias* **15**: 284–90.

Department of Health. (2001) *The National Service Framework for Older People.* London: Department of Health.

Department of Health. (2009) *Living Well with Dementia: A National Dementia Strategy.* London: Department of Health.

Eggert GM, Friedman B, Zimmer JG. (1990) Models of intensive case management. In: Reif L, Trager B (eds). *Health care of the aged: needs, policies and services.* New York: The Haworth Press.

Eloniemi-Sulkava U, Notkola IL, Hentinen M *et al.* (2001) Effects of supporting community-living demented patients and their caregivers: a randomized trial. *Journal of the American Geriatrics Society* **49**: 1282–7.

Gaugler JE, Kane RL, Kane RA, Newcomer R. (2005) Early community-based service utilization and its effects on institutionalization in dementia caregiving. *The Gerontologist* **45**: 177–85.

Glendinning C, Challis D, Fernández J-L *et al.* (2008) *Evaluation of the Individual Budgets Pilot Programme Final Report.* University of York, York: Social Policy Research Unit. Available from: www.pssru.ac.uk/pdf/IBSEN.pdf.

Her Majesty's (HM) Government. (2008) *Putting people first: a shared vision and commitment to the transformation of adult social care.* London: HM Government.

Howe A, Kung F. (2003) Does assessment make a difference for people with dementia? The effectiveness of the Aged Care Assessment Teams. *International Journal of Geriatric Psychiatry* **18**: 205–10.

Hughes J, Sutcliffe C, Challis D. (2005) Social work. In: Burns A (ed). *Standards in dementia care.* London: Taylor and Francis.

Hunter S, Brace S, Buckley G. (1990) The interdisciplinary assessment of older people at entry into long-term institutional care: lessons for the new community care arrangements. *Research Policy and Planning* **11**: 2–9.

Lindesay J, Herzberg J, Collighan G *et al.* (1996) Treatment decisions following assessment by multidisciplinary psychogeriatric teams. *Psychiatric Bulletin* **20**: 78–81.

Minkman M, Ligthart S, Huijsman R. (2009) Integrated dementia care in The Netherlands: a multiple case study of case management programmes. *Health and Social Care in the Community* **17**: 485–94.

Ministry of Health Welfare and Sports. (2008) *Caring for people with dementia*, DLZ/KZ-U-2853804. The Hague: Ministry of Health Welfare and Sports.

Moriarty JM. (1999) Use of community and long-term care by people with dementia in the UK: a review of some issues in service provision and carer and user preferences. *Aging and Mental Health* **3**: 311–19.

Moriarty J, Webb S. (2000) *Part of their lives: community care for older people with dementia.* Bristol: The Policy Press.

Norwegian Ministry of Health and Care Services. (2007) *Dementia Plan 2015, Making the Most of Good Days, Subplan of Care Plan 2015.* Oslo: Norwegian Government Administration Services Distribution Services.

O'Shea E, O'Reilly S. (1999) *An Action Plan for Dementia, Report Number 54.* Dublin: National Council on Ageing and Older People.

Peet S, Castleden C, Potter J, Jagger C. (1994) The outcome of a medical examination for applicants to Leicestershire homes for older people. *Age and Ageing* **23**: 65–8.

Republique Francaise. (2008) National Plan for "Alzheimer and Related Diseases" 2008–2012. Available from: www.plan-alzheimer.gouv.fr/medias/m/cms/article/alzheimer/9/8/8/8/89/plan-alzheimer-2008-2012-en-couleur.pdf.

Sharma S, Aldous J, Robinson M. (1994) Assessing applicants for part 3 accommodation: is a formal clinical assessment worthwhile? *Public Health* **108**: 91–7.

Social Services Inspectorate/Social Work Services Group (SSI/ SWSG). (1991) *Care management and assessment: managers guide*. London: HMSO.

Tucker S, Baldwin R, Hughes J *et al*. (2009) Integrating mental health services for older people in England – from rhetoric to reality. *Journal of Interprofessional Care* **23**: 341–54.

Weiner K, Stewart K, Hughes J *et al*. (2002) Care management arrangements for older people in England: key areas of variation in a national study. *Ageing and Society* **22**: 419–39.

Weiner K, Hughes J, Challis D, Pederson I. (2003) Integrating health and social care at the micro level: Health care professionals as care managers for older people. *Social Policy and Administration* **37**: 498–515.

21

Occupational therapy in dementia care

ALISSA WESTPHAL

21.1 INTRODUCTION

Occupational therapy (OT) is concerned with a person's ability to undertake meaningful and required occupations and roles. The profession is built on the philosophical belief that functioning in meaningful and purposeful occupations and roles is necessary throughout life for maintaining health and well-being (AOTA, 2008). Historically, the paradigms underpinning the profession have evolved with paradigms recognizing occupational functioning as arising from a systemic and dynamic relationship between the attributes of the person, the physical, social and cultural environment and occupation (Letts *et al.*, 2003). Physical and psychiatric conditions often disrupt this relationship. Occupational therapists (OTs) use rehabilitative and adaptive approaches to address occupational performance issues and maximize the functioning (Hopkins and Smith, 1993; Fisher, 2006a).

Dementia is a condition that causes skill loss resulting in deteriorating occupational functioning. The disease trajectory, while progressive, differs for each person and is frequently accompanied by additional functional difficulties caused by age-related physical conditions and behavioural and psychological symptoms of dementia (BPSD) (see Chapter 8, Neuropsychiatric aspects of dementia and Chapter 9, Measurement of behaviour disturbance, non-cognitive symptoms and quality of life). Those with dementia are commonly supported by caregivers who themselves experience difficulty during the disease progression. The applicability of OT philosophy to dementia care has been questioned due to its focus on health, competency and independence (Perrin *et al.*, 2008). Despite this, OT paradigms provide a framework for understanding and responding to the complex and progressive occupational dysfunction that is unique to the experience of each person with dementia and their caregivers (Letts *et al.*, 2003).

21.2 OCCUPATIONAL THERAPY ROLE

The role of OT in caring for people with dementia varies according to the specific care setting, presenting issues, severity of the person's dementia and the cultural context. Roles can include:

- maximizing the person's independence in everyday activities through modifications of the activity, environment and approach and, where required, use of adaptive equipment;
- maintaining the person's sense of self-worth and supporting their identity through facilitating their engagement in meaningful and interesting activities and roles;
- facilitating recovery of skills, for example physical functioning;
- recommending supports that allow the person to remain in their preferred care environment or alternate accommodation when required;
- minimizing risk and maximizing safety of the person's occupational performance;
- addressing BPSD using non-pharmacological approaches;
- contributing to diagnostic formulation and assessment of disease progression;
- developing and reviewing activity programmes and environments that support the needs of people with dementia in a group residential setting;

- supporting and building the capacities of caregivers and services to effectively care for people with dementia;
- developing evidence to inform and advance clinical practice;
- contributing to the development of policy in areas of health and ageing.

The OT process involves assessment, treatment planning, implementation and evaluation. Best practice advocates the engagement of both the person with dementia and their caregiver(s) throughout this process (Strong, 2003).

21.3 ASSESSMENT

21.3.1 Purpose and process of the occupational therapy assessment

Assessment is a major role of OT and the first step in assisting the person with dementia to be as independent as possible. The goal of assessment is to gain a comprehensive understanding of the impact of dementia on the person's daily functioning and on their caregiver (Letts *et al.*, 2003). Completion of OT assessments can provide specific information in the following areas:

1. Body systems and functions of the person:
   - cognitive function: memory, judgement, problem solving, concentration, behaviour regulation;
   - perceptual and sensory function: visual, auditory, proprioceptive sensation, stereognosis and praxis;
   - motor function: balance, mobility and transfers, hand function, co-ordination;
   - communication skills: verbal and non-verbal social skills, receptive and expressive dysphasia;
   - psychological state: mood, anxiety and motivation.
2. The environment:
   - physical, social, cultural and spiritual characteristics: contrasts, temperature, accessibility, level of sensory stimulation, lighting, design, furnishings, cues, personalization, language use, values, expectations, supports, knowledge, tolerance and flexibility.
3. Occupational functioning:
   - pre-morbid history: interests, routines, personality, meaningful activities, roles;
   - personal activities of daily living (PADLs), domestic activities of daily living (DADLs) and community activities of daily living (CADLs): eating, dressing, grooming, bathing, toileting, medication management, home and money management, leisure, telephone use, driving and transport;
   - task issues: demands, complexity, sequencing, environmental context, cues, and familiarity;
   - risk issues: risks to the person with dementia, caregiver and others associated with occupational dysfunction;
   - current occupational preferences: interests, roles, routines and meaningful activities.
4. The caregiver:
   - knowledge: understanding of the person they are caring for and dementia-related changes;

- caring role: difficulties, changes, motivation and concerns;
- communication and approach.

OT assessment facilitates identification of the person and caregivers needs and intervention priorities. While overlapping at times, the information gathered complements that obtained by other professional disciplines providing a unique picture of the impact of the dementia on the person's activities of daily living (ADL) and leisure performance (Fossey, 2001).

The focus of assessment changes with disease progression, reflecting the changing needs of the person and caregiver (Zgola, 1999) from one focused on maintenance of ADL performance within the home to assessment of PADL performance to enable access to appropriate care and supports.

OT assessment information is collected through interviews, observation and standardized assessments. No single assessment measures all areas of interest. Instead the OT chooses the most appropriate tools. Understanding the presenting issues and the person's background, including their level of education, pre-morbid functioning and roles and cultural history, are necessary to inform selection and interpretation of assessment tools. Finally, developing a trusting and supportive relationship, adapting communication and approach, focusing on abilities and engaging the caregiver to assist with the assessment process and maximizing the accuracy of the results.

21.3.1.1   INTERVIEW

Interviews provide a foundation for identification of areas requiring assessment allowing the OT to gain an understanding of the life story of the person with dementia. Interviews may be conducted with the person with dementia, their caregivers, family members and other relevant persons. Caregivers and family members are frequently interviewed in order to obtain a collateral history and understand their views on the person's functioning. Building rapport, basic counselling skills, use of interpreters, adapting communication in response to communication deficits are commonly used during interviews to assist in developing therapeutic relationships and obtaining information. Interviews may be used instead of observation or standardized assessments when time or funding prohibit more comprehensive assessments.

21.3.1.2   OBSERVATIONS

The functioning of a person with dementia may be observed when participating in daily living and leisure activities that are relevant to them. Observational assessments provide a flexible approach to identifying functional performance issues (Alexander, 1994) and may be completed at the pace and manner in which the person is able or accustomed. Where possible, OTs complete observations of functional performance within environmental contexts familiar to the person, often during home visits. This aims to minimize the person's anxiety, their need to learn new skills and maximize their orientation.

21.3.1.3 STANDARDIZED TESTS

Assessment tools are often used by occupational therapists in addition to the aforementioned methods to:

- gain an objective and measurable picture of a person's performance in particular areas, including BPSD;
- assess the severity of cognitive or occupational dysfunction compared to a normative group;
- establish a baseline measure of functioning to which subsequent assessments may be compared;
- evaluate the efficacy of specific interventions.

A wide range of tools exist for use with people who have dementia. They can typically be divided into cognitive, functional performance, environmental, risk, quality of life, caregiver and behavioural assessments. A selection of assessments commonly reported in the occupational therapy literature is shown in **Table 21.1**.

21.4 INTERVENTION

OT interventions focus on maximizing functioning primarily using adaptive or compensatory, rather than rehabilitative, approaches. Interventions are individualized in response to differences in the presenting issues and goals, the stage of the person's dementia and the results of the completed assessment. Ongoing review of OT interventions is required to ensure they best address the issues being experienced by and needs of the person with dementia and their caregiver.

21.4.1 The use of activities

Activity interventions aim to preserve the person's dignity and self-esteem by successfully engaging them in meaningful and purposeful activity that provides continuity with their occupational history, interests, roles and motivations. Knowledge about the person, including their retained abilities, allows the OT to modify and provide activities that best fit their skills from the earlier to late stages of dementia. General principles for activity interventions gleaned from literature include the following:

- Familiar and novel activities (Perrin *et al.*, 2008). Familiar activities provide continuity and familiarity for the person with dementia, allowing them to participate using well-learned skills. On the other hand, novel activities have no associated preconceived expectations of performance potentially providing 'failure free' experiences.
- Simplifying activity demands and structure (Hellen, 1998). Reducing the number of steps in an activity, providing assistance only where needed, and limiting choices to match the person's abilities all support successful occupational performance.
- Temporal adjustments (Pool, 2008). Allow the person to set the pace and provide activities within a familiar routine. When this is not possible due to time limitations, priority should be given to those which are most important to the person.

- Engage multiple senses (Pool, 2008). Activities that engage the senses become increasingly important with disease progression, affording opportunities for engagement for those with severely impaired cognitive and communication skills.
- The experience and variety (Hellen, 1998; Truscott, 2004). Activities provide opportunities for sharing experiences, reminiscing, building friendship, pleasure, expressing emotions and being creative. The focus of activities shifts to the experience of 'doing' rather than the product or outcome. Variety of activity opportunities remains important.
- Physical activity (Eggermont and Scherder, 2006). Access to indoor and outdoor opportunities for physical activity can assist in maintaining physical and mental functioning and managing some BPSD.
- Individualized (Robert Dooley and Hinojosa, 2004). All effort should be made to tailor activities to be continuous with the person's life story and needs.

21.4.2 Environment adaptations

Environmental adaptations involve changes to the physical, social and organizational/institutional environments of the person with dementia and their carers. Modifying environments can maximize the person's occupational performance by providing accessible opportunities for engagement, compensating for skill deficits, utilizing strengths, minimizing risk and managing BPSD (Cooper and Day, 2003; Brawley, 2006). Furthermore, environmental interventions are applicable across various care settings throughout the disease trajectory.

Outcomes of research on environmental interventions have been mixed (Gitlin *et al.*, 2003). Small sample sizes, methodological flaws, variations in study end points and intensity and types of environmental interventions make it difficult to establish definitive empirical evidence. Environmental intervention principles include:

- Promoting comfort (Calkins, 2005). Preferred temperature, familiar furnishings and objects, appropriate pressure care and familiar caregivers provide comfort.
- Optimal sensory stimulation (Calkins, 2004; Calkins, 2005). Sensory stimulation can be altered to meet the needs of the person through changing location or amount of sensory stimulation, for example noise present in the immediate environment.
- Contrasts and lighting (Brawley, 2006). Maximizing contrast between items can optimize orientation to and awareness of objects. Conversely, minimizing contrasts can be used to camouflage or reduce cueing. Glare, shadows, poor lighting levels and sudden lighting changes should be addressed.
- Cueing and shaping engagement (Cooper and Day, 2003; Marcy-Edwards *et al.*, 2005; Brawley, 2006). Signs, labels, clocks, calendars, structured routine, strong contrasts, development of activity-specific areas, task-related items placed in the task environment, walking

Table 21.1 Assessment tools used by occupational therapists in dementia care.

Assessment tool	Area(s) assessed											Additional details
	Cognitive and perceptual skills	PADLs	DADLs	CADLs	Leisure	Environment	Quality of life and care	Carergiver	BPSD	Other	Translations available	
Mini-Mental State Examination (Folstein et al., 1975)	✓										✓	Screening tool covering orientation, memory, registration, attention and calculation, recall, and language
Hierarchical Dementia Scale (Cole and Dastoor, 1996)	✓									✓	✓	Assesses impairment and preserved function in 19 domains to identify strategies that maximize functioning
Lowenstein Occupational Therapy Cognitive Assessment for Geriatric Population (Elazer et al., 1996)	✓											19 subtests covering five areas: orientation, memory, perception, visuomotor organization and thinking operations
Allen Cognitive Levels Assessment (Allen and Allen, 1987)	✓										✓	Assesses the person's ability to complete leather-lacing tasks of increasing difficulty
Assessment of Motor and Process Skills (Fisher, 2006b)		✓	✓	✓							✓	Motor and process skills assessed during ADL performance (choice of 85 ADLs). Specialized training required to use tool
Domestic and Community Skills Assessment (Collister and Alexander, 1991)		✓	✓	✓						✓		Two sections: an interview of the person and their caregiver and assessment of ADL performance (17 items)
Assessment of Living Skills and Resources (Williams et al., 1991)			✓	✓						✓		Self-report assessment. Measures task performance and resources (11 ADLs)

(Continued over)

Table 21.1 Assessment tools used by occupational therapists in dementia care. (continued)

Assessment tool	Area(s) assessed											Additional details
	Cognitive and perceptual skills	PADLs	DADLs	CADLs	Leisure	Environment	Quality of life and care	Carergiver	BPSD	Other	Translations available	
Barthel Index (Mahoney and Barthel, 1965)		✓								✓	✓	Also assesses mobility using a brief index of independence (10 items)
Functional Independence Measure (Guide from the Uniform Data Set for Medical Rehabilitation, 1993)		✓								✓	✓	Also assesses communication, mobility and social cognition (18 items). Specialized training required to use tool
Pool Activity Level Instrument (Pool, 2008)	✓				✓					✓		Assesses the level of the person's abilities, engagement and life history. Used to develop a plan for engagement in activities
Structured Assessment of Independent Living Skills (Mahurin et al., 1991)	✓	✓	✓	✓						✓		Also assesses social interaction (50 items)
Activities of Daily Living Questionnaire (Johnson et al., 2004)		✓	✓	✓	✓					✓		Also assesses communication skills (28 items)
Daily Activities Questionnaire (Oakley et al., 1991)		✓	✓	✓								Level of dependency in 12 areas of functioning assessed
Kitchen Task Assessment (Baum and Edwards, 1993)			✓									Assesses the person's ability to cook pudding from a commercial packet mix
Lawton Instrumental Activities of Daily Living Scale (Lawton and Brody, 1969)		✓	✓	✓							✓	Interview-based rating of independence in 14 ADL domains
Bristol Activities of Daily Living Scale (Bucks et al., 1996)		✓	✓	✓	✓							Carer-rated assessment of 20 ADL areas including orientation and communication

(Continued over)

Measure	Description
Functional Activities Questionnaire (Pfeffer et al., 1992)	Provides a rating of incapacitation in ADLs
Interview of deterioration in daily activities in dementia scale (Teunisse and Derix, 1997)	20 ADL areas assessed based on interview
Canadian Occupational Performance Measure (Law et al., 1991)	Assesses the person's perceived satisfaction and performance of daily performance during an interview
Safety Assessment Scale (Poulin de Courval et al., 2006)	Short (19 items) and long (71 items) versions. Assesses behavioural and environmental risks to the person with dementia in nine domains
Dementia Care Mapping (Bradford Dementia Group, 1997)	Assesses quality of care within care environments such as nursing homes
Home Environment Assessment Protocol (Gitlin et al., 2002)	Caregiver interview and structured observation of up to eight areas of the home (192 items rated). Hazards, adaptations, orientation and comfort assessed
Zarit Carer Burden Interview (Zarit et al., 1980)	Assesses caregivers perception of burden (22 statements)
Expanded Group Activity Form (Thorgrimsen et al., 2002: expanded from Bender et al., 1987)	Evaluates the participation of people with dementia in a group environment
Revised Memory and Behaviour Problems Checklist (Teri et al., 1992)	Frequency rating of 24 items related to depressive, disruptive and memory-related behaviours

tracks, furniture placement, photos and objects that are personally familiar to the person can support the person's orientation to and engagement in activities. Removing or disguising objects can be used to reduce cueing or use of objects where engagement is not desired or is unsafe.

- Simplification (Calkins, 2004). Reducing clutter and distractions can minimize the complexity of the environment, reducing the demands placed on the person.
- Privacy (Brawley, 2006). Provision of privacy during PADLs and other activities remains crucial to caring for the person with dementia.

OTs prescribe and recommend adaptive equipment to optimize the person's functioning, address safety concerns and reduce caregiver burden. Examples of adaptive equipment include: shower stools, grab rails, non-slip mats, hand-held showers, commode chairs, contrasting toilet seats, modified clothing, large calendars, talking clocks, modified telephones (large and photo buttons), contrasting crockery and napery, modified cutlery, specialized seating, medication dispensing packs, personal alert alarms, isolation switches for ovens and stoves, stove dial covers and smoke and gas detectors.

21.4.3 Working with families and carers

Caregivers have a crucial role in facilitating the person's occupational performance. This role changes with disease progression. Interventions with caregivers aim to reduce care burden by:

- building caregiver capacities to understand, care for and support continued engagement of the person with dementia in meaningful activities;
- supporting caregiver to attend to their occupational roles and needs.

Elements of the OT intervention process with caregivers include: flexibility, affording choice, making small changes gradually, providing education and information, encouraging caregiver breaks, drawing on their experiences as an expert on the person with dementia, validating their experience and re-adjusting interventions based on the caregiver's feedback (Josephsson et al., 2000; Graff et al., 2003; Gitlin and Corcoran, 2005; Egan et al., 2006). This process minimizes excess disability by assisting caregivers, often through role play or modelling, to learn skills and generate strategies to more effectively match their communication, approach and assistance to the person's abilities. Finally, OTs assist in minimizing disruption to the caregiver's occupational identity by encouraging use of support services and engagement in meaningful activities (Hasselkus and Murray, 2007).

21.4.4 Managing BPSD

The emergent paradigms for explaining and treating BPSD view these symptoms as arising from unmet needs, difficulties coping with stress and reinforced learning (O'Connor et al., 2009; see Chapter 8, Neuropsychiatric aspects of dementia and Chapter 9, Measurement of behaviour disturbance, non-cognitive symptoms and quality of life). Current OT paradigms based on systems theory encapsulate these models providing OTs with a comprehensive framework for assessing and intervening non-pharmacologically with BPSD. The professional paradigm also affords understanding of the BPSD in the context of the person's occupational identity. OT interventions typically follow the principles outlined earlier. Additional principles include:

- Utilization of the BPSD. Some behavioural symptoms can be effectively utilized. Pacing may be provided with a purpose through engaging the person in physical activities such as sweeping, going for a walk outside or cleaning windows. Similarly, an apron customized to include multi-sensory opportunities may be used to reduce clothing removal due to 'fiddling' with shirt buttons where discomfort is not the triggering issue. Finally, where the BPSD can be understood in the context of the person's previous occupational identity, 'jobs' may be provided that address this need. For example, tactile floor tiles may be laid out for the person who previously was a tiler and now crawls around feeling the floor's surface.
- Refocusing attention. Providing a person with an alternative purposeful activity that is not reliant on cognitive processing or placing them in an alternative environment can assist in distracting and shifting their behaviour away from the BPSD.
- Environmental placement. Many environments engender particular behaviours. For example, libraries, churches and baby nurseries are areas associated with quieter activity. Environments can be manipulated to promote or cue alternative behaviours. In some cases, positioning in the environment can cue BPSD. For example, for a person who has difficulty sitting long enough to consume their meal, facing them away from changes in visual stimuli (people walking by) can assist in reducing cues that encourage them to get up and walk.

Thorough assessment is always required when faced with BPSD. Reversible causes should always be treated and interventions should be individualized, address risk and support the caregiver in understanding, responding and coping with the BPSD. Finally, OTs should regularly review interventions to ensure they are current and address the issues of concern.

21.5 CONCLUSION

While the specific role of the OT differs across settings and based on the severity of the person's dementia and presenting issues, occupational dysfunction remains a common theme. OTs are uniquely skilled in assessing and providing individualized and responsive interventions that address performance issues and BPSD experienced by the person with dementia. Addressing these issues assists in optimizing functioning and maximizing the quality of life of the person and their caregiver.

REFERENCES

Alexander K. (1994) Occupational therapy. In: Chiu E, Ames A (eds). *Functional psychiatric disorders of the elderly.* Cambridge: Cambridge University Press, 522–43.

Allen CK, Allen RE. (1987) Cognitive disabilities: measuring the social consequences of mental disorders. *Journal of Clinical Psychiatry* **48**: 185–9.

American Occupational Therapy Association – AOTA. (2008) Occupational therapy practice framework: domain and process, 2nd edn. *The American Journal of Occupational Therapy* **62**: 625–83.

Baum C, Edwards DF. (1993) Cognitive performance in senile dementia of Alzheimer's type: the kitchen task assessment. *The American Journal of Occupational Therapy* **47**: 431–6.

Bender M, Norris A, Bauckham P. (1987) *Group work with the elderly.* Bicester, UK: Winslow.

Bradford Dementia Group. (1997) *Evaluating Dementia Care: The DCM Method,* 7th edn. Bradford: University of Bradford.

Brawley EC. (2006) *Design innovations for ageing and Alzheimer's: Creating caring environments.* Hoboken, NJ: John Wiley & Sons.

Bucks RS, Ashworth DL, Wilcock GK, Seigfried K. (1996) Assessment of activities of daily living in dementia: Development of the Bristol activities of daily living scale. *Age and Ageing* **25**: 113–20.

Calkins MP. (2004) Articulating environmental press in environments for people with dementia. *Alzheimer's Care Quarterly* **5**: 165–72.

Calkins MP. (2005) Environments for late-stage dementia. *Alzheimer's Disease Quarterly* **6**: 71–5.

Collister L, Alexander K. (1991) *The Occupational Therapy Domestic and Community Skills Assessment (DACSA) Research Edition.* Melbourne: Latrobe University.

Cole MG, Dastoor DP. (1996) The Hierarchic Dementia Scale: Conceptualisation. *International Psychogeriatrics* **8**: 205–12.

Cooper BA, Day K. (2003) Therapeutic design of environments for people with dementia. In: Letts L, Rigby P, Steward D (eds). *Using environments to enable occupational performance.* Thorofare, NJ: Slack, 253–68.

Elazer B, Itzkovitch M, Katz N. (1996) *LOTCA-G A geriatric version for assessing elderly. A manual and test kit.* Pequannock, NJ: Maddak.

Egan M, Hobson S, Fearing VG. (2006) Dementia and occupation: A review of the literature. *The Canadian Journal of Occupational Therapy* **73**: 132–40.

Eggermont LH, Scherder EJ. (2006) Physical activity and behaviour in dementia: a review of the literature and implications for psychosocial intervention in primary care. *Dementia* **5**: 411–28.

Fisher AG. (2006a) *Assessment of motor and process skills. Volume 1: Development, standardisation and administration manual,* 6th edn. Fort Collins, CO: Three Star Press.

Fisher AG. (2006b) *Assessment of motor and process skills. Volume 2: Users manual,* 6th edn. Fort Collins, CO: Three Star Press.

Folstein MF, Folstein SE, McHugh PR. (1975) Mini-Mental State: A practical method for grading cognitive status of patients for the clinician. *Journal of Psychiatric Research* **12**: 189–98.

Fossey E. (2001) Effective interdisciplinary teamwork: an occupational therapy perspective. *Australasian Psychiatry* **9**: 232–5.

Gitlin L, Liebman J, Winter J. (2003) Are environmental interventions effective in the management of Alzheimer's disease and related disorders?: A synthesis of the evidence. *Alzheimer's Care Quarterly* **4**: 85–107.

Gitlin LN, Schinfeld S, Winter L et al. (2002) Evaluating home environments of people with dementia: interrater reliability and validity of the Home Environmental Assessment Protocol (HEAP). *Disability and Rehabilitation* **24**: 59–71.

Gitlin LN, Corcoran MA. (2005) *Occupational therapy and dementia care: The environmental skill-building program for individuals and families.* Bethesda, MD: American Occupational Therapy Association.

Graff MJL, Vernooij-Dassen MJFJ, Hoefnagels WHL et al. (2003) Occupational therapy at home for older individuals with mild to moderate cognitive impairments and their primary caregivers: A pilot study. *Occupational Therapy Journal of Research* **23**: 155–64.

Guide from the Uniform Data Set for Medical Rehabilitation. (1993) *Adult FIM, Version 4.* Buffalo, NY: State University of New York.

Hasselkus BR, Murray BJ. (2007) Everyday occupation, well-being and identity: The experience of caregivers in families with dementia. *The American Journal of Occupational Therapy* **61**: 9–20.

Hellen CR. (1998) *Alzheimer's disease: Activities-focused care,* 2nd edn. Woburn, MA: Butterworth-Heinemann.

Hopkins A, Smith H. (1993) *Willard and Spackman's occupational therapy,* 8th edn. Philadelphia, PA: J.B. Lippincott Co.

Johnson N, Barion A, Rademaker A et al. (2004) The activities of daily living questionnaire: A validation study in patients with dementia. *Alzheimer's Disease and Associated Disorders* **18**: 223–30.

Josephsson S, Backman L, Nygard L, Borell L. (2000) Non professional caregivers' experience of occupational performance on the part of relatives with dementia: Implications for caregiver program in occupational therapy. *Scandinavian Journal of Occupational Therapy* **7**: 61–6.

Law M, Polatajko H, Pollok N et al. (1991) *Canadian occupational performance measure.* Toronto: Canadian Association of Occupational Therapists.

Lawton MP, Brody EM. (1969) Assessment of older people: self-maintaining and instrumental activities of daily living. *The Gerontologist* **9**: 179–86.

Letts L, Baum C, Permutter M. (2003) Person-environment-occupation assessment with older adults. *Occupational Therapy Practice* **2**: 27–33.

Marcy-Edwards D, Grant NK, Slater S. (2005) The exploration of self-determined behaviour and activity vignettes: A descriptive exploratory study. *Alzheimer's Disease Quarterly* **6**: 35–51.

Mahoney F, Barthel D. (1965) Functional evaluation: the Barthel Index. *Maryland State Medical Journal* **2**: 61–5.

Mahurin R, DeBettignies B, Pirozzolo F. (1991) Structured assessment of independent living skills: Preliminary report of a performance measure of functional abilities in dementia. *Journal of Gerontology* **46**: 58–66.

Oakley F, Sutherland T, Hill JL *et al.* (1991) The daily activities questionnaire: a functional assessment for people with Alzheimer's disease. *Physical and Occupational Therapy in Geriatrics* **10**: 67–81.

O'Connor DW, Ames D, Gardner B, King M. (2009) Psychosocial treatments of behavioural symptoms in dementia: a systematic review of reports meeting quality standards. *International Psychogeriatrics* **21**: 225–40.

Perrin T, May H, Anderson E. (2008) *Wellbeing in dementia care: An occupational approach for therapists and carers*, 2nd edn. Philadelphia, PA: Churchill Livingstone, Elsevier.

Pfeffer RI, Kurosaki TT, Harrah CH *et al.* (1992) Measurement of functional activities in older adults in the community. *Journal of Gerontology* **37**: 323–9.

Pool J. (2008) *The Pool Activity Level Instrument for Occupational Profiling: A practical resource for carers of people with cognitive impairment*, 3rd edn. London: JKP.

Poulin de Courval L, Genlinas I, Gauthier S *et al.* (2006) Reliability and validity of the Safety Assessment Scale for people with dementia living at home. *The Canadian Journal of Occupational Therapy* **73**: 67–75.

Robert Dooley N, Hinojosa J. (2004) Improving quality of life for persons with Alzheimer's disease and their family caregivers: Brief occupational therapy intervention. *The American Journal of Occupational Therapy* **58**: 561–9.

Strong J. (2003) Seeing beyond the clouds: Best practice and occupational therapy. *The Canadian Journal of Occupational Therapy* **70**: 197–9.

Teri L, Traux P, Logsdon R *et al.* (1992) Assessment of behavioural problems in dementia: The revised memory and behaviour problems checklist (RMBPC). *Psychology and Ageing* **7**: 622–31.

Teunisse S, Derix MMA. (1997) The interview for deterioration in daily living activities in dementia: Agreement between primary and secondary caregivers. *International Psychogeriatrics* **9** (Suppl. 1): 155–62.

Thorgrimsen L, Kennedy L, Douglas C *et al.* (2002) The group activity form: is it valid and reliable? *The British Journal of Occupational Therapy* **65**: 283–7.

Truscott M. (2004) Adapting leisure and creative activities for people with early stage dementias. *Alzheimer's Care Quarterly* **5**: 92–102.

Williams J, Drinka T, Greenberg J *et al.* (1991) Development and testing of the Assessment of Living Skills and Resources (ASLAR) in elderly community-dwelling veterans. *Gerontologist* **31**: 84–91.

Zarit SH, Reever KE, Bach-Peterson J. (1980) Relatives of the impaired elderly: correlates of feeling of burden. *The Gerontologist* **20**: 649–55.

Zgola J. (1999) *Care that works: A relationship approach to persons with dementia*. Baltimore, MD: Johns Hopkins University Press.

22

The role of the speech and language therapist in the assessment and management of the person with dementia

BRONWYN MOORHOUSE

22.1 INTRODUCTION

Communication is integral to successful living (Lubinski, 1991), however in dementia its breakdown is well documented. In 1991, Bourgeois reviewed dementia articles in journals of the American Speech-Language-Hearing Association (ASHA) (Bourgeois, 1991). These articles focused on how cognitive-linguistic profiles influence dementia diagnosis. People with dementia, who live for up to 20 years after diagnosis, also need help with communication to optimize quality of life (Bourgeois, 2002). Moreover, in dementia, communication difficulties predict problem behaviours which in turn affect caregiver burden (Savundranayagam et al., 2005). In the past 15 years, research exploring how to optimize interactions in dementia has emerged (Ripich et al., 2000; Haight et al., 2006; Alm et al., 2007). A dynamic interplay exists between executive and language dysfunction in dementia (Byrne and Orange, 2005). Hence, speech and language therapists (SLTs) (speech pathologists) should work with other disciplines in assessing and managing this interplay. This chapter outlines cognitive-linguistic deficits seen in dementia and assessments SLTs use to examine these. It also explores how SLTs can help people with dementia, significant others and care staff, to participate in real-life communication. As eating and swallowing often decline in dementia (Logemann, 2003), the SLT's role in managing these processes will also be outlined.

22.2 COGNITIVE-LINGUISTIC AND OROMOTOR CHANGES IN DEMENTIA

Reduced language capacity in normal ageing is subtle. There is no loss of phonologic or syntactic knowledge, while grammar simplification and increased time required for word finding and understanding complex (written) language are seen mainly in later old age (75+ years) (Bayles and Tomoeda, 2007). Conversely, Reisberg et al. (1999) used the term retrogenesis to describe parallels between language acquisition and language loss in Alzheimer's disease (AD). Fried-Oken et al. (2000) noted that most research into communication and dementia relates to AD. Nonetheless they concluded that many language changes in AD also occur with other dementias. The following sections outline these changes according to Global Deterioration Scale (GDS) stages (Reisberg et al., 1982). Information particular to vascular dementia (VaD), dementia with Lewy bodies (DLB) and frontotemporal dementia (FTD) will then be outlined.

22.2.1 Early/mild stages AD (geriatric depression scales 3 and 4)

Word finding difficulties are common in early AD (Bourgeois, 2002), affecting most recently acquired low frequency words (Haak, 2002). Conversation is vague and semantically empty

(Bayles and Tomoeda, 2007). Usually communication is successful for brief interactions, but breaks down if lengthy (Haak, 2002). Language comprehension is sometimes intact (Bayles, et al. 1992) or may decline for longer grammatically complex sentences (Clark, 1995), or material needing inference (Fried-Oken et al., 2000) or abstraction (Haak, 2002). Poor memory and executive function impact use of conversational rules around repetition, topic maintenance and turn taking (Watson et al., 1999). Phrases are often aborted, but output may also be verbose (Bayles and Tomoeda, 2007). Oral reading, reading comprehension, (Bayles et al., 1992) spelling and writing are often relatively spared, but written passage generation is poor (Haak, 2002).

22.2.2 Middle/moderate stage AD (geriatric depression scale 5)

Communicative intent and general message frameworks are still evident, however utterances are depleted of content words (Haak, 2002), less concise and more repetitious with reference errors abounding (Bayles and Tomoeda, 2007). Due to pervasive lexical retrieval difficulty, indefinite labels (e.g. 'thing') often replace content words (Bourgeois, 2002) and the person may withdraw or speak excessively (Clark, 1995). Automatic and social phrases are retained, but the person often forgets what they wish to say (Haak, 2002) or repeatedly asks the same questions (Byrne and Orange, 2005). Paraphasias and confabulations appear and discourse breakdown increases with poor propositional topic development, difficulty changing topic and maintaining discourse flow (Mentis et al., 1995; Fried-Oken et al., 2000). Expression and comprehension of complex grammar (e.g. embedded clauses or passives) is poor and abstract interpretation is lost, while understanding of one- (Haak, 2002) and sometimes two-stage (Fried-Oken et al., 2000) commands is preserved. Reading aloud and writing mechanics are relatively spared, but reading comprehension and writing are often limited to single words (Haak, 2002) and accuracy is reduced (Bayles et al., 1992).

22.2.3 Late/severe stage AD (geriatric depression scales 6 and 7)

Initially, use of automatic and social phrases may continue (Haak, 2002). Utterances often contain strings of non-words with occasional real words interspersed, however message form, simple grammar and intonation are basically present (Bayles and Tomoeda, 2007). There is failure to obey speaker–listener conversational discourse roles and sometimes difficulty initiating speech, articulatory breakdowns and dysphagia (Clark, 1995). Eventually the person becomes completely mute (Bourgeois, 2002), although conceptual knowledge may be preserved until very late (Fried-Oken et al., 2000). People also fail to comprehend spoken or written language (Bayles and Tomoeda, 2007) relying on non-verbal cues and emotion (Haak, 2002). Vocalizations may become disruptive – sometimes due to failure to access specific words for basic needs and emotions (Bourgeois,

2002). Resistance may reflect failure to understand verbal direction.

22.2.4 Vascular dementia

VaD occurs following multiple small infarcts which occur progressively. Unlike AD, deterioration is usually stepwise with new deficits becoming evident suddenly after each new infarct (Tomoeda, 2001). As such, individual deficit profiles (depending on infarct locations) are often less uniform across language areas than with AD (Hopper and Bayles, 2001). Nonetheless, Vuorinen et al. (2000) found little difference, on average, in deficit level across comprehension, naming and description tasks between individuals with mild to moderate AD versus VaD. Powell et al. (1988) also reported greater motoric speech involvement in VaD (e.g. dysarthria and intonation changes).

22.2.5 Dementia with Lewy bodies

DLB may be the second most common dementia after AD (Hopper and Bayles, 2001), but many people with DLB also have AD lesions (McKeith et al., 1995). Most commonly reported characteristics are insidious onset, beginning with forgetfulness, then word finding, verbal fluency and calculation difficulties and then other cognitive skills (McKeith et al., 1995). Fluctuating cognition (with periods of lucidity in early to mid stages), often mild extrapyramidal features (e.g. dysarthria and dysphagia) and a more rapid progression than AD are also observed (Tomoeda, 2001).

22.2.6 Frontotemporal dementia

FTD is an umbrella term for neurodegenerative conditions causing language and/or behavioural decline (Grossman, 2002). Personality change and bizarre affect are often seen in this condition. Primary progressive aphasia (PPA) is another type of FTD. Described by Mesulam (Mesulam 1982; Mesulam, 2001) as a slowly progressive aphasia without generalized dementia, aphasic symptoms slowly increase in number and severity with sparing of non-language executive skill for at least two years post-onset. Despite initial divergent presentations in PPA, evidence suggests a progression towards non-fluency and eventual mutism at an earlier stage than in AD (Kertesz et al., 2003).

Semantic dementia (SD) and progressive non-fluent aphasia (PNFA) are both forms of PPA (Hodges et al., 2008). In SD phonology, syntax and speech fluency are initially spared, while naming, single word comprehension and semantic association tasks are impaired (Gorno-Tempini et al., 2004). Initially, semantic paraphasias and then more general terms are frequently substituted for specific names (Hodges and Patterson, 2007) with phonological, syntactic and morphological processing deficits often emerging with disease progression (Bright et al., 2008). PNFA usually begins with word finding difficulties or speech dysfluency (Narvid and Gorno-Tempini, 2008), however it progresses to reduced output (particularly for self-generated connected speech) and impaired articulatory precision (Patterson *et al.*, 2006), sometimes described as apraxia of speech (Gorno-Tempini *et al.*, 2008). True agrammatism is not a feature, as normal ratios of verbs to nouns and function to content words have been observed (Graham *et al.*, 2004). Dysarthria is also sometimes reported with FTLD, occurring much more commonly with non-fluent than fluent PPA (Clark *et al.*, 2005).

Gorno-Tempini and colleagues (2004) also used the term 'logopenic' to describe a progressive aphasia of 'intermediate' fluency. Spontaneous speech is halting with word finding pauses and phonemic paraphasias. Motor speech and grammar are spared. Due to a proposed phonological loop (working memory) disorder, repetition and sentence comprehension are impaired regardless of syntactic complexity while single word comprehension is spared (Gorno-Tempini *et al.*, 2008).

22.3   COGNITIVE-LINGUISTIC ASSESSMENTS USED IN DEMENTIA

When undertaking comprehensive dementia assessment, SLTs need to consider the World Health Organization's (WHO) International Classification of Functioning, Disability and Health (ICF) (WHO, 2001). The ICF has two parts. The first part comprises the components 'body function and structure' and 'activities and participation'. Assessing body function impairment (e.g. anomia) is important for diagnosis and investigation of underlying deficit patterns (Bourgeois and Hickey, 2009). The ICF provides a framework to move beyond solely assessing impairments which fail to fully explain heterogeneous communicative performance in dementia. Evaluating people's capacity to undertake an activity along with rating actual activity performance in their environment is an important precursor to intervention (Byrne and Orange, 2005). Personal traits including low hearing, or vision (Tomoeda, 2001) or cultural differences (Lydall-Smith *et al.*, 1996) should also be allowed for. Environmental and personal factors which are components of Part 2 of the ICF will be considered below.

22.3.1   ICF body function and structure focused assessments

In diagnosing presence and type of dementia, individual profiles of cognitive-linguistic functioning ideally form part of a memory clinic evaluation (Ames *et al.*, 1992). Accurate early dementia diagnosis is crucial in identifying strengths and weaknesses for optimal informational counselling, some interventions and effective care plan development. It also allows for establishment of baselines for intervention effects or decline over time (Tomoeda, 2001). Appropriate cognitive-linguistic normative data help to distinguish those with early dementia from the 'worried well' (Bryan *et al.* 2001).

Perhaps the best known cognitive-linguistic assessment in this area is the Arizona Battery for Communication

Disorders of Dementia (ABCD) (Bayles and Tomoeda, 1993). It assesses mild to moderate dementia across five constructs: linguistic comprehension, linguistic expression, verbal memory, visuospatial skills and mental status. It has norms from 86 people with probable AD (McKhann *et al.*, 1984) and 86 normal elderly, and takes 60–90 minutes to administer. Subtest summary scores are averaged to gain (high normal, low normal, mildly impaired or moderately impaired) construct profiles useful in identifying relative strengths (Bourgeois and Hickey, 2009). Although developed in the US, ABCD norms have also been found appropriate with UK (Armstrong *et al.*, 1996) and Australian (Moorhouse *et al.*, 1999) samples. ABCD administration time in poorly resourced clinics may be excessive. Story Retelling and Word Learning subtests are most sensitive to dementia (Tomoeda, 2001). The Boston Naming Test has also been found to detect early dementia (Stevens *et al.*, 1992). The Barnes Language Assessment (BLA) (Bryan *et al.*, 2001) assesses mild, moderate and sometimes severe dementia in 40–60 minutes. It examines expression, comprehension, reading and writing, memory and executive functions using items adapted from existing tests and has descriptive performance statistics for 43 normal elderly and 43 people suspected of having a non-specific dementia.

SLTs also have a crucial role in detailed assessment of PPA important for differential diagnosis and appropriately targeted education, support and intervention (Nickels and Croot, 2009). Some tests are specifically tailored to assess PPA, such as 'Repeat and Point' which has been shown to differentiate SD from PNFA (Hodges *et al.*, 2008). It uses ten concrete nouns of varying lengths. Each noun must be repeated (difficult for those with PNFA) and then target pictures identified from an array of six semantic foils (difficult for those with SD). The Cambridge Semantic Memory Battery (Hodges and Patterson, 2007) comprises 64 items (living and man-made) used across a range of tasks probing input to and output from a central semantic knowledge base in SD. More general aphasia assessments are also used to examine levels of language breakdown in PPA (Bright *et al.*, 2008; Jokel *et al.*, 2009).

22.3.2   ICF activity and participation focused assessments

'Activity' and 'participation' focused assessments are useful for understanding how individual deficit patterns translate to specific skills (e.g. capacity to initiate a conversation) and how those skill sets are used to participate in real life (e.g. actually performing in a conversation). They are somewhat overlapping constructs and hence will be grouped together (Byrne and Orange, 2005).

Some studies assessing pragmatic skills in dementia use conversational analysis (CA) to examine phenomena such as 'trouble indicating behaviour' (TIB) and patterns and types of conversational repair trajectory (Watson *et al.*, 1999). The Profile of Pragmatic Impairment in Communication (PPIC) has ten scales assessing literal content, general participation in conversation, quality and quantity of conversational content, internal and external relevance, clarity of expression, social style, subject matter and aesthetics of communication in people with dementia. It examines literal and intended meaning (implicature). Adequate reliability and validity have been shown on seven PPIC scales (exceptions being subject matter, quality and social style) (Hayes *et al.*, 2004). Despite the ecological validity of such assessments, they are extremely time-consuming for clinicians (Bourgeois and Hickey, 2009).

The Functional Linguistic Communication Inventory (FLCI) (Bayles and Tomoeda, 1994) and the Communication Outcome Measure of Functional Independence (COMFI) (Santo Pietro and Boczko, 1997) examine pragmatic skills more time efficiently. The FLCI assesses functional communication in moderate to severe AD. It rates ability to greet, answer questions, reminisce and participate in conversations (which may identify intervention stimuli and cues) and takes 30 minutes to administer (Bourgeois and Hickey, 2009). The COMFI is a standardized scale assessing behaviours observed during meals in care settings. It rates psychosocial interaction, cognition, communication and conversational initiation and maintenance, along with participation in the tasks of cooking and eating breakfast and socializing with others.

22.4   OPTIMIZING COMMUNICATION IN DEMENTIA

Byrne and Orange (2005) discuss advantages of the ICF in terms of its comprehensive approach to communication intervention in dementia. Isolated impairment-based interventions (e.g. naming work) do not consider ICF activity limitations (e.g. cannot initiate conversations) or participation restrictions (e.g. does not socialize) stemming from interaction of impairments with environmental and personal factors. Conversely, use of approaches such as functional communication or environmental adaptation without considering impairments that either underlie functional communication changes or underscore need for environmental modifications and supports is equally problematic. Interventions described below often lack the comprehensive approach facilitated by the ICF framework. Others span different components, so are placed where they fit best. In selecting interventions, individuals' and carers' needs, interests and desired outcomes must be addressed (Bourgeois and Hickey, 2009).

22.4.1   ICF function and structure focused interventions

One impairment-based approach to restoring aspects of communication involves relearning or maintenance of ability to name specific word groups or learn key information in early to middle dementia. Spaced retrieval (SR) (involving rehearsal and recall at gradually increasing intervals) (Abrahams and Camp, 1993; Brush and Camp, 1998), repeated exposure and questioning (by students) about related semantic properties (Arkin, *et al.*, 2000) or coaching on picture description, word association, simple discourse role-plays and word category assignments (Arkin and Mahendra,

2001) facilitated performance on specific tasks with some maintenance over several weeks (Abrahams and Camp, 1993). Brush and Camp (1998) reported some use of learned information to achieve speech-language goals while Arkin and Mahendra (2001) reported no change on discourse meaningfulness or the ABCD, but significantly higher ratios of different nouns to total nouns at post-test. Further objective outcome measurement for such interventions are required to determine whether functional gains are made.

Given relative sparing of executive function in PPA, aphasia therapy strategies may be useful in optimizing communication. Most studies have targeted naming skills and, for some time, have demonstrated gains (Bier *et al.*, 2009; Heredia *et al.*, 2009; Jokel *et al.*, 2009). Recent work, however, has suggested that acquisition and retention patterns may vary according to PPA type (Newhart *et al.*, 2009). In reviewing studies in this area, Croot *et al.* (2009) found that despite consistent gains on training items, generalization to non-treated items and functional communication was more limited.

22.4.2   ICF activity and participation focused interventions

These interventions aim primarily to optimize functional communication of the person with dementia. Clark and Witte (1991) advocated training in early AD in use of adaptive strategies – for example saying 'Please repeat exactly what you just said' or 'Give me a little time. I'm having trouble finding the exact words' or 'I forgot what we were discussing'. They also suggested strategies to assist self-cueing (e.g. using circumlocution or semantically related words) and teaching of a script strategy for simple storytelling (e.g. theme, characters, setting and events) to improve cohesion and topic maintenance. Clark in an unpublished research paper (Enhancement of communication adequacy in early stage Alzheimer's disease patients. Hunter College of CUNY, New York, 1988) (cited in Clark and Witte, 1991) used these strategies with eight people with mild to moderate AD. Carers reported maintained or increased functional communication. Aphasia test scores were stable for six months.

Group programmes in later dementia which use residual communication strengths with interesting tangible stimuli may also be beneficial. Santo Pietro and Boczko (2001) used intact procedural memories to facilitate communication in residents with mild-moderate to moderate-severe AD. 'Breakfast Clubs' held each working day for 12 weeks involved members using greetings, discussing and choosing food for breakfast, helping one another prepare ingredients, setting the table, general conversation, cleaning up and saying goodbye. SLTs provided visual and semantic cues, paired choices and trigger phrases to help members indicate choices and ingredients required. Participants improved significantly on the ABCD and had more self-initiated topic comments per session, more cross-conversation exchanges and increased initiation of procedural memories. Matched controls in a conversation group showed either no gains or slight declines over this period.

22.4.3   Environmental supports to communication

Byrne and Orange (2005) conclude that inclusion of 'environment' as a core ICF feature reflects a conceptual shift from individuals needing to 'fit in' with society to the environment being modified to accommodate them. The 'environment' includes communication partner support or other devices or props to aid interaction.

Conversation is collaborative. Where one partner has AD, the other can use strategies to optimize interaction (Kessler et al., 2001). People with mild AD should be encouraged to speak even when having word finding difficulties and should be urged to use spared communicative abilities to reinforce self-worth – for example reading to a grandchild or writing letters to friends (Haak, 2002). When optimizing comprehension in dementia, the partner should match language complexity to individual levels (Haak, 2002), initially, using slightly slower speech and reduced information (Bourgeois, 2002) and with progression, conversing about tangible things, simplifying vocabulary, using non-verbal cues and restating messages when not understood (Bayles and Tomoeda, 2007) or forgotten (Enderby, 2002). Before starting, it helps to orient to topic and then maintain and extend it (Kessler et al., 2001). In middle to late dementia, questions with alternatives (e.g. 'do you want fish or chicken?'), short utterances and names (rather than pronouns) are useful (Haak, 2002). Demonstration to aid comprehension, avoidance of sarcasm and innuendo, use of native language and familiar wording (e.g. respectful title or maiden name) also promote conversation. When confusion occurs, carers should re-introduce themselves (Haak, 2002).

Santo Pietro (2002) emphasized the importance of the SLT's role in training trainers or care staff in use of effective communication strategies using a 'teaching by modeling' paradigm and use of role-play rather than formal lectures. On site, short training modules also need to include information about environmental supports and barriers to effective communication. Santo Pietro also stressed the need to evaluate real world training outcomes. The FOCUSED programme for carers emphasizes strategies based on an interactive discourse model – F-face to face, O-orient to conversation topic, C-continue the topic, U-unstick communication blocks, S-structure questions, E-exchange conversation and D-direct short sentences (Ripich and Wykle, 1996). Presented over several sessions, it involves role-play, discussion and home assignments. Ripich et al. (2000) found that six months post-training, when planning a menu together, 22 FOCUSED trained carers asked significantly more yes/no and choice questions (associated with a higher percentage of successful communication outcomes) to partners with early to middle AD than controls.

Wong et al. (2009) targeted use of residual (automatic) verbal and non-verbal abilities along with props in a discourse-based intervention with an individual with SD. The communication partner was educated to interpret underlying non-verbal messages and facilitate multi-modal message delivery. They found the individual then continued to participate in conversation despite disease progression.

Bourgeois (1992) explored the introduction of personalized memory wallets to enhance communication in six people with mild to moderate AD. She trained carers in wallet use with role-play. Wallets contained individualized simple written information, drawings and photographs. Carers used the wallet daily across 4 or 5 days with participants to facilitate discussion about 'day', 'family' and 'yourself'. During training and maintenance, participants made more novel topic statements and fewer ambiguous utterances. A further three participants also appeared to benefit from wallet use even with minimal carer training. Most participants used their wallets spontaneously to initiate conversations. Similarly, Baker (2001) reported on SLTs compiling life story books (LSBs) for people with severe dementia and some (verbal or non-verbal) language skills. They trained relatives and staff, for example in presentation speed and cueing. After six months, carer reports indicated more focused and shared conversation, revived spousal involvement and changed staff attitudes towards the person. Staff also had greater understanding of the SLT's role and interest in future collaborations. Haight et al. (2006) evaluated outcomes when care staff (who had 10 hours of training) used LSBs with 15 people with dementia. Intervention was for 1 hour each week over 8 weeks with significantly improved scores compared with controls on depression, mood, mental status and communication scales.

Alm et al. (2004) used a generic computerized interactive reminiscence presentation of 'entertainment', 'recreation' and 'local Dundee life' (with text, photos, graphics, sound and film recordings) to facilitate conversation between nine people with mild to moderate dementia and care staff. Compared with a book, this device allowed more flexibility in presentation order, greater search speed for specific items and a more engaging multimedia format for individuals struggling to initiate interactions. General observations indicated that most videos and photos and all songs cued conversation and that people with dementia could usually use the touch screen. Carers reported enhanced conversation enjoyment. After developing an updated system entitled CIRCA, Alm et al. (2007) compared nine people with moderate to severe dementia and their carers with a further nine matched pairs undertaking traditional reminiscence activities. The CIRCA group carers improved significantly more with asking direct questions and offering subject and materials choice while those with dementia improved significantly more on making these choices and with amount of information and memories shared. Conversational contributions and control of direction were also more equal with CIRCA. CIRCA's hypermedia structure provided a varied and failure-free environment while still prompting personal memories with generic content.

Because more primitive senses of smell and taste may be relatively preserved in later dementia, stimulation of these senses via spice jars, scratch and sniff books, ethnic foods or texture can also aid comprehension or trigger conversation (Lubinski, 1991; Bourgeois, 2002). Having a pet or a toy present may also facilitate communication (Hopper et al., 1998). Use of space is important, for example placing chairs and beds appropriately for comfortable interaction or using round tables for meals (Morse and Intrieri, 1997). The environment should also be set up (e.g. colour coded) so people can find their way to spaces where they can interact (Lubinski, 1991).

Fried-Oken (2008) outlined three treatment goals for augmentative and alternative communication (AAC) use in PPA, compensating for progressive language loss (rather than skill recovery), starting early while the person can still learn to use AAC and including key communication partners in training. Initially, SLTs may develop individually tailored communication books with specific information, questions and text or gestures (e.g. 'yes', 'no') to reduce communication breakdown. As PPA progresses, SLTs need to work with individuals and partners to develop appropriate low tech AAC devices such as talking photo albums, easy to use electronic devices and 'Talking Mats' (see below). In latter stages, when there is minimal functional language, partners can support participation by carrying conversation content and presenting limited choices to indicate needs. Any AAC system must also be appropriate and adaptive to individual life changes (Garret and Lasker, 2005). Fried-Oken *et al.* (2000) discussed use of AAC to facilitate communication in late dementia and suggested intervention over time would best meet complex and changing needs. They also asserted that cognitive-linguistic strengths and weaknesses would need to be carefully assessed to develop optimal AAC input and/or output systems.

Talking Mats are an innovative interviewing method which supports people with limited communication in giving information, making decisions or setting goals. Topics are presented in a structured fashion to support comprehension and expression. Three sets of pictorial symbols (topic, options and visual scale) backed with Velcro (for placement on a mat) are used. The person places relevant options under the visual scale (happy, unsure, not happy) which is recorded for further reference and conversation. Murphy *et al.* (2005) found that the use of Talking Mats assisted seven people with dementia and limited or no speech express views on themes of activities, people, environment and self, not only by supporting communication, but also by reducing memory load.

In late dementia, SLTs can also work with carers to make 'personal communication dictionaries' (PCDs) to foster interactions – even with non-intentional communicators. This tool was originally developed for early communicators (Siegel and Wetherby, 2000). Compilation of a communication dictionary requires careful observation and documentation of an individual's consistent non-verbal behaviours, for example when wanting something. Carers can also record observations in categories – 'What Fred does' (e.g. Takes your hand and pulls it towards his mouth), 'What it might mean' (e.g. 'I'm hungry or thirsty'), 'What you should do' (e.g. Give food or drink if appropriate). PCDs are especially useful when carers do not know the person. They should be easily accessible for reference and amendment. They may also help familiar carers to structure observations to best meet the person's needs.

22.4.4   Personal and environmental barriers to communication

Just as carers can act as facilitators, if they fail to use optimal strategies, they can create unnecessary barriers to communication (Byrne and Orange, 2005). Other insidious barriers equally deserve SLTs' attention. Problems with hearing and vision should be corrected optimally, background noise limited and lighting optimized (Enderby, 2002). People should be treated with dignity and cultural sensitivity (Lydall-Smith *et al.*, 1996). Poor management of medical conditions and drug regimes can also affect communication negatively (Clark, 1995). Although physical space is often limited and opportunities for solitude or intimacy rare, socialization can also be minimal (Lubinski, 1991). Some attitudes should also be challenged, for example ignoring those with severe communication issues (Lubinski, 1991). Barriers in use of AAC include the person or family's lack of acceptance, poor matching of AAC systems with communicators' abilities and lack of contextual practice, appropriately trained communication partners or opportunities (because others anticipate needs) (Fried-Oken, 2008).

22.5   EATING IN DEMENTIA

In mid to late dementia, individuals often demonstrate weight loss, malnutrition and/or dehydration. Bourgeois and Hickey (2009) stress that SLTs must consider dysphagia along with other environmental and personal factors impacting upon problems above, for example bland institutional food, poor eating environment and limited staff skills or availability for optimal mealtime assistance. Not only should SLTs assess oropharyngeal function to reduce choking and aspiration risk (e.g. by modifying consistencies or positioning; Gillick and Mitchell, 2002), but they should also consider environmental modification for optimal eating, for example presenting more appealing food (one course at a time) or drink and training staff in optimal assistance measures. SLTs may use instrumental examinations where pharyngeal dysphagia is suspected (Logemann, 2003), however people with advanced dementia often cannot co-operate with such procedures (Gillick and Mitchell, 2002). Bourgeois and Hickey (2009) also argue that people may not cope with change of environment necessary for videofluoroscopy, however having the usual carer present barium substances sometimes ameliorates this situation. Where a person can no longer swallow safely or rejects food or drink, a percutaneous endoscopic gastrostomy (PEG) tube is sometimes inserted to administer liquid food directly into the stomach (Gillick and Mitchell 2002). Although many consider withholding food to be cruel, people appear to experience little thirst or hunger at life's end (Bourgeois and Hickey, 2009). PEG limitations include diarrhoea and nausea in 10 per cent of people, tubes frequently being pulled out and failure to enhance survival or comfort (Gillick and Mitchell, 2002; Logemann, 2003) with aspiration continuing to contribute to mortality (Dharmarajan and Unnikrishnan, 2004). If there is no medical living will, guardians should decide based on what people would choose for themselves. As part of a team, SLTs should provide family with clear information regarding PEGs versus other options (e.g. mouth swabs or ice chips) so they can make the best decision for their relative (Gillick and Mitchell, 2002).

22.6   CONCLUSIONS

In recent years, knowledge about SLTs' role in assessing and managing dementia has increased – especially for PPA, contribution of the ICF to promoting communicative participation in people with dementia and the use of AAC to optimize communication. Technological advances assisting communication have also been made and there is greater understanding of issues around eating in dementia. There is still need for further work in these areas and for growth in the evidence base for efficacy of SLT interventions. Single case investigations require collection of lengthy baseline as well as intervention data, while group studies require strict selection criteria and well-matched control groups (Lum, 2001). People with dementia-associated communication problems are the profession's fastest growing clinical population (ASHA, 2005). Nonetheless, in 2002, Bryan and Maxim observed that in the previous ten years, there had only been a very small rise in the numbers of SLTs specializing in dementia (Bryan and Maxim, 2002). In a more recent Royal College of Speech and Language Therapists' press release (RCSLT, 2007), it was still noted that most people with dementia in the UK are denied access to SLT services. Similarly, a Speech Pathology Australia (SPA, 2003) briefing paper indicated inadequate numbers of SLTs to meet needs of people over 65. Prejudices need to be overcome and SLT services provided on the basis of clinical need rather than diagnosis (RCSLT, 2005). Given growing evidence for efficacy of SLT involvement in dementia, advances outlined above and population trend imperatives, professional associations need to continue lobbying governments for appropriate levels of service.

REFERENCES

Alm N, Astell A, Ellis M et al. (2004) A cognitive prosthesis and communication support for people with dementia. *Neuropsychological Rehabilitation* 14: 117–34.

Alm N, Dye R, Gowans G et al. (2007) A communication support system for older people with dementia. *Computer* 40: 35–41.

American Speech-Language-Hearing Association. (2005) The Roles of Speech–Language Pathologists Working With Individuals With Dementia-Based Communication Disorders: *Position statement.* Available from www.asha.org/policy.

Ames D, Flicker L, Helme R. (1992) A memory clinic at a geriatric hospital: Rationale, routine and results from the first 100 patients. *The Medical Journal of Australia* 156: 618–22.

Armstrong L, Bayles K, Borthwick S, Tomoeda C. (1996) Use of the Arizona Battery for Communication Disorders of Dementia in the UK. *European Journal of Disorders of Communication* 31: 171–80.

Arkin S, Rose C, Hopper T. (2000) Implicit and explicit learning gains in Alzheimer's patients: Effects of naming and information retrieval training. *Aphasiology* 14: 723–42.

Arkin S, Mahendra N. (2001) Discourse analysis of Alzheimer's patients before and after intervention: Methodology and outcomes. *Aphasiology* 15: 533–69.

Abrahams JP, Camp CJ. (1993) Maintenance and generalization of object naming training in anomia associated with degenerative dementia. *Clinical Gerontologist* 12: 57–72.

Baker J. (2001) Life story books for the elderly mentally ill. *International Journal of Language and Communication Disorders,* 36 (Suppl.): 185–7.

Bayles KA, Tomoeda CK. (1993) *The Arizona Battery for communication disorders of dementia.* Austin, TX: Pro-Ed.

Bayles KA, Tomoeda CK. (1994) *Functional linguistic communication inventory.* Austin, TX: Pro-Ed.

Bayles KA, Tomoeda CK. (2007) *Cognitive-communication disorders of dementia.* San Diego, CA: Plural Publishing.

Bayles KA, Tomoeda CK, Trosset MW. (1992) Relation of linguistic communication abilities of Alzheimer's patients to stage of disease. *Brain and Language* 42: 454–72.

Bier N, Macoir J, Gagnon L et al. (2009) Known, lost, and recovered: Efficacy of formal-semantic therapy and spaced retrieval method in a case of semantic dementia. *Aphasiology* 23: 210–35.

Bourgeois MS. (1991) Communication treatment for adults with dementia. *Journal of Speech and Hearing Research* 34: 831–44.

Bourgeois MS. (1992) Evaluating memory wallets in conversations with persons with dementia. *Journal of Speech and Hearing Research* 35: 1344–57.

Bourgeois MS. (2002) Where is my wife and when am I going home? The challenge of communicating with persons with dementia. *Alzheimer's Care Quarterly* 3: 132–44.

Bourgeois MS, Hickey EM. (2009) *Dementia: From diagnosis to management: A functional approach.* Hove: Taylor and Francis.

Bright P, Moss HE, Stamatakis EA, Tyler LK. (2008) Longitudinal studies of semantic dementia: The relationship between structural and functional changes over time. *Neuropsychologia* 46: 2177–88.

Brush JA, Camp CG. (1998) Using spaced retrieval as an intervention during speech-language therapy. *Clinical Gerontologist* 19: 51–64.

Bryan K, Maxim J. (2002) Letter to the editor. *International Journal of Language and Communication Disorders* 37: 215–22.

Bryan K, Binder J, Dann C et al. (2001) Development of a screening instrument for language in older people. *Ageing and Mental Health* 5: 371–8.

Byrne K, Orange JB. (2005) Conceptualizing communication enhancement in dementia for family caregivers using the WHO-ICF Framework. *Advances in Speech-Language Pathology* 7: 187–202.

Clark DG, Charuvastra A, Miller BL et al. (2005) Fluent versus nonfluent primary progressive aphasia: A comparison of clinical and functional neuroimaging features. *Brain and Language* 94: 54–60.

Clark LW, Witte K. (1991) Nature and efficacy of communication management in Alzheimer's disease. In: Lubinski R (ed.). *Dementia and communication.* Philadelphia: B.C. Decker, 238–56.

Clark LW. (1995) Interventions for persons with Alzheimer's disease: Strategies for maintaining and enhancing communicative success. *Topics in Language Disorders* 15: 47–65.

Croot K, Nickels L, Laurence F, Manning M. (2009) Impairment and activity/participation directed interventions in progressive language impairment: clinical and theoretical issues. *Aphasiology* **23**: 125–60.

Dharmarajan TS, Unnikrishnan D. (2004) Tube feeding in the elderly. The technique, complications and outcome. *Postgraduate Medicine* **115**: 51–4, 58–61.

Enderby P. (2002) Promoting communication skills with people who have dementia. In: Stokes G, Goudie F (eds). *The essential dementia care handbook*. Bicester, UK: Speechmark, 102–8.

Fried-Oken M, Rau MT, Oken BS. (2000) AAC and dementia. In: Beukleman D, Yorkston K, Reichle J (eds). *Augmentative and alternative communication for adults with acquired neurological disorders*. Baltimore: Paul H Brooks, 375–405.

Fried-Oken M. (2008) Augmentative and alternative communication treatment for persons with primary progressive aphasia. *Perspectives on Augmentative and Alternative Communication* **17**: 99–104.

Garret KL, Lasker JP. (2005) Adults with severe aphasia. In: Beukleman D, Mirenda P (eds). *Augmentative and alternative communication: Supporting children and adults with complex communication needs*. Baltimore: Paul H Brooks, 467–504.

Gillick MR, Mitchell SL. (2002) Facing eating difficulties in end stage dementia. *Alzheimer's Care Quarterly* **3**: 227–32.

Gorno-Tempini ML, Dronkers NF, Rankin KP *et al.* (2004) Cognition and anatomy in three variants of primary progressive aphasia. *Annals of Neurology* **55**: 335–46.

Gorno-Tempini ML, Brambati SM, Ginex V *et al.* (2008) The logopenic variant of primary progressive aphasia. *Neurology* **71**: 1227–34.

Graham N, Patterson K, Hodges J. (2004) When more yields less: Speaking and writing deficits in nonfluent progressive aphasia. *Neurocase* **10**: 141–55.

Grossman M. (2002) Frontotemporal dementia: A review. *Journal of the International Neuropsychological Society* **8**: 566–83.

Haak NJ. (2002) Maintaining connections: Understanding communication from the perspective of persons with dementia. *Alzheimer's Care Quarterly* **3**: 116–31.

Haight BK, Gibson F, Michel Y. (2006) The Northern Ireland life review/life storybook project for people with dementia. *Alzheimer's and Dementia* **2**: 56–8.

Hayes S-J, Niven B, Godfrey H, Linscott R. (2004) Clinical assessment of pragmatic language impairment: A generalisability study of older people with Alzheimer's disease. *Aphasiology* **18**: 693–714.

Heredia CG, Sage K, Ralph MAL, Berthier ML. (2009) Relearning and retention of verbal labels in a case of semantic dementia. *Aphasiology* **23**: 192–209.

Hodges JR, Patterson K. (2007) Semantic dementia: A unique clinopathological syndrome. *Lancet Neurology* **6**: 1004–14.

Hodges JR, Martinos M, Woollams AM *et al.* (2008) Repeat and point: Differentiating semantic dementia from progressive non-fluent aphasia. *Cortex* **44**: 1265–70.

Hopper T, Bayles KA, Tomoeda CK. (1998) Using toys to facilitate communicative function in individuals with Alzheimer's disease. *Journal of Medical Speech Language Pathology* **6**: 73–80.

Hopper T, Bayles KA. (2001) Management of neurogenic communication disorders associated with dementia. In: Chapey R (ed.). *Language intervention strategies in aphasia and related neurogenic communication disorders*, 4th edn. Philadelphia: Lippincott, Williams and Wilkins, 829–46.

Jokel R, Cupit J, Rochon E, Leonard C. (2009) Relearning lost vocabulary in nonfluent progressive aphasia with MossTalk Words. *Aphasiology* **23**: 175–91.

Kertesz A, Davidson W, McCabe P *et al.* (2003) Primary progressive aphasia: Diagnosis, varieties, evolution. *Journal of the International Neuropsychological Society* **9**: 710–19.

Kessler T, Croot K, Togher L. (2001) Strategies to facilitate communication with a person with dementia of the Alzheimer type. In: Wilson L, Hewat S (eds). *Proceedings of the 2001 Speech Pathology Australia National Conference*. Melbourne, 20–23 May: 27–34.

Logemann JA. (2003) Dysphagia and dementia. *ASHA Leader* **8**: 1–14.

Lubinski R. (1991) Environmental considerations for elderly patients. In: Lubinski R (ed.). *Dementia and communication*. Philadelphia: B.C. Decker, 257–73.

Lum C. (2001) *Scientific thinking in speech and language therapy*. London: Lawrence Erlbaum.

Lydall-Smith S, Moorhouse B, Gilchrist J. (1996) *Culturally appropriate dementia assessment*. Canberra: Commonwealth of Australia.

McKeith IG, Galasko GK, Wilcock GK, Byrne EJ. (1995) Lewy body dementia – Diagnosis and treatment. *British Journal of Psychiatry* **167**: 709–17.

McKhann G, Drachman D, Folstein M *et al.* (1984) Clinical diagnosis of Alzheimer's disease: Report of the NINCDS-ADRDA work group under the auspices of Department of Health and Human Services task force on Alzheimer's disease. *Neurology* **34**: 939–44.

Mentis M, Briggs-Whittaker J, Gramigna GD. (1995) Discourse topic management in senile dementia of the Alzheimer type. *Journal of Speech and Hearing Research* **38**: 1054–66.

Mesulam MM. (1982) Slowly progressive aphasia without generalized dementia. *Annals of Neurology* **11**: 592–8.

Mesulam MM. (2001) Primary progressive aphasia. *Annals of Neurology* **49**: 425–32.

Moorhouse B, Douglas J, Pannacio J, Steel G. (1999) Use of the Arizona Battery for Communication Disorders of Dementia in an Australian context. *Asia Pacific Journal of Speech, Language and Hearing* **4**: 93–107.

Morse J, Intrieri R. (1997) 'Talk to me' Patient communication in a long-term care facility. *Journal of Psychosocial Nursing* **35**: 34–43.

Murphy J, Tester S, Hubbard G, Downs M. (2005) Enabling frail older people with a communication difficulty to express their views: The use of Talking Mats as an interview tool. *Health and Social Care in the Community* **13**: 95–107.

Narvid J, Gorno-Tempini ML. (2008) Frontotemporal lobar degeneration. In: Cappa SF, Abutalebi J, Demonet JF *et al.* (eds). *Cognitive neurology: A clinical textbook*. Oxford: Oxford University Press, 229–50.

Newhart M, Davis C, Kannan V et al. (2009) Therapy for naming deficits in two variants of primary progressive aphasia. *Aphasiology* 23: 823–34.

Nickels L, Croot K. (2009) Progressive language impairments: Intervention and management (Editorial). *Aphasiology* 23: 123–4.

Patterson K, Graham NL, Lambon Ralpha MA, Hodges JR. (2006) Progressive non-fluent aphasia is not a progressive form of (non-fluent) post stroke aphasia. *Aphasiology* 20: 1018–34.

Powell AL, Cummings JL, Hill MA, Benson DF. (1988) Speech and language alterations in multi-infarct dementia. *Neurology* 38: 717–19.

Reisberg B, Ferris SH, De Leon MJ, Crook T. (1982) The global deterioration scale for assessment of primary degenerative dementia. *American Journal of Psychiatry* 139: 1136–9.

Reisberg B, Franssen EH, Hasan SM et al. (1999) Retrogenesis: Clinical, physiologic and pathologic mechanisms in brain ageing Alzheimer's and other dementing processes. *European Archives of Psychiatry and Clinical Neuroscience* 249 (Suppl. 3): 28–36.

Ripich DN, Wykle ML. (1996) *Alzheimer's disease communication guide: The FOCUSED programme for caregivers.* San Antonio: The Psychological Corporation.

Ripich DN, Ziol E, Fritsch T, Durand EJ. (2000) Training Alzheimer's Disease caregivers for successful communication. *Clinical Gerontologist* 21: 37–56.

Royal College of Speech and Language Therapists. (2005) Speech and language therapy provision for people with dementia. *RCSLT position paper.* Available from: www.rcslt.org/resources/publications/dementiapaper.pdf.

Royal College of Speech and Language Therapists. (2007). Communication must be at centre of new dementia strategy: *RCSLT Press release* (8 August 2007). Available from: www.rcslt.org/news/press_releases/newdemntiastrategy

Santo Pietro MJ, Boczko F. (1997) *Communication outcome measure of functional independence (COMFI Scale).* Vero Beach FL: Speech Bin.

Santo Pietro MJ, Boczko F. (2001) The breakfast club. *Alzheimer's Care Quarterly* 2: 56–60.

Santo Pietro MJ. (2002) Training nursing assistants to communicate effectively with people with Alzheimer's disease: A call for action. *Alzheimer's Care Quarterly* 3: 157–64.

Savundranayagam MY, Hummert ML, Montgomery RJ. (2005) Investigating the effects of communication problems on caregiver burden. *The Journals of Gerontology Series B: Psychological Sciences and Social Sciences* 60: S48–55.

Siegel E, Wetherby A. (2000) Nonsymbolic communication. In: Snell M, Brown F (eds). *Instruction of students with severe disabilities*, 5th edn. Upper Saddle River, NJ: Prentice Hall, 409–51.

Speech Pathology Australia. (2003) Aged Care. *SPA Briefing Paper.* Available from: www.speechpathologyaustralia.org.au/library.

Stevens S, Pitt B, Nicholl C et al. (1992) Language assessment in a memory clinic. *International Journal of Geriatric Psychiatry* 7: 45–51.

Tomoeda CK. (2001) Comprehensive assessment for dementia: A necessity for differential diagnosis and management. *Seminars in Speech and Language* 22: 275–89.

Vuorinen E, Laine M, Rinne J. (2000) Common pattern of language impairment in vascular dementia and in Alzheimer's disease. *Alzheimer Disease and Associated Disorders* 14: 81–6.

Watson CM, Chenery HJ, Carter MS. (1999) An analysis of trouble and repair in the natural conversations of people with dementia of the Alzheimer's type. *Aphasiology* 13: 195–218.

Wong SB, Anand R, Chapman SB et al. (2009) When nouns and verbs degrade: facilitating communication in semantic dementia. *Aphasiology* 23: 286–301.

World Health Organisation. (2001) International Classification of Functioning, Disability and Health, Retrieved July 8 2009. Available from: www3.who.int/icf/icftemplate.cfm

23

The role of physiotherapy in the management of dementia

IRENE SMITH LASSEN

23.1 INTRODUCTION

Physiotherapy (PT) is based on the comprehensive and theoretical model of a correlation between motor function and psychosocial development and function in each individual. The human being is a dynamic whole in which interactions occur between biomechanical, neuromuscular, psychomotor and mental functions, between body and mind.

Physiotherapists working in the field of dementia focus their approach on assessment of the body, evaluation of the type and level of strain and resources in the patient and treatment of the physical problems and conditions. Information about physical function contributes to diagnosis and therapy.

Since dementia is highly prevalent among elderly people, patients often have various somatic illnesses, neurological or musculoskeletal problems that may affect their motor function and state of mind. On the other hand these physical conditions may be reinforced by their mental and cognitive dysfunction.

Due to great variation in symptoms in patients with dementia, the PT must be directed to the individual functional ability in order to stimulate and support the patient in achieving a sense of well-being and as much control as possible over their life.

Physiotherapy interventions for people with dementia can take many forms depending on the severity of the illness and the purpose of the contribution, but physical activity should be provided to minimize physical and mental decline. Exercise is associated with improving both cognition and physical performance (Stevens and Killeen, 2006; Christofoletti et al., 2007).

In early dementia, the object of PT is promoting awareness of the body and its possibly hidden resources, working consciously with experiences of the body as a part of the whole identity.

Later in the course, PT can aim at decreasing anxiety and depressive symptoms that may accompany progression of the disease.

Gradually, as the dementia develops and the patient's functions decline, treatment focuses on activating the patient and establishing an environment that maintains and motivates movement and activities of daily living (ADLs).

23.2 THE DEMENTIA SYMPTOMS

Dementia produces a decline in intellectual functioning and usually some interference with personal ADLs. The motor functions are affected in almost every patient in the late stages but in some types of dementia also earlier in the course.

There is a close relationship between gait and cognition, and subtle disturbances in gait can be observed in ageing and in subtypes of dementia that are not known for prominent motor disturbances (Scherder et al., 2007). A thorough study with a large population detected that affected balance and gait function, especially walking speed, may be early dementia symptoms (Li Wang et al., 2006). The most complicated motor functions deteriorate first, whereas the more simple physical tasks (e.g. grip function) are preserved till late in the course.

Depression and anxiety are common reactions to the experience of failing functions. Having depression is not just a matter of the mind but also affects the body. Patients with depression in comparison with non-depressed people have more muscular tension, pain complaints, negative attitude towards own physical ability, restraint breathing and less flexibility and freedom in movements (Jacobsen et al., 2006). These symptoms are easily mixed up with and mistaken for symptoms following somatic illnesses and physical decline due to ageing. In combination with the depressive symptoms, a higher level of anxiety appears, causing pain, provoking tension and unpleasant bodily symptoms.

Due to affected perceptual and sensory function patients frequently have difficulties following instructions and performing ADLs, but cover up their problems.

Agitated and restless behaviour is observed in some patients, especially when perceiving multiple environmental stimuli, while other patients may live a sedentary lifestyle and reach the limit of their physical ability simply in the performance of normal ADLs. Inactivity results in increasing dependency on the help of others.

The physical functions are not debilitated concurrently with the other functions and this creates an area in which patients may achieve an experience of remaining resources and a feeling of success, adding quality to their lives.

23.3   ASSESSMENT

The assessment of the body includes observations and specific tests (e.g. Berg Balance Scale, Timed Up and Go Test, and Katz Index of ADL) and is aiming at identifying the impact of the dementia on the patient's way of moving and breathing, the manner of posture, balance and the muscular tension and strength. Differentiation between natural ageing processes and dementia processes pose unique challenges.

Patients with cognitive impairments are often unable to verbally express discomfort and acknowledge pain. Attention must be paid to assessing pain using observational methods (Buffum et al., 2007).

Collateral information may be gathered from relatives and nursing staff about the patient's personality and earlier interests focusing on physical activity.

23.4   INTERACTION

The importance of interaction between patient and physiotherapist is a central feature in clinical practice and studies have focused on the most important factors for successful treatment. Thornquist (1991) indicates the importance of how the physiotherapist continuously uses her body to communicate. She also points to the problem of interpreting body language as an observer, since a gesture or a posture is dependent on the specific context. Self-experience and clinical experience develops knowledge in the cognitive, affective

and psychomotor domains, and when working with demented people one has to deal with all these domains. According to Watzlawick et al. (1967), all behaviour in an interactional situation has message value and is thereby communication. Even nonsense, silence, withdrawal, immobility (postural silence) or any other form of denial is a communication.

Establishing and maintaining contact focusing on the patient's resources are important aspects in the interaction and are considered vital for outcome (Gyllensten et al., 2000). These might, however, be complicated in the treatment of dementia patients if their motivation fluctuates. Clinical experience and reflecting on communication and the therapeutic process are important tools in interaction and alliance formation.

The sooner in the dementia course that physiotherapy is implemented, the easier it will be to develop an alliance with the patient, which can be maintained over years.

23.5   INTERVENTION

23.5.1   Body awareness therapy

In recent decades, there has been an increasing acknowledgement of how the mind and the body influence each other, and the use of the treatment modality of body awareness therapy (BAT) has been steadily growing within PT practice.

In BAT one uses movements, breathing, massage and awareness to try to restore balance, flexibility and the unity of body and mind working with the resources of the body as a whole. The therapist encourages the patient to move in more optimal ways, using both body and words to guide them. The relation to the ground, vertical balance in the centre line, centring of movements and co-ordination from the solar plexus area, breathing, flow and mental presence and awareness are seen as important aspects trained in basic BAT (Gyllensten, 2001). The movements in BAT are quite simple, fundamental and easy to learn, which makes them very suitable for dementia patients who often lack the ability to understand and perform more complicated exercises. BAT is inspired by Tai Chi and the slow, rhythmic pace of the functionally based Tai Chi-like exercises is recommended in Alzheimer's disease (AD) (Klein, 2008).

Basic BAT consists of movements of the body as a whole in lying, sitting, standing and walking positions. The work usually starts with stretching exercises on the floor or on a couch and breathing exercises aimed at letting go of old compensations and control of the breathing and just letting it be. One progresses to the sitting or standing position and here the work of becoming more aware and in contact with the antigravity muscles continues. The three basic co-ordinations starting in the trunk are practised: flexion-extension around the centre of movement in the solar plexus area, rotation around the vertical axis and trunk rotation and counter-rotation as seen in walking (Roxendal, 1987).

Focusing on activating health-promoting resources rather than on physical symptoms and limitations, BAT is a useful way of thinking and approach in treatment of dementia patients. The features of dementia are disturbances of cognitive functions and the sensorium as well as changes in physical functions, and by initiating BAT in an early stage the basic elements of the movement skills are stimulated and may help the patient maintain functional ability and an experience of identity.

23.5.2   Massage and touching

Treatment is often supplemented by massage. Physical touch stimulates mental and physiological processes. Massage reduces muscle tension, and rhythmical stroking of the skin has a medical effect in consequence of secreting oxytocin: reduced pain sensitivity, anxiety level, blood pressure and pulse, indicating a calm well-being (Uvnäs-Moberg, 2004).

People have a lifelong need for physical touch, and massage is an important way of communication. Touching is an intimate kind of contact that creates a connection between people (Montagu, 1986). Through the hands, the therapist is in contact with respiration, emotionality, movements, tension and changes in tension in the patient. BAT holds special massage techniques that can activate both postural and autonomous reflexes (Mattson, 1998). Tactile skin stimulation evokes a more distinct sensation of the body and its centre, diverting attention from unpleasant thoughts and emotions and is suggested as a non-pharmacological treatment for agitation and motor restlessness. Studies provide support for the efficacy of massage and touch, including reflexology as a treatment of behavioural and emotional conditions (Viggo Hansen et al., 2006; Hodgson and Andersen, 2008) and acupressure is an efficacious method for decreasing agitation behaviours in patients with dementia (Yang et al., 2007).

Elderly dementia patients are in physical contact with nursing staff when washing, dressing, feeding and personal hygiene are taken care of but beyond that, massage can be given with the one purpose that they have a positive bodily experience. The caregivers can profitably be instructed in therapeutic touching techniques to make the nursing situations mutually pleasant. Nursing attendants providing tender touch to nursing home residents reported that most of the residents enjoyed receiving gentle massage, and this type of treatment improved communication with the residents (Sansone and Schmitt, 2000).

23.5.3   Decreasing anxiety and depressive symptoms

Clinical experience in PT treatment of depression and anxiety shows that patients benefit from BAT, including calming massage and relaxation techniques.

Several studies show that physical activity has a positive effect on the mental state, decreasing anxiety and depressive symptoms. Physical training should be individualized and supervised, including aerobic training and progressive resistance training (Singh et al., 1997; Lawler and Hopker, 2001). Blumenthal et al. (1999) found that exercise training in older

depressed patients accelerated the effect of medical treatment and follow up showed a significant decrease in depressive symptoms and fewer relapses. Moderate intensity, chair-based exercise has reduced negative affect in moderate and severe dementia, and both immediate changes and long-term effects of exercise have been revealed (Edwards et al., 2008). There is a positive effect of exercise on mood, and Williams and Tappen (2007) found that patients with AD were in a better mood after a four-month programme of comprehensive exercise compared with walking alone or social conversation.

23.5.4   Mobility and physical activity

Physical ability deteriorates with age, and the physiological and pathological responses to ageing have a direct effect on movement and function. A number of age-induced changes that affect movement or function can be prevented, slowed down or even reversed by exercises (Trew, 1997).

Patients with dementia should be given opportunities for goal-directed movements in a plain and systematic way to maintain mobility and transfer skills (Oddy, 1998). Movement/mobility/transfer can be defined as movements that enable the patient to perform ADLs and to move around in his habitual environment. The results of goal-directed physical training on impaired elderly people with dementia are significant improvements on the ability to walk and transfer, mobility and balance (Toulotte et al., 2003).

A study providing physiotherapy, including a music and movement group, body awareness and functional mobility training, also showed significant improvement on mobility skills of elderly people with severe dementing illness (Pomeroy, 1993).

From clinical experience, weight resistance training is an effective, structured method to mobilize physical resources. Records should be kept to motivate the patients, showing progress and illustrating what they are capable of doing.

Training and maintaining mobility skills can postpone the time when the dementia patient needs personal care and social services. Regular physical exercise should be provided in all dementia stages.

Studies have shown that exercise slowed and reversed disability in some ADLs and may retard the rate of progression of cognitive symptoms of dementia (Stevens and Killeen, 2006). Even significant reduction in behavioural problems, such as wandering, physical and verbal abuse and sleep disorders, has been reported after a moderate intensity exercise programme (Landi et al., 2004).

23.5.5   Communication

To initiate a movement or a transfer, the dementia patient needs to understand the purpose. Approaching the patient slowly from in front prevents him from being surprised or scared, and a friendly smile while keeping a distance can make him feel safe. Commands must be short, concise and simple, instructing the patient in positive phrases. In an explanation the words must accurately describe what is to be done. Demonstrating the movement using gestures, signs and touching may clarify to the patient how to move in the right way and in the right direction. Throughout the session it is important to observe facial expression and body language to receive an impression of how the patient responds to the treatment.

Strategies for helping patients in daily activities are essential to promote mobility. Nursing staff and relatives often lack knowledge about techniques for activating the patient, but through instructions from a physiotherapist they can help arrange facilities creating a safe, stimulating environment drawing on the patient's resources. Guidance and advice for the practical daily care of people with dementia are described in detail by Oddy (1998).

23.5.6 Group activity

In some psychogeriatric wards and nursing homes, movement groups are practised and have proven useful to dementia patients with similar mobility levels. The activity must be structured in a calm, secure atmosphere with adequate lightning, no interrupting background noises and no big empty spaces around the circle in which the patients are placed. Music can be applied to give rhythm and an opportunity to join in the tunes. The patients may not remember the activity from one session to another and must be prepared and invited to participate.

Words and movements applied to the session must be recognizable for the patients: movements that are related to ADLs and awaken memories. The elements are simple exercises stimulating muscle strength, mobility, balance, body awareness and spatial perception. Long instructions must be avoided. For recognition and predictability, several repetitions are carried out for each exercise and the programme is repeated from one session to another comprising:

- mobility training: simple, soft movements related to ADL functions performed in a moderate speed and with the sufficient time during and in between the exercises;
- light aerobic training in order to increase the patient's circulation and staying power;
- simple balance, stability and strength exercises, for example weight transfer sideways sitting on chairs and pushing a medical ball around the circle;
- body awareness and spatial exercises in which the physiotherapist designates the specific body part and direction for the movement;
- non-verbal interaction between the patients by rolling, throwing and kicking a ball or a balloon.

Mobility groups have both medical and economic benefits. The social contact of the group is essential to prevent isolation and a passive life that usually follow reduced motor skills. The patients dare more in the group and, through visual stimulation, it is easier for them to revive the pleasure of movements. Staying in good physical shape may reduce the consumption of medicine and medical costs. In this way, it is possible to add quality of life to the patients.

23.6   SUMMARY

The dementia population is a large and diverse group of patients who present various symptoms of illness, different somatic illnesses, and varying function levels. Treatment must be based on individual ability, capacity and interest. A PT assessment contributes to a broader view of the patient, and, with the therapist's knowledge of the human body and the declining functions due to ageing and dementia, attention can be focused on preventing the consequences and mobilizing existing physical possibilities. Patients benefit from the simplicity of basic BAT applied in individual treatment and exercise groups, activating physical resources and maintaining their motor skills. Positive bodily sensations can be evoked while the dementia causes loss of functions; promoting mobility and stimulating ADLs increases the patients' ability to cope with the dementia. The quality of life gained through physical training results in both personal and economic benefit and physical exercise should be considered in future preventive strategies for dementia.

REFERENCES

Blumenthal JA, Babyak MA, Moore KA et al. (1999) Effects of exercise training on older patients with major depression. *Archives of Internal Medicine.* **159**: 2349–56.

Buffum MD, Hutt E, Chang VT et al. (2007) Cognitive impairment and pain management: review of issues and challenges. *Journal of Rehabilitation Research and Development.* **44**: 315–29.

Christofoletti G, Oliani MM, Gobbi S, Stella F. (2007) Effects of motor intervention in elderly patients with dementia: an analysis of randomized controlled trials. *Topics in Geriatric Rehabilitation.* **23**: 149–54.

Edwards N, Gardiner M, Ritchie DM et al. (2008) Effect of exercise on negative affect in residents in special care with moderate to severe dementia. *Alzheimer Disease and Associated Disorders.* **22**: 362–8.

Gyllensten AL, Gard G, Hansson L, Ekdahl C. (2000) Interaction between patient and physiotherapist in psychiatric care – reflecting the physiotherapist's perspective. *Advances in Physiotherapy.* **2**: 157–67.

Gyllensten AL. (2001) *Basic body awareness therapy. Assessment, treatment and interaction.* Sweden: Lund University.

Hodgson NA, Andersen S. (2008) The clinical efficacy of reflexology in nursing home residents with dementia. *Journal of Alternative and Complementary Medicine.* **14**: 269–75.

Jacobsen LN, Lassen IS, Friis P, Licht R. (2006) Bodily symptoms in patients with severe depression. *Nordic Journal of Psychiatry.* **60**: 294–8.

Klein PJ. (2008) Tai Chi Chuan in the management of Parkinson's disease and Alzheimer's disease. *Medicine and Sport Science.* **52**: 173–81.

Landi F, Russo A, Bernabei R. (2004) Physical activity and behaviour in the elderly: a pilot study. *Archives of Gerontology and Geriatrics Supplement.* **9**: 235–41.

Lawler DA, Hopker SW. (2001) The effectiveness of exercise as an intervention in the management of depression: systematic review and meta-regression analysis of randomised controlled trials. *British Medical Journal.* **322**: 763–7.

Li Wang MS, Larson EB, Bowen JD, van Belle G. (2006) Performance-based physical function and future dementia in older people. *Archives of Internal Medicine.* **166**: 1115–20.

Mattson M. (1998) *Body awareness, applications in physiotherapy.* Sweden: Umeaa University.

Montagu A. (1986) *Touching – the human significance of the skin.* New York: Harper and Row.

Oddy R. (1998) *Promoting mobility for people with dementia; a problem-solving approach.* London: Age Concern.

Pomeroy VM. (1993) The effect of physiotherapy input on mobility skills of elderly people with severe dementing illness. *Clinical Rehabilitation.* **17**: 163–70.

Roxendal G. (1987) *Ett Helhetsperspektiv – Sjukgymnastik i Framtiden* (A holistic perspective – physiotherapy in the future). Lund: Studentlitteratur.

Sansone P, Schmitt L. (2000) Providing tender touch massage to elderly nursing home residents: a demonstration project. *Geriatric Nursing.* **21**: 303–8.

Scherder E, Eggermont L, Swaab D et al. (2007) Gait and ageing and associated dementa; its relationship with cognition. *Neuroscience and Biobehaviour Review.* **31**: 485–97.

Singh NA, Clements KM, Fiatarone MA. (1997) A randomized controlled trial of progressive resistance training in depressed elders. *Journal of Gerontology Series A: Biological Sciences and Medical Sciences.* **52**: M27–35.

Stevens J, Killeen M. (2006) A randomised controlled trial testing the impact of exercise on cognitive symptoms and disability of residents with dementia. *Contemporary Nurse.* **21**: 32–40.

Thornquist E. (1991) Body communication is a continuous process. *Scandinavian Journal of Primary Health Care.* **9**: 191–6.

Toulotte C, Fabre C, Dangemont B et al. (2003) Effects of physical training on the physical capacity of frail, demented patients with a history of falling: a randomised controlled trial. *Age and Ageing.* **32**: 67–73.

Trew M. (1997) The effects of age on human movement. In: Trew M, Everett T (eds). *Human movement. An introductory text.* New York: Churchill Livingstone, 119–28.

Uvnäs-Moberg K. (2004) *The oxytocin factor. Tapping the hormone of calm, love, and healing.* New York: Da Capo Press Inc.

Viggo Hansen N, Jørgensen T, Ørtenblad L. (2006) Massage and touch for dementia. *Cochrane Database Systematic Review.* **18**: CD004989.

Watzlawick P, Weakland JH, Jackson D. (1967) *Pragmatics of human communication. A study of interactional patterns, pathologies and paradoxes.* New York: WW Norton.

Williams CL, Tappen RM. (2007) Effect of exercise on mood in nursing home residents with Alzheimer's disease. *American Journal of Alzheimers Disease and Other Dementia.* **22**: 389–97.

Yang MH, Wu SC, Lin JG, Lin LC. (2007) The efficacy of acupressure for decreasing agitated behaviour in dementia: a pilot study. *Journal of Clinical Nursing.* **16**: 308–15.

Therapeutic effects of music in people with dementia

LINDA A GERDNER AND RUTH REMINGTON

> Awake, arise, listen to the song of life … At first all may seem confusion … but wait, strive to catch the deeper melody, for the song it's there.
>
> Excerpt from *A Song of Life* by Albert J Atkins in 1905

24.1 BEHAVIOURAL AND PSYCHOLOGICAL SYMPTOMS OF DEMENTIA

Over 80 per cent of people with dementia (PWD) will eventually display agitated behaviours (Ellison, 2008). Agitation interferes with care delivery and social interaction, ultimately having a negative impact on the person's quality of life (Léger *et al.*, 2002). Management of these behaviours has been identified as a major stressor to health-care professionals (Brodaty *et al.*, 2003). For these reasons, much of the research that has evaluated the effects of music in PWD has focused on agitation as the primary outcome variable.

The presentation of music can be grouped into the following three categories: classical music or music believed to be calming/relaxing, individualized or preferred music, and music activities implemented by a certified music therapist.

24.2 CLASSICAL MUSIC OR MUSIC BELIEVED TO BE CALMING/RELAXING

Goddaer and Abraham (1994) hypothesized that 'relaxing' music would buffer the 'general noise level' found in dining rooms in long-term care facilities, thus exerting a calming effect which would reduce the frequency of agitated behaviours in 29 people with severe cognitive impairment. Baseline data were collected during week one. Music was played in the dining room daily during the noon meal during week two. Music was removed during week three and reintroduced during week four. A modified version of the Cohen–Mansfield Agitation inventory (CMAI) was used to measure the dependent variable. Significant reductions were observed on the cumulative incidence of total agitated behaviours (63.4 per cent), as well as the cumulative incidence of physically non-aggressive behaviours (56.3 per cent) and verbally agitated behaviours (74.5 per cent).

The findings of this study were replicated using a smaller sample of subjects ($n = 10$) residing in a special care unit (Denny, 1997). Classical music was played from 11.45 a.m. to 1.15 p.m. daily during weeks two and four in the dining room during the noon meal. A modified version of the CMAI was used to measure the dependent variable.

Tabloski and colleagues (1995) used a quasi-experimental design with a convenience sample of 20 cognitively impaired nursing home residents to measure the effects of Kobialka's recording of Pachelbel's Canon in D on the frequency of agitation. The dependent variable was measured using the Agitated Behaviour Scale (ABS; Corrigan, 1989). Agitation was assessed 15 minutes prior to the intervention, during the 15-minute presentation of music, and throughout the 15 minutes following the presentation of music. The intervention and assessment process was repeated approximately 1 week later. Repeated measure analysis of variance (R-ANOVA) revealed a statistically significant reduction in agitated behaviours during ($p < 0.01$) and after the music intervention ($p < 0.05$).

Remington (2002) used a four group, repeated measures experimental design to compare the effects of hand massage (HM) and calming music (CM) on the frequency of agitation in PWD. Agitated nursing home residents were randomly assigned to one of four groups ($n = 17$ each): (1) CM, (2) HM, (3) simultaneous implementation of CM and HM, or (4) control. A new age arrangement of Pachelbel's Canon in D was selected for its calming qualities, such as a slow tempo of 52 beats per minute (instead of 88 to 108 beats per minute in the original orchestral arrangement), soft dynamic levels and repetitive themes. The music did not contain recognizable lyrics or melodies that might evoke emotional responses. Each group received 10 minutes of the identified intervention with the control receiving no intervention. The number of occurrences (frequency) and types of agitated behaviours were recorded for 10 minutes on four occasions using a modified version of the CMAI immediately before the intervention, during the intervention, immediately following the intervention and again 1 hour following the intervention. Findings report a statistically significant reduction in agitated behaviours across all three experimental groups when compared to the control group.

Using a repeated measures design, Thompson *et al.* (2005) compared the effect of music (Vivaldi's Four Seasons, Winter) on language fluency in healthy older adults ($n = 16$) and older adults with dementia ($n = 16$). Subjects were asked to name as many examples of items in a category as they could within 1 minute. Each subject was tested both with music playing and without. Both the healthy subjects and the subjects with dementia demonstrated a similar small but significant improvement in performance when music was played.

24.3   INDIVIDUALIZED MUSIC

Individualized music is defined as music that has been integrated into the person's life and is based on personal preference (Gerdner, 1992). Extensive clinical experience in combination with research findings (Gerdner, 1992) led to the development of a mid-range theory of individualized music intervention for agitation (IMIA; Gerdner, 1997). Elements of the mid-range theory include: cognitive impairment, progressively lowered stress threshold, agitation and individualized music. Cognitive impairment results in a decreased ability to receive and process stimuli, resulting in a progressive decline in the person's stress threshold (Hall and Buckwalter, 1987). Dysfunctional behaviours such as agitation occur when the stress threshold is exceeded (Hall and Buckwalter, 1987). Music may be used as a means of communicating with this population, even in the advanced stages of dementia when the person has difficulty or an inability to understand verbal language and has a decreased ability to interpret environmental stimuli. It is theorized that the presentation of individualized music (carefully selected music, based on personal preference) will provide an opportunity to stimulate remote memory. This changes the focus of attention and provides an interpretable stimulus, overriding stimuli in the environment that is meaningless or confusing. The elicitation of memories associated with positive feelings will have a soothing effect on the person with dementia, which in turn will prevent or alleviate agitation (Gerdner, 1997).

The propositions of this theory were tested using an experimental repeated measures pre-test–post-test crossover design to compare the immediate and residual effects of individualized music to classical 'relaxation' music relative to baseline on the frequency of agitated behaviours in PWD. Thirty-nine subjects were recruited from six long-term care facilities (LTCFs). An interview guide was used to obtain specific information on the subject's musical preference and to identify the importance of music in the subject's life prior to the onset of dementia. If cognitive impairment precluded the subject from completing the form, a family member provided the information. Group A ($n = 16$) received individualized music for 6 weeks followed by a 2-week 'washout' period and 6 weeks of classical relaxation music. Group B ($n = 23$) received the same protocol but in reverse order. Music interventions were presented for 30 minutes, twice a week. A modified version of the CMAI was used to measure the dependent variable. A repeated measures analysis of variance with Bonferroni post hoc test showed a significant reduction in agitation during and following the presentation of individualized music compared to classical music (Gerdner, 2000).

These efforts have resulted in an expanding body of research to support the use of this intervention for the management of agitation in PWD (Ragneskog *et al.*, 2001; Janelli *et al.*, 2002; Suzuki *et al.*, 2004; Sung *et al.*, 2006; Sung *et al.*, 2008; Park and Pringle-Specht, 2009).

Japanese researchers (Suzuki *et al.*, 2004) expanded these efforts by adding functional and biophysiological measures, as well as behavioural outcome measures. The study included ten subjects with dementia who received individualized or preferred music twice a week for 8 weeks. During the corresponding time period, 13 subjects participated in a comparison intervention (games, drawing, pasting pictures). Analysis, comparing baseline to 1-week post intervention scores, found that subjects in the experimental group had a statistically significant improvement in the 'language' subscale of the Mini-Mental State Examination (MMSE) and a statistically significant reduction in 'irritability' as measured by the Multidimensional Observational Scale. In addition, there was a significant reduction in stress index as measured by a salivary chromogranin A (CgA) following session 16. The authors concluded, 'the changes in CgA levels supported Gerdner's mid range theory'. No significant findings occurred in the control group across outcome measures.

Given its efficacy when implemented by research staff, it is important to evaluate the effectiveness of individualized music when implemented by trained staff and family members. As a beginning, Gerdner (2005) conducted a pilot study using a mixed methodology that included both quantitative and qualitative measures. Following appropriate training, staff and family played individualized music for eight PWD living in LTCF. The intervention was implemented over a 4-week period. Individualized music was played daily for 30 minutes at a prescribed time (prior to the estimated 'peak level' of agitation). The mean rate of compliance was 86.3 per cent. In addition, staff administered music on an as-needed basis (when the PWD first began exhibiting signs of agitation). Agitation was measured using a modified version of the CMAI. A statistically significant reduction in agitation was found during the immediate presentation of music, with an overall reduction in agitation found on day shift during weeks 1–8 and on evening shift during weeks 5–8. Staff and family interviews provided convergent validity to quantitative findings. In addition, staff and family reported that individualized music provided a catalyst for meaningful interaction between the PWD and others.

Researchers in Taiwan evaluated nursing staff ($n = 17$) knowledge and adherence to the evidence-based guideline for individualized music. Initial training included an interactive educational programme. Ongoing reminders, a local opinion leader and an audit checklist were used to facilitate and monitor continued adherence to the intervention protocol. Comparison of pre- and post-test scores found a statistically significant improvement ($p < 0.001$) in knowledge of the intervention following the training session with a mean compliance of 72 per cent (Sung et al., 2008). In addition, this study evaluated residents' responses to individualized music as measured by the CMAI (Sung et al., 2006). An experimental group ($n = 32$) received individualized music for 30 minutes, twice per week over 6 weeks, while the control group ($n = 25$) received the usual care with no music. The experimental group had a statistically significant reduction in overall agitation ($t = -2.19$, $p < 0.05$) and physically non-aggressive behaviours ($t = -3.75$, $p < 0.0001$) compared to the control group.

Park and Pringle-Specht (2009) trained 15 family members caring for an older adult with dementia in the home environment on the use of the evidence-based guideline for individualized music (Gerdner, 2007). Outcome measures included the modified CMAI. A quasi-experimental design was used in which individualized music was implemented twice a week for 2 weeks. There was a significant reduction in agitation during the intervention period ($p < 0.05$) compared to baseline and post-intervention periods.

24.3.1 Evidence-based guideline

An evidence-based guideline for the implementation of individualized music by professional health-care providers has been developed and refined over time (Gerdner, 1996, updated 1999, 2001a; Gerdner, 2007a). An evidence grade schema accompanies this guideline. The schema is used to assign a specific grade based on the strength and type of evidence for each recommendation within the guideline. A simplified version of the protocol was developed for consumers (family caregivers) (Gerdner, 2001b; Gerdner, 2007b).

The guideline describes the assessment criteria for use of pre-recorded music for the purpose of alleviating agitation in PWD. The guideline also includes a recommendation for assessing the temporal patterning of agitation so that the timing of the intervention can be tailored to maximize the effects and benefits of the intervention.

24.4 MUSIC THERAPY

Whereas the music interventions described above can be utilized by professional and lay caregivers, music therapy is a discipline in its own right. A music therapist receives advanced training in music, psychology, physiology and music therapy techniques and completes a clinical internship in a college degree programme (Parker, 2009). Music therapy is presented to individuals or groups. Social interaction becomes an important part of the music session. The therapist interacts with group members through singing, eye contact and conversation between songs. Participants benefit from the social stimulation from others in the group.

Familiar group singing during the sun-downing period, late afternoon and early evening, improved mood and social behaviour in four nursing home residents with moderate dementia who exhibited sun-downing syndrome (Lesta and Petocz, 2006). Subjects' mood and social behaviour were assessed before, during and after a 30-minute group singing intervention, using a facility constructed behaviour assessment chart and a mood and social behaviour tool developed by the investigators. The authors concluded that the increased positive social interaction exhibited by the subjects supports Kitwood's (1997) theory of personhood.

A group music therapy intervention reduced agitation in nursing home residents with dementia. Twenty subjects were assigned to receive either 50 minutes of music therapy three times per week for 15 weeks, or no experimental intervention. The experimental group demonstrated a significant reduction in agitated behaviours (Choi et al., 2009).

In a randomized clinical trial, Guetin and colleagues (2009) investigated the effect of individualized music therapy sessions on anxiety and depression in adults with mild to moderate dementia. Subjects were randomly assigned to the treatment group ($n = 15$) receiving weekly sessions of individualized music therapy, or the control group receiving weekly reading sessions for 16 weeks. The individualized music therapy sessions used music of a style chosen by each subject. Subjects in the experimental group were exposed to a 20 minute sequence with a progressive reduction in rhythm, frequency and volume followed by a 're-enlivening' phase. Subjects were assessed for measures of anxiety (Hamilton Scale) and depression (Geriatric Depression Scale) at weeks 1, 4, 16 and 24. Results indicated that anxiety was significantly improved in the music therapy group at week 4 ($p = 0.002$) and week 16 ($p = <0.001$). The effect was sustained for 8 weeks after withdrawal of the intervention ($p = 0.0002$). A non-significant difference in depression was reported for weeks 4 and 8, however a significant reduction in depression from baseline was observed in the music therapy group by week 24 ($p = 0.03$). Although the sample appeared small, it was determined by power analysis to be adequate for a level of significance of 0.05 and power of 0.9.

Ziv and colleagues (2007) examined the effect of background music on both positive and negative behaviours in a

Non-pharmacological therapies to manage behavioural and psychological symptoms of dementia: what works and what doesn't

GILL LIVINGSTON AND CLAUDIA COOPER

25.1 INTRODUCTION

The neuropsychiatric symptoms of dementia (see Chapter 8, Neuropsychiatric aspects of dementia and Chapter 9, Measurement of behaviour disturbance, non-cognitive symptoms and quality of life) (also known as behavioural and psychological symptoms of dementia (BPSD)) include disturbed perception, thought, mood or behaviour (Finkel et al., 1996). Clinically significant neuropsychiatric symptoms occur in about one-third of people with mild and two-thirds with more severe dementia in the community, so effective treatment is a clinical priority (Lyketsos et al., 2000; Ryu et al., 2005). The prevalence of these symptoms rises to about 80 per cent of people with dementia in 24-hour care, so management in these settings is particularly important (Lawlor, 2000; Margallo-Lana et al., 2001). Neuropsychiatric symptoms contribute significantly to caregiver burden (Coen et al., 1997) institutionalization (O'Donnell et al., 2004) and cost of care, and are persistent (Ryu et al., 2005).

Several cluster analyses have been used to define subgroups of neuropsychiatric symptoms – most commonly agitation, psychosis and mood disorder (Ballard et al., 2008). They may have different aetiologies (Bruen et al., 2008), and require different management. Good practice recommendations suggest that non-pharmacological interventions should usually be first-line treatment with management of medical causes (e.g. pain, delirium), followed by environmental causes (such as excess noise; Yaffe, 2007). If the dementia itself is the underlying problem these strategies may not be effective.

Neuropsychiatric symptoms are often treated with psychotropic medications (see Chapter 27, Drug treatments for the behavioural and psychiatric symptoms of dementia). Major concerns have been raised about their safety (particularly antipsychotics; Wang et al., 2005; Schneider et al., 2006) and efficacy (antipsychotics, carbamazepine and cholinesterase inhibitors; Trinh et al., 2003; Schneider et al., 2005; Sink et al., 2005; Howard et al., 2007). Psychological and psychosocial interventions have fewer risks attached, although there is infrequent good evidence of efficacy.

This chapter examines the evidence for each therapy and discusses what works, what does not and what needs more evidence. We draw on evidence from a systematic review (Livingston et al., 2005), to which we refer readers for more details of the papers reviewed, as well as the more recent literature.

25.2 BEHAVIOURAL MANAGEMENT AND COGNITIVE THERAPIES

25.2.1 Behavioural management techniques with patients

In one randomized controlled trial (RCT), 44 participants with dementia received manual guided treatment for the patient and caregiver, and 43 a problem-solving treatment only for the caregiver (Teri et al., 1997). Both interventions were equally successful in improving depressive symptoms immediately and at six-month follow up (Teri, 1994; Teri et al., 1997). Two smaller RCTs also had positive results (Suhr et al., 1999; Benedict et al., 2000). In one, participants had significantly fewer neuropsychiatric symptoms, two months after being taught progressive muscle relaxation. In the other, the behaviour of patients with multiple sclerosis-associated dementia improved with a cognitive behaviour intervention. Two other RCTs employed behavioural management techniques (BMTs). One used a complex intervention that included a variety of techniques (e.g. life review, sensory stimulation, single-word commands and problem-oriented strategies), and was ineffective (Beck et al., 2002). The second used a token economy, which was more effective in reducing 'bizarre' behaviour in patients with severe dementia, but less effective than a milieu treatment (Mishara, 1978).

There was consistent evidence from the larger RCTs that BMTs reduced depressive symptoms and the effects lasted for months, suggesting they are a promising intervention.

25.2.2 Teaching caregivers BMT

Several very disparate studies in terms of outcomes, follow-up length and controls trained caregivers in BMT. One RCT compared BMT with drug management (haloperidol or trazodone) and placebo and found no difference in agitation or global outcome at 16 weeks (Teri et al., 2000). Similarly, teaching BMT to caregivers did not reduce psychotropic drug use or symptom frequency at one year follow up (Weiner et al., 2002). Combined exercise and BMT led to significant improvements in depression at three months but not at two years (Teri et al., 2003). In a smaller pilot RCT, BMT was taught to caregivers with the aim of reducing stimulation in response to specific stressors they identified (Huang et al., 2003). The study compared an intervention of written materials with a home training programme. Care recipients in the second group were less aggressive, but this finding should be interpreted cautiously, as the study was small and raters were not blind to the intervention status.

An excellent, adequately powered RCT trained 'community consultants' to use a structured manual based intervention (the Star–C treatment) (Teri et al., 2005b). These consultants were primary care health workers rather than research professionals, increasing the trial's clinical relevance. The consultants had eight sessions with 95 individual patient/caregiver dyads at home, teaching them to monitor behavioural problems, understand behaviour management and modify antecedents or consequences. They also concentrated on improving caregiver communication, increasing pleasant events and enhancing caregiver support. There were significant improvements, maintained at six months, in caregiver mood and care recipient neuropsychiatric symptoms.

The evidence that the Star–C treatment, and that BMT with caregivers and exercise training with patients, helps neuropsychiatric symptoms is strong, but it is unclear which were the active components. Other findings are inconsistent and it is unclear that solely teaching BMT's principles to

caregivers is efficacious in managing neuropsychiatric symptoms.

25.2.3 Teaching caregivers to change their behaviour

Ten studies (including nine RCTs) evaluated psychoeducation, teaching family caregivers to change their interactions with relatives with dementia. In an RCT of an educational programme for family caregivers, comprising supportive counselling, psychoeducation and training in management strategies, patients' institutionalization rates decreased (Eloniemi-Sulkava et al., 2001). The effect continued for three months but not two years. A smaller trial examining the intervention's effects with individual families found significant improvements at six months in mood and ideational disturbance (McCallion et al., 1999a). One RCT, with 144 people, compared a group intervention to treatment as usual. The difference in neuropsychiatric symptoms at 16 weeks approached significance (Herbert et al., 2003). In a further trial, primarily powered for caregiver's mental health, neuropsychiatric symptoms improved immediately after 12 weeks training in stress management, dementia education and coping skills but no longer reached significance three months later (Marriott et al., 2000). A pilot RCT, with limited power, involved psychoeducation, instruction to caregivers on how to change their interactions with the patient, or both (Burgener et al., 1998). The difference in patients' behaviour at six months again approached significance. Another study examining the effects of caregiver psychoeducation in working with nursing home residents to enhance social activities and self-care; resulted in decreased agitation after six months (Wells et al., 2000).

We can confidently recommend behavioural management techniques providing psychoeducation to caregivers about changing their interactions with patients, because of consistent evidence from excellent, large RCTs and other studies, and the effects last for months.

25.3 DEMENTIA–SPECIFIC THERAPIES

25.3.1 Reminiscence therapy

Reminiscence therapy is a group intervention using material from the past, such as photos or music, to stimulate memory, and help create identity and intimacy. Only two small studies have been carried out. One RCT had ten participants and reported non-significant behavioural improvements when reminiscence therapy was preceded by reality orientation, but not vice versa (Baines et al., 1987). A second, with 20 participants, compared it to both Snoezelen and participants agitation pre- and post-test (Baillon et al., 2004). Neither arm showed a significant improvement in agitation. Similarly, other studies found no benefit of reminiscence therapy (Livingston et al., 2005).

There is no good evidence of benefit from reminiscence therapy for neuropsychiatric symptoms and some evidence of lack of efficacy.

25.3.2   Validation therapy

Validation therapy works on the philosophy of individual uniqueness, in order to help people with dementia resolve conflicts, by validating their feelings rather than concentrating on facts. There is one RCT comprising 88 patients with dementia that compares validation therapy to usual care or a social contact group (Toseland *et al.*, 1997). At one year follow up, there was no difference in outcome from blinded ratings in nursing time or in psychotropic medication and restraint usage. The only other comparison study found no change in behaviour in five patients who served as their own comparisons (Morton and Bleathman, 1991). A Cochrane review of validation therapy in dementia also found insufficient evidence from RCTs to draw conclusions about validation therapy's efficacy for people with dementia (Neal and Barton Wright, 2003).

There is thus no good evidence of benefit for neuropsychiatric symptoms and some evidence of lack of efficacy.

25.3.3   Reality orientation therapy

This is based on the idea that impaired orientation handicaps people with dementia so reminders can improve functioning. There are two RCTs. The stronger ($n = 57$) found no immediate benefit of reality orientation therapy, compared to active ward orientation (Hanley *et al.*, 1981). The smaller trial ($n = 10$) was unconvincing (Baines *et al.*, 1987).

There is no good evidence of benefit of reality orientation therapy and some evidence of lack of efficacy.

25.3.4   Cognitive stimulation therapy

Cognitive stimulation therapy (CST), derived from reality orientation, uses information processing through themed activities to engage people with dementia while providing a group's social benefits. Its main purpose is cognitive but it might benefit neuropsychiatric symptoms. Three of four RCTs of CST (Quayhagen *et al.*, 1995; Quayhagen *et al.*, 2000; Romero and Wenz, 2001; Spector *et al.*, 2001) showed some positive results, although the studies used different follow-up endpoints (immediately after therapy to nine months after therapy). There were early behaviour improvements but by nine months no significant difference was found. One study showed reduced depression, and another showed improvement in quality of life but not mood (Spector *et al.*, 2001; Spector *et al.*, 2003). The final study did not report whether behavioural differences were significant (Quayhagen *et al.*, 2000).

There is inconsistent evidence that CST improves aspects of neuropsychiatric symptoms immediately and for months afterwards.

25.4   EDUCATING STAFF TO MANAGE BEHAVIOURAL PROBLEMS

Seven RCTs investigated staff education in the treatment of neuropsychiatric symptoms. A recent large cluster RCT included 324 people with dementia in residential care who were assigned to either person-centred care, dementia care mapping (both were taught to the staff), or usual care (Chenoweth *et al.*, 2009). Both interventions improved agitation compared with usual care after the four-month treatment phase and over a four-month follow up.

Other studies found similar results. Teaching communication skills reduced patients' aggression at three months and depression at six months (McCallion *et al.*, 1999b); education about dementia and management strategies reduced physical restraint use (Testad *et al.*, 2002) and education about dementia, communication and management strategies with reflective and case-based learning decreased agitation immediately and 20 weeks later (Deudon *et al.*, 2009). The Star programme, discussed above, teaches staff behavioural principles and the residents in the intervention programme showed a significant decrease in affective and other neuropsychiatric symptoms compared to controls (Teri *et al.*, 2005a). A similar pilot study found improvements in non-affective behavioural symptoms (Lichtenberg *et al.*, 2005). Staff education to implement dementia-specific therapies was ineffective (Schrijnemaekers *et al.*, 2002).

Training staff in 24-hour care settings about dementia, respecting the person as an individual, and communication and sometimes behavioural skills is effective in alleviating patient mood disturbance, agitation and aggression immediately and over months.

25.5   PSYCHOSOCIAL INTERVENTIONS

25.5.1   Sensory enhancement

25.5.1.1   MUSIC/MUSIC THERAPY

These interventions (see Chapter 24, Therapeutic effects of music in people with dementia) can be an activity or part of other activities, such as mealtimes or bath times. Of 25 music/music therapy interventions investigating the effect on neuropsychiatric symptoms, seven were small RCTs. All found improvements in apathy, agitation or disruptive behaviour during or immediately after the session with no longer-term effects (Groene, 1993; Lord and Garner, 1993; Korb, 1997; Clark *et al.*, 1998; Gerdner, 2000; Holmes *et al.*, 2006; Garland *et al.*, 2007).

There is consistent evidence that music therapy decreases agitation during sessions and immediately after. There is no evidence that music therapy is useful for longer term treatment of agitation.

25.5.1.2   SNOEZELEN THERAPY/MULTISENSORY STIMULATION

Snoezelen therapy/multisensory stimulation (MSS) combines relaxation and exploration of sensory stimuli, such as lights and sounds, in specially designed rooms for 30–60 minutes, based on the idea that neuropsychiatric symptoms may result from sensory deprivation. There are seven RCTs. The largest recruited 136 patients with moderate to severe dementia randomized to MSS or a control activity (Baker *et al.*, 2003). There was no difference between them on effects on behaviour or mood, and communication/interaction in the short term or up to one month post-intervention. This large trial followed two promising small trials which found (as did other studies) that disruptive or agitated behaviour briefly improved in or outside the treatment setting, but there was no effect after the treatment had stopped (Livingston *et al.*, 2005).

There is very good evidence that Snoezelen has no long-term effects and the immediate effects are no different to those recorded in control activity groups.

25.5.1.3　OTHER SENSORY STIMULATION

There are five RCTs of other sensory stimulation therapies for agitation in dementia. Four weeks of aromatherapy improved agitation compared to placebo in residents with severe dementia (Ballard *et al.*, 2002). A well-designed trial compared hand massage with music, or massage plus music (Remington, 2002). Agitation decreased for an hour after the massage. An RCT of 51 residents with dementia in long-term care found no difference in aggression but decreased agitation immediately in the therapeutic touch group versus simulated therapeutic touch or usual care but not after 24 hours (Hawranik *et al.*, 2008). A smaller RCT comparing 22 patients to 18 controls in a sensory integration programme that emphasized bodily responses found no efficacy (Robichaud *et al.*, 1994). A recent RCT meta-analysis of non-pharmacological treatments found that sensory interventions, defined as aromatherapy, hand massage and a thermal bath, were an effective intervention immediately for agitation (Kong *et al.*, 2009).

There is evidence for short-term benefits of sensory stimulation in agitation but no evidence for sustained usefulness.

25.5.1.4　SIMULATED PRESENCE THERAPY

This involves playing positive autobiographical memories that are audiotaped (usually by a relative) over the phone. RCTs found no or very little improvement in agitated or withdrawn behaviours (Miller *et al.*, 2001; Garland *et al.*, 2007; Zetteler, 2008).

There is very limited evidence that this intervention works immediately and none for longer term efficacy.

25.5.1.5　VISUALLY COMPLEX ENVIRONMENTS

Nine studies investigated the effects of complex or distracting visual patterns near or on the exit (Livingston *et al.*, 2005). Most were in institutions, extremely small, with 12 or fewer participants and no control group.

Although there are no RCTs of attempts to reduce wandering in either domestic or ward environment (Hermans *et al.*, 2007), there is a consistent effect that a complex environment which makes the exit less clear decreases attempts to leave.

25.5.2　Structured activity

25.5.2.1　THERAPEUTIC ACTIVITY PROGRAMMES

There are six RCTs of therapeutic activities. In a small RCT, therapeutic activities at home were associated with significant decreases in agitation (Fitzsimmons and Buettner, 2002). Another study found that small group discussion and being carried on a bicycle pedalled by volunteers alleviated patients' depression but not agitation at 10 weeks (Buettner and Fitzsimmons, 2002). Four RCTs found no effects of puzzle play and games (three studies) or structured activity (one study) on social interaction, mood and behaviour (Lord and Garner, 1993; Lawton *et al.*, 1998; Baker *et al.*, 2001; Baker *et al.*, 2003).

All the non-RCT studies of therapeutic activities found that activities were ineffective or harmful (Livingston *et al.*, 2005). Weekly activity groups led by nursing assistants found no behavioural changes but a reduction in the use of restraints and drugs; suggesting perhaps that interaction changed the way the staff reacted with patients, rather than their behaviour (Martichuski *et al.*, 1996).

Therapeutic activity encompassed disparate interventions. It is not clear whether they were tailored to individuals' understanding level. Overall, the evidence is inconsistent and inconclusive.

25.5.2.2　MONTESSORI ACTIVITIES

These emphasize the importance of clinician observation to ensure that activity is appropriate. It progresses from simple to complex activities. Three small non-RCTs totalling 32 participants found no change in depression and agitation (Livingston *et al.*, 2005).

There is no evidence to use this intervention.

25.5.2.3　EXERCISE

Exercise as an intervention for neuropsychiatric symptoms was examined in five studies. A well-conducted RCT found no effects on behaviour when one caregiver walked, or walked and talked with two residents (Cott *et al.*, 2002). A Psychomotor Activation Program (PAP) RCT involved 134 residents in 11 'group care' homes (Hopman-Rock *et al.*, 1999). PAP comprises sporting activities such as ball playing and hockey sitting down. There was a trend for behaviour to improve, but the high drop-out due to illness considerably reduced power. Three non-RCTs reported some decrease in agitation or abusive behaviour (Namazi *et al.*, 1994; Holmberg, 1997; Landi *et al.*, 2004).

Not all exercise is the same. Walking up and down corridors seems ineffective, whereas a more varied programme of activity in a social environment requires further research.

25.6　WHAT WORKS, WHAT DOES NOT AND WHAT NEEDS MORE EVIDENCE?

Summarizing the evidence, there are several psychological and behavioural treatment for which we have excellent evidence of efficacy in alleviating neuropsychiatric symptoms immediately and over the longer term.

25.6.1   Immediate and longer term treatment

We can be confident that teaching family carers how to react to neuropsychiatric symptoms; coping strategies including ensuring they have emotional support; and the principles of BMT is effective in managing neuropsychiatric symptoms. It is, however, unclear whether the whole package is essential. In contrast, teaching the principles of BMT to caregivers as a sole intervention is of doubtful efficacy. However, professionals (as opposed to families) using principles of BMT with people with dementia decreases depressive symptoms.

As with family carers, there is excellent evidence that training staff in 24-hour care settings about dementia, respecting the person as an individual, communication and sometimes behavioural skills is effective in alleviating patient mood disturbance, agitation and aggression immediately and over months.

25.6.2   Immediate treatment

There is very consistent evidence that sensory treatments are immediately calming – including music, aromatherapy and hand massage, but there are no long-term benefits. Snoezelen may fall in to the same category but is practically difficult, may be less efficacious and certainly has no additional benefit.

25.6.3   What does not work

There is no evidence that the dementia-specific therapies reminiscence therapy, reality orientation and validation therapy help neuropsychiatric symptoms and some evidence that they do not.

25.6.4   What needs more evidence

There is some promise in exercise (probably in a social setting), therapeutic activity and cognitive stimulation, but more evidence is needed. Visually altering the environment also shows promise in reducing people trying to exit, although it is unclear whether this reduces agitation or just the ability to find the exit.

Overall we judge that effective tools are available to treat neuropsychiatric symptoms in dementia but the systems are not yet in place where they can be routinely available. Finding ways in which management strategies can be effectively and efficiently delivered must now be a high priority.

REFERENCES

Baillon S, Van Diepen E, Prettyman R *et al.* (2004) A comparison of the effects of Snoezelen and reminiscence therapy on the agitated behaviour of patients with dementia. *International Journal of Geriatric Psychiatry* **19**: 1047–52.

Baines S, Saxby P, Ehlert K. (1987) Reality orientation and reminiscence therapy. A controlled cross-over study of elderly confused people. *British Journal of Psychiatry* **151**: 222–31.

Baker R, Bell S, Baker E *et al.* (2001) A randomized controlled trial of the effects of multi-sensory stimulation (MSS) for people with dementia. *British Journal of Clinical Psychology* **40**: 81–96.

Baker R, Holloway J, Holtkamp CCM *et al.* (2003) Effects of multi-sensory stimulation for people with dementia. *Journal of Advanced Nursing* **43**: 465–77.

Ballard CG, O'Brien JT, Reichelt K *et al.* (2002) Aromatherapy as a safe and effective treatment for the management of agitation in severe dementia: The results of a double-blind, placebo-controlled trial with Melissa. *Journal of Clinical Psychiatry* **63**: 553–8.

Ballard C, Day S, Sharp S *et al.* (2008) Neuropsychiatric symptoms in dementia: Importance and treatment considerations. *International Review of Psychiatry* **20**: 396–404.

Beck CK, Vogelpohl TS, Rasin JH *et al.* (2002) Effects of behavioral interventions on disruptive behavior and affect in demented nursing home residents. *Nursing Research* **51**: 219–28.

Benedict RHB, Shapiro A, Priore R *et al.* (2000) Neuropsychological counseling improves social behavior in cognitively-impaired multiple sclerosis patients. *Multiple Sclerosis* **6**: 391–6.

Bruen PD, McGeown WJ, Shanks MF *et al.* (2008) Neuroanatomical correlates of neuropsychiatric symptoms in Alzheimers disease. *Brain* **131**: 2455–63.

Buettner LL, Fitzsimmons S. (2002) AD-venture program: therapeutic biking for the treatment of depression in long-term care residents with dementia. *American Journal of Alzheimer's Disease and Other Dementias* **17**: 121–7.

Burgcncr SC, Bakas T, Murray C *et al.* (1998) Effective caregiving approaches for patients with Alzheimer's disease. *Geriatric Nursing* **19**: 121–6.

Chenoweth L, King MT, Jeon YH *et al.* (2009) Caring for Aged Dementia Care Resident Study (CADRES) of person-centred care, dementia-care mapping, and usual care in dementia: a cluster-randomised trial. *Lancet Neurology* **8**: 317–25.

Clark ME, Lipe AW, Bilbrey M. (1998) Use of music to decrease aggressive behaviors in people with dementia. *Journal of Gerontological Nursing* **24**: 10–17.

Coen R, Swanwick G, O'Boyle C *et al.* (1997) Behaviour disturbance and other predictors of caregiver burden in Alzheimer's Disease. *International Journal of Geriatric Psychiatry* **12**: 331–6.

Cott CA, Dawson P, Sidani S *et al.* (2002) The effects of a walking/talking program on communication, ambulation, and functional status in residents with Alzheimer disease. *Alzheimer Disease and Associated Disorders* **16**: 81–7.

Deudon A, Maubourguet N, Gervais X *et al.* (2009) Non-pharmacological management of behavioural symptoms in nursing homes. *International Journal of Geriatric Psychiatry* **24**: 1386–95.

Eloniemi-Sulkava U, Notkola IL, Hentinen M *et al.* (2001) Effects of supporting community-living demented patients and their caregivers: a randomized trial. *Journal of the American Geriatrics Society* **49**: 1282–7.

Finkel S, Costa e Silva J, Cohen G *et al.* (1996) Behavioral and psychological signs and symptoms of dementia: a consensus statement on current knowledge and implications for research and treatment. *International Psychogeriatrics* **8**: 497–500.

Fitzsimmons S, Buettner LL. (2002) Therapeutic recreation interventions for need-driven dementia-compromised behaviors in community-dwelling elders. *American Journal of Alzheimer's Disease and Other Dementias* **17**: 367–81.

Garland K, Beer E, Eppingstall B *et al.* (2007) A comparison of two treatments of agitated behavior in nursing home residents with dementia: Simulated family presence and preferred music. *American Journal of Geriatric Psychiatry* ; **15**: 514–21.

Gerdner LA. (2000) Effects of individualized versus classical 'relaxation' music on the frequency of agitation in elderly persons with Alzheimer's disease and related disorders. *International Psychogeriatrics* **12**: 49–65.

Groene RW. (1993) Effectiveness of music therapy. 1:1 intervention with individuals having senile dementia of the Alzheimer's type. *Journal of Music Therapy* **30**: 138–57.

Hanley IG, McGuire RJ, Boyd WD. (1981) Reality orientation and dementia: a controlled trial of two approaches. *British Journal of Psychiatry* **138**: 10–14.

Hawranik P, Johnston P, Deatrich J. (2008) Therapeutic touch and agitation in individuals with Alzheimer's disease. *Western Journal of Nursing Research* **30**: 417–34.

Herbert R, Levesque L, Vezina J *et al.* (2003) Efficacy of a psychoeducative group program for caregivers of demented persons living at home: a randomized controlled trial. *Journal of Gerontology Series B – Psychological Sciences and Social Sciences* **58**: S58–67.

Hermans DG, Htay UH, McShane R. (2007) Non-pharmacological interventions for wandering of people with dementia in the domestic setting. *Cochrane Database of Systematic Reviews* **1**: CD005994.

Holmberg SK. (1997) Evaluation of a clinical intervention for wanderers on a geriatric nursing unit. *Archives of Psychiatric Nursing* **11**: 21–8.

Holmes C, Knights A, Dean C *et al.* (2006) Keep music live: music and the alleviation of apathy in dementia subjects. *International Psychogeriatrics* **18**: 623–30.

Hopman-Rock M, Staats PGM, Tak ECPM *et al.* (1999) The effects of a psychomotor activation programme for use in groups of cognitively impaired people in homes for the elderly. *International Journal of Geriatric Psychiatry* **14**: 633–42.

Howard RJ, Juszczak E, Ballard CG *et al.* (2007) Donepezil for the treatment of agitation in Alzheimer's disease. *New England Journal of Medicine* **357**: 1382–92.

Huang HL, Shyu YI, Chen MC *et al.* (2003) A pilot study on a home-based caregiver training program for improving caregiver self-efficacy and decreasing the behavioral problems of elders with dementia in Taiwan. *International Journal of Geriatric Psychiatry* **18**: 337–45.

Kong EH, Evans LK, Guevara JP. (2009) Nonpharmacological intervention for agitation in dementia: A systematic review and meta-analysis. *Aging and Mental Health* **13**: 512–20.

Korb C. (1997) The influence of music therapy on patients with a diagnosed dementia. *Canadian Journal of Music Therapy* **5**: 26–54.

Landi F, Russo A, Bernabei R. (2004) Physical activity and behavior in the elderly: A pilot study. *Archives of Gerontology and Geriatrics* **9**: 235–41.

Lawlor B. (2000) Managing behavioural and psychological symptoms in dementia. *British Journal of Psychiatry* **181**: 463–5.

Lawton MP, Van Haitsma K, Klapper J *et al.* (1998) A stimulation-retreat special care unit for elders with dementing illness. *International Psychogeriatrics* **10**: 379–95.

Lichtenberg PA, Kemp-Havican J, MacNeill SE *et al.* (2005) Pilot study of behavioral treatment in dementia care units. *Gerontologist* **45**: 406–10.

Livingston G, Johnston K, Katona C *et al.* (2005) Systematic review of psychological approaches to the management of neuropsychiatric symptoms of dementia. *American Journal of Psychiatry* **162**: 1996–2021.

Lord TR, Garner JE. (1993) Effects of music on Alzheimer patients. *Perceptual and Motor Skills* **76**: 451.

Lyketsos CG, Steinberg M, Tschanz JT *et al.* (2000) Mental and behavioral disturbances in dementia: findings from the Cache County Study on Memory and Aging. *American Journal of Psychiatry* **157**: 708–14.

McCallion P, Toseland RW, Freeman K. (1999a) An evaluation of a family visit education program. *Journal of the American Geriatrics Society* **47**: 203–14.

McCallion P, Toseland RW, Lacey D *et al.* (1999b) Educating nursing assistants to communicate more effectively with nursing home residents with dementia. *Gerontologist* **39**: 546–58.

Margallo-Lana M, Reichelt K, Hayes P *et al.* (2001) Longitudinal comparison of depression, coping, and turnover among NHS and private sector staff caring for people with dementia. *British Medical Journal* **322**: 769–70.

Marriott A, Donaldson C, Tarrier N *et al.* (2000) Effectiveness of cognitive-behavioural family intervention in reducing the burden of care in carers of patients with Alzheimer's disease. *British Journal of Psychiatry* **176**: 557–62.

Martichuski DK, Bell PA, Bradshaw B. (1996) Including small group activities in large special care units. *Journal of Applied Gerontology* **15**: 224–37.

Miller S, Vermeersch PE, Bohan K *et al.* (2001) Audio presence intervention for decreasing agitation in people with dementia. *Geriatric Nursing* **22**: 66–70.

Mishara BL. (1978) Geriatric patients who improve in token economy and general milieu treatment programs: a multivariate analysis. *Journal of Consulting and Clinical Psychology* **46**: 1340–8.

Morton I, Bleathman C. (1991) The effectiveness of validation therapy in dementia – a pilot study. *International Journal of Geriatric Psychiatry* **6**: 327–30.

Namazi KH, Gwinnup PB, Zadorozny CA. (1994) A low intensity exercise/movement program for patients with Alzheimer's disease: The TEMP-AD protocol. *Journal of Aging and Physical Activity* **2**: 80–92.

Neal M, Barton Wright P. (2003) Validation therapy for dementia. *Cochrane Database of Systematic Reviews* 3: CD001394.

O'Donnell B, Drachman D, Barned H. (2004) Incontinence and troublesome behaviour predict institutionalisation in dementia. *Journal of Geriatric Psychiatry and Neurology* 5: 45–52.

Quayhagen MP, Quayhagen M, Corbeil RR *et al.* (1995) A dyadic remediation program for care recipients with dementia. *Nursing Research* 44: 153–9.

Quayhagen MP, Quayhagen M, Corbeil RR *et al.* (2000) Coping with dementia: evaluation of four nonpharmacologic interventions. *International Psychogeriatrics* 12: 249–65.

Remington R. (2002) Calming music and hand massage with agitated elderly. *Nursing Research* 51: 317–25.

Robichaud L, Hebert R, Desrosiers J. (1994) Efficacy of a sensory integration program on behaviors of inpatients with dementia. *American Journal of Occupational Therapy* 48: 355–60.

Romero B, Wenz M. (2001) Self-maintenance therapy in Alzheimer's disease. *Neuropsychological Rehabilitation* 11: 333–55.

Ryu SH, Katona C, Rive B *et al.* (2005) Persistence of and changes in neuropsychiatric symptoms in Alzheimer disease over 6 months – The LASER-AD study. *American Journal of Geriatric Psychiatry* 13: 976–83.

Schneider LS, Dagerman KS, Insel P *et al.* (2005) Risk of death with atypical antipsychotic drug treatment for dementia: meta-analysis of randomized placebo-controlled trials. *Journal of the American Medical Association* 294: 1934–43.

Schneider LS, Dagerman K, Insel PS. (2006) Efficacy and adverse effects of atypical antipsychotics for dementia: Meta-analysis of randomized, placebo-controlled trials. *American Journal of Geriatric Psychiatry* 14: 191–210.

Schrijnemaekers V, van Rossum E, Candel M *et al.* (2002) Effects of emotion-oriented care on elderly people with cognitive impairment and behavioral problems. *International Journal of Geriatric Psychiatry* 17: 926–37.

Sink KM, Holden KF, Yaffe K. (2005) Pharmacological treatment of neuropsychiatric symptoms of dementia – A review of the evidence. *Journal of the American Medical Association* 293: 596–608.

Spector A, Orrell M, Davies S *et al.* (2001) Can reality orientation be rehabilitated? Development and piloting of an evidence-based programme of cognition-based therapies for people with dementia. *Neuropsychological Rehabilitation* 11: 377–9.

Spector A, Thorgrimsen L, Woods B *et al.* (2003) Efficacy of an evidence-based cognitive stimulation therapy programme for people with dementia: Randomised controlled trial. *The British Journal of Psychiatry* 183: 248–54.

Suhr J, Anderson S, Tranel D. (1999) Progressive muscle relaxation in the management of behavioural disturbance in Alzheimer's disease. *Neuropsychological Rehabilitation* 9: 31–44.

Teri L. (1994) Behavioral treatment of depression in patients with dementia. *Alzheimer Disease and Associated Disorders* 8 (Suppl 3): 66–74.

Teri L, Logsdon RG, Uomoto J *et al.* (1997) Behavioral treatment of depression in dementia patients: a controlled clinical trial. *Journals of Gerontology. Series B. Psychological Sciences and Social Sciences* 52: 159–66.

Teri L, Logsdon RG, Peskind E *et al.* (2000) Treatment of agitation in AD: a randomized, placebo-controlled clinical trial. *Neurology* 55: 1271–8.

Teri L, Gibbons L, McCurry S *et al.* (2003) Exercise plus behavioral management in patients with Alzheimer's Disease A randomised controlled trial. *Journal of the American Medical Association* 290: 2015–22.

Teri L, Huda P, Gibbons L *et al.* (2005a) STAR: A dementia-specific training program for staff in assisted living residences. *Gerontologist* 45: 686–93.

Teri L, McCurry SM, Logsdon R *et al.* (2005b) Training community consultants to help family members improve dementia care: A randomized controlled trial. *Gerontologist* 45: 802–11.

Testad I, Aarsland D, Aasland AM. (2002) The effect of staff training on the use of restraint in dementia: A single-blind randomised controlled trial. *Neurobiology of Aging* 23: 175.

Toseland RW, Diehl M, Freeman K *et al.* (1997) The impact of validation group therapy on nursing home residents with dementia. *Journal of Applied Gerontology* 16: 31–50.

Trinh NH, Hoblyn J, Mohanty SU *et al.* (2003) Efficacy of cholinesterase inhibitors in the treatment of neuropsychiatric symptoms and functional impairment in Alzheimer disease – A meta-analysis. *Journal of the American Medical Association* 289: 210–16.

Wang PS, Schneeweiss S, Avorn J *et al.* (2005) Risk of death in elderly users of conventional vs. atypical antipsychotic medications. *New England Journal of Medicine* 353: 2335–41.

Weiner MF, Tractenberg RE, Sano M *et al.* (2002) No long-term effect of behavioral treatment on psychotropic drug use for agitation in Alzheimer's disease patients. *Journal of Geriatric Psychiatry and Neurology* 15: 95–8.

Wells DL, Dawson P, Sidani S *et al.* (2000) Effects of an abilities-focused program of morning care on residents who have dementia and on caregivers. *Journal of the American Geriatrics Society* 48: 442–9.

Yaffe K. (2007) Treatment of neuropsychiatric symptoms in patients with dementia. *New England Journal of Medicine* 357: 1441–3.

Zetteler J. (2008) Effectiveness of simulated presence therapy for individuals with dementia: A systematic review and meta-analysis. *Aging and Mental Health* 12: 779–85.

26

A predominantly psychosocial approach to behaviour problems in dementia: treating causality

MICHAEL BIRD

26.1 INTRODUCTION AND CONCEPTUAL BACKGROUND

There are frequent injunctions to try psychosocial methods first when treating challenging behaviour associated with dementia (e.g. Howard *et al.*, 2001; Sink *et al.*, 2005), mainly because meta-analyses over two decades show that psychotropic medications, in particular anti-psychotics, have modest effects and frequent side-effects (Schneider *et al.*, 1990; Sink *et al.*, 2005; Schneider *et al.*, 2006). Unfortunately, the clinician seeking a ready-made psychosocial equivalent faces a problem. First, reviews of what are often presented as standardized approaches, such as Snoezelen or staff education, conclude that some show promise but that evidence for their effectiveness is weak (e.g. Landreville *et al.*, 2006; O'Connor *et al.*, 2009). Second, psychosocial interventions are not analogous to medication, and it is misleading to present them as such. Even methods which appear conceptually close (e.g. bright-light therapy) can only be effective in interaction with significant input from other psychosocial modalities, such as the dementia-specific interpersonal skills required to keep participants engaged.

The search for a 'magic pill' (Sink *et al.*, 2005), whether pharmacological or psychosocial, appears to be based on a model which posits standard treatments such as music therapy or risperidone for standard syndromes. The syndromes are usually defined by check-lists such as the Cohen-Mansfield Agitation Inventory (Cohen-Mansfield *et al.*, 1989) or Neuropsychiatric Inventory (Cummings *et al.*, 1994). The consequence is a diverse array of behavioural phenomena clustered under a single label such as behavioural and psychological symptoms of dementia (BPSD) or agitation, and

that the behaviour alone becomes the target of treatment. The problem with this simplistic model, and a major reason why standardized psychopharmacological and psychosocial methods have modest effects, is that it takes little account of the complexities of aetiology. There is abundant evidence that the causes of challenging behaviour in dementia are very diverse and case-specific and, equally, that multiple factors cause behaviour to be perceived as 'challenging' by individual family carers or care staff.

With regard to causal factors of behaviour, though certain phenomena are strongly associated with specific diagnoses (e.g. gorging food in fronto-temporal dementia; Hodges, 2007), only a fraction of the behaviours encountered in everyday practice can be explained by focal brain lesions. There are multiple other causal factors both internal and external to the patient, many of which have nothing to do with dementia *per se*, and which vary from case to case. As a consequence, the same causal factors can produce different behaviours (Moniz-Cook *et al.*, 2001a), or the same behaviour can have different causes. For example, the aetiology of sleep disturbance or night-wandering can be due to staff waking residents up (Schnelle *et al.*, 1999); excessive sleep during the day (Ancoli-Israel *et al.*, 1989); being unable to find the toilet at night (Ersser *et al.*, 1999); the person's premorbid night-time regimes (Bird and Moniz-Cook, 2007); or changes in staff schedules (Cohen-Mansfield *et al.*, 1992).

Extreme variability applies equally to the reasons carers are distressed by the behaviour; there is not a one-to-one relationship between disturbed behaviour and carer distress. Faced with the same behaviour by the same person in residential care, one nurse can see it as extreme, another as no problem (Bird *et al.*, 2007). This is a critical factor because it is usually care-giver distress and failure to cope which leads to referral to health professionals and makes a given situation a 'case'. It is therefore an obvious, though often ignored, clinical target to help resolve the case.

This is not to say that dementia is not a causal factor. Its effects play a part in most cases, for example reduced emotional control, cognitive impairment making it difficult to make sense of the world, and increasingly circumscribed ways of expressing distress. But the effects of dementia, which are not usually amenable to change, rarely cause the behaviour by themselves. They interact with other causal factors – many of which are adjustable – to produce the behaviour. It is the job of the clinician to identify and address causes which are amenable to change.

If a complex interaction of behaviour causes and caregiver factors create a case, it means that standard psychopharmacological or psychosocial strategies will only be effective in a limited number of situations – exactly as the literature shows. Accordingly, the focus of this chapter is the idiosyncratic case-specific approach. The first published case-specific trial was by Hinchliffe et al. (1995), using patients still living at home. More recently, there has been a surge in such trials, most in residential care where more florid behaviours occur. Case-specific studies generally have more robust methodology than most trials of standard psychosocial therapies, and show better results.

Fossey et al. (2006) achieved reductions in anti-psychotic use in residential care. Davison et al. (2006) obtained reductions in frequency and perceived severity of behaviour, staff burden and frequency of GP call-outs. Cohen-Mansfield et al., (2007) found significant reductions in disturbed behaviour and increases in participant affect relative to a control group. Bird et al. (2007) compared a case-specific approach in residential care, using predominantly but not exclusively psychosocial methods, with a control group treated predominantly with psychotropic medication. Both approaches took the same number of clinical visits and produced equivalent reductions in staff stress and behaviour frequency and severity, but the case-specific approach involved much fewer medication changes and drug side effects. In addition, all but one participant could be treated in situ while more than 20 per cent of the control group spent extended periods as psychogeriatric in-patients. Use of antipsychotics declined in the case-specific group and increased in the control group. The difference in approach could not be explained by patient or behaviour variables.

Case-specific studies, by definition, recognize that many factors feed into challenging behaviour, for example delirium or pain, insensitive personal care, depression, boredom (e.g. Cohen-Mansfield et al., 2007) and that causal factors should be treated first. Many writers in the psychopharmacological literature (e.g. Sink et al., 2005) also urge treatment of causal factors before using psychotropic medication, though the main focus is on medical/physical causes with everything else lumped into a vague entity called 'environmental'. The remainder of this chapter is therefore a brief guide to the main medical/physical and psychosocial domains which must be assessed in order to identify and address adjustable causes of challenging behaviour in dementia.

26.2   INTRODUCTION TO ASSESSMENT: UNDERSTANDING THE BEHAVIOUR

If challenging behaviour is the end product of interactions between causal variables idiosyncratic to each case, clinicians must come armed not with pre-conceived answers like behaviour therapy or anti-psychotics, but with a bagful of questions. Answers to these questions can often be obtained from those who know the patient best, for example family members, friends and direct care staff in residential facilities. The latter are often ignored even though they are exposed most often to the behaviour. Some will already have devised techniques which will form part of the intervention, so it is doubly absurd to exclude them. In residential care, progress and doctors' notes, including medication sheets, will provide important information. Another essential source is the person with dementia, using direct discussion where possible, focused attention (e.g. to the content of vocalizations), behavioural observation and behavioural experiments.

The purpose of assessment is to determine the nature and causes of the problem and, concurrently, to devise an intervention package which addresses factors most amenable to change. There are multiple potential causal factors, anything from constipation to staff morale. For the purposes of this chapter, they are clustered into four assessment domains, first, the behaviour. Once enough is known about the behaviour and its context, three potential causal areas must be investigated: the person with dementia, the quality of care and carer characteristics, and the physical sensory and social environment (see **Table 26.1**). Note that these are artificial divisions. Each area can interact with any other, and many other categorizations are possible. Most clinicians who used the case-specific approach quickly develop a gestalt – focusing with increasing efficiency on the main issues once the behaviour has been analysed.

26.2.1   The behaviour

Detailed assessment of the behaviour is critical. Understanding its characteristics, context and effects helps the clinician to decide whether intervention is necessary and, if so, which potential causal domains to examine first (see **Table 26.2**).

26.2.1.1   NATURE, SEVERITY, RISK

The clinician needs to know what the person with dementia is actually doing to have caused the referral. Terms like 'agitation' provide absolutely no information. Even the term 'aggression' means little. It can range from dangerous physical attacks to swearing at an insensitive staff member during personal care, in which case the intervention is likely to focus on the care-giver. Asked about a case of repetitive questions, a domestic staff member said:

> He keeps asking (expletive) stupid questions a million times a day, and it's driving me up the (expletive) wall.

This is a much more precise and clinically useful description of a behaviour and its effects than anything found in a behaviour

Table 26.1 Assessment domains.

The behaviour	What the person is actually doing to cause distress, who is distressed, severity and risk, how long it has been going on and the situations in which it occurs
The person with dementia	Physical medical and psychosocial characteristics of the person manifesting the behaviour
Quality of care and carer characteristics	Quality of care and characteristics of those providing it (e.g. dementia knowledge and skills, attitude, level of burnout/willingness to change, level of support available)
Physical, sensory, social environment	Aspects of the physical and social environment which may impinge on the individual (e.g. glare, noise, facilities like toilet or room difficult to find, uncongenial room or table-mates)

Table 26.2 Suggested domains to address first based on characteristics of the behaviour.

Behaviour characteristics	Suggested causal domains to investigate
Relatively sudden onset or exacerbation	*Person with dementia* (e.g. delirium or other medical problems, medication changes, recent undetected injury)
	Quality of care/carer characteristics (e.g. new staff member with deficient skills or sensitivity; staff shortages making care more hurried)
	Physical/sensory or social environment (e.g. recent change of room, change in furniture layout, loss of another resident)
Increase in severity at certain times of day	*Person with dementia* (e.g. escalating pain, boredom)
	Quality of care/carer characteristics (e.g. staff at handover discussing going home at handover; less skilled night staff)
	Physical/sensory or social environment (e.g. absent or inadequate orientation cues at night; busy noisy times such as meals; high or low temperature at certain times of day)
Only occurs in personal care or when particular parts of the body are touched or in specific body positions	*Person with dementia* (e.g. physical problems such as pain; modesty/fear – perceives it as assault)
	Quality of care/carer characteristics (e.g. ignorance of or insensitivity to patient's emotional response, failure to talk the patient through the procedure; ignorance of pain or lack of care when touching painful areas)
Only some staff stressed by the behaviour	*Quality of care/carer characteristics* (e.g. behaviour only occurs with them because they lack the skills; those stressed lack knowledge of dementia, or the fact that behaviour has causes; those stressed perceive that the patient is suffering but feel unable to help)
Occurs only in certain areas	*Physical/sensory or social environment* (e.g. noisy or confusing areas; glare; points where walking surface changes; too many people or too much activity there)
Occurs only with some staff	*Quality of care/carer characteristics* (e.g. carers noisy, confrontational, hurried, rough or otherwise unskilled; patient dislikes these staff because they are reminded of incidents or people in the past)
Behaviour appears mild but carers significantly distressed	*Carer characteristics* (e.g. carer has limited knowledge of or tolerance for common phenomena in dementia; carer is depressed or burnt out)

check list, and certainly more useful than 'chronic psycho-motor agitation', which was what it said on the referral form.

At this stage, some estimate of frequency and severity may help. Frequency estimates will usually be unreliable and will differ widely between staff in residential care (McCann *et al.*, 1997; Bird *et al.*, 2007) but, collectively, they give some idea of impact, and it is important from the outset to be listening to and empathizing with those facing the behaviour every day. It is also useful in assessing risk. Though cases of severe harm to the patient or others are relatively rare, it is sometimes necessary to ensure immediate safety. This can include specialing, locking doors, some degree of sedation (but only until the case is properly assessed) or referral to an in-patient unit.

26.2.1.2 DISTRESS OR DANGER TO THE PERSON WITH DEMENTIA

Many disturbed behaviours are manifestations of distress by the person with dementia (Cohen-Mansfield *et al.*, 2007). Sensitive care staff often know whether the patient is suffering, and reasonable hypotheses can also be formed through observation of facial expressions, body posture or from what the patient says. For example, pain and depression are common causes of challenging behaviour (Cohen-Mansfield and Werner, 1999), as are fear or anger about physical intrusion during intimate personal care. Even if the person with dementia does not appear distressed, consequences can cause distress or danger. Examples include: wandering near busy roads or entering other people's rooms and being assaulted; premature admission to residential care; being evicted from a facility; or being chemically or physically restrained.

26.2.1.3   DISTRESS OR DANGER TO OTHERS

This essential issue is a missing component in many challenging behaviour texts. There is clearly an obligation to treat if the behaviour is a manifestation of distress, or its consequences cause distress or danger to the person with dementia. If it is not and, equally, it does not cause significant distress or danger to others, it is not challenging behaviour and should be left alone other than, if necessary, explaining the reasoning to carers.

Bizarre behaviour is not necessarily the same as challenging behaviour, yet there are many phenomena associated with dementia that are often classified as agitated, such as repeatedly sorting clothing or seeing one's mother in a mirror. It is essential to establish whether it is a problem for anybody. For example, a dysphasic patient referred to the author because of 'constant muttering' turned out to be saying the Rosary. The intervention consisted of showing staff that the muttering was not directed at them, that the patient was not in distress and that the behaviour was a source of comfort. 'Treating' behaviour simply because it challenges the clinician's perception of what is normal risks producing non-benign outcomes, especially if psychotropic medication is used.

If there is significant distress among caregivers, it is important to discover who is distressed, how much and why. As already discussed, caregivers vary widely in their emotional response to the same phenomena and, in a significant number of cases, it is sufficient to deal with their concerns alone (see 26.3, Assessing and addressing causal domains).

26.2.1.4   ONSET

Relatively sudden onset or escalation of the behaviour is most commonly a sign of underlying physical or medical phenomena, and it is essential that current status, including the medication regime, be investigated by a dementia-literate medical practitioner or nurse. Some psychogeriatric teams in Australia will not take a referral for challenging behaviour without a full medical work up. However, it worth asking caregivers whether recent psychosocial changes coincided with changes in behaviour. Examples include death or discharge of another resident, changes in staff shifts and changes to the physical environment.

26.2.1.5   CONTEXT

In many texts, the 'who-where-when' questions occur at the start of assessment and the traditional A-B-C model is often presented here. Such formulations fail to acknowledge the complexity of this field, where physical, mental and cognitive health boundaries become increasingly blurred and where the

behaviour and attributes both of the person with dementia and those who provide care interact. In many cases, it will not be possible to determine a pattern based on obvious external events. Nevertheless, understanding the environmental context of the behaviour is important, with the clinician looking for patterns. Short-term monitoring sheets can be used, but questioning carers (in residential care as many staff as possible) can usually provide this information in a much richer context. Key questions include whether the behaviour occurs only at certain times of day, only in particular places or situations or only with some care staff and not others.

26.3   ASSESSING AND ADDRESSING CAUSAL DOMAINS

It is important to reiterate that divisions between the domains used in this chapter are artificial and they usually interact. For example, even a single within-patient cause (e.g. arthritic joint pain making the patient lash out during personal care) may involve not only a within-patient solution in the form of more regular pain relief, but also addressing quality of care and carer characteristics (e.g. helping staff identify which joints are affected and developing empathy and skills to minimize pain during the task).

26.3.1   The person with dementia

There are many within-person correlates of disturbed behaviour, such as level of dementia, which are not adjustable. However, even they provide important information; including helping decide which interventions are feasible or helping to understand the behaviour.

26.3.1.1   FIXED FACTORS: BACKGROUND, CAPACITY

A broad history is nearly always required. It is important, not only for the clinician to see beyond the dementia but, in residential care in particular, to help staff perceive the patient as a person more than the sum of their behaviours.

Social and medical background frequently also provides information about the origins of the behaviour and what is possible. To illustrate, pre-morbid sleep patterns can be difficult to switch after the onset of dementia and may have to be worked around, for example arranging for a resident to be kept up late (e.g. Bird and Moniz-Cook, 2007). Discovering that a resident violently resisting personal care had suffered pre-morbid cleanliness-related obsessive compulsive disorder indicated that the behaviour was unlikely to change, so the intervention was directed at improving staff skills and confidence (Bird, 2005). Learning that a woman who screamed during bathing was manifesting panic based on known pre-morbid trauma helped staff to change their approach and largely eliminate the behaviour (Woods and Bird, 1998). Discovering that a retired trawler man attacked others due to his belief that wearing green was unlucky helped staff to largely resolve the problem (Moniz-Cook et al., 2001a).

Retained capacity may be seen as a factor which, though not fixed, is not likely to improve and it is important to assess, for example, the ability to communicate or retain new information (Bird, 2001). This will help determine whether it is possible to work directly with the patient or if all work must be done through family carers or staff in residential care. Formal neuropsychological testing may provide this information, but it is usually more useful to try talking with the patient or use behavioural experiments. For example, in the Woods and Bird (1998) case above, we discovered that this patient could have her hair washed at a salon without panic. Behavioural experiments with a man who sexually assaulted staff in the shower showed that he would refrain if provided with a reward (Bird et al., 1998).

26.3.1.2   WITHIN–PATIENT FACTORS AMENABLE TO ADJUSTMENT

The most common adjustable within-patient causes relate to medical/physical problems, including pain or discomfort, constipation and other common causes of delirium such as drug interactions, dehydration and infections (Cohen-Mansfield and Werner, 1999; Sink et al., 2005). These phenomena can be missed even by geriatricians (Cohen-Mansfield and Lipson, 2002), so clinicians must develop diagnostic awareness regardless of discipline. Discomfort is common. Many patients have ill-fitting clothes, dentures or shoes and, in later stages of dementia, many are left in unchanged positions (if this is suspected, clinicians may try assuming the posture and experiencing the discomfort of holding it unchanged for more than 10 minutes, many patients in residential care are not moved for periods of up to 2 hours; Beck et al., 1998).

Critical to assessment is observation and a history from the family and nursing home notes which provide clues about sources of pain and discomfort (e.g. a propensity to headaches, evidence of a knee reconstruction or long-term back pain). While interventions are primarily medication-based, psychosocial methods are important adjuncts, particularly for pain and discomfort. For example, a case of intrusive wandering precipitated by escalating knee pain was ameliorated both by regular analgesics instead of pro re nata (PRN; as required) and developing ways to induce this somewhat bossy resident to rest in the middle of the day (Bird, 2005). A case of screaming was partially ameliorated by staff providing regular bed turns and ensuring the patient was not dehydrated (Bird and Moniz-Cook, 2007). The resident also had post-traumatic stress disorder related to the Holocaust, so another part of the intervention was making staff aware of this and changing their responses from exasperation to empathy. This illustrates, again, the interaction between within-patient and other domains.

26.3.1.3   MENTAL ILLNESS

Cases already mentioned show that mental illness can be a causal factor for challenging behaviour. The best data are available on depression and it should be remembered that apathy qualifies as challenging behaviour though it is often ignored because it causes few problems to others. Anxiety disorders, delusions and hallucinations are also common (Cohen-Mansfield and Werner, 1997; Cohen-Mansfield and Werner, 1999; Menon et al., 2001). Diagnosis and treatment, particularly in the later stages of dementia, is complex and beyond the scope of this chapter, though clinicians need to be attuned to causal factors such as pain, delirium (Cohen-Mansfield and Taylor, 1998) or lack of social interaction (Ice, 2002). Readers should refer to Chapter 8, Neuropsychiatric aspects of dementia, Chapter 25, Non-pharmacological therapies to manage behavioural and psychological symptoms of dementia: what works and what doesn't and Chapter 74, Depression with cognitive impairment for discussion of causal factors for, and treatment of, affective and psychotic disorders in dementia. In any but the earlier stages of dementia, a talking cure is rarely possible, though there is a slowly expanding literature on psychosocial treatments for affective disorders in dementia (e.g. Teri et al., 2005; Eggermont and Scherder, 2006).

For psychiatric phenomena, the clinician can try obvious means such as reassurance for distressing hallucinations. In a case referred to the author, a nursing home resident's paranoid delusions were ameliorated by helping her to engage in activity with other residents, including some of whom she was suspicious. However psychopharmacological treatment remains the mainstay. Because there are often serious side effects for benzodiazepines, mood stabilizers, antipsychotics and even antidepressants (Sink et al., 2005), and many people with dementia stay on psychotropic medications for years whether they need them or not, it is essential that wherever possible prescribing is undertaken, or at least closely monitored, by dementia-literate medical practitioners, such as geriatricians or psychogeriatricians.

26.3.1.4   BUT IS IT MENTAL ILLNESS?

It is essential not to mistake the effects of cognitive impairment for mental illness. Explanations of 'hallucinations' as misidentifications or perceptual problems, and of 'paranoia' as suspicion due to memory problems (Burns et al., 1990), can reduce unnecessary neuroleptic use. For example, a new resident referred for 'paranoid delusions' and assaulting staff was actually suffering a memory problem. She had forgotten giving away her possessions before being admitted and therefore believed that staff had stolen them. She was helped partly by posting in a prominent place a large reminder of what had happened to her possessions (Bird, 1998).

That case illustrates an important point. Anxiety, fear, despair or frustration lie behind many disturbed behaviours in people, usually with no psychiatric history, who are losing the capacity to make sense of the world, or communicate their needs (Cohen-Mansfield and Werner, 1997; Berg et al., 1998). Overuse of psychiatric templates can be prevented by clinicians spending time observing disturbed behaviour and considering the experience of the person manifesting the behaviour. Exploration of the meaning of behaviour (e.g. Cohen-Mansfield and Werner, 1997) is rare. In an important Swedish study (Edberg et al., 1996; Edberg et al., 1999), a critical component in changing staff practices from task-oriented to person-centred care was helping them consider what the resident's life was like. In the case of the woman (previous paragraph) who forgot where her possessions were, another intervention component was helping staff understand the multiple losses involved in coming into residential care, thus changing their responses from angry denials of stealing to empathy.

26.3.2   Quality of care and carer characteristics

After medical and physical problems, the way care is delivered is probably the most common adjustable causal factor in challenging behaviour. The care environment is inseparable from carer characteristics, which determine both the quality of the care – itself related to the development of disturbed behaviour (Hallberg and Norberg, 1993; Hallberg and Norberg, 1995) and to whether a given carer finds the behaviour 'challenging' (Moniz-Cook et al., 2000; Moniz-Cook et al., 2001b).

26.3.2.1   QUALITY OF CARE AS A CAUSAL FACTOR

The most frequent care situation leading to challenging behaviour is intimate personal tasks: bathing, toileting, dressing/undressing and feeding (Bridges-Parlet et al., 1994; Beck et al., 1998; Moniz-Cook et al., 2003). A common method to assess and address these problems in residential care is observation of different staff undertaking the task and sharing information among them. Alternatively, either with people at home or in residential care, a skilled clinician can attempt the task to assess the problems. For example, during showering, flinching or lashing out when certain body parts are handled may suggest pain. Facial expression can show fear or outrage at what the patient perceives as assault. Problems in feeding can be due to an interaction between staff not having enough time to help all those in their care and the person with dementia having eating difficulties. Referral to relevant health professionals, for example oral health specialists or speech pathologists, should be considered.

When developing interventions in residential care, however poor the facility, there is usually at least one staff member who encounters fewer problems than others in providing care and should be seen as an expert. The difference between the way they and others approach the task will often suggest both the causes of the problem and potential solutions. In some cases, trial and error will be required and it helps if there is such an expert within the facility (or an expert on the clinical team) to model the process. In the case of pre-morbid obsessive compulsive disorder (OCD) described previously, two staff who had known the resident longest demonstrated to demoralized carers how they accomplished showering despite difficulties and provided encouragement and supervision (Bird, 2005). Some staff can care effectively for certain residents but not others and sometimes only a few staff can develop the necessary skills, so information about flexibility in rostering is useful.

Some interventions are very simple. For example, a patient who was violent each night when woken up for a toilet visit was cured by persuading night staff not to wake her up (Bird, 2003). Routine practices such as these, or making all residents eat at tables, or with people they may not like, are rarely questioned. Namazi and Johnson (1996) noted that a person's lifelong preferences, routines and habits rarely accorded with that of the nursing home.

Another causal factor in the care environment is lack of care leading to boredom and, in some cases, depression and apathy. There is evidence that, in residential care, few staff engage socially with residents with dementia for extended periods and some do not engage at all. Most social contact takes place in personal care (e.g. Ice, 2002), and interactions if they occur at all are short and often negative (Burgio et al., 2001). Many residents spend most of their time doing nothing. For example, Voelkl et al. (1995) found that 40 per cent of patients in residential care did not participate in any activity other than routine care over a 1-week period. Reasons for staff socially neglecting residents include lack of time, inclination, permission or peer pressure (Edberg et al., 2008), so any intervention attempting to ameliorate this common cause of disturbed behaviour must take these factors into account.

If boredom is a factor, it is essential to work with carers to devise ways to increase activities which give some pleasure and can be realistically maintained after the clinician has withdrawn. Some families can afford to pay for carers to undertake activity or use community services. Most residential care facilities have diversional therapists, but their resources are often limited to group activities. Ingenuity is required, gathering information about past pleasures which can be adapted, looking at the activity literature and, often, engagement of volunteers, family members or local organizations.

Overall, there is a wide range of ways care practices contribute to problems; only the most common can be presented here. If intervention at this level is required, it is necessary to assess how flexible the rosters are and what resources are available for extra support, such as specialing a patient, extra equipment or referral to an allied health professional. Although there are some facilities where only a masochist would attempt to change care practices, attention paid to building rapport with both senior and care staff usually pays off.

26.3.2.2   CARER CHARACTERISTICS

Assessment of carer characteristics includes their knowledge of dementia, caring skills, knowledge of, attitude to and level of distress related to the individual patient and level of burnout or motivation to change. This information is best acquired informally during the assessment of the behaviour which, as already discussed, must largely be gathered from those providing the care. It is critical information because the nature of nurse–patient interactions, itself a product of attitudes and other carer variables, is associated with disturbed behaviour (Edberg et al., 1999). Accordingly, change in care practices can only occur if some of these characteristics are addressed.

Structured support and education programmes have demonstrated clear benefits for family members dealing with challenging behaviour, including more effective management of behaviour problems and concomitant delayed entry into residential care (Teri, 1999). In institutions, programmes which have addressed staff attitude and care practices have not only improved staff morale and coping (Berg *et al.*, 1994; Moniz-Cook *et al.*, 1998), but have also reduced problem behaviour (Rovner *et al.*, 1996; Bird *et al.*, 2007; Bird *et al.*, 2009), patient dependence (Baltes *et al.*, 1994) and use of antipsychotic medication (Fossey *et al.*, 2006). A composite programme in Sweden addressing staff emotional and attitudinal variables and clinical practice increased staff empathy and resident-specific skills, improved the quality of personal care and thereby reduced difficult behaviour and improved both staff and patient well-being (Edberg *et al.*, 1996; Edberg *et al.*, 1999).

26.3.2.3   CARER DISTRESS

Understanding emotional responses of carers to the behaviour is critical because, in a significant minority of cases, the behaviour can be left alone and carer distress becomes the sole clinical target. There is plenty of room for movement because there is wide variability between home carers and also between care staff in how they perceive a given behaviour (Moniz-Cook *et al.*, 2001b; Bird *et al.*, 2007), and their emotional response is often determined by remediable factors which have nothing to do with the specific patient or dementia. These include depression in family carers or lack of knowledge of dementia (Hinchliffe *et al.*, 1995; de Vugt *et al.*, 2004), or level of support for staff in residential care (Baillon *et al.*, 1996; Moniz-Cook *et al.*, 2000). The purpose of direct intervention at this level is to help those care-givers who are distressed by the behaviour to acquire the knowledge, skills or confidence to cope with it. Twenty per cent of cases were resolved in this way in the intervention study by Bird *et al.* (2009) but it is often ignored, with all attention focused on 'treating' the behaviour.

Even if carer distress is only part of the clinical target, many situations will involve working through family carers or staff as co-therapists (Teri 1999; Teri *et al.*, 2005) and it is often necessary to address that distress before attempting an intervention requiring their input. For example, it was necessary to work first on the anger of a carer whose confrontational response to her husband's obsessive toileting was exacerbating the problem (Bird *et al.*, 1998). Equally, support will be required during an intervention. In a difficult case of violent resistance in personal care (Bird, 2005), it was necessary to establish good rapport with staff and allow them to vent their distress before helping them look at the case objectively. The sources of staff distress and therefore part of the clinical target were: a sense of hopelessness and lack of support; a strong sense of duty of care untempered by awareness of their rights; lack of knowledge about the resident including her degree of abdominal pain; and lack of appreciation about the level of family guilt.

Interventions aimed at carer attitudes, emotional responses or practices require the development of subtle clinical skills, particularly in residential care, where there will be varying levels of skill, insight, flexibility, motivation and,

sometimes, desire to sabotage (Bird *et al.*, 2009). Listening to and responding to staff distress appears relatively rare (Edberg *et al.*, 2008) but, if carer concerns are not listened to, and they have no input to the development of the intervention package, there will be little rapport or compliance. Skilfully applied, what is essentially psychotherapy with the care system becomes a collaborative exercise with those who best know the person with dementia. On the other hand, failure to work with the care system by, for example, masquerading as an expert and simply telling staff what to do, or writing a functional analysis intervention and leaving it with the Director of Nursing, will usually fail.

26.3.3   The physical/social/sensory environment

Although many texts concentrate on the physical environment, the clinical experience of the author suggests that medical/physical problems and quality of care/carer characteristics are the most common remediable casual factors in challenging behaviour. However, physical, sensory and social phenomena can sometimes be both causal and ameliorating factors in challenging behaviour, usually relating to the presence or absence of stimuli. Assessment may take the form of asking carers to monitor whether the behaviour takes place in specific areas, or relates to increases or decreases in sensory stimuli. Observation and behavioural experiments may help assessment, testing hypothesis with the patient if possible, or by the clinician 'putting themselves in the patient's shoes'.

Examples of modification of precipitating factors in the environment include reduction of incontinence by visual, auditory or situational cues (Bird *et al.*, 1995), screaming by room relocation (Meares and Draper, 1999) or relocation from the bathroom to a local salon for hair care (Woods and Bird, 1998), and self-harm by removal of precipitating cues (Bird *et al.*, 1998). Some interventions in the physical or sensory environment can address causes which fall in other domains, such as deficiencies in the care regime. Examples include: 'white noise' (waterscape sounds) or social interaction reducing verbal disruption (Burgio *et al.*, 1996; Cohen-Mansfield and Werner, 1997); bright light reducing motor restlessness (Haffmans *et al.*, 2001); music reducing physical aggression (Clark *et al.*, 1998); personalized tapes made by family members reducing agitation (Woods and Ashley, 1995); and cued recall of more adaptive behaviour for a variety of problems (Bird *et al.*, 1995). For further coverage of factors relating to the physical environment, see Day *et al.* (2000).

26.4   CONCLUSION

The multi-factorial nature of behaviour problems in aetiology and other contextual variables which determine treatment choice, make most cases inappropriate for standardized pharmacological or psychosocial interventions. There is no magic pill for challenging behaviour in dementia (Sink *et al.*, 2005) and, accordingly, no substitute for thorough assessment and modification of likely causal factors.

Unfortunately, both clinical experience and the high rate of inappropriate prescribing for behaviour problems suggests that many clinicians think only of answers, often in a kind of scattergun approach. If enough pellets are fired, something may hit the target. The development and evaluation of standardized techniques is important but only as a means of adding to the tool kit from which the health worker can select the most appropriate combination of techniques after holistic assessment – not before it.

For a given behaviour in any given case, these techniques will be selected from a very diverse range. To illustrate, entirely dependent on the causal information uncovered by assessment, the range of interventions for a screaming case might include: providing regular analgesics; doing nothing about the behaviour and instead addressing carer issues; transferring the patient to a facility sensible enough to have a soundproof room or installing double-glazing; changing rosters so that only certain nurses perform intimate personal care; transmitting soothing sounds through headphones; engaging a volunteer to sit holding the patient's hand; or rationalizing polypharmacy or prescribing antidepressants or antipsychotics.

This example illustrates that psychosocial and pharmacological approaches are not mutually exclusive; both need to form part of the tool-kit. The relationship between them is not one of competition and recommendations to always use psychosocial methods first (e.g. Peisah and Brodaty, 1994; Sink et al., 2005) are incorrect. Though treating causal factors strongly shifts the balance in favour of psychosocial methods (Bird et al., 2007; Bird et al., 2009), if the most appropriate treatment for causes such as depression, pain or infections is psychotropic or other medication, it should be tried first. In some cases, antipsychotics may be the treatment of choice, for example where hallucinations are causing distress and neuroleptic malignancy syndrome is not present, or where there is simply no other alternative.

Usually, however, there are alternatives and they are much more likely to be visible when the clinician looks beyond the referred problem to its causes, including the reasons the behaviour is perceived as a problem. Unfortunately, despite frequent calls for more research into psychosocial alternatives or adjuncts to psychopharmacology for behaviour problems in dementia (e.g. Herrmann, 2001; Margallo-Lana et al., 2001), the research effort remains limited. It is largely undertaken by a finite number of enthusiasts around the world, largely dependent upon charitable and government grants because, by definition, psychosocial research is never going to be funded by the pharmaceutical industry.

In the meantime, there are glimmerings of hope. As well as an increasing number of trials, use of the case-specific approach for challenging behaviour in dementia is growing – in Australia at least – funded by the Australian Government under its *Dementia Behaviour Management and Advisory Service* initiative.

REFERENCES

Ancoli-Israel S, Parker L, Sinaee R et al. (1989) Sleep fragmentation in patients from a nursing home. *Journal of Gerontology: Medical Sciences* **44**: 8–21.

Baillon S, Scothern G, Neville PG, Boyle A. (1996) Factors that contribute to stress in care staff in residential homes for the elderly. *International Journal of Geriatric Psychiatry* **11**: 219–26.

Baltes M, Neumann E, Zank S. (1994) Maintenance and rehabilitation of independence in old age: An intervention program for staff. *Psychology and Aging* **9**: 179–88.

Beck C, Frank L, Chumbler N et al. (1998) Correlates of disruptive behavior in severely cognitively impaired nursing home residents. *Gerontologist* **38**: 187–98.

Berg A, Hansson U, Hallberg I. (1994) Nurses' creativity, tedium and burnout during one year of clinical supervision and implementation of individually planned nursing care: Comparisons between a ward for severely demented patients and a similar control ward. *Journal of Advanced Nursing* **20**: 742–9.

Berg A, Hallberg I, Norberg A. (1998) Nurses' reflections about dementia care, the patients, the care and themselves in their daily caregiving. *International Journal of Nursing Studies* **35**: 271–82.

Bird M. (1998) Clinical use of preserved learning capacity in dementia. *Australasian Journal on Ageing* **17**: 161–6.

Bird M. (2001) Behavioural difficulties and cued recall of adaptive behaviour in dementia: Experimental and clinical evidence. *Neuropsychological Rehabilitation* **11**: 357–75.

Bird M. (2003) Psychiatric and behavioural problems: Psychosocial approaches. In: Mulligan R, Van der Linden M, Juillerat A-C (eds). *The clinical management of early Alzheimer's disease: A handbook*. New Jersey: Erlbaum, 143–67.

Bird M. (2005) A predominantly psychosocial approach to behaviour problems in dementia: treating causality. In: Burns A, O'Brien J, Ames D (eds). *Dementia*, 3rd edn. London: Edward Arnold, 499–509.

Bird M, Moniz-Cook E. (2007) Challenging behaviour in dementia: A psychosocial approach to intervention. In: Woods B, Clare L (eds). *Handbook of the clinical psychology of ageing*. Chichester, UK: Wiley, 571–94.

Bird M, Alexopoulos P, Adamowicz J. (1995) Success and failure in five case studies: Use of cued recall to ameliorate behaviour problems in senile dementia. *International Journal of Geriatric Psychiatry* **10**: 5–11.

Bird M, Llewellyn-Jones R, Smithers H et al. (1998) Challenging behaviours in dementia. *Australasian Journal on Ageing* **17**: 10–15.

Bird M, Llewellyn-Jones RH, Korten A, Smithers H. (2007) A controlled trial of a predominantly psychosocial approach to BPSD: Treating causality. *International Psychogeriatrics* **19**: 874–91.

Bird M, Llewellyn-Jones R, Korten A. (2009) An evaluation of the effectiveness of a case-specific approach to challenging behaviour associated with dementia. *Aging and Mental Health* **13**: 73–83.

Bridges-Parlet S, Knopman D, Thompson T. (1994) A descriptive study of physically aggressive behavior in dementia by direct observation. *Journal of the American Geriatrics Society* **42**: 192–7.

Burgio L, Scilley K, Hardin J *et al.* (1996) Environmental 'White Noise': An intervention for verbally agitated nursing home residents. *Journal of Gerontology: Psychological Sciences* **51B**: P364–73.

Burgio L, Allen-Burge R, Roth D *et al.* (2001) Come talk with me: Improving communication between nursing home assistants and nursing home residents during care routines. *The Gerontologist* **41**: 449–60.

Burns A, Jacoby R, Levy R. (1990) Psychiatric phenomena in Alzheimer's Disease: Disorders of behaviour. *British Journal of Psychiatry* **157**: 86–94.

Clark M, Lipe A, Bilbrey M. (1998) Use of music to decrease aggressive behaviors in people with dementia. *Journal of Gerontological Nursing* **24**: 10–17.

Cohen-Mansfield J, Lipson S. (2002) Pain in cognitively impaired nursing home residents: How well are physicians diagnosing it? *Journal of the American Geriatrics Society* **50**: 1039–44.

Cohen-Mansfield J, Taylor L. (1998) The relationship between depressed affect, pain and cognitive function: A cross-sectional analysis of two elderly populations. *Aging and Mental Health* **2**: 313–18.

Cohen-Mansfield J, Werner P. (1997) Management of verbally disruptive behaviors in nursing home residents. *The Journals of Gerontology* **52A**: M369–77.

Cohen-Mansfield J, Werner P. (1999) Longitudinal predictors of non-aggressive agitated behaviors in the elderly. *International Journal of Geriatric Psychiatry* **14**: 831–44.

Cohen-Mansfield J, Marx M, Rosenthal A. (1989) A description of agitation in a nursing home. *Journals of Gerontology: Medical Sciences* **44**: M77–84.

Cohen-Mansfield J, Marx M, Werner P, Freedman L. (1992) Temporal patterns of agitated nursing home residents. *International Psychogeriatrics* **4**: 197–206.

Cohen-Mansfield J, Libin A, Marx MS. (2007) Non-pharmacological treatment of agitation: a controlled trial of systematic individualized intervention. *The Journal of Gerontology* **62A**: 908–16.

Cummings J, Mega M, Gray K *et al.* (1994) The Neuropsychiatric Inventory: Comprehensive assessment of psychopathology in dementia. *Neurology* **44**: 2308–14.

de Vugt M, Stevens F, Aalten P *et al.* (2004) Do caregiver management strategies influence patient behaviour in dementia? *International Journal of Geriatric Psychiatry* **19**: 85–92.

Davison T, Hudgson C, McCabe M *et al.* (2006) An individualized psychosocial approach for 'treatment resistant' behavioural symptoms of dementia among aged care residents. *International Psychogeriatrics* **19**: 859–73.

Day K, Carreon D, Stump C. (2000) The therapeutic design of environments for people with dementia: A review of the empirical research. *The Gerontologist* **40**: 397–416.

Edberg A-K, Hallberg I, Gustafson L. (1996) Effects of clinical supervision on nurse-patient cooperation quality. *Clinical Nursing Research* **5**: 127–49.

Edberg A-K, Norberg A, Hallberg I. (1999) Mood and general behavior of patients with severe dementia during one year of supervised, individualized planned care and systematic clinical

supervision. Comparison with a similar control group. *Aging and Clinical Experimental Research* **11**: 395–403.

Edberg A-K, Bird M, Richards D *et al.* (2008) Strain in nursing care of people with dementia: Nurses' experience in Australia, Sweden and United Kingdom. *Aging and Mental Health* **12**: 236–43.

Eggermont L, Scherder E. (2006) Physical activity and behaviour in dementia: A review of the literature and implications for psychosocial intervention in primary care. *Dementia: The International Journal of Social Research and Practice* **5**: 411–28.

Ersser S, Wiles A, Taylor H *et al.* (1999) The sleep of older people in hospital and nursing homes. *Journal of Clinical Nursing* **8**: 360–8.

Fossey J, Ballard C, Juszczak E *et al.* (2006) Effect of enhanced psychosocial care on antipsychotic use in nursing home residents with severe dementia: Cluster randomised trial. *British Medical Journal* **332**: 756–8.

Haffmans P, Sival R, Lucius S *et al.* (2001) Bright light therapy and melatonin in motor restless behaviour in dementia: A placebo-controlled study. *International Journal of Geriatric Psychiatry* **16**: 106–10.

Hallberg I, Norberg A. (1993) Strain among nurses and their emotional reactions during one year of systematic supervision combined with the implementation of individualized care. *Journal of Advanced Nursing* **18**: 1860–75.

Hallberg I, Norberg A. (1995) Nurses' experiences of strain and their reactions in the care of severely demented patients. *International Journal of Geriatric Psychiatry* **10**: 757–66.

Herrmann N. (2001) Recommendations for the management of behavioural and psychological symptoms of dementia. *Canadian Journal of Neurological Science* **28**: S96–107.

Hinchliffe A, Hyman I, Blizard B, Livingston G. (1995) Behavioural complications of dementia – Can they be treated? *International Journal of Geriatric Psychiatry* **10**: 839–47.

Hodges J. (2007) *Frontotemporal dementia syndromes*. Cambridge: CUP.

Howard R, Ballard C, O'Brien J, Burns A. (2001) Guidelines for the management of agitation in dementia. *International Journal of Geriatric Psychiatry* **16**: 714–71.

Ice G. (2002) Daily life in a nursing home: Has it changed in 25 years? *Journal of Aging Studies* **16**: 345–59.

Landreville P, Bedard A, Verreault R *et al.* (2006) Non-pharmacological intervention for aggressive behaviour in older adults living in long term care facilities. *International Psychogeriatrics* **18**: 47–74.

McCann J, Gilley D, Hebert L *et al.* (1997) Concordance between direct observation and staff rating of behaviour in nursing home residents with Alzheimer's disease. *Journal of Gerontology* **52**: P63–72.

Margallo-Lana M, Swann A, O'Brien J *et al.* (2001) Prevalence and pharmacological management of behavioural and psychological symptoms amongst dementia sufferers living in care environments. *International Journal of Geriatric Psychiatry* **16**: 39–44.

Meares S, Draper B. (1999) Treatment of vocally disruptive behaviour of multi-factorial aetiology. *International Journal of Geriatric Psychiatry* **14**: 285–90.

Menon A, Gruber-Baldini A, Hebel J *et al.* (2001) Relationship between aggressive behaviours and depression among nursing home residents with dementia. *International Journal of Geriatric Psychiatry* **16**: 139–46.

Moniz-Cook ED, Agar S, Silver M *et al.* (1998) Can staff training reduce behavioural problems in residential care for the elderly mentally ill? *International Journal of Geriatric Psychiatry* **13**: 149–58.

Moniz-Cook ED, Woods R, Gardiner E. (2000) Staff factors associated with perception of behaviour as 'challenging' in residential and nursing homes. *Aging and Mental Health* **4**: 48–55.

Moniz-Cook ED, Woods R, Richards K. (2001a) Functional analysis of challenging behaviour in dementia: the role of superstition. *International Journal of Geriatric Psychiatry* **16**: 45–56.

Moniz-Cook ED, Woods R, Gardiner E *et al.* (2001b) The Challenging Behaviour Scales (CBS): Development of a new scale for staff caring for older people in residential and nursing homes. *British Journal of Clinical Psychology* **40**: 309–22.

Moniz-Cook ED, Stokes G, Agar S. (2003) Difficult behaviour and dementia in nursing homes; Five cases of psychosocial intervention. *International Journal of Clinical Psychology and Psychotherapy* **10**: 197–208.

Namazi K, Johnson B. (1996) Issues related to behavior and the physical environment: bathing cognitively impaired patients. *Geriatric Nursing* **17**: 234–8.

O'Connor D, Ames D, Gardner B, King M. (2009) Psychosocial treatments of behavior symptoms in dementia: A systematic review of reports meeting quality standards. *International Psychogeriatrics* **21**: 225–40.

Peisah C, Brodaty H. (1994) Practical guidelines for the treatment of behavioural complications of dementia. *The Medical Journal of Australia* **161**: 558–64.

Rovner B, Steele C, Folstein M. (1996) A randomized trial of dementia care in nursing homes. *Journal of the American Geriatrics Society* **44**: 7–13.

Schneider J, Pollock V, Lyness A. (1990) A meta-analysis of controlled trials of neuroleptic treatment in dementia. *Journal of the American Geriatrics Society* **38**: 553–63.

Schneider J, Daegerman K, Insel P. (2006) Efficacy and adverse effects of atypical antipsychotics for dementia: Meta-analysis of randomized, placebo-controlled trials. *American Journal of Geriatric Psychiatry* **14**: 191–210.

Schnelle JF, Alessi CA, Al-Samarrai NR *et al.* (1999) The nursing home at night: effects of an intervention on noise, light and sleep. *Journal of the American Geriatrics Society* **47**: 430–8.

Sink KM, Holden FH, Yaffe K. (2005) Pharmacological treatment of neuropsychiatric symptoms of dementia: a review of the evidence. *Journal of the American Medical Association* **293**: 596–608.

Teri L. (1999) Training families to provide care: Effects on people with dementia. *International Journal of Geriatric Psychiatry* **14**: 110–19.

Teri L, McKenzie G, LaFazia D. (2005) Psychosocial treatment of depression in older adults with dementia. *Clinical Psychology: Science and Practice* **12**: 303–16.

Voelkl J, Fries B, Galeck A. (1995) Predictors of nursing home residents' participation in activity programs. *Gerontologist* **35**: 44–51.

Woods P, Ashley J. (1995) Stimulated presence therapy: Using selected memories to manage problem behaviors in Alzheimer's disease patients. *Geriatric Nursing* **16**: 9–14.

Woods R, Bird M. (1998) Non-pharmacological approaches to treatment. In: Wilcock G, Bucks R, Rockwood K (eds). *Diagnosis and management of dementia: A manual for memory disorders teams.* Oxford: OUP, 311–31.

Drug treatments for the behavioural and psychiatric symptoms of dementia

ANNA BURKE AND PIERRE N TARIOT

27.1 INTRODUCTION

Merriam *et al.* (1988) asserted that Alzheimer's disease (AD) is 'the most widely encountered cause of psychiatric pathology associated with a specific neuropathological substrate'. This is consistent with phenomenological studies and literature reviews, which generally converge on the conclusion that roughly 90 per cent of patients with dementia will develop significant behavioural problems at some point in their illness (Tariot and Blazina, 1993). The 'behavioural and psychological signs and symptoms of dementia' (Finkel *et al.*, 1996) do not typically meet criteria for discrete psychiatric disorders. They do, however, tend to occur in clusters of signs and symptoms that may vary among patients and over time (Tariot and Blazina, 1993). Examples of these clusters are provided in **Table 27.1**, based on a review of published studies regarding psychopathological changes in dementia performed in 1993. With experience, these clusters of signs and symptoms can be both predicted and recognized, and can be used as guideposts in the selection of appropriate therapy.

This chapter will focus on agitation, which Cohen-Mansfield and Billig (1986) defined as 'inappropriate verbal, vocal or motor activity unexplained by apparent needs or confusion'. Cohen-Mansfield and Billig (1986) empirically categorized agitated behaviours into three key groups:

1. disruptive but not aggressive (e.g. attempts to leave, robes and disrobes, repeated complaints or questions);
2. socially inappropriate (e.g. disrobing or urinating in public); or
3. aggressive (e.g. physical, such as hitting, slapping, or verbal, such as obscenities or name-calling).

As **Table 27.1** indicates, half or more of patients with dementia show some feature of agitation at some point in the course of their illness.

27.2 A RATIONAL APPROACH

This chapter proposes a systematic general approach to the evaluation and management of agitation that is based on an elaboration of prior work (Leibovici and Tariot, 1988; Tariot *et al.*, 1995a; Tariot, 1996; Tariot and Schneider, 1998; Loy *et al.*, 1999; Tariot, 1999); key aspects are described below:

Define target symptoms. Review the available evidence and delineate the patient's behaviour pattern, for example

Table 27.1   Summary of literature regarding psychopathology of dementia (percentage of patients affected among studies reviewed).

		Range	Median
1.	Disturbed affect/mood	0–86	19
2.	Disturbed ideation	10–73	33.5
3.	Altered perception		
	Hallucinations	21–49	28
	Misperceptions	1–49	23
4.	Agitation		
	Global	10–90	44
	Wandering	0–50	18
5.	Aggression		
	Verbal	11–51	24
	Physical	0–46	14.3
	Resistive/unco-operative	27–65	44
6.	Anxiety	0–50	31.8
7.	Withdrawn/passive behaviour	21–88	61
8.	Vegetative behaviours		
	Sleep	0–47	27
	Diet/appetite	12.5–77	34

Adapted from Tariot and Blazina (1993).

'wanders without an apparent destination, calls out repeatedly, bites and kicks during care'.

Establish or revisit medical diagnoses. It is almost a truism in geriatrics that delirium is a frequent cause of incident agitation and must always be suspected. Common culprits include respiratory or urinary infections, dehydration, occult trauma, electrolyte disturbances or side effects of medications. Such medical problems should be treated specifically and the patient monitored carefully, ideally without the need for other medications.

Establish or revisit neuropsychiatric diagnoses. It is also possible that the disturbed behaviour may reflect a long-standing, recurrent or new onset discrete psychiatric disorder. When a specific disorder is identified, it should be specifically treated and monitored.

Assess and reverse aggravating factors. Examples might include deficits in hearing or vision, or an environment that is too dark, noisy or cold. Disrupted daily routines may present a remediable factor. It is important to look hard for environmental triggers.

Adapt to specific cognitive deficits. Some patients may be able to respond to verbal reassurance and redirection, whereas others may not. Pain or distress may need to be inferred from behaviour or facial expression. Some may need constant environmental cueing to organize their behaviour. It is important to identify each patient's cognitive strengths and weaknesses, attempting to capitalize on residual strengths and avoid weaknesses.

Identify relevant psychosocial factors. It may be easy to overlook the fact that a patient with dementia may be suffering anxiety, sadness, denial or fury in response to major and minor life events. In some long-term care facilities, for instance, moving from one unit to another can be associated with perceived loss of status, as well as

contact with familiar people. It is easy to overlook this as a precipitant of 'agitation'.

Educate caregivers. Caregivers can learn that change in behaviour usually has meaning, and that the behaviours can occur in discernible patterns. This helps caregivers interact in a more supportive manner. In the process, they can be taught to employ essential behaviour management principles, learning, for instance, that their own behaviour is a major determinant of the patient's behaviour. Caregivers can be trained to identify common triggers as well as consequences of agitated behaviour, and work with health professionals to attempt to minimize the triggers and maximize more positive circumstances.

If the behavioural disturbance is grossly aggressive or disruptive, and frankly dangerous, it may be necessary to use antipsychotics or benzodiazepines on an emergency basis, preferably by mouth but sometimes parenterally. In rare cases, hospitalization is needed. Once the emergency is under control, it is imperative to pay attention to the basics outlined above.

27.3   DEVELOPMENT OF THE PSYCHOBEHAVIOURAL METAPHOR

For persisting non-emergent problems where non-pharmacological interventions have been exhausted, we adopt an approach that begins with a definition of a target symptom pattern that is at least roughly analogous to a drug-responsive syndrome. We refer to this as the 'psychobehavioural metaphor' (Leibovici and Tariot, 1988). We then match the dominant target symptoms (the metaphor) to the most relevant drug class. For example, in the case of a verbally and physically agitated patient who is also irritable, negative, has become socially withdrawn and appears dysphoric, we might first undertake a trial of an antidepressant. Conversely, if the patient showed 'agitation' in the context of increased motor activity, loud and rapid speech and lability of affect, we might consider early use of a mood stabilizer. The 'aggressive' patient whose hostile actions are associated with delusions is likely to be treated first with an antipsychotic. Although this approach to drug selection is face-valid, there is limited empirical support for it (Devanand, 2000; Lyketsos *et al.*, 2000; Tariot *et al.*, 2001; Tariot *et al.*, 2002; De Deyn *et al.*, 2003). Thus, the validity of the approach that we have endorsed for some years, and that reflected in most consensus guidelines (Rabins *et al.*, 1997; Doody *et al.*, 2001; Alexopoulos *et al.*, 2005), has not been established empirically. Furthermore, the use of medications to treat any aspect of psychopathology is not recognized by the US Food and Drug Administration and would thus be considered 'off-label'.

The approach adopted in this chapter more or less reflects the position of the American Geriatrics Society and American Association for Geriatric Psychiatry consensus statement (2005) with respect to the use of target symptoms to guide selection of drug class. We emphasize selection of a medication with at least some empirical evidence of efficacy and with the highest likelihood of tolerability and safety. We observe some general rules such as starting with low doses and escalating slowly, assessing target symptoms as well as toxicity and discontinuing the medication if it is harmful or ineffective. Even when a medication is helpful at subtoxic doses, an empirical trial is often performed in reverse and the patient monitored for recurrence of the problem. This type of approach is actually mandated in the nursing home setting in the United States by Federal regulations created in 1987. Sometimes several medications need to be tried in series before a successful one is identified; sometimes combinations are warranted; sometimes no medication is found that is helpful. We hold the view that best practice includes routine use of cholinesterase inhibitors and/or memantine in most patients with AD as well as certain other dementias, meaning that psychotropic use occurs against this backdrop. Evidence suggests that cholinesterase inhibitors and/or memantine may be of benefit in reducing agitated/aggressive behaviours in patients with AD or possibly delaying their emergence (Birks *et al.*, 2000; Trinh *et al.*, 2003; Cummings *et al.*, 2006; Wilcock *et al.*, 2000). Trials conducted with these agents were aimed at obtaining regulatory approval and not informing clinical practice regarding issues such as the advantages or disadvantages of one agent versus the other for relief of behavioural symptoms, or of using psychotropics in combination with these agents. Practice will outstrip evidence for the foreseeable future.

Table 27.2   Selected current pharmacological treatments for agitation in dementia.

Drug and class	Suggesting starting[a] and (maximal) daily dose (mg/d)
Antipsychotics	
Traditional	
Haloperidol	0.25–0.5 (2–4)
Thioridazine	12.5–25 (50–100)
Thiothixene	0.5–1 (2–4)
Atypical	
Clozapine	6.25–12.5 (25–100)
Olanzapine	2.5 (5–10)
Quetiapine	25 (50–200)
Risperidone	0.5 (1–2)
Aripiprazole	5 (15)
Ziprasidone	Unknown
Anxiolytics and sedatives	
Benzodiazepines	
Alprazolam	0.5 (1–2)
Lorazepam	0.5 (2–4)
Oxazepam	10 (40–60)
Non-benzodiazepines	
Zolpidem	2.5 (5)
Buspirone	10 (30–60)
Antidepressants	
Trazodone	25–50 (200–300)
SSRIs	
Citalopram	10 (20)
Fluoxetine	10 (20)
Sertraline	25–50 (100–200)
Anticonvulsants	
Carbamazepine	50–100 (300–500)
Divalproex	125–375 (500–1500)
β-blockers	
Propranolol	20 (50–100)
Others	
Selegiline	10
Oestradiol/progesterone	0.625/2.5

Adapted from Loy *et al.* (1999).
[a]Suggestions are based on published data as well as anecdotal experience, and should be regarded accordingly.
SSRI: selective serotonin reuptake inhibitors.

practice. Much of the older literature was reviewed in the third edition of this book (Profenno *et al.*, 2005); this chapter builds on that and some of our earlier work (Loy *et al.*, 1999; Tariot, 1999; Rosenquist *et al.*, 2000; Profenno and Tariot, 2004). **Table 27.2** provides an overview of individual agents and typical starting doses, based on a mixture of data and clinical experience.

27.4   SPECIFIC CLASSES OF PSYCHOTROPICS

The remainder of this chapter reviews the most relevant classes of agents and specific agents within those classes, focusing on information from approximately the last five years and on older studies that remain crucial guides to

27.5   CONVENTIONAL ANTIPSYCHOTICS

Within the context of the 'metaphor' approach, antipsychotics would be used first for treatment of agitation that included psychotic features. In reality, antipsychotics have been used and studied in patients with a wide range of psychopathology. There are two main classes of antipsychotics: so-called conventional antipsychotics and the newer atypical agents. Prior reviews of the conventional agents have concluded that the effects of these agents were consistent but modest, and that no single agent was better than another (Wragg and Jeste, 1989; Schneider *et al.*, 1990; see **Table 27.3**).

Lanctôt *et al.* (1998) performed a meta-analysis including some studies that were less rigorous than those included in the Schneider *et al.* (1990) meta-analysis. These authors also concluded that type and potency of agent did not influence response. They reported an average therapeutic effect (antipsychotic versus placebo) of 26 per cent, with placebo response rates ranging from 19 to 50 per cent. Side effects occurred more often on drug than placebo (mean difference 25 per cent). These meta-analyses did not include five more recent studies (Devanand *et al.*, 1998; De Deyn *et al.*, 1999; Allain *et al.*, 2000; Teri *et al.*, 2000; Tariot *et al.*, 2002). The data from these newer studies generally conform to the results of the meta-analyses. Lonergan *et al.* (2002) conducted a pooled analysis of five randomized controlled trials (RCTs) of haloperidol versus placebo that included two studies not incorporated in the above meta-analysis, which found decreased aggression but no significant improvement in agitated symptoms overall among haloperidol-treated patients. There was a noteworthy increase in adverse side effects, such as rigidity and bradykinesia, compared to placebo.

Reviews regarding conventional agents cite side effects including akathisia, parkinsonism, tardive dyskinesia, sedation, peripheral and central anticholinergic effects, postural hypotension, cardiac conduction defects and falls (Lanctôt *et al.*, 1998; Lonergan *et al.*, 2002). Based on limited efficacy and a high likelihood of toxicity, Lonergan *et al.* concluded by recommending that haloperidol be used sparingly, on a case by case basis, with monitoring of side effects. Most of these data come from short-term controlled trials; evidence regarding long-term safety is generally lacking. Data available from other elderly populations, however, indicate that caution is warranted. For instance, rates of tardive dyskinesia are five- to six-fold greater in older than in younger populations after treatment with conventional agents (Jeste *et al.*, 1995). For practical purposes, side effects typically guide selection of these agents when used in patients with dementia. A clinical issue that is of particular importance is dementia with co-occurring extrapyramidal disorders such as dementia with Lewy bodies (DLB), where occasional extraordinary sensitivity to conventional agents is seen (Ballard *et al.*, 1998). For all these reasons, it was hoped that atypical antipsychotics would have special utility in patients with dementia.

27.6   ATYPICAL ANTIPSYCHOTICS

27.6.1   Clozapine

Only anecdotes and case reports are available; none are new since our previous chapter was written. Individual patients showed partial improvement in agitation or psychosis, whereas others developed side effects including sedation and anticholinergic effects. While not mentioned specifically in these reports, agranulocytosis and seizures have been reported in other populations, the former requiring regular haematological testing for months. Dose-response issues are unresolved. In using this medication, we err on the side of caution by starting at 6.25 or 12.5 mg/day. Based on the relative lack of motor toxicity encountered with clozapine, a case can be made to select this agent preferentially in patients with dementia and extrapyramidal disorders. However, in view of the lack of information regarding dose-response, the risk of side effects and the lack of controlled data regarding efficacy and tolerability, most clinicians are likely to choose from among the newer atypical agents first (see **Table 27.4**).

27.6.2   Risperidone

The earliest exploratory studies indicated that doses in the range of 0.5–2 mg/day might be best tolerated, with dose-related risk of motor toxicity (especially in patients with extrapyramidal disorders). Sedation, peripheral oedema and orthostatic hypotension were sometimes reported. Use of risperidone can result in increased prolactin levels in other populations, although the clinical significance of this in dementia patients is uncertain. We do not routinely check serum prolactin levels, and would only take action in response to elevated levels associated with symptoms associated with its use (e.g. galactorrhoea in women, sexual dysfunction in men) or with symptoms indicative of a possible hypothalamic tumour (e.g. diplopia). The earlier open trials and case series indicated that risperidone may decrease agitation, aggression or psychosis in patients with dementia, spawning more definitive trials. Three large multicentre RCTs of risperidone have been completed in nursing home patients with relatively severe dementia (De Deyn *et al.*, 1999; Katz *et al.*, 1999; Brodaty *et al.*, 2003) and one in outpatients (Mintzer *et al.*, 2004). A meta-analysis of results from these four studies revealed that risperidone significantly reduced measures of agitation and/or psychosis in comparison with placebo (Schneider *et al.*, 2006). Risperidone-treated patients displayed positive effects on measures of psychosis. The main side effects in these trials were somnolence, extrapyramidal symptoms, abnormal gait and peripheral oedema in addition to cerebrovascular adverse events (CVAEs) and death described later.

In the aggregate, these risperidone studies comprise the largest placebo-controlled, multicentre studies ever conducted of any form of treatment for agitation or aggression associated with dementia. A conservative interpretation of the available evidence would be that the efficacy of risperidone is roughly equivalent to that of haloperidol. The tolerability of risperidone appears to be better, with low-moderate risk of dose-related parkinsonism and sedation and numerically higher rates of peripheral oedema and sedation in patients treated with risperidone versus placebo.

In 2003, the FDA issued a warning titled 'Cerebrovascular Adverse Events, Including Stroke, in Elderly Patients with Dementia' prompting concerns regarding the drug's safety. It

Table 27.3 Conventional antipsychotics.

Study	Diagnosis	N	Design	Dose (mg/day) duration	Response	Adverse effects
Haloperidol						
Schneider et al., 1990	Dementia	252 (in 7 DB, PC trials in primary dementia)	Meta-analysis of 33 neuroleptic trials	2.5–4.6, haloperidol, 3–8 weeks	Little benefit beyond placebo across all neuroleptics; average effect 18 per cent greater than placebo	Not reported
Devanand et al., 1998	AD	71	Randomized DB, PC, parallel group	2–3 or 0.5–0.75, 6 weeks	Decreased psychosis, aggression, agitation with higher dose only, 55–60 per cent response versus 25–35 per cent low dose response versus 25–30 per cent placebo	Moderate–severe EPS at high dose (20 per cent)
Christensen and Benfield, 1998	Organic mental syndrome	48	Randomized crossover to alprazolam	Mean 0.64, 6 weeks	No difference between treatments on CGI, SCAG	None seen at this low dose
De Deyn et al., 1999	AD, vascular, mixed	344	Randomized MC, DB, parallel group risperidone or placebo	Mean 1.2, 13 weeks	Significantly greater improvement for haloperidol versus placebo on BEHAVE-AD and CMAI, decreased physical and verbal aggression (72 per cent risperidone versus 69 per cent haloperidol versus 61 per cent placebo on BEHAVE-AD)	EPS 22 per cent, somnolence (18 per cent haloperidol versus 4 per cent placebo)
Allain et al., 2000	AD, VaD, mixed	306	Randomized MC, DB, PC, parallel group	100–300 tiapride or 2–6 haloperidol, 21 days	Significantly improved CGI and MOSES irritability/ aggressiveness subscore for both drugs compared to placebo, no differences between drugs	Less EPS with tiapride than haloperidol

(Continued over)

Table 27.3 Conventional antipsychotics. (continued)

Study	Diagnosis	N	Design	Dose (mg/day) duration	Response	Adverse effects
Teri et al., 2000	AD	149	Randomized DB, PC, parallel group	1.8 haloperidol, 200 trazodone, or behaviour management techniques, 16 weeks	Reduced agitation not significantly different between treated and placebo groups	Less EPS with behaviour management techniques
Tariot et al., 2002	Probable AD with psychosis	284	Randomized, PC, DB versus quetiapine (n = 94 on haloperidol)	Mean 1.89, 8 weeks	No change in psychosis, some decrease in agitation	EPS, sedation
				Perphenazine mean 6.5 mg/d	Agitation/aggression, lability tension significantly improved on cit versus placebo but not perphenazine versus placebo	No differences in SEs
Pollock et al., 2002	AD, VaD, mixed		Randomized, PC, DB perphenazine versus citalopram	Citalopram mean 20 mg/d 17 days	Response rate NR. Significant improvement in total numbers score on cit versus placebo but not perphenazine	

AD, Alzheimer's disease; BEHAVE-AD, Behavioral Pathology in Alzheimer's Disease Rating Scale; CMAI, Cohen-Mansfield Agitation Inventory; DB, double blind; CGI, Clinical Global Impression; EPS, extrapyrimidal symptoms; MC, multicentre; MOSES, Multidimensional Observation Scale for Elderly Subjects; NR, not reported; PC, placebo controlled; SCAG, Sandoz Clinical Assessment–Geriatric Scale.

Table 27.4 Atypical antipsychotics.

Study drug	Diagnosis	N	Design	Dose (mg/day) duration	Response	Adverse effects
Olanzapine						
Satterlee et al., 1995	AD	238	Randomized, MC, PC, DB	1–8, 8 weeks	No benefit versus placebo	None reported versus placebo
Street et al., 2000	AD, moderate–severe	206	Randomized, MC, PC, DB, parallel group	5, 10 and 15, 6 weeks	Decreased agitation, delusions, hallucinations on NPI-NH at 5 and 10 (but not 15) mg/day versus placebo	Dose-dependent sedation, abnormal gait
Street et al., 2001	AD	105	Open as f/u to previous 6 week DB trial	Flexible 5–15, 18 weeks	Significantly improved agitation and other symptoms by NPI-NH and other scales	Somnolence, accidental injury, rash
Meehan et al., 2002	AD, VaD or mixed with acute agitation	272	Randomized, MC, PC, DB	IM 5, 2.5 or 1 lorazepam, 2 h and prn × 2 within 20 h	Decreased agitation at 2 and 24 h	No significant difference between placebo and any active treatment
Quetiapine						
Tariot et al., 2000a	Various psychotic disorders	184	Open, MC	12.5–800 (median 137.5), 52 weeks	Significant decreases in BPRS total and CGI severity	Somnolence (31 per cent), accidental injury (24 per cent), dizziness (17 per cent)
Scharre and Chang, 2002	AD	10	Open	50–150 (mean = 100), 12 weeks	Improved NPI for delusions and agitation or aggression	Drowsiness (40 per cent), weight gain (40 per cent)
Davis and Baskys, 2002	LBD	10	Open	25–150 (50 mg modal), 12 weeks	Significant reduction in total NPI and agitation subscales of NPI and BPRS	No significant increase in EPS
Tariot et al., 2002	Probable AD with psychosis	284	Randomized, DB, PC versus haloperidol (n = 91 on quetiapine)	Mean 100, 8 weeks	No change in psychosis, some decrease in agitation	Sedation

(Continued over)

Table 27.4 Atypical antipsychotics. (continued)

Study drug	Diagnosis	N	Design	Dose (mg/day) duration	Response	Adverse effects
Zhong, 2007	AD, VaD or mixed with agitation	333	Randomized, DB, PC	Fixed dose 100, 200, 10 weeks	Significant reduction of agitation at 200 mg/d in overall dementia group and in AD subgroup. Trend only at 100 mg/d	Sedation (ir 6.5 per cent of placebo, 11.3 per cent 100 mg/d, and 17.6 per cent 200 mg/d groups). Lethargy (in 5.4 per cent of placebo, 7.3 per cent of 100 mg/ d, and 12.0 per cent of 200 mg/d groups)
Risperidone						
Herrmann, 1998b	AD, vascular, Lewy body	22	Case reports	Mean 1.5, 1 week–10 months	Improvement CGI (17)	EPS (11), sedation (1), drooling (1)
Lavretsky and Sultzer, 1998	AD, vascular, PD, PSP, mixed	15	Open (concurrent psychotropics allowed)	0.5–3, 9 weeks	Decreased agitation (in all 15)	Sedation (5), akathisia (1)
Risperidone						
De Deyn et al., 1999	AD, vascular, mixed dementia	344	Randomized MC, DB, parallel group versus placebo or haloperidol	Mean 1.1, 13 weeks	Decreased physical and verbal aggression (72 per cent risperidone versus 69 per cent haloperidol versus 61 per cent for placebo)	EPS not different from placebo, somnolerce (12 per cent risperidone versus 4 per cent placebo)
Katz et al., 1999	AD, vascular, mixed dementia	625	Randomized MC, PC, DB, parallel group (lorazepam, benztropine and chloral hydrate allowed PRN)	0.5, 1.0, 2.0, 12 weeks	Dose-dependent decrease in aggression and psychosis, significant at 1 and 2 (but not 0.5 mg/day)	Somnolence, EPS 21 per cent (on 2 mg/day, compared to 12 per cent on placebo), mild peripheral edema in some
Brodaty et al., 2003	AD, VD, mixed	345	Randomized, MC, PC, DB	Mean 1.0, 12 weeks	Significant reductions in CMAI total aggression score and BEHAVE-AD aggressiveness	Somnolence, UTI
Mintzer et al., 2004	AD	473	Randomized, PC, DB	0.5–1.5 mg, 8 weeks	No difference on CGI-C and BEHAVE between placebo and risperidone	Somnolence

(Continued over)

Study	Diagnosis	n	Design	Dose/duration	Efficacy	Adverse events
Suh et al., 2007	AC, VD, mixed	120	Randomized, DB, crossover	0.5–1.5 mg risperidone or haloperidol 18 weeks	Improvement in total and subscale scores of the BEHAVE-AD-K, the total and subscale scores of the CMAI-K, and CGI-C was greater with risperidone than with haloperidol	Less EPS in risperidone group
Aripiprazole						
De Deyn et al., 2003	AD	108	Randomized, PC, DB	Mean 10 mg, 10 weeks	No significant drug-placebo difference on primary endpoint. Some secondary measures showed drug-placebo differences at some time points	Somnolence (in 1 per cent of placebo and 8 per cent of drug groups)
Breder, 2007	AD	487	Randomized, PC, DB	2, 5, 10, 10 weeks	Significant drug-placebo difference on primary endpoint in 10 mg/d group. Significant effects on CGI-S and total BPRS in 10 mg/d group; significant effects in 5 and 10 mg/d groups on CMAI	No significant differences in rates of AEs across groups
Alexopoulos et al., 2004	AD	256	Randomized, PC, DB	Mean 8.6 mg/d, 10 weeks	No significant drug-placebo difference on primary endpoints	Somnolence (4 per cent in placebo and 14 per cent in aripip groups)

AD, Alzheimer's disease; BEHAVE-AD, Behavioral Pathology in Alzheimer's Disease Rating Scale; BPRS, Brief Psychiatric Rating Scale; CGI, Clinical Global Impression; CMAI, Cohen-Mansfield Agitation Inventory; DB, double blind; EPS, extrapyrimidal symptoms; LBD, Lewy body disease; MC, multicentre; NPI, Neuropsychiatric Inventory; NPI-NH, Neuropsychiatric Inventory – Nursing Home version; PC, placebo controlled; PRN, *pro re nata* (as needed); VaD, vascular dementia.

referred to CVAEs (e.g. stroke, transient ischaemic attack), including fatalities, reported in patients (mean age 85 years; age range 73–97) in trials of risperidone in elderly patients with dementia-related psychosis and/or agitation. In placebo-controlled trials, a significantly higher incidence of CVAEs was noted in patients treated with risperidone compared to those treated with placebo. Risperidone was associated with a three-fold increased risk of serious CVAEs compared with placebo. Soon after, a similar warning was applied to olanzapine and aripiprazole. The increased risk for CVAEs was determined from research clinical trials and is based on unbiased estimates. However, the construct 'CVAEs' was defined after the trials were completed and was based on spontaneously reported adverse events and interpretation of the risk was limited by the fact that the studies were not designed to investigate a causal link with CVAEs (Burke and Tariot, 2009).

27.6.3　Olanzapine

Studies suggest benefit of olanzapine in treating agitation in patients with dementia. A 6-week, randomized, parallel-group, multicentre study of olanzapine in 206 nursing home residents with dementia and agitation and/or psychosis was completed using fixed doses of 5, 10 and 15 mg/day versus placebo (Street et al., 2000). In patients receiving 5 and 10 mg/day, significant improvement in agitation and aggression compared to placebo was seen, and patients receiving 5 mg/day also demonstrated significant improvement compared to placebo in broader assessments of psychopathology. Sedation and postural instability were observed at all doses in at least 25 per cent of subjects. Some of the patients from this trial received follow-up open-label, flexible-dose treatment for 18 weeks; results were consistent with the findings from an earlier paper (Street et al., 2001).

Meehan et al. (2002) studied acute treatment of agitation with intramuscular olanzapine in 272 inpatients or nursing home residents with AD and/or vascular dementia (VaD). Olanzapine was superior to placebo in treating agitation at 2 and 24 hours. Adverse events were not significantly different between groups. At present, this formulation has not been marketed in the United States.

A cautionary note is warranted when considering using this agent in dementia patients. In January 2004, Eli Lilly issued a warning of increased incidence of CVAEs in dementia patients treated with olanzapine. The medication has also been widely criticized for its potential to cause metabolic syndrome, at least in younger populations. Limited data in the elderly come chiefly from the Clinical Antipsychotic Trial of Intervention Effectiveness-AD (CATIE-AD) trial.

27.6.4　Quetiapine fumarate

Two open trials and a case series with quetiapine within a dose range of 25–800 mg/d suggested possible behavioural benefits for agitation (Tariot et al., 2000; Davis and Baskys, 2002; Scharre and Chang, 2002). A 10-week multicentre

placebo-controlled trial of quetiapine versus haloperidol was conducted in elderly nursing home patients with psychosis that was operationally defined. These criteria were implemented prior to the development of clinical criteria for the psychosis of AD proposed recently (Jeste and Finkel, 2000). This trial is notable in that it may have been the first large placebo-controlled study of antipsychotics in patients with dementia selected because of the presence of psychotic symptoms. Flexible doses of the medication were permitted; the mean daily dose of haloperidol was 2 mg/day at endpoint, while that of quetiapine was approximately 120 mg/day. None of the treatment groups differed with respect to reduction in measures of psychosis, which was the primary outcome of the trial, whereas there was evidence of reduced agitation on some measures with both haloperidol and quetiapine treatment but not placebo. Tolerability of quetiapine was superior to that of haloperidol, however evidence of improvement in agitation was inconsistent.

Zhong et al. (2007) found quetiapine to be effective at 200 mg/day on most measures of agitation associated with dementia with an inconsistent effect of 100 mg/day. Unlike a prior study (Ballard et al., 2005), no worsening in cognitive measures was noted, but sedation was seen in a substantial minority of patients.

27.6.5　Ziprasidone and aripiprazole

There are no geriatrics-specific studies of ziprasidone in the elderly and none in patients with dementia. However, case reports have suggested both oral and injectible forms of the medication may be well tolerated and of some benefit in the treatment of agitation in this population.

Results from a placebo-controlled trial of aripiprazole in 208 outpatients meeting new clinical criteria for psychosis of AD (Jeste and Finkel, 2000) have been presented in abstract form (De Deyn et al., 2003). The medication was generally well tolerated, with numerically more frequent sedation in the active treatment group. The primary outcome, a measure of psychosis, did not show a difference between drug and placebo although there was some behavioural benefit on secondary measures. A multicentre, randomized, double-blind, placebo-controlled trial of three fixed doses of aripiprazole (2, 5 and 10 mg) for the treatment of psychosis in patients with AD indicated that 10 mg daily was safe and efficacious, revealing significant improvement in psychosis, agitation and clinical global impression (Mintzer et al., 2007). In addition, a recent secondary analysis of CATIE-AD data showed that weight gain occurred in women, with olanzapine and quetiapine in particular, and unfavourable changes in HDL cholesterol and girth were evident with olanzapine (Zheng et al., 2009).

27.6.6　Atypicals: summary

The data indicate that atypical antipsychotics as a class are likely better tolerated than typical antipsychotics and at least as efficacious. There appear to be modest differences within the class of atypicals in terms of effectiveness, tolerability and side-effect profile. To address this further, the National Institute of Mental Health (NIMH) conducted the CATIE-AD, which was designed to compare the effectiveness of atypical antipsychotic medications and placebo in patients with AD and psychosis or agitated/aggressive behaviour (Schneider et al., 2006). The study included 421 outpatients with AD and psychosis or agitated/aggressive behaviour. In the first phase of the trial, patients were assigned randomly to masked, flexible-dose treatment with olanzapine, quetiapine, risperidone or placebo for up to 36 weeks. Phase 1 study results have been published (Schneider et al., 2006). The primary measure of effectiveness, time-to-discontinuation for any reason, was not significantly different between the treatment conditions, with median treatment durations of 8.1 weeks for olanzapine, 5.3 weeks for quetiapine, 7.4 weeks for risperidone and 8.0 weeks for placebo. The median time-to-discontinuation due to lack of efficacy was significantly longer with olanzapine and risperidone (22.1 and 26.7 weeks, respectively) versus quetiapine and placebo (9.1 and 9.0 weeks, respectively). However, patients treated with atypicals displayed a shorter time to discontinuation due to adverse events or drug intolerability compared with placebo. Time to discontinuation due to intolerability favoured placebo and quetiapine. Discontinuations due to intolerability occurred in 24 per cent of patients receiving olanzapine, 18 per cent receiving risperidone, 16 per cent receiving quetiapine and 5 per cent receiving placebo. Safety findings were generally consistent with reports of prior studies. Although the trial has frequently been misinterpreted as showing that these medications are ineffective, a more accurate analysis reveals that there is a high rate of adversity that offsets evidence of efficacy, but that a minority of patients also show clinical benefit without toxicity.

Secondary analyses of CATIE-AD phase I data were consistent with a 2006 Cochrane Collaboration review of placebo-controlled trials, which concluded that risperidone and olanzapine may improve aggression compared to placebo and that risperidone may improve psychosis relative to placebo (Ballard and Waite, 2006) In the CATIE-AD trial, patients receiving risperidone demonstrated improvement in a variety of behavioural ratings compared to placebo at the time of discontinuation in phase 1 (Sultzer et al., 2008). Patients taking olanzapine had improvements on measures of hostility and suspiciousness, but demonstrated a worsening of depressive symptoms compared to placebo (Sultzer et al., 2008).

During the past decade, atypical antipsychotics have largely replaced typical agents in the treatment of psychosis, aggression and agitation in patients with dementia because of perceived greater tolerability and lesser, but still increased, risk for acute extrapyramidal symptoms (EPS), and because of the documented lower risk for tardive dyskinesia (TD) compared to typical agents (Jeste et al., 1999; Stanniland and Taylor, 2000; Ritsner et al., 2004; Gill et al., 2005; Burke and Tariot, 2009). On the other hand, most of these drugs have other acute and subacute side effects in elderly people, such as sedation, postural hypotension and, in some cases, falls, especially at higher doses. There have been no large-scale published studies of antipsychotic-associated diabetes, obesity and dyslipidaemia among patients with dementia,

although this a major concern in younger populations. In addition, impairment of cognitive test scores, gait disturbance and anticholinergic effects have been reported in some instances. A recent meta-analysis also demonstrated a significant increase in respiratory tract and urinary tract infections and peripheral oedema in people treated with risperidone as compared with placebo (Ballard and Waite, 2006).

In 2005, a US Food and Drug Administration warning highlighted a significant increase in mortality risk for patients with AD treated with atypical antipsychotic drugs compared with individuals receiving placebo in 17 RCTs. It stated that elderly patients with dementia-related psychosis treated with atypical antipsychotic drugs are at an increased risk of death compared to placebo. The analyses of these trials revealed a risk of death in the drug-treated patients of between 1.6 and 1.7 times that seen in of the placebo-treated group. Although the causes of death were varied, most of the deaths appeared to be either cardiovascular (e.g. heart failure, sudden death) or infectious (e.g. pneumonia) in nature.

Subsequent studies, mainly involving large public databases, have found similar or even higher death rates among elders receiving conventional antipsychotics, which has resulted in a second broader black box warning for all antipsychotics in 2008. Several recent studies aimed at assessing mortality risk in patients receiving atypical antipsychotics (Ballard et al., 2009; Ray et al., 2009) confirm an elevated risk.

Mounting evidence of possible serious adverse effects of these medications underscores the need for caution when considering use of atypicals. Careful evaluation of the risks and benefits of treatment is warranted, including assessment of the level of distress and risk of injury to the patient as a result of insufficiently treated agitated behaviours. Treatment of patients with dementia should emphasize non-pharmacological approaches, including carefully investigating for possible delirium and for social or environmental factors that lead to interventions that capitalize on the patient's residual strengths. The placebo response rate in clinical trials of antipsychotics in dementia is quite high (30–40 per cent), underscoring the notion that nonspecific factors (e.g. enhanced attention) can be therapeutic in this population. However, atypicals remain a valid consideration when other interventions have proven insufficient.

27.7   BENZODIAZEPINES

According to the 'metaphor' approach adopted in this chapter, we would consider these agents first for patients with prominent anxiety. Since features of anxiety and depression overlap extensively in any case, and particularly in patients with dementia, many physicians opt to use an antidepressant rather than a benzodiazepine if medication is needed. Benzodiazepines have been used for agitation associated with dementia, in several studies that have been reviewed previously (Patel and Tariot, 1991; Loy et al., 1999). Most of these showed a reduced level of agitation with short-term therapy. There have been very few studies in the past decade, none of which was placebo-controlled. In the aggregate these studies suggest that agitation associated with anxiety, sleep problems and motor tension might be most likely to respond. Some earlier studies in which benzodiazepines were compared to traditional antipsychotics suggested that antipsychotics might be superior.

Prior reviews indicate that side effects occur commonly with benzodiazepines, including sedation, ataxia, falls, confusion, anterograde amnesia, lightheadedness, paradoxical agitation, as well as tolerance and withdrawal syndromes (Patel and Tariot, 1991). It is because of this safety profile that we reserve the use of benzodiazepines for situational disturbances, such as dental procedures, for as-needed use or situations where routine use has been attempted and found to be convincingly safe. Drugs such as lorazepam and oxazepam tend to be selected first because they have straightforward metabolism and relatively short half-lives.

27.8 BUSPIRONE

There have been no placebo-controlled, double-blind RCTs of this agent. Reduced agitation has been reported in some open trials that we have summarized previously (Loy et al., 1999; Rosenquist et al., 2000), using doses in the range of 10–60 mg/day. The medication has the advantage of generally good tolerability, with the exception of headache, nervousness and dizziness in a modest percentage of patients. There is no evidence regarding tolerance or paradoxical effects in this population.

27.9 ANTIDEPRESSANTS

We would consider using this class of agents first in patients with agitation accompanied by evidence of depressive features as described in the introduction. There is some evidence linking impulsivity to disordered serotonergic function

(Coccaro, 1996), lending support to the use of serotonergic agents. They have also probably been more widely assayed because of their good tolerability profile and widespread use in other psychiatric disorders.

Trazodone was one of the first studied (**Table 27.5**). There has been only one published double-blind, placebo-controlled study, showing no relative benefit of trazodone over haloperidol or placebo in outpatients with dementia and agitation (Teri et al., 2000). The trial also included a non-blinded behaviour management arm; this also showed no relative benefit. Among the non-placebo-controlled studies, doses typically reported ranged from 50 to 400 mg/day, occasionally higher. Irritability, anxiety, restlessness and depressed affect have been reported to improve, along with sleep disturbance. Reported side effects include sedation, orthostatic hypotension and delirium. The most rigorous among these compared trazodone (mean dose about 220 mg/day) with haloperidol (mean dose 2.5 mg/day) (Sultzer et al., 1997). Agitation improved equally in both patient groups, although tolerability was reported to be better in the trazodone group. The Expert Consensus Guideline (Alexopoulos et al., 2005) favours the use of trazodone to treat sleep disturbance primarily, relegating it to second- or third-line use for 'mild' agitation. A typical starting dose would be 25 mg/day, with maximum doses usually of 100–250 mg/day.

Data regarding selective serotonin reuptake inhibitors (SSRIs) are summarized in **Table 27.6**. Nyth and Gottfries (1990) performed a review of controlled studies of citalopram, which suggest some beneficial behavioural effects. Results from two open trials support this conclusion (Ragneskog et al., 1996; Pollock et al., 1997).

A double-blind, placebo-controlled study compared citalopram and perphenazine with placebo in patients with various dementia diagnoses, probable AD and DLB being the more common diagnoses, who had at least one symptom of psychosis or behavioural disturbance. Eighty-five hospitalized patients were treated after 3 days of dose escalation

Table 27.5   Antidepressants.

Study	Diagnosis	N	Design	Dose (mg/day) duration	Response	Adverse effects
Trazodone						
Sultzer et al., 1997	Dementia	28	Randomized DB parallel haloperidol	50–250, 9 weeks	Decreased agitation for both; trazodone better for verbal aggression, oppositional and repetitive behaviours	Sedation (1), imbalance (1); 1/3 fewer dropouts in trazodone group
Teri et al., 2000	AD	149	Randomized DB, PC, parallel group	1.8 haloperidol, 200 trazodone, or behaviour management techniques, 16 weeks	Reduced agitation not significantly different between treated and placebo groups	Less EPS with behaviour management techniques

AD, Alzheimer's disease; DB, double blind; EPS, extrapyramidal symptoms; PC, placebo controlled.

Table 27.6 Antidepressants: selective serotonin reuptake inhibitors.

Study	Diagnosis	N	Design	Dose (mg/day) duration	Response	Adverse effects
Citalopram						
Nyth and Gottfries, 1990	AD, vascular	98	DB, PC	10–30, 4 weeks	Decreased emotional blunting, confusion, irritability, anxiety, mood, restlessness	Confusion (2), dizziness (1), sedation (1)
Nyth et al., 1992	Dementia (29)	149	DB, PC	10–30, 6 weeks	Decreased anxiety, fear, panic, depressed mood in all	Tiredness (18), problem concentrating (9), apathy (8), dizziness (7), sedation (11), tension (11)
Ragneskog et al., 1996	AD (55), vascular dementia (30), alcoholic dementia (5), NOS (3)	123	Open, 2 centres	20–40, 1–12 months	Decreased CGI or Gottfries–Brane-Steen (GBS) for irritability, depression (60 per cent), restlessness, anxiety	Tiredness (15); dizziness (14); drowsiness, sleep disturbances, restlessness (4), aggression (3), anxiety (2)
Pollock et al., 1997	AD	15	Open	20, 2 weeks	Decreased agitation, hostility, delusions, disinhibition	Drop-outs from nausea (1), myoclonus (1)
Pollock et al., 2002	Inpatient AD, VaD, mixed, or other not specified	85	Randomized DB, PC, parallel group	20 citalopram or 6.5 mean perphenazine, up to 17 days	Significantly improved agitation for citalopram versus placebo	Similar scores among all groups
Pollock et al., 2007	Inpatient vascular dementia, DLB, AD, mixed	103	Randomized DB, PC	20–40 mg citalopram or 1–2 mg risperidone, 12 weeks	Decreased agitation and psychosis in both risperidone and citalopram group	Side effect burden was higher in risperidone group
Fluoxetine						
Auchus and Bissey-Black, 1997	AD	15	DB, PC parallel group versus haloperidol	20, 6 weeks	Neither more effective than placebo for agitation	Anxiety, nervousness, confusion, tremor
SertraLine						
Burke et al., 1997	AD, NOS dementia	19	Chart review	50, variable duration	Improved on CGIC (10/11 AD: 4/8 NOS)	None reported
Paroxetine						
Ramadan et al., 2000	AD or VaD	15	Open	10–40, three months	Verbal agitation reduced	Weight gain (5), diarrhea (1), worsened EPS (1)

AD, Alzheimer's disease; DB, double blind; CGI, Clinical Global Impression; DLB, dementia with Lewy bodies; EPS, extrapyramidal symptoms; PC, placebo controlled; NOS, not otherwise specified; VaD, vascular dementia.

with doses of 20 mg/day citalopram or 0.1 mg/kg per day of perphenazine for up to 14 days. Both citalopram and perphenazine demonstrated significant improvement compared with placebo for agitation, lability and psychosis. Side effects were similar in the three treatment groups (Pollock *et al.*, 2002). Similarly, a 12 week RCT of non-depressed patients with dementia hospitalized due to behavioural disturbances evaluated the efficacy of citalopram versus risperidone for the treatment of behavioural disturbances and psychotic symptoms associates with dementia (Pollock *et al.*, 2007). The study concluded that agitation and psychotic symptoms improved in both groups, but did not differ significantly between the groups. However, the lack of a placebo comparator limits interpretation of the clinical significance of these findings. The side-effect burden was significantly increased in the risperidone group.

An abstract from the CATIE-AD trial addressed the effectiveness of citalopram versus atypical antipsychotics and reported no differences in time to all-cause discontinuation for any antipsychotic versus citalopram (Schneider *et al.*, 2008). Times to discontinuation due to lack of efficacy or intolerability also did not differ by treatment group. Patients showed generally mild improvement on rating scales during treatment but changes did not differ significantly between antipsychotics and citalopram.

No benefit of administration has been reported yet for fluoxetine or fluvoxamine, and only anecdotes have been published regarding other SSRIs, all suggesting possible benefit, at least in individual patients. Although overall, evidence for efficacy of SSRIs is inconsistent.

Gastrointestinal distress, loss of appetite and weight, sedation, insomnia, sexual dysfunction and occasional paradoxical agitation can occur with serotonergic agents, although, as a group, they tend to be well tolerated. Because of the suggestion of benefit and the relatively benign side-effect profile, consensus statements endorse their use in some cases (Alexopoulos *et al.*, 2005).

27.10 ANTICONVULSANTS

From a clinical perspective, we might consider the use of anticonvulsants first in patients with features of mania, as well perhaps in those with prominent impulsivity, lability or episodic severe aggression. Evidence regarding these agents was summarized in earlier versions of this book; we will review it briefly here (see also **Table 27.7** and **Table 27.8**). Carbamazepine at doses of about 300 mg/day showed benefit in some, but not all, small controlled trials for treatment of agitation (Tariot *et al.*, 1994; Tariot *et al.*, 1995b; Tariot *et al.*, 1998; Olin *et al.*, 2001). Although tolerability was acceptable in these trials, side effects seen in other populations, such as rashes, sedation, hematologic abnormalities, hepatic dysfunction and altered electrolytes, would be more likely to be evident with widespread use of carbamazepine in the elderly (Tariot *et al.*, 1995b). Further, it has considerable potential for significant drug–drug interactions. Our view is that it has a limited role in this population, but the findings suggested that it might be beneficial to examine other, potentially safer, anticonvulsants.

Valproic acid, also available as the enteric-coated derivative, divalprocx sodium, is approved by the US FDA for the treatment of acute mania associated with bipolar disorder. Preliminary studies suggested that valproate may be effective and safe for the treatment of agitation associated with dementia and justified further studies. The first randomized, placebo-controlled, parallel group study of this agent was 6 weeks in duration, and suggested (but did not prove) benefit (Porsteinsson *et al.*, 2001) at a mean divalproex sodium dose of 826 mg/day (mean level 46 µg/day. Serious adverse events occurred at a rate of 10 per cent in both the drug and placebo groups, with milder side effects occurring more frequently in the drug group, chiefly consisting of sedation, gastrointestinal distress, and ataxia, typically rated as mild, and the expected decrease in average platelet count (about 20 000/mm^3). An open label extension study

Table 27.7 Anticonvulsants: carbamazepine.

Study	Diagnosis	N	Design	Dose (mg/day) duration	Response	Adverse effects
Tariot *et al.*, 1994	AD, vascular dementia	25	Crossover, PC (some other psychotropics permitted)	300 modal, 5 weeks	Decreased agitation (16 versus 4 placebo)	Tics (1), sedation
Tariot *et al.*, 1998	Dementia	51	Randomized PC (no psychotropics except chloral hydrate as needed)	300 modal, 6 weeks	Improved on CGI (20/26); also improved on OAS, BPRS, BRSD	Ataxia (nine versus three placebo), disorientation (4 versus 0 placebo), tics (1), sedation
Olin *et al.*, 2001	AD	21	Randomized, DB, PC	388, 6 weeks	Improved BPRS hostility item	Diarrhoea more common with active treatment

AD, Alzheimer's disease; BPRS, Brief Psychiatric Rating Scale; BRSD, CERAD Behavioral Rating Scale for Dementia; CGI, Clinical Global Impression; OAS, Overt Aggression Scale; PC, placebo controlled.

Table 27.8 Anticonvulsants: divalproex.

Study	Diagnosis	N	Design	Dose (mg/day) plasma level (µg/ml) duration	Response	Adverse effects
Herrmann, 1998	AD, LBD, VaD	16	Open	750–2500 (mean = 1331), (mean level = 459 µM/l), 5–34 weeks	Improved on CMAI, BEHAVE-AD (11)	Sedation, ataxia, diarrhoea (1)
Kunik et al., 1998	Dementia	13	Retrospective review (concurrent BDZs, antipsychotics)	500–1750 (mean = 846), (mean level = 48), duration variable	Decreased physical not verbal agitation and aggression on CMAI (10)	None reported; drug interaction with phenytoin noted (1)
Porsteinsson et al., 2001	AD, vascular dementia, mixed dementia	56	Randomized PC (no psychotropics except chloral hydrate as needed)	375–1375 (mean = 826), (mean level = 45), 6 weeks	Decreased agitation by BPRS and CGI	Sedation and nausea, vomiting or diarrhoea
Tariot et al., 2001	AD and/or VaD with secondary mania	172	Randomized, DB, PC, parallel-group	1000 median	Significant improvement on CMAI verbal agitation subscale	Somnolence, thrombocytopenia
Sival et al., 2002	AD, VaD, other and mixed dementia	42	Randomized, DB, PC, crossover	480 (mean level = 41), 3 weeks active treatment	No change in aggressive behaviour compared to placebo	Small increase in incidence of adverse events compared to placebo
Porsteinsson et al., 2003	AD, VaD, mixed dementia	46	Open extension	250–1500 (mean = 851), (mean level = 47), 6 weeks	Decreased agitation by BPRS and CGI	Fall, sedation, and nausea, vomiting or diarrhoea

AD, Alzheimer's disease; BEHAVE-AD, Behavioral Pathology in Alzheimer's Disease Rating Scale; BPRS, Behavioral Pathology in Alzheimer's Disease Rating Scale; CGI, Behavioral Pathology in Alzheimer's Disease Rating Scale; CMAI, Cohen-Mansfield Agitation Inventory; LBD, Lewy body disease; PC, placebo controlled; VaD, vascular dementia.

(Porsteinsson *et al.*, 2003) confirmed the findings from the placebo-controlled phase of the trial.

A randomized, double-blind, placebo-controlled, cross-over study of valproate 480 mg/day for 3 weeks was conducted in patients with dementia and aggressive behaviour (Sival *et al.*, 2002). No significant differences in aggressive behaviour in this short-term trial were seen between placebo and active treatments according to the primary outcome measure; there was a trend to improvement in measures of aggression; and there were significant effects on restless, melancholic, and anxious behaviours. There were no drug-placebo differences in rate or type of adverse events.

The first multicentre, placebo-controlled, 6-week RCT of divalproex sodium was conducted in 172 nursing home residents with dementia and agitation who also met criteria for secondary mania. A target dose of 20 mg/kg/day was reached in 10 days (Tariot *et al.*, 2001). This titration rate and dose resulted in sedation in about 20 per cent of the drug-treated group and a relatively high dropout rate, leading to premature discontinuation of the study ($n = 100$ completers). There were no significant drug-placebo differences in change in manic features, but there was a significant effect of drug on agitation. Sedation occurred in 36 per cent of the drug group versus 20 per cent of the placebo group, and mild thrombocytopenia affected 7 per cent of the drug group and none of the placebo-treated patients. The results from this trial were used to amend the Package Insert information, cautioning against use of similar doses and/or titration rates in the elderly.

A later double-blind, placebo-controlled 6 week RCT in 153 nursing home patients with AD complicated by agitation was conducted by the Alzheimer's Disease Cooperative study (ADCS) (Tariot *et al.*, 2005). This trial showed similar safety and tolerability findings as the previous valproate studies, but failed to show benefit over placebo in the treatment of agitation associated with dementia. This study was the largest to prospectively address agitation as the primary outcome.

There has also been hope that, based on putative neuroprotective effects, valproate administration might be therapeutic for long-term treatment of AD. For this reason, the ADCS conducted a placebo-controlled trial of low doses (about 10 mg/kg/day) divalproex sodium in 313 people with AD not yet complicated by agitation or psychosis. The treatment period was two years, with a 2 month placebo washout at the end of double-blind treatment. The primary outcome was survival until incident agitation or psychosis; key secondary measures addressed measures of cognitive, functional and global progression of dementia. Preliminary results have been presented in abstract form (Tariot *et al.*, unpublished abstract, ICAD 2009). There was no clinical benefit of active treatment for any of the outcomes.

There are no controlled studies of the newer anticonvulsants including lamotrogine, gabapentin and topiramate. There are a few case reports and case series suggest benefit with gabapentin (Regan and Gordon, 1997; Hawkins *et al.*, 2000; Herrmann *et al.*, 2000; Roane *et al.*, 2000; Megna *et al.*, 2002).

Evidence regarding the efficacy of anticonvulsants in the treatment of agitation associated with dementia appears is sparse, conflicting and inconclusive. Further study might clarify the clinical role for this class of agents, but at present the data do not support common use. Nevertheless, some consensus statements suggest a possible role as a second- or third-line treatment for agitation and aggressive behaviours in patients with dementia. We would only consider this approach if other treatments had failed.

27.11   SELEGILINE

Also known as L-deprenyl, selegiline relatively selectively inhibits monoamine oxidase (MAO) type B at doses up to 10 mg/day, while non-selectively inhibiting MAO A and B at higher doses. It has primarily been used in the treatment of motor dysfunction patients with Parkinson's disease, but there are a surprising number of clinical reports in patients with dementia. In many cases, the agent was assessed as a possible disease modifier or cognition-enhancing agent, rather than as treatment for behaviour per se. In a meta-analysis, Tolbert and Fuller (1996) reported that all uncontrolled studies of this agent in dementia that addressed behavioural changes indicated beneficial behavioural effects of selegiline, whilst 2/5 double-blind, placebo-controlled studies reported somewhat positive behavioural effects. A different meta-analysis of 11 randomized placebo-controlled double-blind trials found that four trials indicated positive behavioural effects (Birks and Flicker, 1998). Since the overall evidence of behavioural efficacy is limited, selegiline is not likely to be a first, or even second, choice for the treatment of agitation. Its role as a neuroprotective agent or cognitive enhancer in dementia has yet to be fully clarified.

27.12   α AND β-ADRENERIC AGENTS

Beta-blocking agents have not been subject to rigorous study. Most of the evidence comes from open trials conducted more than ten years ago (Rosenquist *et al.*, 2000). Doses used are typically below 100 mg/day for propranolol. A recent study evaluating the efficacy of the β-adrenergic antagonist propranolol for treatment-resistant disruptive behaviours and overall behavioural status in nursing home residents AD (Peskind *et al.*, 2005) illustrated moderate benefits. Short-term propranolol augmentation treatment appeared modestly effective and well tolerated for overall behavioural status in patients with disruptive behaviours. Propranolol may be helpful specifically for aggression and uncooperativeness. However, the usefulness of propranolol in this very old and frail population was limited by the high frequency of relative contraindications to β-blocker treatment

Adverse reactions of β-blockers include bradycardia, hypotension, potential worsening of congestive heart failure or asthma, reduced adrenergic response to hypoglycaemia in patients with diabetes, sedation, increased confusion, psychosis, depression and increased atrioventricular block. It is unclear what role this class of medication has in the treatment of agitation associated with dementia at this point. If it is to be attempted at all, we would argue that it should occur only after safer and more conventional therapies have failed, and only with careful monitoring for side effects.

Prazosin, a nonsedating medication used for hypertension and benign prostatic hypertrophy, antagonizes NE effects at brain postsynaptic α-1 adrenoreceptors. A recent small, double-blind, placebo-controlled, parallel group study examined the efficacy and tolerability of prazosin for behavioural symptoms in patients with agitation/aggression in AD (Wang et al., 2009). Subjects received doses between 1 and 6 mg daily using a flexible dose algorithm. Those receiving prazosin displayed a significant improvement in behavioural symptoms as compared to the placebo group with no significant increase in adverse effects. These encouraging preliminary results require confirmation in larger controlled studies.

27.13   LITHIUM

There are no controlled studies of this agent for agitation in dementia; there are at most some case series published in the 1980s (Rosenquist et al., 2000). The limited literature suggests that occasional patients showed improvement, but toxicity was common, including worsening of extrapyramidal syndromes, ataxia and confusion. Since the therapeutic index is so narrow, we find it hard to justify using this agent in a patient lacking a syndromal diagnosis of bipolar disorder. Even then, we are more inclined to use anticonvulsants first. If we choose lithium, close monitoring is in order.

27.14   CHOLINERGIC THERAPIES

As summarized by Cummings (2000), there is evidence that cholinergic agents, especially cholinesterase inhibitors, may have modest clinically relevant psychotropic effects in some patients with dementia. For the most part, the studies were not designed to address behavioural outcomes as the primary goal. A review of 24 trials involving nearly 5800 participants found benefits of treatment noted on measures of activities of daily living and behaviour in patients receiving donepezil (Birks, 2006). The effects of donepezil, galantamine and rivastigmine in people with mild, moderate or severe dementia due to AD were also supported in a review of ten double-blind, placebo-controlled RCTs (Birks and Harvey, 2006). The reviewers found no differences in efficacy between study medications. A meta-analysis of 29 parallel-group or cross-over, placebo-controlled RCTs of outpatients diagnosed with mild to moderate AD meant to quantify the efficacy of cholinesterase inhibitors for neuropsychiatric and functional outcomes found that cholinesterase inhibitors had a modest beneficial impact. No difference in efficacy among various cholinesterase inhibitors was observed (Trinh et al., 2003).

Citing preliminary studies which were conducted in patients displaying baseline low levels of psychopathology associated with dementia, Cummings et al. (2006) conducted an exploratory analysis of data pertaining to the efficacy of donepezil treatment of patients with severe behavioural disturbances. The results of these analyses suggest that donepezil reduces behavioural symptoms, particularly mood disturbances and delusions, in patients with AD with relatively severe psychopathology.

By way of overview, there have not been a sufficient number of prospective RCTs specifically addressing whether cholinesterase inhibitor therapy definitely mitigates symptoms already present, or delays emergence of symptoms in those not yet afflicted. In the aggregate, the data available suggest that these salutary effects may exist. Since best practice is to treat most people with AD with these agents anyway, there seems to be little reason to refrain from using them as first-line therapy for treatment of non-emergent psychopathology in people with AD.

27.15   MEMANTINE

Memantine is a non-competitive inhibitor of N-methyl-D-aspartate (NMDA) receptors that may permit normal memory formation but blocks their excitotoxic activation (Winblad et al., 2002). Memantine was approved for treatment of moderate to severe AD, alone or in addition to cholinesterase inhibitors, on the basis of three placebo-controlled trials (Winblad and Poritis, 1999; Reisberg et al., 2003; Tariot et al., 2004). A review of double-blind, parallel group, placebo-controlled, RCTs of memantine in people with dementia (McShane et al., 2006) reported a slight decrease in development of agitation in patients taking memantine. This effect was slightly larger, but still small, in moderate to severe AD. There was no evidence about whether memantine had an effect on agitation which is already present. A significant advantage for memantine over placebo was also supported by a pooled analysis of three studies of patients with symptoms of aggression/agitation, delusions and hallucinations (Wilcock et al., 2008).

As with the overview of the behavioural effects of cholinesterase inhibitors, the available data suggest, but do not prove, that memantine therapy will reduce behavioural symptoms or delay their emergence. Since it is indicated for treatment of moderate-severe AD, there is little reason not to deploy it in such patients and observe whether behavioural symptoms are improved.

27.16   HORMONAL THERAPY

There are no definitive studies of hormonal agents, which are sometimes used when more conventional therapies fail. The available literature was summarized by Rosenquist et al. (2000). The anecdotal evidence is by no means conclusive, and only suggests that these agents might occasionally be helpful particularly in patient displaying sexual disinhibition. Controlled studies would be extremely useful.

27.17   SUMMARY

Humane treatment of patients with dementia includes vigorously addressing the kinds of behavioural and psychological signs and symptoms that are likely to occur. The main emphasis should be on non-pharmacological approaches, including carefully investigating for possible delirium and searching hard for social or environmental interventions that capitalize on the patient's residual strengths. It is indeed this process of attempting to 'find what works' that makes treatment in this population so fascinating, as well as challenging.

Psychotropics should be reserved for cases where other, simpler interventions have been attempted and deemed inadequate. We advocate a target symptom-based approach, which matches the most salient target symptoms to a relevant drug class. Although there is no compelling empirical support for this approach, it has the advantage of being face-valid and logical, which are reassuring features when one is a consultant in a confusing situation.

Much of the available data do in fact indicate that antipsychotics as a group can show benefit for agitation associated with psychotic features. However, these medications are not without risk. Mounting evidence as to the cerebrovascular adverse effects and other potentially deadly side effects of both conventional and atypical antipsychotics has overshadowed evidence of their efficacy. Although they remain an indispensible treatment for patients displaying severely agitated and psychotic behaviours, this increasing safety data emphasized the need for vigilance when evaluating appropriate treatment options.

Emerging data regarding alternative treatment options for agitated behaviours such as antidepressant therapy is promising, but still limited. The available literature regarding non-antipsychotic medication includes anticonvulsants, anxiolytics and a variety of other agents with less foundation. As data accrue regarding these therapies, we will have a clearer sense of exactly how and when they should be deployed. In the meantime, clinicians are obliged to deal as thoughtfully as possible with patients on a case-by-case basis, attempting first and foremost to avoid toxicity of therapies intended to help.

REFERENCES

Alexopoulos GS, Streim J, Carpenter D, Docherty JP. (2004) Expert consensus panel for using antipsychotic drugs in older patients. Using antipsychotic agents in older patients. *Journal of Clinical Psychiatry* **65** (Suppl. 2): 5–99.

Alexopoulos GS, Jeste DV, Chung H *et al.* (2005) The expert consensus guideline series. Treatment of dementia and its behavioral disturbances. Introduction: methods, commentary, and summary. *Postgraduate Medicine* **Spec No**: 6–22.

Allain H, Dautzenberg PH, Maurer K *et al.* (2000) Double blind study of tiapride versus haloperidol and placebo in agitation and aggressiveness in elderly patients with cognitive impairment. *Psychopharmacology (Berlin)* **148**: 361–6.

American Geriatrics Society; American Association for Geriatric Psychiatry. (2005) Consensus statement on improving the quality of mental health care in U.S. nursing homes: management of depression and behavioral symptoms associated with dementia. *Journal of the American Geriatrics Society* **51**: 1287–98.

Auchus AP, Bissey-Black C. (1997) Pilot study of haloperidol, fluoxetine, and placebo for agitation in Alzheimer's disease. *Journal of Neuropsychiatry and Clinical Neurosciences* **9**: 591–3.

Ballard C, Waite J. (2006) The effectiveness of atypical antipsychotics for the treatment of aggression and psychosis in Alzheimer's disease. *Cochrane Database of Systematic Reviews* (1): CD003476.

Ballard C, Grace J, McKeith I, Holmes C. (1998) Neuroleptic sensitivity in dementia with Lewy bodies and Alzheimer's disease. *Lancet* **351**: 1032–3.

Ballard C, Margallo-Lana M, Juszczak E *et al.* (2005) Quetiapine and rivastigmine and cognitive decline in Alzheimer's disease: randomized double blind placebo controlled trial. *British Medical Journal* **330**: 874–87.

Ballard C, Hanney ML, Theodoulou M *et al.* (2009) The dementia antipsychotic withdrawal trial (DART): long-term follow-up of randomised placebo controlled trial. Available from: www.thelancet.com/neurology Jan 9.

Birks J. (2006) Cholinesterase inhibitors for Alzheimer's disease. *Cochrane Database of Systematic Reviews* (1): CD005593.

Birks J, Flicker L. (1998) The efficacy and safety of selegiline for the symptomatic treatment of Alzheimer's disease: a systematic review of the evidence (Cochrane review). The Cochrane Library, Issue 2. Oxford: Update Software.

Birks J, Harvey RJ. (2006) Donepezil for dementia due to Alzheimer's disease. *Cochrane Database of Systematic Reviews* (1): CD001190.

Birks J, Grimley Evans J, Iakovidou V, Tsolaki M. (2004) Rivastigmine for Alzheimer's disease. *Cochrane Database of Systematic Reviews* (4): CD001191.

Brodaty H, Ames D, Snowdon J *et al.* (2003) A randomized placebo-controlled trial of risperidone for the treatment of aggression, agitation, and psychosis of dementia. *Journal of Clinical Psychiatry* **64**: 134–43.

Burke AD, Tariot PN. (2009) Atypical antipsychotics in the elderly: a review of therapeutic trends and clinical outcomes. *Expert Opinion on Pharmacotherapy* **10**: 2407–14.

Burke WJ, Dewan V, Wengel SP *et al.* (1997) The use of selective serotonin reuptake inhibitors for depression and psychosis complicating dementia. *International Journal of Geriatric Psychiatry* **12**: 519–25.

Christensen DB, Benfield WR. (1998) Alprazolam as an alternative to low-dose haloperidol in older, cognitively impaired nursing facility patients. *Journal of the American Geriatrics Society* **46**: 620–5.

Coccaro EF. (1996) Neurotransmitter correlates of impulsive aggression in humans. *Annals of the New York Academy of Sciences* **794**: 82–9.

Cohen-Mansfield J, Billig N. (1986) Agitated behaviors in the elderly. I. A conceptual review. *Journal of the American Geriatrics Society* **34**: 711–21.

Cummings JL. (2000) Cholinesterase Inhibitors: A new class of psychotropic compounds. *American Journal of Psychiatry* **157**: 4–16.

Cummings JL, McRae T, Zhang R. (2006) Donepezil-Sertraline Study Group. Effects of donepezil on neuropsychiatric symptoms in patients with dementia and severe behavioral disorders. *American Journal of Geriatric Psychiatry* 14: 605–12.

Cummings JL, Schneider E, Tariot PN *et al.* (2006) Behavioral effects of memantine in Alzheimer disease patients receiving donepezil treatment. *Neurology* 67: 57–63.

Davis P, Baskys A. (2002) Quetiapine effectively reduces psychotic symptoms in patients with Lewy body dementia: an advantage of the unique pharmacological profile? *Brain Aging* 2: 49–53.

De Deyn PP, Rabheru K, Rasmussen A *et al.* (1999) A randomized trial of risperidone, placebo, and haloperidol for behavioral symptoms of dementia. *Neurology* 53: 946–55.

De Deyn PP, Jeste DV, Auby P *et al.* (2003) Aripiprazole in dementia of the Alzheimer's type. Poster presented at 16th Annual Meeting of American Association for Geriatric Psychiatry, March.

Devanand DP. (2000) Depression in dementia. In: Qizilbash N, Schneider L, Chui H *et al.* (eds). *Evidence-based dementia: A practical guide to diagnosis and management.* Oxford: Blackwell Science Ltd.

Devanand DP, Marder K, Michaels KS *et al.* (1998) A randomized, placebo-controlled, dose-comparison trial of haloperidol for psychosis and disruptive behaviors in Alzheimer's disease. *American Journal of Psychiatry* 155: 1512–20.

Doody RS, Stevens JC, Beck C *et al.* (2001) Practice parameter: Management of dementia (an evidence-based review) Report of the Quality Standards Subcommittee of the American Academy of Neurology. *Neurology* 56: 1154–66.

Finkel SI, Costa e Silva J, Cohen G *et al.* (1996) Behavioral and psychological signs and symptoms of dementia: a consensus statement on current knowledge and implications for research and treatment. *International Psychogeriatrics* 8 (Suppl. 3): 497–500.

Gill SS, Rochon PA, Herrmann N *et al.* (2005) Atypical antipsychotic drugs and risk of ischaemic stroke: population based retrospective cohort study. *British Medical Journal* 330: 445.

Hawkins JW, Tinklenberg JR, Sheikh JI *et al.* (2000) A retrospective chart review of gabapentin for the treatment of aggressive and agitated behavior in patients with dementias. *American Journal of Geriatric Psychiatry* 8: 221–5.

Herrmann N. (1998) Valproic acid treatment of agitation in dementia. *Canadian Journal of Psychiatry* 43: 69–72.

Herrmann N, Rivard MF, Flynn M *et al.* (1998) Risperidone for the treatment of behavioral disturbances in dementia: a case series. *Journal of Neuropsychiatry and Clinical Neurosciences* 10: 220–3.

Herrmann N, Lanctot K, Myszak M. (2000) Effectiveness of gabapentin for the treatment of behavioral disorders in dementia. *Journal of Clinical Psychopharmacology* 20: 90–93.

Jeste DV, Finkel SI. (2000) Psychosis of Alzheimer's disease and related dementias. Diagnostic criteria for a distinct syndrome. *American Journal of Geriatric Psychiatry* 8: 29–34.

Jeste DV, Caligiuri MP, Paulsen JS *et al.* (1995) Risk of tardive dyskinesia in older patients. A prospective longitudinal study of 266 outpatients. *Archives of General Psychiatry* 52: 756–65.

Jeste DV, Lacro JP, Bailey A *et al.* (1999) Lower incidence of tardive dyskinesia with risperidone compared with haloperidol in older patients. *Journal of the American Geriatrics Society* 47: 716–19.

Katz I, Jeste DV, Mintzer JE *et al.* (1999) Comparison of risperidone and placebo for psychosis and behavioral disturbances associated with dementia: a randomized, double-blind trial. *Journal of Clinical Psychiatry* 60: 107–15.

Kunik ME, Puryear L, Orengo CA *et al.* (1998) The efficacy and tolerability of divalproex sodium in elderly demented patients with behavioural disturbances. *International Journal of Geriatric Psychiatry* 13: 29–34.

Lanctôt KL, Best TS, Mittmann N *et al.* (1998) Efficacy and safety of neuroleptics in behavioral disorders associated with dementia. *Journal of Clinical Psychiatry* 59: 550–61.

Lavretsky H, Sultzer D. (1998) A structured trial of risperidone for the treatment of agitation in dementia. *American Journal of Geriatric Psychiatry* 6: 127–35.

Leibovici A, Tariot PN. (1988) Agitation associated with dementia: a systematic approach to treatment. *Psychopharmacology Bulletin* 24: 49–53.

Lonergan E, Luxenberg J, Colford J. (2002) Haloperidol for agitation in dementia. *Cochrane Database of Systematic Reviews* (2): CD002852.

Loy R, Tariot PN, Rosenquist K. (1999) Alzheimer's disease: behavioral management. In: Katz IR, Oslin D, Lawton MP (eds). *Annual Review of Gerontology and Geriatrics: Psychopharmacologic Interventions in Late Life* 19: 136–94.

Lyketsos CG, Sheppard JM, Steele CD *et al.* (2000) Randomized, placebo-controlled, double-blind clinical trial of sertraline in the treatment of depression complicating Alzheimer's disease: initial results from the Depression in Alzheimer's Disease study. *American Journal of Psychiatry* 157: 1686–9.

McShane R, Areosa Sastre A, Minakaran N. (2006) Memantine for dementia. *Cochrane Database of Systematic Reviews* (2): CD003154.

Meehan KM, Wang H, David SR *et al.* (2002) Comparison of rapidly acting intramuscular olanzapine, lorazepam, and placebo: a double-blind, randomized study in acutely agitated patients with dementia. *Neuropsychopharmacology* 26: 494–504.

Megna JL, Devitt PJ, Sauro MD, Dewan MJ. (2002) Gabapentin's effect on agitation in severely and persistently mentally ill patients. *Annals of Pharmacotherapy* 36: 12–16.

Merriam AE, Aronson MK, Gaston P *et al.* (1988) The psychiatric symptoms of Alzheimer's disease. *Journal of the American Geriatrics Society* 36: 7–12.

Mintzer J, Weiner M, Greenspan A et al. (2004) Efficacy and safety of a flexible dose of risperidone versus placebo in the treatment of psychosis of Alzheimer's disease. Poster presented at the International College of Geriatric Psychopharmacology; Oct 14–17. Basel, Switzerland.

Mintzer JE, Tune LE, Breder CD et al. (2007) Aripiprazole for the treatment of psychoses in institutionalized patients with Alzheimer dementia: a multicenter, randomized, double-blind, placebo-controlled assessment of three fixed doses. American Journal of Geriatric Psychiatry 15: 918–31.

Nyth AL, Gottfries CG. (1990) The clinical efficacy of citalopram in treatment of emotional disturbances in dementia disorders. A Nordic multicentre study. British Journal of Psychiatry 157: 894–901.

Nyth AL, Gottfries CG, Lyby K et al. (1992) A controlled multicenter clinical study of citalopram and placebo in elderly depressed patients with and without concomitant dementia. Acta Psychiatrica Scandinavica 86: 138–45.

Olin JT, Fox LS, Pawluczyk S et al. (2001) A pilot randomized trial of carbamazepine for behavioral symptoms in treatment-resistant outpatients with Alzheimer's disease. American Journal of Geriatric Psychiatry 9: 400–5.

Patel S, Tariot PN. (1991) Pharmacologic models of Alzheimer's disease. Psychiatric Clinics of North America 14: 287–308.

Peskind ER, Tsuang DW, Bonner LT et al. (2005) Propranolol for disruptive behaviors in nursing home residents with probable or possible Alzheimer disease: a placebo-controlled study. Alzheimer Disease and Associated Disorders 19: 23–8.

Pollock BG, Mulsant BH, Sweet R et al. (1997) An open pilot study of citalopram for behavioral disturbances of dementia. Plasma levels and real-time observations. American Journal of Geriatric Psychiatry 5: 70–78.

Pollock BG, Mulsant BH, Rosen J et al. (2002) Comparison of citalopram, perphenazine, and placebo for the acute treatment of psychosis and behavioral disturbances in hospitalized, demented patients. American Journal of Psychiatry 159: 460–5.

Pollock BG, Mulsant BH, Rosen J et al. (2007) A double-blind comparison of citalopram and risperidone for the treatment of behavioral and psychotic symptoms associated with dementia. American Journal of Geriatric Psychiatry 15: 942–52.

Porsteinsson AP, Tariot PN, Erb R et al. (2001) Placebo-controlled study of divalproex sodium for agitation in dementia. American Journal of Geriatric Psychiatry 9: 58–66.

Porsteinsson AP, Tariot PN, Jakimovich LJ et al. (2003) Valproate therapy for agitation in dementia: open-label extension of a double-blind trial. American Journal of Geriatric Psychiatry 11: 434–40.

Profenno LA, Tariot PN. (2004) Pharmacologic management of agitation in Alzheimer's disease. Dementia and Geriatric Cognitive Disorders 17: 65–77.

Profenno LA, Jakimovich L, Holt CJ et al. (2005) A randomized, double-blind, placebo-controlled pilot trial of safety and tolerability of two doses of divalproex sodium in outpatients with probable Alzheimer's disease. Current Alzheimer Research 2: 553–8.

Rabins P, Blacker D, Bland W et al. (1997) Practice guideline for the treatment of patients with Alzheimer's disease and other dementias of late life. American Journal of Psychiatry 154: 1–39.

Ragneskog H, Eriksson S, Karlsson I, Gottfries CG. (1996) Long-term treatment of elderly individuals with emotional disturbances: an open study with citalopram. International Psychogeriatrics 8: 659–68.

Ramadan FH, Naughton BJ, Bassanelli AG. (2000) Treatment of verbal agitation with a selective serotonin reuptake inhibitor. Journal of Geriatric Psychiatry and Neurology 13: 56–9.

Raskind MA, Cyrus PA, Ruzicka BB, Gulanski BI. (1999) The effects of metrifonate on the cognitive, behavioral, and functional performance of Alzheimer's disease patients. Metrifonate Study Group. Journal of Clinical Psychiatry 60: 318–25.

Ray WA, Chung C, Murray K et al. (2009) Atypical antipsychotic drugs and the risk of sudden cardiac death. New England Journal of Medicine 360: 225–35.

Regan WM, Gordon SM. (1997) Gabapentin for behavioral agitation in Alzheimer's disease. Journal of Clinical Psychopharmacology 17: 59–60.

Reisberg B, Doody R, Stöffler A et al. (2003) Memantine in moderate-to-severe Alzheimer's disease. New England Journal of Medicine 348: 1333–41.

Ritsner M, Gibel A, Perelroyzen G et al. (2004) Quality of life outcomes of risperidone, olanzapine, and typical antipsychotics among schizophrenia patients treated in routine clinical practice: a naturalistic comparative study. Journal of Clinical Psychopharmacology 24: 582–91.

Roane DM, Feinberg TE, Meckler L et al. (2000) Treatment of dementia-associated agitation with gabapentin. Journal of Neuropsychiatry and Clinical Neuroscience 12: 40–43.

Rosenquist K, Tariot P, Loy R. (2000) Treatments for behavioural and psychological symptoms in AD and other dementias. In: O'Brien J (ed.). Dementia. London: Edward Arnold, 571–602.

Satterlee WG, Reams SG, Burns PR et al. (1995) A clinical update in olanzapine treatment in schizophrenia and in elderly Alzheimer's disease patients. Psychopharmacology Bulletin 31. Abstract.

Scharre DW, Chang SI. (2002) Cognitive and behavioral effects of quetiapine in Alzheimer's disease patients. Alzheimer Disease and Associated Disorders 16: 128–30.

Schneider LS, Pollock VE, Lyness SA. (1990) A meta-analysis of controlled trials of neuroleptic treatment in dementia. Journal of the American Geriatrics Society 38: 553–63.

Schneider LS, Dagerman K, Insel PS. (2006) Efficacy and adverse effects of atypical antipsychotics for dementia: meta-analysis of randomized, placebo-controlled trials. *American Journal of Geriatric Psychiatry* **14**: 191–210.

Schneider LS, Tariot PN, Dagerman KS *et al.* (2006) Effectiveness of atypical antipsychotic drugs in patients with Alzheimer's disease. *New England Journal of Medicine* **355**: 1525–38.

Schneider LS, Tariot PN, Lyketsos CG *et al.* (2008) National Institute of Mental Health Clinical Antipsychotic Trials of Intervention Effectiveness (CATIE): Alzheimer disease trial methodology. *American Journal of Geriatric Psychiatry* **9**: 346–60.

Sival RC, Haffmans PM, Jansen PA *et al.* (2002) Sodium valproate in the treatment of aggressive behavior in patients with dementia – a randomized placebo controlled clinical trial. *International Journal of Geriatric Psychiatry* **17**: 579–85.

Stanniland C, Taylor D. (2000) Tolerability of atypical antipsychotics. *Drug Safety* **22**: 195–214.

Street JS, Clark WS, Gannon KS *et al.* (2000) Olanzapine treatment of psychotic and behavioral symptoms in patients with Alzheimer disease in nursing care facilities: a double-blind, randomized, placebo-controlled trial. The HGEU Study Group. *Archives of General Psychiatry* **57**: 968–76.

Street JS, Clark WS, Kadam DL *et al.* (2001) Long-term efficacy of olanzapine in the control of psychotic and behavioral symptoms in nursing home patients with Alzheimer's dementia. *International Journal of Geriatric Psychiatry* **16** (Suppl. 1): S62–70.

Suh GH, Son HG, Ju YS *et al.* (2004) A randomized, double-blind, crossover comparison of risperidone and haloperidol in Korean dementia patients with behavioral disturbances. *American Journal of Geriatric Psychiatry* **12**: 509–16.

Sultzer DL, Gray KF, Gunay I *et al.* (1997) A double-blind comparison of trazodone and haloperidol for treatment of agitation in patients with dementia. *American Journal of Geriatric Psychiatry* **5**: 60–69.

Sultzer DL, Davis SM, Tariot PN *et al.* (2008) Clinical symptom responses to atypical antipsychotic medications in Alzheimer's disease: phase 1 outcomes from the CATIE-AD effectiveness trial. *American Journal of Psychiatry* **165**: 844–54.

Tariot PN. (1996) Treatment strategies for agitation and psychosis in dementia. *Journal of Clinical Psychiatry* **57** (Suppl. 14): 21–9.

Tariot PN. (1999) Treatment of agitation in dementia. *Journal of Clinical Psychiatry* **60** (Suppl. 8): 11–20.

Tariot PN. (2003) Valproate use in neuropsychiatric disorders in the elderly. *Psychopharmacology Bulletin* **37** (Suppl. 2): 116–28.

Tariot PN, Blazina L. (1993) The psychopathology of dementia. In: Morris J (ed.). *Handbook of dementing illnesses.* New York: Marcel Dekker, 461–75.

Tariot PN, Schneider LS. (1998) Nonneuroleptic treatment of complications of dementia: applying clinical research to practice. In: Nelson JC (ed.). *Geriatric psychopharmacology.* New York: Marcel Dekker, 427–53.

Tariot PN, Erb R, Leibovici A *et al.* (1994) Carbamazepine treatment of agitation in nursing home patients with dementia: a preliminary study. *Journal of the American Geriatrics Society* **42**: 1160–6.

Tariot PN, Schneider LS, Katz IR. (1995a) Anticonvulsant and other non-neuroleptic treatment of agitation in dementia. *Journal of Geriatric Psychiatry and Neurology* **8** (Suppl. 1): S28–39.

Tariot PN, Frederiksen K, Erb R *et al.* (1995b) Lack of carbamazepine toxicity in frail nursing home patients: a controlled study. *Journal of the American Geriatrics Society* **43**: 1026–9.

Tariot PN, Erb R, Podgorski CA *et al.* (1998) Efficacy and tolerability of carbamazepine for agitation and aggression in dementia. *American Journal of Psychiatry* **155**: 54–61.

Tariot PN, Salzman C, Yeung PP *et al.* (2000) Long-term use of quetiapine in elderly patients with psychotic disorders. *Clinical Therapeutics* **22**: 1068–84.

Tariot PN, Schneider L, Mintzer J *et al.* (2001) Safety and tolerability of divalproex sodium for the treatment of signs and symptoms of mania in elderly patients with dementia: results of a double-blind, placebo-controlled trial. *Current Therapeutic Research* **62**: 51–67.

Tariot P, Schneider L, Katz I *et al.* (2002) Quetiapine in nursing home residents with Alzheimer's dementia and psychosis. *American Journal of Geriatric Psychiatry* **10**: 93.

Tariot PN, Farlow MR, Grossberg GT *et al.*, Memantine Study Group. (2004) Memantine treatment in patients with moderate to severe Alzheimer disease already receiving donepezil: a randomized controlled trial. *JAMA* **291**: 317–24.

Tariot PN, Raman R, Jakimovich L *et al.* (2005) Divalproex sodium in nursing home residents with possible or probable Alzheimer's disease complicated by agitation: a randomized controlled trial. *American Journal of Geriatric Psychiatry* **13**: 942–9.

Teri L, Logsdon RG, Peskind E *et al.* (2000) Treatment of agitation in AD: a randomized, placebo-controlled clinical trial. *Neurology* **55**: 1271–8.

Tolbert SR, Fuller MA. (1996) Selegiline in treatment of behavioral and cognitive symptoms of Alzheimer disease. *Annals of Pharmacotherapy* **30**: 1122–9.

Trinh NH, Hoblyn J, Mohanty S, Yaffe K. (2003) Efficacy of cholinesterase inhibitors in the treatment of neuropsychiatric symptoms and functional impairment in Alzheimer disease: a meta-analysis. *Journal of American Medical Association* **289**: 210–16.

Wang LY, Shofer JB, Rohde K *et al.* (2009) Prazosin for the treatment of behavioral symptoms in patients with Alzheimer disease with agitation and aggression. *American Journal of Geriatric Psychiatry* **17**: 744–51.

Wilcock GK, Ballard CG, Cooper JA, Loft H. (2008) Memantine for agitation/aggression and psychosis in moderately severe to severe Alzheimer's disease: a pooled analysis of 3 studies. *Journal of Clinical Psychiatry* **69**: 341–8.

Winblad B, Poritis N. (1999) Memantine in severe dementia: results of the 9M-Best Study (Benefit and efficacy in severely demented patients during treatment with memantine). *International Journal of Geriatric Psychiatry* **14**: 135–46.

Winblad B, Mobius HJ, Stoffler A. (2002) Glutamate receptors as a target for Alzheimer's disease – are clinical results supporting the hope? *Journal of Neural Transmission. Supplementum* **62**: 217–25.

Wooltorton E. (2002) Risperidone (Risperdal): increased rate of cerebrovascular events in dementia trials. *Canadian Medical Association Journal* **167**: 1269–70.

Wragg RE, Jeste DV. (1989) Overview of depression and psychosis in Alzheimer's disease. *American Journal of Psychiatry* **146**: 577–87.

Zheng L, Mack WJ, Dagerman KS. (2009) Metabolic changes associated with second-generation antipsychotic use in Alzheimer's disease patients: The CATIE-AD Study. *American Journal of Psychiatry* **166**: 583–90.

Zhong KX, Tariot PN, Mintzer J *et al.* (2007) Quetiapine to treat agitation in dementia: a randomized, double-blind, placebo-controlled study. *Current Alzheimer Research* **4**: 81–93.

28

Psychological approaches for the practical management of cognitive impairment in dementia

ANNE UNKENSTEIN

28.1 INTRODUCTION

A psychological approach to the management of cognitive impairment in dementia aims to promote the best possible quality of life for both people with dementia and their carers, by offering positive, individualized and effective management. With the growing emphasis on early diagnosis of dementia, there are increasing opportunities to provide psychological interventions from the earliest stages of dementia. This chapter focuses on practical and personalized strategies. Assessment and feedback processes are outlined and specific techniques for managing cognitive impairment in early, moderate and later stage dementia are described.

28.2 FACTORS INFLUENCING MANAGEMENT OF COGNITIVE IMPAIRMENT IN DEMENTIA

Each person who has dementia is unique. The way the person presents results from a complex interaction of brain disease, personality, biography, health and social psychology (Kitwood, 1993). Each person needs to be treated as an individual. An approach that might prove successful for one person may prove ineffective for another (Woods and Bird, 1999). There is no single correct approach to the management of cognitive impairment in dementia. The help that is relevant can vary considerably.

There is a great deal of variation in cognitive function in dementia according to the stage of dementia and different causes and patterns of brain pathology. Dementia does not imply global impairment of brain function. There will nearly always be some retained abilities. It is important to identify these cognitive strengths and use them positively. Interventions can draw on retained skills in order to bypass weaknesses.

Cognitive impairment is just one aspect of dementia. People with dementia also experience changes in behaviour, emotional control, personality and self-care. These changes need to be taken into account when working on strategies for cognitive impairment. A team approach with agreement about realistic goals and consistent strategies is recommended. Carers need to be included in management planning. Wherever the person with dementia lives, carers will be involved. They may be relatives, friends, neighbours or health professionals.

Not all of the person's symptoms are directly due to brain disease. People with dementia are very sensitive to their physical and psychological environment. Dementia is sometimes first suspected when a person experiences a change to his/her usual environment, such as moving to a new house or the death of a spouse. It is important to be aware of environmental factors that may adversely affect cognitive function and make appropriate changes to the environment in order to enhance cognitive abilities.

Health factors can exacerbate any cognitive impairment. Sensory impairment, especially of vision and hearing, can adversely affect cognitive function. People with dementia commonly experience anxiety, distress and depression. Confusion can also be increased during acute or chronic illness and with any physical discomfort or pain. Alcohol, some medications and fatigue may cause transient exaggeration of cognitive impairment. It is necessary to be alert to any superimposed health problems and to control these to help people maintain maximum function.

Progressive decline in cognitive function is characteristic of dementia. Management strategies need to be flexible and adapted over time. Assessment at regular intervals will allow for the development of realistic expectations. The aim of any strategies employed is to maintain as high a level of function as possible by helping the individual to better utilize remaining function.

28.3 ASSESSMENT

A thorough assessment is required in order to design an individualized approach to management of cognitive impairment. This should include assessment of the person's medical and psychological status and assessment of cognition. Assessment of the person's health is important, as there may be additional treatable medical conditions.

It is beneficial to interview the carers to gain information about the person's personality, interests, home environment and the history of events leading up to the assessment. Information about strategies that the carers have already tried and their willingness to provide support can also be gathered.

A neuropsychological assessment (see Chapter 7, Neuropsychological assessment of dementia) provides a basis for individual intervention. It allows for a focus on strengths by outlining abilities that remain unaffected, and also outlines areas of cognitive impairment to be managed. Serial neuropsychological assessment can be used to monitor progression of symptoms over time. It can provide an objective viewpoint to the carers and to the person with dementia with regard to the progression of symptoms. Part of the assessment is to check the attitude of the person to their symptoms, as this will influence choice of strategies.

The assessment phase will identify the problem but it is important to go beyond this phase for better management of cognitive impairment. It is beneficial to share the information gathered with the person with dementia and their carers.

28.4 FEEDBACK AFTER PSYCHOLOGICAL ASSESSMENT

A feedback session following psychological assessment can serve many purposes. It provides information about how the disease is affecting aspects of cognitive function in order to improve understanding. While it is important to acknowledge areas of loss, a positive approach can be maintained by highlighting what the person can still do.

The carers are often the people who provide ongoing management of the person with cognitive impairment. Feedback can empower carers by acknowledging the success they have had with strategies that they have already tried. It can also provide emotional support and practical help and assistance. Carers have access to a lot of general information about dementia (e.g. Draper, 2004; Ladd and Rand, 2006). However, specific information that is more relevant to their particular situation can be provided in a feedback session.

Feedback usually includes the person with dementia, but can be given to carers alone where appropriate. The psychologist can provide a description of the person's cognitive strengths and weaknesses. This information is then used to help carers make sense of behaviour that otherwise would seem to suggest that the person is purposefully being annoying. For example, by outlining the different types of memory and how each is affected, it becomes easier to understand why a person can recall information from their remote past but not what was said 2 minutes ago. Furthermore, if carers know that the person has memory impairment they are more likely to understand why the person persistently repeats the same question or forgets to pass on a phone message. It can be reinforced that this is not done deliberately. Behaviour is thus reinterpreted as related to brain disease and not purposeful or intended. This information is also useful when it comes to management of cognitive impairment. For example, if carers know that forgetfulness is due to memory loss from brain disease they are more likely to understand that the person is unlikely to learn by repetition. They are also more likely to use strategies that avoid reliance on intact memory ability.

A feedback session offers an opportunity to ask the person with dementia and the carers how the cognitive problems manifest themselves in everyday life. This information can be used to make strategies realistic and relevant to the life of the person with dementia (Wilson, 2002).

A written reminder of what was discussed during the feedback session can be useful. Both the person with dementia and the carers may forget what was discussed, especially if they are just coming to terms with the diagnosis.

An initial discussion of strategies to help manage cognitive impairment can be included in a feedback session. The types of strategies employed will vary according to the person's individual situation and the cause and stage of dementia.

28.5 EARLY STAGE DEMENTIA – MEMORY STRATEGIES

In early dementia the most significant cognitive impairment is typically in memory function. Impairment of new learning is most prominent, including acquisition and retention of new information. At this stage, people with dementia may forget what you have just told them, forget where they have put something, repeat the same thing as if they have not said it before or have difficulty learning how to use something new.

At this stage, the person often remains aware of cognitive losses and may be motivated to seek methods to compensate for them. The person is usually living in the family home. Initial strategies therefore focus on the individual with increasing involvement of family carers over time. The aim is to maintain as much independence as possible and to promote confidence in remembering. Family members and friends need to avoid taking over responsibilities too soon.

Many of the strategies that are used by people experiencing normal memory change with ageing are useful at this stage (see Sargeant and Unkenstein (2001), for a detailed description of memory strategies). It is important to ask people whether they are already using any memory aids before explaining the use of memory strategies. People should be encouraged to draw on strategies that they have used in the past. They will be more likely to use strategies if they are already familiar with them (Kotler-Cope and Camp, 1990). Everyone has different preferences. Some people like to use diaries, while others prefer a notice board.

People need not just one technique, but a whole range of strategies. It is important to find out the typical things a person tends to forget and work out strategies that will suit these specific situations and be usable for that person. Strategy use will vary according to differing interests, lifestyles and home environments. A home visit can be useful to help tailor strategies to particular situations.

The emphasis is on practical compensatory techniques, which avoid challenging the person's lost memory function. For example, rather than asking a question that relies on intact memory function such as 'What show did you watch on television last night?', rephrase the question to 'Did you enjoy the show that you watched last night?' If people become repetitive it may be best to try distracting them with another topic of conversation. Enhancing familiarity is also beneficial. Developing a regular routine and doing things at a set time of the day or week will reduce the load on memory.

Memory strategies can be thought of as internal or external. Internal strategies involve some form of internal mental manipulation, for example, mentally retracing one's steps to remember where an object was left. External strategies involve using some sort of external aid, for example a note pad for writing a list, or a diary. They can also involve making changes to the environment, for instance, having designated locations in which to store particular items.

Internal strategies focus on enhancing encoding and retrieval processes. The emphasis is on making more efficient use of current cognitive capacity. A motivated individual with early stage dementia may employ simple internal strategies. These strategies typically involve one of three main features: focusing attention, adding meaning to the information to be remembered, or reducing the amount of information to be remembered. Simple internal strategies such as ensuring understanding, associating new information with information that is known well, and visualization may be useful for motivated individuals with early dementia.

When people with dementia are supported with repeated training sessions, they can learn and retain new information using specific learning methods. One technique that has been found to assist learning is spaced retrieval, which requires people to recall information over increasingly longer periods of time. This is sometimes combined with other learning techniques, such as the errorless learning approach, where

people are not allowed to commit errors when they are receiving memory training (Bourgeois et al., 2003; Clare, 2008).

Some well-known internal strategies or mnemonic techniques, such as the method of loci and peg word systems, are quite complex. These techniques require considerable remaining cognitive capacity including new learning and motivation for success. People with early stage dementia usually do not have the motivation or learning ability required to use these techniques (Grandmaison and Simard, 2003).

External strategies aim to compensate for memory impairment by reducing the demand on a person's memory. They are generally easier to use and more suitable for everyday remembering than internal strategies. They may involve written reminders, storage of objects in specially designated places, technical memory devices and reminders from other people.

Written reminders assist with remembering locations of objects, a task that has to be done, appointments, shopping items, messages, names and instructions. Calendars, diaries, notebooks, notepads, noticeboards, sticky notes and computers are all useful. Having a pen or pencil attached reduces the load on memory even further. Such written aids should not only be readily visible and accessible but should also be in close proximity to the to-be-remembered activity. For example, a shopping list pad on the refrigerator door, or instructions for how to operate a piece of equipment permanently displayed on that equipment.

External memory strategies can assist with orientation in early stage dementia. It is helpful to mark off the days as they pass on a calendar, or use a flip-top desk calendar and turn each day over as it passes. Newspapers can also serve as prompts. Clocks should be positioned in places where they are readily seen and ideally should have day and date built in.

Storing objects in specially designated places can help with remembering the location of objects, a task that has to be done, or something to be taken out. For example, keys can be stored near the front door of the house. This makes it easy to pick up the keys when leaving the house and to get into the habit of putting them back when returning.

Leaving objects in visible locations can act as a reminder to do something. Medications can be left somewhere obvious in the kitchen if they are to be taken with meals. Objects that a person needs to take out with them can be located in a special place near the front door, such as a hall table.

A useful storage device for managing medications is a dosette box, divided into compartments that relate to the day of the week or time of the day into which a set number of tablets can be placed. The box has to be filled at weekly or other intervals, but is simple to use and lets people know whether they have taken the necessary tablets.

Basic alarms are useful to help people remember something they have to do. A common example is an oven timer used as a reminder to turn the oven off. Many household objects have built in memory aids. Modern telephones have a system that enables storage of frequently used numbers that can then be dialled by pressing only one appropriately labelled button. Automatic shut-off devices on electrical and gas appliances, such as stovetops, kettles or lights can be installed. These devices turn the power off after a period of time if the appliances are left on. More complex electronic memory aids can be useful for motivated and insightful individuals but may require training to know how to operate them. They usually rely on other cognitive processes remaining intact and may not suit the person with early stage dementia.

Reminders from other people can provide an excellent memory back-up system. Family members can provide telephone reminders or leave notes in a regular and prominent location. Reminders need to be specific. For example, a note saying 'back in 5 minutes' does not provide enough information. The person with dementia needs to know when the person will return (Twining, 1991).

People with mild to moderate dementia can be trained to use internal and external memory strategies in group programmes (Mate-Kole et al., 2007; Kurz et al., 2009). This typically involves an extended programme over several weeks in a group format that includes training in the use of memory strategies, relaxation techniques and stress management. People with dementia have been shown to improve in aspects of cognition and behaviour after attending these groups. See Sitzer et al (2006) for a review of the efficacy of cognitive training in dementia.

28.6   MODERATE DEMENTIA – WORKING WITH CARERS

As dementia progresses, people can experience increasing memory loss, language difficulties and specific disorders such as apraxia. They may be unable to function independently outside the home and require increasing assistance with tasks of personal care. They could be living in their own home or supported accommodation. By this stage the person's insight into their cognitive losses usually has diminished.

With little awareness of their difficulties and increased cognitive impairment, it becomes difficult to work on strategies with the person with dementia alone. The management of cognitive impairment therefore becomes focused on working in collaboration with family members or other carers. Carers know the person best and often come up with strategies that work well for that person. Carers can provide reminders for the person, encourage the person to use external memory aids and make appropriate changes to the environment. Without this assistance the person is unlikely to make use of memory strategies. By this stage strategies for other areas of cognitive impairment are also required. Providing support and information to the carers can help to further tailor strategies to make them suit the individual's current cognitive strengths and weaknesses.

Carers will need to become increasingly involved in the use of external memory strategies and can assist with setting up a designated 'memory centre' in a visible location in the home environment (Sargeant and Unkenstein, 2001). Here the carer could hang a whiteboard on which the day, date and daily schedule is written or a clock with the day and date on it. A pin board next to the whiteboard can be used to display other important information. The carer may need to keep

reminding the person to check the memory centre. Carers can also develop 'communication books'. For this, a notebook is left in a special location where visitors can write messages. The person can be encouraged to check this book regularly as a reminder of who has visited recently.

These strategies are a form of reality orientation, an approach that emphasizes the use of external cues and structures to assist the person in maintaining contact with the environment (see Woods (2002) for a review of reality orientation). Carers can help to provide personalized reality orientation, by identifying to which realities the person needs or desires to be oriented. A structured programme of reality orientation and cognitive stimulation for people with dementia can improve memory and functional abilities (Spector et al., 2003). Typically, a structured stimulation programme would consist of several weeks of group intervention sessions.

Carers can continue to encourage a regular routine of familiar activities. Sudden unexplained changes or unfamiliar activities could cause the person distress. Carers can help the person focus on activities that are familiar and based on previous interests, such as gardening, walking the dog or other household tasks. Drawing on the continued strength of memories of procedures and lifetime memories can provide meaningful activity. Carers at accommodation facilities can find out about the person's past likes, dislikes, lifestyle and life interests from family members. This information and any old photos available can be recorded in a book that can be used as a cue for discussion and reminiscence (see Woods et al. (2005) for a review of reminiscence).

A familiar environment will reduce the demand on the person's memory. Unnecessary changes such as rearranging furniture should be avoided. If changes have to be made, they should be introduced slowly, with explanation.

Carers may need assistance with strategies for other areas of cognitive impairment. For example, the person at this stage may experience apraxia, an inability to carry out routine patterns of voluntary movement. A common problem caused by apraxia is difficulty with dressing. Helping the carer to understand that a person can sometimes dress automatically, but has difficulty when the movement comes under conscious control, is useful. To remove the degree of voluntary focus from the action, avoid giving the person direct instructions about performing the task. Specific techniques include distracting the person's attention from the task, imitation, laying the clothes out in the order in which the person likes to put them on and giving reassurance and praise for each successful step. See Holden (1995) for strategies for other specific cognitive disorders.

28.7   LATER STAGE DEMENTIA – ENVIRONMENTAL ADAPTATION

In the later stages of dementia, people experience marked confusion and widespread cognitive disturbance. Most people with advanced dementia are living in supported accommodation with professional carers. Strategies for management of cognitive impairment need to be focused more on the environment in which the person is living. Adaptations are made to the environment rather than expecting the individual to change. Visiting the person's residence allows one to observe environmental cues, how they might best be used and/or changed and how new ones might be introduced (Kapur, 1995).

At this stage people become dependent on their environment to support them. Making adaptations to the environment can enhance feelings of security and help people cope with their confusion and disorientation. A 'dementia friendly environment' provides orientation strategies that help to reduce confusion and promote independence (Davis et al., 2009). When one first moves into a new residence there is often a settling in period. An unfamiliar and new environment can increase confusion. It helps to make the environment as familiar as possible. Possessions, such as photos, objects and furniture can be put in the person's room.

A routine and daily timetable should be emphasized. Orientation information or cues can lessen confusion. For example, having access to a window helps a person to tell the time of the day and the weather. A good sensory environment with adequate light is important. Making each part of a large place unique in some way is useful for orientation to the environment. Colour and furniture can highlight difference. Smaller spaces are less confusing than large.

Clear labelling throughout the accommodation facility can further lessen confusion. Way-finding cues can be marked on the floor or walls with coloured lines or arrows. Individual rooms can be clearly labelled. Large uppercase print with black against white is often best for older people (Kapur, 1995). Pictures may be more easily understood than written labels (e.g. a picture of a toilet on the toilet doors). Carers can wear name badges, with their first name only, that are large enough to read. People will require continued instruction as to how to use these orientation aids.

To maximize cognitive function it helps to simplify the environment to avoid the person becoming overwhelmed. If there is excessive stimulation then confusion may be exacerbated. It helps to remove distractions, keep noise levels down and not have too many people around (Robinson et al., 2001).

It is often difficult to communicate with the individual with this stage of dementia. Using an empathic, validating approach that displays respect and sensitivity to feelings can help to ensure understanding.

28.8   CONCLUSION

Improving the practical management of cognitive impairment in dementia using a psychological approach is just one part of the challenge to maintain maximum function throughout the course of the illness (Kitwood, 1993). For any symptom of dementia, the first step involves investigating what may be causing the person to present in that particular way. Multidisciplinary assessment will establish whether there are any environmental factors that can be altered or health factors that can be treated in order to enhance the individual's function. Effective management strategies that are relevant to the stage

of dementia and other individual variables can be developed using a collaborative approach involving the person with dementia, carers and health professionals.

REFERENCES

Bourgeois M, Camp C, Rose M et al. (2003) A comparison of training strategies to enhance use of external aids by persons with dementia. Journal of Communication Disorders 36: 361–78.

Clare L. (2008) Neuropsychological rehabilitation and people with dementia. Hove: Psychology Press.

Davis S, Byers S, Nay R, Koch S. (2009) Guiding design of dementia friendly environments in residential care settings. Considering the living experiences. Dementia 8: 185–203.

Draper B. (2004) Dealing with dementia: A guide to Alzheimer's disease and other dementias. Crows Nest, NSW: Allen and Unwin.

Grandmaison E, Simard M. (2003) A critical review of memory stimulation programs in Alzheimer's disease. Journal of Neuropsychiatry and Clinical Neuroscience 15: 130–44.

Holden U. (1995) Ageing, neuropsychology and the 'new' dementias. London: Chapman and Hall.

Kapur N. (1995) Memory aids in the rehabilitation of memory disordered patients. In: Baddeley AD, Wilson BA, Watts FN (eds). Handbook of memory disorders. Chichester: John Wiley & Sons, 533–56.

Kitwood T. (1993) Person and process in dementia. International Journal of Geriatric Psychiatry 8: 541–5.

Kotler-Cope S, Camp CJ. (1990) Memory interventions in aging populations. In: Lovelace E (ed). Aging and cognition: Mental processes, self-awareness and interventions. North Holland: Elsevier Science Publications, 231–61.

Kurz A, Pohl C, Ramsenthaler M, Sorg C. (2009) Cognitive rehabilitation in patients with mild cognitive impairment. International Journal of Geriatric Psychiatry 24: 163–8.

Ladd K, Rand E. (2006) Living with Alzheimer's and other dementias: After the diagnosis. South Yarra: Michelle Anderson Publishing.

Mate-Kole C, Fellows R, Said P et al. (2007) Use of computer assisted and interactive cognitive training programmes with moderate to severely demented individuals: A preliminary study. Aging and Mental Health 11: 485–95.

Robinson A, Spencer B, White L. (2001) Understanding difficult behaviours. Some practical suggestions for coping with Alzheimer's disease and related illnesses. Ann Arbor, MI: The Alzheimer's Program, Eastern Michigan University.

Sargeant D, Unkenstein A. (2001) Remembering well: How memory works and what to do when it doesn't. St Leonards, NSW: Allen and Unwin.

Sitzer D, Twamley E, Jeste D. (2006) Cognitive training in Alzheimer's disease: a meta-analysis of the literature. Acta Psychiatrica Scandinavica 114: 75–90.

Spector A, Thorgrimsen L, Woods B et al. (2003) Efficacy of an evidence-based cognitive stimulation therapy programme for people with dementia. *British Journal of Psychiatry* **183**: 248–54.

Twining C. (1991) *The memory handbook: A practical guide to understanding and managing early dementia.* Bicester: Winslow Press.

Wilson BA. (2002) Management and remediation of memory problems in brain-injured adults. In: Baddeley AD, Wilson BA, Watts FN (eds). *Handbook of memory disorders.* Chichester: John Wiley & Sons, 655–82.

Woods B. (2002) Reality orientation: a welcome return? *Age and Ageing* **31**: 155–6.

Woods B, Bird M. (1999) Non-pharmacological approaches to treatment. In: Wilcock G, Bucks R, Rockwood K (eds). *Diagnosis and management of dementia: A manual for memory disorders teams.* Oxford: Oxford University Press, 311–31.

Woods B, Spector AE, Jones CA *et al.* (2005) Reminiscence therapy for dementia. *Cochrane Database of Systematic Reviews* (1): CD001120.

Sexuality and dementia

JOE STRATFORD AND JAMES WARNER

29.1 INTRODUCTION

Dementia and its relationship with sexuality raises many significant medical, ethical, cultural and relationship issues. Our sexuality is one of the most basic elements of our humanity. With an ageing population and associated increases in numbers of individuals affected by dementia, this relationship will only increase in its relevance. This chapter addresses some of these complex issues and reviews this most challenging and wide-ranging area.

29.2 SEXUALITY AND AGEING

Whilst attempts have been made to try and dispel the myth that older people are asexual, disappointing evidence indicates that the true message is only partially accepted. A stark illustration of this is identified by Bouman *et al.* (2006) in making reference to two recent United Kingdom Department of Health directives: The National Service Framework (NSF) for Older People and the National Sexual Health Strategy (NSHS). Bouman *et al.* highlight how the NSF does not mention sexual health and the NSHS does not discuss older people. Ironically, one of the NSF's explicit aims is to 'root out age discrimination'. The implication seems to be that older people and sexual health is simply not a sufficiently important issue to be included in such directives.

29.2.1 Sexual activity in older people

In the 1940s and 1950s (Kinsey *et al.*, 1948; Kinsey *et al.*, 1953) undertook some of the earliest population surveys into sexual behaviour and attitudes. Despite this, and perhaps representative of the time, the samples only included three women and just two men over the age of 80.

Although sexual activity appears to decline with advancing age (Schiavi *et al.*, 1990; Kaiser, 1996), sexual activity does not stop, at least among many older individuals. One study of people attending a community centre in the USA (age range 42–82) found over two-thirds reported having a sexual partner (Wiley and Bortz, 1996). Over 90 per cent of this (self-selected) sample, including those over 70, desired sexual activity at least once a week, although less than half achieved this. In a large US study, Lindau and colleagues (2007) studied over 3000 older adults (age range 57–85) and found that whilst 84 per cent of the 57–64-year-olds reported sexual activity in the last 12 months, 39 per cent of the 75–85-year-olds were still active.

Although levels of sexual activity may decrease with age, there is evidence that the elderly are becoming more sexually active. In a large Swedish study stretching over a 30-year period looking at trends, Beckman *et al.* (2008) studied four cohorts of 70-year-old community-dwelling older people. Over 1500 subjects were assessed at four separate intervals (1970–71, 1976, 1992 and 2000), each assessment being identical although each assessed a different cohort of 70-year-olds. Sexual activity (defined as intercourse within the last 12 months) in males increased from 47 per cent in 1970–71 to 66 per cent in 2000. In females, the increase was from 12 to 34 per cent over the same time.

Overall, older women are less likely to be sexually active than older men. This may be in part due to the decreased likelihood of women being in a spousal or intimate relationship, often as a result of separation or bereavement. For both sexes, sexual activity is also related to physical health.

Those who rate their health as poor are less likely to be sexually active than those who rate their health as very good or even excellent (Lindau *et al.*, 2007).

Sexual activity does not always have to mean sexual intercourse. As people age, intimacy with a partner appears to be expressed in less vigorous ways and there may be physiological reasons behind this. Touching, holding hands, hugging and kissing seem to assume greater importance when compared to activities such as intercourse or masturbation (Ginsberg *et al.*, 2005).

29.2.2   Sexual dysfunction in older people

Psychosexual dysfunction in late life can arise as a result of a number of factors. In males these can include erectile disorders, delayed ejaculation and longer refractory times (Masters, 1986; Carbone and Seftel, 2002). In women, reduced vaginal lubrication can lead to associated dypareunia (Howard *et al.*, 2006). Across both sexes, decreased levels of sex hormones may also lead to a general loss of sexual drive (Masters and Johnson, 1981).

Despite the increasing availability of medications to directly treat sexual difficulties such as erectile dysfunction, many drugs prescribed for pre-existing medical conditions can cause impotence or lack of libido (Kessel, 2001). Certain medical conditions can either directly or indirectly have an adverse impact on sexual functioning. Specific diagnoses such as diabetes, urogential tract conditions or cancer can directly inhibit sexual performance, whilst the presence of pain or ill health in any form can reduce libido (Howard *et al.*, 2006).

29.2.3   Sexuality and residential care settings

Sexuality and its associated activities can be argued as being as important in residential facilities as anywhere else. The expression of this sexuality is particularly challenging in such institutions for a variety of reasons (Bauer *et al.*, 2009). The move into institutional residential care inevitably leads to a loss of privacy, especially where personal care and supervision are required (Bouman *et al.*, 2006).

Much of the evidence related to sexuality and its expression in residential facilities is mixed. There seems to be a huge variation in attitudes to this issue dependent on what kind of facility and which staff group is being assessed (Bouman *et al.*, 2006). Bouman and colleagues investigated staff attitudes toward sexuality in later life in a number of UK nursing and residential homes. The mean scores across the board revealed a positive and permissive attitude towards the issue. However, greater negative and restrictive attitudes to sexuality were held by care assistants compared with nurses and by those with less than five years' experience than by more experienced staff. Interestingly, nurses in nursing homes displayed significantly more negative attitudes towards sexuality compared with colleagues working in residential homes (Bouman *et al.*, 2007).

29.3   EFFECTS OF DEMENTIA ON SEXUALITY AND SEXUAL BEHAVIOUR

The onset of dementia may have a significant effect on the sex life of the individual and their partner, although the evidence base for such changes in sexual behaviour in dementia remains small. Wright (1991) undertook a controlled study of the impact of Alzheimer's disease (AD) on marital relationships. Eight of the 30 (27 per cent) couples of the dementia-affected group were sexually active, compared with 14 of the 17 (82 per cent) controls. In those individuals still sexually active, compared with controls, sex took place more often in couples where one partner had dementia.

Derouesné *et al.* (1996), in a survey of 135 married couples, one of whom had possible or probable AD, found that 80 per cent of spouses reported a change in patient's sexual activity. This was not linked to the degree of cognitive impairment or the gender of the patient. Eloniemi-Sulkava *et al.* (2002) questioned the spousal caregivers of 42 demented patients over a seven-year period. At the onset of dementia, 32 (76 per cent) of couples engaged in regular sexual intercourse. By the seventh year, 7 (28 per cent) of couples continued to engage in such activity. Whilst 25 caregivers (60 per cent) reported negative behavioural changes in the sexual side of the marriage, 4 (10 per cent) reported positive changes. In most studies of this type sexual demands and activity seem to decrease following the onset of dementia. However, there does appear to be a small proportion of cases where such demands increase. This would be especially true of those dementias characterized by disinhibited behaviours such as frontal lobe dementias.

29.3.1   Effects on the individual

Dementia has a profound effect upon any individual. Many aspects of it are likely to diminish sexual interest and ability to engage in a sexual relationship. There are few published studies on the impact of dementia on sexual function. Zeiss *et al.* (1990), in an uncontrolled survey of 55 men with AD, found that 53 per cent reported erectile dysfunction. This was not related to age, degree of cognitive impairment or medication. The high rate of erectile disorder in partners of patients with dementia may be due to the additional stress placed upon the relationship by the diagnosis (Litz *et al.*, 1990). In their Finnish study of 42 couples, Eloniemi-Sulkava *et al.* (2002) found that 34 (81 per cent) of caregivers reported a decrease in the libido of their demented spouse. So far there are no published studies that examine the prevalence of female sexual dysfunction in the context of dementia.

29.3.2   Effect on the partnership

Dementia leads to an inexorable change in the nature of most relationships, but none is more poignant than that between partners. Partners of individuals with dementia become carers as the disease process robs an individual of their autonomy. This can lead to such carers being vulnerable to depression and anxiety as carer burden increases (see Chapter 2, The lived experience of dementia, Chapter 15, Family carers of people with dementia and Chapter 16, One caregiver's view). Apparent lack of interest, wandering, forgetting technique, incontinence and poor self-care are also likely to have an adverse effect on a couple's sex life. Despite this there has been relatively little research in this area (Baikie, 2002). Although not all dementia-affected couples experience a change in sexual activity, an altered sexual relationship is a difficulty many couples face after the onset of dementia. The diagnosis should not be assumed to herald cessation of an active sex life, and couples should be encouraged to think and act flexibly in order to adjust to the impact of the disorder (Davies et al., 1998).

Partners of individuals with dementia may confine themselves to celibacy at a time when the rewards of caring for the patient are becoming increasingly scarce. Some partners who retain their sex drive may seek sexual satisfaction elsewhere, through masturbation, visiting prostitutes or longer-term relationships outside the partnership. This may lead to guilt, especially if the patient is still living at home. This is a particularly difficult area to manage as partners are understandably reticent to talk about this. If they do, it is vital to have a non-judgemental, supportive approach. Partners will often blame themselves for the cessation of a sexual relationship. Counselling about the reasons for the patient's altered sex drive and an explanation that this is related to the dementia may help to reassure partners. It is important to stress to patients and carers that a lack of sexual activity should not preclude physical intimacy, and that physical intimacy such as cuddling is unlikely to result in sexually inappropriate behaviour by the patient (Davies et al., 1992).

29.3.3 Ethical issues of sexual relationships

People with dementia should have a right to express their sexual feelings and this should be no different to the rest of society. The difficulty which arises within the context of dementia relates to firstly whether the expression of such feelings conflicts with the basic rights of those affected by such activity but, also importantly, whether the issue of capacity has been considered.

Capacity is not an all-or-nothing concept. It can vary over time and is decision-specific. The same would apply to the capacity for an individual to engage in a sexual relationship. Due to its sensitive and complex nature, the capacity of a demented individual to enter into a sexual relationship could be difficult to establish. In an attempt to address this, Lichtenberg and Strzepek (1990) developed a structured assessment technique to aid decisions about patients' ability to consent to sexual relationships. It includes sections addressing the patient's awareness of the relationship, their ability to avoid exploitation and an assessment of their awareness of any potential risks which could arise from it.

29.3.4 Inappropriate sexual activity

There is no clear consensus on what constitutes inappropriate sexual activity in the context of dementia. As Series and Dégano (2005) note, the decision of when a particular behaviour becomes abnormal needs to be based on a judgement of what is normal or appropriate for an individual in a particular situation. This may differ according to the environment or on the level of risk or discomfort to others. Despite this lack of consensus, a reasonably large body of evidence has developed in recent years examining the nature and range of sexually inappropriate behaviour in dementia. The terms 'hypersexuality' and 'sexual disinhibition' are also often used interchangeably.

Despite this lack of consensus, behaviours which are often cited in the literature include: making explicit sexual comments, inappropriate touching of one's own genitals or the genitals/breasts of others. Inappropriate disrobing or masturbation in public areas right through to attempted intercourse with a non-consenting other have all been described. Prevalence rates of such behaviour vary between 2 per cent (Devanand et al., 1992) and 25 per cent (Szasz, 1983) depending on the study and the criteria used. Burns et al. (1990) reported disinhibition to be present in 7 per cent of a sample of 178 patients with AD. In this study there was no difference between males and females. However, Black et al. (2005) in their review, state that these behaviours are more common in males. Patients with AD have been reported as being less likely to present with such behaviour when compared with other types of dementia (Zeiss et al. 1996), although Tsai et al. (1999), in their study of 133 patients with dementia, found no such differences between dementias of various types.

The aetiology behind hypersexuality within dementia can be multifactorial. Frontal lobe damage and temporal lobe dysfunction, leading to the Kluver–Bucy syndrome (Kluver and Bucy, 1937) have been associated with such behaviours. In addition, drugs such as alcohol and other sedatives can produce behavioural and sexual disinhibition in both healthy individuals and those with dementia. L-dopa can also cause hypersexuality in people with Parkinson's disease. Social factors such as the misinterpretation of cues and pre-morbid patterns of sexual activity may also all play a part in the development of sexually inappropriate behaviour (Series and Dégano, 2005).

29.3.5 Summary

Given the extensive evidence of the frequency and importance of sex among older community-dwelling and care-home residents, as well as the physiological impact of ageing on sexual function, assessment of the impact of the diagnosis on the sexual life of the individual with dementia, their spouse or partner and wider contacts, becomes paramount. Ongoing reviews are necessary as dementia progresses, as difficulties may wax and wane as cognitive problems progress or with the advent of behavioural and psychological symptoms of dementia. Discussions about sexual difficulties should be initiated by clinicians, as people are often reluctant to volunteer to talk about their sex life. Older people may feel that sexual disorders are part of the ageing process, or that they are not a priority if they or their partner has dementia.

If a sexual problem is suspected, then taking a history in a confident but sensitive manner can be very helpful.

29.4   ASSESSMENT

Most people faced with a sexual problem probably will discuss it first with their general practitioner (GP), although many individuals are reticent about this and prefer an entrée in the guise of a physical complaint (d'Ardenne, 1988). Whilst few studies exist about older people communicating their sexual difficulties, Gott and Hinchliff (2003) studied the barriers to seeking treatment for sexual problems in primary care. In their sample of 55 subjects between the ages of 50 and 92, they found that patients cited specific demographic characteristics of the GP as reasons for not seeking treatment. Patients preferred a GP of their own gender and an older doctor was seen as being preferable to someone less likely to have experienced such difficulties themselves.

There is also evidence that it is not just the reluctance of patients which acts as a barrier to seeking help. Dogan et al. (2008) examined the attitudes and knowledge of 87 Turkish medical doctors towards the sexuality of older people. Sixty-nine per cent of respondents felt that they had limited information and knowledge regarding sexual health issues in older people. Kleinplatz (2008) argues that doctors should ask – and be trained to ask – every patient, regardless of age about any sexual problems being experienced.

Taking a psychosexual history is a delicate task that requires sensitivity and timing. With older patients it may take more than one interview, and is probably best left altogether until a rapport has been established. People respond to an open interviewing style, irrespective of their generation. Opinions differ about how to take a psychosexual history, particularly about whether to interview people separately or together. The presence of dementia can clearly complicate this process and much will depend on the severity of the cognitive impairment. Where the dementia is mild to moderate, it is probably perhaps best to see the couple together and then see the informant alone.

As with many other clinical scenarios in medicine, the taking of a comprehensive medical and psychosexual history may reveal clues as to the aetiology of the particular problem. It is likely however, that the issues are multifactorial involving various organic, psychological and relationship elements. An understanding and appreciation of these factors together with a degree of flexibility on the part of the clinician is required in the management of such difficulties.

29.5   MANAGEMENT

29.5.1   Managing common sexual dysfunction

Erectile disorder (ED) may be treated by behavioural and/or pharmacological approaches. Sensate focus (Masters and Johnson, 1966) is a graded programme of behavioural exercises that involves the couple engaging in mutual erotic exercise stopping short of intercourse. This change in focus of the sexual act away from the intercourse may help reduce spectatoring (self-monitoring of erectile capacity) and performance anxiety. Applying this technique requires commitment and may be difficult for individuals with dementia.

Oral phosphodiesterase inhibitors such as sildenafil (Viagra) are an oral treatment for ED which is effective in most patients. Older age does not appear to be a contra-indication per se, although these drugs should be avoided in patients with cardiovascular or hepatic disease, recent stroke and those on vasodilators (especially nitrates). Vaginal discomfort during intercourse is often related to atrophy and dryness of the vaginal mucosa, secondary to low oestrogen levels. Initially, these may respond to simple water-based lubricants or topical oestrogen creams.

29.5.2   Managing inappropriate behaviours

Any strategy to manage sexually inappropriate behaviour needs to begin with a comprehensive assessment of the behaviour. This will involve a description of the behaviour but also a consideration of the frequency and context. Another important consideration is how much of a problem this behaviour presents and to whom, as well as a comprehensive risk assessment (Series and Dégano, 2005).

Specific interventions to reduce such unwanted behaviours have been suggested (Jensen, 1989; Howell and Watts, 1990). Most rely on behavioural modification, including removing reinforcement during the undesired behaviour and increasing reinforcement of appropriate alternative behaviours. The utility of these approaches has not been established.

29.5.3   Pharmacological approaches

Despite the most comprehensive assessment and detailed behavioural management strategies, some sexually disinhibited behaviour can continue, leading to the prescription of medication. Currently no medication has been licensed either in the UK (Series and Dégano, 2005) or in the USA (Kettl, 2008) for this specific purpose. While there have been no double-blind, placebo-controlled trials for any of the drugs used to combat such symptoms, their use has been reported in the literature and exists mainly in the form of case reports or series. A summary is outlined below.

29.5.3.1   HORMONAL APPROACHES

These agents decrease serum testosterone levels with the aim of reducing sexual drive, although the extent to which serum testosterone correlates with hypersexual behaviour is not clear (Levitsky and Owens, 1999). Cyproterone acetate (CPA) is a progestogen and exerts its effect by both inhibiting testosterone release and blocking androgen receptors. Haussermann et al. (2003) describe the successful reduction in inappropriate sexual behaviour following treatment with CPA. Huertas et al. (2007) conducted a study comparing CPA against haloperidol, admittedly looking at non-sexual aggressive behaviours. Twenty-four patients completed the study which revealed a significant reduction in such behaviours favouring the CPA.

Medroxypreogesterone acetate (MPA) acts in a similar manner to CPA although it is less potent in its mode of action (Guay, 2008). Again, case reports show favourable outcomes targeting inappropriate sexual behaviour in the context of dementia (Cooper, 1987).

Luteinizing hormone releasing hormone (LHRH) analogues such as leuprorelin, triptorelin and goserelin inhibit gonadotrophin release suppressing ovarian and testicular hormone production and result in a 'chemical castration' (Guay, 2008). Amadeo (1996) found beneficial effects of leuprorelin in three subjects with dementia exhibiting sexual disinhibition. Ott (1995) also reports the successful treatment of a demented patient with Kluver–Bucy syndrome.

Oestrogens such as diethylstilbestrol (DES) have also been used in this context. They act by reducing luteinizing hormone (LH) and follicle stimulating hormone (FSH) which, in turn, leads to a reduction in testosterone production (Black et al., 2005). Lothstein et al. (1997) reported marked improvements in behaviour in 38 out of 39 demented subjects who were exhibiting sexually inappropriate behaviour, when treated with DES.

Other drugs with anti-androgenic properties such as cimetidine (a histamine H2 blocker), ketoconazole (an antifungal) and spironolactone (a potassium-sparing diuretic) have also been studied. Wiseman et al. (2000) reported on 20 demented patients with sexually inappropriate behaviour. Fourteen of the 20 patients responded favourably to the cimetidine while the remaining six responded to combinations of cimetidine and ketoconazole, spironolactone, or both.

The use of medication to hormonally suppress the libido is a controversial issue in itself but these medications (especially CPA and oestrogens) carry significant side effects in the form of cardiovascular and thromboembolic risks which require careful consideration.

29.5.3.2 ANTIDEPRESSANTS

Medications which enhance serotonin activity, such as the selective serotonin reuptake inhibitors (SSRIs), are thought to act by not only their negative effect on the libido but also via their anti-obsessional properties (Series and Dégano, 2005). They also have the advantage of being well tolerated and safe compared to other drugs. Leo and Kim (1995) also found that clomipramine – a tricyclic antidepressant but with significant serotonergic properties – was effective in treating two dementia patients exhibiting sexual disinhibition.

29.5.3.3 ANTIPSYCHOTICS

Antipsychotics have been used in attempts to manage a variety of challenging behaviours within the context of dementia, not just sexually disinhibited behaviour. These drugs exert their anti-libidinal effect through dopamine receptor blockade (Black et al., 2005) but have been the subject of significant debate given their potential side effects (O'Brien, 2008). Macknight and Rojas-Fernandez (2000)

report the beneficial use of quetiapine in an 85-year-old man with dementia and parkinsonism who presented with excessive masturbation 'to the point of self-injury'. The patient had previously been tried on CPA and paroxetine with no success. Within 2 days of the quetiapine being commenced, the sexual behaviours had improved with no worsening of his parkinsonism. Dhikav et al. (2007) also report the successful treatment of a 70-year-old man with AD and sexual disinhibition following the introduction of olanzapine.

29.5.3.4 CHOLINESTERASE INHIBITORS

It might be reasonable to predict that cholinesterase inhibitors (ChEIs) should also have an important role in managing these behaviours. At present however, the situation remains unclear. While Alagiakrishnan et al. (2003) report the improvement of sexually inappropriate behaviour in a 72-year-old female given rivastigmine, Freymann et al. (2005) found that such behaviour did not respond to donepezil and was actually made worse by galantamine, in a 78-year-old male with dementia. The patient was subsequently commenced on carbamazepine which led to a 90 per cent improvement in the behaviour.

29.5.3.5 OTHER MEDICATIONS

In addition to those described above, case reports of beneficial effects of other medications including gabapentin (Alkhalil et al., 2003), buspirone (Tiller et al., 1998) and pindolol (Jensen, 1989) exist.

29.5.4   Ethical issues of drug management

There are complex ethical considerations when drugs are used to combat sexually inappropriate behaviour in patients who are unable to provide informed consent. Central to this issue is the concept of human rights, those belonging both to the perpetrator and those on the receiving end of such behaviour. Any medication decision must be made in the light of an assessment of risk to all parties and involving all relevant individuals. This decision should form part of a multidisciplinary care plan which should be reviewed at regular individuals.

29.6   SEXUAL ABUSE

Although much has been written about elder abuse, there is scant recognition of the potential of sexual abuse in older people with dementia. Estimates of the prevalence of all forms of elder abuse vary, but one study found rates of 16 per cent of a survey of 126 patients in a geriatric psychiatry service had experienced some abuse (Vida et al., 2002). There was a trend for individuals with dementia to experience more elder abuse although sexual abuse was not specifically classified in this study.

Burgess and Phillips (2006) found in a study of 284 cases of elder abuse that 60 per cent had been diagnosed with some form of dementia. Such patients presented with symptoms of distress rather than verbal disclosures and disappointingly, perpetrators of such abuse were less likely to be arrested or charged if the elderly individual had dementia.

It is clear that individuals with dementia are vulnerable to many forms of exploitation or sexual abuse in a variety of settings. This abuse can be perpetrated by a variety of individuals who have dealings with the patient within or outside the family. Marriage, for example, may be a means to effect this abuse (Peisah et al., 2008). People with dementia may be physically frail and unable to resist sexual advances; when it does occur, they may not be able to report it. This already complex issue is also exacerbated by a lack of definitions and awareness among health professionals and the public.

29.7   CONCLUSIONS

Clearly, the impact of dementia upon the sexuality of an individual has profound implications for the patient, their partner and all those involved in caring for them. When difficulties do occur, they can be significant and a comprehensive assessment of all the relevant factors needs to be considered. If specific management is required, then this needs to take account of sometimes complex ethical issues such as capacity, consent and basic human rights. Professionals of all disciplines need to be alert to these problems and offer support and help when necessary.

REFERENCES

Alagiakrishnan K, Sclater A, Robertson D. (2003) Role of cholinesterase inhibitor in the management of sexual aggression in an elderly demented woman. *Journal of the American Geriatric Society* 51: 1326.

Alkhalil C, Hahar N, Alkhalil B et al. (2003) Can gabapentin be a safe alternative to hormonal therapy in the treatment of inappropriate sexual behavior in demented patients? *International Urology and Nephrology* 35: 299–302.

Amadeo M. (1996) Antiandrogen treatment of aggressivity in men suffering from dementia. *Journal of Geriatric Psychiatry and Neurology* 9: 142–5.

Baikie E. (2002) The impact of dementia on marital relationships. *Sexual and Relationship Therapy* 17: 289–99.

Bauer M, Nay R, McAuliffe L. (2009) Catering to love, sex and intimacy in residential aged care: what information is provided to consumers? *Sexuality and Disability* 27: 3–9.

Beckman N, Waern M, Gustafson D, Skoog I. (2008) Secular trends in self reported sexual activity and satisfaction in Swedish 70 year olds: cross sectional survey of four populations, 1971–2001. *British Medical Journal* 337: 151–4.

Black B, Muralee S, Tampi RR. (2005) Inappropriate sexual behaviours in dementia. *Journal of Geriatric Psychiatry and Neurology* 18: 155–62.

Bouman WP, Arcelus J, Benbow SM. (2006) Nottingham study of sexuality and ageing (NoSSA I). Attitudes regarding sexuality and older people: A review of the literature. *Sexual and Relationship Therapy* 21: 149–61.

Bouman WP, Arcelus J, Benbow SM. (2007) Nottingham study of sexuality and ageing (NoSSA II). Attitudes of care staff regarding sexuality and residents: A study in residential and nursing homes. *Sexual and Relationship Therapy* 22: 45–61.

Burgess AW, Phillips SL. (2006) Sexual abuse, trauma and dementia in the elderly: a retrospective study of 284 cases. *Victims and Offenders* 1: 193–204.

Burns A, Jacoby R, Levy R. (1990) Psychiatric phenomena in Alzheimer's disease. IV: Disorders of behaviour. *British Journal of Psychiatry* 157: 86–94.

Carbone DJ, Seftel AD. (2002) Erectile dysfunction: diagnosis and treatment in older men. *Geriatrics* 57: 18–24.

Cooper AJ. (1987) Medroxyprogesterone acetate (MPA) treatment of sexual acting out in men suffering from dementia. *Journal of Clinical Psychiatry* 48: 368–70.

d'Ardenne P. (1988) Talking to patients about sex. *The Practitioner* 232: 810–12.

Davies HD, Zeiss AM, Tinklenberg JR. (1992) 'Til death do us part: intimacy and sexuality in the marriages of Alzheimer's patients. *Journal of Psychosocial Nursing and Mental Health Services* 30: 5–10.

Davies HD, Zeiss AM, Shea EA, Tinklenberg JR. (1998) Sexuality and intimacy and Alzheimer's patients and their partners. *Sexuality and Disability* 16: 193–203.

Derouesné C, Guigot J, Chermat V et al. (1996) Sexual behavioural changes in Alzheimer disease. *Alzheimer Disease and Associated Disorders* 10: 86–92.

Devanand DP, Brockington CD, Moody BJ et al. (1992) Behavioural syndromes in Alzheimer's disease. *International Psychogeriatrics* 4 (Suppl. 2): 161–84.

Dhikav V, Anand K, Aggarwal N. (2007) Grossly disinhibited sexual behavior in dementia of Alzheimer's type. *Archives of Sexual Behavior* 36: 133–4.

Dogan S, Demir B, Eker E, Karim S. (2008) Knowledge and attitudes of doctors toward the sexuality of older people in Turkey. *International Psychogeriatrics* 20: 1019–27.

Eloniemi-Sulkava U, Notkola IL, Hämäläinen K et al. (2002) Spouse caregivers' perceptions of influence of dementia on marriage. *International Psychogeriatrics* 14: 47–58.

Freymann N, Michael R, Dodel R, Jessen F. (2005) Successful treatment of sexual disinhibition in dementia with carbamazepine – a case report. *Pharmacopsychiatry* 38: 144–5.

Ginsberg TB, Pomerantz SC, Kramer-Feeley V. (2005) Sexuality in older adults: behaviours and preferences. *Age and Ageing* 34: 475–80.

Gott M, Hinchliff S. (2003) Barriers to seeking treatment for sexual problems in primary care: a qualitative study with older people. *Family Practice* 20: 690–5.

Guay DRP. (2008) Inappropriate sexual behaviours in cognitively impaired older individuals. *American Journal of Geriatric Pharmacology* 6: 269–88.

Haussermann P, Goecker D, Beier K et al. (2003) Low-dose cyproterone acetate treatment of sexual acting out in men with dementia. International Psychogeriatrics 15: 181–6.

Howard JR, O'Neill S, Travers C. (2006) Factors affecting sexuality in older Australian women: sexual interest, sexual arousal, relationships and sexual distress in older Australian women. Climacteric 9: 355–67.

Howell T, Watts DT. (1990) Behavioral complications of dementia: a clinical approach for the general internist. Journal of General Internal Medicine 5: 431–7.

Huertas D, López-Ibor Aliño JJ, Molina JD et al. (2007) Antiaggressive effect of cyproterone versus haloperidol in Alzheimer's disease: A randomized double-blind pilot study. Journal of Clinical Psychiatry 68: 439–44.

Jensen CF. (1989) Hypersexual agitation in Alzheimer's disease. Journal of the American Geriatrics Society 37: 917.

Kaiser FE. (1996) Sexuality in the elderly. Urologic Clinics of North America 23: 99–109.

Kessel B. (2001) Sexuality and the older person. Age and Ageing 30: 121–4.

Kettl P. (2008) Inappropriate behavior in long-term care. Annals of Long Term Care 16: 29–35.

Kinsey A, Pomeroy W, Martin C. (1948) Sexual behaviour in the human male. Philadelphia: Saunders.

Kinsey A, Pomeroy W, Martin C, Gebhard P. (1953) Sexual behaviour in the human female. Philadelphia: Saunders.

Kleinplatz PJ. (2008) Sexuality and older people. British Medical Journal 337: 121–2.

Kluver H, Bucy PC. (1937) Psychic blindness and other symptoms following biltateral temporal lobectomy in rhesus monkeys. American Journal of Physiology 119: 352–3.

Leo RJ, Kim KY. (1995) Clomipramine treatment of paraphilias in elderly demented patients. Journal of Geriatric Psychiatry and Neurology 8: 123–4.

Levitsky AM, Owens NJ. (1999) Pharmacologic treatment of hypersexuality and paraphilias in nursing home residents. Journal of the American Geriatrics Society 47: 231–4.

Lindau ST, Schumm LP, Laumann EO et al. (2007) A study of sexuality and health among older adults in the United States. New England Journal of Medicine 357: 762–74.

Lichtenberg PA, Strzepek DM. (1990) Assessments of institutionalized dementia patients' competencies to participate in intimate relationships. The Gerontologist 30: 117–20.

Litz BT, Zeiss AM, Davies HD. (1990) Sexual concerns of male spouses of female Alzheimer's disease patients. The Gerontologist 30: 113–16.

Lothstein LM, Fogg-Waberski J, Reynolds P. (1997) Risk management and treatment of sexual disinhibition in geriatric patients. Connecticut Medicine 61: 609–18.

Macknight C, Rojas-Fernandez C. (2000) Quetiapine for sexually inappropriate behavior in dementia. Journal of the American Geriatric Society 48: 707.

Masters WH. (1986) Sex and ageing – expectations and reality. Hospital Practice 21: 175–98.

Masters WH, Johnson VE. (1966) Human sexual response. Boston: Little and Brown.

Masters WH, Johnson VE. (1981) Sex and the ageing process. Journal of the American Geriatrics Society 29: 385–90.

O'Brien J. (2008) Antipsychotics for people with dementia. British Medical Journal 337: 64–5.

Ott BR. (1995) Leuprolide treatment of sexual aggression in a patient with dementia and the Kluver-Bucy syndrome. Clinical Neuropharmacology 18: 443–7.

Peisah C, Brodaty H, Bridger M. (2008) Abuse by marriage: the exploitation of mentally ill older people. International Journal of Geriatric Psychiatry 23: 883–8.

Schiavi RC, Schreiner-Engel P, Mandeli J et al. (1990) Healthy aging and male sexual function. American Journal of Psychiatry 147: 766–71.

Series H, Dégano P. (2005) Hypersexuality in dementia. Advances in Psychiatric Treatment 11: 424–31.

Szasz G. (1983) Sexual incidents in an extended care unit for aged men. Journal of the American Geriatric Society 31: 407–11.

Tiller JWG, Dakis JA, Shaw JM. (1998) Short-term buspirone treatment in disinhibition with dementia. Lancet 2: 510.

Tsai S-J, Hwang J-P, Yang C-H et al. (1999) Inappropriate sexual behaviours in dementia: a preliminary report. Alzheimer Disease and Associated Disorders 13: 60–62.

Vida S, Monks RC, Des Rosiers P. (2002) Prevalence and correlates of elder abuse and neglect in a geriatric service. Canadian Journal of Psychiatry 47: 459–67.

Wiley D, Bortz WM. (1996) Sexuality and ageing – usual and successful. Journal of Gerontology 51: M142–6.

Wiseman SV, McAuley JW, Freidenberg GR et al. (2000) Hypersexuality in patients with dementia: possible response to cimetidine. Neurology 54: 2024.

Wright LK. (1991) The impact of Alzheimer's disease on the marital relationship. The Gerontologist 31: 224–37.

Zeiss AM, Davies HD, Wood M, Tinklenberg JR. (1990) The incidence and correlates of erectile problems in patients with Alzheimer's disease. Archives of Sexual Behaviour 19: 325–31.

Zeiss AM, Davies HD, Tinklenberg JR. (1996) An observational study of sexual behaviour in demented male patients. Journals of Gerontology 51: M325–9.

Residential care for people with dementia

JOHN SNOWDON AND NITIN PURANDARE

30.1 A GLOBAL PERSPECTIVE ON RESIDENTIAL CARE PROVISION

Availability of residential long-term care (LTC) facilities for people with dementia and physical disabilities varies from country to country, and within countries. In many areas of the world, relatively little funding is allocated to the LTC sector. Even between developed nations there is considerable variation in the types, organization, funding and policies of residential facilities. Hence caution needs to be exercised when considering generalizations about how residential care is or should be provided for people with dementia.

Ribbe et al. (1997) noted that there are no universally accepted definitions for the different LTC services. They compared provision of residential care in ten developed countries, based on an understanding that nursing homes provide nursing care 24 hours per day, while residential homes provide personal care and social involvement for people unable to manage adequately at home, but who need no more nursing than visiting nurses can offer. They found that, in spite of having similar age distributions, the proportion of those aged 65 years or more in the Netherlands who were in nursing homes was half that found in the United States, but the proportion in residential homes was four times higher. In France, nobody was in a nursing home but 4 per cent of the elderly were in residential homes. In 2004, of those over 65 years in the United States, 3.63 per cent were in nursing homes, in a total nursing home resident population of 1.49 million (National Nursing Home Survey, 2004).

Worldwide, the population of older people, especially the very old, is expected to rise considerably. There is a steep rise in the prevalence of dementia in late old age. In Japan, a doubling of the proportion of people aged over 80 years, from 2.8 to 5.7 per cent, was expected to occur between 1993 and 2010, with a further rise to 9.7 per cent by 2025. Substantial rises in the proportion aged over 80 years are occurring in many countries (Ribbe et al., 1997). The fact that the worldwide number of people with dementia is anticipated to increase from 24.3 million in 2001 to over 81.1 million by 2040 (Ferri et al., 2005) has startling implications regarding funding, policies and planning of LTC for people with dementia. In the UK, the demand for LTC beds is expected to rise from 450 000 in 2000 to 1.1 million in 2051, with quadrupling of the annual LTC cost from £12.9 billion to £53.9 billion (Wittenberg et al., 2004).

30.2 PREVALENCE OF DEMENTIA IN LTC FACILITIES

Researchers in diverse countries have reported varying rates of dementia in LTC facilities. A recent review of 30 studies, dating back to 1986, noted a median prevalence of 58.6 per cent (Conn et al., 2009). A large UK study found that 62 per cent of LTC residents had dementia (Matthews and Dening, 2002). Recent nursing home studies have shown rates of 69.5 per cent in Helsinki (Hosia-Randell and Pitkälä, 2005), 78 per cent in Sydney (Brodaty et al., 2001) and 80.5 per cent in Norway (Selbaek et al., 2007). The proportions with Alzheimer's disease (AD), vascular dementia (VaD), mixed, dementia with Lewy bodies (DLB), frontotemporal dementia (FTD), alcoholic, traumatic or other types of dementia has not usually been reported. Cases of young onset dementia (including FTD and HIV) are relatively uncommon in nursing homes but may well require special attention because of a greater incidence of behavioural problems or the difficulty of providing age-appropriate activities and involvement.

The prevalence of dementia in residential homes has generally been reported as lower than that in nursing homes, though in Maryland (United States) the difference was small. There, 67.7 per cent of assisted living residents (74 per cent response rate) fulfilled criteria for dementia and an additional 6.6 per cent had clinically significant cognitive dysfunction (Rosenblatt et al., 2004). Small facilities had higher percentages with dementia (81 versus 63 per cent). Some 83 per cent of those with dementia had exhibited neuropsychiatric symptoms in the previous month. Residents with dementia required twice the amount of staff time given to those without dementia.

A report commissioned by Alzheimer's Australia illustrates the huge economic impact of dementia, and its potential workforce demands (Access Economics, 2009). The cost implications of the projected increase in need for LTC of people with dementia are considerable. Of 230 000 people with dementia in a population of 21 million in Australia in 2008, 90 200 were living in residential care facilities, cared for by 78 000 full-time equivalent (FTE) staff. There were 0.9 and 0.8 FTEs per high care (nursing home) and low care (residential home) resident, respectively. Modelling in the report suggested that, in the absence of changes of policy or other arrangements, there will be a shortage of 71 000 FTEs within two decades. There is already difficulty recruiting staff skilled in dementia care, partly attributable to unattractive rates of pay, and this has an obvious impact on the quality of care provided in LTC facilities.

The quality of care in US nursing homes in the last three decades has been described as poor, largely attributable to inadequate staffing and a poor mix of skills (Harrington, 2001). This is in spite of legislation (the Omnibus Budget Reconciliation Act, 1987; OBRA-87), brought in to ensure higher standards of care and the development of best practice guidelines. The government was said to be reluctant to impose higher standards for staffing because of concerns over cost. Furthermore, Harrington (2001) commented that fraud and financial mismanagement were widespread throughout the nursing home industry.

To provide good care in such facilities, 'one must battle against nihilism, cynicism and resistance to change which is often present in geriatric institutions' (Conn, 2007). OBRA-87 mandated formal psychiatric assessments of nursing home residents suspected of having mental disorders, but it was observed that this further entrenched a pattern of relative neglect of patients with dementia in formal mental health services planning (Borson et al., 1997). It is evident that money alone cannot ensure a high standard of dementia care in LTC facilities – though it can help. Factors that can contribute to good care will be discussed later in this chapter.

30.3 BEHAVIOURAL AND PSYCHOLOGICAL SYMPTOMS OF DEMENTIA IN LTC FACILITIES

The prevalence of behavioural and psychological symptoms of dementia (BPSD) in nursing homes varies between 24 and 93 per cent in the United States (Beck and Shue, 1994; Gruber-Baldini et al., 2004). Selbaek et al. (2007) reported that 65.2 per cent of residents in Norwegian nursing homes exhibited one or more clinically significant behavioural symptoms, and that frequency of delusions, hallucinations, aggression/agitation, apathy, disinhibition and aberrant motor behaviour increased with progression of dementia. An English study reported that 79 per cent of residents with dementia in both nursing and residential homes had clinically significant BPSD (Margallo-Lana et al., 2001).

Brodaty et al. (2001) reported that 80 per cent of nursing home residents showed behavioural disturbances, with people who did not have dementia being rated nearly as highly on behavioural disturbance scales as those with dementia. This raises questions about the relative importance of organic and environmental factors in development of BPSD. Brodaty et al. (2001) found a three-fold difference in the prevalence of different BPSD across nursing homes, but size accounted for only 3 per cent of the variance. The extent of the difference is difficult to explain. Some nursing homes may be reluctant to accept 'difficult' referrals. The study did find greater functional incapacity to be associated with increased rates of behavioural disturbance, including aggressiveness.

In assisted living facilities, 49 per cent of residents with dementia were observed to exhibit one or more behavioural symptoms at least once weekly, 19 per cent showing aggressive and 34 per cent physically non-aggressive behaviour (Gruber-Baldini et al., 2004). Rates were higher in facilities with fewer residents.

Brodaty et al. (2001) noted positive associations between ratings of behavioural disturbance and psychosis and depression. Wancata et al. (2003) reported that 38 per cent of newly admitted residents with dementia had marked or severe non-cognitive symptoms of dementia, including 30 per cent with depressive symptoms and 12.7 per cent with 'aggressive-psychotic symptoms'; one-third remitted from these symptoms within six months. Menon et al. (2001) analysed data from residents with dementia newly admitted to Maryland nursing homes. Nursing staff observed physical aggressive behaviours in 10.5 per cent and verbal aggressive behaviours in 10.4 per cent. The rates varied with degree of cognitive impairment, with physical aggression displayed by 15 per cent of those with severe dementia and 2.4 per cent with mild dementia, and verbal aggression by 13 and 5.4 per cent, respectively. They found that those manifesting physical or verbal aggression (mainly those with more severe cognitive impairment) were more likely to be rated as depressed.

Studies have found the prevalence of depression in LTC facilities to be much higher than that reported among older people living at home. Depression levels were somewhat higher in nursing homes than in residential homes (Snowdon and Fleming, 2008). Of residents newly accommodated in Maryland nursing homes (assessed 21–65 days after admission, thus minimizing the effect of relocation stress on results), 23.6 per cent of demented and 22.3 per cent of non-demented subjects were recorded as depressed (Kaup et al., 2007). Among those with dementia, depression in residential homes was not significantly less prevalent than in nursing homes (Gruber-Baldini et al., 2005). Most residents with anxiety symptoms are also depressed (Parmelee et al., 1993).

Evers *et al.* (2002) drew attention to the high prevalence of major depression among residents in the last six months of life, both those with dementia and those without.

Among nursing home residents, the evidence regarding an association of depression with cognitive impairment is unclear. Some have observed no association (Katz and Parmelee, 1994). Others have reported depression to be more prevalent among those with mild to moderate dementia (Evers *et al.*, 2002; Jones *et al.*, 2003). In contrast, Teresi *et al.* (2001) diagnosed major depression in 5.8 per cent of nursing home residents with little or no cognitive impairment, but in 22.8 per cent of those with moderate to severe dementia. Gruber-Baldini *et al.* (2005), examining scores on the Cornell Scale for Depression in Dementia (Alexopoulos *et al.*, 1988) among residents of nursing homes and residential homes, found that participants with depression were more likely to be severely or very severely cognitively impaired. The association of behavioural symptoms with Cornell Scale scores was significant, though it was much stronger among those with dementia in residential homes. Barca *et al.* (2008), who conducted a factor analysis of ratings on the Cornell, noted that scores on the mood subscale did not differ across varied levels of dementia severity, but on the other four subscales increases were associated with severity of dementia. In an earlier factor analysis (Kurlowicz *et al.*, 2002), a clear separation had been noted between somatic/vegetative features and a 'core depression factor', raising questions about the scale's validity in a population with high levels of dementia, medical illness and/or functional disability. Some symptoms of depression as rated by the Cornell overlap with those of dementia. Nursing home resident scores on the Cornell Scale and on the Neuropsychiatric Inventory (Cummings *et al.*, 1994) correlated highly ($r = 0.7$; Barca *et al.*, 2009). Apathy (which needs to be distinguished from depression) is common early in AD and becomes more severe as cognitive impairment worsens.

Examination of the factors associated with depression, agitation and other behavioural and mental disorders in LTC facilities is relevant to discussions concerning optimal management, interventions and therapy for these disorders. For example, depression among residents with dementia has been reported as more common in for-profit than not-for-profit nursing homes (Gruber-Baldini *et al.*, 2005). To what extent are depressive symptoms a result of demoralizing situations and circumstances? To what extent is disruptive behaviour attributable to neurobiochemical or structural brain changes, maybe interacting with environmental factors? Outcome studies exploring whether medications, psychological therapies or environmental adjustments appear to be related to reduction in symptoms will provide clues. The finding that, in a one-year study of residents with dementia in LTC facilities, 45 per cent of agitation cases, nearly 60 per cent with delusions and over 60 per cent of depression cases resolved independently of pharmacological treatment (Ballard *et al.*, 2001), should provoke consideration of what factors specific to LTC situations contribute to development of these conditions. This also highlights the self-limiting course of certain BPSD, and therefore the propriety of regular reviews of medication, with attempts to cease unnecessary prescriptions.

The fact that, in a LTC facility in California for people with cognitive impairment, 40 residents scored >12 on the Cornell Scale soon after admission, but that only six of them were still depressed after six months (in contrast to worse outcomes elsewhere), raises questions about factors that maintain depressive symptoms (Payne *et al.*, 2002). Commenting on a decrease in depressive symptoms from 41.3 to 28.9 per cent during the first six months of admission to Dutch nursing homes, Smalbrugge *et al.* (2006) suggested that adaptation to pre-admission factors, facilitated by the nursing home environment, may explain the fall. When the prevalence does not fall (as in the study by Scocco *et al.*, 2006), reasons should be sought.

30.4   RECOGNITION OF DEPRESSION IN CASES OF DEMENTIA IN LTC FACILITIES

Cohen *et al.* (2003) have commented on the evidence (e.g. Bagley *et al.*, 2000) that depression in nursing homes is frequently overlooked and undertreated. They found that in spite of using the minimum data set (MDS) in US nursing homes, 75 per cent of major depressive disorders and 87 per cent of all types of depression escaped recognition; further, only 33 per cent of those identified as depressed were treated with antidepressants. These authors showed that use of the Cornell Scale resulted in a significant increase in the percentage of residents given antidepressants. Before screening, only 16 per cent of patients who scored 5 or more on the Cornell Scale were prescribed antidepressants, whereas after routine screening was introduced 36 per cent were given antidepressants. They recommended mandatory screening, and suggested that referrals to staff psychiatrists of all those scoring 5 or more on the Cornell Scale would not impose an undue burden on them.

The American Geriatrics Society and American Association of Geriatric Psychiatry (2003a), in a consensus statement, recommended that residents should be screened for depressive symptoms within the first 2–4 weeks of admission to an LTC facility, and subsequently at least every six months. Use of the Cornell Scale was supported for residents with moderate or severe dementia, and of the Geriatric Depression Scale (Yesavage *et al.*, 1983) for residents with no more than mild to moderate cognitive impairment. However, limitations should be recognized, as discussed in the previous section. Somatic items comprise 37 per cent of the Cornell. The prevalence of depression may be overestimated in patients with physical problems. Kurlowicz *et al.* (2002) called for research to establish whether an intrapsychic subscale of the Cornell may be more useful than the global scale for measuring depression among those with dementia, physical illness and/or disability. Greenberg *et al.* (2004) found that in palliative care cases the psychiatrist's diagnostic assessments did not correspond well with Cornell Scale scores, and concluded that there was no scale valid and reliable enough to effectively ascertain depression in the most severely demented patients. A short form of the Geriatric Depression Scale (GDS-15), validated by Herrmann *et al.* (1996), has been found useful in screening for depression among residents with only mild to moderate cognitive impairment (Gerety *et al.*, 1994), and in such cases correlates more closely than does the Cornell with psychiatrist assessments on other depression rating scales, such as the Montgomery Åsberg Depression Rating Scale (MADRS; Montgomery and Åsberg, 1979; Snowdon and Fleming, 2008). Even if such scales are not valid in all cases, use of the GDS-15 and/or Cornell, as appropriate, in LTC facilities, is strongly recommended, with the intention that, if pointers to depression are identified, staff and doctors will be prompted to discuss possible causation and appropriate interventions.

30.5 MANAGEMENT OF DEMENTIA IN LTC FACILITIES

Prevention and management of dementia, BPSD and depression in cases of dementia are discussed in Chapter 8, Neuropsychiatric aspects of dementia, Chapter 9, Measurement of behaviour disturbance, non-cognitive symptoms and quality of life, Chapter 23, The role of physiotherapy in the management of dementia, Chapter 24, Therapeutic effects of music in people with dementia, Chapter 25, Non-pharmacological therapies to manage behavioural and psychological symptoms of dementia: what works and what doesn't and Chapter 58, Prevention of Alzheimer's disease. Aspects specific to care in LTC facilities will be discussed here.

Little will be said about short-term residential care ('respite') because of the dearth of relevant data and studies. It has proved effective in reducing the subjective burden and depression experienced by family caregivers of people with dementia (Donath *et al.*, 2009). However, studies around the world have shown low utilization of such care, even when caregivers were well aware of its availability.

30.5.1 Physical and social environment and staff training

First, it is appropriate to re-emphasize the importance of environment and of care arrangements in relation to prevention or development of mood and behaviour disturbance. Guidelines are available (e.g. American Geriatrics Society and American Association for Geriatric Psychiatry, 2003b; Conn and Gibson, 2007) to advise on how, and in what settings, optimal care can be provided. Koopmans (2005) recommends accommodating residents at similar stages of dementia together, but notes that a drawback is the need to move them when their dementia progresses. Others advocate ageing in place. There is also an argument for housing people with early-onset dementia together. The major need surely is to look at the needs of the individual and what suits that person best.

As stated earlier, funding varies between jurisdictions, both in relative amount and how it is allocated. However, Conn and Gibson (2007) pointed out that countries that have residential care facilities for older people commonly face challenges that include 'inadequate staffing levels, lack of staff training regarding mental health issues, ageing and poorly designed LTC homes, failure to identify and assess residents in a timely fashion, inappropriate use of psychotropic medications, and limited availability of mental health consultants'.

Management of dementia in LTC settings is optimized by having available a multidisciplinary team that can co-ordinate care. Facility-based staff members may take on mental health interest roles, such as recognition and co-ordination of management of depression, and may be designated to have a role liaising with doctors and visiting mental health professionals. Some LTC facilities make arrangements for a consultation-liaison old age mental health service to be accessible to work with facility staff and primary care doctors in dealing with the range of psychiatric and behavioural problems associated with dementia. An Australian model for dealing with challenging behaviours blended clinical consultation with staff training and educational interventions (Turner and Snowdon, 2009). A UK study found that few LTC facilities had visits from psychologists or social workers, and only one-third received visits from old age psychiatrists (Purandare *et al.*, 2004).

Citing Canadian national guidelines relating to mental health issues in LTC homes, Conn and Gibson (2007) discussed organizational and systems issues. The first concerned LTC homes developing the physical and social environment as a therapeutic milieu through the intentional use of design principles. Verbeek *et al.* (2009) declared that traditional institutional care has been arranged according to the medical model, with emphasis given to the treatment of the underlying pathology. They contended that this model has become outmoded. They said that a shift towards a psychosocial model has occurred, this approach being person-centred and aimed at supporting the well-being and remaining strengths of older people with dementia.

It has been recognized that a facility's architectural and physical environment influences dementia care, and studies have suggested that small, domestic-style environments are beneficial for older people with dementia. Verbeek *et al.* (2009) reviewed and compared 11 concepts, from various countries, that have adopted a home-like philosophy of care in a small-scale context. They referred to CADE units in Australia, the Cantou in France, Group Living and Small-scale Living in Sweden and the Netherlands and Belgium, Green Houses in the United States, and comparable concepts developed in Japan, Canada, the UK and the United States. In all of the 11, residents are encouraged to participate in the household as far as possible, with activities (such as cooking) being planned according to residents' wishes. Residents are stimulated, encouraged and supported, with an emphasis on autonomy and choice. Care staff function as part of the household, and thus need to have skills and attitudes that suit the philosophy. In Green Houses, staff (certified nursing assistants) receive 120 hours of additional training for an expanded universal role, that includes cooking, cleaning, laundry, shopping and more (Ragsdale and McDougall, 2008).

The Green House model of care was developed by Dr William Thomas, who had introduced the Eden Alternative in the 1990s. This model aimed to reduce loneliness, boredom and helplessness among nursing home residents. To enhance quality of life, nursing home staff were encouraged to integrate plants, animals and children into the daily life of residents.

Impetus towards developing the above ideas may have been accelerated by reports such as that from Sloane *et al.* (1991). They found that the development of specialized dementia units (whether areas within nursing homes or entire facilities) apparently led to less use of physical restraints but no reduction in the use of pharmacological restraint.

30.5.2 Psychotherapeutic approaches and person–centred care

A person-centred approach argues that much of what is described as 'challenging behaviour' is a rational response to an untenable situation, and can be a response to unmet physical or social needs (Downs *et al.*, 2005). Cohen-Mansfield (2001) suggested an environmental vulnerability model and a behavioural and learning model. Non-pharmacological treatments for behavioural disturbance, based on these models, are discussed in Chapter 23, The role of physiotherapy in the management of dementia and Chapter 24, Therapeutic effects of music in people with dementia. Snoezelen and aromatherapy are examples of strategies used by nursing home staff to reduce agitation. Chenoweth *et al.* (2009) have presented evidence of the effectiveness of dementia-care mapping and person-centred care in reducing agitation among residents of LTC facilities.

It has been stated that most agitated behaviours of people with dementia are manifestations of unmet needs (Camp *et al.*, 2002). The goals of treatment should be to uncover and address such needs; the person has been unable to fulfil them because of a combination of perceptual problems, communication difficulties and an inability to manipulate the environment through appropriate channels (Camp *et al.*, 2002). Cohen-Mansfield (2001) categorized non-pharmacological interventions, but Cody *et al.* (2002) detailed some of the challenges to their use in nursing homes. They even suggested (and this was long after OBRA-87 was introduced) that staff members often see the sedating effects of psychotropic drugs as desirable – and might prefer their use to resident activity. Attitudes and the quality of care in LTC facilities are largely determined by the leadership, example and training provided in those facilities, in addition to their design and philosophy.

There is good reason to examine factors that might be responsible for demoralization among LTC residents who become depressed. Higher levels of mastery and greater satisfaction with available social support have been shown to have effects in lessening depression and in buffering the adverse impact of disability (Jang *et al.*, 2002). Blanchard *et al.* (2009) have discussed the processes of adjustment needed to overcome the multiple losses of function, abilities, roles and relationships that may occur in old age. They referred to construction and consolidation of a new understanding of oneself, with emergence of meaning to life, goals and something to hope for. Losses in one domain are compensated for through strengths in other domains. The relevance to LTC facility care is striking.

Another model (Restore, Empower, Mobilize) for brief individual psychotherapy to treat depression in long-term care residents with mild to moderate dementia has been presented by Carpenter *et al.* (2002).

Bharucha *et al.* (2006) reviewed 18 studies of psychotherapy provided in LTC settings. A majority showed benefits on instruments measuring depression, hopelessness, self-esteem, perceived control and on other variables. They commented that a perception that psychotherapy is a 'medical' intervention is a serious obstacle because of the lack of availability of consultants to do this work. They suggested the possibility of psychiatric nurse practitioners being trained as depression care managers or masters-level mental health care specialists, who could also provide staff training in the management of 'difficult' patients and co-ordinate group therapy.

30.5.3 Psychotropic medications

The use of antipsychotic medication to suppress behavioural disruption has varied between countries and over time. Extensive comparisons will not be presented here. However, a major catalyst for discussions leading to OBRA-87 was concern about misuse of psychotropic medication in US nursing homes. Introduction of federal antipsychotic drug regulations led to a 36 per cent reduction in prescriptions for neuroleptics in Baltimore nursing homes over six months (Rovner *et al.*, 1992), and other studies (cited by Hughes *et al.*, 2000) showed comparable results. Data from various countries showed that in the mid-1990s over 20 per cent of residents in Iceland, Italy and Sweden, but only 14.4 per cent of US nursing home residents, were taking antipsychotic drugs (Hughes *et al.*, 2000).

In Sydney nursing homes in 1993, 27.4 per cent of residents were taking typical antipsychotic medication regularly, while ten years later, 23.6 per cent were given antipsychotics regularly, one-third typical and two-thirds atypical (Snowdon *et al.*, 2006). Two-thirds of those given antipsychotics had dementia or cerebral disease and not schizophrenia (Snowdon *et al.*, 2005). The percentage of residents regularly taking anxiolytics fell progressively over the ten years (8.6 to 4.1 per cent), and similarly there was a fall in regular hypnotic use (26.6 to 11.3 per cent). The use of antidepressants increased, but not as much as in US nursing homes (Snowdon *et al.*, 2006). The changes have been attributed to increased availability of best practice information in Sydney. At the same time in Norway, 21.8 per cent of nursing home residents were taking antipsychotics, 24.5 per cent anxiolytics, 30.6 per cent hypnotics and 39.5 per cent antidepressants (Barca *et al.*, 2009). Antipsychotics were more commonly prescribed for those with severe dementia, reflecting the fact that psychotic and aggressive symptoms increase with severity of dementia (Selbaek *et al.*, 2007). In Sweden, 26.3 per cent of residents of LTC facilities for older people were taking antipsychotics, use being higher among those with aggressive, verbally disruptive and wandering behaviour (Lövheim *et al.*, 2006). In Helsinki in 2003, a remarkable 43.3 per cent of residents with dementia and 41 per cent of those without were given antipsychotics, while 41.4 per cent of those with dementia and

51.9 per cent of those without were given antidepressants (Hosia-Randell *et al.*, 2005), and there was high use of anxiolytics and hypnotics. In Dutch nursing homes, antipsychotic and antidepressant drugs were more often prescribed for residents with severe dementia, while anxiolytics and sedatives had no association with dementia stage (Nijk *et al.*, 2009). Both antipsychotic and anxiolytic use were associated with agitation.

The use of other types of medication in managing screaming, hypersexuality and other behavioural problems has been discussed elsewhere in this book, as has the use of anticholinesterase inhibitors. Frequency of use of the latter in nursing homes varies markedly between countries.

It is relevant to note that the evidence showing effectiveness of antidepressants in both community (Roose *et al.*, 2004) and LTC (Snowden *et al.*, 2003) settings is limited, and that a systematic review found no clear evidence for efficacy of antidepressants in dementia (Bains *et al.*, 2009). Depression levels reduced in only one-third of depressed residents treated with antidepressants for two months (Boyle *et al.*, 2004). Several studies showed that residents with dementia responded less well than those without dementia (Snowden *et al.*, 2003). Depression among residents with dementia develops in response to a complex mix of factors, some ongoing, so that non-response to antidepressants may seem understandable. When symptoms are common to both depression and dementia, difficulty suppressing symptoms may be because antidepressants have no effect on the underlying dementia (Purandare *et al.*, 2001).

30.6   STANDARDS OF CARE IN LTC FACILITIES

Useful advice on standards to be achieved in nursing home care has been provided by Koopmans (2005). Physicians specially trained in nursing home medicine are employed by Dutch nursing homes, with a ratio of one doctor per 100 patients. Availability of doctors and specialists to visit or work in LTC facilities varies between jurisdictions, as does the availability of psychologists. Standards of care are largely dependent on staffing, and how well the staff work with residents. Standards regarding regular screening of mood, behaviour, physical function and use of medication are desirable, and capacity to respond to special needs should be one of the standards. Dufey and Hope (2005) have listed a number of standards for nurses to achieve when caring for people with dementia.

30.7   PALLIATIVE CARE

Hertogh (2005a) has discussed issues to be addressed during end-of-life care, which in due course applies to most people living in nursing homes. Quality of life needs to be assessed. Provision of high quality palliative care in the nursing home setting is essential (Engel *et al.*, 2006); next-of-kin are generally opposed to the use of feeding tubes. Advance directives should be discussed with a care provider at the time of admission. However, Hertogh (2005a) pointed out that

euthanasia in cases of dementia is almost an unthinkable option due to impaired cognitive skills and inability of such patients to provide informed consent. Opiates are frequently used in Dutch nursing homes for symptom control, but the administration of medications specifically intended to cause death was found to be uncommon (2 per cent; van der Steen *et al.*, 2005). These issues are also discussed in Chapter 37, Care and management of the patient with advanced dementia.

30.8   GOOD CARE

Hertogh (2005b) has discussed elements of an 'ethic of care' in LTC for people with dementia. Caregivers are encouraged to move beyond a simple custodial approach to caring, and focus on the residual abilities and subjective experiences rather than functional deficits of people with dementia. The ethic of care 'allows criticism of a society that is too unilaterally oriented towards the maxims of individual autonomy and independence'. Central to the ethic are safety and self-esteem. Caregivers should afford people with dementia meaningful choices that allow them to enhance their self-esteem and personhood. Good care recognizes the fear and anxiety experienced by people with dementia due to loss of control and progressive threatening of their identity. They need a safe haven where they can feel 'at home' and secure.

'Bringing together of functional caring and empathetic treatment is exactly what defines the specific competency needed for caregiving in dementia'. There is also a need to care for the carers and attention to the morale of those working and living in LTC facilities. Adequate funding for well integrated care is vital.

REFERENCES

Access Economics. (2009) Making choices. Future dementia care: projections, problems and preferences. Report for Alzheimer's Australia. Available from: www.alzheimers.org.au

Alexopoulos GS, Abrams RC, Young RC, Shamoian CA. (1988) Cornell Scale for depression in dementia. *Biological Psychiatry* 23: 271–84.

American Geriatrics Society and American Association for Geriatric Psychiatry. (2003a) Consensus statement on improving the quality of care in US nursing homes: management of depression and behavioral symptoms associated with dementia. *Journal of the American Geriatrics Society* 51: 1287–98.

American Geriatrics Society and American Association for Geriatric Psychiatry. (2003b) The American Geriatrics Society and American Geriatric Psychiatry recommendations for policies in support of quality mental health care in U.S. nursing homes. *Journal of the American Geriatrics Society* 51: 1299–304.

Bagley H, Cordingley L, Burns A *et al.* (2000) Recognition of depression by staff in nursing and residential homes. *Journal of Clinical Nursing* 9: 445–50.

Bains J, Birks J, Dening T. (2009) Antidepressants for treating depression in dementia. *The Cochrane Database of Systematic Reviews* (3): CD003944.

Ballard CG, Margallo-Lana M, Fossey J *et al.* (2001) A 1-year follow-up study of behavioral and psychological symptoms in dementia among people in care environments. *Journal of Clinical Psychiatry* **62**: 631–6.

Barca ML, Selbaek G, Laks J, Engedal K. (2008) The pattern of depressive symptoms and factor analysis of the Cornell Scale among patients in Norwegian nursing homes. *International Journal of Geriatric Psychiatry* **23**: 1058–65.

Barca ML, Selbaek G, Laks J, Engedal K. (2009) Factors associated with depression in Norwegian nursing homes. *International Journal of Geriatric Psychiatry* **24**: 417–25.

Beck CK, Shue VM. (1994) Interventions for treating disruptive behavior in demented elderly people. *Nursing Clinics of North America* **29**: 143–55.

Bharucha AJ, Dew MA, Miller MD *et al.* (2006) Psychotherapy in long-term care: a review. *Journal of the American Medical Directors Association* **7**: 568–80.

Blanchard M, Serfaty M, Duckett S, Flatley M. (2009) Adapting services for a changing society: a reintegrative model for old age psychiatry (based on a model proposed by Knight and Emanuel, 2007). *International Journal of Geriatric Psychiatry* **24**: 202–6.

Borson S, Loebel JP, Kitchell M *et al.* (1997) Psychiatric assessments of nursing home residents under OBRA-87: should PASARR be reformed? *Journal of the American Geriatrics Society* **45**: 1173–81.

Boyle VL, Roychoudhury C, Beniak R *et al.* (2004) Recognition and management of depression in skilled-nursing and long-term care settings. Evolving targets for quality improvement. *American Journal of Geriatric Psychiatry* **12**: 288–95.

Brodaty H, Draper B, Saab D *et al.* (2001) Psychosis, depression and behavioural disturbances in Sydney nursing home residents: prevalence and predictors. *International Journal of Geriatric Psychiatry* **16**: 504–12.

Camp CJ, Cohen-Mansfield J, Cepezuti EA. (2002) Use of nonpharmacologic interventions among nursing home residents with dementia. *Psychiatric Services* **53**: 1397–401.

Carpenter B, Ruckdeschel K, Ruckdeschel H, Van Haitsma K. (2002) R-E-M psychotherapy: a manualized approach for long-term care residents with depression and dementia. *Clinical Gerontologist* **25**: 25–49.

Chenoweth L, King MT, Jeon Y-H *et al.* (2009) Caring for aged dementia care resident study (CADRES) of person-centred care, dementia-care mapping, and usual care in dementia: a cluster-randomised trial. *Lancet Neurology* **8**: 317–25.

Cody M, Beck C, Svarstad BL. (2002) Challenges to the use of nonpharmacologic interventions in nursing homes. *Psychiatric Services* **53**: 1402–6.

Cohen CI, Hyland K, Kimhy D. (2003) The utility of mandatory depression screening of dementia patients in nursing homes. *American Journal of Psychiatry* **160**: 2012–17.

Cohen-Mansfield J. (2001) Nonpharmacologic interventions for inappropriate behaviors in dementia: a review, summary and critique. *American Journal of Geriatric Psychiatry* **9**: 361–81.

Conn DK. (2007) Mental health issues in long-term care facilities. In: Conn DK, Herrmann N, Kaye A *et al.* (eds). *Practical psychiatry in the long-term care home. A handbook for staff*, 3rd edn. Toronto: Hogrefe & Huber, 11.

Conn DK, Gibson M. (2007) Guidelines for the assessment and treatment of mental health issues. In: Conn DK, Herrmann N, Kaye A *et al.* (eds). *Practical psychiatry in the long-term care home. A handbook for staff*, 3rd edn. Toronto: Hogrefe and Huber, 267–78.

Conn D, Seitz D, Purandere N. (2009) Epidemiology of psychiatric disorders in long-term care. Report presented at the International Psychogeriatric Association's 14th Biennial Congress, Montreal.

Cummings JL, Mega M, Gray K *et al.* (1994) The Neuropsychiatric Inventory: assessing psychopathology in dementia patients. *Neurology* **44**: 2308–14.

Donath C, Winkler A, Grabel E. (2009) Short-term residential care for dementia patients: predictors for utilization and expected quality from a family caregiver's point of view. *International Psychogeriatrics* **21**: 703–10.

Downs M, Brooker D, Bruce E. (2005) The practice of person-centred dementia care: UK. In: Burns A (ed). *Standards in dementia care*. Abingdon: Taylor & Francis, 13–19.

Dufey A-F, Hope K. (2005) Recognizing and delivering quality nursing care for people with dementia. In: Burns A (ed.). *Standards in dementia care*. Abingdon: Taylor & Francis, 155–63.

Engel SE, Kiely DK, Mitchell SL. (2006) Satisfaction with end-of-life care for nursing home residents with advanced dementia. *Journal of the American Geriatrics Society* **54**: 1567–72.

Evers MM, Samuels SC, Lantz M *et al.* (2002) The prevalence, diagnosis and treatment of depression in dementia patients in chronic care facilities in the last six months of life. *International Journal of Geriatric Psychiatry* **17**: 464–72.

Ferri CP, Prince M, Brayne C *et al.* (2005) Global prevalence of dementia: a Delphi consensus study. *Lancet* **366**: 2112–17.

Gerety MB, Williams JW, Mulrow CD *et al.* (1994) Performance of case-finding tools for depression in the nursing home: influence of clinical and functional characteristics and selection of optimal threshold scores. *Journal of the American Geriatrics Society* **42**: 1103–9.

Greenberg L, Lantz MS, Likourezos A *et al.* (2004) Screening for depression in nursing home palliative care patients. *Journal of Geriatric Psychiatry and Neurology* **17**: 212–18.

Gruber-Baldini AL, Boustani M, Sloane PD, Zimmerman S. (2004) Behavioural symptoms in residential care/assisted living facilities: prevalence, risk factors, and medication management. *Journal of the American Geriatrics Society* **52**: 1610–17.

Gruber-Baldini AL, Zimmerman S, Boustani M *et al.* (2005) Characteristics associated with depression in long-term care residents with dementia. *Gerontologist* **45**: 50–55.

Harrington C. (2001) Residential nursing facilities in the United States. *British Medical Journal* **323**: 507–10.

Herrmann N, Mittmann N, Silver IL *et al.* (1996) A validation study of the Geriatric Depression Scale short form. *International Journal of Geriatric Psychiatry* **11**: 457–60.

Hertogh CMPM. (2005a) End-of-life care and medical decision-making in patients with dementia. In: Burns A (ed). *Standards in dementia care*. London: Taylor & Francis, 339–53.

Hertogh CMPM. (2005b) Towards a more adequate moral framework: elements of an 'ethic of care' in nursing home care for people with dementia. In: Burns A (ed). *Standards in dementia care*. London: Taylor & Francis, 371–7.

Hosia-Randell H, Pitkälä K. (2005) Use of psychotropic drugs in elderly nursing home residents with and without dementia in Helsinki, Finland. *Drugs and Aging* 22: 793–800.

Hughes CM, Lapane KL, Mor V *et al.* (2000) The impact of legislation on psychotropic drug use in nursing homes: a cross-national perspective. *Journal of the American Geriatrics Society* 48: 931–7.

Jang Y, Haley WE, Small BJ, Mortimer JA. (2002) The role of mastery and social resources in the associations between disability and depression in later life. *Gerontologist* 42: 807–13.

Jones RN, Marcantonio ER, Rabinowitz T. (2003) Prevalence and correlates of recognized depression in U.S. nursing homes. *Journal of the American Geriatrics Society* 51: 1404–9.

Katz IR, Parmelee PA. (1994) Depression in elderly patients in residential care settings. In: Schneider LS, Reynolds CF, Lebowitz BD, Friedhoff AJ (eds). *Diagnosis and treatment of depression in late life*. Washington: American Psychiatric Press, 437–61.

Kaup BA, Loreck D, Gruber-Baldini AL *et al.* (2007) Depression and its relationship to function and medical status, in nursing home admissions. *American Journal of Geriatric Psychiatry* 15: 438–42.

Koopmans RTCM. (2005) Standard of care for dementia in nursing homes: the Dutch experience and views. In: Burns A (ed). *Standards in dementia care*. London: Taylor & Francis, 143–53.

Kurlowicz LH, Evans LK, Strumpf NE, Maislin G. (2002) A psychometric evaluation of the Cornell Scale for depression in dementia in a frail, nursing home population. *American Journal of Geriatric Psychiatry* 10: 600–08.

Lövheim H, Sandman P-O, Kallin K *et al.* (2006) Relationship between antipsychotic drug use and behavioral and psychological symptoms of dementia in old people with cognitive impairment living in geriatric care. *International Psychogeriatrics* 18: 713–26.

Margallo-Lana M, Swann A, O'Brien J *et al.* (2001) Prevalence and pharmacological management of behavioural and psychological symptoms amongst dementia sufferers living in care environments. *International Journal of Geriatric Psychiatry* 16: 39–44.

Matthews FE, Dening TR. (2002) Prevalence of dementia in institutional care. *Lancet* 360: 225–6.

Menon AS, Gruber-Baldini AL, Hebel JR *et al.* (2001) Relationships between aggressive behaviors and depression among nursing home residents with dementia. *International Journal of Geriatric Psychiatry* 16: 139–46.

Montgomery SA, Åsberg M. (1979) A new depression scale designed to be sensitive to change. *British Journal of Psychiatry* 134: 382–9.

National Nursing Home Survey, 2004. Accessed July 7, 2009. Available from: www.cdc.gov/nchs/nnhs.htm.

Nijk RM, Zuidema SU, Koopmans RTCM. (2009) Prevalence and correlates of psychotropic drug use in Dutch nursing-home patients with dementia. *International Psychogeriatrics* 21: 485–93.

Parmelee PA, Katz IR, Lawton MP. (1993) Anxiety and its association with depression among institutionalized elderly. *American Journal of Geriatric Psychiatry* 1: 46–58.

Payne JL, Sheppard J-M, Steinberg M *et al.* (2002) Incidence, prevalence, and outcomes of depression in residents of a long-term care facility with dementia. *International Journal of Geriatric Psychiatry* 17: 247–53.

Purandare N, Burns A, Craig S *et al.* (2001) Depressive symptoms in patients with Alzheimer's disease. *International Journal of Geriatric Psychiatry* 16: 960–4.

Purandare N, Burns A, Challis D, Morris J. (2004) Perceived mental health needs and adequacy of service provision to older people in care homes in the UK: a national survey. *International Journal of Geriatric Psychiatry* 19: 549–53.

Ragsdale V, McDougall GJ. (2008) The changing face of long-term care: looking at the past decade. *Issues in Mental Health Nursing* 29: 992–1001.

Ribbe MW, Ljunggren G, Steel K *et al.* (1997) Nursing homes in 10 nations: a comparison between countries and settings. *Age and Ageing* 26: 3–12.

Roose SP, Sackheim H, Krishnan KRR *et al.* (2004) Antidepressant pharmacotherapy in the treatment of depression in the very old: a randomized, placebo-controlled trial. *American Journal of Psychiatry* 161: 2050–9.

Rosenblatt A, Samus QM, Steele CD *et al.* (2004) The Maryland assisted living study: prevalence, recognition, and treatment of dementia and other psychiatric disorders in the assisted living population of Central Maryland. *Journal of the American Geriatric Society* 52: 1618–25.

Rovner BW, Edelman BA, Cox MP, Shmuely Y. (1992) The impact of antipsychotic drug regulations on psychotropic prescribing practices in nursing homes. *American Journal of Psychiatry* 149: 1390–2.

Scocco P, Rapattoni M, Fantoni G. (2006) Nursing home institutionalization: a source of eustress or distress for the elderly? *International Journal of Geriatric Psychiatry* 21: 281–7.

Selbaek G, Kirkevold O, Engedal K. (2007) The prevalence of psychiatric symptoms and behavioural disturbances and the use of psychotropic drugs in Norwegian nursing homes. *International Journal of Geriatric Psychiatry* 22: 843–9.

Sloane PD, Mathew L, Scarborough M *et al.* (1991) Physical and pharmacologic restraint of nursing home patients with dementia. Impact of specialized units. *Journal of the American Medical Association* 265: 1278–82.

Smalbrugge M, Jongenelis L, Pot AM *et al.* (2006) Incidence and outcome of depressive symptoms in nursing home patients in the Netherlands. *American Journal of Geriatric Psychiatry* 14: 1069–76.

Snowdon J, Fleming R. (2008) Recognising depression in residential facilities: an Australian challenge. *International Journal of Geriatric Psychiatry* 23: 295–300.

Snowden M, Sato K, Roy-Byrne P. (2003) Assessment and treatment of nursing home residents with depression or behavioral symptoms associated with dementia: a review of the literature. *Journal of the American Geriatrics Society* 51: 1305–17.

Snowdon J, Day S, Baker W. (2005) Why and how antipsychotic drugs are used in 40 Sydney nursing homes. *International Journal of Geriatric Psychiatry* 20: 1146–52.

Snowdon J, Day S, Baker W. (2006) Current use of psychotropic medication in nursing homes. *International Psychogeriatrics* 18: 241–50.

Teresi J, Abrams R, Holmes D et al. (2001) Prevalence of depression and depression recognition in nursing homes. *Social Psychiatry and Psychiatric Epidemiology* 36: 613–20.

Turner J, Snowdon J. (2009) An innovative approach to behavioral assessment and intervention in residential care: a service evaluation. *Clinical Gerontologist* 32: 260–75.

Van der Steen JT, van der Wal G, Mehr DR et al. (2005) End-of-life decision making in nursing home residents with dementia and pneumonia: Dutch physicians' intentions regarding hastening death. *Alzheimer Disease and Associated Disorders* 19: 148–55.

Verbeek H, van Rossum E, Zwakhalen SMG et al. (2009) Small, homelike care environments for older people with dementia: a literature review. *International Psychogeriatrics* 21: 252–64.

Wancata J, Benda N, Meise U, Windhaber J. (2003) Non-cognitive symptoms of dementia in nursing homes: frequency, course and consequences. *Social Psychiatry and Psychiatric Epidemiology* 38: 637–43.

Wittenberg R, Comas-Herrera A, Pickard L, Hancock R. (2004) Future demand for long-term care in the UK: a summary of projections of long-term care finance for older people to 2051. Joseph Rowntree Foundation. Future costs of long-term care for older people, Findings Ref: 944. York, UK: JRF.

Yesavage JA, Brink TL, Rose TL et al. (1983) Development and validation of a geriatric depression screening scale: a preliminary report. *Journal of Psychiatric Research* 17: 37–49.

31

Design and dementia

JUNE ANDREWS AND COLM CUNNINGHAM

31.1 WHY ATTENTION TO BUILDING DESIGN AND TECHNOLOGY IS VITAL FOR THE PERSON WITH DEMENTIA

Good 'dementia-friendly' design and technology maximizes the independence of the person with dementia and reduces the burden of care for families or health and social care workers. It can reduce the cost of care by delaying institutionalization and reducing adverse incidents in care settings. In addition, because the best practice recommendation may even be less expensive than what the architect or project manager would otherwise propose, the financial savings can start even before the project is operational.

Dementia is a symptom of an underlying disease process. The 'dementia' is the extent to which that process (e.g. Alzheimer's disease or vascular disease) makes the person less able to remember or learn things or work things out, and cope with the stress cause by reduction in that capacity. The majority of people with dementia are older, or very old, and their capacity to deal with the common changes of ageing is reduced by their cognitive impairment and understandable stress, much of which is environmental. Their stress response may often be behaviour that is disturbing to those around them.

For any individual, the extent to which the disease causes 'dementia' or reduction in capacity varies. This variation is affected by a number of factors, including the behaviour of people who interact with the patient or client and other physical illnesses or fatigue. One crucial, frequently ignored factor is the environment.

Solutions to this are based on three elements.

1. Research involving people with dementia.
2. Extrapolation from sensory and physical impairment research.

3. Sharing examples of good practical solutions based on an understanding of cognitive impairment.

31.2 HOW THE BUILT ENVIRONMENT AFFECTS THE PERSON WITH DEMENTIA

31.2.1 Impaired memory

When you do not remember where you are, it is as if you are in the building for the first time. You may ask people where you are, and why, and try to get out to see if you can get your bearings from a more familiar landmark. If people stop you getting out, you will probably become very stressed and redouble your efforts. The dementia-friendly building aims to compensate for this. You do not have to remember or be told where anything is. You can see everywhere important that you need to go.

31.2.2 Impaired reasoning

Anyone can momentarily forget where they are or how to use an everyday object. Usually we can work it out. In the dementia-friendly building you get help with this. For example, the soap, tap, flush handle and the paper holder in the toilet will be very easy to understand, an objective best achieved by using familiar or traditional designs.

31.2.3 Impaired learning

Because of the learning problem, the person with dementia goes through the same effort again and again to work things out. Dementia-friendly design provides lots of cues to support any residual learning capacity. Design cues can help with finding places, but it also helps with where not to go. An example is the hazard of frequent exiting through the fire escape door in the absence of a fire. Design can make this less likely and can balance the high risk of someone getting lost with the hypothetical risk of the fire door not being found by staff and visitors in a real fire.

31.2.4   Ordinary changes of ageing

The majority of people with dementia are old or very old, and they will have many common age related problems with a reduced capacity to learn or work out how to compensate. The building needs to compensate on their behalf. If the person needs help with mobility, they may forget to use the call assist button. A technology such as a passive infrared beam can alert carers to the fact that the person is on the move, and they can go to help in good time.

31.2.5   High levels of stress

It is sad to contemplate the possible level of stress created in anyone by never knowing where they are or why they are there, and never reaching the stage of being even vaguely familiar with the strange environment in which they find themselves. This is made worse by meaningless noise and activity. The building design can conceal background tasks like delivery of laundry, and reduce unavoidable noises. Incorporating outdoor spaces for recreation and exercise also reduces stress.

31.3   SOME PRACTICAL IMPLICATIONS

Assessing the designs for a planned building or evaluating the changes that can be made to an existing building can identify important ways in which the environment can be changed to actively assist the person with dementia. The use of a tool to inform these decisions is important to ensure that evidence and not just opinion informs the outcome of these critical decisions (Cunningham, 2009), for example Cunningham et al.'s (2008) design audit tool can be used to audit health services, care homes and a range of other premises. There are some basic ideas that can be incorporated in any minor change or decor choice in any setting, but it is advisable to consult an architect or designer who has been trained in dementia-friendly principles for any large project, and for commissioners to be at least familiar with the basic principles to ensure value for money and a reduction in running costs while achieving the best outcome for residents and staff.

31.3.1   At home

The person with dementia who has lived in the same place for a long time will be most comfortable if supported there with the minimum of change. Because the person with dementia

has poor short-term memory, they may not remember agreeing to, or witnessing any 'improvement' you or their family make. Instead they may rationalize the change by assuming they've been robbed, or that someone is trying to annoy them by moving things round, or that they are not even in the right house. So you have to balance the possible benefit of your change against the more certain risk that it will be disconcerting. The safest and most productive change is to improve the level of lighting throughout the house (Pollock et al., 2007). You must increase the power of all light fittings, clear bushes from outside windows, clean the windows and make sure curtains and blinds can be moved right back to let in daylight. Low energy light bulbs must be replaced regularly as their luminosity fades. It is important to consider that assistive technology is increasingly available and affordable (Kerr et al., 2010) and can extend the time that the person can remain in their own home. For example, a person with dementia may forget they have left a tap running. If there is a flood they can end up being displaced to an unfamiliar setting while home repairs are undertaken. Use of a flood detector built in to an alert system, or an adapted plug that allows water to drain away by being triggered by the weight of water above, can help reduce the risk of a costly and potentially permanent move.

31.3.2   In hospitals and care homes

It is never too soon in a new build to consider incorporating dementia-friendly features, as simple changes in the architectural plan can improve the building at no extra cost (Dementia Services Development Centre, 2007). Examples of what design might do include the following.

31.3.2.1   NIGHT CARE

Problem – The person with dementia might not sleep well at night and may fall, or give rise to disruption of others.

Solutions – due to the yellowing of the ageing eye, the day/night cycle can be disrupted because of poor daylight exposure during daylight hours (Koncelik, 2003). A garden or bright daylight access can help to reset the clock. Space and quiet available in the daytime can support meaningful activity to create healthy fatigue by bedtime. Reduced noise levels and slowed activity at bedtime can promote falling off to sleep (Kerr et al., 2008). Vision panels in bedroom doors and extraneous lights offer poor support for carers who wish to observe the resident at night, but can wake the person up and unhelpfully tempt them out of their room. Passive infrared sensors can warn staff, if necessary, that the person is awake and moving about, and can switch on the bathroom light to cue the person to use the toilet and go back to bed. The positioning of the bed head so that the lavatory pan can be seen is crucial for this. The use of vibrating pagers for call alerts can reduce the meaningless noise of buzzers in the night (and day). One of the simplest design and technology changes to assist people with dementia at night is the use of an analogue clock set to the right time. One of the first things any of us does when we wake is to check the time. The current generation of older people with dementia may have forgotten what a digital clock is and therefore be unable to tell the time (Fleming *et al.*, 2008). An appropriately positioned and well lit analogue clock can reduce the need for someone with dementia to get up to orientate themselves.

31.3.2.2   HYGIENE

Problem – the person with dementia may not use the toilet appropriately and may thus require extra help with bathing and dressing.

Solutions – incontinence can be caused by not getting to the toilet in time, so make sure that the floor coverings are smooth, mat and self-coloured to encourage the person with dementia to walk more swiftly to the right place (Perritt *et al.*, 2005). Make the toilet door easy to find with bright contrasting colour to the surrounding wall and signage at low height, so the person does not have to look up (Cunningham *et al.*, 2008). The sign should include words and pictures that make sense to the generation using, i.e. the matchstick man/woman symbol is a relatively new identifier for the toilet and may be overlooked. Inside the toilet, ensure the fixtures and fittings are culturally appropriate and recognizable in traditional designs and contrasting colours. This may currently mean offering a bar of green soap and a cotton towel, against strict infection control guidance, but some independent cleansing is better than the person not washing their hands at all.

If a bath becomes necessary, the design of the bathroom is key. Shiny surfaces and floors can cause visual problems leading to falls. Mirrors can cause distress as the person may not recognize their reflection. Designing the home so that the bathroom has to be used as a store for shiny metal lifting equipment and boxes of continence pads reduces the capacity of the person to work out where they are and why they are there, giving rise to resistance to the idea of being undressed. Laying out of clothes in the order they are to be put on is made easier if there is a place to do that in the bathroom.

31.3.2.3   UNWANTED EXITING AND WALKING

Problem – There is a perceived danger that the person will walk into danger, or cause a nuisance

Solution – The design solution depends on the reason for this being a problem. There are design solutions that help with the need for staff to know where everyone is all the time, the need for residents to burn off energy to reduce their own stress and the need for families to feel that their relative is safe.

The use of discrete electronic equipment can assist with monitoring movement with minimum use of staff time and with the minimum use of restraint. Unwanted exiting requires all hazardous exits to be made less attractive to the casual observer. This includes the use of lighting and floor covering and paint work to conceal them and to make the approach to these areas less interesting. Vision panels in exit doors offer a window into a more interesting world than where the resident is. Turn their attention the other way. A safe garden is a good alternative for the inquisitive, as long as it is fulfilling and interesting. If it is not, it will not work and you will soon know.

Any design features which reduce stress will help. Making the purpose of the room clear and obvious and keeping the size at a domestic scale my help. High levels of noise, and low levels of light have both been shown to make people with dementia restless. Designing in the ability to locally control the temperature allows staff to support the person to find one individual place that suits them. Pain may be a root cause of restlessness and a really comfortable quiet place to sit would help (McClean and Cunningham, 2007).

Exercise is one of the few interventions in dementia for which there is strong evidence, and designing a good place where dance, or music and movement can easily be organized, in addition to outside activities, may reduce the pacing behaviour. The purpose of the pacing may be a futile attempt of the person to find their own room, and there are many design solutions that will make this easier for them. The lack of everyday household spaces and objects means that anxious old people, with no motivation to do anything or who spend the whole day running their hands across tabletops, have nowhere familiar to do what they have always done to pass the time. Given a kitchen, they can happily spend hours keeping the surfaces clean or mopping the sink. Yet few units provide even the rudiments of a kitchen, except for the occupational therapy activity kitchen and then it is behind closed doors and only available to certain patients at certain times. Washing poles and a line in the garden with an adjacent sink, some grass to cut or an old car in the garden to tinker with can be planned into the design.

31.4   CONCLUSIONS

It is possible to design buildings that help people with dementia to function at their best. Buildings where people with dementia live are also where staff and families spend much of their lives. Good design can help staff in their very complex and challenging work and make families more comfortable with visiting and supporting. Perhaps the most important message of the building is that people with dementia and the staff who care for them are valued and respected. This is a crucial message given the increasing numbers of people who will be living and working in these environments. Providing people with dementia with the opportunity to make good decisions with a positive outcome, by design environments that compensate for their impairments, will enhance the quality of their lives.

REFERENCES

Cunningham C. (2009) Auditing design for dementia. *Journal of Dementia Care* 3: 31–2.

Cunningham C, Marshall M, McManus M *et al.* (2008) *Design for people with dementia: Audit tool.* University of Stirling: Dementia Services Development Centre.

Dementia Services Development Centre. (2007) *Best practice in design for people with dementia pack.* University of Stirling: Dementia Services Development Centre.

Fleming R, Crookes P, Sum S. (2008) A review of the empirical literature on the design of physical environments for people with dementia. Australia: Dementia Collaborative Research Centres, Australia. Available in print in the UK as part of *'Design for people with dementia: Audit tool.* University of Stirling: Dementia Services Development Centre. Last accessed September 30, 2009. Available from: www.dementia.unsw.edu.au/DCRCweb.nsf/resources/DCRC1+Products+3/$file/Design+of+Environment+Literature+Review.pdf.

Koncelik J. (2003) The human factors of ageing. In: Scheidt RJ, Windley P (eds). *Physical environments and ageing.* Canada: Hawthorn Press.

Kerr B, Cunningham C, Martin S. (2010). *Telecare and dementia Using telecare effectively in the support of people with dementia.* University of Stirling: Dementia Services Development Centre.

Kerr D, Wilkinson H, Cunningham C. (2008) *Supporting older people in care homes at night.* Joseph Rowntree Foundation. Last accessed September 30, 2009. Available from: www.jrf.org.uk/publications/supporting-older-people-care-homes-night.

McClean W, Cunningham C. (2007) *Pain in older people with dementia: A practice guide.* University of Stirling: Dementia Services Development Centre.

Perritt M, McCune ED, McCune SL. (2005) Research Informs Design: Empirical findings suggest recommendations for carpet pattern and texture. *Alzheimer's Care Quarterly* 6: 300–5.

Pollock R, McNair D, McGuire B, Cunningham C. (2007) *Designing lighting for people with dementia.* University of Stirling: Dementia Services Development Centre.

32

Legal issues and dementia

ROBIN JACOBY

32.1 JURISDICTIONS

An international book, such as this one, cannot possibly cover all the different jurisdictions in which its readers work. This chapter will, therefore, address the issues that are general to many legal systems. This is easier for anglophone ones (the UK, Commonwealth, United States, and for the time being Hong Kong) which have a common tradition incorporating much common law – law made by judges' precedent as opposed to statute law made by legislatures – and even share some court rulings, such as the famous Banks v Goodfellow judgement (see below under 32.3.3, Capacity to make a will). However, francophone jurisdictions (France, francophone Africa and the Territoires d'Outre-Mer) share a completely different basis, the Napoleonic Code, which has also left its mark on German law; whereas the Netherlands and to an extent South Africa have a tradition of Roman Dutch law. As this book is in English and the author is not familiar with Napoleonic or Roman Dutch law, with regret, focus is mainly on the Anglophone system.

32.2 CAPACITY

Most of the legal issues that arise in dementia centre on the affected person's mental capacity or competence. British English tends to use competence in a non-legal context and capacity in a legal one, whereas with American English it is the other way round. In this chapter the words will be considered interchangeable and have effectively the same meaning. Also, to avoid repetition, mental capacity should be understood, although the adjective may be omitted.

The most important fact about capacity is that it is task or function specific. In other words, we must talk about the capacity to do something specified. The logical implication is that capacity, or lack of it, to do one thing does not necessarily mean the capacity, or lack of it, to do another. For example, a person with dementia may no longer be competent to manage his financial affairs, but may be competent to donate power of attorney (see below under 32.3.1 Management of financial affairs).

Capacity is not only task specific, but also time specific. A person must be competent to do the task at the time he is required to do it, irrespective of whether he was incompetent before or afterwards. For example, someone with dementia could be in hospital with a serious illness that causes delirium and renders him incompetent to make a will. He is given antibiotics, the delirium remits, and he has the capacity to make the will.

In many cases where dementia is concerned, capacity can be considered situation dependent, by which it is meant that a person with borderline capacity for a task may be tilted towards capacity and away from incapacity by optimizing the situation. A quiet side-room instead of a noisy general hospital ward; adequate time set aside for an assessment; sitting opposite the patient so that he can lip-read and hear better are not only standard requirements for any examination of an older person, but may also maximize the chance that he will be competent to make the decision that is needed.

The second most important fact about capacity is that, like innocence, in law it is presumed until proven otherwise. Judging by the study of Markson et al. (1994) this is not understood by all members of the medical profession. In a survey of 2100 physicians, surgeons and psychiatrists, 72 per cent erroneously considered that dementia automatically conferred incapacity, 66 per cent thought the same for depression and 71 per cent for psychosis, although it has to be said that psychiatrists responded more correctly than the others.

32.2.1   General requirements for capacity

Although capacity is task specific, and sometimes certain legal tests have to be applied, for example for testamentary capacity (see below under 32.3.3 Capacity to make a will), some general requirements can be outlined. **Box 32.1** gives the criteria of Applebaum and Grisso (1998) which are among the best.

The United Kingdom Parliament effectively incorporated these criteria into its Mental Capacity Act (2005) which states at Section 3(1) 'For the purposes of Section 2, a person is unable to make a decision for himself if he is unable:

- to understand the information relevant to the decision;
- to retain the information;
- to use or weigh that information as part of the process of making the decision; or
- to communicate his decision (whether by talking, using sign language or any other means)'.

Box 32.1 Requirements for capacity

To make a competent decision a person must be able to:

- Understand information relevant to the decision
- Use the information rationally. e.g. make a risk/benefit comparison
- Appreciate the situation and its consequences
- Communicate the choice or decision

After Applebaum and Grisso (1998).

32.3   SPECIFIC CAPACITIES

32.3.1   Management of financial affairs

The capacity to manage one's financial affairs is the paradigm case of task specificity, for two reasons: first, thresholds vary with the complexity of the task; and second, competence to make a general decision, such as whether to donate power of attorney, may accompany incompetence to make specific financial decisions, for example whether to sell particular shares on the stock market. As regards varying thresholds, consider the theoretical case of two people with exactly the same degree of dementia. The first has an occupational pension from which his rent and utility bills are paid by direct debit from his bank account, and a small amount of money in a savings account. He is assessed by an old age psychiatrist who judges him competent to manage his limited financial affairs. The second person is a millionaire with a variety of share portfolios, joint trusts and other complex financial instruments. The same psychiatrist judges him to be incompetent to manage his affairs.

For people who are deemed to lack the capacity to manage their financial affairs, there are legal mechanisms to have it

done for them. Where the person with dementia has had foresight, most countries have legislated for some sort of power of attorney (PoA). However, someone making a PoA must have the legal capacity to do so. In essence, this boils down to being able to understand that, if the donor becomes incompetent, the attorney ('attorney' here and elsewhere in this chapter does, of course, mean the person nominated in a power of attorney, and not necessarily a lawyer; attorneys are most commonly spouses or adult offspring), after whatever process the particular jurisdiction requires, will have the power to do anything with the donor's finances that he himself could have done prior to losing capacity. As mentioned in the preceding paragraph, someone who retains the capacity to donate PoA may at the same time lack the capacity to manage his affairs. This was endorsed in an English High Court ruling in the landmark case of two elderly women with dementia (Re K and Re F, 1988). The implication of the ruling is that the PoA must be implemented and the attorney take over management of the affairs as soon as the PoA is executed by the donor.

For people with dementia who have not donated PoA when competent to do so and who are no longer competent to manage their affairs, different countries have different mechanisms for appointing someone to take over management on their behalf. Clearly, donating a PoA has the advantage of choice over the sometimes cumbersome mechanisms of court-appointed managers. However, there is little doubt that PoAs are sometimes abused, often by adult offspring, who cream off the assets for their own advantage. For a review of elder maltreatment, see Hirsch and Vollhardt (2008).

32.3.2   Capacity to refuse medical treatment

People with dementia are mostly old and are, therefore, at high risk of co-morbid physical illness, often requiring at least consideration of potentially hazardous interventions, such as surgery. Any medical treatment given against his will to a person competent to decide for himself constitutes an assault in law. It is, therefore, essential to determine whether a person with dementia retains the capacity to decide on treatment. If he does retain that capacity he also retains the right to decline treatment.

To determine whether the person with dementia has the requisite capacity, the criteria of Applebaum and Grisso (1988) are generally applicable (**Box 32.1**) which are essentially the same as the England and Wales Mental Capacity Act 2005. If the patient is judged to be lacking the capacity and has not written an advance directive (see above under 32.2.1 General requirements for capacity), many jurisdictions confer on medical staff the best interest obligation. That is to say that a doctor may go ahead with treatment provided the treatment is necessary and is in the best interest of the patient.

32.3.2.1   ADVANCE DIRECTIVES

Advance directives (sometimes called living wills) are statements made by people, competent to make them, about their medical treatment should they lose their mental capacity to decide on it. Since no person can dictate to a doctor what treatment he must give, advance directives are in effect advance refusals of treatment. They may be divided into three types:

1. an instruction directive;
2. a proxy directive;
3. a values directive.

An instruction directive is, as the name implies, a specific instruction. For example, if I lose irreversibly my mental capacity, by reason of dementia, to care for my basic nutritional and hygiene needs, and I no longer recognize any of my close family, I do not wish to have any medical or surgical treatment that could prolong my life. Instruction directives are the most common type of advance directive and appear quite straightforward. They are recognized as legally binding in many jurisdictions. However, it is still the case that relatively few people make them. For those who do make them at a young age and forget about them, there is a potential problem, as medical intervention preferences change with advancing age towards wanting treatment rather than refusing it. Furthermore, people, especially non-medical, cannot envisage every eventuality. For example, there could be medical treatments that prolong life but significantly reduce suffering. For this reason, a proxy advance directive might be preferred.

A proxy directive might run as follows. If, by reason of dementia, I lose irreversibly my mental capacity to care for my basic nutritional and hygiene needs, and I no longer recognize any of my close family, I wish my spouse to decide on any medical or surgical treatment because I know that s/he will act in my best interests. As a general rule, proxy directives taking this form are not legally valid, but the Mental Capacity Act 2005 in England and Wales has introduced a new Lasting Power of Attorney which permits a donor to give his attorney the power to make health-care decisions on his behalf. Doubtless there are other jurisdictions that have made similar legal provisions.

The third type of advance directive is a values directive in which the person making it gives a statement of his values and asks that his doctors adhere to them if he becomes incompetent. For example, he might state these lines by the poet Arthur Hugh Clough are a statement of my beliefs and should be taken into account if I become incompetent:

Thou shalt not kill
But need'st not strive
Officiously
To keep alive.

As far as this author is aware, no jurisdiction would consider this a legally binding advance directive but, if a person with dementia who is no longer competent to decide on treatment has made such a statement, it must surely be best practice for his medical team to take it into account in considering how to act in his best interests. Indeed, even if such an explicit statement has not been made, it is best practice for medical and nursing staff to try and ascertain from relatives what the patient's values were before he lost capacity and to take them into account.

32.3.3 Capacity to make a will

In countries where the Napoleonic Code is the basis for law disposition of one's estate after death is restricted to a considerable extent, and offspring cannot normally be excluded. In anglophone jurisdictions, there is testamentary freedom, provided the testator is mentally competent to make a will. Spouses or children may be disinherited in favour of such as a mistress or an animal charity, although in some jurisdictions, for example England and Wales, provision must be made for those spouses or children who are still financially dependent on the testator.

Unlike other capacities, testamentary capacity is governed in most Anglophone jurisdictions by the Banks v Goodfellow judgement (1870) given by Lord Chief Justice Cockburn, the relevant part of which states:

> It is essential ... that a testator shall understand the nature of the act and its effects; shall understand the extent of the property of which he is disposing; shall be able to comprehend and appreciate claims to which he ought to give effect; and with a view to the latter object no disorder of mind shall poison his affections, pervert his sense of right and prevent the exercise of his natural faculties – that no insane delusion shall influence his Will in disposing of the property and bring about a disposal of it which, if the mind had been sound, would not have been made.

This judgement can be simplified into four limbs which are set out in **Box 32.2**.

Many people with dementia are able to understand the nature and consequences of the act of making a will. Conversely, if they are not, then it is all but inconceivable that they would be able to satisfy the other limbs of the Banks v Goodfellow test.

It is not necessary for a testator (female, testatrix) to appreciate the extent of their estate down to the last penny (cent), but to have a general grasp. However, the more complex the estate, the higher the threshold of capacity on this limb of the legal test. For example, let us take again our theoretical case of two individuals with exactly the same degree of dementia. The first may be able to understand that he owns his house, has a few shares and a few thousand dollars in the bank and would, therefore, have sufficient

---

Box 32.2 The Banks v Goodfellow test simplified

A testator must be able to:

- Understand the nature and consequences of the act of making a will
- Appreciate the extent of his estate
- Know who might have a claim on his bounty (both those to be included and excluded)
- Have no mental disorder and no insane delusion directly affecting the above

appreciation of his estate. The second may, however, lack the capacity to appreciate his estate because it consists of live business interests, complex trusts, joint insurance policies, cross-national share portfolios and foreign properties. Nevertheless, it is possible to maximize capacity on this limb of the Banks v Goodfellow test, as discussed below under assessment of testamentary capacity.

The capacity to appreciate the moral claims of those who might expect to benefit from the testator's bounty is the one that is most frequently contested after the testator's death. Common scenarios are the disinheritance of one child in favour of another, or of a caregiver or charity. The grounds on which such wills are challenged clearly vary, but allegations include the following: inability to recall relatives; false beliefs about relatives or others; delirium supervening on dementia; and undue influence, frequently by a caregiver.

Undue influence is extremely difficult to prove in some jurisdictions, notably the UK and some Commonwealth countries, because it is necessary to prove coercion in contentious probate cases, although paradoxically it is not necessary in the equity jurisdiction which deals with *inter vivos* contracts – those made when people are alive. Thus, for example, it is easier to prove undue influence in the case of a person with dementia who is prevailed upon to sell his house at an absurd knock-down price to an unscrupulous caregiver, than to prove it if he leaves the caregiver the house in his will. It is the common experience of old age psychiatrists that their dementia patients are not only vulnerable to undue influence, but actually are so influenced. However, it is another thing to prove it in a court of law. In the United States, where the difference between probate and equity jurisdictions does not exist, it is much easier to prove undue influence. The issue of undue influence is discussed in detail by Peisah *et al.* (2009).

Psychiatrists are called upon to assess testamentary capacity in two situations: prospective, i.e. before the patient dies; and retrospective, i.e. after death. There would be fewer retrospective cases if lawyers were to observe the so-called golden rule formulated by Lord Templeman (Kenward v Adams 1975) which (paraphrased) recommends that lawyers drawing up wills for elderly persons should always seek a medical opinion on the testator's capacity, however embarrassing it may be to propose it to their client. Golden rule assessments are discussed by Jacoby and Steer (2007) and Shulman *et al.* (2009). As with any assessment of capacity, examinations of prospective testators should attempt to maximize capacity by an unhurried approach in a nonthreatening atmosphere. If the potential testator cannot give a full enough account of his estate, it is legitimate to give him the information, the examiner having been briefed beforehand by the lawyer, and to ask him to commit it to memory. If he can do this for a sufficient length of time to make competent decisions fulfilling the other limbs of the Banks v Goodfellow test, then his appreciation of his property may be adequate. It is vital for the doctor to understand, however, that the decision on whether this or any other aspect of the Banks v Goodfellow test is fulfilled rests solely with the court. The doctor's role is to give his opinion in order to assist the court in reaching its decision.

Retrospective assessments of the testamentary capacity of testators whose wills are subject to legal challenge is more complex because opinions have to be given on the basis of surviving documents and not examination of the testator himself. Furthermore, there are nearly always witness statements from the opposing sides that contradict each other. It is not within either the remit or the expertise of a psychiatrist to decide which statements are true or not, for this is also the sole prerogative of the court. Although the psychiatrist may be instructed by lawyers acting for one or other party, his obligation is exclusively to the court and for which he must provide an independent opinion. Prospective and retrospective assessments of testamentary capacity are discussed in full by Posener and Jacoby (2008).

Most jurisdictions require a testator to have full capacity when he gives instructions to his lawyer for drawing up his will and when he executes it, i.e. signs it in the presence of witnesses. Given that some lawyers move at a less than rapid pace to engross a will once instructions have been given, there are sometimes cases where the testator loses the necessary capacity between instructions and execution. In such cases the will might be valid if the testator can appreciate that he is signing a will drawn up on his previous instructions (based on the case of Parker v Felgate, 1883).

32.3.4   Capacity to decide residence

Problems arise when people with dementia either lack the insight to determine or deny the risks attendant on independent life at home. Different countries have different laws on involuntary committal to another place of residence, but the psychiatrist or community nurse may need to take a variety of general factors into account when dealing with such situations. First, relatives may have a more restrictive agenda than is warranted. They may want a move to institutional care when the person could remain at home with adequate support, for reasons such as guilt, infantilization, inability or unwillingness to provide support themselves or a lack of understanding of the nature of dementia. It is this author's view that psychiatrists do not always need to play safe and err on the side of involuntary removal from home. In his experience, disagreements can often be resolved and agreement reached by patient face-to-face discussion with the various parties and mutual acceptance of risk. Furthermore, some jurisdictions allow for objections to home care on the part of the person with dementia legally to be overcome so that, if necessary, the patient's home can be entered without permission to provide care.

32.3.5   Capacity to litigate and stand trial

Few people with dementia are likely to litigate. In the UK, the capacity to litigate is based on the decision in the case of Masterman-Lister (2002). A statement, now removed, from the Official Solicitor's website in the UK went as follows: '… to have capacity to litigate a person must have capacity to understand, absorb and retain information (including advice) relevant to the matter in question, sufficiently to enable him or her to make decisions based upon such information. This includes the ability to weigh information (and advice) in the balance as part of the process of understanding and acting on any advice'. It is not difficult to see that this accords to a considerable extent with the general statements about capacity made above under 32.2.1 General requirements for capacity. In the UK, if a person with dementia lacks the capacity to litigate he may be represented by the Official Solicitor. Other countries, of course, have their own agents for such purposes.

Capacity to stand trial is termed (dis)ability in relation to trial or fitness to plead in the UK; whereas in the United States it is competence to stand trial. It is a more important issue than capacity to litigate because a small but significant number of dementia sufferers commit offences, some serious, including homicide. In the UK the criteria for fitness to plead are shown in **Box 32.3**.

Box 32.3 Fitness to plead in the UK

To be fit to plead a defendant must be able to:

- Understand the nature of the charge
- Understand the meaning of entering a plea
- Understand the consequences of entering a plea
- Be able to instruct lawyers
- Understand the details of the evidence
- Follow the proceedings in court so as to make a proper defence, including challenging a juror

---

In the United States the criteria for competence to stand trial are based on the case of Dusky v United States (1960) which states that the defendant requires 'sufficient present ability to consult with his attorney with a reasonable degree of rational understanding – and whether he has a rational as well as factual understanding of the proceedings against him'. It is difficult to make general statements about what happens in practice because of the variation in worldwide jurisdictions, but in the UK the authorities are keen to divert dementia sufferers away from the criminal justice system at least for less serious offences, such as shop-lifting. For more serious offences fitness to plead does become an issue. Grubin (1991) studied 286 people in England and Wales who had been declared unfit to plead between 1976 and 1988. Ten out of 286 (3.4 per cent) were found to be suffering from dementia, six of whom died in hospital whilst still considered unfit to plead. Heinik *et al.* (1994) studied a group of elderly offenders referred by courts to a forensic unit in Israel for psychiatric evaluation. Of the 17 with a diagnosis of dementia, several of whom had committed violent offences, nine were considered incompetent to stand trial, and the same number were considered incompetent to be sentenced. So in summary, of the small proportion of people with dementia who commit serious criminal offences, many are unfit or incompetent to stand trial and few, if any, recover sufficiently to face trial.

REFERENCES

Applebaum P, Grisso T. (1998) Assessing patients' capacities to consent to treatment. *New England Journal of Medicine*. **319**: 1635–8.

Grubin DH. (1991) Unfit to plead in England and Wales, 1976 1988: a survey. *British Journal of Psychiatry*. **158**: 540–8.

Heinik J, Kimhi R, Hes J. (1994) Dementia and crime: a forensic psychiatry unit study in Israel. *International Journal of Geriatric Psychiatry*. **9**: 491–4.

Jacoby R, Steer P. (2007) How to assess capacity to make a will. *British Medical Journal*. **335**: 155–7.

Hirsch RD, Vollhardt BR. (2008) Elder maltreatment. In: Jacoby R, Oppenheimer C, Dening T, Thomas A (eds). *The Oxford textbook of old age psychiatry*. Oxford: Oxford University Press, 731–45.

Markson LJ, Kern DC, Annas GJ, Glantz LH. (1994) Physician assessment of patient competence. *Journal of the American Geriatrics Society*. **42**: 1074–80.

Peisah C, Finkel S, Shulman K et al. (2009) The wills of older people: risk factors for undue influence. *International Psychogeriatrics*. **21**: 7–15.

Posener H, Jacoby R. (2008) Testamentary capacity. In: Jacoby R, Oppenheimer C, Dening T, Thomas A (eds). *The Oxford textbook of old age psychiatry*. Oxford: Oxford University Press, 753–60.

Shulman KI, Peisah C, Jacoby R et al. (2009) Contemporaneous assessment of testamentary capacity. *International Psychogeriatrics*. **21**: 433–9.

Legal cases

Banks v. Goodfellow [1870] 5. LR QB 549

Dusky v. United States [1960] 362 US 402.

Kenward v. Adams [1975] *The Times* (London) 29 November.

Masterman-Lister v. Brutton & Co., [2002] EWHC 417 (QB)

Parker v. Felgate [1883] 8 PD. 171

Re K and Re F [1988] *All England Law Reports*, p. 358

33

Driving and dementia

DESMOND O'NEILL

33.1 INTRODUCTION

Driving has become an almost indispensable part of everyday life for older people worldwide, with falling use of public transportation and increasing personal affluence leading to greater access to the personal car (OECD, 2001). These trends are particularly noticeable in rural areas, where the proportion of older people tends to be higher and where public transport is less accessible.

Despite increasing levels of age-related disease and disability, older drivers in general compensate and adapt to their changing circumstances, and are the safest demographic group on the roads, with even the oft-quoted increased crash rate per kilometre disappearing when allowance is made for distance travelled (Langford et al., 2008). This, and increasing awareness of the negative effects of driving cessation (Arcury et al., 2005; Freeman et al., 2006), have led to an attitudinal shift among clinicians to consider mobility as the primary concern in driving assessment, with due regard for safety to the same extent as other demographic groups (Martin et al., 2009).

The US Transportation Research Board, the Organization for Economic Cooperation and Development and the European Conference of Ministers for Transport have all prepared reports on ageing and transport (CEMT, 2001; OECD, 2001; US Department of Transportation, 2003). Drivers in Finland, the UK, Ireland and the United States report health as the primary cause of driving cessation, usually without a formal consultation to ensure maximal remediation (Persson, 1993; Rabbitt et al., 1996; Hakamies-Blomqvist and Wahlstrom,

1998; O'Neill et al., 2000). While the knowledge base is still slender, the issues involved have major practical, ethical and societal implications for patients, family carers and health professionals. There are widely differing agendas on the part of those involved: the patient, the carers, the physician, the statutory licensing authority and the insurance companies.

Dementia is a largely age-related disorder, and the developed world is experiencing an exponential rise in the proportion of older drivers among the driving population. In the United States only 5.9 per cent of drivers were over 60 in 1940; this had increased to 7.4 per cent by 1952 and to 11.4 per cent by 1960 (McFarland et al., 1964). Older drivers should comprise 39 per cent of the driving population in the USA by 2050 (Malfetti, 1985). Over one-third of those aged over 80 in 1990 drove at least once a year in Ontario, Canada (Chipman et al., 1998). In the UK, there was an increase of 600 per cent in the number of women drivers over the age of 65 between 1965 and 1985 (Department of Transport, 1991). Although most drive personal automobiles, this is not exclusively the case. On the one hand, licensing regulations for drivers of public service vehicles and heavy transport vehicles is nearly always more restricted and uses a more algorithmic approach than for drivers of personal automobiles. On the other hand, those who develop dementia at a younger age are more likely to be driving heavy goods or public service vehicles, and the abolition of mandatory retirement age in the United States has resulted in school bus drivers being able to continue into their mid-eighties, and there has been litigation concerning this group.

33.2   WHAT PUBLIC HEALTH ISSUES ARISE WITH OLDER DRIVERS?

One of the most important, and under-recognized, public health hazards arising from dementia is the consequences of loss of mobility for those who stop driving (Taylor and Tripodes, 2001). One key question about the ageing of the driving population is whether they add significantly to hazard on the roads. This question is symptomatic of an ageist approach to older driver issues; it is likely that the predominant problem is that older people give up driving without sufficient remediation (White and O'Neill, 2000). The crash rate for older drivers for a given period of time is considerably lower than for the driving population as a whole (Gebers et al., 1993). Many safety experts defend older drivers as a relatively safe group (Evans, 1988) and in some road tests healthy older drivers perform better than younger controls (Gebers et al., 1993). The increased crash rate per distance driven noted in older populations in comparison to middle-aged controls is not only academic while older people continue to drive a lower mileage; it also is a product of driving a low mileage, which is itself intrinsically risky. If younger and older people who drive a low mileage are compared, this apparent increase disappears (Hakamies-Blomqvist et al., 2002). Low mileage exposes them to more dangers per mile than high-mileage drivers as they encounter disproportionately more intersections, congestion, confusing visual environments, signs and signals (Janke, 1991), yet older drivers cope at least as well with this.

Crashes involving older people are more likely to be fatal, by a factor of 3.5 in two-car accidents (Klamm, 1985), reflecting the increased frailty and reduced reserve of older adults, while raising suspicions that automobile design may not be tailored for maximum safety of this group (Schieber, 1994; Li et al., 2003). Opposing these trends is the fact that the accident rates for young adults often arise from behaviour that leads to high-risk situations; older drivers tend to avoid high-risk situations (Planek et al., 1968) and have the lowest proportion of crashes while under the influence of alcohol (National Center for Statistics and Analysis: National Highway Traffic Safety Administration, 1995).

Janke (1994) has suggested an interpretation of these apparently contradictory findings. A group's average crash rate per year may be considered as an indicator of the degree of risk posed to society by that group, whereas the average accident rate per mile indicates the degree of risk posed to individual drivers in the group when they drive, as well as their passengers. The increased risk to individual drivers is most likely due to age-related illnesses, particularly neurodegenerative and vascular diseases (O'Neill, 1992; Johansson et al., 1997).

33.3   IS DRIVING WITH DEMENTIA A PUBLIC HEALTH HAZARD?

The precise contribution of dementia to overall crash hazard is uncertain. Although Johansson et al. (1997) suggested a major role for dementia as cause of crashes among older

drivers on neuropathological grounds, subsequent interviews with families did not reveal significant problems with memory or activities of daily living (Lundberg et al., 1999). The Stockholm group also showed that older drivers with a high level of traffic violations had a high prevalence of cognitive deficits (Lundberg et al., 1998). Retrospective studies of dementia and driving from dementia clinics tend to show a high risk (Friedland et al., 1988; Lucas-Blaustein et al., 1988; O'Neill, 1993b), whereas those which are prospective and look at the early stages of dementia show a less pronounced risk pattern. In the first two years of dementia, the risk approximates that of the general population (Drachman and Swearer, 1993; Carr et al., 2000). The most carefully controlled study of crashes and dementia showed no increase in crash rates for drivers with dementia (Trobe et al., 1996). Likely causes of this finding include lower annual mileage and restriction of driving by the patient, family and physicians.

Extrapolating from special populations may skew risk predictions. For example, epilepsy, for which most countries have relatively clear-cut guidelines, would seem to pose a clear threat to driving ability as viewed from a clinic setting. Recent population-based studies suggest that the increased risk is relatively low (Hansotia and Broste, 1991; Drazkowski, 2003). In a population renewing their licences in North Carolina, the lowest decile had a relative crash risk of 1.5 in the three years previous to the cognitive testing (Stutts et al., 1998). A somewhat reassuring finding from this cohort is that those with the poorest scores for visual and cognitive function also drove less and avoided high-risk situations (Stutts, 1998). A reasonable conclusion from these studies is that dementia among drivers is not yet a public health problem. Although increasing numbers of older drivers may change this situation, it is also possible that 'Smeed's law' will operate, whereby increasing numbers of drivers among a defined population are associated with a drop in fatality rates per car (Hakamies-Blomqvist et al., 2005).

33.4   IS THERE A ROLE FOR SCREENING OLDER POPULATIONS OF DRIVERS?

Despite the lack of convincing evidence for an older driver 'problem', ageist policies in many jurisdictions have led to screening programmes for older drivers. In the absence of reliable and sensitive assessment tools, this approach is flawed, as illustrated by data from Scandinavia (Hakamies-Blomqvist et al., 1996). In Finland, there is regular age-related medical certification of fitness to drive, whereas Sweden has no routine medical involvement in licence renewal. There is no reduction in the number of older people dying in car crashes in Finland but an increase in the number of those dying as pedestrians and cyclists, possibly due in part to unnecessarily removing drivers from their cars. A more minimalist and less medical approach using very simple measures, such as a vision test and a written skill examination, may be more helpful (Levy et al., 1995); unfortunately this approach is also associated with a reduction in the number of older drivers, a possible negative health impact (Levy et al., 1995). Another approach is opportunistic health screening, perhaps of those older drivers with traffic violations (Johansson *et al.*, 1996). It remains to be seen whether these and other screening policies reduce mobility among older people, a practical and civil rights issue of great importance. Another problem is the uncertainty about the outcome of screening, as there is currently a limited repertoire.

33.5 PHYSICIANS AND DRIVING ASSESSMENT

Another problem is the relative ignorance of physicians about the effects of illness on driving. Some of this relates to the predominantly negative tone of much of the medical regulations for driving (White and O'Neill, 2000), and it is likely that doctors are insufficiently aware of health care interventions that have been shown to improve driving comfort and safety: examples exist for arthritis, stroke and cataract (van Zomeren *et al.*, 1987; Jones *et al.*, 1991; Monestam and Wachtmeister, 1997). Doctors are unaware of the driving habits of their patients when prescribing drugs that may affect driving (Cartwright, 1990) and also have a patchy knowledge of medical regulations for driving (Strickberger *et al.*, 1991; O'Neill *et al.*, 1994). As the regulations are rarely based on evidence-based criteria and are negatively presented, this 'failure' by doctors to acquaint themselves with the regulations may reflect a healthy cynicism about the current official medical fitness criteria. There may also be an element of ageism by which doctors may assume that older patients do not drive: a review of dementia from the UK seemed to take this attitude (Almeida and Fottrell, 1991), whereas US reviewers have been aware of the high number of older drivers for years (Winograd and Jarvik, 1986).

Drivers may not only be unaware, but also may wilfully ignore medical advice and regulations. In many countries they continue to drive despite failing to comply with regulations for diabetes, visual disease and automatic implantable cardioverter defibrillators (Frier *et al.*, 1980; Eadington and Frier, 1988; McConnell *et al.*, 1991; Finch *et al.*, 1993). However, there is no evidence that this under-reporting results in any increased crash risk!

We have little information on advice given to drivers with dementia by family physicians or physicians at specialist clinics for the evaluation of dementia. This would be of interest because of the wide range of answers given for patients with life-threatening arrhythmias (Strickberger *et al.*, 1991). In any event, a major shift of emphasis is required by health care professionals to consider driving ability in the functional assessment of older people.

The procedures for intervention after the opportunistic detection of illnesses relevant to driving vary widely. In the UK, the doctor's duty is to inform the patient that he/she must contact the Driver and Vehicle Licencing Authority (DVLA); direct contact by the doctor with the DVLA is only allowed if there is evidence of continued driving which constitutes a hazard to others, and if persuasion through other family members and carers has been unsuccessful. This contrasts with the position in several states in the United States and provinces in Canada where the doctor is bound by law to report patients with certain illnesses to the licensing authorities. This disparity is confusing, but cross-national comparisons may prove a boon to researchers who wish to establish the most appropriate methods for screening and reporting of age-related diseases.

33.6 ASSESSMENT PROCEDURES

A systematic inclusion of a question on transport and driving is now mandatory in comprehensive assessment of patients with memory problems (Adler and Silverstein, 2008), and should identify whether or not the patient drives (Bradley *et al.*, 2000); this is important in view of the relatively low assessment of driving in primary care (Pimlott *et al.*, 2006). The placing of driving issues in an appropriate therapeutic context is the most important task. Rather than focussing on the difficult case of patients who present late with impaired driving ability and insight, we must recognize that the assessment of dementia provides the potential for a range of interventions, one of the most important of which is the establishment of a framework for advance planning in a progressive disease. We need to start a process which encompasses an assessment, a commitment to maximizing mobility, but also an awareness-raising process for the patient and carers that the progression of the disease will inevitably result in a loss of driving capacity. This latter component has been termed a modified Ulysses contract, after the hero made his crew tie him to the mast on the condition that they did not heed his entreaties to be released when seduced by the song of the sirens (Howe, 2000). Developing this process incorporates some new stances in dementia care, in particular of diagnostic disclosure in at least general terms – the patient who drives needs to be told that he/she has a memory problem that is likely to progress and hamper driving ability. In general, carers are fearful of diagnosis disclosure, but older people seem to want to be told if they have this illness. There is evidence such a process may facilitate driving cessation, by enhancing a therapeutic dimension to disease diagnosis and advance planning (Bahro *et al.*, 1995). It forms the basis of a useful patient and carer brochure from the Hartford Foundation (2000) which is available online. This type of approach also seems to have worked with older, visually-impaired drivers (Owsley *et al.*, 2003).

The most useful model of assessment is that of an assessment cascade (see **Figure 33.1**).

Not all levels will be required by all patients: a patient with a homonymous hemianopia is barred from driving throughout the EU, and referral to a social worker to plan alternative transportation is appropriate. Equally, a mild cognitive defect may only require a review by the physician and occupational therapist (OT). The overall interdisciplinary assessment should attempt to provide solutions to both maintaining activities and exploring transport needs. An on-road test may be helpful as it may demonstrate deficits to a patient or carer who is ambivalent about the patient stopping driving. At a therapeutic level, team members may be able to help patients come to terms with losses associated with stopping driving. The OT

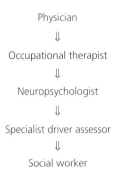

Physician
⇓
Occupational therapist
⇓
Neuropsychologist
⇓
Specialist driver assessor
⇓
Social worker

Figure 33.1 An assessment cascade.

may be able to maximize activities and function and help focus on preserved areas of achievement, whereas the social worker can advise on alternative methods of transport.

The assessment of fitness to drive should only take place after a thorough evaluation of the underlying medical condition(s). Dementia may coexist with other conditions that affect driving ease and ability. Important components of the history and examination of theoretical relevance to the driving task are medication and alcohol use (Doege and Engelburg, 1986), perception, cognitive status and psychomotor ability. Perception is probably more important than vision. Cognition may be usefully measured by the physician using one of the many brief mental status schedules (O'Neill, 1993a), and the elements of general clinical assessment of older drivers for medical fitness to drive are now described on both sides of the Atlantic (Carr, 1993; O'Neill, 1993a; O'Neill, 1993b). Although the Mini-Mental State Examination (MMSE; see Chapter 6, Screening and assessment instruments for the detection and measurement of cognitive impairment) correlates with driving performance (Odenheimer et al., 1994; Fitten et al., 1995; Fox et al., 1997), it is not sufficiently sensitive or specific to be used as a determinant of driving ability (Lundberg et al., 1997).

The basic thrust of the assessment is to catalogue and remedy pathologies that may be relevant to driving: vision, cognitive function, neurological and musculoskeletal disorders, as well as conditions that may give rise to transient loss of consciousness, such as diabetes and syncope. In any one illness there may be multiple facets that affect driving: in Parkinson's disease, this includes motor, cognitive and affective aspects. Each component needs to be maximally remedied before a final decision is made.

The patient's own assessment of driving should be assessed, and a promising approach is the Adelaide Self-Efficacy Scale (George et al., 2007). It is encouraging that self-assessed driving skills in mild cognitive impairment seem preserved (Okonkwo et al., 2009). A collateral (witness) history of driving abilities is important, given the often collaborative nature of driving in later life (Vrkljan and Polgar, 2007), but cognisant of the conflict of interest of a spouse who does not drive (Adler et al., 2000).

Medication review is important: some medications may improve driving skills (antidepressants, anti-inflammatories, and possibly cholinesterase inhibitors (ChEIs; Daiello et al., 2008)), while others pose hazards – in the case of neuroleptics, almost certainly as a marker of the nature and severity of the underlying illness (Brunnauer et al., 2004). The significance of benzodiazepines is uncertain (O'Neill, 1998).

33.7   FURTHER ASSESSMENT

In cases of very mild or very severe cognitive impairment, the judgement may be relatively easy and require little supplementary testing. For those falling in between, the precise nature of the further evaluation is not yet standardized, but neither is the neuropsychological evaluation of dementia. Physicians may need to invoke the assistance of a driving specialist centre, the components of which are medical, OT, sometimes neuropsychology, and specialist driving assessors. A first effort may be made with a suitably trained OT (Ranney and Hunt, 1997).

The choice of tests will be relatively arbitrary and, as in any memory clinic where doctors will familiarize themselves with the battery of tests carried out by the OT or psychologist in the local area, it is likely that good communication between professionals and familiarity with the chosen tests is as important as the precise tests chosen. The relatively poor clinical utility of cognitive scales in determining fitness to drive (Molnar et al., 2007) relates to their lack of congruity to current models of driving behaviour and capabilities (Fuller, 2005). This does not mean that cognition should not be assessed, but rather that such measures should be integrated with other factors, including an assessment of insight/anosagnosia, judgement skills and strategic thinking.

While a number of screening and evaluation test batteries have been proposed, it makes more sense to choose some core areas of interest, and to allow some room for clinical judgements on areas such as judgement and impulsiveness. The task is rendered more complex by the sophistication of models of driving, which do not conform easily to traditional cognitive test batteries. At least five main types of model have been explored: psychometric, motivational, hierarchical controls, information processing and error theory (O'Neill, 1996). At a minimum, a test battery should contain a general measure of overall cognitive function, a dementia grading and include tests of attention, particularly visual attention, information processing and perception. Some matching to dementia type will be appropriate (e.g. attention in subcortical dementias, judgement in frontotemporal dementia).

Specific tests that shown statistical (but not clinically useful!) correlation with driving ability in more than one study include the MMSE, the Trail Making Test (Maag, 1976; Janke and Eberhard, 1998; Mazer et al., 1998; Stutts et al., 1998), and a range of tests of visual attention (Klavora et al., 1995; Duchek et al., 1998; Marottoli et al., 1998; Owsley et al., 1998; Trobe, 1998), including the Useful Field of View, a composite measure of pre-attentive processing, incorporating speed of visual information processing, ability to ignore distractors (selective attention) and ability to divide attention (Owsley et al., 1991). A range of other tests have been assessed in single studies (including traffic sign recognition; Carr et al., 1998) and a comprehensive review is available from the US National Highway Traffic Safety Administration (Staplin et al., 1999). In conjunction with the clinical assessment and collateral history, these tests will help to decide which patients require on-road testing, as well as those who are likely to be dangerous to test (Fox *et al.*, 1997)!

The use of simulators to assess the driving capabilities of patients with dementia has not been widely accepted, but is a potentially useful research tool (Uc and Rizzo, 2008). Simulators may have a more important role in driver rehabilitation of those with neurological disease (Akinwuntan *et al.*, 2005). Older people may be more prone to motion sickness in driving simulators (Golding, 2006).

33.8   ON-ROAD TESTING

If this assessment is inconclusive, an on-road assessment is advisable. In the UK, assessments are available from the Forum group of driver assessment centres. In the US, the Association of Driver Rehabilitation Specialists (ADED, www.aded.net) can provide a list of suitably qualified driving assessors. It is important to emphasize to the patient that this test is not the driving test used for learner drivers. Rather, this is an assessment to gain insight into both the capabilities and difficulties of the driver. A good relationship with a specialist driving assessor is important to the assessment process. The assessor will require a full clinical report, and may use a scoring system for on-road testing of patients with dementia. These include the Washington University Road Test (Hunt *et al.*, 1997) and the Alberta Road Test (Dobbs *et al.*, 1998). The authors of the latter have classified the errors made by drivers with dementia into categories of increasing significance, providing a basis for future studies.

33.9   DECISION–MAKING AND INTERVENTIONS

If the assessment points to safe driving practice, the decision to continue driving entails several components. These are:

- duration before review;
- possible restriction;
- driving accompanied;
- licensing authority reporting relationship;
- insurance reporting responsibility.

As dementia is progressive, any declaration of fitness to drive should be subject to regular review; one study suggests that a review period of six months is probably reasonable (Duchek *et al.*, 2003); sooner if any deterioration is reported by the carer. It is also important to advise patients and their families of the predicted decline in driving ability on an individual basis, although three years from when the disease becomes clinically obvious may be a reasonable group average (Breen *et al.*, 2007). Nevertheless, some patients with mild and slowly progressive dementia appear to retain driving skills for longer than this (Ott *et al.*, 2008). Given evidence that the crash rate is reduced if the driver is accompanied (Bédard *et al.*, 1996), it may be sensible to restrict driving to when there is someone else in the car, using the co-pilot syndrome (Shua-Haim and Gross, 1996). There

is preliminary evidence that drivers with restricted driving licences have lower crash rates (Caragata Nasvadi and Wister, 2009). Patients should be advised to avoid traffic congestion as well as driving at night and in bad weather. The patient and carers should acquaint themselves with local driver licensing authority requirements as well as the policy of their motor insurance company. All this should be recorded in the medical notes. Except for jurisdictions where there is mandatory reporting of drivers with dementia, there is no obligation on the doctor to break medical confidentiality in these cases.

33.10   WHEN DRIVING IS NO LONGER POSSIBLE

If the assessment supports driving cessation, patients and carers should be told, and a social worker consulted to help maximize transportation options. Giving up driving can have a big effect on lifestyle. Forty-two per cent of older people think that driving is a right as opposed to 27 per cent who think that it is a privilege (AA Foundation for Road Safety Research, 1988). However, normal older drivers accept that their physician's advice would be very influential in deciding to give up driving (AA Foundation for Road Safety Research, 1988) and many patients with dementia respond to advice from families or physicians (Adler and Kuskowski, 2003).

For those who resist persuasion, removal of a driving licence represents a potential breach of civil rights (Reuben *et al.*, 1988). The way we deal with driving reflects how we help patients to deal with the reality of the deficits caused by dementia. A more positive approach has been suggested whereby the issue of driving is treated as a part of a therapeutic programme. A case was described whereby the patient's feelings and fears about giving up driving were explored with him (Bahro *et al.*, 1995). The intervention was designed with the patient as collaborator rather than patient and by dealing with the events at an emotional rather than at an intellectual level. The patient was able to grieve about the disease and in particular about the loss of his car. This in turn enabled him to redirect his attention to other meaningful activities that did not involve driving. Although this approach may be hampered by the dementia, it reflects a more widespread trend towards sharing the diagnosis of dementia with the patient.

If this approach is unsuccessful, confidentiality may have to be broken for a small minority of cases. Most professional physician associations accept that the principle of confidentiality is covered to a degree by a 'common good' principle of protecting third parties when direct advice to the patient is ignored (General Medical Council, 1985; Retchin and Anapolle, 1993). Removal of the driving licence is not likely to have much effect on these patients, and the vehicle may need to be disabled or removed (Donnelly and Karlinsky, 1990).

In the event of a decision to advise cessation of driving, advice from a social worker is helpful in planning strategies for alternative modes of travel. The availability of transport resources within the family or of high-quality alternative transportation are helpful (Freund, 2007), as may be provision of support groups for driving cessation (Dobbs *et al.*, 2009). This may be difficult in rural settings.

33.11   THE FUTURE

Several developments may attenuate the problems of the older driver with dementia. At a population level, preventive strategies for dementia may lessen the burden of cognitive disability, and strictures on the prescribing of agents such as long-acting benzodiazepines may reduce crash susceptibility. Improvements in highway design, signage and Intelligent Transportation Systems may make travel safer for all. Improved assessment procedures may also maintain transport options (Martin *et al.*, 2009).

For the individual, we do not know whether ChEI therapy can help driving skills in early Alzheimer's disease. There is also a suggestion that cognitive training with useful field of view can help driving skills in non-demented older adults (Ball and Owsley, 1994); this form of cognitive rehabilitation may be useful. Finally, older drivers can benefit from environmental and technological cueing (Dingus *et al.*, 1997); developments in this technology may benefit drivers with cognitive impairment.

REFERENCES

AA Foundation for Road Safety Research. (1988) *Motoring and the older driver.* Basingstoke: AA Foundation for Road Safety Research.

Adler G, Kuskowski M. (2003) Driving cessation in older men with dementia. *Alzheimer Disease and Associated Disorders* 17: 68–71.

Adler G, Silverstein NM. (2008) At-risk drivers with Alzheimer's disease: recognition, response, and referral. *Traffic Injury Prevention* 9: 299–303.

Adler G, Rottunda S *et al.* (2000) Caregivers dependent upon drivers with dementia. *Journal of Clinical Geropsychology* 6: 83–90.

Akinwuntan AE, De Weerdt W, Feys H *et al.* (2005) Effect of simulator training on driving after stroke: a randomized controlled trial. *Neurology* 65: 843–50.

Almeida J, Fottrell E. (1991) Management of the dementias. *Reviews in Clinical Gerontology* 1: 267–82.

Arcury TA, Preisser JS, Gesler WM, Powers JM. (2005) Access to transportation and health care utilization in a rural region. *Journal of Rural Health* 21: 31–8.

Bahro M, Silber E, Box P, Sunderland T. (1995) Giving up driving in Alzheimer's disease – an integrative therapeutic approach. *International Journal of Geriatric Psychiatry* 10: 871–4.

Ball K, Owsley C. (1994) Predicting vehicle crashes in the elderly: who is at risk? In: Johansson K, Lundberg C (eds). *Aging and driving.* Stockholm: Karolinska Institutet, 1–2.

Bradley EH, Bogardus Jr ST, van Doorn C *et al.* (2000) Goals in geriatric assessment: are we measuring the right outcomes? *Gerontologist* 40: 191–6.

Breen DA, Breen DP, Moore JW *et al.* (2007) Driving and dementia. *British Medical Journal* 334: 1365–9.

Bédard M, Molloy M, Lever J. (1996) Should demented patients drive alone? *Journal of the American Geriatrics Society* 44: S9.

Brunnauer A, Laux G, Geiger E, Moller HJ. (2004) The impact of antipsychotics on psychomotor performance with regards to car driving skills. *Journal of Clinical Psychopharmacology* 24: 155–60.

Caragata Nasvadi G, Wister A. (2009) Do restricted driver's licenses lower crash risk among older drivers? A survival analysis of insurance data from British Columbia. *Gerontologist* 49: 474–84.

Carr DB. (1993) Assessing older drivers for physical and cognitive impairment. *Geriatrics* 48: 46–8, 51.

Carr DB, LaBarge E, Dunnigan K, Storandt M. (1998) Differentiating drivers with dementia of the Alzheimer type from healthy older persons with a Traffic Sign Naming test. *Journal of Gerontology: Biological Sciences and Medical Sciences* 53: M135–9.

Carr DB, Duchek J, Morris JC. (2000) Characteristics of motor vehicle crashes of drivers with dementia of the Alzheimer type (Friedland, Koss *et al.*). *Journal of American Geriatrics Society* 48: 18–22.

Cartwright A. (1990) Medicine taking by people aged 65 or more. *British Medical Bulletin* 46: 63–76.

CEMT. (2001) *Report on transport and ageing of the population.* Paris: CEMT.

Chipman ML, Payne J, McDonough P. (1998) To drive or not to drive: the influence of social factors on the decisions of elderly drivers. *Accident; Analysis and Prevention* 30: 299–304.

Daiello LA, Festa EK *et al.* (2008) Cholinesterase inhibitors improve visual attention in drivers with Alzheimer's disease. *Alzheimer's and Dementia* 4 (Supplement 1): T498.

Department of Transport. (1991) *The older driver: Measures for reducing the number of casualties among older people on our roads.* London: Department of Transport.

Dingus TA, Hulse MC, Mollenhauer MA *et al.* (1997) Effects of age, system experience, and navigation technique on driving with an advanced traveler information system. *Human Factors* 39: 177–99.

Dobbs AR, Heller RB, Schopflocher D. (1998) A comparative approach to identify unsafe older drivers. *Accident; Analysis and Prevention* 30: 363–70.

Dobbs BM, Harper LA *et al.* (2009) Transitioning from driving to driving cessation: The role of specialized driving cessation support groups for individuals with dementia. *Topics in Geriatric Rehabilitation* 25: 73–86.

Doege TC, Engelburg AL. (eds) (1986) *Medical conditions affecting older drivers.* Chicago: American Medical Association.

Donnelly RE, Karlinsky H. (1990) The impact of Alzheimer's disease on driving ability: a review. *Journal of Geriatric Psychiatry and Neurology* 3: 67–72.

Drachman DA, Swearer JM. (1993) Driving and Alzheimer's disease: the risk of crashes. *Neurology* 43: 2448–56.

Drazkowski JF, Fisher RS, Sirven JI *et al.* (2003) Seizure-related motor vehicle crashes in arizona before and after reducing the driving restriction from 12 to 3 months. *Mayo Clinic Proceedings* 78: 819–25.

Duchek JM, Hunt L, Ball K et al. (1998) Attention and driving performance in Alzheimer's disease. Journal of Gerontology: Psychological Sciences and Social Sciences 53: 130–41.

Duchek JM, Carr DB, Hunt L et al. (2003) Longitudinal driving performance in early-stage dementia of the Alzheimer type. Journal of the American Geriatrics Society 51: 1342–7.

Eadington DW, Frier BM. (1988) Type 1 diabetes and driving experience: an eight-year cohort study. Diabetic Medicine 6: 137–41.

Evans L. (1988) Older driver involvement in fatal and severe traffic crashes. Journal of Gerontology 43: S186–93.

Finch NJ, Leman RB, Kratz JM, Gillette PC. (1993) Driving safety among patients with automatic implantable cardioverter defibrillators. Journal of the American Medical Association 270: 1587–8.

Fitten LJ, Perryman KM, Wilkinson CJ et al. (1995) Alzheimer and vascular dementias and driving. A prospective road and laboratory study. Journal of the American Medical Association 273: 1360–5.

Fox GK, Bowden SC, Bashford GM, Smith DS. (1997) Alzheimer's disease and driving: prediction and assessment of driving performance. Journal of the American Geriatrics Society 45: 949–53.

Freeman EE, Gange SJ, Munoz B, West SK. (2006) Driving status and risk of entry into long-term care in older adults. American Journal of Public Health 96: 1254–9.

Freund K. (2007) Independent Transportation Network: supporting transportation in later life. Irish Ageing Studies Review 1: 13–24.

Friedland RP, Koss E, Kumar A et al. (1988) Motor vehicle crashes in dementia of the Alzheimer type. Annals of Neurology 24: 782–6.

Frier BM, Matthews DM, Steel JM, Duncan LJ. (1980) Driving and insulin-dependent diabetes. Lancet 1: 1232–4.

Fuller R. (2005) Towards a general theory of driver behaviour. Accident, Analysis and Prevention 37: 461–72.

Gebers MA, Romanowicz PA, McKenzie DM. (1993) Teen and senior drivers. Sacramento: California Department of Motor Vehicles.

General Medical Council. (1985) Professional conduct and discipline: Fitness to practice. London: General Medical Council.

George S, Clark M, Crotty M. (2007) Development of the Adelaide driving self-efficacy scale. Clinical Rehabilitation 21: 56–61.

Golding JF. (2006) Motion sickness susceptibility. Autonomic Neuroscience: Basic and Clinical 129: 67–76.

Hakamies-Blomqvist L, Wahlstrom B. (1998) Why do older drivers give up driving? Accident; Analysis and Prevention 30: 305–12.

Hakamies-Blomqvist L, Johansson K, Lundberg C. (1996) Medical screening of older drivers as a traffic safety measure – a comparative Finnish-Swedish Evaluation study. Journal of the American Geriatrics Society 44: 650–3.

Hakamies-Blomqvist L, Ukkonen T et al. (2002) Driver ageing does not cause higher accident rates per mile. Transportation Research Part F, Traffic Psychology and Behaviour 5: 271–4.

Hakamies-Blomqvist L, Wiklund M, Henriksson P. (2005) Predicting older drivers' accident involvement – Smeed's law revisited. Accident; Analysis and Prevention 37: 675–80.

Hansotia P, Broste SK. (1991) The effect of epilepsy or diabetes mellitus on the risk of automobile accidents. New England Journal of Medicine 324: 22–6.

Hartford Foundation. (2000) At the crossroads: a guide to Alzheimer's disease, dementia and driving. Hartford, CT: Hartford Foundation.

Howe E. (2000) Improving treatments for patients who are elderly and have dementia. Journal of Clinical Ethics 11: 291–303.

Hunt LA, Murphy CF, Carr D et al. (1997) Reliability of the Washington University Road Test. A performance-based assessment for drivers with dementia of the Alzheimer type. Archives of Neurology 54: 707–12.

Janke MK. (1991) Accidents, mileage, and the exaggeration of risk. Accident; Analysis and Prevention 23: 183–8.

Janke MK. (1994) Age-related disabilities that may impair driving and their assessment. Sacramento: California Department of Motor Vehicles.

Janke MK, Eberhard JW. (1998) Assessing medically impaired older drivers in a licensing agency setting. Accident; Analysis and Prevention 30: 347–61.

Johansson K, Bronge L, Lundberg C et al. (1996) Can a physician recognize an older driver with increased crash risk potential? Journal of the American Geriatrics Society 44: 1198–204.

Johansson K, Bogdanovic N, Kalimo H et al. (1997) Alzheimer's disease and apolipoprotein E e4 allele in older drivers who died in automobile accidents [letter]. Lancet 349: 1143–4.

Jones JG, McCann J, Lassere MN. (1991) Driving and arthritis. British Journal of Rheumatology 30: 361–4.

Klamm ER. (1985) Auto insurance: needs and problems of drivers 55 and over. In: Malfetti JL (ed.) Drivers 55+: Needs and problems of older drivers: Survey results and recommendations. Falls Church, VA: AAA Foundation for Road Safety, 87–95.

Klavora P, Gaskovski P, Martin K et al. (1995) The effects of Dynavision rehabilitation on behind-the-wheel driving ability and selected psychomotor abilities of persons after stroke. American Journal of Occupational Therapy 49: 534–42.

Langford J, Bohensky M, Koppel S, Newstead S. (2008) Do older drivers pose a risk to other road users? Traffic and Injury Prevention 9: 181–9.

Levy DT. (1995) The relationship of age and state license renewal policies to driving licensure rates. Accident; Analysis and Prevention 27: 461–7.

Levy DT, Vernick JS, Howard KA. (1995) Relationship between driver's license renewal policies and fatal crashes involving drivers 70 years or older. Journal of the American Medical Association 274: 1026–30.

Li G, Braver ER, Chen LH. (2003) Fragility versus excessive crash involvement as determinants of high death rates per vehicle-mile of travel among older drivers. Accident; Analysis and Prevention 35: 227–35.

Lucas-Blaustein MJ, Filipp L, Dungan C, Tune L. (1988) Driving in patients with dementia. Journal of the American Geriatrics Society 36: 1087–91.

Lundberg C, Johansson K, Ball K et al. (1997) Dementia and driving – an attempt at consensus. Alzheimer Disease and Associated Disorders 11: 28–37.

Lundberg C, Hakamies-Blomqvist L, Almkvist O, Johansson K. (1998) Impairments of some cognitive functions are common in crash-involved older drivers. Accident; Analysis and Prevention 30: 371–7.

Lundberg C, Johansson K, Bogdanovic N et al. (1999) Follow-up of Alzheimer's disease and apolipoprotein E e4 allele in older drivers who died in automobile accidents. In: O'Neill D (ed.) The older driver, health and mobility. Dublin: ARHC Press.

Maag F. (1976) [Practical driving tests–experiences and resulting problems]. Beitrage zur Gerichtlichen Medizin 34: 111–15.

McConnell RA, Spall AD, Hirst LH, Williams G. (1991) A survey of the visual acuity of Brisbane drivers. Medical Journal of Australia 155: 107–11.

McFarland RA, Tune GS, Welford AT. (1964) On the driving of automobiles by older people. Journal of Gerontology 19: 190–7.

Malfetti JL (ed.) (1985) Drivers 55 plus: Needs and problems of older drivers: Survey results and recommendations. Washington, DC: AAA Foundation for Road Safety.

Marottoli RA, Richardson ED, Stowe MH et al. (1998) Development of a test battery to identify older drivers at risk for self-reported adverse driving events. Journal of the American Geriatrics Society 46: 562–8.

Martin AJ, Marottoli R, O'Neill D. (2009) Driving assessment for maintaining mobility and safety in drivers with dementia. Cochrane Database of Systematic Reviews (1): CD006222.

Mazer BL, Korner-Bitensky NA, Sofer S. (1998) Predicting ability to drive after stroke. Archives of Physical Medicine and Rehabilitation 79: 743–50.

Molnar FJ, Marshall SC, Man-Song-Hing M et al. (2007) Acceptability and concurrent validity of measures to predict older driver involvement in motor vehicle crashes: an Emergency Department pilot case-control study. Accident; Analysis and Prevention 39: 1056–63.

Monestam E, Wachtmeister L. (1997) Impact of cataract surgery on car driving: a population based study in Sweden. British Journal of Ophthalmology 81: 16–22.

National Center for Statistics and Analysis: National Highway Traffic Safety Administration. (1995) Traffic Safety Facts 1994: Older population. Washington, DC: National Highway Traffic Safety Administration.

O'Neill D. (1992) Physicians, elderly drivers and dementia. Lancet 339: 41–3.

O'Neill D. (1993a) Brain stethoscopes: the use and abuse of brief mental status schedules. Postgraduate Medical Journal 69: 599–601.

O'Neill D. (1993b) Illness and elderly drivers. Journal of the Irish College of Physicians and Surgeons 14–16.

O'Neill D. (1996) The older driver. Reviews in Clinical Gerontology 6: 295–302.

O'Neill D. (1998) Benzodiazepines and driver safety. Lancet 352: 1324–5.

O'Neill D, Crosby T, Shaw A et al. (1994) Physician awareness of driving regulations for older drivers. Lancet 344: 1366–7.

O'Neill D, Bruce I et al. (2000) Older drivers, driving practices and health issues. Clinical Gerontology 10: 181–91.

Odenheimer GL, Beaudet M, Jette AM et al. (1994) Performance-based driving evaluation of the elderly driver: safety, reliability, and validity. Journal of Gerontology 49: M153–9.

OECD. (2001) Ageing and transport: Mobility needs and safety issues. Paris: OECD.

Okonkwo OC, Griffith HR, Vance DE et al. (2009) Awareness of functional difficulties in mild cognitive impairment: a multidomain assessment approach. Journal of the American Geriatrics Society 57: 978–84.

Ott BR, Heindel WC, Papandonatos GD et al. (2008) A longitudinal study of drivers with Alzheimer disease. Neurology 70: 1171–8.

Owsley C, Ball K, Sloane ME et al. (1991) Visual/cognitive correlates of vehicle accidents in older drivers. Psychology and Aging 6: 403–15.

Owsley C, Ball K, McGwin Jr G et al. (1998) Visual processing impairment and risk of motor vehicle crash among older adults. Journal of the American Medical Association 279: 1083–8.

Owsley C, Stalvey BT, Phillips JM. (2003) The efficacy of an educational intervention in promoting self-regulation among high-risk older drivers. Accident; Analysis and Prevention 35: 393–400.

Persson D. (1993) The elderly driver: deciding when to stop. Gerontologist 33: 88–91.

Pimlott NJ, Siegel K, Persaud M et al. (2006) Management of dementia by family physicians in academic settings. Canadian Family Physician 52: 1108–9.

Planek TW, Condon ME, Fowler RC. (1968) An investigation into problems and opinions of older drivers. Chicago: National Safety Council.

Rabbitt P, Carmichael A, Jones S, Holland C. (1996) When and why older drivers give up driving. Basingstoke: AA Foundation for Road Safety Research.

Ranney TA, Hunt LA. (1997) Researchers and occupational therapists can help each other to better understand what makes a good driver: two perspectives. Work 8: 293–7.

Retchin SM, Anapolle J. (1993) An overview of the older driver. Clinics in Geriatric Medicine 9: 279–96.

Reuben DB, Silliman RA, Traines M. (1988) The aging driver. Medicine, policy, and ethics. Journal of the American Geriatrics Society 36: 1135–42.

Schieber F. (1994) High-priority research and development needs for maintaining the safety and mobility of older drivers. Experimental Aging Research 20: 35–43.

Shua-Haim JR, Gross JS. (1996) The co-pilot driver syndrome [see comments]. Journal of the American Geriatrics Society 44: 815–17.

Staplin L, Lococo KH, Stewart J, Decina LE. (1999) Safe Mobility for Older People Notebook. DOT HS 808 853. Washington, DC: National Highway Traffic Safety Administration.

Strickberger SA, Cantillon C, Friedman PL. (1991) When should patients with lethal ventricular tachyarrhythmias resume driving? Annals of Internal Medicine 115: 560–3.

Stutts JC. (1998) Do older drivers with visual and cognitive impairments drive less? Journal of the American Geriatrics Society 46: 854–61.

Stutts JC, Stewart JR, Martell C. (1998) Cognitive test performance and crash risk in an older driver population. Accident; Analysis and Prevention 30: 337–46.

Taylor BD, Tripodes S. (2001) The effects of driving cessation on the elderly with dementia and their caregivers. Accid; Analysis and Prevention 33: 519–28.

Trobe JD. (1998) Test of divided visual attention predicts automobile crashes among older adults (editorial). *Archives of Ophthalmology* **116**: 665.

Trobe JD, Waller PF, Cook-Flannagan CA *et al.* (1996) Crashes and violations among drivers with Alzheimer disease. *Archives of Neurology* **53**: 411–16.

Uc EY, Rizzo M. (2008) Driving and neurodegenerative diseases. *Current Neurology and Neuroscience Reports* **8**: 377–83.

US Department of Transportation. (2003) *Safe mobility for a maturing society: challenges and ooportunities.* Washington, DC: US Department of Transportation.

van Zomeren AH, Brouwer WH, Minderhoud JM. (1987) Acquired brain damage and driving: a review. *Archives of Physical Medicine and Rehabilitation* **68**: 697–705.

Vrkljan BH, Polgar JM. (2007) Driving, navigation, and vehicular technology: experiences of older drivers and their co-pilots. *Traffic Injury Prevention* **8**: 403–10.

White S, O'Neill D. (2000) Health and relicencing policies for older drivers in the European Union. *Gerontology* **46**: 146–52.

Winograd CH, Jarvik LF. (1986) Physician management of the demented patient. *Journal of the American Geriatrics Society* **34**: 295–308.

Quality of life in dementia: conceptual and practical issues

BETTY S BLACK AND PETER V RABINS

34.1 INTRODUCTION

A fundamental goal of care for individuals with dementia is the maximization of their quality of life over the illness course. A major challenge is determining what makes life as good as possible in the face of this chronic, progressive illness that impacts every aspect of life. The importance of this goal is reflected by the increasing focus of research on quality of life (QoL) in dementia that has occurred over the past two decades. This chapter examines how QoL in dementia is conceptualized and measured, what we are learning about it, and how future research may advance understanding of this sometimes elusive concept.

QoL is an individual's state of being that is determined by the evaluation of important aspects of life based on a set of values, goals, experiences and culture. While there is general agreement that QoL is a multi-dimensional concept, there is no consensus on how to define it or on what aspects of life should be considered when appraising QoL. For example, the World Health Organization defines QoL as 'the individual's perceptions of their position in life in the context of the culture and value system in which they live, and in relationship to their goals, expectations, standards and concerns' (WHO QoL Group, 1995). However, as Faden and German (1994) note, there are multiple valid and competing conceptions of the good life, that the meaning of QoL changes over the course of a lifetime, and that adaptation to circumstances at the moment affects one's perception of QoL.

Health-related QoL (HRQoL), a more narrow concept, focuses on aspects of life that are affected by a person's health

conditions and the treatment of those conditions (Kane, 2003). Though more specific than QoL, HRQoL is also a multi-dimensional concept that refers to one's social, psychological and physical well-being consonant with the individual's values and culture. This construct is broader than concepts such as mood or function and is of interest because its primary focus is on individuals' subjective global assessment of their situation as opposed to measures that assess standardized outcomes such as depression or activities of daily living. Although HRQoL is conceptualized as a broad construct, most researchers have concluded that it is constructed of several domains, most commonly physical health, psychological well-being, function and social activity (Patrick and Erickson, 1993).

Lawton (1997), one of the most influential forces in how QoL is conceptualized and measured, argued that QoL can and should be assessed both subjectively and objectively. He defined QoL as 'the multi-dimensional evaluation, by both intrapersonal and social-normative criteria, of the person-environment system of the individual' (Lawton and Herzog, 1991). He believed that there is a need for a frame of reference against which an individual's subjective assessment can be compared and that often there are consensual standards of quality (Lawton, 1997). Lawton suggested that subjective aspects of QoL (e.g. psychological well-being) and objective domains (e.g. physical safety) should be assessed in parallel to examine congruence and incongruence between the two approaches.

While HRQoL is conceptualized as a global construct and often examined using generic instruments, such as the

Quality of Well-being (QWB) scale (Kaplan and Bush, 1982) and the SF-36 (Ware and Sherbourne, 1992), many researchers have taken the approach of developing instruments specific to certain diseases because those diseases' characteristics have a significant impact on measurement of the construct. This approach can be particularly advocated for dementia because the disorder ultimately robs a person of the ability to express oneself owing to the progressive debilitating nature of most dementias and because of the unique value placed on thought and cognition. Ettema *et al.* (2005b) define dementia-specific QoL as 'the multi-dimensional evaluation of the person-environment system of the individual, in terms of adaptation to the perceived consequences of the dementia'. They contend that successful adaptation to the effects of the disease will lead to a sense of well-being.

Examining QoL can contribute uniquely to assessing the effectiveness of interventions to treat people with dementia. Agencies that approve pharmacological agents have chosen to emphasize cognitive improvement as a necessary attribute for drugs approved to treat cognitive disorders. However, these diseases also impair function and social capacity. Therefore, it is plausible that effective treatments might improve the non-cognitive aspects of dementia more than the cognitive aspects, and non-biological interventions may affect well-being more than medications (Whitehouse, 2006). Thus, measuring QOL has unique potential for examining treatment outcomes.

34.2   GOALS OF MEASURING QUALITY OF LIFE

While the goals of examining QoL have positive intents, the idea of measuring QoL has also garnered criticisms. Jennings (2000) outlined some objections to the construct of QoL, beginning with the claim that it is so vague and so prone to misapplication that it is either useless or dangerous. Another objection is that it attempts to measure aspects of human existence that are ineffable and unmeasurable. Third, the construct can be seen as narrowing rather than expanding individual values since it claims to define a norm or a narrow view of QoL. Finally, the term has within it an implication of judgement. Jennings concludes, however, that the value of this construct is that it can be used to improve aspects of life of the disenfranchised and that if the term's drawbacks are kept in mind they can be minimized. He suggests that QoL has the strength of setting positive goals which counteracts its negative application as a ranking of individuals or comparison of the states of individuals. Ultimately, both Jennings (2000) and Hughes (2003) concluded that the examination of QoL in people with dementia emphasizes those with the disease and that this strength counteracts the concept's inherent drawbacks.

Measuring QoL can serve several important purposes. Determining QoL increases basic understanding of the impact that dementia has on individuals over the course of their illness (Kerner *et al.*, 1998). Beyond specific aspects of the dementia syndrome, such as cognitive and functional impairments, QoL provides a more global indicator of how dementia influences well-being. Because dementia affects many people, has multiple causes and is non-linear in progression, QoL provides a common language for evaluating interventions' effects (Mack and Whitehouse, 2001). As new therapies become available, reliable measures of QoL are important for comparing drugs in terms of benefits and side effects, and for comparing non-pharmacological interventions with each other or with drugs (Rabins and Kasper, 1997). QoL can be a key consideration in evaluating service programmes or care institutions (Brooker, 2005; Kazui *et al.*, 2008) and in developing clinical guidelines (NICE, 2006). For those whose lives have been altered by moving to long-term care facilities (LTCFs), Kane (2003) believes that we have a moral responsibility to understand and to improve QoL in LTCFs. QoL is also a major consideration in advanced dementia when decision makers are often faced with choosing between aggressive interventions or palliative approaches to care (Taylor *et al.*, 2008). Finally, QoL issues must be kept in mind when allocating scarce resources at both the individual and societal levels (Whitehouse *et al.*, 1997; Brod *et al.*, 1999; Selai and Trimble, 1999; Banerjee and Wittenberg, 2009).

34.3   CHALLENGES IN MEASURING QUALITY OF LIFE IN DEMENTIA

The assessment of QoL in people with dementia presents several conceptual and practical challenges (Rabins and Kasper, 1997). The first is whether there are domains of QoL that are unique to dementia as opposed to other illnesses. Some of the hallmarks of dementia are that it impairs memory, it can affect attention, insight, judgement, problem solving, behaviour, personality, communication skills, and it can lead to other non-cognitive symptoms (Rabins *et al.*, 2006). This constellation of possible features unique to dementia can markedly influence QoL. As Howard and Rockwood (1995) note, Alzheimer's disease (AD), the leading cause of dementia, has many manifestations, not all of which are present in all patients. They emphasize the need to employ QoL measures that discriminate between patterns of symptoms throughout the illness. An individual's environment also has an influence on functioning and opportunities for social interaction which impact HRQoL. Measures of QoL must be sensitive to the settings where people with dementia reside or receive care.

A second issue relates to the subjective nature of the construct. In the earlier stages of dementia when symptoms are mild to moderate and individuals can conceptualize this construct and express opinions, the determination of self-rated QoL is most appropriate and informative. There is great interest in capturing the perspectives of those who have dementia; there is clear evidence that it is feasible to assess QoL directly from those in the mild to moderate stages (Logsdon and Teri, 1997; Brod *et al.*, 1999; Logsdon *et al.*, 2000; Selai *et al.*, 2001a; Selai *et al.*, 2001b; Trigg *et al.*, 2007a); and there is some support for seeking self-rated QoL from individuals with more severe impairments (Hoe *et al.*, 2005; James *et al.*, 2005). However, since some individuals lose the capacity to self-assess QoL, they must either be excluded from measurement or methods must be used whereby other knowledgeable individuals can provide an indication of their QoL.

Reliance on others to determine an individual's QoL raises important concerns and questions. Does another person have the right to make judgements about an individual's state of well-being? If so, who is the most appropriate person to serve as a proxy rater of QoL? One of the most consistent findings in the literature on QoL in dementia is that proxy ratings are generally lower than self ratings. A noted exception to this is the finding by Ready and colleagues (2006) that greater patient insight is associated with higher caregiver ratings than patient ratings. Concordance between patient and proxy responses are influenced by the nature of their relationship, the amount of time spent together, the degree of objective-ness of the questions, the patient's level of impairment and the proxy's well-being (Brod et al., 1999; Logsdon et al., 2002; Snow et al., 2005; Banerjee et al., 2006; Karlawish et al., 2008b; Conde-Sala et al., 2009). Proxy ratings have the drawback of filtering a subjective measure though the opi-nion of another who may or may not share relevant values. This limitation may be unavoidable, especially for those with advanced dementia. However, measures consisting of items that describe observable behaviours and expressions can help to minimize this limitation (Rabins and Kasper, 1997).

A third major issue is establishing acceptable psycho-metric properties of instruments that measure QoL in a disorder which renders some individuals unable to con-ceptualize the construct. Establishing the validity of a mea-sure is a challenge when there is no universally accepted definition of QoL and any definition is subject to individual interpretation and values (Rabins and Kasper, 1997). While criterion validity may not be possible, most developers seek to establish face and content validities by demonstrating the relevance and comprehensiveness of their instrument. Relia-bility of a measure can more readily be established by demonstrating that its items have internal consistency, that it has good repeatability across administrations and that its use by multiple observers produces similar results. Another psychometric challenge for QoL instruments in dementia is to demonstrate responsiveness or sensitivity to meaningful change. This is a critical characteristic for its usefulness as an outcome measure.

Hughes (2003) identifies three somewhat similar problems in the assessment of QoL in dementia. One is the determi-nation of domains, second is the subjective-objective pro-blem, and third is how QoL should be assessed in the incapacitated person. Hughes identifies the construct of 'personhood' as an ethical solution to these dilemmas. In defining a person as a 'situated embodied agent', he suggests that both prior and current values and wishes of the person should be considered and that a person's social context of family, friends, neighbours and values be incorporated.

34.4 APPROACHES TO MEASURING QUALITY OF LIFE

Numerous approaches have been used to assess QoL in people with dementia. Differences relate to the type of

instrument used (generic versus disease-specific), the scope of the instrument (a single item versus multiple domains), the type of scores the measure produces, and the method used to collect data. The approach selected by an investigator depends on several factors. First, the purpose for measuring QoL may determine whether a generic or disease-specific instrument is most appropriate. While a disease-specific QoL measure is most sensitive to the unique characteristics of dementia and its impact on people's lives, it cannot be used to compare the well-being of individuals who have dementia with that of people who have other illnesses. Naglie (2007) notes that generic measures can be classified as health profiles or utility measures and can be helpful for health policy decision-making. If QoL is used as an outcome measure, it is important to consider whether the instrument's content will provide an appropriate measure of effectiveness of the ther-apy, intervention or programme being examined. Since most agree that QoL is multi-dimensional, investigators wanting to examine relationships between an intervention and particular aspects of QoL may prefer an instrument that provides subscale scores reflecting specific QoL domains rather than one that provides a single summary score. Instruments also vary in how items are scored. In many cases, the items of an instrument contribute equally to either a subscale score or the total score, while other measures have weighted scores based on the assumption that the issues reflected by different items vary in their contribution to the individual's QoL.

Characteristics of the study sample can influence the choice of methods and instruments. Some instruments have been designed to assess QoL of people across the illness course. These usually rely on proxy raters, such as family members or formal health-care providers, so that individuals with advanced dementia can be included along with those who are less impaired. This approach is useful for minimizing missing data in longitudinal studies if participants are likely to lose the ability to self-assess as the illness progresses. Proxy rated instruments can vary in whether the proxy is asked to respond based on what they think the person's QoL is or based on what they think the person with dementia would say. Other instruments have been developed for those with mild to moderate dementia who are likely to be able to self-assess their QoL or participate in the assessment process along with a knowledgeable informant. Some measures focus on QoL in people with late-stage dementia, often relying on formal caregivers as proxy raters or observers.

Lawton (1997) rejected the idea that there can be only one scale of QoL since life is composed of many facets. He argued that for clinical and research purposes it is important to know the separate content and salience values for each of the domains that compose QoL. Beyond the subjective measure of QoL involving self-report, he described two types of objective measures of QoL that deal with observable phe-nomena (Lawton, 1997). First are attribute ratings, which are characteristics rated based on the rater's familiarity with or observation of the person's typical behaviour over a period of time. Instruments examining attributes (functional health, behavioural symptoms, social interaction and affect) are typically rated by a family member or health-care provider. The second type of objective measure is direct observation and coding of ongoing behaviour, which can include behaviours of people with dementia, their displays of affect and interactions with care providers, or aspects of the environment. Trained researchers typically complete observational measures.

Concerns about the high cost of care associated with dementia have increasingly led to reliance on utility-based measures of QoL that are used to conduct cost-effectiveness analyses (Naglie *et al.*, 2006). Generic utility instruments provide a global measure of an individual's preference for a health state using a single number usually ranging from 0 (representing death) to 1 (representing perfect health) and allow for the evaluation of interventions in terms of their cost per quality-adjusted life year (QALY; Naglie, 2007). Thus, QALY is a measure of disease burden that incorporates both the quality and quantity of life lived and is based on the relative desirability ('utility') of different outcomes (Knapp and Mangalore, 2007). When aggregated over time, a measure of QALY can range from less than 0 (states worse than death) to 1. Utilities can be obtained directly from individuals or from health indices that incorporate a health state classification system and a set of population-derived weights that produce a utility score. Methods commonly used for establishing preferences from individuals are the visual analogue scale (VAS), the standard gamble (SG), and the time trade-off (TTO) approaches (Knapp and Mangalore, 2007). Two frequently used indexes for measuring health preferences are the EuroQoL Group's EQ-5D (Rabin and de Charro, 2001) and the Health Utility Index (HUI) (Horsman *et al.*, 2003), both of which have been used to assess QoL in individuals who have dementia (Jonsson *et al.*, 2006; Naglie *et al.*, 2006; Karlawish *et al.*, 2008b; Kavirajan *et al.*, 2009; Miller *et al.*, 2009). While the EQ-5D measures health states according to five dimensions (mobility, self-care, usual activities, pain/discomfort and anxiety/depression), a recent version of the HUI (HUI3) is based on eight attributes (vision, hearing, speech, ambulation, dexterity, emotion, cognition and pain). Knapp and Mangalore (2007) discuss the advantages and disadvantages of using the QALY measurement approach.

34.5 MEASURES OF QUALITY OF LIFE IN DEMENTIA

While many investigators choose to use generic measures to examine QoL in dementia, the nine instruments described below and summarized in **Table 34.1** are examples of disease-specific measures for assessing QoL in people with dementia. This is not an exhaustive list, but it includes many of the instruments represented in the current literature on QoL in dementia, and it illustrates the variability that exists in the content and data collection methods of dementia-specific QoL instruments. Other instruments used to measure dementia-related QoL that are not described in detail here are the Pleasant Events Schedule-Alzheimer's Disease (PES-AD; Logsdon and Teri, 1997), the Quality of Life Assessment Schedule (Selai *et al.*, 2001b), the Quality of Life Questionnaire for Dementia (Terada *et al.*, 2002) and the Bath Assessment of Subjective Quality of Life in Dementia (Trigg *et al.*, 2007a). For additional reviews of generic and disease-specific instruments,

see Salek *et al.* (1998), Walker *et al.* (1998), Selai and Trimble (1999), Demers *et al.* (2000), Ready and Ott (2003), Ettema *et al.* (2005a), Schölzel-Dorenbos *et al.* (2007) and Banerjee *et al.* (2009). An online database of QoL instruments that includes descriptive information and notes the existence of any translations is available at www.proqolid.org.

34.5.1 Activity and Affect Indicators of Quality of Life

Albert *et al.* (1996) and Albert *et al.* (2000) developed the Activity and Affect Indicators of Quality of Life (AAIQOL) by adapting two existing measures to assess QoL related to the domains of activity and affect as rated by caregivers. The 53-item PES-AD (Logsdon and Teri, 1997) was reduced to 15 items, which are used to determine the frequency of, opportunity for and enjoyment of activities that take place either outside the home (five items) or indoors (ten items). Affect is measured using Lawton's Affect Rating scale (Lawton, 1994), which consists of three positive affects (pleasure, interest, contentment) and three negative affects (anger, anxiety, depression). The frequency of each affect in the previous 2 weeks is determined based on a 5-point scale. A composite QoL indicator is then constructed by combining the affect and activity indicators. While the developers have reported that reliability and validity of the AAIQOL are acceptable (Albert *et al.*, 1996) and that it can be used in clinical and community-based samples, they suggest that the affect measure may be a less reliable indicator of QoL when reported by proxies (Albert *et al.*, 2000). While the AAIQOL has been referred to by some investigators as the 'AAL-AD' (Dooley and Hinojosa, 2004), the 'QOL in AD' (Zimmerman *et al.*, 2005) and the 'QOL-D' (Sloane *et al.*, 2005), the developers prefer the title used here.

34.5.2 Alzheimer Disease-Related Quality of Life (ADRQL) measure

The Alzheimer Disease-Related Quality of Life (ADRQL) is a proxy rated measure of QoL of individuals who have AD or other types of dementia for use across all levels of disease severity (Rabins *et al.*, 2000). It was developed using an iterative process involving input from health-care providers, informal caregivers and a national panel of experts in dementia research and treatment. The original ADRQL contains 47 items reflecting five domains (social interaction, awareness of self, enjoyment of activities, feelings and mood, response to surroundings) that describe primarily observable behaviours. It is administered as a structured interview to a formal or informal care provider who has extensive knowledge of the person with dementia in the previous 2 weeks, with response choices of 'agree' or 'disagree' for each item. One assumption underlying the ADRQL's development was that the included items and domains vary in their contribution to the concept of QoL. By developing preference weights for items, these differences were incorporated into the measure, and the preference weights were used to assign a scale value to each ADRQL item. Summary scores ranging

Table 34.1 Dementia-specific measures of quality of life.

Instrument	Content/domains	Respondent	Patient population	Items
Activity and Affect Indicators of Quality of Life (AAIQOL)	Activity Positive affect Negative affect	Proxy – formal or informal caregiver	Mild to severe	21
Alzheimer Disease-Related Quality of Life (ADRQL)	Social interaction Awareness of self Enjoyment of activities Feelings and mood Response to surroundings	Proxy – formal or informal caregiver	Mild to severe	40
Cornell-Brown Scale (CBS) for Quality of Life in Dementia	Negative affectivity Physical complaints Positive affectivity Satisfaction	Clinician with patient's and caregiver's input	Mild to moderate	19
Dementia Care Mapping (DCM)	Well-being Ill-being Personal detractions	Trained observer	Moderate to severe	24
Dementia Quality of Life (DQoL)	Self-esteem Positive affect/humour Negative affect Feelings of belonging Sense of aesthetics	Patient	Mild to moderate	29
DEMQOL, DEMQOL-Proxy	Daily activities/looking after self Health and well-being Cognitive functioning Social relationships Self-concept	Patient, proxy	Mild to moderate, mild to severe	28 31
QUALIDEM	Care relationship Positive affect Negative affect Restless tense behaviour Positive self image Social relations Social isolation Feeling at home Having something to do	Professional caregiver	Moderate to severe	37
Quality of Life-AD (QoL-AD)	Physical condition Mood Interpersonal relationships Ability to participate in meaningful activities Financial situation Overall assessment of self Life quality as a whole	Patient, proxy or both	Mild to moderate	13
Quality of Life in Late Stage Dementia (QUALID)	Activity Affect	Proxy	Severe	11

from 0 to 100 are calculated for each domain and for the overall QoL score; higher scores reflect a higher QoL. The ADRQL has good reliability and validity (Black *et al.*, 2000; Gonzalez-Salvador *et al.*, 2000) and is responsive to change (Lyketsos *et al.*, 2003; Missotten, *et al.*, 2007). A 40-item version of the ADRQL now has been recommended by the developers based on analyses of data from three residential settings demonstrating improved psychometric properties over the original version (Kasper *et al.*, 2009). The 40-item

ADRQL can be derived from the original 47 items and reflects the same five QoL domains.

34.5.3 Cornell–Brown Scale for quality of life in dementia

Ready *et al.* (2002) developed the Cornell–Brown Scale (CBS) by modifying the Cornell Scale for Depression (Alexopoulos *et al.*, 1988). The CBS was developed based on the idea that high QoL is indicated by the presence of positive affect, satisfaction, self-esteem and the relative absence of negative affect. It includes 19 bipolar items in four categories (negative affectivity, physical complaints, positive affectivity and satisfaction) that yield a single QoL score. The CBS is completed by a clinician after a joint semi-structured interview with the patient and caregiver. Based on information obtained regarding the previous month, each item is rated on a 5-point scale from −2 to +2. Reliability and validity have been demonstrated in a sample of outpatients with either dementia or mild cognitive impairment, with similar properties based on data from the mild and the more severely impaired halves of the sample (Ready *et al.*, 2002).

34.5.4   Dementia Care Mapping approach

Kitwood and Bredin (1994) devised the Dementia Care Mapping (DCM) method for evaluating the quality of care and well-being of people with dementia in residential care settings. The DCM methodology is based on the social-psychological theory of dementia care (Kitwood and Bredin, 1992), which holds that much of the decline among those with dementia is a consequence of social and environmental factors. DCM is a structured, observational method in which the well-being or ill-being (WIB) of patients is rated based on signs from the patient and the behaviour of staff toward them Trained observers also record any personal detractors (PDs), which are any episodes that could lead to a reduction in self-esteem for the person with dementia. Typically, five to ten residents are rated every 5 minutes over 6 hours using 24 activity categories and indicators of social withdrawal. WIB values, which range from −5 (ill-being) to +5 (well-being), can be aggregated to determine an overall WIB score for the group and for each individual. Reviews have described the extensive use of DCM and summarized evidence of its reliability, validity and responsiveness to change (Beavis *et al.*, 2002; Brooker, 2005). DCM has undergone several changes since its inception (Brooker and Surr, 2006), and other investigators have tried to simplify the process and reduce the resources required to implement this method (Fulton *et al.*, 2006). Despite the limitations associated with the use of DCM (Beavis *et al.*, 2002; Thornton, 2004; Sloane, 2007), it is unique among the measures used to assess QoL in dementia in that it also serves to examine some elements of quality of care and is used as a tool for practice development.

34.5.5   Dementia Quality of Life (DQoL) instrument

Brod and colleagues (1999) developed the Dementia Quality of Life (DqoL), which was designed to be administered to people with mild to moderate dementia. It is a 29-item instrument developed through an iterative process involving a literature review, focus groups, pilot testing and statistical examination of its psychometric properties. Screening questions assess the individual's comprehension of the response format. The DQoL consists of items rated on a 5-point visual

scale that form five subscales (self-esteem, positive affect/humour, negative affect, feelings of belonging, sense of aesthetics). The developers have reported good internal consistency, reliability and construct validity and suggest that reliable data can be obtained from individuals with Mini-Mental State Examination (MMSE) scores >12.

34.5.6   DEMQOL and DEMQOL–Proxy measures

The DEMQOL and DEMQOL-Proxy were devised by Smith and colleagues (2007) to assess HRQoL in all stages of dementia severity. These instruments were developed via a multi-stage process beginning with the development of a conceptual framework that includes five domains (daily activities/looking after self, health and well-being, cognitive functioning, social relationships, self-concept; Smith *et al.*, 2005a). The DEMQOL is a 28-item instrument administered to persons with mild to moderate dementia, and the DEM-QOL-Proxy is a 31-item caregiver questionnaire regarding patients with mild to severe dementia; higher scores indicate better QoL. The authors, who report satisfactory psychometric properties on these measures, recommend that both instruments be used together, although the DEMQOL cannot be used with individuals who have severe cognitive impairment (i.e. MMSE scores <10).

34.5.7   QUALIDEM measure

Ettema *et al.* (2007a) and Ettema *et al.* (2007b) developed the QUALIDEM to assess QoL in individuals with dementia living in residential care. Content of the QUALIDEM is based on an iterative process that involved a literature review, qualitative research methods, field testing and psychometric analyses. It is a multi-dimensional scale, rated by professional caregivers, that consists of 37 items describing observable behaviour and making up nine subscales (Koopmans *et al.*, 2009). The subscale scores are linearly transformed to range from 1 to 100, with higher scores reflecting a better QoL. The developers report that 18 of the QUALIDEM items comprising six subscales are applicable for measuring QoL in the final phase of dementia. The QUALIDEM is reported to have satisfactory reliability and validity for use in research and practice. The authors strongly discourage the calculation of a total score since the subscales differ in content and distinct subscale information would be lost.

34.5.8   Quality of Life-AD measure

The Quality of Life-AD (QoL-AD) was developed by Logsdon and colleagues (2000) to assess QoL as perceived by both the patient and their caregiver. The content of the QoL-AD was derived based on a review of literature on QoL of older adults and other chronically ill populations and the input of patients, caregivers and experts in the fields of geriatrics and gerontology. The QoL-AD consists of 13 items used to assess seven aspects of the patient's QoL (physical condition, mood, interpersonal relationships, participation in activities, financial situation, overall assessment of self, life quality as a whole). An interviewer administers the QoL-AD to patients with mild to moderate illness, and caregivers complete the measure in the form of a questionnaire. Each item is rated by the patient and by the caregiver on a 4-point scale, from 1 (poor) to 4 (excellent). Total scores as rated by each person range from 13 to 52. A weighted composite score is calculated by giving greater weight to the patient's rating than the caregiver's rating. The developers (Logsdon et al., 2000; Logsdon et al., 2002) report that the QoL-AD has good reliability and validity, and it is responsive to change (Spector et al., 2003; Karlawish et al., 2004). The QoL-AD is a widely used instrument that frequently serves as an indicator of concurrent validity for other dementia-specific and generic measures of QoL.

34.5.9 Quality of Life in Late Stage Dementia scale

Weiner and colleagues (2000) developed the Quality of Life in Late Stage Dementia Scale (QUALID) to assess QoL in people with late-stage dementia residing in institutional settings. The scale items were selected from the affect and activity measure (the AAIQOL) devised by Albert et al. (1996). A group of clinicians experienced in assessing people with AD selected the items by consensus to measure QoL in people with late-stage dementia in long-term care. The QUALID, which is administered as a structured interview, contains 11 items reflecting observable behaviours rated by frequency on a 5-point Likert scale by a nursing home technician who had at least 30 hours of exposure to the resident in the previous week. Scores range from 11 to 55; lower scores reflect a better QoL. The developers report that the QUALID has good internal consistency, adequate construct validity and is responsive to change (Weiner et al., 2000; Martin-Cook et al., 2005).

34.6 CORRELATES OF QUALITY OF LIFE IN DEMENTIA

With the establishment of the validity of disease-specific measures of QoL and the identification of predictors of well-being in people with dementia, researchers have identified a few fairly consistent correlates of QoL across studies, while other relationships are less clear. In a review of findings based on dementia-specific measures, Banerjee and colleagues (2009) suggest that there is little relationship between severity of cognitive impairment and HRQoL. They cite several studies (Logsdon et al., 2002; Smith et al., 2005a; Fuh and Wang, 2006; Vogel et al., 2006) that have found little or no association between cognitive function and QoL, but they note exceptions to this too, such as a study by Edelman et al. (2005) that found QoL-AD scores significantly worsening as MMSE scores decreased. Other research findings reveal that the relationship between cognitive function and QoL is variable. Some investigators identify significant correlations

(Samus, 2005; Winzelberg et al., 2005; Samus, 2006; Falk et al., 2007), others report no significance between the two factors (Trigg et al., 2007b; Karlawish et al., 2008a; Missotten et al., 2008), and still others report that their findings differ based on the person's level of cognitive impairment (mild versus moderate; Matsui et al., 2006) or on who rates the person's QoL (self versus proxy; Edelman et al., 2004a). Banerjee et al. (2009) note that, while staff ratings of QoL usually show higher correlations with cognitive function than self-reports or family caregiver reports, the absolute level of correlation is generally low, suggesting that QoL and cognition are independent constructs.

Investigators often find that activities of daily living (ADL) impairments or greater physical dependency are associated with diminished QoL in persons with dementia (Albert et al., 2000; Gonzalez-Salvador et al., 2000; Logsdon et al., 2002; Hoe et al., 2005; Ettema et al., 2007b; Conde-Sala et al., 2009), but there are exceptions to these findings. Neither Fuh and Wang (2006) nor Matsui and colleagues (2006) found an association between QoL measures and ADL impairments, while others report findings in which proxy ratings of QoL are associated with functional status but self ratings are not (Edelman et al., 2004b; Edelman et al., 2005). Thus, studies do not reveal a clear pattern in the relationship between QoL and functional status.

One of the most consistent findings in people with dementia is the relationship between symptoms of depression and lower QoL (Smith et al., 2005b; Banerjee et al., 2006; Vogel et al., 2006; Ettema et al., 2007b; Trigg et al., 2007b). In some studies, this is reflected by both self and proxy ratings of QoL (Logsdon et al., 2002; Shin et al., 2005; Snow et al., 2005). A partial exception to this relationship was reported by Hoe et al. (2005) who found that individuals with severe dementia had QoL-AD scores significantly associated with the mood scale on the Health Status Questionnaire, but not with the Cornell Scale for Depression in Dementia or the depression or anxiety subscales of the Hospital Anxiety and Depression Schedule. The generally strong relationships among dementia, depression and QoL highlight the importance of diagnosis and treatment of depression, especially in LTCFs where depression is common.

The relationship between behavioural disorders and poor QoL in people with dementia has been widely reported (Samus, 2005; Banerjee et al., 2006; Samus, 2006; Hoe et al., 2007). In a review, Banerjee and colleagues (2009) cite studies in which behavioural disorders are associated with decreased QoL based on staff and caregiver ratings but not based on self ratings (Logsdon et al., 2002; Hoe et al., 2005; Banerjee et al., 2006; Hoe et al., 2006). They suggest that these differences may be due to either the patient's lack of insight due to dementia or differential appraisals of the impact that these disorders have for the individuals with dementia compared to proxies. However, some investigators have found significant relationships between individuals' behavioural disturbances and their QoL as rated by both the caregiver and the patient (Matsui et al., 2006; Hurt et al., 2008), and others have found that these disorders are significantly associated with lower QoL for both patients and caregivers (Shin et al., 2005; Conde-Sala et al., 2009). Researchers have also found significantly lower QoL in individuals with dementia taking psychotropic medications

(Albert *et al.*, 1996; Gonzalez-Salvador *et al.*, 2000; Ballard *et al.*, 2001; Falk *et al.*, 2007). However, since these are cross-sectional studies, it is unclear whether medications adversely affect QoL or whether lower QoL is due to the psychiatric and behavioural problems being treated.

A limited number of longitudinal cohort studies have examined change in QoL, and some of these have identified specific correlates of change. Lyketsos and colleagues (2003) identified a small but significant mean change in ADRQL scores over two years in a residential setting, with lower baseline scores being the only significant predictor of change in residents' QoL. In a 12-month follow-up examination of QoL-AD scores in a randomized controlled trial (RCT), Karlawish *et al.* (2004) found that declines in functional status were more strongly associated with diminished QoL than with declines in cognition. Zimmerman and colleagues (2005) conducted a six-month follow up of QoL-AD scores in the Dementia Care project and found a small but significant worsening in QoL associated with greater cognitive impairment and depression. In an examination of the psychometric properties of the ADRQL, Kasper *et al.* (2009) found a significant decline in QoL among those in a community-based sample who had increases in ADL impairments over one year. Other investigators found no significant mean change in QoL after periods ranging from six months to two years (Hoe *et al.*, 2005; Selwood *et al.*, 2005; Missotten *et al.*, 2007). However, even in studies that report little or no mean change in QoL, sizable proportions of their samples show either increases or decreases in QoL over time (Lyketsos *et al.*, 2003; Selwood *et al.*, 2005; Missotten *et al.*, 2007). Further research is needed to better understand what leads to these fluctuations in QoL.

34.7   QUALITY OF LIFE AS AN OUTCOME MEASURE

Relatively few published trials have examined QoL as an outcome measure of dementia interventions (Takeda *et al.*, 2006; Schölzel-Dorenbos *et al.*, 2007; Banerjee *et al.*, 2009), particularly with the use of dementia-specific measures. To date, QoL measures are more commonly used in non-pharmacological studies than in pharmacological trials. Donepezil trials conducted by Rogers *et al.* (1996), Rogers *et al.* (1998a) and Rogers *et al.* (1998b) demonstrated improvement in QoL. However, the QoL changes observed were not always significant or seen in the intervention group, and the rating scales had not been validated for use in dementia. Using the QoL-AD, Aisen *et al.* (2003) found that non-steroidal anti-inflammatory drugs had no effect on either cognition or QoL; and Lu *et al.* (2006) showed that testosterone replacement therapy improved QoL in AD, but had no significant effect on cognition. In an examination of the QUALID's responsiveness based on secondary analysis from a study that showed no differences between olanzapine and risperidone for treating behavioural disturbances, QoL was significantly related to improvements in neuropsychiatric symptoms and inversely related to the drugs' adverse effects (Martin-Cook *et al.*, 2005). Finally, phase 1 of the CATIE-AD trial of three atypical anti-psychotics showed some

improvement in clinical symptoms, but the interventions had no effect on cognition or QoL (Sultzer *et al.*, 2008).

Studies examining non-pharmaceutical interventions and their effects on QoL have focused on both those with dementia and their caregivers. A series of reports examined the impact of cognitive stimulation therapy (CST; Spector *et al.*, 2003; Knapp *et al.*, 2006; Woods *et al.*, 2006). Spector and colleagues (2003) found that a 14-session CST programme had a significant positive impact on MMSE and QoL-AD scores of people with dementia; Knapp *et al.* (2006) determined there was a high probability that CST is more cost-effective than treatment as usual; and Woods *et al.* (2006) reported that changes in cognitive function mediate the effects of CST in improving QoL. Using DCM in an RCT, aromatherapy with Melissa oil improved QoL and reduced agitation in individuals with severe dementia (Ballard *et al.*, 2002). Lai and colleagues (2004) also used DCM and found that reminiscence therapy had a significant impact on WIB scores for nursing home residents with dementia in the intervention group. In another reminiscence-based partially masked RCT, Politis *et al.* (2004) found a significant reduction in apathy but no clear improvement in QoL. Other investigators have found that community-based occupational therapy improves patients' QoL and their informal caregivers' well-being (Dooley and Hinojosa, 2004; Graff *et al.*, 2007). Teri and colleagues (2005) used the QoL-AD in an RCT to determine whether community consultants to family caregivers could reduce mood and behaviour problems in people with AD. Their STAR-C training programme significantly reduced behaviour problems and improved QoL for the patients and benefited the caregivers by significantly improving measures of depression, burden and reactivity to the patients' behaviour problems. While other RCTs (Logiudice *et al.*, 1999) have successfully focused on improving caregiver well-being, it is beyond this chapter's scope to examine that research. However, since efforts to maximize caregivers' QoL are of equal importance, caregiver QoL should be included as an outcome measure, particularly in community-based studies (Schölzel-Dorenbos *et al.*, 2007).

34.8   QUESTIONS AND ISSUES FOR THE FUTURE

Examining QoL in dementia is an important means of understanding the experience of people with these disorders, determining the efficacy and effectiveness of pharmacological and non-pharmacological approaches to care, and evaluating and improving care practices. Substantial advances have occurred over the past two decades in the study of QoL in dementia, especially recently. This work serves as a foundation for understanding QoL, but additional progress is needed in several areas, including measurement issues, identifying correlates of QoL and predictors of change, and assessing the impact of interventions on patients' well-being.

Reliable and valid dementia-specific instruments are now available to measure QoL across the spectrum of disease severity. Many of these instruments are available in multiple languages, and some have been validated across cultures. They reflect different conceptualizations of this construct and rely on varied methods for data collection to provide indicators of QoL. For some of these measures, limited or no data are available on their responsiveness, a psychometric property that is critical for determining the impact of therapeutic interventions. Related to this are the questions of how should users interpret changes in QoL scores, and what is a minimally important difference or a clinically significant change in scores (Naglie, 2007; Schölzel-Dorenbos et al., 2007). Addressing these issues in future research will facilitate greater reliance on QoL as an outcome measure in clinical trials.

There is a consensus on the importance of obtaining self-assessed QoL from individuals who are capable of conceptualizing this construct and responding meaningfully to assessment items. The value of this approach is highlighted by the consistent differences that are seen between self-rated and proxy-rated measures of QoL, differences that may be attributable to characteristics of the person with dementia, the proxy informant and/or the QoL instrument. This indicates that the perspectives of the person with dementia and the carer differ and suggests that proxy ratings cannot be substituted directly for self ratings. Clarification of criteria are needed for including self-ratings to maximize the use and validity of self-assessment; and guidance is needed to determine the most appropriate proxy for those who cannot self-assess (Naglie, 2007). Further research should determine the aspects of cognitive impairment that affect the effectiveness of self-rated QoL measures and what factors confound QoL ratings provided by patients, informal caregivers and professional care providers.

Most published research on QoL in dementia is based on cross-sectional data; little is known about the natural history of QoL in dementia (Banerjee et al., 2009) or how change occurs in QoL (Selwood et al., 2005). Longitudinal studies show that decline in QoL is not inevitable with disease progression and that QoL may be as likely to improve with time as it is to diminish. More prospective studies are needed with larger, representative samples, conducted over longer periods of time to identify causal relationships and mediating factors for individuals with dementia (Banerjee et al., 2009). Studies also need to include control groups of older, cognitively intact adults to help identify the impact that dementia has on HRQoL and its change over time. Because our knowledge of QoL near the end of life in dementia is limited (Koopmans et al., 2009), studies are needed to determine the impact that care settings, approaches to symptom management and end-of-life care decision-making have on QoL.

We anticipate that interest in and the importance of maximizing QoL will increase in the future as the numbers of individuals with dementia grow and as investigators seek to identify effective therapies to assist those with this disorder and their caregivers.

REFERENCES

Aisen P, Schafer K, Grundman M et al. (2003) Effects of rofecoxib or naproxen vs placebo on Alzheimer disease progression: a randomized controlled trial. Journal of the American Medical Association 289: 2819–26.

Albert S, Castillo-Castanada C, Jacobs D et al. (2000) Proxy-reported quality of life in Alzheimer's patients: comparison of clinical and population-based samples. In: Albert S, Logsdon R (eds). Assessing quality of life in Alzheimer's disease. New York: Springer, 69–80.

Albert SM, Del Castillo-Castaneda C, Sano M et al. (1996) Quality of life in patients with Alzheimer's disease as reported by patient proxies. Journal of the American Geriatrics Society 44: 1342–7.

Alexopoulos GS, Abrams RC, Young RC, Shamoian CA. (1988) Cornell scale for depression in dementia. Biological Psychiatry 23: 271–84.

Ballard C, O'Brien J, James I et al. (2001) Quality of life for people with dementia living in residential and nursing home care: the impact of performance on activities of daily living, behavioral and psychological symptoms, language skills, and psychotropic drugs. International Psychogeriatrics 13: 93–106.

Ballard C, O'Brien J, Reichelt K, Perry E. (2002) Aromatherapy as a safe and effective treatment for the management of agitation in severe dementia: The results of a double-blind, placebo-controlled trial with Melissa. Journal of Clinical Psychiatry 63: 553–8.

Banerjee S, Wittenberg R. (2009) Clinical and cost effectiveness of services for early diagnosis and intervention in dementia. International Journal of Geriatric Psychiatry 24: 748–54.

Banerjee S, Smith SC, Lamping DL et al. (2006) Quality of life in dementia: More than just cognition. An analysis of associations with quality of life in dementia. Journal of Neurology, Neurosurgery, and Psychiatry 77: 146–8.

Banerjee S, Samsi K, Petrie CD et al. (2009) What do we know about quality of life in dementia? A review of the emerging evidence on the predictive and explanatory value of disease specific measures of health related quality of life in people with dementia. International Journal of Geriatric Psychiatry 24: 15–24.

Beavis D, Simpson S, Graham I. (2002) A literature review of dementia care mapping: methodological considerations and efficacy. Journal of Psychiatric and Mental Health Nursing 9: 725–36.

Black BS, Rabins PV, Kasper JD. (2000) Alzheimer Disease Related Quality of Life (ADRQL) User's Manual. Baltimore, MD: DEMeasure.

Brod M, Stewart AL, Sands L, Walton P. (1999) Conceptualization and measurement of quality of life in dementia: The Dementia Quality of Life Instrument (DQoL). The Gerontologist 39: 25–35.

Brooker DJ. (2005) Dementia Care Mapping: A review of the research literature. Gerontologist 45: 11–18.

Brooker DJ, Surr C. (2006) Dementia Care Mapping (DCM): Initial validation of DCM 8 in UK field trials. International Journal of Geriatric Psychiatry 21: 1018–25.

Conde-Sala JL, Garre-Olmo J, Turro-Garriga O et al. (2009) Factors related to perceived quality of life in patients with Alzheimer's disease: The patient's perception compared with that of caregivers. International Journal of Geriatric Psychiatry 24: 585–94.

Demers L, Oremus M, Perrault A et al. (2000) Review of outcome measurement instruments in Alzheimer's Disease drug trials: Psychometric properties of functional and quality of life scales. *Journal of Geriatric Psychiatry and Neurology* **13**: 170–80.

Dooley NR, Hinojosa J. (2004) Improving quality of life for persons with Alzheimer's disease and their family caregivers: Brief occupational therapy intervention. *American Journal of Occupational Therapy* **58**: 561–9.

Edelman P, Fulton BR, Kuhn D. (2004a) Comparison of dementia-specific quality of life measures in adult day centers. *Home Health Care Services Quarterly* **23**: 25–42.

Edelman P, Kuhn D, Fulton BR. (2004b) Influence of cognitive impairment, functional impairment and care setting on Dementia Care Mapping results. *Aging and Mental Health* **8**: 514–23.

Edelman P, Fulton BR, Kuhn D, Chang C-H. (2005) A comparison of three methods of measuring dementia-specific quality of life: Perspectives of residents, staff, and observers. *The Gerontologist* **45**: 27–36.

Ettema TP, Dröes RM, de Lange J *et al.* (2005a) A review of quality of life instruments used in dementia. *Quality of Life Research* **14**: 675–86.

Ettema TP, Dröes RM, de Lange J *et al.* (2005b) The concept of quality of life in dementia in the different stages of the disease. *International Psychogeriatrics* **17**: 353–70.

Ettema TP, Dröes RM, De Lange J *et al.* (2007a) QUALIDEM: Development and evaluation of a dementia specific quality of life instrument: Scalability, reliability and internal structures. *International Journal of Geriatric Psychiatry* **22**: 549–56.

Ettema TP, Dröes RM, de Lange J *et al.* (2007b) QUALIDEM: Development and evaluation of a dementia specific quality of life instrument: Validation. *International Journal of Geriatric Psychiatry* **22**: 424–30.

Faden R, German PS. (1994) Quality of life: considerations in geriatrics. *Clinics in Geriatric Medicine* **10**: 541–51.

Falk H, Persson LO, Wijk H. (2007) A psychometric evaluation of a Swedish version of the Quality of Life in Late-Stage Dementia (QUALID) scale. *International Psychogeriatrics* **19**: 1040–50.

Fuh JL, Wang SJ. (2006) Assessing quality of life in Taiwanese patients with Alzheimer's disease. *International Journal of Geriatric Psychiatry* **21**: 103–7.

Fulton BR, Edelman P, Kuhn D. (2006) Streamlined models of dementia care mapping. *Aging and Mental Health* **10**: 343–51.

Gonzalez-Salvador T, Lyketsos CG, Baker A *et al.* (2000) Quality of life in dementia patients in long-term care. *International Journal of Geriatric Psychiatry* **15**: 181–9.

Graff MJL, Vernooij-Dassen MJM, Thijssen M *et al.* (2007) Effects of community occupational therapy on quality of life, mood health status in dementia patients and their caregivers: A randomized controlled trial. *Journal of Gerontology: Medical Sciences* **62**: 1002–9.

Hoe J, Katona C, Roch B, Livingston G. (2005) Use of the QOL-AD for measuring quality of life in people with severe dementia-the LASER-AD study. *Age and Ageing* **34**: 130–5.

Hoe J, Hancock G, Livingston G, Orrell M. (2006) Quality of life of people with dementia in residential care homes. *British Journal of Psychiatry* **188**: 460–4.

Hoe J, Katona C, Orrell M, Livingston G. (2007) Quality of life in dementia: Care recipient and caregiver perceptions of quality of life in dementia: the LASER-AD study. *International Journal of Geriatric Psychiatry* **22**: 1031–6.

Horsman J, Furlong W, Feeny D, Torrance G. (2003) The Health Utilities Index (HUI): concepts, measurement properties and applications. *Health and Quality of Life Outcomes* **1**: 1–13.

Howard K, Rockwood K. (1995) Quality of life in Alzheimer's disease. *Dementia* **6**: 113–16.

Hughes J. (2003) Quality of life in dementia: an ethical and philosophical perspective. *Expert Reviews in Pharmacoeconomics Outcomes Research* **3**: 525–34.

Hurt C, Bhattacharyya S, Burns A *et al.* (2008) Patient and caregiver perspectives of quality of life in dementia. *Dementia and Geriatric Cognitive Disorders* **26**: 138–46.

James BD, Xie SX, Karlawish JHT. (2005) How do patients with Alzheimer disease rate their overall quality of life? *American Journal of Geriatric Psychiatry* **13**: 484–90.

Jennings B. (2000) A life greater than the sum of its sensations: Ethics, dementia, and the quality of life. In: Albert S, Logsdon R (eds). *Assessing quality of life in Alzheimer's disease.* New York: Springer.

Jonsson L, Andreasen N, Kilander L *et al.* (2006) Patient- and proxy-reported utility in Alzheimer disease using the EuroQoL. *Alzheimer Disease and Associated Disorders* **20**: 49–55.

Kane RA. (2003) Definition, measurement, and correlates of quality of life in nursing homes: Toward a reasonable practice, research, and policy agenda. *The Gerontologist* **43**: 28–36.

Kaplan RM, Bush JW. (1982) Health-related quality of life measurement for evaluation research and policy analysis. *Health Psychology* **1**: 61–80.

Karlawish J, Lu M, Logsdon R *et al.* (2004) How much do 12 month changes in cognition and function influence changes in mild to moderate patients and caregivers ratings of patient quality of life? *Neurobiology of Aging* **25**: S325.

Karlawish JH, Zbrozek A, Kinosian B *et al.* (2008a) Preference-based quality of life in patients with Alzheimer's disease. *Alzheimer's and Dementia* **4**: 193–202.

Karlawish JHT, Zbrozek A, Kinosian B *et al.* (2008b) Caregivers' assessments of preference-based quality of life in Alzheimer's disease. *Alzheimer's and Dementia* **4**: 208–11.

Kasper JD, Black BS, Shore AD, Rabins PV. (2009) Evaluation of the validity and reliability of the Alzheimer disease-related Quality of Life Assessment Instrument. *Alzheimer Disease and Associated Disorders* **23**: 275–84.

Kavirajan H, Hays R, Vassar S, Vickrey B. (2009) Responsiveness and construct validity of the Health Utilities Index in patients with dementia. *Medical Care* **47**: 651–61.

Kazui H, Harada K, Eguchi YS *et al.* (2008) Association between quality of life of demented patients and professional knowledge of care workers. *Journal of Geriatric Psychiatry and Neurology* **21**: 72–78.

Kerner DN, Patterson TL, Grant I, Kaplan RM. (1998) Validity of the quality of well-being scale for patients with Alzheimer's disease. *Journal of Aging and Health* **10**: 44–61.

Kitwood T, Bredin K. (1992) Towards a theory of dementia care: personhood and well-being. *Aging and Society* **12**: 269–87.

Kitwood T, Bredin K. (1994) *Evaluating dementia care: the DCM method*, 6th edn. University of Bradford: Bradford Dementia Research Group.

Knapp M, Mangalore R. (2007) The trouble with QALYs.... *Epidemiologia e Psichiatria Sociale* 16: 289–93.

Knapp M, Thorgrimsen L, Patel A et al. (2006) Cognitive stimulation therapy for people with dementia: cost-effectiveness. *British Journal of Psychiatry* 188: 574–80.

Koopmans RTCM, van der Molen M, Raats M, Ettema TP. (2009) Neuropsychiatric symptoms and quality of life in patients in the final phase of dementia. *International Journal of Geriatric Psychiatry* 24: 25–32.

Lai C, Chi I, Kayser-Jones J. (2004) A randomized controlled trial of a specific reminiscence approach to promote the well-being of nursing home residents with dementia. *International Psychogeriatrics* 16: 33–49.

Lawton MP. (1994) Quality of life in Alzheimer disease. *Alzheimer Disease and Associated Disorders* 8: 138–50.

Lawton MP. (1997) Assessing quality of life in Alzheimer Disease research. *Alzheimer Disease and Associated Disorders* 11: 91–99.

Lawton MP, Herzog RA. (1991) Special research methods for gerontology. *International Journal of Aging and Human Development* 33: 113–18.

Logiudice D, Waltrowicz W, Brown K et al. (1999) Do memory clinics improve the quality of life of carers? A randomized pilot trial. *International Journal of Geriatric Psychiatry* 14: 626–32.

Logsdon RG, Teri L. (1997) The Pleasant Events Schedule-AD: psychometric properties and relationship to depression and cognition in Alzheimer's disease patients. *The Gerontologist* 37: 40–45.

Logsdon R, Gibbons L, McCurry S. (2000) Quality of life in Alzheimer's disease patients. In: Albert S, Logsdon R (eds). *Assessing quality of life in Alzheimer's disease*. New York: Springer Publishing Company.

Logsdon RG, Gibbons LE, McCurry SM, Teri L. (2002) Assessing quality of life in older adults with cognitive impairment. *Psychosomatic Medicine* 64: 510–19.

Lu P, Masterman D, Mulnard R et al. (2006) Effects of testosterone on cognition and mood in male patients with mild Alzheimer disease and healthy elderly men. *Archives of Neurology* 63: 177–85.

Lyketsos CG, Gonzalez-Salvador T, Chin JJ et al. (2003) A follow-up study of change in quality of life among persons with dementia residing in a long-term care facility. *International Journal of Geriatric Psychiatry* 18: 275–81.

Mack JL, Whitehouse PJ. (2001) Quality of life in dementia: State of the art - report of the international working group for harmonization of the dementia drug guidelines and the Alzheimer's Society satellite meeting. *Alzheimer Disease and Associated Disorders* 15: 69–71.

Martin-Cook K, Hynan LS, Rice-Koch K et al. (2005) Responsiveness of the Quality of Life in Late-Stage Dementia scale to psychotropic drug treatment in late-stage dementia. *Dementia and Geriatric Cognitive Disorders* 19: 82–5.

Matsui T, Nakaaki S, Murata Y et al. (2006) Determinants of the quality of life in Alzheimer's disease patients as assessed by the Japanese version of the Quality of Life- Alzheimer's Disease Scale. *Dementia and Geriatric Cognitive Disorders* 21: 182–91.

Miller E, Schneider L, Resenheck R. (2009) Assessing the relationship between health utilities, quality of life, and health services use in Alzheimer's disease. *International Journal of Geriatric Psychiatry* 24: 96–105.

Missotten P, Squelard G, Ylieff M et al. (2008) Relationship between quality of life and cognitive decline in dementia. *Dementia and Geriatric Cognitive Disorders* 25: 564–72.

Missotten P, Ylieff M, Di Notte D et al. (2007) Quality of life in dementia: A 2-year follow-up study. *International Journal of Geriatric Psychiatry* 22: 1201–7.

Naglie G. (2007) Quality of life in dementia. *Canadian Journal of Neurological Sciences* 34: S57–61.

Naglie G, Tomlinson G, Tansey C et al. (2006) Utility-based quality of life measures in Alzheimer's disease. *Quality of Life Research* 15: 631–43.

NICE. (2006) *Dementia: Supporting people with dementia and their carers in health and social care*. London: National Institute for Health and Clinical Excellence.

Patrick DL, Erickson P. (1993) Concepts of health-related quality of life. In: Patrick DL, Erickson P (eds). *Health status and health policy*. New York: Oxford University Press, 76–112.

Politis A, Vozzella S, Mayer L et al. (2004) A randomized, controlled, clinical trial of activity therapy for apathy in patients with dementia residing in long-term care. *International Journal of Geriatric Psychiatry* 19: 1087–94.

Rabin R, de Charro F. (2001) EQ-5D: A measure of health status from the EuroQol Group. *Annals of Medicine* 33: 337–43.

Rabins PV, Kasper JD. (1997) Measuring quality of life in dementia: Conceptual and practical issues. *Alzheimer Disease and Associated Disorders* 11: 100–4.

Rabins P, Kasper J, Kleinman L et al. (2000) Concepts and methods in the development of the ADRQL: An instrument for assessing health-related quality of life in persons with Alzheimer's disease. In: Albert S, Logsdon R (eds). *Assessing quality of life in Alzheimer's disease*. New York: Springer, 51–68.

Rabins PV, Lyketsos CG, Steele CD. (2006) *Practical dementia care*, 2nd edn. New York: Oxford University Press.

Ready RE, Ott BR. (2003) Quality of life measures for dementia. *Health and Quality of Life Outcomes* 1: 1–9.

Ready RE, Ott BR, Grace J, Fernandez I. (2002) The Cornell–Brown Scale for quality of life in dementia. *Alzheimer Disease and Associated Disorders* 16: 109–15.

Ready RE, Ott BR, Grace J. (2006) Insight and cognitive impairment: Effects on quality-of-life reports from mild cognitive impairment and Alzheimer's disease patients. *American Journal of Alzheimer's Disease and Other Dementias* 21: 242–8.

Rogers SL, Friedhoff LT, Group TDS. (1996) The efficacy and safety of donepezil in patients with Alzheimer's disease: results of a US multicenter, randomized, double-blind, placebo-controlled trial. *Dementia* 7: 293–303.

Rogers S, Doody R, Mohs R et al. (1998a) Donepezil improves cognition and global function in Alzheimer disease: a 15-week, double-blind, placebo-controlled study. *Archives of Internal Medicine* 158: 1021–31.

Rogers S, Farlow M, Doody R et al. (1998b) A 24-week, double-blind, placebo-controlled trial of donepezil in patients with Alzheimer's disease. Neurology 50: 136–45.

Salek SS, Walker MD, Bayer AJ. (1998) A review of quality of life in Alzheimer's Disease: Part 2: Issues in assessing drug effects. Pharmacoeconomics 14: 613–27.

Samus Q. (2005) The association of neuropsychiatric symptoms and environment with quality of life in assisted living residents with dementia. Gerontologist 45: 19–26.

Samus Q. (2006) Correlates of caregiver-related quality of life in assisted living: The Maryland Assisted Living Study. Journal of Gerontology: Psychological Sciences 61: P311–14.

Schölzel-Dorenbos CJ, Ettema TP, Bos J et al. (2007) Evaluating the outcome of interventions on quality of life in dementia: Selection of the appropriate scale. International Journal of Geriatric Psychiatry 22: 511–519.

Selai C, Trimble MR. (1999) Assessing quality of life in dementia. Aging and Mental Health 3: 101–11.

Selai C, Vaughan A, Harvey RJ, Logsdon RG. (2001a) Using the QOL-AD in the UK. International Journal of Geriatric Psychiatry 16: 537–42.

Selai CE, Trimble MR, Rossor MN, Harvey RJ. (2001b) Assessing quality of life in dementia: Preliminary psychometric testing of the Quality of Life Assessment Schedule (QOLAS). Neuropsychological Rehabilitation 11: 219–43.

Selwood A, Thorgrimsen L, Orrell M. (2005) Quality of life in dementia – a one-year follow-up study. International Journal of Geriatric Psychiatry 20: 232–7.

Shin I, Carter M, Masterman D et al. (2005) Neuropsychiatric symptoms and quality of life in Alzheimer disease. American Journal of Geriatric Psychiatry 13: 469–74.

Sloane P. (2007) Dementia care mapping as a research tool. International Journal of Geriatric Psychiatry 22: 580–9.

Sloane PD, Zimmerman S, Williams CS et al. (2005) Evaluating the quality of life of long-term care residents with dementia. The Gerontologist 45: 37–49.

Smith S, Lamping D, Banerjee S et al. (2005a) Measurement of health-related quality of life for people with dementia: Development of a new instrument (DEMQOL) and an evaluation of current methodology. Health Technology Assessment 9: 112.

Smith SC, Murray J, Banerjee S et al. (2005b) What constitutes heath-related quality of life in dementia? Development of a conceptual framework for people with dementia and their carers. International Journal of Geriatric Psychiatry 20: 889–95.

Smith SC, Lamping DL, Banerjee S et al. (2007) Development of a new measure of health-related quality of life for people with dementia: DEMQOL. Psychological Medicine 37: 737–46.

Snow A, Dani R, Souchek J et al. (2005) Comorbid psychosocial symptoms and quality of life in patients with dementia. American Journal of Geriatric Psychiatry 13: 393–401.

Spector A, Thorgrimsen L, Woods B et al. (2003) Efficacy of an evidence-based cognitive stimulation therapy programme for people with dementia. British Journal of Psychiatry 183: 248–54.

Sultzer DL, Davis SM, Tariot PN et al. (2008) Clinical symptom responses to atypical antipsychotic medications in Alzheimer's Disease: phase 1 outcomes from the CATIE-AD effectiveness trial. American Journal of Psychiatry 165: 844–54.

Takeda A, Loveman E, Clegg A et al. (2006) A systematic review of the clinical effectiveness of donepezil, rivastigmine and galantamine on cognition, quality of life and adverse events in Alzheimer's disease. International Journal of Geriatric Psychiatry 21: 17–28.

Taylor HA, Black BS, Rabins PV. (2008) Deciding in the best interest of clients with dementia: The experience of public guardians. Journal of Clinical Ethics 19: 120–6.

Terada S, Ishizu H, Fujisawa Y et al. (2002) Development and evaluation of a health-related quality of life questionnaire for the elderly with dementia in Japan. International Journal of Geriatric Psychiatry 17: 851–8.

Teri L, McCurry S, Logsdon R, Gibbons L. (2005) Training community consultants to help family members improve dementia care: A randomized controlled trial. The Gerontologist 45: 802–11.

Thornton A. (2004) Dementia Care Mapping reconsidered: Exploring the reliability and validity of the observational tool. International Journal of Geriatric Psychiatry 19: 718–26.

Trigg R, Jones RW, Skevington SM. (2007a) Can people with mild to moderate dementia provide reliable answers about their quality of life? Age and Ageing 36: 1–7.

Trigg R, Skevington S, Jones R. (2007b) How can we best assess the quality of life of people with dementia? The Bath Assessment of Subjective Quality of Life in Dementia (BASQID). The Gerontologist 47: 789–97.

Vogel A, Mortensen E, Hasselbalch S et al. (2006) Patient versus informant reported quality of life in the earliest phases of Alzheimer's disease. International Journal of Geriatric Psychiatry 21: 1132–8.

Walker MD, Salek SS, Bayer AJ. (1998) A review of quality of life in Alzheimer's Disease: Part 1: Issues in assessing disease impact. Pharmacoeconomics 14: 499–530.

Ware JE, Sherbourne CD. (1992) The MOS 36-item short-form health survey (SF-36). Medical Care 30: 473–83.

Weiner MF, Martin-Cook K, Svetlik DA et al. (2000) The quality of life in late-stage dementia (QUALID) scale. Journal of the American Medical Directors Association 1: 114–16.

Whitehouse P. (2006) Quality of life: The bridge from the cholinergic basal forebrain to cognitive science and bioethics. Journal of Alzheimer's Disease 9: 447–53.

Whitehouse PJ, Orgogozo J-M, Becker RE et al. (1997) Quality-of-life assessment in dementia drug development: Position paper from the International Working Group on Harmonization of Dementia Drug Guidelines. Alzheimer Disease and Associated Disorders 11: 56–60.

WHO QoL Group. (1995) WHO Quality of Life-100. Geneva: World Health Organization Division of Mental Health.

Winzelberg G, Williams C, Preisser J et al. (2005) Factors associated with nursing assistant quality-of-life ratings for residents with dementia in long-term care facilities. The Gerontologist 45: 106–14.

Woods B, Thorgrimsen L, Spector A, Royan L, Orrell M. (2006) Improved quality of life and cognitive stimulation therapy in dementia. Aging and Mental Health 10: 219–26.

Zimmerman S, Sloane PD, Williams CS et al. (2005) Dementia care and quality of life in assisted living and nursing homes. The Gerontologist 45: 133–46.

35

Ethical issues and dementia

JULIAN HUGHES

35.1 INTRODUCTION

Maurice O'Connor Drury, a psychiatrist, noted down many of his conversations with his friend and former teacher the philosopher Ludwig Wittgenstein. Thus, in 1947:

> You must always be puzzled by mental illness. The thing I would dread most, if I became mentally ill, would be your adopting a common sense attitude; that you could take it for granted that I was deluded.

> Drury (1981)

I want to use this idea in connection with dementia. Drury later published a collection of lectures in which he encouraged the thought that we should see that there is a mystery at the heart of mental illness: '… there will always be in psychiatry the realm of the inexplicable' (Drury, 1973). I want to suggest that our response to the ethical issues that arise in connection with dementia should be understood, in some sense, as reflecting the 'inexplicable' or puzzle raised by mental illness.

The different issues that arise for family carers of people with dementia, which cause ethical concerns, are legion (Baldwin et al., 2004). Each such issue (from confidentiality to truth-telling to wandering to research) deserves considerable thought, but there are unifying themes. I have lumped them together under four headings: destigmatizing dementia, diagnosis, decision-making and domestic concerns. (The topic of dying could be added, but is dealt with in Chapter 36, End-of-life decisions and dementia and Chapter 37, Care and management of the patient with advanced dementia.) Each heading might be regarded as mundane, in the sense of raising purely practical or procedural matters but, in each case, I want

to suggest that there is also a puzzle, something that points in the direction of the inexplicable. This might give us the right perspective to negotiate the ethical difficulties that arise in connection with dementia.

35.2 DESTIGMATIZING DEMENTIA

A great deal is spoken about the stigma that attends dementia. It should be regarded broadly. It is not just that services for people with dementia often take a low priority, nor is it just that expenditure on research on dementia is lower than it ought to be, nor is it simply that people with dementia on a medical ward might be regarded as a nuisance if they wander and so forth. Stigma is also obvious in everyday encounters, where people with dementia can be treated in ways that signal they are regarded as a nuisance: by the general public, but also by professionals making off-hand remarks (Alzheimer's Society, 2008). At a personal level, people with dementia and their carers report how friends stop visiting once the diagnosis is known (see Chapter 2, The lived experience of dementia). Insidiously, the stigma is internalized, so that many people with dementia also feel they are useless. Even those who care the most, family and friends, can end up acting in ways that undermine the standing of the person with dementia.

Sabat has captured this tendency by using the phrase 'malignant positioning' (Sabat, 2006). This draws on the earlier work of Tom Kitwood and his talk of 'malignant social psychology' (Kitwood, 1997). The person loses abilities to do even everyday things, not because of organic brain pathology, but because of societal responses. Then the person not only has to put up with the brain pathology, but also with the social and psychological environment in which people accept it is inevitable that he or she will be incompetent. This is not 'malignant' because the people concerned are evil, but because – by undermining the person's sense of self – the effects of the brain disease are compounded. Taking over tasks, presuming the person does not understand, talking over the person, ignoring or infantilizing – these are all ways in which the person can be positioned negatively.

The insidious thing is that much of this can seem perfectly ordinary. It is accepted that the person with dementia may no longer have meaningful contributions to make. The focus becomes their cognitive impairment and presumed general incompetence. The end result is a lack of real respect for the person because of, what Post (2006) has called, our 'hyper-cognitive' society.

This brings us to the crux of the first ethical theme, which underlies the issue of stigma in many of its guises, namely that, in some sense, it is presumed (it is the taken-for-granted 'common sense attitude' that Wittgenstein dreaded perhaps) that the person has been lost in dementia. Thus people talk about the loss of the biographical self and the continuance of the purely biological self in dementia, with all of the ethical ramifications that this entails. Stigma actually both encourages and stems from the thought that the person is no longer a person. We need to plant, or reaffirm, the idea that the person persists in a variety of ways that should remain morally compelling.

Kitwood (1997) emphasized the importance of person-centred care as a way to affirm the person as a person, to show that he or she remains valued as an individual with a unique perspective and social environment; this in turn has led to dementia care mapping, an observational practice that is intended to improve the quality of care (Brooker, 2007). There is now a host of work to attest to the continued possibilities for people (as persons) with dementia. The Dementia Advocacy and Support Network, for instance, an open access website run by people with dementia for people with dementia, contains lists of books written by people with dementia charting their experience (see www.dasninterna-tional.org). There is also the observation of 'lucid episodes', when people with dementia who have not spoken in a coherent way for some while, suddenly say something that is completely lucid and relevant (Normann et al., 1998). Then there is the possibility that more attention to communication might help to maintain the person's standing as a self, that contact can be made with people even in the severe stages of the disease (Allan and Killick, 2010). Communication has been key to the development of the work of Sabat, who has shown convincingly that in moderate to severe dementia people still convey meaning (Sabat and Harré, 1994). Subsequently, Sabat (2001) has been able to expand his critique of a narrow view of dementia to show how selfhood can be maintained by various means.

This takes us on to the second justification for the idea that the person persists in a variety of ways. This is a philosophical justification and it depends on seeing personhood not just in terms of cognitive abilities, but also in terms of emotional, volitional, bodily and psychosocial aspects, where (indeed) the possibilities for personhood are not circumscribed. Crucially, personhood is situated in place, culture, history, personal narrative, moral and spiritual fields, family and social networks and so forth (Hughes, 2001; Hughes et al., 2006). The upshot is that personhood, even in severe dementia, can be held by others. Furthermore, this theoretical stance turns out to have practical application in the work of Sabat (2001) and others (e.g. Stokes, 2000). In brief, the psychosocial environment turns out to be potent, which reflects puzzling aspects of our standing as people; for it implies that in some mysterious way we exist in communion with others. The Zulu notion of our interconnectedness, ubuntu, is apposite: a person is a person among others (Battle, 1997).

Our first ethical theme, therefore, is that of stigma. The mundane attitude is to regard stigma as almost inevitable given the nature of this brain disease; but the corrective is to see the possibilities of personhood, which help to reveal something inexplicable. For what it is to be a person cannot be pinned down. In a puzzling way, our mutual inter-dependency and our bodily situated nature as human beings mean that part of our reality is held in being by others.

35.3   DIAGNOSIS

The second theme concerns several issues to do with diagnosis. At the mundane level, there is the issue of whether or not to tell the person the diagnosis. Even though practice is not uniform, in the literature the consensus seems to be that people should be told the diagnosis honestly (Bamford et al., 2004). This then raises an issue about how to tell people the diagnosis (Whitehouse et al., 2004). Part of the worry is that telling people the diagnosis might cause upset, anxiety and, in a small proportion, suicidal thoughts and actions (Haw et al., 2009). In fact, the risk of suicide, which is low overall for people with dementia, is increased soon after diagnosis; one putative risk factor is mild cognitive impairment (MCI; Haw et al., 2009).

While on the face of it there is little here that needs to raise insurmountable ethical concerns, in practice it remains the case that discerning whether, when and how to tell someone the diagnosis remains difficult. This reflects the need to understand people individually, so that the success of diagnostic disclosure will depend on the quality of the therapeutic alliance, which may have to be established relatively quickly. The nature of real empathy has an inexplicability about it that is puzzling. Establishing a deeper relationship, especially in the context of dementia, will not always be straightforward. So telling the diagnosis will not always be uncontroversial and may be ethically problematic.

Other ethical and philosophical concerns are raised in connection with the 'diagnosis' of MCI, which has already been mentioned in connection with suicide. Once again, the problem can be regarded in a 'common sense' way. When a person has dementia, the diagnosis should be made in order for the person to access appropriate help and support; and this should not be delayed, because help will be required. The next step in the (mundane) argument is to say that the sooner help can be given the better. Indeed, if a pre-dementia stage could be defined, it might be that help could be given even sooner, which would be a good thing if it alleviates suffering (incidentally, it might also increase profits for drug companies). MCI is now regarded as the pre-dementia phase and there is intense interest in trying to find a treatment that works in this phase that might put off or prevent the illness from progressing.

The scientific standing of MCI is now seemingly well established (see Chapter 43, Mild cognitive impairment: a historical perspective, Chapter 44, Clinical characteristics of mild cognitive impairment and Chapter 45, Managing the patient with mild cognitive impairment). However, the worry about the 'diagnosis' of MCI being given to people where this leads to anxious uncertainty is real, as is the stigma. In a qualitative study, Corner and Bond (2006) described the case of Rose, who was given the 'diagnosis' of something that was 'very mild, not really dementia'. Her husband, Ron, put matters in this way:

> When we were told that Rose had this dementia we were just devastated, that's the only word for it. Our world came crashing down around us and … we cried for days. We couldn't bring ourselves to talk to … the kids … or anyone about it. It was too shameful for Rose. She didn't want anyone to know. … That was oh, eighteen months ago now, and really she's no different to then. But every time she's even a bit forgetful, we're thinking "Is this it then?", even though we're not quite sure what "it" is or will be. … We've just been turned upside down by it. … You picture these people who are vegetables … it's horrific'.

It has to be recognized, too, that MCI is a construct and one that reflects different values and serves a number of possible social purposes (Graham and Ritchie, 2006; Moreira *et al.*, 2008). Others have questioned not only MCI, but the diagnosis of Alzheimer's disease (AD) itself (Whitehouse and George, 2008). It can be argued that any diagnosis requires an evaluative decision, being not just a matter of facts, but of facts and values (Fulford, 1989). This suggests that the biological and clinical standing of MCI should not be accepted too readily without further consideration of its value commitments. It raises important questions about the values that underpin our ascriptions of normal and abnormal ageing. MCI raises broader themes to do with how we see our lives in old age. This realization raises a question about labels as such and, in particular, in connection with AD:

> … perhaps it is time to reflect on the individual and social advantages and disadvantages of these labels on the continuum of cognitive aging. The process of social deconstruction (i.e. ending AD as a label) cannot eliminate the suffering that accompanies the loss of cognitive capacity … We need to imagine different, perhaps wiser, visions and values about aging processes in our brains that respect our limits as mortal creatures and as scientists. Perhaps by pursuing this exercise in humility we can recognize that, although some suffering may be inevitable in life, the stories we tell about brain aging can dramatically affect the quality of our lives and of our deaths.

Whitehouse (2006)

We might 'take it for granted' that a diagnosis has to be made, but there is a normative judgement involved in deciding that anything is a disease (Sadler, 2005). When we are considering age-related disorders, the normative judgement turns out to be about our lives as such, about what constitutes normal and abnormal ageing and about how this is to be determined. While this neither seems as if it ought to be decided on the basis of fact, nor is it clearly a matter of fact. In which case, it needs to be negotiated. It needs, however, to be negotiated in a way that is useful to the people involved. But what is and is not MCI, or even AD, cannot simply be 'taken for granted'; rather we should be puzzled by the ways in which our normative decisions about diagnoses shape our lives, but are shaped by them too.

35.4 DECISION-MAKING

There is much that could be said about decision-making. Many carers give descriptions of how difficult it is to take over from the person with dementia. When taking over is done too soon it amounts to Sabat's 'malignant positioning', where the person with dementia is regarded as incompetent. But it can also be said that the issue of incompetence is, actually, the core ethical difficulty in dementia. In England and Wales, the legal approach to these difficulties is set out in the Mental Capacity Act 2005 (MCA). The central plank of this approach is to establish whether or not the person has capacity and, if the person lacks capacity, then decisions must be made in the person's best interests. The mundane view is simply to believe that following the legal algorithms suggested by the MCA might be enough to ensure that the right thing is done.

However, in practice it turns out that none of these steps is straightforward (Hughes, 2007). One element in judging capacity, for instance, is that the person should be able to weigh matters up. But this overlooks the extent to which we all weigh things from different perspectives, using different scales. In any case, one of the basic principles of the MCA is that people should be allowed to make unwise decisions; but where a lack of wisdom ends and a failure to weigh up properly begins is not clear. Moreover, it is not self-evident that decision-making capacity is wholly a matter of cognitive skills; it may, for instance, involve emotion too (Charland, 1998).

Meanwhile, the concept of 'best interests' is also highly problematic, because it can be decided subjectively or objectively and no decision about someone's best interests can be regarded as impervious to challenge. Although it is sometimes stated that I can know my own best interests, this depends on a stipulative definition, namely that my own best interests are whatever I say they are. If this definition is accepted, then (as long as I can state them) my best interests are clear. But why should the definition be accepted, if (for instance) I say that my best interests are served by my continuing to drink alcohol when I'm already drunk? How much more complex, then, if my best interests have to be determined when I cannot state them, but where I might already have made some relevant statements, for instance in an advance directive (Hughes and Sabat, 2008)?

The mundane point is that decision-making for people with cognitive impairment is a matter of following legally prescribed procedures; but the corrective is to see that (in addition to the legal steps) ethical, value-laden, emotionally-driven, evaluative decisions must also be made. The complexity that then emerges, which causes us to puzzle when faced by decisions that look as if they should be routine, is related to the complexity that surrounds personhood, where some features of our lives are perhaps cognitively inexplicable.

35.5   DOMESTIC CONCERNS

The fourth ethical theme is to do with care and accommodation. The environment matters for people with dementia. This includes the social environment where communication, verbal and non-verbal, helps to define the quality of the social space. The mundane ethical issue is not without great significance: how should people with dementia be looked after? Especially given demographic predictions, it becomes imperative that action is taken to improve the standards of accommodation and care; in addition there should be different types of care so that people have real choices. Whether this includes care at home in the community or care in institutional settings, there is a moral imperative that the quality of care should be good. Partly on account of stigma, much of what passes for dementia care takes place away from public view and, at least in the UK, standards can be unacceptably low (Ballard et al., 2001).

The manner in which it is decided that people require long-term care also needs consideration. This brings to the fore the underlying moral concern, which is (once again) that people should be regarded personally, that is, as individual people. And, as we have already discussed, this requires that we accept the broad view of personhood in dementia (Hughes, 2001). Hence, when decisions have to be made – often acting in the person's best interests – they should be made with a broad perspective. Details of the person's values and previous wishes, as well as their current inclinations, need to be taken into account; but so do the views of others involved in the person's care.

Once again, the corrective turns out to be the notion of personhood, which should induce a sense of puzzlement (because decisions cannot be taken for granted) in all those determined to do the right thing. A sense, too, of outrage if people are being looked after in conditions that do not encourage dignity or the possibility of living life as fully as possible. The inclination to care should itself be taken to gesture at something inexplicable: even in frail and heavily dependent lives there is something worthwhile that has a natural tendency to draw from us instincts of compassion and genuine (ethical) concern.

35.6   CONCLUSION

I have discussed some of the ethical issues that arise in dementia. I have suggested that our response to the ethical issues can be understood as reflecting puzzling aspects of our humanity, which at least point in the direction of the inexplicable. It is our standing as people in the normative, evaluative human world, even when we have dementia, which seems fundamental. And looking in the direction of what it is to be a person – where this reveals not only our desire for autonomy, but also our inevitable dependency – should help to give us the right perspective and allow us to negotiate the numerous ethical difficulties that arise in connection with dementia (Hughes and Baldwin, 2006).

REFERENCES

Allan K, Killick J. (2010) Communicating with people with dementia. In: Hughes JC, Lloyd-Williams M, Sachs GA (eds). *Supportive care for the person with dementia*. Oxford: Oxford University Press, 217–25.

Alzheimer's Society. (2008) *Out of the shadows*. London: Alzheimer's Society.

Baldwin C, Hope T, Hughes J et al. (2004) Ethics and dementia: the experience of family carers. *Progress in Neurology and Psychiatry* **8**: 24–8.

Ballard C, Fossey J, Chithramohan R et al. (2001) Quality of care in private sector and NHS facilities for people with dementia: cross sectional survey. *British Medical Journal* **323**: 426–7.

Bamford C, Lamont S, Eccles M et al. (2004) Disclosing a diagnosis of dementia: a systematic review. *International Journal of Geriatric Psychiatry* **19**: 151–69.

Battle M. (1997) *Reconciliation – The Ubuntu theology of Desmond Tutu*. Cleveland, Ohio: The Pilgrim Press.

Brooker D. (2007) *Person-centred dementia care: making services better*. London: Jessica Kingsley.

Charland LC. (1998) Appreciation and emotion: theoretical reflections on the MacArthur Treatment Competence Study. *Kennedy Institute of Ethics Journal* **8**: 359–76.

Corner L, Bond J. (2006) The impact of the label of mild cognitive impairment on the individual's sense of self. *Philosophy, Psychiatry, and Psychology* **13**: 3–12.

Drury MO'C. (1973) *The danger of words*. London and New York: Routledge and Kegan Paul.

Drury MO'C. (1981) Conversations with Wittgenstein. In: Rhees R (ed.) *Ludwig Wittgenstein: personal recollections*. Oxford: Blackwell, 112–89.

Fulford KWM. (1989) *Moral theory and medical practice*. Cambridge: Cambridge University Press.

Graham JE, Ritchie K. (2006) Mild cognitive impairment: ethical considerations for nosological flexibility in human kinds. *Philosophy, Psychiatry, and Psychology* **13**: 31–43.

Haw C, Harwood D, Hawton K. (2009) Dementia and suicidal behavior: a review of the literature. *International Psychogeriatrics* **21**: 440–53.

Hughes JC. (2001) Views of the person with dementia. *Journal of Medical Ethics* **27**: 86–91.

Hughes JC. (2007) Ethical issues and health care for older people. In: Ashcroft RE, Dawson A, Draper H, McMillan JR (eds). *Principles of health care ethics*, 2nd edn. Chichester: John Wiley and Sons, 469–74.

Hughes JC, Baldwin C. (2006) *Ethical issues in dementia care: making difficult decisions*. London: Jessica Kingsley.

Hughes JC, Sabat SR. (2008) The advance directive conjuring trick and the person with dementia. In: Widdershoven GAM, McMillan J, Hope T, van der Scheer L (eds). *Empirical ethics in psychiatry*. Oxford: Oxford University Press, 123–40.

Hughes JC, Louw SJ, Sabat SR. (eds) (2006) *Dementia: mind, meaning, and the person*. Oxford: Oxford University Press.

Kitwood T. (1997) *Dementia reconsidered: the person comes first*. Buckingham: Open University Press.

Moreira T, Hughes JC, Kirkwood T *et al*. (2008) What explains variations in the clinical use of mild cognitive impairment (MCI) as a diagnostic category? *International Psychogeriatrics* **20**: 697–709.

Normann HK, Asplund K, Norberg A. (1998) Episodes of lucidity in people with severe dementia as narrated by formal carers. *Journal of Advanced Nursing* **28**: 1295–300.

Post SG. (2006) *Respectare*: moral respect for the lives of the deeply forgetful. In: Hughes JC, Louw SL, Sabat SR (eds). *Dementia: mind, meaning, and the person*. Oxford: Oxford University Press, 223–34.

Sabat SR. (2001) *The experience of Alzheimer's disease: Life through a tangled veil*. Oxford: Blackwell.

Sabat SR. (2006) Mind, meaning, and personhood in dementia: the effects of positioning. In: Hughes JC, Louw SL, Sabat SR (eds). *Dementia: mind, meaning, and the person*. Oxford: Oxford University Press, 287–302.

Sabat SR, Harré R. (1994) The Alzheimer's disease sufferer as a semiotic subject. *Philosophy, Psychiatry, and Psychology* **1**: 145–60.

Sadler JZ. (2005) *Values and psychiatric diagnosis*. Oxford: Oxford University Press.

Stokes G. (2000) *Challenging behaviour in dementia: a person-centred approach*. Bicester: Winslow Press.

Whitehouse PJ. (2006) Demystifying the mystery of Alzheimer's as late, no longer MCI. *Philosophy, Psychiatry, and Psychology* **13**: 87–8.

Whitehouse PJ, George DR. (2008) *The myth of Alzheimer's: what you aren't being told about today's most dreaded diagnosis*. New York: St. Martin's Press.

Whitehouse P, Frisoni GB, Post S. (2004) Breaking the diagnosis of dementia. *Lancet Neurology* **3**: 124–8.

to the basic principles of medical ethics, namely beneficence and non-maleficence. Since in most cases physicians would be guided by these basic principles, why would we wish to deviate from them in someone with severe dementia?

Thinking in this way suggests the doctrine of ordinary and extraordinary means. Thus, we are not morally bound to use those means that would be regarded as extraordinary in the sense that they are unlikely to work and might be burdensome. On the whole, we wish to keep people with severe dementia out of acute hospitals, but some treatments (e.g. for fractures) may be effective in terms of relieving pain and distress. Nevertheless, in someone who is already immobile through severe dementia, surgery intended to enable the person to walk would be otiose.

Withholding and withdrawing treatment will also often require the exercise of a number of virtues. Compassion is a basic virtue in health care, but there is also the virtue of fidelity. If, for instance, we know that the person has particular religious beliefs, we are true to the person by ensuring that these are not transgressed. Similarly, the virtues of bravery and steadfastness are required in the face of pressure, for instance, to admit someone to an acute hospital where palliative care in the person's own environment would be the best option. These decisions often require a form of selfless courage. It is certainly not always easy to be virtuous.

36.3.3   Artificial nutrition and hydration

It has been accepted for some years that the available evidence suggests that tube feeding in dementia is not appropriate. Tube feeding in advanced dementia does not produce its intended goals. It does not reduce the risk of aspiration pneumonia, nor of malnutrition; nor does it encourage survival, prevent pressure sores, decrease the risk of other infections, increase functional status or comfort. Meanwhile, for people with dementia there is a significant mortality associated with percutaneous endoscopic gastrostomy (PEG) tube insertion. Hence, there seems to be no ethical reason to pursue artificial nutrition and hydration in people with severe dementia. There may, however, be exceptions, where the cause of the dysphagia is thought to be temporary, rather than evidence that the dementia has reached the severe stage in which dysphagia becomes increasingly common.

An expert group (Gillette Guyonnet et al., 2007) pointed out that the consequences of weight loss and altered nutritional status are important. Poor nutrition can itself worsen cognitive impairment; it leads to a loss of independence and institutionalization; and it is associated with mortality. In general, hand-feeding is probably more appropriate at the end of life, where this also provides the potential benefits of human contact. Yet, it may be that nutritional status requires much greater consideration in the milder stages of dementia in order to avoid later consequences, which tend to worsen quality of life.

36.3.4   Antibiotics

One of the great pioneers of palliative care for people with dementia is Ladislav Volicer (Volicer and Hurley, 1998). He helped to establish the view that antibiotic use in severe dementia might do no more good than simple analgesia and antipyretics and might even do harm. More recently (van der Steen et al., 2002a), pneumonia was associated with considerable discomfort, which was worse in those people with dementia from whom antibiotics were withheld; who, however, were the group in whom pneumonia was worse at baseline. A study by the same Dutch group showed that most physicians tended to treat pneumonias with antibiotics: 69 per cent with curative and 8 per cent with palliative intentions (van der Steen et al., 2002b). In those 23 per cent of patients with more severe dementia, more severe pneumonia, where the patients had poorer food and fluid intake and more evidence of dehydration, antibiotics were withheld. Thus, physicians seemed to be making judgements about whether or not infections were terminal.

There is, therefore, some similarity between the issues raised in connection with artificial nutrition and hydration and those raised by the use of antibiotics. There is the general casuistic point, which is that cases have to be judged individually, with the particularities taken into consideration. This emphasizes the overarching importance of the virtue of practical wisdom, which contributes to the background (external) horizon with which our patterns of practice must cohere. The Aristotelian virtue of practical wisdom, or phronesis, is also understood as prudence: keeping in view the broader aims of treatment and applying them to the particular case at hand.

36.3.5   Advance care planning

One of the cornerstones of palliative and supportive care is advance care planning. Particularly in dementia it would seem to be an extremely good idea that people should set out their thoughts, which may be general as in an advance statement, or may be particular as in an advance refusal of treatment. In many ways, the issues that I have discussed above are complicated precisely because we do not know the wishes of the person concerned. So we have to rely on clinical judgements about what might be in the person's best interests, or we are thrown back on proxy decision-making by friends and family. Advance care planning at least gives us some indication as to the wishes of the person him or herself. However, advance directives are problematic (Hughes, 2008; Hughes and Sabat, 2008). The main issue is to do with the applicability of any advance directive. The issue of validity, whether the advance directive was actually made by the person concerned, is obviously extremely important. But applicability is harder to judge. Things may have changed between the advance directive being made and the circumstances arising in which it should or should not be put into effect. One of the things that may well have changed is the person concerned. There is, then, a tension between the person's previous wishes and what might be their present wishes. An ethical approach would seem to be a pattern of practice that tries to establish some balance between the person's previous and present wishes. A sensible tactic is to involve those close to the person whose views should carry considerable weight.

Advance care planning involves more than advance directives. It may be that the person has appointed an attorney to make decisions about their health and general welfare. Even so, this does not absolve health-care professionals from making their own judgements concerning what might be best for their patients. It may be that those holding a power of attorney require more information or advice in order for them to make the best decision for the person concerned. And, albeit rarely, it may be that legal measures should be pursued if the attorney's decisions are deemed malicious. Nonetheless, in general it would seem to be worthwhile to encourage some form of advance care planning and the sooner the process is started in dementia the better (Hertogh, 2006; Gillick, 2010). Having said this, the tensions implicit in advance care planning have to be acknowledged. Given the complexity of the decisions that are faced, advance care planning has to be a mutual endeavour involving the patient and the clinician, but also probably involving close (usually family) carers. Under such circumstances, the tension is between whether the clinician should be, to some degree, paternalistic; or whether they should honour the person's autonomous decisions (Hertogh, 2010). Once again, it might be that the notion of patterns of practice helps. Under what circumstances do I simply follow the wishes of my patient? Under what circumstances do I take control and act in their best interests? Under what circumstances is it honest, prudent and true to the patient to do his or her bidding and under what circumstances is it not?

36.4 CONCLUSION: THE AUTHENTIC CADENCE

This last question raises again the issue of dying and how we might make the end ring true. The issue of assisted dying – euthanasia or physician-assisted suicide – inevitably arises, although why this should be considered for people with dementia when it has not become a reality for other people is both a puzzle and a worry. People sometimes argue against assisted dying that, if it were legal, older people would feel in some way obliged to consider it. This argument tends to be given short shrift; so it is ironic that it is then suggested that people with dementia have some sort of duty to die because of the pressures caused by our ageing societies. The advocates of assisted dying appeal to autonomy and dignity. But those who oppose them point to basic instincts around caring and against the dismantling of prohibitions that have underpinned civil society. After all, none of us is wholly autonomous; and there is a type of dignity that reflects our standing as human beings as such. To contemplate the intentional killing of people with dementia raises ethical concerns, even for those who might otherwise support such moves (Hertogh *et al.*, 2007).

A pattern of practice around the very end of life that is to be authentic must square with our other practices of care in which the aim is not death, but life. Of course, death has to be accepted as part of the reality of life. But the aim of palliative and supportive care is to make life as good as possible while neither hastening nor postponing death. If the virtues are about living well, they are also about dealing with death in a way that shows fortitude, honesty, courage and charity. To suggest that human flourishing should have as its aim the extinction of innocent human life does not ring true when this is compared with the possibilities and implications inherent to care and compassion. The authentic cadence in dementia is, after all, often soft: a fading away rather than a dramatic ending – a natural peace rather than an inflicted death.

REFERENCES

Cipher DJ, Clifford PA. (2004) Dementia, pain, depression, behavioral disturbances, and ADLs: toward a comprehensive conceptualization of quality of life in long-term care. *International Journal of Geriatric Psychiatry* 19: 741–8.

Gillette Guyonnet GS, Abellan Van Kan G, Alix E *et al.* (2007) IANA (International Academy on Nutrition and Aging) expert group: weight loss and Alzheimer's disease. *The Journal of Nutrition, Health and Aging* 11: 38–48.

Gillick MR. (2010) Advance care planning: an American view. In: Hughes JC, Lloyd-Williams M, Sachs GA (eds). *Supportive care for the person with dementia*. Oxford: Oxford University Press, 263–70.

Herr K, Coyne PJ, Key T *et al.* (2006) Pain assessment in the nonverbal patient: position statement with clinical practice recommendations. *Pain Management Nursing* 7: 44–52.

Hertogh CM. (2006) Advance care planning and the relevance of a palliative care approach in dementia. *Age and Ageing* 35: 553–5.

Hertogh C. (2010) Advance care planning and palliative care in dementia: a view from the Netherlands. In: Hughes JC, Lloyd-Williams M, Sachs GA (eds). *Supportive care for the person with dementia*. Oxford: Oxford University Press, 271–80.

Hertogh CMPM, de Boer ME, Dröes R-M, Eefsting JA. (2007) Would we rather lose our life than lose our self? Lessons from the Dutch debate on euthanasia for patients with dementia. *American Journal of Bioethics* 7: 48–56.

Hughes JC. (ed.) (2006a) *Palliative care in severe dementia*. London: Quay Books.

Hughes JC. (2006b) Patterns of practice: a useful notion in medical ethics? *Journal of Ethics in Mental Health* 1: 1–5. Available via www.jemh.ca

Hughes JC. (2008) Assessment of competency and advance directives. In: Stoppe G (eds). *Competence assessment in dementia*. Wien, New York: Springer-Verlag, 77–84.

Hughes JC, Sabat SR. (2008) The advance directive conjuring trick and the person with dementia. In: Widdershoven GAM, McMillan J, Hope T, van der Scheer L (eds). *Empirical ethics in psychiatry*. Oxford: Oxford University Press, 123–40.

Hughes JC, Robinson L, Volicer L. (2005) Specialist palliative care in dementia. *British Medical Journal* 330: 57–8.

Hughes JC, Jolley D, Jordan A, Sampson EL. (2007) Palliative care in dementia: issues and evidence. *Advances in Psychiatric Treatment* 13: 251–60.

Jordan A, Lloyd-Williams M. (2010) Distress and pain in dementia. In: Hughes JC, Lloyd-Williams M, Sachs GA (eds). *Supportive care for the person with dementia*. Oxford: Oxford University Press, 129–37.

Louw SJ, Hughes JC. (2005) Moral reasoning – the unrealized place of casuistry in medical ethics. *International Psychogeriatrics* **17**: 149–54.

Pointon B. (2007) Who am I? – the search for spirituality in dementia. A family carer's perspective. In: Coyte ME, Gilbert P, Nicholls V (eds). *Spirituality, values and mental health*. London: Jessica Kingsley, 114–20.

Robinson L, Hughes JC, Daley S *et al.* (2005) End-of-life care and dementia. *Reviews in Clinical Gerontology* **15**: 135–48.

Sampson EL, Ritchie CW, Lai R *et al.* (2005) A systematic review of the scientific evidence for the efficacy of a palliative care approach in advanced dementia. *International Psychogeriatrics* **17**: 31–40.

Sampson EL, Gould V, Lee D, Blanchard MR. (2006) Differences in care received by patients with and without dementia who died during acute hospital admission: a retrospective case note study. *Age and Ageing* **35**: 187–9.

Sampson EL, Blanchard MR, Jones L *et al.* (2009) Dementia in the acute hospital: prospective cohort study of prevalence and mortality. *British Journal of Psychiatry* **195**: 61–6.

Shega JW, Sachs GA. (2010) Offering supportive care in dementia: reflections on the PEACE programme. In: Hughes JC, Lloyd-Williams M, Sachs GA (eds). *Supportive care for the person with dementia*. Oxford: Oxford University Press, 33–44.

Small N, Downs M, Froggatt K. (2006) Improving end-of-life care for people with dementia – the benefits of combining UK approaches to palliative care and dementia care. In: Miesen BML, Jones GMM (eds). *Care-giving in dementia – research and application*, Volume 4. London and New York: Routledge, 365–92.

Small N, Froggatt K, Downs M. (2007) *Living and dying with dementia: dialogues about palliative care*. Oxford: Oxford University Press.

van der Steen JT, Ooms ME, Ader HJ *et al.* (2002a) Withholding antibiotic treatment in pneumonia patients with dementia: a quantitative observational study. *Archives of Internal Medicine* **162**: 1753–60.

van der Steen JT, Ooms ME, Mehr DR *et al.* (2002b) Severe dementia and adverse outcomes of nursing home-acquired pneumonia: evidence for mediation by functional and pathophysiological decline. *Journal of the American Geriatrics Society* **50**: 439–48.

Volicer L, Hurley A. (1998) *Hospice care for patients with advanced progressive dementia*. New York, NY: Springer Publishing Company.

Zwakhalen SM, Hamers JPH, Abu-Saad HH, Berger MPF. (2006) Pain in elderly people with severe dementia: a systematic review of behavioural pain assessment tools. *BMC Geriatrics* **6**: 3.

Care and management of the patient with advanced dementia

PETER V RABINS AND BETTY S BLACK

37.1 INTRODUCTION

Many of the distinctions among the illnesses that cause the syndrome of dementia become blurred or disappear in advanced or late stage dementia for several reasons. First, neuropathological abnormalities become so widespread that almost all brain systems that subserve cognition and function become impaired. A second and related issue is that the widespread involvement of subcortical or 'downstream' structures and systems results in widespread and near total dysfunction of 'upstream' cognitive and motor systems that are not directly involved by neuropathology. Thus, this chapter will approach late stage or advanced dementia as a single or common end point of all the dementias even though some distinctions, for example the frequency of myoclonus and seizures, do persist. Thus, while knowledge of the unique aspects of specific diseases plays a prominent role in the care of people with dementia in the earlier stages of the dementia, this is usually not the case in late-stage dementia (Robinson *et al.*, 2006).

37.2 IMPAIRMENTS ARISING DIRECTLY FROM THE DEMENTIA

Gait disorder resulting from pyramidal, extrapyramidal, accessory motor, visuo-spatial and executive function disorder greatly increases the risk of falls in those who are still ambulatory. Most individuals eventually become unable to ambulate without assistance and many become fully bed-bound no matter what steps are taken whatever the aetiology. For parallel reasons, many individuals develop generalized spasticity and rigidity and experience a marked limitation in the ability to generate spontaneous movement. These impairments predispose to skin breakdown and the development of pressure or decubitus ulcers.

Disordered swallowing also becomes almost universal due to primary involvement of bulbar and cortico-bulbar tracts. Sometimes referred to as a dyspraxia of swallowing, this limits oral intake, impairs normal swallowing, and leads to malnutrition, aspiration of food and secretions into the lungs and aspiration pneumonia. Weight loss and loss of muscle mass, compounded by loss of subcutaneous tissue and immune system impairment, increase the risk of developing frailty and a cascade of declining health that includes increased risk of fracture and the development of skin breakdown.

Loss of meaningful speech due to impaired motor control of speech, apraxia of speech and aphasia markedly impairs the ability to communicate. These impairments not only cause an inability to report recent events or to describe pain or depression but can also result in a distancing of the patient from care providers and loved ones because speech is so crucial to interpersonal communication. Inability to verbally report pain is a particular challenge. As a result, pain should be included in the differential diagnosis of restlessness, calling out, directed or random striking out and distressed facial appearance. Gaze palsies, apraxia of eye movement and severe visuo-spatial impairment result in the patient's not looking at people in the environment and an inability to look at feeding utensils or other environmental activities. This further impairs social connectedness with people and increases the risk of falling, poor oral intake and social isolation.

Seizures occur in 10 per cent of people with Alzheimer's disease (AD) and are more common in vascular dementia. Myoclonus, the sudden contraction of large muscle groups results in jerking movement of the limbs, trunk and head. It rarely presents a safety risk but can be frightening to the patient and their carers.

Neuropsychiatric and behavioural symptoms remain common in late-stage disease. In a recent study of 123 individuals with late stage disease, Kverno et al. (2008) reported a high prevalence of aggression or agitation (50.4 per cent), depression (45.5 per cent) and withdrawal and lethargy (43.1 per cent). Determining symptom precipitants and aetiology becomes even more challenging in late-stage patients due to the physical and cognitive impairments described above. Hallucinations and delusions may require pharmacotherapy if associated with distress or risk of harm, but can often be treated with non-pharmacologic approaches.

37.3   CO-MORBID MEDICAL ILLNESS

Multi-system medical problems are common due to the advanced age of most individuals as well as the dementia. The majority of patients in one series had problems with skin (95.1 per cent), nutrition/hydration (85.4 per cent), the gastrointestinal system (80.5 per cent), infection (79.7 per cent), genitourinary or gynaecologic systems (73.2 per cent), pain (63.4 per cent) or the musculoskeletal system (61.0 per cent; Black et al., 2006).

37.4   UNIQUE ETHICAL DILEMMAS

Ethical dilemmas present throughout the course of dementia and are discussed in Chapter 35, Ethical issues and dementia and Chapter 36, End-of-life decisions and dementia. One challenge of late-stage care is that even when individuals have previously expressed wishes for end-stage or terminal care, those expressions of wishes are usually separated by many months or years from the actual event and the person has lost all possibility of comprehending and therefore participating in revising or changing their wishes in consideration of circumstances they had not foreseen. In the United States, unique criteria for hospice care eligibility have been developed as a result of the assumed difficulty in estimating six month life expectancy (the primary criterion of hospice benefits). Almost half of individuals with late-stage dementia die from pneumonia, with aspiration being the genesis in a majority of cases. This raises the question of whether and when pneumonia should be treated with antibiotics in late-stage disease, whether scientifically unproven steps should be taken to limit the risk of aspiration and questions about the placement of PEG tubes in patients no longer able to swallow or maintain adequate calorie intake. The purpose and efficacy of medications for the cognitive symptoms of dementia and for chronic medical conditions such as anti-coagulants, lipid-lowering agents and cognition enhancement also deserves attention. Hospice care services for people with dementia have become more available in many countries in recent years and provide an important care option for many individuals (Rabins et al., 2006).

REFERENCES

Black B, Finucane T, Baker A et al. (2006) Health problems and correlates of pain in nursing home residents with advanced dementia. *Alzheimer Disease and Associated Disorders* **20**: 283–90.

Kverno K, Rabins P, Blass D et al. (2008) Prevalence and treatment of neuropsychiatric symptoms in advanced dementia. *Journal of Gerontological Nursing* **34**: 8–15.

Rabins PV, Lyketsos CG, Steele CD (2006) Terminal Care. In: *Practical dementia care*, 2nd edn. London and New York, Oxford University Press, 241–50.

Robinson L, Hughes J, Daley S et al. (2006) End-of-life care and dementia. *Reviews in Clinical Gerontology* **15**: 135–48.

38

Alzheimer associations and societies

HENRY BRODATY AND MARIKA DONKIN

38.1 INTRODUCTION

Alzheimer disease associations are voluntary organizations that advocate on behalf of people with dementia and their carers. The growth in these associations has been brought about by the quantum leap of public awareness about Alzheimer's disease (AD) and related disorders, particularly in developed countries. The rise in public awareness has occurred as a result of a number of converging factors.

The first is the landmark study of Blessed *et al.* (1968) that identified AD as a disease. Prior to this study, the symptoms of AD had been considered part of normal ageing and AD itself regarded as a relatively rare condition.

The second factor is the 'greying' of the world's population, age being the major risk factor for dementia. Average life expectancy in developed countries is currently greater than 75 years for males and 80 years for women (Central Intelligence Agency, 2009). At least 8 per cent of the world's population is aged 65 years and older, and in the UK people aged 65 years and over comprise 16 per cent of the population (Central Intelligence Agency, 2009). In Sweden, this figure has reached over 18 per cent (Central Intelligence Agency, 2009). There are estimated to be over 35 million people with dementia worldwide in 2010, rising to 65 million by 2030 and 115 million by 2050 (Alzheimer's Disease International, 2009a).

Third, there has been increasing public awareness of dementia and AD, and resultant interest in and fear of the disease. This has been fuelled by publicized cases of prominent people who have developed dementia (e.g. Ronald Reagan, Margaret Thatcher, Rita Hayworth, Charles Bronson and Charlton Heston) and medical breakthroughs, including discovery of contributing factors and trials of new treatments. Research activity is the fourth factor, including molecular biology, epidemiology, genetic studies and social and psychological research aimed at improving diagnosis and assessment, discovering preventative factors and treatments for dementia and determining the impact on carers and ways to reduce their burden and stress levels. The final factors the breakdown of traditional family structures, the changing roles of women and adult children and changing values have reduced the moral obligation to care for older members of the community. This has increased pressure on governments and health-care systems to support the needs of people with dementia and their carers.

Being a carer of a person with dementia is very stressful, and it is known that carers experience higher levels of psychological distress and lower levels of self-efficacy and subjective well-being than both non-carers and carers of people with other types of diseases and disabilities (Pinquart and Sorensen, 2003; see Chapter 2, The lived experience of dementia, Chapter 15, Family carers of people with dementia and Chapter 16, One caregiver's view). Carers seek each other out for support and company, and as a result Alzheimer associations around the world have grown. In developed counties such as the UK, US and Australia, Alzheimer associations have been a powerful voice for promoting carers' and care recipients' needs.

The remainder of this chapter is divided into three sections. The first outlines the concepts of support groups and reviews the empirical evidence for their effectiveness, the second and third describe the functioning of Alzheimer's associations nationally and internationally.

38.2 SUPPORT GROUPS

Support groups, also called self-help groups, are gatherings of people who come together with a common problem or goal to provide support to members, share their experiences, problems, ideas and strategies, learn and gather information about a topic and encourage each other to take care of their own health and well-being (Alzheimer's Disease International, 2000). Alzheimer's support groups are available for most chronic conditions since the rise of the self-help movement in the late twentieth century, and clinicians should be aware of them and be able to provide their patients and their family with relevant information about them. Professionals and advocates for the people affected by the condition are often involved in their development. Alzheimer support groups came about as people with dementia and their families saw the condition as being largely ignored.

The advantages of support groups such as the Alzheimer Association include:

- support, both emotional and practical;
- education;
- universalization – a sense of belonging and not being alone;
- identity and a sense of purpose.

However, they are not appropriate for everyone – some people may feel uncomfortable sharing their feelings in a group setting. Support groups are distinct from group psychotherapy sessions as members are not viewed as patients. Support group sessions are not clinical and are not necessarily led by a professional such as a psychologist. The group leader may be a professional or someone who is, or has been, a carer for a person with dementia. Professionally led groups tend to be more formally structured. Professional group leaders have relevant qualifications and training, whereas peer group leaders tend to rely more on their own experience. Either way, a group leader needs to have appropriate skills, which include public speaking, encouraging participation and ensuring everyone gets heard, listening without judging, ensuring the group's rules and values are respected and identifying individuals requiring more support and making suggestions, for example for professional counselling (Alzheimer's Disease International, 2000). Particularly for peer group led groups, it may be appropriate to have two leaders so that if a member requires individual support during a session, or if the leader becomes unavailable, e.g. if caring responsibilities need attention, the group does not become leaderless (Alzheimer's Disease International, 2000).

Emerging technology has allowed for support to be provided in ways other than face to face, such as by telephone or the Internet. This is important for reaching isolated carers, and to allow for carers to access support at any time of the day or night.

38.2.1   Alzheimer support groups

Alzheimer support groups are usually provided for carers, but increasingly there are groups designed specifically for people with (early stage) dementia, or for both affected people and their families. Alzheimer support groups tend to be led by health professionals such as social workers and/or carers, and to meet monthly at the same location for 1–2 hours. The

structure and content varies between groups, and they may be highly structured with set discussion topics, videos and guest speakers or unstructured to allow for more informal interaction. There are groups that are located next to day centres that have activities for patients while their carers attend the support group. Anecdotally, it is known that some carers benefit greatly from support groups and attend regularly for months or years (Ebenstein, 2004). Others try them and find that they are unsuitable, and others may attend irregularly, during a particularly stressful time or only when specifically invited. Carers who never attend may feel that they have sufficient informal social or formal support (e.g. counselling) or may be unaware of the existence of such groups or how to gain access to them.

Telephone and online support groups and education networks are becoming more common and are advantageous as they can be used by a broader range of individuals at a time and location that is suitable to the individual. Interventions include: conference calling among family members of dementia patients; telephone support systems with automated messages; stress monitoring and advice; respite calls for care recipients; on-line discussion groups; electronic reminder services; computer-based forums and question and answer sessions (Internet and non-Internet based networks); email; electronic encyclopaedias and libraries; and computer-based decision support modules (Cassie and Sanders, 2008; Powell et al., 2008).

Like carers, people with dementia often need support and people to talk to who are going through the same experiences, especially in the early stages of the illness. Support groups for people with dementia are fewer in number than those for carers. The presumption that people with dementia are unable to benefit from support group interventions due to a lack of awareness of their disease and its implications is erroneous. There is growing awareness that groups can be important forms of support, in particular for people with early stage dementia, but that they require careful planning and should be led by trained facilitators (Alzheimer's Disease International, 2003). Examples include the on-line 'virtual' group 'Dementia Advocacy Support Network International' (www.dasninternational.com) and 'Memory Club' a support group for people with early stage dementia and their carers (Zarit et al., 2004). Following the example in the Netherlands, Alzheimer associations in the UK and Australia have developed 'Alzheimer cafés' for people with early stage dementia and their families. The purpose of these gatherings is to provide social and emotional support, and a forum for informal advice and consultations with staff from the associations (Bailey and Moriarty, 2006; Mather, 2006). People with early stage dementia have been successfully integrated into these programmes and anecdotal evidence (participant numbers and comments) indicates that they enjoy the sessions and find them beneficial (Mather, 2006).

38.2.2   The efficacy of support groups

Participation in support groups has been reported to have a positive impact on the well-being of carers. Specifically, it has been associated with lower levels of carer burden (Parker *et al.*, 2008), higher subjective well being (Pinquart and Sorensen, 2006), better self-reported general health (Javadpour *et al.*, 2008), higher morale (Gonyea, 1990), enhanced competence and empowerment (Chan and O'Connor, 2008) and increased used of formal support services (Ebenstein, 2004).

The findings regarding the efficacy of support groups are equivocal, as many studies have shown no significant positive effects. Parker and colleagues (2008) performed a systematic review of carer interventions, including three support group interventions. One study reported significant reductions in distress and improvements in quality of life for participants who attended a support group led by a nurse over a period of 12 weeks (Fung and Chein, 2002). The sessions included psychological support, education and problem solving. Telephone- and Internet-based support interventions have been found to enhance carers' and care recipients' quality of life and independent living skills (Eisdorfer *et al.*, 2003; Topo, 2009). In the other two studies reviewed by Parker and colleagues, support group participation had no significant effect on participants' depression or self-esteem scores (Pillemer and Suitor, 2002) or on neuropsychiatric symptoms of the participants' care recipients (Senanarong *et al.*, 2004). In Pinquart and Sorenson's (2006) systematic review, only one of the support group interventions (number of support interventions reviewed not specified) resulted in a significant positive effect on one outcome measure, subjective well being. The Befriending and Costs of Caring (BECCA) long-term randomized controlled trial (RCT) of support for 236 carers by volunteers in London and East Anglia had no effect on carers' quality of life, anxiety, loneliness, perceived support or positive affect at six, 15 or 24 months follow up (Charlesworth *et al.*, 2008).

Support groups are most likely to have positive effects on carer burden, depression and quality of life if they include a counselling component and discussion of individualized strategies to assist carers with care-recipient problem behaviours, rather than only providing education and general training (Selwood *et al.*, 2007). Groups led by professionals tend to produce greater improvement in participants' psychological functioning, while peer-led groups increase informal support networks and feelings of self-efficacy (Toseland *et al.*, 1989). Carer variables are also important. Support group participation is likely to be more beneficial for carers whose social networks do not include people who understand their experiences and for carers who are more stressed, are dissatisfied with their caregiving role, are employed and have care recipients who are more apathetic or in nursing homes (Cuijpers *et al.*, 1996; Pillemer and Suitor, 2002).

Many carers do not attend support groups, either because of barriers or by choice. A major barrier to carer attendance at support groups, reported by 80 per cent of carers, is that they had not received advice encouraging them to attend (Molinari *et al.*, 1994). The two main ways support groups build and maintain membership is through general public awareness and outreach to individuals who share the group's concern but are not currently attending (Wituk *et al.*, 2002). Groups tend to be more successful when they have specific strategies to target and recruit potential members (Wituk

et al., 2002). It is also the responsibility of health professionals such as GPs to provide carers with information about support groups. Communication problems (including use of jargon, lack of face-to-face contact) between the carers and health professionals can impede such referrals (Bruce *et al.*, 2002; Carpentier *et al.*, 2008). These findings suggest that improved communication between carers and health professionals and active outreach by support groups may facilitate their use.

38.2.3 The impact of cultural factors

In anglophone countries such as the United States, Australia and the UK, ethnic minority groups are under-represented in the use of community services such as support groups (Henderson *et al.*, 1993; Chan and O'Connor, 2008). While it is unclear why carers from minority groups are less likely to attend support groups, a number of contributing factors may be the diverse interpretations of dementia and the stigma attached to the disease in some cultures, programmes may be culturally insensitive or non-inclusive in their approach, and minority group experiences and expectations may differ from the other 'mainstream' participants (Chan and O'Connor, 2008). For instance, Diaz (2002) reported that ethnic minority groups found it difficult to relate to mainstream support group practice norms such as questioning authority and discussing conflict and feelings towards caregiving (Diaz, 2002).

Despite these limitations, there is evidence that diverse cultural groups can benefit from participating in support groups. Confirming the results of previous studies (e.g. Leung *et al.*, 1993), Fung and Chein (2002) found that Chinese people, who have culturally defined caregiving roles based on the notion of filial piety and are traditionally said to be uncomfortable discussing personal problems, were able to express their feelings and difficulties openly in a support group environment with other carers who had similar experiences, and reported significant reductions in distress levels compared to controls (Fung and Chein, 2002). Further research is required to determine whether similarly positive outcomes would be found for other cultural minorities.

Support groups can be made more appropriate and attractive to a range of cultures through:

- active outreach by groups to culturally diverse communities;
- group leaders addressing from the outset the reluctance of some cultures to 'speak out' about negative feelings about the caregiving role, normalizing feelings of guilt and reframing traditional beliefs about speaking out (Chan and O'Connor, 2008);
- recruiting and training ethnic support group leaders;
- finding a culturally neutral site for the group to meet;
- letting the participants decide the form of the group (Henderson, 1992; Henderson *et al.*, 1993).

Over half the people with dementia globally live in low and middle income countries (Alzheimer's Disease International, 2009a). Health-care and community services for people with dementia and their carers are lacking in developing countries, as is research in this area (Javadpour *et al.*, 2008). A number of recent studies have trialled supportive interventions for family carers. A Thai intervention including support group participation helped to decrease neuropsychiatric symptoms of care recipients and had a small effect on reducing carer distress (Senanarong *et al.*, 2004). In a small study from Iran, 29 female carers attended 8-weekly sessions in a support group conducted by a trained senior psychiatry resident involving education and interactive group activities based on the Alzheimer's Association Guidelines for Carers (Javadpour *et al.*, 2008). Post-intervention scores showed highly significant reductions (from pre-intervention scores) in perceived stress and general health of carers and the neuropsychiatric symptoms of their care recipients (Javadpour *et al.*, 2008). There was no longitudinal follow up and additional research would help to consolidate these findings.

38.2.4   Special support groups

People with younger onset dementia, gay couples affected by dementia, people with uncommon forms of dementia, people in second (or later marriages) or people who are very prominent in their community and their families may find that mainstream support groups are unsuitable for them (Moore, 2002; Chaston *et al.*, 2004; Arai *et al.*, 2007). Some Alzheimer associations (for example Alzheimer's Australia and the UK Alzheimer's Society) have developed support groups tailored specifically for groups such as those with younger onset dementia and those in the early stages of dementia multicultural carers, male carers, adult children of people with dementia and people with frontotemporal dementia and Pick's Disease (Alzheimer's Australia, 2005; Alzheimer's Australia, 2009; Frontier Frontotemporal Dementia Research Group, 2009; Pick's Disease Support Group, 2009). The US Alzheimer's Association has online support groups for Spanish-speaking carers and carers who have lost their care recipient (Alzheimer's Association, 2009a).

38.3   ALZHEIMER ASSOCIATIONS

The main aim of all Alzheimer associations (also called Alzheimer's associations or societies) is to improve the quality of life for people with dementia and their families (www.alz.co.uk/adi/). While these associations are called 'Alzheimer's' they encompass the spectrum of different dementias and many were previously known as 'Alzheimer's disease and related disorders associations'. Over 70 national Alzheimer associations around the world are members of the umbrella organization Alzheimer's Disease International (ADI).

Associations vary in their governance and service provision. Associations may be centralized with a national body and branches through the country (e.g. UK) or may have a federated structure, with autonomous organizations in each state or province which join together to form a national body (e.g. Canada, Australia). While membership is open to anyone with an interest in dementia, associations mainly cater

for carers and people with dementia. Many people working in the dementia area also join as do those who wish to lend their support. Most associations strive to have a broad cross-section of the 'dementia community' on their boards – consumers, i.e. carers and if possible people with dementia, service providers, doctors and people with influence who are interested from the general community. It is generally considered desirable that carers or people with dementia constitute at least half the board.

Standard services provided by Alzheimer associations are support groups, free-phone telephone help lines, telephone counselling, information via the web, education, training, public awareness, media campaigns and public advocacy. Additionally, associations may provide in-person counselling, drop-in centres, speaker panels, opportunities for volunteers and funding for research. Associations strive to raise awareness of dementia, reduce stigma, and influence policy and politicians through lobbying and advocacy. In the past, associations faced a conflict between being supporters and advocates for people with dementia and their families versus being direct service providers. Over time, many associations have taken on service roles in addition to their support and advocacy roles, for example running a day centre (e.g. Pakistan) or nursing home (e.g. Tasmania, Australia).

38.3.1   Information

Provision of information is one of the most important aims of Alzheimer associations. They assist people with dementia, their families, carers, health professionals, governments and members of the public to obtain information about the disease, how and where to get help, how to manage legal issues and problem behaviours and how to access community and health services. Sources of information provided by associations include websites, fact sheets, research summaries, newsletters, information sessions, information provision at support group meetings and telephone 'hotlines'. To be able to offer these services, associations require an office, access to appropriate technology and staff or volunteers. Collaboration between physicians and Alzheimer associations can improve the quality and quantity of information provided to people with dementia and their carers (Fortinsky *et al.*, 2002).

38.3.2   Support

Emotional and practical support offered through carer groups (see 38.2 Support groups) or individually through in-person or telephone counselling. The support groups are the backbone of any association. (Support groups may also be offered by residential facilities and other care providers, usually not-for-profit and religious organizations.)

38.3.3   Training

Alzheimer associations co-ordinate and run training and education programmes for people with dementia, their carers and health professionals. Often people who manage and care for people with dementia both at home and in health-care settings are untrained or undertrained, and rely on programmes developed by Alzheimer associations. Even though education alone has limited benefits (Brodaty, 1994; Brodaty et al., 1994; Marriott et al., 2000; see Chapter 23, The role of physiotherapy in the management of dementia), it is an integral part of any intervention for people with dementia and their families and for health professionals. Education combined with counselling improves carer depression, burden, social support and self-efficacy (Belle et al., 2006; Mittelman et al., 2006; see Chapter 15, Family carers of people with dementia and Chapter 23, The role of physiotherapy in the management of dementia).

The UK Alzheimer's Society runs a number of training programmes designed for people with dementia and informal and professional carers that cover topics including introduction to dementia care, ideas for activities for people with dementia, diet and nutrition, improving communication, facilitating the move to residential care and dealing with grief and other emotions, as well as 'train the trainer' programmes. They are run at various locations throughout the UK (other than Scotland), and for an additional fee can be tailored for an individual workplace and run in-house (such as a nursing home). The society also publishes training materials that can be downloaded from the website or ordered online (Alzheimer's Society, 2009c).

Alzheimer's Australia has developed Dementia and Memory Community Centres located throughout the country, that provide community information services about dementia and preventative strategies, carer education courses, conferences for families and professionals, and awareness-raising activities. The Australian Government funds Alzheimer's Australia to deliver *Living With Memory Loss* programmes in every Australian state and territory for people with early stage dementia and their carers, involving dementia education, information about treatment options and services, strategies and emotional support. They are run in 2 hour sessions over a period of 7 weeks. Three hundred and thirty-nine carers and 231 people with dementia from 41 groups participated in an evaluation of the programme. Significant improvement in general mental health scores, more positive perceptions of the caregiving role and decreased stress from problem behaviours were evident for carers either immediately or three months after the programme. A sample of carers who indicated clinically significant depression scores at the start showed significantly reduced depression scores following the programme. Depression scores for participants with dementia were significantly reduced at the three-month follow up, and those with clinical symptoms demonstrated significant reduction in depression symptoms at the end of the programme, at the three-month follow up and, for those who continued, at the 15-month follow up (Bird et al., 2005).

The USA Alzheimer's Association offers a number of professional training programmes for formal care workers and workshops for informal carers, such as 'Foundations of Dementia Care' and 'Activity Based Dementia Care'. Available programmes vary by state. In Cleveland, Ohio, primary care physicians collaborated with the Cleveland chapter of the Alzheimer's Association to provide individualized education

to family caregivers and capable care recipients regarding dementia care and available services in the community. In an evaluation study involving 44 participants who completed the full intervention, the programme led to enhanced self-efficacy for managing dementia symptoms and accessing community services and high levels of satisfaction (Fortinsky et al., 2002). The Alzheimer Association has also developed on-line professional training programmes available to anyone with access to the Internet. These are *CARES: A Dementia Caregiving Approach for Direct Care Workers* and *Dementia Care Training for Team Leaders*. The CARES programme is a ten module, 10 hour on-line interactive tool designed for nurses, social workers and other professionals who work with people with dementia. It covers issues relating to caring for, communicating with and engaging people with dementia in meaningful activity. Dementia Care Training for Team Leaders provides guidance for those who supervise people who care for dementia patients, such as nursing home administrators and unit coordinators but not basic care issues. These resources can be purchased through the USA Alzheimer's Association website (Alzheimer's Association, 2009b).

Alzheimer associations in low and middle income countries are increasingly developing training programmes to raise awareness and educate family carers and health-care workers about dementia. The Alzheimer's and Related Disorders Society of India launched a Comprehensive Dementia Care Program in Cochin in 2004. The ten month training programme includes nursing, community health and welfare and the challenges of geriatric nursing in the field of dementia (Alzheimer's and Related Disorders Society of India, 2009). The Lanka Alzheimer's Foundation in Sri Lanka runs periodic workshops and in-house training programmes for formal and informal carers on a one-to-one basis (Lanka Alzheimer's Foundation, 2009). More information about interventions in developing countries is given below under section 38.4 Alzheimer's Disease International.

38.3.4 Services

Services that are used by carers include home care, day care, in-home (sitting), residential respite and permanent care. Carers have different needs, and finding the right solution can help to reduce carer stress and depression and delay or make institutionalization of the care recipient less likely (Callahan et al., 2006; Mittelman et al., 2006). Meeting the service needs of carers is difficult because of limited resources, and most countries around the world lack adequate services. In Canada, for example, there is no single agency with the ultimate responsibility for organizing dementia care services, and each community has developed its own selection, resulting in fragmented, unco-ordinated service provision (Jaglal et al., 2007).

Despite the demands on dementia carers and their high levels of stress and burden, even when services are available, their use by carers is low (Brodaty et al., 2005). Impediments to using services were perceived lack of need, resistance to accepting help, not having enquired, lack of knowledge, lack of availability, previous bad experiences, ineligibility and cost (Brodaty et al., 2005). Many carers who denied needing services displayed other indications of need, such as low levels of life satisfaction and satisfaction with their role and high levels of feelings of resentment and overload (Brodaty *et al.*, 2005). Alzheimer associations have an important role in providing, enhancing and facilitating use of services for people with dementia and their families. They can also inform governments how to deliver and monitor services with reasonable standards of care at economic cost.

38.3.5   Research

Research on AD and dementia is critical, but in most countries research is under-funded in relation to disease burden or completely lacking. For example, in Australia, funding for research on dementia relative to disease burden is 50 per cent of that for cancer (Low *et al.*, 2008). In the UK, the government invests eight times more in cancer than dementia research (Alzheimer's Society, 2009a). The World Alzheimer Report highlighted that worldwide research funding is skewed to diseases with high levels of mortality, such as cancer and heart disease, while those with high levels of disease burden are under-resourced (Alzheimer's Disease International, 2009a). Alzheimer associations act as advocacy groups to exert pressure on funding bodies and governments to make funds available for research. Additionally, they provide researchers with access to people with dementia and their families and give advice on research projects, particularly about the carer perspective. The UK Alzheimer's Society has a large public involvement in dementia research, investing over £6 million, funding over 100 projects at universities and other institutions, and working in partnership with the scientific community and people affected by dementia. The Quality Research in Dementia network of 80 community volunteers works with scientists to set the research agenda and award grants to ensure the best projects which are likely to have the biggest impact receive funding (Alzheimer's Society, 2009a). The Alzheimer's Association in the United States facilitates dementia research by offering research grants, publishing a bimonthly peer-reviewed journal, Alzheimer's and Dementia: The Journal of the Alzheimer's Association and convening a Research Roundtable, a consortium of Alzheimer Association staff, advisors, scientists, academics and government agencies. The Roundtable facilitates the development and implementation of new dementia treatments and sponsors the association grants (Alzheimer's association, 2009c).

Researchers help Alzheimer associations by advising, contributing to publications, submitting research ideas for funding consideration and delivering presentations.

38.3.6   Public awareness

Alzheimer associations help raise public awareness about dementia which increases public interest and coverage in the media and fosters recognition of dementia as a priority area of concern. This is achieved through publications, courses, training materials, funding and contributing to research and conferences and posting information on websites. Some Alzheimer associations are also involved in lobbying politicians and forming links with professional associations.

In response to a movement run by Alzheimer Europe and its member organizations, on December 16, 2008 the Council of the European Union adopted a set of conclusions on public health strategies to combat neurodegenerative disease associated with ageing, in particular AD, that included recognizing that these diseases constitute a 'priority for action' (Alzheimer Europe, 2006; Council of the European Union, 2008). The UK Alzheimer's Society runs campaigns that help to raise public awareness, gain funding and lobby politicians. Currently there are campaigns dedicated to accessing anti-dementia medications through the National Health Service, increasing access to high quality services and influencing candidates at the next general elections about such issues (Alzheimer's Society, 2009b). People assist by attending rallies, emailing members of parliament, and signing petitions (Alzheimer's Society, 2009b). In February 2009, the Alzheimer's Society worked with England's Department of Heath to develop the first ever English National Dementia Strategy, designed to increase public awareness, ensure early diagnosis and improve interventions, with specific proposals including the introduction of a dementia specialist in every hospital and care home and for mental health teams to assess people with dementia (Department of Health, 2009).

38.3.7   Fund raising

Alzheimer associations are charities or not-for-profit organizations. Funding comes from member fees, donations and fund-raising activities organized by the associations, and in some countries, government grants. In many countries, the government does not contribute, or the amount given is inadequate (Alzheimer's Society, 2009a). The grant itself is important because of the recognition the money offers. Most funding comes from individuals, trusts, industry and legacies. In 2007/08, 50 per cent of the UK Alzheimer's Society's funding came from donations, fundraising and legacies (Alzheimer's Society, 2008). Associations need to use the money they obtain efficiently and budget carefully. Accountability is maintained through financial reporting in annual reports. Every association requires someone with financial experience to help guide it. A fund-raising strategy and clear aims also assist the process.

38.4   ALZHEIMER'S DISEASE INTERNATIONAL

Alzheimer's Disease International (ADI), the International Federation of Alzheimer's Disease and Related Disorders Societies, was formed in Washington in 1984 with four founding members. This has grown over 70 member associations, primarily in the Americas, Northern, Western and Southern Europe, and the Asia Pacific (see **Figure 38.1**). Four paid staff (and many volunteers) are responsible for ADI's administration, including an executive director, finance and technology manager, membership and events manager and an administrator. The governance structure includes a

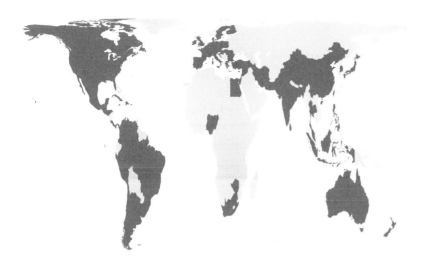

Figure 38.1 Map of the world with those countries belonging to ADI shown in dark grey. (Source: Alzheimer's Disease International, member countries map 2009. Reprinted by kind permission of Alzheimer's Disease International.)

council made up of a representative from each member association that meets annually and elects a board, led by the chairman. Funding comes from membership fees, conference fees, donations and investments.

To become a member, a national association must fulfil the following criteria:

- uphold the primary aim of the association, being to support people with dementia and their carers;
- have a board of directors that represents the views of family carers, professional carers, medical professionals and people with dementia;
- be recognized as the main organization for people with dementia and their carers in the country, and to work closely with health and social services and related organizations;
- undertake a range of services for family carers and people with dementia, for instance a telephone helpline, support groups, dissemination of public information and education and development of branches/groups around the country;
- be financially viable and have sufficient funds to meet expenses;
- send one representative to each ADI conference and council meeting and appropriate regional meetings;
- pay the annual membership fee;
- be an active member of ADI by referring to ADI on the website, observing World Alzheimer's Day, using the ADI logo on materials and reflecting ADI's message consistently.

ADI's main aim is to build and strengthen member associations by facilitating the sharing of expertise and resources. Another important aim is to encourage the formation of associations in countries where they do not exist. To address these aims, ADI has developed the Alzheimer university training programme. These are a series of workshops that aim to strengthen associations by focusing on issues fundamental to running an organization (such as organizational structure, relationships between staff and volunteers, strategic planning and information technology). For new and emerging associations, workshops are designed to help them develop the skills to set up an association,

including identifying aims, fundraising, recruiting volunteers, running support groups, raising awareness and providing information (Alzheimer's Disease International, 2005). These are held over 3 days annually in London or in association with regional meetings; ADI financially supports participants to attend.

ADI disseminates information and acts as a resource point. It issues a regular newsletter, fact sheets and publications on a number of issues relevant to people with dementia, their carers and Alzheimer associations. Publications are available on the website (www.alz.co.uk), and most are available in English and Spanish. Links to websites that provide dementia information in a variety of other languages are also provided.

ADI hosts an international conference annually. It is a multi-disciplinary event and delegates include staff and volunteers from Alzheimer Associations, people with dementia and their families, clinicians, researchers and scientists. Topics include emerging dementia research (for instance about prevention and treatment), dementia care, national strategies, services and training. Presentations become available on the website following the conference.

ADI has close associations with the World Health Organization (WHO) (officially since 1996), the International Psychogeriatric Association, World Psychiatric Association and the World Federation of Neurology. The pharmaceutical industry seeks ADI's advice about dementia treatment and consumer needs. ADI and WHO collaborated to produce a caregiver publication, the WHO provide speakers for ADI conferences and the organizations work together to achieve funding for projects. WHO also supported the launch of ADI's World Alzheimer's Day in 1994. Held annually on 21 September, associations around the world mark World Alzheimer's Day by holding 'memory walks', open days, lectures, training courses and entertainment designed to raise awareness about dementia. ADI supplies its members with a bulletin that has a special focus each year and materials to which they can add their own information, then download, print and distribute. ADI also provides its member countries with materials and ideas for activities that they can adapt to their culture and language.

In addition, regional groupings have been formed for Ibero-Latin America and Asia-Pacific which hold their own annual conferences and produce publications relevant to their zone. Europe has an independent organization, Alzheimer Europe (www.alzheimer-europe.org) which has a close collaborative relationship with ADI.

The 10/66 Dementia Research Group (www.alz.co.uk/1066) is ADI's research arm. This collaboration of researchers from developed and developing countries carries out research into dementia and ageing in low and middle income countries. The 10/66 name derives from the fact that less than 10 per cent of all population-based research into dementia is directed toward the 66 per cent of all people with dementia who live in developing countries, and was formed to redress the balance. Funding for the 10/66 group comes partly from ADI and mostly from grants; it has endorsement from WHO. Since its establishment in 1998, 10/66 has published the results of pilot studies in 28 centres in India, China, southeast Asia, Latin America, Nigeria and Russia and RCTs of caregiver interventions in Russia, India, Venezuela, Peru, Dominican Republic and China. It has also published qualitative studies in India and population-based epidemiological studies in eight Latin American countries. As of September 14, 2009, there were 38 publications covering methods, case identification, validation, prevalence, caregivers, behavioural problems and health policy (Alzheimer's Disease International, 2009b).

The aim of the pilot studies was to develop and validate an education- and culture-fair dementia diagnostic algorithm to be used in older populations with little formal education (Prince et al., 2003; Prince et al., 2008) and to obtain information about care arrangements for people with dementia (Prince, 2004), the impact of caring on their carers and common behavioural problems (The 10/66 Dementia Research Group, 2004).

The RCT interventions were designed to provide basic education about dementia and specific training on managing problem behaviours targeted at the main carer but also involving other family members (Dias et al., 2008; Gavrilova et al., 2008; see Chapter 15, Family carers of people with dementia).

The qualitative research studies used focus groups and open-ended interviews to investigate knowledge and beliefs about dementia in developing countries. There is a lack of awareness in these countries that dementia is an organic brain disease and symptoms are often thought to be a normal part of ageing (Shaji et al., 2003). The epidemiological studies involve surveys of all residents aged 65 years and older with sample sizes of at least 2000 in each participating Latin American country, with an ultimate total sample of 25 000. Data are being collected on dementia diagnoses, mental disorders, health, socio-demographic factors, risk factors, care arrangements, carer strain and health service utilization (The 10/66 Dementia Research Group, 2008a). A follow-up study, currently being undertaken using these data to assess risk factors for dementia and mortality, will be completed in 2010 (The 10/66 Dementia Research Group, 2008b).

While the 10/66 studies are its major research commitment, ADI is also involved in other research projects. The Stroud Symposia, a collaboration between the Stroud Centre at Columbia University, ADI and the Institute of Psychiatry collects information about the experiences of people with dementia and their carers, in an effort to improve their quality of life (see www.stroudsymposia.org). Member associations actively support medical research in their countries and ADI's medical and scientific advisory panel provide expert advice and act as international ambassadors for ADI.

38.5   CONCLUSION

Alzheimer associations are a major support for people with dementia and their families. They are a key part of the awareness, political and societal processes to destigmatize dementia, to assure adequate services and to improve the quality of life of those living with dementia. Alzheimer's associations are an important therapeutic intervention in their own right and should be part of the armamentarium of clinicians helping those who live with dementia. Empirical research supporting their benefits is limited mainly by logistic difficulties. However, a plethora of anecdotal reports demonstrate their benefits and the rise and development of associations around the world are testimony to their value.

REFERENCES

Alzheimer's and Related Disorders Society of India. (2009) *Comprehensive dementia care program at Cochin*. Retrieved 16 September, 2009. Available from: www.alzheimer.org.in/

Alzheimer's Association. (2009a) *Alzheimer's Association online community*. Retrieved 20 August 2009. Available from: www.alzheimers.infopop.cc/eve

Alzheimer's Association. (2009b) *Professional training and education programs*. Retrieved 22 September 2009. Available from: http://www.alz.org/professionals_and_researchers_education.asp

Alzheimer's Association. (2009c) *Researchers*. Retrieved 22 September, 2009. Available from: www.alz.org/professionals_and_researchers_researchers.asp

Alzheimer's Australia. (2005) *Next steps: Younger onset dementia*. Australian Capital Territory, Alzheimer's Australia.

Alzheimer's Australia. (2009) *Services and support*. Retrieved 20 August, 2009. Available from: www.alzheimers.org.au/content.cfm?categoryid=9

Alzheimer's Disease International. (2000) *Starting a self-help group*. London: Alzheimer's Disease International.

Alzheimer's Disease International. (2003) *How to include people with dementia in the activities of Alzheimer associations*. London: Alzheimer's Disease International.

Alzheimer's Disease International. (2005) *The Alzheimer University*, Retrieved 2 September, 2009, Available from: www.alz.co.uk/adi/alzuni.html

Alzheimer's Disease International. (2009a) *World Alzheimer report*. London: Alzheimer's Disease International.

Alzheimer's Disease International. (2009b) *10/66 publications*. Retrieved 22 September, 2009. Available from: www.alz.co.uk/1066/1066_publications.php

Alzheimer Europe. (2006) *Making dementia a public health priority*, 2006. Retrieved 2 September, 2009. Available from: www.dementia-in-europe.eu/

Alzheimer's Society. (2008) *Annual review 2007/08*. London: Alzheimer's Society, 1–24.

Alzheimer's Society. (2009a) *Our research programme*. Retrieved August 20, 2009a. Available from: www.alzheimers.org.uk/site/scripts/documents_info.php?categoryID=200294&documentID=347

Alzheimer's Society. (2009b) *Campaign: Championing the rights of people with dementia*. Retrieved 1 September, 2009b. Available from: www.alzheimers.org.uk/site/scripts/documents.php?categoryID=200149

Alzheimer's Society. (2009c) *Training*. Retrieved 19 September, 2009c. Available from: www.alzheimers.org.uk/site/scripts/documents.php?categoryID=200307

Arai A, Matsumoto T, Ikeda M, Arai Y. (2007) Do family caregivers perceive more difficulty when they look after patients with early onset dementia compared to those with late onset dementia. *International Journal of Geriatric Psychiatry* 22: 1255–61.

Bailey J, Moriarty J. (2006) Alzheimer's Society Derby branch: A comprehensive programme of support for people with dementia and their carers. *Dementia: The International Journal of Social Research and Practice* 5: 293–6.

Belle S, Burgio L, Burns R *et al.* (2006) Enhancing the quality of life of dementia caregivers from different ethnic or racial groups. *Annals of Internal Medicine* 145: 727–38.

Bird M, Caldwell T, Maller J, Korten A. (2005) *Alzheimer's Australia Early Stage Dementia Support and Respite Project: Final report on the national evaluation*. Queanbeyan: Australian Government.

Blessed G, Tomlinson BE, Roth M. (1968) The association between quantitative measures of dementia and of senile change in the cerebral grey matter of elderly subjects. *British Journal of Psychiatry* 114: 797–811.

Brodaty H. (1994) Dementia and the family In: Bloch S, Hafner J, Harari E, Szmukler GI (eds). *The family in clinical psychiatry*. Oxford: Oxford University Press, 224–6.

Brodaty H, Roberts K, Peters K. (1994) Quasi-experimental evaluation of an educational model for dementia caregivers. *International Journal of Geriatric Psychiatry* 9: 195–204.

Brodaty H, Green A, Low LF. (2005) Family carers for people with dementia In: Burns A, O'Brien J, Ames D (eds). *Dementia*. London: Hodder Arnold, 117–35.

Bruce DG, Paley GA, Underwood PJ *et al.* (2002) Communication problems between dementia carers and general practitioners: effect on access to community support services. *Medical Journal of Australia* 177: 186–8.

Callahan CM, Boustani MD, Unverzagt FW *et al.* (2006) Effectiveness of collaborative care for older adults with Alzheimer disease in primary care: a randomized controlled trial. *Journal of the American Medical Association* 295: 2148–57.

Carpentier N, Pomey MP, Contreras R, Olazabal I. (2008) Social care interface in early-stage dementia: practitioners' perspectives on the links between formal and informal networks. *Journal of Aging and Health* 20: 710–38.

Cassie KMC, Sanders S. (2008) Familial caregivers of older adults In: Cummings SM, Kropf NP (eds). *Handbook of psychosocial interventions with older adults: Evidence-based approaches*. New York: Haworth Press, 293–320.

Central Intelligence Agency. (2009) *The world factbook*. Retrieved 26 June 2009. Available from: www.cia.gov/library/publications/the-world-factbook.html

Chan SM, O'Connor DL. (2008) Finding a voice: The experiences of Chinese family members participating in family support groups. *Social Work with Groups* 31: 117–35.

Charlesworth G, Shepstone L, Wilson E *et al.* (2008) Befriending carers of people with dementia: randomised controlled trial. *British Medical Journal* 336: 1295–7.

Chaston D, Pollard N, Jubb D. (2004) Young onset dementia: a case for real empowerment. *Journal of Dementia Care* 12: 24–6.

Council of the European Union. (2008) *Council Conclusions on public health strategies to combat neurodegenerative diseases associated with ageing and in particular Alzheimer's disease*. Brussels: Council of the European Union.

Cuijpers P, Hosman CMH, Munnichs JMA. (1996) Change mechanisms of support groups for caregivers of dementia patients. *International Psychogeriatrics* 8: 575–87.

Department of Health. (2009) *National Dementia Strategy*. Retrieved 16 September, 2009. Available from: www.dh.gov.uk/en/SocialCare/Deliveringadultsocialcare/Olderpeople/NationalDementiaStrategy/index.htm

Dias A, Dewey ME, D'Souza J *et al.* (2008) The effectiveness of a home care program for supporting caregivers of persons with dementia in developing countries: a randomised controlled trial from Goa, India. *Plos One* 3: e2333.

Diaz TP. (2002) Group work from an Asian Pacific Island perspective: Making connections between group worker ethnicity and practice. *Social Work with Groups* 25: 43–60.

Ebenstein H. (2004) The relationship between caregiver support groups and the market framework of caregiving. *Journal of Gerontological Social Work* 44: 127–49.

Eisdorfer C, Czaja S, Loewenstein D *et al.* (2003) The effect of a family therapy and technology-based intervention on caregiver depression. *The Gerontologist* 43: 521–31.

Fortinsky RH, Unson CG, Garcia RI. (2002) Helping family caregivers by linking primary care physicians with community-based dementia care services. *Dementia: The International Journal of Social Research and Practice* 1: 227–40.

Frontier Frontotemporal Dementia Research Group. (2009) *Events – Carer Support Group*. Retrieved 16 September, 2009. Available from: www.ftdrg.org/events/

Fung W, Chein W. (2002) The effectiveness of a mutual support group for family caregivers of a relative with dementia. *Archives of Psychiatric Nursing* 16: 134–44.

Gavrilova SI, Ferri CP, Mikhaylova N *et al.* (2008) Helping carers to care: The 10/66 Dementia Research Group's randomized control trial of a caregiver intervention in Russia. *International Journal of Geriatric Psychiatry* 24: 347–54.

Gonyea JG. (1990) Alzheimer's disease support group participation and caregiver well-being. *Clinical Gerontologist* 10: 17–34.

Henderson JN. (1992) The power of support: Alzheimer's disease support groups for minority families. *Aging* 363–364: 24–8.

Henderson JN, Gutierrez-Mayka M, Garcia J, Boyd S. (1993) A model for Alzheimer's disease support group development in African-American and Hispanic populations. *The Gerontologist* 33: 409–14.

Jaglal S, Cockerill R, Lemieux-Charles L et al. (2007) Perceptions of the process of care among caregivers and care recipients in Dementia Care Networks. American Journal of Alzheimer's Disease and Other Dementias 22: 103–11.

Javadpour A, Ahmadzadeh L, Bahredar MJ. (2008) An educative support group for female family caregivers: impact on caregivers psychological distress and patient's neuropsychiatry symptoms. International Journal of Geriatric Psychiatry 24: 469–71.

Lanka Alzheimer's Foundation. (2009) Training for carers. Retrieved 16 September, 2009. Available from: www.alzlanka.org/index.php?option=com_content&task=view&id=44&Itemid=28

Leung M, Wong J, Siu VT. (1993) The emergence of a self-help association for relatives of the mentally disturbed in Hong Kong. In: Pearson V (ed.). Psychiatric rehabilitation: The Asian experience. Hong Kong: Center for Social Science Research, Hong Kong University, 415–32.

Low LF, Gomes L, Brodaty H. (2008) Australian Dementia Research: current status, future directions? Sydney: Dementia Collaborative Research Centre, Paper 16.

Marriott A, Donaldson C, Tarrier N, Burns A. (2000) Effectiveness of cognitive-behavioural family intervention in reducing the burden of care in carers of patients with Alzheimer's disease. British Journal of Psychiatry 176: 557–62.

Mather L. (2006) Memory Lane Café: Follow-up support for people with early stage dementia and their families and carers. Dementia: The International Journal of Social Research and Practice 5: 290–3.

Mittelman MS, Haley WE, Clay OJ, Roth DL. (2006) Improving caregiver well-being delays nursing home placement of patients with Alzheimer disease. Neurology 67: 1592–9.

Molinari V, Nelson N, Shekelle S, Crothers MK. (1994) Family support groups of the Alzheimer's assocation: an analysis of attendees and non-attendees. Journal of Applied Gerontology 13: 86–98.

Moore W. (2002) Lesbian and gay elders: connecting care providers through a telephone support group. Journal of Gay and Lesbian Social Services 14: 23–41.

Parker D, Mills S, Abbey J. (2008) Effectiveness of interventions that assist caregivers to support people with dementia living in the community: A systematic review. International Journal of Evidence-Based Healthcare 6: 137–72.

Pick's Disease Support Group. (2009) The Pick's Disease Support Group. Retrieved 16 September, 2009. Available from: alzheimers.org.uk/site/scripts/documents_info.php?categoryID=200171&documentID=167

Pillemer K, Suitor J. (2002) Peer support for Alzheimer's caregivers. Research on Aging 24: 171–92.

Pinquart M, Sorensen S. (2003) Differences between caregivers and noncaregivers in psychological health and physical health: a meta-analysis. Psychology and Aging 18: 250–67.

Pinquart M, Sorensen S. (2006) Helping caregivers of persons with dementia: which interventions work and how large are their effects? International Psychogeriatrics 18: 577–95.

Powell J, Chiu T, Eysenbach G. (2008) A systematic review of networked technologies supporting carers of people with dementia. Journal of Telemedicine and Telecare 14: 154–6.

Prince M. (2004) 10/66 Dementia Research Group. Care arrangements for people with dementia in developing countries. International Journal of Geriatric Psychiatry 19: 170–7.

Prince M, Acosta D, Chiu H et al. (2003) Dementia diagnosis in developing countries: a cross-cultural validation study. Lancet 361: 909–17.

Prince MJ, de Rodriguez JL, Noriega L et al. (2008) The 10/66 Dementia Research Group's fully operationalised DSM-IV dementia computerized diagnostic algorithm, compared with the 10/66 dementia algorithm and a clinician diagnosis: a population validation study. BMC Public Health 8: 219.

Selwood A, Johnston K, Katona C et al. (2007) A systematic review of the effect of psychological interventions on family caregivers of people with dementia. Journal of Affective Disorders 101: 75–89.

Senanarong V, Jamjumras P, Harmphadungkit K et al. (2004) A counseling intervention for caregivers: effect on neuropsychiatric symptoms. International Journal of Geriatric Psychiatry 19: 781–8.

Shaji KS, Smitha K, Praveen Lal K, Prince MJ. (2003) Caregivers of people with Alzheimer's disease: a qualitative study from the Indian 10/66 Dementia Research Network. International Journal of Geriatric Psychiatry 18: 1–6.

The 10/66 Dementia Research Group. (2004) Behavioural and psychological symptoms of dementia in developing countries. International Psychogeriatrics 16: 1–19.

The 10/66 Dementia Research Group. (2008a) Population-based epidemiological studies (prevalence phase). Retrieved 2 September, 2009. Available from: www.alz.co.uk/1066/pop_based_ep_studies_prevalence_phase.php

The 10/66 Dementia Research Group. (2008b) Population-based epidemiological studies (incidence phase). Retrieved 2 September, 2009. Available from: www.alz.co.uk/1066/pop_based_ep_studies_incidence_phase.php

Topo P. (2009) Technology studies to meet the needs of people with dementia and their caregivers: A literature review. Journal of Applied Gerontology 28: 5–37.

Toseland RW, Rossiter CM, Labrecque MS. (1989) The effectiveness of peer-led and professionally led groups to support family caregivers. The Gerontologist 29: 465–71.

Wituk SA, Shepherd MD, Warren M, Meissen G. (2002) Factors contributing to the survival of self-help groups. American Journal of Community Psychology 30: 349–66.

Zarit SH, Femia EE, Watson J et al. (2004) Memory club: a group intervention for people with early stage dementia and their care partners. Gerontologist 44: 262–9.

Health economic aspects of dementia

ANDERS WIMO, LINUS JÖNSSON AND BENGT WINBLAD

39.1 INTRODUCTION

A highly prevalent group of disorders such as dementia present a challenge for any health care and social support system. The combination of costly care (Ernst and Hay, 1994; Winblad et al., 1997), difficulties in funding health care and an important contribution by informal caregivers focus on the basics in any health economic analysis and put the costs of dementia and cost effectiveness of dementia care into focus. It has been debated whether 'the welfare state' will be able to care for the increasing number of elderly people in general (OECD, 1996), and with dementia in particular (Lovestone, 2002). However, in the light of the enormous economic impact of dementia, it is surprising that the health economics of dementia have such a small scientific base (Jonsson et al., 2000; Gray, 2002; SBU, 2008). The first (and only) basic textbook in this field (Wimo et al., 1998a) was published in 1998 and reviewers have stressed the need for further studies (Jonsson et al., 2000; Shukla et al., 2000; Grutzendler and Morris, 2001; Lamb and Goa, 2001; NICE, 2001; Clegg et al., 2002; Gray, 2002; Lyseng-Williamson and Plosker, 2002; Olin and Schneider, 2002; Wolfson et al., 2002; Birks and Harvey, 2006; Jonsson, 2003; Lyseng-Williamson and Plosker, 2003; Leung et al., 2003; SBU, 2008; Jönsson and Wimo, 2009; NICE, 2009).

39.2 PERSPECTIVE

An important purpose of economic evaluation is that it should serve as a tool for decision making regarding allocation of scarce resources (Drummond et al., 2004). There are many 'players and payers' involved in delivery and financing of dementia care. Therefore, it is essential to define the perspective of any pharmacoeconomic analysis. The viewpoint may be a county council, a municipality, the public sector in general, an insurance company, a family member or a patient. The main cost drivers are costs of living (in its wide context, including also care in nursing homes) and informal caring (Wimo and Winblad, 2003b). There is a complex interaction between those who finance the care and those who may benefit from the results of interventions. Therefore, the detection of suboptimal incentives is an essential part of the economic analysis. Limiting the economic analysis only to the health-care sector or the public sector excludes substantial components from the analysis. Thus, a societal perspective where all relevant costs are included regardless of where they occur and regardless of who pays is often to be preferred.

39.3 COSTS

Any resource has an alternative use to a certain cost with foregone benefits. This cost is the opportunity cost which is recommended in economic evaluations. Although easy in theory, the opportunity cost approach is problematic to apply in dementia. Costs are also by tradition divided into direct costs (of resources used) and indirect costs (of resources lost due to, for example, mortality, morbidity and production losses). Direct costs are often presented in two ways: direct medical costs (e.g. hospital care, clinic visits, drugs, etc.) and direct non-medical costs (e.g. social/home services, nursing home care). Informal care is often regarded as an indirect cost although this is not always obvious since many caregivers are retired.

39.4   FAMILY MEMBERS AND INFORMAL CARE

Informal carers (mostly spouses or children) are of great importance in dementia care. An informal carer is often part of a 'dementia family'. In that sense, their situation can be analysed in terms of, for example, burden, quality of life, coping, stress, social network and morbidity (Max et al., 1995; Jansson et al., 1998; Schulz and Beach, 1999; Wimo et al., 1999b; Almberg et al., 2000).

They are also often providers of an extensive amount of unpaid informal care (Rice et al., 1993; Stommel et al., 1994; Langa et al., 2001; Moore et al., 2001; Wimo et al., 2002; Nordberg et al., 2005), which constitute a great part of the societal costs.

Measuring caregiver time is problematic. Support in personal activities of daily living (ADLs) and instrumental activities of daily living (IADLs) are well-defined activities. However, a substantial part of caregiver activities is linked to supervision to manage behavioural symptoms or to prevent dangerous events (Wimo et al., 2002). The assessments of supervision and surveillance in terms of minutes and hours may, however, be difficult.

Two other important factors are care productivity and joint production. A formal caregiver is probably more efficient and takes less time to support ADL tasks than an informal caregiver. This must be considered if a replacement approach is used. Joint production means that the patient and the caregiver are doing things together (e.g. shopping).

Costing informal care is also a complicated and controversial issue (Koopmanschap, 1998; Jonsson et al., 2000; van den Berg et al., 2006). There are two frequently used methods, the opportunity cost approach and the replacement cost approach.

Whether the caregiver is paid or not is not of interest for the economic valuation. Payment has an impact on the distribution of the economic burden, but not on the total societal cost. The relevant cost is the opportunity cost and thus, the question is to identify the alternative use of the caregiver's time. If the alternative is working in the labour market, the cost for informal care should be valued to the production loss due to absence from work.

However, more problematic is the costing of leisure time and caregiver time during retirement. There is no consensus how this should be performed. The cost for the caregiver's time may the value of the time used as leisure time (Karlsson et al., 1998). However, there is no such market price available. Willingness to pay approaches – for example the contingent valuation method (Johannesson et al., 1992) are options and a study with this approach has recently been published (Gustavsson et al., 2010).

With the replacement cost approach it is assumed that the informal carer should be replaced with a professional carer in

a 1:1 ratio. The informal caregiver's time and the professional caregiver's time are regarded as perfect substitutes. However, we do not know if there actually will be a complete replacement with a professional carer.

39.5   TYPES OF STUDIES AND DESIGN ASPECTS

39.5.1   Descriptive studies

Cost description (CD) describes only the costs (no outcome) of a single treatment/care, without making any comparison between alternative treatments. Thus, CD cannot give any support in priority discussions, but presents a framework for how costs are calculated (see **Box 39.1**).

Cost of illness (COI) studies are also descriptive. The COI is equal to what these resources would have been used for if there had been no case of illness (the opportunity cost). Two approaches can be used: an incidence approach or a prevalence approach. With the incidence approach the costs for new cases are estimated where both the annual costs and future (discounted) costs are included. In the prevalence approach the costs for all cases during, for example, a year are estimated – both for those who have dementia already and for new cases occurring during the year in question (Lindgren, 1981; Rice et al., 1985). Only exceptionally have both approaches shown the same results. The choice of approach depends on the purpose of the study; if the aim is to illustrate the economic consequences of interventions, the incidence approach is preferable. If the idea is to estimate the economic burden during a defined year, the prevalence approach is the best option.

Another issue is whether to use use a top-down or a bottom-up approach. In the 'top-down' approach the total national cost for a specific resource is distributed on different diseases. The 'bottom-up' method starts from a defined subgroup with, for example, dementia, and registers all cost of illness related to it, followed by an extrapolation to the total dementia population. It is problematic to compensate for co-morbidity and net costs may be difficult to estimate. It is also

---

Box 39.1 Different kinds of health economic studies

Descriptive studies
CD: Cost Description
COI: Cost of Illness

Evaluation studies
CA: Cost Analysis (incomplete evaluation)
CMA: Cost Minimisation Analysis
CEA: Cost Effectiveness Analysis
CBA: Cost Benefit Analysis
CUA: Cost Utility Analysis
CCA: Cost Consequence Analysis

important to specify the included cost categories (e.g. is cost of informal care included?). In an estimate of the worldwide societal costs of dementia, resulting in a total cost of $US 315 billion in 2005, we included direct costs ($US 210 billion) and costs of informal care ($US 105 billion) (Wimo *et al.*, 2007b). It is obvious that dementia care is costly, but the great range in cost figures in **Table 39.1** illustrates that the costing approaches vary in studies and that the cost levels vary between countries.

There is also a strong association between costs and functional decline (Quentin *et al.*, 2009). In a population-based Swedish COI study with a bottom-up approach, where costs were expressed in terms of the Clinical Dementia Rating (CDR) the cost ratio between severe dementia and no decline was 6.5 (**Table 39.2**). The proportion of net costs (costs assumed to only due to dementia) and gross costs (costs including co-morbidities) was about 80 per cent.

39.5.2   Economic evaluations

In a cost analysis (CA), only the costs of different therapies are compared (not outcomes). Thus, a CA is an incomplete economic evaluation. A complete economic evaluation includes the incremental costs and outcomes and comparisons between different treatment alternatives. In a cost minimization analysis (CMA) the effects of different treatments are assumed to be equivalent and the analysis is focused on to identify the cheapest therapy. The value of CMA is questioned, since the assumption of similar treatment effects is problematic (Briggs and O'Brien, 2001).

In a cost-effectiveness analysis (CEA), the effect is expressed as a nonmonetary quantified unit, such as the cost per nursing home admission averted. A cost benefit analysis (CBA) expresses all costs and outcomes in monetary units, for example dollars or euros. Few attempts have been made to apply CBA to dementia. It has, however, been argued that CBA approaches such as 'willingness to pay' could be of value (Wimo *et al.*, 2002). In a cost utility analysis (CUA) the effect is expressed as utilities, such as quality adjusted life years (QALYs; Torrance, 1997).

It is important to include a discussion of uncertainty in economic evaluations (Briggs and O'Brien, 2001) and important factors should be varied in a sensitivity analysis.

In a cost consequence analysis (CCA), cost and outcomes are analysed and presented separately. The value of CCA is under discussion (Winblad *et al.*, 1997) since results may be difficult to interpret and the selection of outcomes may be biased.

39.6   THE NEED FOR MODELLING

An intervention in dementia may influence the course of the disease. Therefore, an economic evaluation has to take into account impacts on costs and outcomes during the whole lifespan. Most clinical studies last for 6–12 months. Due to practical and ethical issues, single studies covering the whole disease period will probably never be undertaken. One option to determine long-term effects is to extend ongoing studies. In randomized controlled trials (RCTs) it is difficult to maintain the original design for many years, but open follow up studies have been used for cholinesterase inhibitors (Knopman *et al.*, 1996; Geldmacher *et al.*, 2003; Wallin *et al.*, 2004). However, there are several drawbacks, such as selection bias, patients lost to follow up and problems defining

Table 39.1   Cost of illness studies expressed as $US 2005 (currency conversions to $US by PPPs (purchasing power parities), time transformations by CPI (consumer price index)); source for PPP and CPI: OECD, data on file: www.oecd.org). Figures are rounded off.

Country	Annual costs per patient US$ 2005	Cost categories included	Source
World	10 800	D, IC	Wimo *et al.* (2007b)
USA	60 400	D, IC	Ernst and Hay (1994)
Canada	14 900	D, IC	Ostbye and Crosse (1994)
EU27	23 400	D, IC	Wimo *et al.* (2008)
Europe	12 200	D	Andlin-Sobocki *et al.* (2005)
Belgium	16 300	D, IC	Scuvee-Moreau *et al.* (2002)
Denmark	11 900	D	Kronborg Andersen *et al.* (1999)
Finland	37 000	D, IC	François *et al.* (2004)
France	6 800	D, IC	Souetre *et al.* (1995)
France	25 500	D, IC	Rigaud *et al.* (2003)
Germany	13 400	D	Schulenberg and Schulenberg (1998)
Ireland	11 200	D, IC	O'Shea and O'Reilly (2000)
Nordic	15 600	D, IC	Jonsson *et al.* (2006b)
Italy	58 200	D, IC	Cavallo and Fattore (1997)
Spain	30 700	D, IC	Boada *et al.* (1999)
Spain	33 900	D	Atance Martinez *et al.* (2004)
Sweden	30 300	D, IC	Jonsson *et al.* (2006b)
Sweden	42 200	D, IC	Wimo *et al.* (2007a)
The Netherlands	11 800	D	Koopmanschap *et al.* (1998)
UK	41 800	DC, IC	Knapp and Prince (2007)

Table 39.2 Societal costs of dementia in Sweden (Wimo *et al.*, 2009) in relation to CDR ($US by PPPs in 2005 level).

CDR	Cognitive decline	Gross costs	Net costs
0	None	7 100	
0.5	Light	19 600	
1	Mild	28 000	20 900
2	Moderate	38 400	31 300
3	Severe	46 300	39 100

controls. Therefore, there is a need for modelling approaches (Buxton *et al.*, 1997). The basic idea is that results from a short core period are extrapolated to a longer period. Inputs from several sources, for example efficacy, costing and progression, are used. Markov models are frequently used for this purpose (Sonnenberg and Leventhal, 1998). Other approaches, such as decision tree models (Weinstein and Fineberg, 1980), survival models (Fenn and Gray, 1999) and discrete events simulation (Caro, 2005) have been used. Thirteen types of models regarding Alzheimer's Disease (AD) have been identified in different studies (Cohen and Neumann, 2008). Discounting of costs (and perhaps outcomes) is recommended. The discount rate is often 3–5 per cent (Siegel *et al.*, 1997), but it can be varied in a sensitivity analysis.

Models are controversial. The use of cognition as the vehicle for costs is questioned (Green, 2007). Long-term effects, such as exhaustion of carers and staff, which do not occur in the core period and symptoms which do not have a linear progressive course, such as behavioural and psychological symptoms of dementia (BPSD; Ferris and Mittelman, 1996), are difficult to model. A model is also linked, implicitly or explicitly, to a specific organization of care.

39.7 OUTCOME MEASURES

Cognition is considered as a mandatory primary efficacy outcome in most dementia trials. For the patient, the cognitive capacity is indeed a relevant outcome since it affects intellectual capacity and thinking. However, other outcomes are probably more important for the caregivers such as ADL-capacity, mood-depression and BPSD. For both patients and caregivers, aspects of quality of life are significant outcomes. For staff, ADL-capacity and BPSD and, in a wider context, care planning are essential.

Surrogate endpoints are in principal regarded as inappropriate to use in cost-effectiveness analysis (Johannesson *et al.*, 1996). The Mini-Mental State Examination (MMSE; Folstein *et al.*, 1975) is often used in dementia studies as well as other measures of cognitive capacity such as the Alzheimer's Disease Assessment Scale – cognitive subscale (ADAS-Cog; Rosen *et al.*, 1984). However, in our view they should be regarded as surrogate endpoints. Since the MMSE is highly correlated with costs (Ernst *et al.*, 1997; Hux *et al.*, 1998; Wimo *et al.*, 1998c; Jonsson *et al.*, 1999b), and also to other, more relevant outcomes, such as ADL-capacity, position in care organization and severity of dementia, it has frequently been used in economic evaluations of dementia. The MMSE

is also used in most longitudinal population-based studies and thus it may be useful as a link between clinical studies and population studies in the discussions of efficacy versus clinical effectiveness. However, delay in progression in terms of severity presents a broader outcome than cognition and severity scales such as the CDR (Berg, 1988) and the Global Deterioration Scale (GDS; Reisberg *et al.*, 1988) or multidimensional instruments such as the Gottfries–Bråne–Steen Scale (GBS; Bråne *et al.*, 2001) are suggested as more relevant for use than cognition.

Postponing or preventing nursing home entry has also been suggested. Knopman *et al.* (1996) indicated that nursing home care can be postponed about one year with tacrine treatment. In a Swedish study (Wallin *et al.*, 2004) of tacrine, the findings were similar. Sano *et al.* (1997) found that vitamin E/selegiline treatment postponed nursing home placement. A study on donepezil indicated an even longer postponement of institutionalization (Geldmacher *et al.*, 2003). However, the situation is more complex regarding caregivers. It may be an advantage that spouses can go on living together, but a prolonged period at home may be more stressful for the caregiver (Max, 1996). This potential risk was, however, not confirmed in the two published RCTs where the amount of informal care was measured (Wimo *et al.*, 2003a; Wimo *et al.*, 2003b).

Quality of life (QoL) of both patients and caregivers is a relevant outcome. Health-related QoL includes several dimensions, such as ADLs, social interaction, perception, pain, anxiety, economic status, etc. One potential problem in QoL assessments is the patient's difficulty to value his/her own health state (Stewart and Brod, 1996). Thus, proxies (mostly caregivers) are often used. Proxies are not necessarily a problem. The US panel for cost-effectiveness recommends that the general public should value health states and in that sense, an indirect measurement is not disqualified (Siegel *et al.*, 1997). If the proxy is a family member, the answers may reflect, in part, the situation and interests of the proxy, which must be considered. Some attributes may be difficult for proxies, such as 'pain', whereas others, such as 'mobility' are less problematic. In a project where proxy-rated and self-rated QoL were used simultaneously, great differences between the two approaches occurred (Jonsson, 2003; Jonsson *et al.*, 2006a).

In principle, two kinds of instruments can be used: diagnosis specific or generic instruments (Bowling, 1995; Spilker, 1996; Salek *et al.*, 1998; Walker *et al.*, 1998).

More or less dementia-specific instruments such as the Dementia Quality of Life instrument (DQoL; Brod *et al.*, 1999), Quality of Life Alzheimer's Disease (QOLAD; Selai *et al.*, 2001; Logsdon *et al.*, 2002) and Quality of Life Assessment Schedule (QOLAS; Selai *et al.*, 2000; Elstner *et al.*, 2001) may be useful in CCA trials but are inappropriate for complete economic evaluations since these instruments not are preference based (Torrance *et al.*, 1996; Siegel *et al.*, 1997).

There is a great number of generic QoL scales, such as the sickness impact profile (Bergner *et al.*, 1981), the Short Form 36 (SF-36; Ware and Sherbourne, 1992), the QLA-scale (Blau, 1977), the Health Utilities Index (HUI; Torrance *et al.*, 1996; Neumann *et al.*, 2000), the EuroQoL/EQ-5D (Coucill *et al.*, 2001) or the Quality of Well-being Scale (QWBS; Kerner *et al.*, 1998). HUI, EQ-5D, QWBS and the caregiver quality of life index (CQLI; Mohide *et al.*, 1988) can be used to calculate QALYs (Torrance, 1997).

QALYs are used in CUA and reflect both quantity and quality of life (Torrance, 1996; Torrance *et al.*, 1996) and give opportunities for comparisons with other diseases. Utilities are expressed as a figure between 0 (death) and 1 (perfect health). Disease-related utilities are also under development, for example in AD (Ekman *et al.*, 2007). QALYs are not uncontroversial (Tsuchiya *et al.*, 2003). Chronic incurable progressive disorders may be misfavoured when compared with surgical treatments, such as cataract surgery or hip replacement surgery.

There are also other approaches, such as disability adjusted life years (DALYs; Allotey *et al.*, 2003) and healthy years equivalents (HYE; Dolan, 2000). However, DALYs focus on productivity more than QoL and HYEs require a great number of health scenarios (Torrance, 1996).

Burden scales, such as the Burden Interview (Zarit *et al.*, 1980) can to some extent be used as indicators of caregiver QoL, but the interplay between patient status, caregiver QoL and burden is complex (Deeken *et al.*, 2003).

The choice of outcome measure in economic evaluation in dementia is not an obvious one. As different outcome measures give different pieces of information, several outcome measures can be used.

39.8   RESOURCE UTILIZATION IN DEMENTIA

The costing process usually consists of two phases; first, resource utilization is expressed in terms of physical units (such as nursing home days) and second, the resource utilization figures are calculated into costs by the use of unit costs for each resource. Resource Utilization in Dementia (RUD; Wimo *et al.*, 1998b) is an example of a framework assessing the use of formal and informal resources, aiming at calculating costs from a societal perspective (**Box 39.2**). RUD has been used in several studies (Wimo *et al.*, 1999a; Wimo *et al.*, 2000; Wimo *et al.*, 2003a; Wimo *et al.*, 2003b).

Box 39.2 Components of a resource utilization battery, RUD (resource utilization in dementia) (Wimo *et al.*, 1998b)

Patient	Caregiver
Accomodation/long term care	Informal care time (for patient)
(Work status)	Work status
Respite care	(Respite care)
Hospital care	Hospital care
Out clinic visits	Out clinic visits
Social service	Social service
Home nursing care	Home nursing care
Day care	Day care
Drug use	Drug use

A comprehensive battery can be time-demanding and thus a short version, the RUD Lite (Wimo and Winblad, 2003b) was developed. It was possible to limit the number of variables in the RUD considerably without losing the societal perspective in the analysis; RUD Lite covers about 95 per cent of the costs resulting from the complete RUD (Wimo and Winblad, 2003b). One part of the RUD is the caregiver time subscale. Other instruments that assess caregiver time are the Caregiver Activities Time Survey (CATS; Clipp and Moore, 1995) and the Caregiver Activity Survey (CAS; Davis *et al.*, 1997).

Since the organization of dementia care varies between countries, any resource use battery must be adapted to the specific situation in a country.

39.9   PHARMACOECONOMIC STUDIES

Even if it would be advantageous to design studies purely for health economic purposes, pharmacoeconomics will probably be part of comprehensive phase III/IV studies (Hill and McGettigan, 1998). It is however, important to refine the methods used (Briggs and O'Brien, 2001). It has also been debated whether pharmacoeconomic aspects are best included in phase III or phase IV studies (Schneider, 1998).

Several pharmacoeconomic evaluations have been published, mainly on the cholinesterase inhibitors (one on memantine) with various approaches. The early tacrine studies focused on costs and they are also based on the same efficacy study (Knapp *et al.*, 1994). Even if treatment seems to be cost saving, the range is large in these studies, from about 1 to 17 per cent, indicating different methodological approaches but also problems. Few studies are empirical (**Table 39.3**) and most evaluations are based on models (**Table 39.4** and **Table 39.5**). The empirical studies are short-term studies with weak statistical power for the cost results. In the donepezil models, Markov models have been used with QALYs or severity (avoided) as outcome, while survival analysis have been used in the rivastigmine models. In the galantamine studies, the assessment of health economics in Alzheimer's disease (AHEAD) concept is used (Caro *et al.*, 2001). In general, the results favour drug use, but sensitivity analyses show a range of results, indicating uncertainty.

Drug trials are often criticized regarding representativeness. Schneider *et al.* (1997) showed that study populations in dementia drug trials only reflect about 7 per cent of a general dementia population. The progression rate of cognition is slower in placebo groups in most clinical studies than in population-based studies. Another issue is whether study populations reflect the dementia care organization to which the results are generalized.

39.10   PROGRAMMES

The term 'non-pharmacological treatment' is commonly used to describe care interventions such as day care, caregiver support, living arrangements and case management. We think this term is inappropriate since in most cases it reflects basic care for people with dementia and therefore we use the

Table 39.3 Randomized controlled trials with empirical pharmacoeconomic data. Costs are expressed as $US 2005 (PPPs).

Drug	Country	Duration	Results US$ 2005[a]	Sensitivity analysis	Source
Donepezil	Nordic	1 year	1210 (ns)	555–1296–1314	Wimo et al. (2003a), Europe
Donepezil	Can., France, Aus	6 months	312 (ns)	73–497	Feldman et al. (2004)
Donepezil	UK	60 weeks	−887 (ns)	Yes, but results not presented	AD2000, Courtney et al. (2004)
Memantine	USA	6 months	7697 ($p < 0.05$)	Yes, but results were not presented	Wimo et al. (2003b), USA
Risperidone (r), olanzapine (o) and quetiapine (q)	USA	9 months	(per month) 187 (r), −9 (o), −193 (q). Overall $p = 0.02$ (placebo lower)	Different WTP-levels	USA, Rosenheck et al. (2007)

[a]A positive value indicates net savings with treatment.

Table 39.4 Cost-analysis models. Costs are expressed as US$ 2005 (PPPs).

Drug	Model length (years)	Cost diff.	Cost diff.[a] (%) versus comparator	Range in sensitivity analysis	Comment	Source
1. Tacrine	4.4	3 029	17.3	113–6595 US$	Costs effects annualized by study's authors	Lubeck et al. (1994)
2. Tacrine	5.3	12 171	7.5	698–26 687 US$		Henke and Burchmore (1997)
3. Tacrine	9	26 303	1.3	0.6–5.2 per cent		Wimo et al. (1997)
4. Rivastigmine	2	2 186[b]	NA	NA	Mild	Fenn and Gray (1999)
	0.5	18[b]	NA	NA		
5. Rivastigmine	2	4 135[b]	NA	NA	All	Hauber et al. (2000b)
	0.5	155[b]	NA	NA		

[a]A positive value indicates net savings with treatment with CHEIs.
[b]The cost for rivastigmine is not included.
NA, not available.

term 'programmes'. The economic literature in this field is sparse and heterogeneous, but some studies have been published (**Table 39.6**). The problem with such studies, besides their heterogeneity, is that study samples often are small, resulting in weak statistical power, wide confidence intervals, etc. Bootstrapping methods can partly compensate for that.

39.11   MILD COGNITIVE IMPAIRMENT

Health economic effects on mild cognitive impairment (MCI) can be divided into short- and long-term effects (Wimo and Winblad, 2003a). In the short-term perspective, an intervention can perhaps result in a reduction of informal care in terms of IADL. Thus it is questionable whether the costs of a drug will be offset from a short-term viewpoint. In the long run, the question will be whether survival is affected and whether there will be any transitions of symptoms and resource use during the course of the dementia. To design

studies to answer these questions is not easy. A synthetic approach with RCTs covering segments of the dementia course, modelling studies and open follow-up studies probably will be needed, resulting in some kind of 'best guess' judgement.

39.12   PHARMACOECONOMICS AND DRUG AUTHORITIES

New drugs go through several steps for drug authorities before entering the market. These steps are not necessarily handled within the same authorities. While the registration process in the European Union is getting harmonized through EMEA (CPMP, 1997), focusing on cognition, ADLs and a global effect (Hill and McGettigan, 1998), decisions about pricing and reimbursement remain on the country level. Furthermore, there may be different forms of budget restrictions on various levels in the care organization. In the

Table 39.5 Cost-effectiveness models. Costs are expressed as $US 2005 (PPPs).

Drug	Model length (years)	Model type	Country	Outcome	Cost diff.[a]	C/E or similar[b]	Range in sensitivity analysis	Source
Donepezil	5	Markov	UK	Severity	-2 591	10 415	1721–18 076	Stewart et al. (1998)
Donepezil	5	Markov	Canada	Severity	877	<0	<0–8577	O'Brien et al. (1999)
Donepezil	5	Markov	Sweden	Severity	417	<0	<0–3309	Jonsson et al. (1999a)
Donepezil	2	Markov	USA	QALYs	89	<0	<0–513 145	Neumann et al. (1999)
Donepezil	2	Markov	Japan	QALYs	249	<0	<0–43 492[c]	Ikeda et al. (2002)
Rivastigmine	2	Survival	Canada	QALYs	429	<0	Treshold analysis different WTPs	Hauber et al. (2000a)
Galantamine	10	AHEAD	Canada	QALYs	762	<0	<0–41 748	Getsios et al. (2001)
Galantamine	10.5	AHEAD	Sweden	NNT FTC[c]	3 142	<0	NA	Garfield et al. (2002)
Galantamine	10.5	AHEAD	USA	NNT FTC	4 100	<0	<0–15 238	Migliaccio-Walle et al. (2003)
Galantamine	10	AHEAD	The Netherlands	QALYs	1 813	<0	<0–5270	Caro et al. (2002)
Galantamine	10	AHEAD	UK	QALYs	-799	14 23	9639–28 920	Ward et al. (2003)
Memantine	2	Markov	UK	QALYs	3 191	<0	<0–239 740	Jones et al. (2004)
Memantine	5	Markov	Finland	Depend.	1 694	<0	<0 in 94 per cent of Monte Carlo simulations	François et al. (2004)
Memantine	5	Markov	Canada	QALYs	13 255	<0	<0 all scenarios	Jonsson (2005)

[a]A positive value indicates net savings with treatment with CHEIs.
[b]A positive value indicates a cost per gained QALY/avoided deterioration in severity; <0 cost savings and a positive outcome.
[c]Number needed to treat to avoid full time care.
NA, not available.

Table 39.6 Economic evaluations of programs (US$ 2005, PPPs).

Program	Design	Country	Duration	Outcome	Results	ICER in base option	Sensitivity analysis or similar	Source
Day care	Prosp. non RCT	Sweden	6 months	Well years	-3303	9815/WY	NA	Wimo et al. (1990)
Day care	Prosp. non RCT	Sweden	1 year	QALYs	4821	Neutral	NA	Wimo et al. (1994)
Caregiver support	Prosp. RCT	Canada	6 months	QALYs	-839	25 299/QALY	NA	Drummond et al. (1991)
Group living	Model	Sweden	8 years	QALYs	10 491	Dominance	<0 in all options	Wimo et al. (1995)
Caregiver support	CBA-Model	Switzerland	?	Monetary		Dominance	<0 in all options	Nocera et al. (2002)
Caregiver support	Model	Finland	5 years	QALYs	3151	Dominance	71 per cent of MC -simulations cost saving and QALY gaining	Martikainen et al. (2004)
Case management	RCT+bootstrapping	The Netherlands	6 months	'Successful treatment'	242	4247/unit	95 per cent versus WTP of 37 800	Melis et al. (2008)
Case management	RCT+bootstrapping	The Netherlands	3 months	'Successful treatment'	2212	Dominance (94 per cent probability)	99 per cent versus WTP of 2200 per 'successful treatment'	Graff et al. (2008)
Case management	RCT+bootstrapping	The Netherlands	1 year	QALYs	82	1750/QALY	72 per cent versus WTP of 50 000	Wolfs et al. (2007)

US, the specific guidelines for antidementia drugs presented by the FDA demand 'clinically meaningful effects' (Leber, 1997).

Drugs used in dementia are rather expensive and the fact that a drug is registered in a country does not mean that the drug will be available for all patients. A European review by Alzheimer Europe in 2006 showed great variability in Europe regarding reimbursement and accessibility to cholinesterase inhibitors (AlzheimerEurope, 2006) and the situation is even more pronounced from a worldwide viewpoint (Suh *et al.*, 2009). The great UK controversy regarding the recommendations from NICE for drug treatment in AD highlights how delicate this issue is (NICE, 2009). The critical question is the reimbursement decisions (Drummond, 2003). For example, in Sweden the cholinesterase inhibitors are reimbursed like other drugs. However, in Sweden the Dental and Pharmaceutical Benefits Agency, TLV, is a central government agency whose remit is to determine whether a pharmaceutical product or dental care procedure should be reimbursed and the drugs used in AD are on the forthcoming agenda. The experiences from Australia and Canada, with drug authorities demanding health economic evaluations as part of the reimbursement decision process, illustrate that this issue is indeed complicated (Hill and McGettigan, 1998). The Canadian Health Technology Assessment Guidelines for Pharmacoeconomics (CCOHTA), focused on meta-analysis and epidemiological data and emphasized the use of cost-benefit and cost-utility analysis (CCOHTA, 1997).

39.13 INTERNATIONAL COMPARISONS

The way care is financed and organized, as well as the relative supply of different forms of care, the general taxation level and the economic strength of countries are factors that make comparisons between countries difficult.

Comparing currencies presents problems. Usual currency exchange rates reflect trade between countries rather than purchasing power. Purchase power parities (PPPs; OECD, www.oecd.org/std/ppp/pps), are probably better to use than exchange rates. Comparisons over time both within and between countries are also linked to uncertainty. Consumer price indices are often used, but an index that reflects changes in the health care sector is better. The Statistical Office of the European Communities, Eurostat presents Harmonized Indices of Consumer Prices (HICPs) for different sectors, i.e. health.

In multinational studies, the results should be aggregated in terms of resource use (and not in monetary terms) from every country. The cost calculations should then be performed in one currency, based on aggregated resource use. However, if there are great differences in care organization between countries, aggregation of resource utilization results may also be problematic. For example, the concept of 'nursing home' can include a wide range of resources in terms of number of staff and their competence, physical environment and technical equipment, leading to different costs. There are also care concepts that are used just in one or few countries such as DOMUS care in the UK (Beecham *et al.*, 1993),

Group Living in Sweden (Wimo *et al.*, 1995) and special care units (SCU) in the US (Maas *et al.*, 1998). Home care may denote social services with poorly qualified staff, but also specific teams focused on dementia. Even if a care organization can be divided roughly into levels (such as nursing home care, intermediate care alternatives, home care), such a simplistic division questions the validity of multinational intervention studies.

39.14 SEVERE DEMENTIA

Several years in the course of dementia are spent in the stage of severe dementia (Winblad *et al.*, 1999). In a model of a Swedish cohort the course of dementia with an estimated survival up to nine years was simulated (Wimo *et al.*, 1998c). About 75 per cent of the total costs occurred in severe dementia, indicating that the total span for benefits during the total course in terms of cost reduction is only 25 per cent, if efficacy is shown only for mild–moderate dementia. The results indicate that severe dementia must be the focus for improved care and research. Many of the instruments we use today for outcome research show floor effects in severe dementia and they are not sufficiently sensitive to detect clinically relevant changes (Winblad *et al.*, 1999). There are studies that have shown positive effects in severe dementia for menatine (Reisberg *et al.*, 2003), donepezil (Winblad *et al.*, 2006) and to some extent galantamine (Burns *et al.*, 2009), but health economic studies for severe dementia are available only for memantine (Wimo *et al.*, 2003b).

39.15 CONCLUSIONS

The health economics of dementia are in an embryonic state, even if the number of published studies is increasing. There is a great need for methodological improvement. In view of the increasing number of people with dementia and existing as well as new drugs in the pipeline, there is also great interest in pharmacoeconomics among the drug authorities in different countries and in the pharmaceutical companies engaged in drug development. The sparse economic literature on different care programmes is a great problem.

REFERENCES

Allotey P, Reidpath D, Kouame A, Cummins R. (2003) The DALY, context and the determinants of the severity of disease: an exploratory comparison of paraplegia in Australia and Cameroon. *Social Science and Medicine* 57: 949–58.

Almberg B, Grafstrom M, Krichbaum K, Winblad B. (2000) The interplay of institution and family caregiving: relations between patient hassles, nursing home hassles and caregivers' burnout. *International Journal of Geriatric Psychiatry* 15: 931–9.

AlzheimerEurope. (2006) *Dementia in Europe Yearbook 2006.* Luxembourg: Alzheimer Europe.

Andlin-Sobocki P, Jonsson B, Wittchen HU, Olesen J. (2005) Cost of disorders of the brain in Europe. *European Journal of Neuroscience.* **12** (Suppl 1): 1–27.

Atance Martinez JC, Yusta Izquierdo A, Grupeli Gardel BE. (2004) [Costs study in Alzheimer's disease]. *Revista Clínica Española* **204**: 64–9.

Beecham J, Cambridge P, Hallam A, Knapp M. (1993) The cost of Domus care. *International Journal of Geriatric Psychiatry* **8**: 827–31.

Berg L. (1988) Clinical Dementia rating (CDR). *Psychopharmacology Bulletin* **24**: 637–9.

Bergner M, Bobbitt RA, Carter WB, Gilson BS. (1981) The Sickness Impact Profile: development and final revision of a health status measure. *Medical Care* **19**: 787–805.

Birks JS, Harvey R. (2006) Donepezil for dementia due to Alzheimer's disease. *Cochrane Database of Systematic Reviews* **25**: CD001190.

Blau TH. (1977) Quality of Life, social indicators and criteria of change. *Professional Psychology* **8**: 464–73.

Boada M, Pena-Casanova J, Bermejo F et al. (1999) [Costs of health care resources of ambulatory-care patients diagnosed with Alzheimer's disease in Spain]. *Medicina Clínica* **113**: 690–5.

Bowling A. (1995) *Measuring Health. A review of quality of life measurement scales.* Philadelphia: Open University Press, Milton Keynes.

Bråne G, Gottfries CG, Winblad B. (2001) The Gottfries–Brane–Steen scale: validity, reliability and application in anti-dementia drug trials. *Dementia and Geriatric Cognitive Disorders* **12**: 1–14.

Briggs AH, O'Brien BJ. (2001) The death of cost-minimization analysis? *Health Economics* **10**: 179–84.

Brod M, Stewart AL, Sands L, Walton P. (1999) Conceptualization and measurement of quality of life in dementia: the dementia quality of life instrument (DQoL). *Gerontologist* **39**: 25–35.

Burns A, Bernabei R, Bullock R et al. (2009) Safety and efficacy of galantamine (Reminyl) in severe Alzheimer's disease (the SERAD study): a randomised, placebo-controlled, double-blind trial. *Lancet Neurology* **8**: 39–47.

Buxton MJ, Drummond MF, van Hout BA et al. (1997) Modelling in economic evaluation: an unavoidable fact of life. *Health Economics* **6**: 217–27.

Caro JJ. (2005) Pharmacoeconomic analyses using discrete event simulation. *Pharmacoeconomics* **23**: 323–32.

Caro JJ, Getsios D, Migliaccio-Walle K et al. (2001) Assessment of health economics in Alzheimer's disease (AHEAD) based on need for full-time care. *Neurology* **57**: 964–71.

Caro JJ, Salas M, Ward A et al. (2002) Economic analysis of galantamine, a cholinesterase inhibitor, in the treatment of patients with mild to moderate Alzheimer's disease in the Netherlands. *Dementia and Geriatric Cognitive Disorders* **14**: 84–9.

Cavallo MC, Fattore G. (1997) The economic and social burden of Alzheimer disease on families in the Lombardy region of Italy. *Alzheimer Disease and Associated Disorders* **11**: 184–90.

CCOHTA. (1997) *Guidelines for economic evaluation of pharmaceuticals: Canada,* 2nd edn. Ottawa: The Canadian Coordinating Office for Health Technology Assessment.

Clegg A, Bryant J, Nicholson T et al. (2002) Clinical and cost-effectiveness of donepezil, rivastigmine, and galantamine for Alzheimer's disease. *A systematic review. International Journal of Technology Assessment in Health Care* **18**: 497–507.

Clipp EC, Moore MJ. (1995) Caregiver time use: an outcome measure in clinical trial research on Alzheimer's disease. *Clinical Pharmacology and Therapeutics* **58**: 228–36.

Cohen JT, Neumann PJ. (2008) Decision analytic models for Alzheimer's disease: state of the art and future directions. *Alzheimers and Dementia* **4**: 212–22.

Coucill W, Bryan S, Bentham P et al. (2001) EQ-5D in patients with dementia: an investigation of inter-rater agreement. *Medical Care* **39**: 760–71.

Courtney C, Farrell D, Gray R et al. (2004) Long-term donepezil treatment in 565 patients with Alzheimer's disease (AD2000): randomised double-blind trial. *Lancet* **363**: 2105–15.

CPMP. (1997) Note for guidance on medical products in the treatment of Alzheimer's disease. London: EMEA.

Davis KL, Marin DB, Kane R et al. (1997) The Caregiver Activity Survey (CAS): development and validation of a new measure for caregivers of persons with Alzheimer's disease. *International Journal of Geriatric Psychiatry* **12**: 978–88.

Deeken JF, Taylor KL, Mangan P et al. (2003) Care for the caregivers: a review of self-report instruments developed to measure the burden, needs, and quality of life of informal caregivers. *Journal of Pain and Symptom Management* **26**: 922–53.

Dolan P. (2000) A note on QALYs versus HYEs. Health states versus health profiles. *International Journal of Technology Assessment in Health Care* **16**: 1220–4.

Drummond MF. (2003) The use of health economic information by reimbursement authorities. *Rheumatology (Oxford).* **42** (Suppl 3): iii60–3.

Drummond MF, Mohide EA, Tew M et al. (1991) Economic evaluation of a support program for caregivers of demented elderly. *International Journal of Technology Assessment in Health Care* **7**: 209–19.

Drummond MF, Sculper MJ, Torrance GW et al. (2004). *Methods for the economic evaluation of health care programmes.* Oxford: Oxford University Press.

Ekman M, Berg J, Wimo A et al. (2007) Health utilities in mild cognitive impairment and dementia: a population study in Sweden. *International Journal of Geriatric Psychiatry* **22**: 649–55.

Elstner K, Selai CE, Trimble MR, Robertson MM. (2001) Quality of Life (QOL) of patients with Gilles de la Tourette's syndrome. *Acta Psychiatrica Scandinavica* **103**: 52–9.

Ernst RL, Hay JW. (1994) The US economic and social costs of Alzheimer's disease revisited. *American Journal of Public Health* **84**: 1261–4.

Ernst RL, Hay JW, Fenn C et al. (1997) Cognitive function and the costs of Alzheimer disease. An exploratory study. *Archives of Neurology* **54**: 687–93.

Feldman H, Gauthier S, Hecker J et al. (2004) Economic evaluation of donepezil in moderate to severe Alzheimer disease. *Neurology* **63**: 644–50.

Fenn P, Gray A. (1999) Estimating long-term cost savings from treatment of Alzheimer's disease. A modelling approach. *Pharmacoeconomics* **16**: 165–74.

Ferris SH, Mittelman MS. (1996) Behavioral treatment of Alzheimer's disease. *International Psychogeriatrics* 8: 87–90.

Folstein MF, Folstein SE, McHugh PR. (1975) "Mini-mental state". A practical method for grading the cognitive state of patients for the clinician. *Journal of Psychiatric Research* 12: 189–98.

François C, Sintonen H, Sulkava R, Rive B. (2004) Cost effectiveness of memantine on moderately severe to severe Alzheimer's disease. A Markov model in Finland. *Clinical Drug Investigation* 24: 373–84.

Garfield FB, Getsios D, Caro JJ et al. (2002) Assessment of Health Economics in Alzheimer's Disease (AHEAD). Treatment with Galantamine in Sweden. *Pharmacoeconomics* 20: 629–37.

Geldmacher DS, Provenzano G, Mcrae T et al. (2003) Donepezil is associated with delayed nursing home placement in patients with Alzheimer's disease. *Journal of the American Geriatrics Society* 51: 937–44.

Getsios D, Caro JJ, Caro G, Ishak K. (2001) Assessment of health economics in Alzheimer's disease (AHEAD): galantamine treatment in Canada. *Neurology* 57: 972–8.

Graff MJ, Adang EM, Vernooij-Dassen MJ et al. (2008) Community occupational therapy for older patients with dementia and their care givers: cost effectiveness study. *British Medical Journal* 336: 134–8.

Gray A. (2002) Health Economics. In: Qizilbash N, Schneider L, Chui H et al. (eds). *Evidence-based dementia practice*. Oxford: Blackwell Publishing.

Green C. (2007) Modelling disease progression in Alzheimer's disease: a review of modelling methods used for cost-effectiveness analysis. *Pharmacoeconomics* 25: 735–50.

Grutzendler J, Morris JC. (2001) Cholinesterase inhibitors for Alzheimer's disease. *Drugs* 61: 41–52.

Gustavsson A, Jonsson L, McShane R et al. (2010) Willingness-to-pay for reductions in care need: estimating the value of informal care in Alzheimer's disease. *International Journal of Geriatric Psychiatry* 25: 622–32.

Hauber AB, Gnanasakthy A, Mauskopf JA. (2000a) Savings in the cost of caring for patients with Alzheimer's disease in Canada: an analysis of treatment with rivastigmine. *Clinical Therapeutics* 22: 439–51.

Hauber AB, Gnanasakthy A, Snyder EH et al. (2000b) Potential savings in the cost of caring for Alzheimer's disease. Treatment with rivastigmine. *Pharmacoeconomics* 17: 351–60.

Henke CJ, Burchmore MJ. (1997) The economic impact of the tacrine in the treatment of Alzheimer's disease. *Clinical Therapeutics* 19: 330–45.

Hill S, McGettigan P. (1998) Drug authorities' policy on the assessment of drugs for dementia. In: Wimo A, Karlsson G, Jönsson B, Winblad B (eds). *The health economics of dementia*. London: Wiley.

Hux MJ, O'Brien BJ, Iskedjian M et al. (1998) Relation between severity of Alzheimer's disease and costs of caring. *Canadian Medical Association Journal* 159: 457–65.

Ikeda S, Yamada Y, Ikegami N. (2002) Economic evaluation of donepezil treatment for Alzheimer's disease in Japan. *Dementia and Geriatric Cognitive Disorders* 13: 33–9.

Jansson W, Almberg B, Grafstrom M, Winblad B. (1998) The Circle Model – support for relatives of people with dementia. *International Journal of Geriatric Psychiatry* 13: 674–81.

Johannesson M, Johansson PO, Jonsson B. (1992) Economic evaluation of drug therapy: a review of the contingent valuation method. *Pharmacoeconomics* 1: 325–37.

Johannesson M, Jonsson B, Karlsson G. (1996) Outcome measurement in economic evaluation. *Health Economics* 5: 279–96.

Jones RW, McCrone P, Guilhaume C. (2004) Cost effectiveness of memantine in Alzheimer's disease: an analysis based on a probabilistic Markov model from a UK perspective. *Drugs & Aging* 21: 607–20.

Jonsson B, Jonsson L, Wimo A. (2000) Cost of dementia. In: May M, Sartorius N (eds). *Dementia. WPA Series evidence and experience in psychiatry*. London: John Wiley and Sons.

Jonsson L. (2003) Pharmacoeconomics of cholineesterase inhibitors in the treatment of Alzheimer's disease. *Pharmacoeconomics* 21: 1025–37.

Jonsson L. (2005) Cost-effectiveness of memantine for moderate to severe Alzheimer's disease in Sweden. *American Journal of Geriatric Pharmacotherapy* 3: 77–86.

Jonsson L, Andreasen N, Kilander L et al. (2006a) Patient- and proxy-reported utility in Alzheimer disease using the EuroQoL. *Alzheimer Disease and Associated Disorders* 20: 49–55.

Jonsson L, Eriksdotter Jonhagen M, Kilander L et al. (2006b) Determinants of costs of care for patients with Alzheimer's disease. *International Journal of Geriatric Psychiatry* 21: 449–59.

Jonsson L, Lindgren P, Wimo A et al. (1999a) The cost-effectiveness of donepezil therapy in Swedish patients with Alzheimer's disease: a Markov model. *Clinical Therapeutics* 21: 1230–40.

Jonsson L, Lindgren P, Wimo A et al. (1999b) Costs of Mini Mental State Examination-related cognitive impairment. *Pharmacoeconomics* 16: 409–16.

Jönsson L. (2003) *Economic evaluation of treatments for Alzheimer's disease. Neurotec*. Stockholm: Karolinska Institutet.

Jönsson L, Wimo A. (2009) The cost of dementia in europe: a review of the evidence, and methodological considerations. *Pharmacoeconomics* 27: 391–403.

Karlsson G, Jonsson B, Wimo A, Winblad B. (1998) Methodological issues in health economics of dementia. In: Wimo A, Jonsson B, Karlsson G, Winblad B (eds). *Health economics of dementia*. London, UK: John Wiley and Sons.

Kerner DN, Patterson TL, Grant I, Kaplan RM. (1998) Validity of the Quality of Well-Being Scale for patients with Alzheimer's disease. *Journal of Aging and Health* 10: 44–61.

Knapp M, Prince M. (2007) *Dementia UK*. London: Alzheimer's Society.

Knapp MJ, Knopman DS, Solomon PR et al. (1994) A 30-week randomized controlled trial of high-dose tacrine in patients with Alzheimer's disease. The Tacrine Study Group. *Journal of the American Medical Association* 271: 985–91.

Knopman D, Schneider L, Davis K et al. (1996) Long-term tacrine (Cognex) treatment: effects on nursing home placement and mortality, Tacrine Study Group. *Neurology* 47: 166–77.

Koopmanschap MA. (1998) Indirect costs and costing informal care. In: Wimo A, Karlsson G, Jonsson B, Winblad B (eds). *The health economics of dementia*. London: John Wiley and Sons.

Koopmanschap MA, Polder JJ, Meerding WJ *et al.* (1998) Costs of dementia in the Netherlands. In: Wimo A, Jonsson B, Karlsson G, Winblad B (eds). *The health economics of dementia*. London: John Wiley and Sons.

Kronborg Andersen C, Sogaard J, Hansen E *et al.* (1999) The cost of dementia in Denmark: the Odense Study. *Dementia and Geriatric Cognitive Disorders* 10: 295–304.

Lamb HM, Goa KL. (2001) Rivastigmine. A pharmacoeconomic review of its use in Alzheimer's disease. *Pharmacoeconomics* 19: 303–18.

Langa KM, Chernew ME, Kabeto MU *et al.* (2001) National estimates of the quantity and cost of informal caregiving for the elderly with dementia. *Journal of General Internal Medicine* 16: 770–8.

Leber P. (1997) Slowing the progression of Alzheimer disease: methodologic issues. *Alzheimer Disease and Associated Disorders.* 11 (Suppl 5): S10–21; discussion S37–9.

Leung GM, Yeung RY, Chi I, Chu LW. (2003) The economics of Alzheimer disease. *Dementia and Geriatric Cognitive Disorders* 15: 34–43.

Lindgren B. (1981) *Costs of illness in Sweden 1964–1975*. Lund: Liber.

Logsdon RG, Gibbons LE, McCurry SM, Teri L. (2002) Assessing quality of life in older adults with cognitive impairment. *Psychosomatic Medicine* 64: 510–9.

Lovestone S. (2002) Can we afford to develop treatments for dementia? *Journal of Neurology, Neurosurgery, and Psychiatry* 72: 685.

Lubeck DP, Mazonson PD, Bowe T. (1994) Potential effect of tacrine on expenditures for Alzheimer's disease. *Medical Interface* 7: 130–8.

Lyseng-Williamson KA, Plosker GL. (2002) Galantamine: a pharmacoeconomic review of its use in Alzheimer's disease. *Pharmacoeconomics* 20: 919–42.

Lyseng-Williamson KA, Plosker GL. (2003) Spotlight on Galantamine in Alzheimer's Disease. *Disease Management, Health Outcomes* 11: 125–8.

Maas ML, Specht JP, Weiler K *et al.* (1998) Special care units for people with Alzheimer's disease. Only for the privileged few? *Journal of Gerontological Nursing* 24: 28–37.

Martikainen J, Valtonen H, Pirttila T. (2004) Potential cost-effectiveness of a family-based program in mild Alzheimer's disease patients. *European Journal of Health Economics* 5: 136–42.

Max W. (1996) The cost of Alzheimer's disease. Will drug treatment ease the burden? *Pharmacoeconomics* 9: 5–10.

Max W, Webber P, Fox P. (1995) Alzheimer's disease. The unpaid burden of caring. *Journal of Aging and Health* 7: 179–99.

Melis RJ, Adang E, Teerenstra S *et al.* (2008) Multidimensional geriatric assessment: back to the future cost-effectiveness of a multidisciplinary intervention model for community-dwelling frail older people. *Journals of Gerontology. Series A, Biological Sciences and Medical Sciences* 63: 275–82.

Migliaccio-Walle K, Getsios D, Caro JJ *et al.* (2003) Economic evaluation of galantamine in the treatment of mild to moderate Alzheimer's disease in the United States. *Clinical Therapeutics* 25: 1806–25.

Mohide EA, Torrance GW, Streiner DL *et al.* (1988) Measuring the wellbeing of family caregivers using the time trade-off technique. *Journal of Clinical Epidemiology* 41: 475–82.

Moore MJ, Zhu CW, Clipp EC. (2001) Informal costs of dementia care: estimates from the National Longitudinal Caregiver Study. *Journals of Gerontology. Series B, Psychological Sciences and Social Sciences* 56: S219–28.

Neumann PJ, Hermann RC, Kuntz KM *et al.* (1999) Cost-effectiveness of donepezil in the treatment of mild or moderate Alzheimer's disease. *Neurology* 52: 1138–45.

Neumann PJ, Sandberg EA, Araki SS *et al.* (2000) A comparison of HUI2 and HUI3 utility scores in Alzheimer's disease. *Medical Decision Making* 20: 413–22.

NICE. (2001) Guidance on the use of donepezil, rivastigmine and galantamine for the treatment of Alzheimer's disease. National Institute for Clinical Excellence (NICE).

NICE. (2009) Donepezil, galantamine, rivastigmine (review) and memantine for the treatment of Alzheimer's disease (amended).

Nocera S, Bonato D, Telser H. (2002) The contingency of contingent valuation. How much are people willing to pay against Alzheimer's disease? *International Journal of Health Care Finance and Economics* 2: 219–40.

Nordberg G, Von Strauss E, Kareholt I *et al.* (2005) The amount of informal and formal care among non-demented and demented elderly persons-results from a Swedish population-based study. *International Journal of Geriatric Psychiatry* 20: 862–71.

O'Brien BJ, Goeree R, Hux M *et al.* (1999) Economic evaluation of donepezil for the treatment of Alzheimer's disease in Canada. *Journal of the American Geriatrics Society* 47: 570–8.

O'Shea E, O'Reilly S. (2000) The economic and social cost of dementia in Ireland. *International Journal of Geriatric Psychiatry* 15: 208–18.

OECD. (1996) Caring for frail elderly people – policies in evolution. In: Hennessy P (ed.). *Social policy studies* 19. Paris: OECD.

Olin J, Schneider L. (2002) Galantamine for Alzheimer's disease. *Cochrane Database of Systematic Reviews* 3: CD001747.

Ostbye T, Crosse E. (1994) Net economic costs of dementia in Canada. *Canadian Medical Association Journal* 151: 1457–64.

Quentin W, Riedel-Heller SG, Luppa M *et al.* (2009) Cost-of-illness studies of dementia: a systematic review focusing on stage dependency of costs. *Acta Psychiatrica Scandinavica* 121: 243–59.

Reisberg B, Ferris SH, De Leon MJ, Crook T. (1988) Global Deterioration Scale (GDS). *Psychopharmacology Bulletin* 24: 661–3.

Reisberg B, Doody R, Stoffler A *et al.* (2003) Memantine in moderate-to-severe Alzheimer's disease. *New England Journal of Medicine* 348: 1333–41.

Rice DP, Hodgson TA, Kopstein AN. (1985) The economic costs of illness: a replication and update. *Health Financing Review* 7: 61–80.

Rice DP, Fox PJ, Max W *et al.* (1993) The economic burden of Alzheimer's disease care. *Health Affairs (Millwood)* 12: 164–76.

Rigaud AS, Fagnani F, Bayle C et al. (2003) Patients with Alzheimer's disease living at home in France: costs and consequences of the disease. *Journal of Geriatric Psychiatry and Neurology* **16**: 140–5.

Rosen WG, Mohs RC, Davis KL. (1984) A new rating scale for Alzheimer's disease. *American Journal of Psychiatry* **141**: 1356–64.

Rosenheck RA, Leslie DL, Sindelar JL et al. (2007) Cost-benefit analysis of second-generation antipsychotics and placebo in a randomized trial of the treatment of psychosis and aggression in Alzheimer disease. *Archives of General Psychiatry* **64**: 1259–68.

Salek SS, Walker MD, Bayer AJ. (1998) A review of quality of life in Alzheimer's disease. Part 2: Issues in assessing drug effects. *Pharmacoeconomics* **14**: 613–27.

Sano M, Ernesto C, Thomas RG et al. (1997) A controlled trial of selegiline, alpha-tocopherol, or both as treatment for Alzheimer's disease. The Alzheimer's Disease Cooperative Study. *New England Journal of Medicine* **336**: 1216–22.

SBU. Dementia. A systematic review. Stockholm, Staten beredning för medicinsk utvärdering (SBU) (The Swedish Council on Technology Assessment in Health Care), 2008.

Schneider L. (1998) Designing phase III trials of anti-dementia drugs with a view towards pharmacoeconomical considerations. In: Wimo A, Jonsson B, Karlsson G, Winblad B (eds). *Health economics of dementia*. London, UK: John Wiley and Sons.

Schneider LS, Olin JT, Lyness SA, Chui HC. (1997) Eligibility of Alzheimer's disease clinic patients for clinical trials. *Journal of the American Geriatrics Society* **45**: 923–8.

Schulenberg J, Schulenberg I. (1998) Cost of treatment and cost of care for Alzheimer's disease in Germany. In: Wimo A, Jonsson B, Karlsson G, Winblad B (eds). *The health economics of dementia*. London: John Wiley and Sons.

Schulz R, Beach SR. (1999) Caregiving as a risk factor for mortality: the Caregiver Health Effects Study. *Journal of the American Medical Association* **282**: 2215–9.

Scuvee-Moreau J, Kurz X, Dresse A. (2002) The economic impact of dementia in Belgium: results of the National Dementia Economic Study (NADES). *Acta Neurologica Belgica* **102**: 104–13.

Selai CE, Elstner K, Trimble MR. (2000) Quality of life pre and post epilepsy surgery. *Epilepsy Research* **38**: 67–74.

Selai C, Vaughan A, Harvey RJ, Logsdon R. (2001) Using the QOL-AD in the UK. *International Journal of Geriatric Psychiatry* **16**: 537–8.

Shukla VK, Otten N, Coyle D. (2000) *Drug treatments for Alzheimer's Disease III. a review of published pharmacoeconomic evaluations*. Ottawa, Canada: Canadian Coordinating Office for Health Technology Assessment (CCOHTA).

Siegel JE, Torrance GW, Russell LB et al. (1997) Guidelines for pharmacoeconomic studies. Recommendations from the panel on cost effectiveness in health and medicine. Panel on cost Effectiveness in Health and Medicine. *Pharmacoeconomics* **11**: 159–68.

Sonnenberg FA, Leventhal EA. (1998) Modeling disease progression with Markov models. In: Wimo A, Jonsson B, Karlsson G, Winblad B (eds). *Health economics of dementia*. London, UK: John Wiley and Sons.

Souetre EJ, Qing W, Vigoureux I et al. (1995) Economic analysis of Alzheimer's disease in outpatients: impact of symptom severity. *International Psychogeriatrics* **7**: 115–22.

Spilker B. (1996) *Quality of life and pharmacoeconomics in clinical trials*. Philadelphia: Lippincott-Raven Publishers.

Stewart A, Brod M. (1996) Measuring health related quality of life in older and demented people. In: Spilker B (ed.) *Quality of life and pharmacoeconomics in clinical trials*. Philadelphia: Lippincott-Raven Publishers.

Stewart A, Phillips R, Dempsey G. (1998) Pharmacotherapy for people with Alzheimer's disease: a Markov-cycle evaluation of five years' therapy using donepezil. *International Journal of Geriatric Psychiatry* **13**: 445–53.

Stommel M, Collins CE, Given BA. (1994) The costs of family contributions to the care of persons with dementia. *Gerontologist* **34**: 199–205.

Suh GH, Wimo A, Gauthier S et al. (2009) International price comparisons of Alzheimer's drugs: a way to close the affordability gap. *International Psychogeriatrics* **21**: 1116–26.

Torrance G. (1996) Designing and conducting cost-utility analysis. In: Spilker B (ed.) *Quality of life and pharmacoeconomics in clinical trials*. Philadelphia: Lippincott-Raven Publishers.

Torrance GW. (1997) Preferences for health outcomes and cost-utility analysis. *American Journal of Managed Care*. **3** (Suppl): S8–20.

Torrance GW, Feeny DH, Furlong WJ et al. (1996) Multiattribute utility function for a comprehensive health status classification system. Health Utilities Index Mark 2. *Medical Care* **34**: 702–22.

Tsuchiya A, Dolan P, Shaw R. (2003) Measuring people's preferences regarding ageism in health: some methodological issues and some fresh evidence. *Social Science and Medicine* **57**: 687–96.

Van den Berg B, Brouwer W, Van Exel J et al. (2006) Economic valuation of informal care: lessons from the application of the opportunity costs and proxy good methods. *Social Science and Medicine* **62**: 835–45.

Walker MD, Salek SS, Bayer AJ. (1998) A review of quality of life in Alzheimer's disease. Part 1: Issues in assessing disease impact. *Pharmacoeconomics* **14**: 499–530.

Wallin AK, Gustafson L, Sjogren M et al. (2004) Five-year outcome of cholinergic treatment of Alzheimer's disease: early response predicts prolonged time until nursing home placement, but does not alter life expectancy. *Dementia and Geriatric Cognitive Disorders* **18**: 197–206.

Ward A, Caro JJ, Getsios D et al. (2003) Assessment of health economics in Alzheimer's disease (AHEAD): treatment with galantamine in the UK. *International Journal of Geriatric Psychiatry* **18**: 740–7.

Ware Jr JE, Sherbourne CD. (1992) The MOS 36-item short-form health survey (SF-36). I. Conceptual framework and item selection. *Medical Care* **30**: 473–83.

Weinstein MC, Fineberg HV. (1980) *Clinical decision analysis*. Philadelphia: W.B. Saunders.

Wimo A, Winblad B. (2003a) Pharmacoeconomics of mild cognitive impairment. *Acta Neurologica Scandinavica*. **179** (suppl): 94–9.

Wimo A, Winblad B. (2003b) Resource utilisation in dementia: RUD Lite. *Brain Aging* **3**: 48–59.

Wimo A, Wallin JO, Lundgren K *et al.* (1990) Impact of day care on dementia patients–costs, well-being and relatives' views. *Family Practice* **7**: 279–87.

Wimo A, Mattsson B, Krakau I *et al.* (1994) Cost-effectiveness analysis of day care for patients with dementia disorders. *Health Economics* **3**: 395–404.

Wimo A, Mattson B, Krakau I *et al.* (1995) Cost-utility analysis of group living in dementia care. *International Journal of Technology Assessment in Health Care* **11**: 49–65.

Wimo A, Karlsson G, Nordberg A, Winblad B. (1997) Treatment of Alzheimer disease with tacrine: a cost-analysis model. *Alzheimer Disease and Associated Disorders* **11**: 191–200.

Wimo A, Jonsson B, Karlsson G, Winblad BE. (1998a) *The health economics of dementia.* London: John Wiley and Sons.

Wimo A, Wetterholm AL, Mastey V, Winblad B. (1998b) Evaluation of the resource utilization and caregiver time in Anti-dementia drug trials – a quantitative battery. In: Wimo A, Jonsson B, Karlsson G, Winblad B (eds). *The health economics of dementia.* London: John Wiley and Sons.

Wimo A, Witthaus E, Rother M, Winblad B. (1998c) Economic impact of introducing propentofylline for the treatment of dementia in Sweden. *Clinical Therapeutics* **20**: 552–66; discussion 550–51.

Wimo A, Johansson L, Von Strauss E, Nordberg G. (1999a) Formal and informal home care to Swedish demented patients, an application of RUD (Resource Utilization in Dementia)(abstract). *International Psychogeriatrics*, **11** (suppl 1): 197.

Wimo A, Winblad B, Grafstrom M. (1999b) The social consequences for families with Alzheimer's disease patients: potential impact of new drug treatment. *International Journal of Geriatric Psychiatry* **14**: 338–47.

Wimo A, Nordberg G, Jansson W, Grafstrom M. (2000) Assessment of informal services to demented people with the RUD instrument. *International Journal of Geriatric Psychiatry* **15**: 969–71.

Wimo A, Von Strauss E, Nordberg G *et al.* (2002) Time spent on informal and formal care giving for persons with dementia in Sweden. *Health Policy* **61**: 255–68.

Wimo A, Winblad B, Engedal K *et al.* (2003a) An economic evaluation of donepezil in mild to moderate Alzheimer's disease: results of a 1-year, double-blind, randomized trial. *Dementia and Geriatric Cognitive Disorders* **15**: 44–54.

Wimo A, Winblad B, Stoffler A *et al.* (2003b) Resource utilisation and cost analysis of memantine in patients with moderate to severe Alzheimer's disease. *Pharmacoeconomics* **21**: 327–40.

Wimo A, Johansson L, Jönsson L. (2007a) Demenssjukdomarnas samhällskostnader och antalet dementa i Sverige 2005 (The societal costs of dementia and the number of demented in Sweden 2005) (in Swedish). In: Socialstyrelsen E (ed.) *Underlag från experter.* Stockholm: SOCIALSTYRELSEN.

Wimo A, Jönsson L, Winblad B. (2007b) An estimate of the total worldwide societal costs of dementia in 2005. *Alzheimer's and Dementia* **3**: 81–91.

Wimo A, Jönsson L, Gustavsson A. (2008) The cost of illness and burden of dementia in Europe. In: Europe A (ed.) *Dementia in Europe Yearbook 2008.* Luxembourg: Alzheimer Europe.

Wimo A, Johansson L, Jonsson L. (2009) [Prevalence study of societal costs for dementia 2000–2005. More demented people – but somewhat reduced costs per person]. *Lakartidningen* **106**: 1277–82.

Winblad B, Hill S, Beermann B *et al.* (1997) Issues in the economic evaluation of treatment for dementia. Position paper from the International Working Group on Harmonization of Dementia Drug Guidelines. *Alzheimer Disease and Associated Disorders* **11**: 39–45.

Winblad B, Wimo A, Mobius HJ *et al.* (1999) Severe dementia: a common condition entailing high costs at individual and societal levels. *International Journal of Geriatric Psychiatry* **14**: 911–4.

Winblad B, Kilander L, Eriksson S *et al.* (2006) Donepezil in patients with severe Alzheimer's disease: double-blind, parallel-group, placebo-controlled study. *Lancet* **367**: 1057–65.

Wolfs CA, Dirksen CD, Kessels A *et al.* (2007) Economic evaluation of an integrated diagnostic approach for psychogeriatric patients: Results of a randomized controlled trial. In: Wolfs CA (ed.) *An integrated approach to dementia. A clinical and economic evaluation (thesis).* Maastricht: Neuropsych Publishers.

Wolfson C, Oremus M, Shukla V *et al.* (2002) Donepezil and rivastigmine in the treatment of Alzheimer's disease: a best-evidence synthesis of the published data on their efficacy and cost-effectiveness. *Clinical Therapeutics* **24**: 862–86; discussion 837.

Zarit SH, Reever KE, Bach-Peterson J. (1980) Relatives of the impaired elderly: correlates of feelings of burden. *Gerontologist* **20**: 649–55.

The global challenge of dementia: what can be done

CLEUSA P FERRI, JIM JACKSON AND MARTIN PRINCE

40.1 GLOBAL CHALLENGE OF DEMENTIA

Demographic ageing has been much more rapid in all regions than first anticipated with a sharp increase in the numbers and proportion of older people in developing countries (World Population Prospects, 2003). In 2005, 20 per cent of the population in high income countries (HICs) was aged over 60 years, and this is predicted to increase to 32 per cent by 2050. This proportion in low and middle income countries (LMICs) was just 8 per cent in 2005 but is expected to rise to 20 per cent by 2050. Chronic non-communicable diseases, which were under-prioritized in the public health agenda for years, are now assuming a greater significance in LMICs.

Co-morbid health conditions are particularly common among older people, with physical conditions affecting different organ systems coexisting with mental and cognitive disorders. Dementia has a disproportionate impact on dependency and disability and yet its global public health importance is still underappreciated. There is a general lack of awareness of Alzheimer's disease (AD) and other dementias as medical conditions, which is accentuated in LMICs, where they are commonly perceived as a normal part of ageing (Patel and Prince, 2001). Lack of awareness directly affects help-seeking behaviour and hence the recognition and management of the condition, which in turn contribute to the burden experienced by family and other carers of people with dementia.

40.1.1 Prevalence

Alzheimer's Disease International (ADI), the umbrella organization for national Alzheimer's associations, convened a panel of international experts in 2004 to review the global evidence on the prevalence of dementia, and to estimate the prevalence of dementia in each world region, the current numbers of people affected, and the projected increases over time. The expert consensus estimated that in 2001, 24.2 million people lived with dementia worldwide and that this amount would double every 20 years with 4.6 million new cases annually (Ferri et al., 2005). Most people (two-thirds) lived in LMICs, a proportion that was projected to increase rapidly with sharper increases estimated for developing than developed regions. These estimates were revised in 2009, when a systematic review of the world literature on the prevalence of dementia was conducted for the World Alzheimer's Report (ADI, 2009). For this occasion, rather than relying on expert consensus only, a quantitative meta-analysis was attempted to synthesize the available evidence for some regions.

Since the Lancet/ADI estimates were published, the global evidence-base has expanded considerably. There have been new studies from Europe (Francesconi et al., 2006; Lobo et al., 2007; Fernandez et al., 2008) and the USA (Plassman et al., 2007), and an explosion of studies from LMICs and other regions and groups previously under-represented in the literature (ADI, 2009). By 2009, 41 per cent (64/158) of dementia prevalence studies had been conducted in LMICs. A very different situation compared to 1998, when the 10/66 Dementia Research Group was founded – its title being derived from the estimate that only 10 per cent of population-based research had been conducted in LMICs, relative to the two-thirds of people with dementia living in those regions.

The updated estimates (ADI, 2009) confirmed the previous projection of numbers doubling every 20 years. Total figures were estimated to be approximately 10 per cent higher than the previous estimates (48.1 million in 2020 and 90.3 million in 2040). Over the next 20 years, the numbers of people with dementia are anticipated to increase by 40 per cent in Europe, 63 per cent in North America, 77 per cent in the southern Latin American cone and 89 per cent in developed Asia Pacific countries. In comparison, the percentage increase is expected to be 117 per cent in East Asia, 107 per cent in South Asia, 134–146 per cent in Latin America and 125 per cent in North Africa and the Middle East.

40.1.2   Burden

The number of people worldwide affected by dementia provides one indicator of the impact of the disorder, without fully capturing the problem for the individual affected, their families and society. The impact of dementia can be understood at three levels:

1. the person with dementia, who experiences ill health, disability, impaired quality of life and reduced life expectancy;
2. the family and friends of the person with dementia, who provide the cornerstone of care and support for the person with dementia;
3. wider society, health and long-term care systems and lost productivity.

The Global Burden of Disease report shows that non-communicable diseases are rapidly becoming the dominant causes of ill health in all developing regions except Sub-Saharan Africa (Fuster and Voute, 2005). Dementia is one of the main causes of disability in later life, but it is important to understand the contribution of dementia, relative to that of other chronic diseases. The estimates contained in the WHO's Global Burden of Disease (GBD) report, first published in 1996 and updated to 2005, provide important evidence in this respect (WHO, 1996; WHO, 2006). These are highly influential in terms of priorities for policymaking and planning at national, regional and international levels. The key indicator is the disability adjusted life year (DALY), a single integrated measure of disease burden calculated as the sum of years lived with disability (YLD) and years of life lost (YLL). In a wide consensus consultation for the Global Burden of Disease report, disability from dementia was accorded a higher disability weight (0.67) than that for almost any other condition, with the exception of severe developmental disorders (WHO, 2004a). A weight of 0.67 signifies that each year lived with dementia entails the loss of two-thirds of one DALY. According to the GBD estimates, dementia contributed 11.2 per cent of all years lived with disability among people aged 60 years and over: more than stroke (9.5 per cent), musculoskeletal disorders (8.9 per cent), cardiovascular disease (5.0 per cent) and all forms of cancer.

The economic costs of dementia are enormous. These include the costs of: (a) 'formal care' – health care, social/community care, respite and long-term residential or nursing home care and (b) 'informal care' – unpaid care by family members including their lost opportunity to earn income.

Wimo *et al.* (2007) attempted to estimate the worldwide cost of dementia in 2005. This amounted to $US 315 billion per year, of which $US 227 billion (72 per cent of the worldwide total) was contributed by HICs and $US 88 billion (28 per cent) by LMICs. This exercise showed that informal care is more used in LMICs, where few formal health or social care services are available. Informal care accounted for 56 per cent of costs in LICs, 42 per cent in MICs and 31 per cent in HICs. Detailed studies of informal costs outside Western Europe and North America are rare, but a study of a sample of 42 AD patients in Denizli, Turkey, found that formal care for the elderly was rare: only 1 per cent of old people in Turkey live in residential care. Families therefore provide most of the care. The average annual cost of care (excluding hospitalization) was $US 4930 for severe cases and $US 1766 for mild ones. Most costs increased with the severity of the disease, although out-patient costs declined. Carers spent 3 hours per day looking after the most severely affected patients (Zencir *et al.*, 2005).

The 10/66 Dementia Research Group has also examined the economic impact of dementia in its pilot study of 706 people with dementia, and their caregivers, living in Latin America, India, China and Nigeria (10/66 Dementia Research Group, 2004). One of the key findings from this study was that caregiving in the developing world is associated with substantial economic disadvantage. A high proportion of carers had to cut back on paid work to care. Many carers needed and obtained additional support, and while this was often informal unpaid care from friends and other family members, paid caregivers were also relatively common. People with dementia were heavy users of health services, and associated direct costs were high. Compensatory financial support was negligible; few older people in developing countries receive government or occupational pensions, and virtually none of the people with dementia in the 10/66 study received disability pensions. Carers were commonly in paid employment, and almost none received any form of carer allowance (10/66 Dementia Research Group, 2004). The combination of reduced family incomes and increased family expenditure on care is obviously particularly stressful in lower income countries where so many households exist at or near to subsistence level. While health-care services are cheaper in LICs, in relative terms families from the poorer countries spend a greater proportion of their income on health care for the person with dementia. They also tend to selectively use the more expensive services of private doctors. Numerous studies have shown that the costs of caring can extend beyond demands on time and money and can affect in the longer term the carer's health and morale.

40.2   WHAT CAN BE DONE?

The increasing global burden of dementia requires strong commitment and leadership from different parts of society, especially from policymakers and health professionals to place dementia higher up in the global health agenda, in order to improve the lives of people with dementia. Dementia has already become a health priority in some countries, including Australia, France, South Korea, England and Scotland. The key elements of these countries' plans are: to raise awareness; to improve diagnosis and treatment and to increase the capacity of health-care systems to respond to the challenge of the increasing number of people with dementia.

Awareness and understanding →	Capacity building →	Risk reduction →	Service development →	Service development
• The public • Health and care service decision makers	• Family carers • Primary healthcare workers • Resource acquisition • Legislative and policy framework	• Diet • Exercise • Social interaction	• Primary care • Community support for families	• Secondary care • Institutional care

Figure 40.1 A graduated approach to dementia service development. Reproduced with permission from Alzheimer Disease International (ADI, 2009).

The key elements for countries with limited resources will differ in its contents and process of implementation and they should start with initiatives that have the maximum impact for as many people as possible. ADI developed a graduated approach for countries with limited resources (ADI, 2009), illustrated in **Figure 40.1**. This focuses initial attention on awareness and understanding and from this, moves on to risk reduction and the underlying issues of capacity building and resource development. Service development starts in primary care, before secondary care can be considered because this will be more equitable, benefiting more people with dementia and their families. It has the potential to prevent or at least delay the need for expensive institutional services that few families can afford.

40.2.1 Increasing awareness – decreasing stigma

Awareness raising and increasing understanding are important to counter the fatalism and stigma that are often associated with dementia. The heart of awareness-raising is to explain that dementia is an illness/disease, that it is not an inevitable consequence of ageing, and that it is worth assisting family carers and people with dementia to live as normal a life as possible for as long as possible. Efforts to increase awareness must be accompanied by health system and service reform, so that help-seeking is met with a supply of better prepared and more responsive services. Awareness-raising and increasing understanding is also essential for all those involved in decision making about dementia services. Without a basic understanding of the nature of the illness, its social and economic consequences and the practical steps that can be taken, it is unlikely that either existing services will be redesigned or enhanced or that new services will be considered.

ADI identified raising awareness of dementia among people in general, carers and health workers as a global priority (Graham and Brodaty, 1997).

1. A critical mass of informed carers can assist awareness-raising, provide advice and support to families, and can work with Alzheimer associations to lobby for more services that better meet their needs.
2. Community solidarity can effect change through support for policies based on equity and justice – equal access to health and social care, and welfare benefits. Aware communities can provide support, and reduce stigma and exclusion of those with dementia and their carers. Policymakers can be held to account by media campaigns and advocacy from committed non-governmental organizations (NGOs). In high income countries awareness is growing rapidly, with the media playing an important part (Prince et al., 2008). Recent evidence-based reports from the UK and Australian Alzheimer associations garnered media attention and were instrumental in making dementia a national priority. Media in LMICs can be receptive to these stories, informing the public and stimulating debate, but efforts are required to alert them to the importance of ageing and dementia, and to build their capacity to report the problem (Prince et al., 2008).
3. Intergenerational solidarity can be promoted through awareness-raising among children and young adults. In many LMICs, children or children-in-law are the most frequent carers for people with dementia (Choo et al., 2003; 10/66 Dementia Research Group, 2004; Dias et al., 2004), and the most likely to initiate help-seeking. A high proportion of people with dementia in LMICs live in multigeneration households with young children, and their carers will have divided responsibilities. Children will be future carers of older parents, and future older people. They are receptive, and easily accessed through schools.
4. The provision of disability pensions and carer benefits will inevitably increase requests for diagnostic assessment.
5. Increasingly the voices of people who have been diagnosed with dementia are being heard, either singly (Taylor, 2007) or collectively (Scottish Dementia Working Group, 2009). By describing their experiences of how it feels to be diagnosed with dementia and their need for supportive services, they are challenging the stigma and the lack of public understanding associated with dementia.

40.2.2 Improving the capacity of existing services

40.2.2.1 RECOGNITION AND DIAGNOSIS

Dementia is a hidden problem, especially in LMICs, with little help-seeking despite the high burden it poses to carers and families. Dementia is in many settings seen as 'normal' ageing and there is reluctance from family, patients and health workers to make a dementia diagnosis as it carries a burden of stigma. However, recognition is the first step in enhancing the capacity of family carers to look after their relative with dementia, and to empower them in their interaction with service providers. It can be boosted by community dissemination of information from government, health-care providers and media. Also, help-seeking can be promoted by proactive case-finding. In India and Brazil, after brief training, community health workers were able to identify likely cases of dementia in the community with a positive predictive value (PPV) of 66 per cent (Shaji et al., 2002a; Ramos-Cerqueira et al., 2005).

Another step in recognizing/diagnosing dementia is testing. Population screening is not considered cost-effective even in high income countries (National Collaborating Centre for Mental Health, 2007). Few trials evaluating dementia screening in primary care have been performed, with little evidence on its benefits and potential harms (Brayne et al., 2007). Selective screening of those for whom there is a prior index of suspicion can be carried out either by cognitive testing, or informant report of cognitive and functional decline. The Mini-Mental State Examination (MMSE) is the most widely used cognitive screen, and adapted versions have been normed for use in many LMICs (Bird et al., 1987; Ganguli et al., 1995; Brucki et al., 2003; Xu et al., 2003; Castro-Costa et al., 2008). However, it takes 10 minutes to administer and is prone to educational and cultural bias (Black et al., 1999; Ng et al., 2007). A systematic review of 16 brief screening assessments identified three (the General Practitioner Assessment of Cognition, Mini-Cog and Memory Impairment Screen), taking less than 5 minutes to administer, that were considered suitable and valid for routine use in general practice, but they have not been validated in poorer settings (Brodaty et al., 2006; see Chapter 6, Screening and assessment instruments for the detection and measurement of cognitive impairment).

In HICs, diagnoses are typically made by specialist dementia services, not widely available in LMICs. The 10/66 Dementia Research Group's culture and education-fair diagnostic protocol is validated across many LMICs, cultures and languages (Prince et al., 2003; Liu et al., 2005), but would need adaptation for routine clinical use. Good practice guidelines (National Collaborating Centre for Mental Health, 2007) advocate a 'dementia screen' to exclude treatable causes of dementia: haematology, biochemistry, thyroid function tests, vitamin B_{12} and folate levels are routinely recommended; testing for syphilis or HIV is indicated only for those at risk. Feasibility and cost-effectiveness needs to be tested in LMICs.

Disclosure of dementia diagnosis is considered by primary care physicians to be the most difficult area of dementia management (Bamford et al., 2004). A recent systematic review identified eight domains of good practice for disclosing dementia diagnosis – preparation; integrating family members; exploring the patient's perspective; disclosing the diagnosis; responding to patient reactions; focusing on quality of life and well-being; planning for the future; and communicating effectively (Lecouturier et al., 2008). The person being assessed should be asked if they and/or others wish to be told the diagnosis. They should then be provided with information about the signs and symptoms of dementia, course and prognosis, available treatments, local care and support services. Medico-legal issues may be discussed, including financial and testamentary capacity and driving safety.

40.2.2.2   PREVENTION

Prevention could in principle be highly cost effective, considering the high cost attached to the care and treatment of those with dementia. With changing lifestyles, exposure levels to cardiovascular disease risk factors are rising rapidly in many LMICs. Recent research suggests that vascular disease predisposes to AD as well as to vascular dementia (Hofman et al., 1997) and primary prevention should focus upon targets suggested by current evidence: risk factors for vascular disease, including hypertension, smoking, type II diabetes and hyperlipidaemia (see Chapter 3, Prevalence and incidence of dementia, Chapter 47, Risk factors for Alzheimer's disease, Chapter 58, Prevention of Alzheimer's disease and Chapter 60, Vascular factors and Alzheimer's disease). There is still a need for more research to identify modifiable risk factors and to establish the risk attributable to different factors across different populations. Although current knowledge is not enough to show how dementia might be prevented in individuals, it does point to how the risk for populations as a whole might be reduced. Dementia should therefore be included in awareness campaigns to reduce the risk of cardiovascular and other chronic diseases.

In comparison with the situation in most HICs, efforts to prevent and control the coming epidemic of cardiovascular and other chronic diseases in most of the LMICs are in their infancy (Epping-Jordan et al., 2005). Advocated measures include the implementation of tobacco-free policies, taxation of tobacco products, comprehensive bans on advertising of tobacco products, salt reduction through voluntary agreements with the food industry and combination drug therapy for those at high risk of cardiovascular disease (Epping-Jordan et al., 2005). The detection and control of hypertension, hyperlipidaemia, diabetes and metabolic syndrome is poorly implemented by overstretched primary care services that struggle to cope with the double burden of historic priorities (maternal, child and communicable diseases) and the increase of chronic disease in adults.

40.2.2.3   IMPROVING TREATMENT

The 10/66 Dementia Research Group's carer pilot study conducted in several developing countries (WHO, 2009) indicated that people with dementia were using primary and secondary care health services. Only 33 per cent of people with dementia in India, 11 per cent in China and South-East Asia and 18 per cent in Latin America had used no health services at all in the previous three months. There was also a heavy use of private medical services, which might be a reflection of the carer's perception of the unresponsiveness of services provided by the government. Many developing countries have in place comprehensive community-based primary care system staffed by doctors, nurses and generic multi-purpose health workers, yet primary healthcare services in LMICs fail older people with dementia as they are clinic-based and preoccupied with simple curative interventions, orientated towards acute rather than chronic conditions (Patel and Prince, 2001; Shaji *et al.*, 2002b; Dias *et al.*, 2004; Prince *et al.*, 2007). A paradigm shift is needed to encompass continuing care and support as part of a wider chronic disease strategy. Given the frailty of many older people with dementia, there is also a need for outreach, assessing and managing patients in their own homes. The WHO Innovative Care for Chronic Conditions framework (Epping-Jordan *et al.*, 2004) makes no mention of dementia, but the principles are highly applicable: a dialogue to build commitment for change; extended, regular health-care contact; a multi-sector approach; centring care on patients and families, supporting patients in the community; and an emphasis on prevention. Dementia care should be an essential component of chronic disease care strategies.

40.2.2.4   REDUCING COSTS OF TREATMENT

Newly developed and effective anti-dementia drugs are likely to be very expensive. Costs of cholinesterase inhibitors (ChEIs) are reimbursed in some countries in Latin American and some provinces in China, and generic ChEIs are available in India (Prince *et al.*, 2009). This is a very active and promising field for drug development and any new disease-modifying agent (Rafii and Aisen, 2009) would raise huge ethical and practical challenges and will need a response on the scale of the Global Fund and PEPFAR initiatives for HIV/AIDS to secure affordability for people in developing countries. This would, of necessity, include strengthening the capacity of primary care to diagnose dementia and deliver treatment and care, as part of wider improvements in primary health care for older people (WHO, 2009). Costs of primary care and community interventions can be minimized through task-shifting to non-specialist and para-professional staff and integration with more broadly-based chronic disease (Epping-Jordan, 2004), disability and elder care programmes (United Nations, 2002; WHO, 2004b).

40.2.3   Delivering efficacious treatment

40.2.3.1   PRACTICE-BASED PROGRAMMES

Although many LMICs aim to have in place comprehensive community-based primary care systems staffed by doctors, nurses and generic multi-purpose health workers, most have insufficient specialists dedicated to dementia care to provide national frontline dementia services (Prince *et al.*, 2009). Initial diagnosis and needs assessment can be conducted in primary care, although specialist input would be desirable. A commitment to continuing care is essential, with regular review, coupled with updated physical health and needs assessments. Practice-based case managers can co-ordinate this process; this collaborative care model has been shown to reduce behavioural and psychological symptoms of dementia

(BPSD) and carer strain in a randomized controlled trial (RCT) in the United States (Callahan *et al.*, 2006). Specialists, where available, can help with advice, inpatient or outpatient review of refractory BPSD, and respite care.

40.2.3.2   COMMUNITY-BASED PROGRAMS

Those with dementia are mostly cared for by their families. The 10/66 pilot study (WHO, 2006) showed that levels of career strain and psychological morbidity are at least as high as in LMICs as in the developed world. Carer support programmes are essential for the management of dementia, and can be delivered by trained community health workers or peer-to-peer by more experienced carers. Carer strain should trigger more intensive intervention comprising, as indicated, psychological assessment and treatment for the carer, respite, and carer education and training. In practice, such interventions, especially in LMICs, may be usefully incorporated into horizontally constructed community-based programmes addressing the generic needs of frail, dependent older people and their carers, whether arising from cognitive, mental or physical disorders (Prince *et al.*, 2009).

Respite care might be an important level of care, as it aims to decrease carer burden and contribute to keeping the person with dementia at home for longer. Despite the satisfaction manifested by carers, there is no clear evidence on its benefits. A systematic review (Lee and Cameron, 2004) which included three RCTs found no evidence of efficacy of respite care for people with dementia or for their caregivers. However, the authors found methodological problems in the trials and suggest that there is a need for more methodologically sound research before any firm conclusion can be drawn. Day care and residential care are often more expensive than targeted home care supplementing family support and care, and is unlikely to be a priority for government investment when the housing conditions of the general population are poor. Nevertheless, even in some of the poorest developing countries, nursing and residential care homes are opening up in the private sector to meet the demand from the growing affluent middle class. Good quality, well-regulated residential care has a role to play in all societies, for those with no family supports and for those where family support capacity is exhausted, both as temporary respite and to provide longer-term care. Nevertheless, overinvestment in residential care reduces the capacity to develop community and home-based support services, especially in settings with poor resources. It is therefore important to balance the development of residential care and community services for people with dementia. Absence of regulation, staff training and quality assurance is a serious concern in developed and developing countries alike. Important priorities would include a system of registration and inspection of homes, training of careworkers, and provision of medical services for residents to create the best possible quality care.

Table 40.1 shows ADI's vision for the pattern of dementia service development (ADI, 2009). It is based on the graduated approach to service development (see **Figure 40.1**) and recognizes that progress depends on available resources.

Table 40.1   Alzheimer's Disease International's vision for the pattern of dementia service development (ADI, 2009).

	Low and middle income countries	High income countries
Awareness and understanding	• Public education – dementia as an illness, not an inevitable part of old age; where to go for help and information • Risk reduction as part of general health promotion • Campaigns against stigma and discrimination	• Public education – dementia as an illness, not an inevitable part of old age; where to go for help and information • Risk reduction as part of general health promotion • Campaigns for early help-seeking and recognition of dementia • Campaigns against stigma and discrimination
Capacity building	• Integrate dementia awareness and understanding into primary health care planning • Education/training for health care professionals, auxiliary health workers and care workers • Information and training for family carers • Integrate dementia into curricula	• National plans for dementia services, from diagnosis to palliative care • Budgets specifically for dementia • Education/training for health care professionals, auxiliary health workers and care workers • Information and training for family carers • Integrate dementia into curricula for healthcare professionals
Services	• Detection and diagnosis in primary health care • Information, advice and support for family carers through auxiliary health workers • Treatment of cognitive impairment with cholinesterase inhibitors where affordable • Care workers employed by families of people with dementia • Advice and support from primary care if behavioural and psychological symptoms of dementia (BPSD) become problematic	• Detection and diagnosis shared between primary and secondary health care • Treatment of cognitive impairment with cholinesterase inhibitors • Post-diagnosis support for people with dementia • Information, advice and support for family carers through self-help groups and specialist dementia workers • Community based services for people with dementia to provide stimulation and help maintain skills whilst providing respite for family carers • Extra support for people with dementia experiencing BPSD including secondary medical care • Continuing care in the person with dementia's own home for as long as possible • High quality care homes for people with dementia no longer able to care for themselves in their own homes • End of life palliative care

We began by stating that the health-care needs of older people have been underprioritized. The full implications of demographic ageing, the prevalence of dementia and their impact on both people with dementia and health-care systems are only just beginning to be recognized. Nevertheless, there are grounds for optimism: some governments have made dementia a national health priority and we have shown that it possible for low and medium income countries to take steps to improve dementia care through primary care and support for people with chronic illnesses. Now is the time for governments to act and learn from their emerging experiences. Future research will play an important role in evaluating new dementia initiatives and filling our gaps in knowledge about prevention and treatment.

REFERENCES

ADI. (2009) World Alzheimer Report. London: Alzheimer Disease International.

Bamford C, Lamont S, Eccles M *et al.* (2004) Disclosing a diagnosis of dementia: a systematic review. *International Journal of Geriatric Psychiatry* **19**: 151–69.

Bird HR, Canino G, Stipec MR *et al.* (1987) Use of the Mini-mental State Examination in a probability sample of a Hispanic population. *Journal of Nervous and Mental Disease* **175**: 731–7.

Black SA, Espino DV, Mahurin R *et al.* (1999) The influence of noncognitive factors on the Mini-Mental State Examination in older Mexican-Americans: findings from the Hispanic EPESE.

Established Population for the Epidemiologic Study of the Elderly. *Journal of Clinical Epidemiology* **52**: 1095–102.

Brayne C, Fox C, Boustani M. (2007) Dementia screening in primary care: is it time? *Journal of the American Medical Association* **298**: 2409–11.

Brodaty H, Low LF, Gibson L, Burns K. (2006) What is the best dementia screening instrument for general practitioners to use? *American Journal of Geriatric Psychiatry* **14**: 391–400.

Brucki SM, Nitrini R, Caramelli P et al. (2003) Suggestions for utilization of the mini-mental state examination in Brazil. *Arquivos de Neuropsiquiatria* **61**: 777–81.

Callahan CM, Boustani MA, Unverzagt FW et al. (2006) Effectiveness of collaborative care for older adults with Alzheimer disease in primary care: a randomized controlled trial. *Journal of the American Medical Association* **295**: 2148–57.

Castro-Costa E, Fuzikawa C, Uchoa E et al. (2008) Norms for the mini-mental state examination: adjustment of the cut-off point in population-based studies (evidences from the Bambui health aging study). *Arquivos de Neuropsiquiatria* **66**: 524–8.

Choo WY, Low WY, Karina R et al. (2003) Social support and burden among caregivers of patients with dementia in Malaysia. *Asia Pacifi. Journal of Public Health* **15**: 23–9.

Dias A, Samuel R, Patel V et al. (2004) The impact associated with caring for a person with dementia: a report from the 10/66 Dementia Research Group's Indian network. *International Journal of Geriatric Psychiatry* **19**: 182–4.

Epping-Jordan JE, Pruitt SD, Bengoa R, Wagner EH. (2004) Improving the quality of health care for chronic conditions. *Quality and Safety in Health Care* **13**: 299–305.

Epping-Jordan JE, Galea G, Tukuitonga C, Beaglehole R. (2005) Preventing chronic diseases: taking stepwise action. *Lancet* **366**: 1667–71.

Fernandez M, Castro-Flores J, Perez-de las HS et al. (2008) Prevalence of dementia in the elderly aged above 65 in a district in the Basque Country. *Revista de Neurologia* **46**: 89–96.

Ferri CP, Prince M, Brayne C et al. (2005) Global prevalence of dementia: a Delphi consensus study. *Lancet* **366**: 2112–7.

Francesconi P, Roti L, Casotto V et al. (2006) Prevalence of dementia in Tuscany: results from four population-based epidemiological studies. *Epidemiologia e Prevenzione* **30**: 237–44.

Fuster V, Voute J. (2005) MDGs: chronic diseases are not on the agenda. *Lancet* **366**: 1512–4.

Ganguli M, Ratcliff G, Chandra V et al. (1995) A Hindi Version of the MMSE: The Development of a Cognitive Screening Instrument for a Largely Illiterate Rural Elderly Population in India. *International Journal of Geriatric Psychiatry* **10**: 367–77.

Graham N, Brodaty H. (1997) Alzheimer's Disease International. *International Journal of Geriatric Psychiatry* **12**: 691–2.

Hofman A, Ott A, Breteler MMB et al. (1997) Atherosclerosis, apolipoprotein E, and prevalence of dementia and Alzheimer's disease in the Rotterdam Study. *Lancet* **349**: 151–4.

Lecouturier J, Bamford C, Hughes JC et al. (2008) Appropriate disclosure of a diagnosis of dementia: identifying the key behaviours of 'best practice'. *BMC Health Services Research* **8**: 95.

Lee H, Cameron M. (2004) Respite care for people with dementia and their carers. *Cochrane Database of Systematic Review* CD004396.

Liu SI, Prince M, Chiu MJ et al. (2005) Validity and reliability of a Taiwan Chinese version of the community screening instrument for dementia. *American Journal of Geriatric Psychiatry* **13**: 581–8.

Lobo A, Saz P, Marcos G et al. (2007) Prevalence of dementia in a southern European population in two different time periods: the ZARADEMP Project. *Acta Psychiatrica Scandinavica* **116**: 299–307.

National Collaborating Centre for Mental Health. (2007) A NICE-SCIE Guideline on supporting people with dementia and their carers in health and social care – National Clinical Practice Guideline Number 42: The British Psychological Society and The Royal College of Psychiatrists.

Ng TP, Niti M, Chiam PC, Kua EH. (2007) Ethnic and educational differences in cognitive test performance on mini-mental state examination in Asians. *American Journal of Geriatric Psychiatry* **15**: 130–9.

Patel V, Prince M. (2001) Ageing and mental health in a developing country: who cares? Qualitative studies from Goa, India. *Psychological Medicine* **31**: 29–38.

Plassman BL, Langa KM, Fisher GG et al. (2007) Prevalence of dementia in the United States: the aging, demographics, and memory study. *Neuroepidemiology* **29**: 125–32.

Prince M, Acosta D, Chiu H et al. (2003) Dementia diagnosis in developing countries: a cross-cultural validation study. *Lancet* **361**: 909–17.

Prince M, Livingston G, Katona C. (2007) Mental health care for the elderly in low-income countries: a health systems approach. *World Psychiatry* **6**: 5–13.

Prince M, Acosta D, Albanese E et al. (2008) Ageing and dementia in low and middle income countries-Using research to engage with public and policy makers. *International Review of Psychiatry* **20**: 332–43.

Prince MJ, Acosta D, Castro-Costa E et al. (2009) Packages of care for dementia in low- and middle-income countries. *PLoS Medicine* **6**: e1000176.

Rafii MS, Aisen PS. (2009) Recent developments in Alzheimer's disease therapeutics. *BMC Medicine* **7**: 7.

Ramos-Cerqueira AT, Torres AR, Crepaldi AL et al. (2005) Identification of dementia cases in the community: a Brazilian experience. *Journal of the American Geriatric Society* **53**: 1738–42.

Scottish Dementia Working Group. Accessed 2 October 2009. Available from: www.sdwg.org.uk.

Shaji KS, Arun Kishore NR, Lal KP, Prince M. (2002a) Revealing a hidden problem. An evaluation of a community dementia case-finding program from the Indian 10/66 dementia research network. *International Journal of Geriatric Psychiatry* **17**: 222–5.

Shaji KS, Smitha K, Praveen Lal K, Prince M. (2002b) Caregivers of patients With Alzheimer's disease: a qualitative study From The Indian 10/66 Dementia Research Network. *International Journal of Geriatric Psychiatry* **18**: 1–6.

Taylor R. (2007) *Alzheimer's from the inside out*. Baltimore, Maryland: Health Professions Press Inc.

The 10/66 Dementia Research Group. (2004) Care arrangements for people with dementia in developing countries. *International Journal of Geriatric Psychiatry* **19**: 170–7.

United Nations. (2002) Report of the Second World Assembly on Ageing, Madrid, 8–12 April 2002. New York: United Nations.

Wimo A, Winblad B, Jonsson L. (2007) An estimate of the total worldwide societal costs of dementia in 2005. *Alzheimer's and Dementia* 3: 81–91.

World Health Organization. (1996) *The Global Burden of Disease: A comprehensive assessment of mortality and disability from diseases, injuries and risk factors in 1990 and projected to 2020.* The Harvard School of Public Health: Harvard University Press.

World Health Organization. (2004a) *Global Burden of Disease 2004 Update: Disability Weights for Diseases and Conditions.* Geneva: World Health Organization.

World Health Organization. (2004b) *Towards age-friendly primary health care.* Geneva: World Health Organization.

World Health Organization. (2006) Neurological disorders: public health challenges, Chapter 3.1 Dementia, 42–55.

World Health Organization. (2009) Maximizing Positive Synergies Collaborative Group. An assessment of interactions between global health initiatives and country health systems. *Lancet* 373: 2137–69.

World Population Prospects. (2003) *The 2002 Revision – Highlights.* New York: United Nations.

Xu G, Meyer JS, Huang Y *et al.* (2003) Adapting mini-mental state examination for dementia screening among illiterate or minimally educated elderly Chinese. *International Journal of Geriatric Psychiatry* 18: 609–16.

Zencir M, Kuzu N, Beser NG *et al.* (2005) Cost of Alzheimer's disease in a developing country setting. *International Journal of Geriatric Psychiatry* 20: 616–22.

Development of a national strategy for dementia: dementia and policy in the UK

SUBE BANERJEE

41.1 INTRODUCTION

For those who are 'in the know', there can be no doubt that dementia is one of the greatest societal challenges that we face as we start the the twenty-first century. Its personal and societal impacts are greater than those health conditions such as cancer and heart disease that preoccupied the last century (Lowin *et al.*, 2001). Dementia is a challenge at international, national, regional and local levels as well as the personal. It is in all ways exceptional in terms of size, cost and current and future impact (Alzheimer's Disease International, 2009) with 35.6 million people with dementia in 2010, and the numbers doubling every 20 years, to 65.7 million in 2030 and 115.4 million in 2050. This is an issue for the developing world as well as the developed; even now around a half of these cases are in Asia and that proportion will rise swiftly. The profound negative impacts of dementia on people with dementia themselves, their families, and in terms of health and social service use, are again not in doubt. Dementia is highly stigmatized and universally feared, with studies suggesting that it is one of the very few illnesses rated as 'worse than death' (Patrick *et al.*, 1994).

The problem is that there are relatively few people 'in the know'. Also, those that are 'in the know' are generally not those with the power to determine the priorities for health services and those making spending decisions. Powerful misconceptions concerning dementia include: it being a normal part of ageing; that there is nothing that can be done to help; and that it is better not to know. These toxic misbeliefs are the norm and are shared by most politicians, policy makers and health administrators as well as the general population. This has resulted in a situation where dementia has been considered an issue that is 'a social issue' outside the remit of health, so allowing health policy makers and providers to abrogate responsibility for assessment, treatment and care.

The direct result of this is that the large majority of people with dementia and their family carers do not benefit from the positive intervention and support that can promote independence and give people with dementia and their family carers good life quality, steering a course in the 7–12 years that they might be living with dementia, that avoids crises and harm and that promotes well-being for all involved. In fact, systems often seem to have been designed perversely to result in the avoidance of diagnosis and the consequent denial of care. So, for example, a fundamental flaw in the current UK system is that only about one-third of people with dementia receive a diagnosis of dementia; and then when they do it is usually late in the disorder, often at a time of crisis when it is too late to prevent the harm that has been caused to the person with dementia and their family (National Audit Office, 2007).

The size of the challenge in terms of need, cost and will required to improve the quality of services requires political priority in order to generate health policy that works for people with dementia. This can be at the level of a hospital, a region, a particular health maintenance organization, or at a national level, depending how health and social care systems are organized. This transformational change is, of course, what researchers and practitioners and Alzheimer's associations across the globe have been trying to achieve for the past 25 years, but with only limited success. However, this is a long game and the evidence base and the political climate has been changed by their actions. There are encouraging signs that systems may be becoming willing to take on their responsibilities for people with dementia rather than shirk them, and one way of doing this is by the generation of national policy on dementia.

In an affecting speech, launching the five-year, €1.6 billion French *Plan Alzheimer* in February 2008, Nicolas Sarkozy expressed an urgent need for change:

> This is a moment awaited by all, I know. I understand the impatience expressed. How could it be otherwise? When the suffering of a loved one affects a whole family, I know we can wait no longer and that every day counts. Today I am launching a five year National Plan for Alzheimer's. This is a lasting State commitment in the battle that we wage against the disease. It is also a personal commitment from me.

Later, in a speech made at the height of the credit crisis in October 2008, he took time to feature Alzheimer's disease as the primary focus for health in the French EU presidency, stating that finding a solution for the challenges posed by dementia was as important as finding a solution for the world's financial problems.

The *Plan Alzheimer* (Republique Française, 2007) has been followed by the *National Dementia Strategy* for England (Department of Health, 2009) and there is similar work completed or in progress in countries and systems as diverse as Australia, Norway, South Korea, India and Denmark. These initiatives vary but generally include a mixture of high level (often five year) strategic planning for quality improvement in dementia care, with specific clinical, social and research commitments. Their scope is comprehensive and their intension is to provide the policy framework for local service development. These documents are therefore political as well as clinical statements. Given the potential transformative effect of such national policy for people with dementia, in this chapter we shall look at the processes by which such a commitment might be encouraged and then developed, with particular reference to the English National Dementia Strategy.

41.2   THE POLICY FRAMEWORK

The realization that all is not well in the health and social care provided for people with dementia has developed clarity and momentum over the past decades. Services for people with dementia are complex, and include primary health care, specialist services in mental health (e.g. old-age psychiatry), care provided in general hospitals (e.g. geriatrics and neurology), as well as social care commissioned and provided by both local authorities, the voluntary and independent sectors and for-profit providers of home care and care homes. Across the world there is no clear idea of which subspecialty of medicine should take the lead in the diagnosis and treatment

of dementia which adds a further element of complexity and confusion. There are examples of excellent dementia care provided for particular groups with dementia or in particular areas but there are no systems where care has been found to be uniformly of high quality.

Strategy and policy evolves but, as the evidence base has grown, so the last decade has seen a growing acknowledgement of the challenge posed by dementia and the need for service improvement. To illustrate the building blocks needed, details of relevant UK reports and policy include *Forget me not: Mental health services for older people* (Audit Commission, 2000). Key findings included:

- only a half of general practitioners (GPs) believed it important to look actively for signs of dementia and to make an early diagnosis;
- less than half of GPs felt that they had received sufficient training in how to diagnose dementia;
- a lack of clear information, counselling, advocacy and support for people with dementia and their family carers;
- an insufficient supply of specialist home care;
- poor quality assessment and treatment, with little joint health and social care planning and working;
- they found little improvement when reviewing change two years later (Audit Commission, 2002).

The National Service Framework for Older People (Department of Health, 2001) included a chapter on mental health and older people including a consideration of dementia, advocating:

- early diagnosis and intervention;
- that National Health Service (NHS) and local authorities should review arrangements for health promotion, early detection and diagnosis, assessment, care and treatment planning, and access to specialist services;
- the provision of 'integrated' and 'comprehensive' services.

Reviewing progress, this appears to have had little positive impact on services for people with dementia and their families (Banerjee *et al.*, 2010).

Everybody's business: Integrated mental health services for older adults: a service development guide (Care Services Improvement Partnership, 2005) – this set out the essentials for a service that works for older people's mental health including:

- memory assessment services to enable early diagnosis of dementia for all;
- integrated community mental health teams whose role includes the management of people with dementia with complex behavioural and psychological symptoms.

This had little effect since there were no levers to mandate such service provision.

Dementia: Supporting people with dementia and their carers in health and social care a joint clinical guideline on the management of dementia (National Institute For Health and

Clinical Excellence and Social Care Institute Of Excellence, 2006) – key recommendations included:

- integrated working across all agencies;
- memory assessment services as a point of referral for diagnosis of dementia;
- assessment, support and treatment (where needed) for carers;
- assessment and treatment of non-cognitive symptoms and behaviour that challenges;
- dementia care training for all staff working with older people;
- improvement of care for people with dementia in general hospitals.

A useful, if unprioritized, list of things that might be done but are generally not done, did not prompt change in services but showed what might be done.

The Dementia UK Report (Knapp *et al.*, 2007) – published by the Alzheimer's Society, the report's key findings included:

- the number of people with dementia in the UK – 700 000;
- the projected number of people with dementia in the UK – doubling in 30 years to 1.4 million;
- the costs of dementia £17 billion per year;
- low level of diagnosis and management of dementia in the UK;
- high variation in activity between areas in the UK;
- the recommendation that dementia should be made an explicit national health and social care priority;
- the need to improve the quality of services provided for people with dementia and their carers.

Positive impact in terms of the government accepting the figures and the need to do something to improve care, with the next two reports formed the priority for making dementia a priority and developing national policy.

Improving services and support for people with dementia (National Audit Office, 2007) – this report by the external auditors of UK governmental spending was profoundly critical of the quality of care received by people with dementia and their families. Its findings included:

- the size and availability of specialist community mental health teams was extremely variable;
- the confidence of GPs in spotting the symptoms of dementia was poor and lower than it had been in 2000 (down to one-third);
- deficiencies in carer support;
- services are not currently delivering value for money to taxpayers or people with dementia and their families;
- that too few people are being diagnosed or being diagnosed early enough;
- early diagnosis and intervention is needed to improve quality of life;
- services in the community, care homes and at the end of life are not delivering consistently or cost-effectively against the objective of supporting people to live

independently as long as possible in the place of their choosing;
- the need for a 'spend to save' approach, with upfront investment in services, for early diagnosis and intervention and improved specialist services, community services and in general hospitals resulting in long-term cost savings from prevention of transition into care homes and decreased length of hospital stay.

Required high level response from government and very much helped in the prioritization of dementia, forming part of the rationale for the National Dementia Strategy.

Improving services and support for people with dementia (Public Accounts Committee, 2008) – NAO reports are followed up by the PAC which is the senior committee of the House of Commons and which holds to account by interrogation the heads of the civil service responsible for government spending, in this case the Department of Health. At the committee's public hearing on 15 October 2007 the NHS Chief Executive and other senior policy-makers from the Department of Health were questioned on the NAO's criticisms, the PAC's subsequent recommendations included:

- dementia should be made a high priority for the NHS and Social Care;
- the need for explicit national ownership and leadership;
- early diagnosis;
- improving public attitudes and understanding;
- co-ordinated care;
- all improvements to benefit carers too;
- improvements in care in care homes;
- improvements in care in general hospitals.

Required high level response from government and very much helped in the prioritization of dementia, forming part of the rationale for the content of the National Dementia Strategy.

The Government's response to the PAC report was to accept virtually all the conclusions and recommendations of the committee, assuring the committee that their findings would be fully addressed in a new National Dementia Strategy. In preparation for this, there was a one-year programme to develop a National Dementia Strategy and implementation plan.

The above demonstrates the development of policy over time. The first four initiatives above had much to commend them in terms of their content but achieved little in the way of tangible benefit for people with dementia and their carers. They can, however, be seen as a necessary set of steps to initiatives 4 to 7 which made the difference between there being a National Dementia Strategy and there not being one.

41.3 MAKING THE CASE FOR A NATIONAL DEMENTIA STRATEGY

So dementia has long been a 'Cinderella' element of health and social care systems, suffering from a triple discrimination coming from that associated with: age, mental disorder and dementia itself. What is it that has allowed Cinderella to come to the ball? In effect, there has been a three way pressure, encapsulated in the policy detailed above, which has acted together to bring dementia out of the shadows and into the minds of the public and politicians.

- First, we have had advances in research, giving solid information of the epidemiology of dementia, increasing understanding of the underlying biological processes, the first set of symptomatic treatments and tantalizing glimpses of future interventions for disease prevention and disease modification.
- Second, across the medical, psychological and social fields people have developed innovative ways of working with people with dementia, emphasizing the personhood of people with dementia and demonstrating the positive good that can be done even without drug treatments to slow, halt or reverse the disease processes.
- Third, the strategic case is made by demographic changes resulting in major growth in the numbers of the oldest old, meaning that the numbers of people with dementia are already large and will grow quickly and predictably. A consequence of this growth is that of a growth in the costs of care for dementia.

Dementia care is complex. It transcends boundaries of health and social care and the roles of family, the voluntary sector and industry in developing treatments and interventions and in providing placements for people with dementia. How then does a health system decide if concerted national action is needed? The following five steps attempt to summarize out the process of development of the argument and evidence that enabled politicians and policy makers to decide that it was of value to develop a national dementia strategy.

41.3.1   Step 1: what are the numbers?

Advances in research into case definition and population-based surveys have given solid information of the epidemiology of dementia. In the UK, the leading voluntary sector advocacy organization for people with dementia and their carers, the Alzheimer's Society, commissioned independent researchers at the Institute of Psychiatry and the London School of Economics to synthesize all available data on the prevalence of dementia using a Delphi approach. This was then used with local and national demographic data to generate a definitive number of people with dementia in the UK (700 000) and in each individual health and social service funding area (Knapp *et al.*, 2007). There is no more powerful tool than locally derived and relevant data.

41.3.2   Step 2: what are the costs?

A primary concern of government is cost. Knowledge about what an illness is already costing and how that money is being spent is very powerful. Using best available national measures of service use in dementia and the costs of services with the numbers generated above can give you the costs of

dementia. The issue of how to cost the work done by family carers is difficult and the status of work forgone in order to care (opportunity costs) is controversial, but a pragmatic approach making the best of data that will have holes in them is needed. In the Dementia UK report this was costed at minimum wage. This yielded a cost of £17 billion per year, a sum equivalent to one-fifth of the whole health budget and more than heart disease, stroke and cancer combined. This helps to gain the attention of policy-makers and politicians. The majority of these costs (£7 billion) were in care home costs for people with dementia.

41.3.3   Step 3: what about the future?

All countries have population projections and the numbers with dementia in the next 20–30 years can be predicted because those people will already have the pathology at work. It is the work of politicians and policy-makers to think strategically, so a measure of future threat is of use. The figures generated above allow for the calculation of projections of the growth in numbers and costs of dementia into the future. In the case of the UK this meant that in just 30 years (i.e. in 2027) there would be a doubling of the numbers of people with dementia to 1.4 million and a trebling of the costs to over £50 billion per year (Lowin *et al.*, 2001). These figures make clear the need for a strategic plan for dementia and strongly support the need for this to be at a national rather than a local level.

41.3.4   Step 4: is it broke?

The old maxim 'if it ain't broke don't fix it' is of importance here. If we have excellent quality diagnostic, treatment and care services for people with dementia and their families then the need is to preserve these and grow them. If, however, we find our services are not 'fit for purpose' then there may be a need for more radical changes. In the UK, an analysis of prescription of anti-dementia medication (prior to recent NICE guidelines) showed the level of UK diagnosis and treatment of people with dementia was generally low with a 24–30-fold variation in activity between highest and lowest activity by area. International comparisons suggested that the UK is in the bottom third of European performance with less than half the activity of France, Sweden, Ireland and Spain (Waldemar *et al.* 2007). These data make the case for the system being 'broke'.

41.3.5   Step 5: they would say that wouldn't they?

Independent corroboration is vital. The data cited above were generated by a pressure group for dementia (the Alzheimer's Society) and researchers dedicated to making the case for dementia. To gain credibility, it is very useful if dispassionate external assessment can come to the same conclusions. In the UK, a vital spur to the government making dementia a national priority were the analyses carried out by the

Government's own auditors, the NAO (2007) and the subsequent enquiry by the UK House of Commons' PAC (2008) described above. These confirmed the findings of the Dementia UK report providing vital external validation.

41.4 DEVELOPING THE STRATEGY

Making dementia a priority is only the first stage. There is then a need to develop what will go into the policy. How does one develop a national strategy for an illness that is so common, and where care can be provided by any combination of health services, social services, family and friends, and the third sector? A further challenge is to deal with the fact that there are potential major problems at all stages in the complex care pathway.

From the start it was decided that the strategy should be designed to address the needs of all people with dementia, no matter of what type, age, ethnic origin or social status. A second important primary decision was to enter into as full a consultation as possible. An External Reference Group (ERG) was convened and chaired independently of the Department of Health by the chief executive of the UK Alzheimer's Society. A further strength was that the many reports over the years that had identified flaws in the system meant that there was a consensus as the areas needing attention from the start. So with the announcement made by ministers that dementia was to be a national priority it was stated that there would be a one year process to develop a national dementia strategy and implementation plan. The overall structure developed as a framework for this work stood up well in the development process. It was structured along three themes:

1. improving public and professional attitudes and understanding of dementia;
2. early diagnosis and intervention for all;
3. good quality care and support at all stages from diagnosis through to the end of life.

Three ERG subgroups worked on these themes, generating a comprehensive report on improving dementia care which informed but did not determine the development of the strategy.

The development included two waves of formal external consultation organized jointly by the Department of Health and the Alzheimer's Society. The first, completed prior to developing the consultation document, involved a nationwide listening and engagement exercise where more than 3000 people were able to contribute to and engage with developing the strategy. The Alzheimer's Society also ran similar events especially for people with dementia and carers and distributed questionnaires, both through the society's branches and on-line. Feedback from all these sources was reviewed to ensure that all views were captured.

A consultation document containing draft proposals was then generated by a Department of Health (DH) strategy working group co-chaired by a senior social services leader and a senior dementia specialist from a health background (Department of Health, 2008). This emphasized the need for joint and integrative approaches throughout. In the second phase, between July and September 2008, the DH held a formal public consultation exercise on the draft proposals for the strategy, receiving over 600 written responses from individuals including those with dementia and their carers, and a wide range of professional and other stakeholder groups. These responses were analysed and informed the development of the final strategy. In addition, 53 regional consultation events were held; over 4000 individuals attended these meetings. Meetings covered the whole country including rural and urban areas, again specific groups were targeted to ensure the views of diverse populations had been included in the development of the strategy such as: people with dementia themselves, people with learning disabilities, people from minority ethnic groups, and older people in prisons and remote and island communities. Officials from the DH attended all these meetings as well as other dementia-related conferences and meetings across the country to publicize the consultation and gather feedback.

This process is clearly time consuming and labour intensive so why bother? The answer to this is that the inclusiveness and comprehensiveness of the development and consultation process for such a strategy lends it both validity and power when moving towards implementation.

41.5 THE STRATEGY

Finally, the National Dementia Strategy was published on February 3, 2009 (Department of Health, 2009). A detailed analysis of the strategy is beyond the scope of this paper. A brief summary is provided below on the 17 interlinked objectives of the final strategy. It attempts to deliver all the elements identified in the development phases discussed above. The strategy is for a five year plan of comprehensive service building and reorganization that requires services in England to transcend existing boundaries between health and social care and the third sector, between service providers and people with dementia and their carers.

It presents a comprehensive critical analysis of the current systems of providing health and social care for people with dementia and their carers which may be of relevance to a wider group of developed health systems, setting out the actions needed to enable people to live well with dementia. The key objectives of the strategy, addressed in more detail in the full document, are presented here, this is not in order of priority but according to the narrative of the strategy which is based on a notional pathway through care:

Objective 1: Improving public and professional awareness and understanding of dementia. Public and professional awareness and understanding of dementia to be improved and the stigma associated with it addressed. This should inform individuals of the benefits of timely diagnosis and care, promote the prevention of dementia, and reduce social exclusion and discrimination. It should encourage behaviour change in terms of appropriate help-seeking and help provision.

Objective 2: Good-quality early diagnosis and intervention for all. All people with dementia to have access to a pathway of care that delivers: a rapid and competent specialist assessment; an accurate diagnosis, sensitively communicated to the person with dementia and their carers; and treatment, care and support provided as needed following diagnosis. The system needs to have the capacity to see all new cases of dementia in the area.

Objective 3: Good-quality information for those with diagnosed dementia and their carers. Providing people with dementia and their carers with good-quality information on the illness and on the services available, both at diagnosis and throughout the course of their care.

Objective 4: Enabling easy access to care, support and advice following diagnosis. A dementia adviser to facilitate easy access to appropriate care, support and advice for those diagnosed with dementia and their carers.

Objective 5: Development of structured peer support and learning networks. The establishment and maintenance of such networks will provide direct local peer support for people with dementia and their carers. It will also enable people with dementia and their carers to take an active role in the development and prioritization of local services.

Objective 6: Improved community personal support services. Provision of an appropriate range of services to support people with dementia living at home and their carers. Access to flexible and reliable services, ranging from early intervention to specialist home care services, which are responsive to the personal needs and preferences of each individual and take account of their broader family circumstances. Accessible to people living alone or with carers, and people who pay for their care privately, through personal budgets or through local authority-arranged services.

Objective 7: Implementing the Carers' Strategy. Family carers are the most important resource available for people with dementia. Active work is needed to ensure that the provisions of the Carers' Strategy are available for carers of people with dementia. Carers have a right to an assessment of their needs and can be supported through an agreed plan to support the important role they play in the care of the person with dementia. This will include good-quality, personalized breaks. Action should also be taken to strengthen support for children who are in caring roles, ensuring that their particular needs as children are protected.

Objective 8: Improved quality of care for people with dementia in general hospitals. Identifying leadership for dementia in general hospitals, defining the care pathway for dementia there and the commissioning of specialist liaison older people's mental health teams to work in general hospitals.

Objective 9: Improved intermediate care for people with dementia. Intermediate care which is accessible to people with dementia and which meets their needs.

Objective 10: Considering the potential for housing support, housing-related services and telecare to support people with dementia and their carers. The needs of people with dementia and their carers should be included in the development of housing options, assistive technology and telecare. As evidence emerges, commissioners should consider the provision of options to prolong independent living and delay reliance on more intensive services.

Objective 11: Living well with dementia in care homes. Improved quality of care for people with dementia in care homes by the development of explicit leadership for dementia within care homes, defining the care pathway there, the commissioning of specialist in-reach services from community mental health teams, and through inspection regimes.

Objective 12: Improved end of life care for people with dementia. People with dementia and their carers to be involved in planning end of life care which recognizes the principles outlined in the Department of Health End of Life Care Strategy. Local work on the End of Life Care Strategy to consider dementia.

Objective 13: An informed and effective workforce for people with dementia. Health and social care staff involved in the care of people who may have dementia to have the necessary skills to provide the best quality of care in the roles and settings where they work. To be achieved by effective basic training and continuous professional and vocational development in dementia.

Objective 14: A joint commissioning strategy for dementia. Local commissioning and planning mechanisms to be established to determine the services needed for people with dementia and their carers, and how best to meet these needs. These commissioning plans should be informed by the World Class Commissioning guidance for dementia developed to support this strategy.

Objective 15: Improved assessment and regulation of health and care services and of how systems are working for people with dementia and their carers. Inspection regimes for care homes and other services that better assure the quality of dementia care provided.

Objective 16: A clear picture of research evidence and needs. Evidence to be available on the existing research base on dementia in the UK and gaps that need to be filled.

Objective 17: Effective national and regional support for implementation of the strategy. Appropriate national and regional support to be available to advise and assist local implementation of the strategy. Good-quality information to be available on the development of dementia services, including information from evaluations and demonstrator sites.

41.6 IMPLEMENTATION

It would be all too easy to believe with the formulation of a strategy that the work is now done. However, the final phase is implementation and that will be a profound challenge. In the UK, decisions on what to invest in lie at a local level with around 150 Primary Care Trusts. Convincing these commissioners that investing in dementia services is 'worth it'

Colour Plate Section

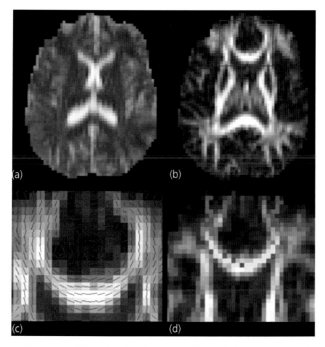

Plate 1 Apparent diffusion coefficient (ADC) and fractional anisotropy (FA). Diffusion tensor imaging provides quantitative measures of (a) ADC and (b) FA. Brighter signal means more average diffusion and more constrained diffusion for ADC and FA respectively. Note that grey and white matter do not differ in ADC but have very different FA values, such that FA provides a map of the myelinated axons of white matter. By calculating the tensor information the direction of diffusion can be determined in each voxel (c), from which tracts can be reconstructed (d). Panel C shows the principal diffusion direction in the region including the genu of the corpus callosum depicted by the red box in panel B. In panel D, a tract of the forceps minor (yellow) has been reconstructed by placing a single 'seed' voxel (blue) in the genu of the corpus callosum.

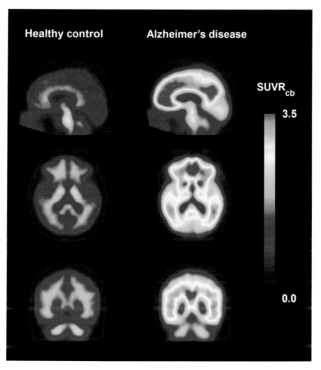

Plate 2 Typical pattern of 11C–PiB binding in AD. Representative parametric sagittal, transaxial and coronal 11C–PiB PET images in control subjects (right column) compared with AD patients (left column). 11C–PiB retention is observed in frontal, temporal and parietal cortices as well as in the posterior cingulate/precuneus areas, with relative sparing of occipital and sensori-motor cortex.

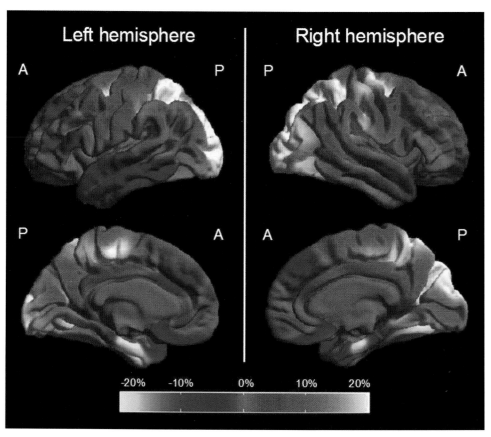

Plate 14 Regional percentage differences in cortical thickness in posterior cortical atrophy (PCA) ($n = 48$) compared with typical amnestic Alzheimer's disease (AD) (tAD; $n = 30$) for the left and right hemisphere (Lehmann *et al.*, 2009). The colour scale represents magnitude of cortical thickness difference. Red and yellow (positive values) represent lower cortical thickness in PCA subjects compared with tAD, whereas dark to light blue (negative values) represents greater cortical thickness.

will be a complex marathon of a race. This will require leadership at a local level as well as at regional and national level. The plan is for local implementation with regional support and national co-ordination in an iterative programme with staged introduction of the 17 elements of the strategy across the country in a logical order. The reality is that with the development of the National Dementia Strategy, the work to truly change things for people with dementia and their carers is only just beginning.

However, the potential benefits of the strategy are worth it. Full implementation of the strategy would mean that all people with dementia and those who care for them would have access to the best possible healthcare and support. We know that early diagnosis, effective intervention and support from diagnosis through the course of the illness can enable people to live well with dementia. We also know that improving health and social care outcomes in dementia in the short and medium term can have significant benefits for society both now and in the future.

The vision is for the positive transformation of dementia services. A system where all people with dementia have access to the care and support they need. A system where the public and professionals alike are well informed; where the fear and stigma associated with dementia have been allayed; and where the false beliefs that dementia is a normal part of ageing and nothing can be done have been corrected. It would be a system where families affected by dementia know where to go for help, what services to expect, and where the quality of care is high and equal wherever they might live. This is a vision worth working for and one that in the large majority of health and social service systems will require national strategy and delivery if it is to become a reality.

REFERENCES

Alzheimer's Disease International. (2009) *World dementia report.* London: ADI.

Audit Commission. (2000) *Forget me not: Mental health services for older people.* London: Audit Commission.

Audit Commission. (2002) *Forget me not 2002: Developing mental health services for older people in England.* London: Audit Commission.

Banerjee S, Graham N, Gurland B. (2010) The Stroud/ADI dementia quality framework: a cross-national population-level framework for assessing the quality of life impacts of services and policies for people with dementia and their family carers. *International Journal of Geriatric Psychiatry* **25**: 249–57.

Care Services Improvement Partnership. (2005) *Everybody's business.* Leeds: Care Services Improvement Partnership.

Department of Health. (2001) *National service framework for older people.* London: Department of Health.

Department of Health. (2008) *Transforming the quality of dementia care – consultation on a national dementia strategy.* London: Department of Health.

Department of Health. (2009) *Living well with dementia: A national dementia strategy.* London: Department of Health.

Knapp M, Prince M, Albanese E *et al.* (2007) *Dementia UK.* London: Alzheimer's Society.

Lowin A, Knapp M, McCrone P. (2001) Alzheimer's disease in the UK; comparative evidence on cost of illness and volume of health services research funding. *International Journal of Geriatric Psychiatry* **16**: 1143–8.

National Audit Office. (2007) *Improving services and support for people with dementia.* London: National Audit Office.

National Institute for Health and Clinical Excellence and Social Care Institute of Excellence. (2006) *Dementia: supporting people with dementia and their carers in health and social care.* London: National Collaborating Centre for Mental Health.

Patrick DL, Starks HE, Cain KC *et al.* (1994) Measuring preferences for health states worse than death. *Medical Decision Making* **14**: 9–18.

Public Accounts Committee. (2008) *Improving services and support for people with dementia.* London: TSO.

Republique Française. (2007) *Plan Alzheimer.* Available from: www.plan-alzheimer.gouv.fr/

Waldemar G, Kieu T, Phung T *et al.* (2007) Access to diagnostic evaluation and treatment for dementia in Europe. *International Journal of Geriatric Psychiatry* **22**: 47–54.

42

The pharmaceutical industry and dementia: how can clinicians, researchers and industry work together ethically for the betterment of people with dementia and their families?

MARTIN M BEDNAR AND LEON FLICKER

42.1 ACADEMIC HEALTH-CARE INVESTIGATORS, THE PHARMACEUTICAL INDUSTRY AND DEMENTIA

If I have seen further it is by standing on ye shoulders of Giants.

Sir Isaac Newton, 1676

42.1.1 The relationship can be productive

The therapeutic advances that have improved the lives of individuals with dementia, most notably Alzheimer's disease (AD), are the culmination of scientific innovation emanating from very distinct sectors of the scientific community. The successful 'handoff' of scientific information seemed, in a sense, well orchestrated albeit not pre-planned. While academic health-care investigators demonstrated a critical deficiency of the neurotransmitter acetylcholine in the brains of AD patients in the 1970s (Davies and Maloney, 1976; Davies and Verth, 1977), the use of available agents such as choline supplements did not have the potency or suitable drug characteristics to meaningfully improve the lives and memory of AD patients. In parallel, the pharmaceutical industry, recognizing the importance of the structural and biochemical derangements in the brains of AD patients, was able to produce a class of therapeutics known as cholinesterase inhibitors (ChEIs). Initial reports (Summers et al., 1986) necessitated a standardized approach to evaluation of dementia drugs (Leber, 1990). After successful multicentre randomized trials (e.g. Davis et al., 1992), tacrine was the first drug that was approved in 1993 by the United States Food and Drug Administration (FDA) and heralded a major advance in the treatment of people with Alzheimer's disease, the ChEIs.

The history of the development of ChEIs inhibitors for the treatment of AD is notable for several reasons. It is an example of rational drug design that has dominated drug development since the 1950s, largely (though not completely) replacing accidental drug discovery that was prevalent in the first half of the twentieth century and the reliance on folklore prior to the twentieth century. It is also an excellent example of how the cross-fertilization of diverse groups of scientists and clinicians within both academia and the pharmaceutical industry, with different skill sets and goals, resulted in a significant therapeutic advance to the benefit of patients. What is clear is that neither group could have accomplished this goal anywhere near as effectively on their own. It is also clear that each group contributed to the success of the other by providing critical data, access to patients and feedback (forward and back translation) over the 15-plus years it took from concept to the first drug approval for AD as well as for the 15-plus years since that first drug approval. This is but one example of many where academia and the pharmaceutical industry have complemented, enriched and enhanced the professional roles of each other for the betterment of society.

The key aspect of the academic investigator–pharma relationship outlined above, defining disease targets (mechanisms) that, in turn, facilitate drug design, has been primarily opportunistic and has not required prospective codified guidelines (rules) for engagement. However, more interdependent activities readily demonstrate points of friction within this success story. Some of these include defining the value, financial and medical, of ChEIs, for a given country or world region or for a particular stage of illness (mild, moderate and severe). This was particularly important with drugs such as tacrine which not only had major financial costs, but large numbers of patients developed hepatotoxicity (Ames et al., 1990). Variable patient access to needed medicines, usually on the basis of cost, is another issue that deserves attention to ensure that needed medicines are available to the patients in need of them.

42.1.2   There is a potential for conflict of interests, particularly with clinician researchers

Another aspect is the question of innovation versus incremental improvement of a medicine or class of medicines, for example pharmacokinetics, route of delivery, safety and efficacy advantages, within this class of therapeutics. Are each of these characteristics truly driving innovation and providing enhanced value for the patient or are they simply strategies used by the pharmaceutical industry to maintain patent protection, market share and revenue? Thus, there may be a key conflict in the academia–pharma relationship: on one hand, pharma's advancement of applied science to create and market new medicines that create shareholder value versus academia's pursuit of advancements in basic and clinical science as well as the fiduciary responsibility of the health-care professional to do what is in the best interest of the patient.

The group of academic researchers who are also active clinicians are particularly prone to a duality of interests, which often are congruent but sometimes conflicting. They have simultaneous duties to develop new medications that will provide their sponsors with an increase in share value, as

well as a responsibility to society to develop better treatments, but also a duty to their patients to provide the best available treatment for that individual. These dual interests frequently coexist without conflict, but sometimes there is conflict between these competing demands.

With this historical backdrop, the path forward should acknowledge that a relationship between academic health-care investigators and the pharmaceutical industry is in the best interest of society and the patient. Each has complementary skill sets (see **Table 42.1**), resources and goals that, if appropriately harnessed, can compensate for knowledge gaps of each party. The key issue is how to effectively and efficiently use these resources, skills and knowledge in a way that acknowledges potential conflicts (both between and within the pharmaceutical industry and academia; see **Table 42.2**), minimizes or eliminates the potential for personal gain to supersede societal benefit and provides the needed transparency.

Thus, it is reasonably certain that the pharmaceutical industry will continue to rely on academic health-care investigators to conduct basic research that better defines the pathophysiology of disease and that identifies new therapeutic targets, paving the way for the development of innovative medicines. Pharma will also continue to look to academic health-care investigators to facilitate access to consenting patients necessary for the conduct of clinical trials for these potential new medicines. A significant perturbation of these 'traditional' roles for the pharmaceutical industry and academia seems both unlikely to occur and of doubtful value.

The current infrastructure of academia does not easily lend itself to creating a new relationship between the pharmaceutical industry and patients or for the academic health-care investigator to translate promising therapeutic targets into new chemical entities. These pertubations are likely to markedly complexify health care and result in ambiguity regarding patient care, the outcome being an inefficient strategy in which no part is well served.

On the other hand, to conclude that the responsibility of the academic health-care investigator to always act in the best interest of the patient is in opposition to the pharmaceutical industry's goal to generate financial value from the creation of new medicines is misleading, but nonetheless frequently cited. The fiduciary responsibility of the academic health-care investigator to their patients actually relies on the interaction of the health-care professional with the pharmaceutical industry to facilitate improvements in health care, including the bidirectional exchange of information regarding translational

Table 42.1   Academia-Pharma: complementary[a] skill sets.

Academia	Pharmaceutical industry
Original basic science idea, e.g. novel receptor, biochemical action	Applied creativity, e.g. drugable chemical series
Research focus allows for digression to follow novel observations that may not be related to the original research question	Rational drug design maintains focus on operationalization
Novel observations typically anecdotal	Rigour of safety and efficacy of a therapeutic must meet regulatory (societal) demands before being marketed

[a]Though not intended to suggest they are mutually exclusive!

Table 42.2   Confounders in the healthcare–pharmaceutical industry relationship.

Does disclosure of conflict of interest by health-care professionals genuinely alleviate the potential of bias or simply serve to remove attention from it (Kassirer, 2009)?

Limited numbers of opinion leaders who sway national and international prescribing. Alternatively, the pharmaceutical industry seeks prominent health-care professionals to improve credibility. The potential for coercion and abuse exist

Loss of potential health-care leaders, the clinician-scientist, due to both reduced funding and the dedicated time to do so (vicious cycle)

Physicians must remain unbiased and devoted to patient care, but they are already influenced by federal constraints, managed care regulations and reimbursement

Primary goals of an academic institution (e.g. physician hours involved with direct patient care, the rise of for-profit academic medical centres and also private practice consortiums that conflict with the traditional charitable/altruistic service of the physician) may not align with the goals of the health-care professional, where publications and grants can be the most significant factor in promotions

The need for the pharmaceutical industry to sponsor/subsidize health-care research, meetings, etc. has increased as traditional sources of funding diminish

Academia-led research does not undergo the same degree of scrutiny as that in the pharmaceutical industry – reverse bias (Doogan, 2009)

The potential for data fraud both by health-care professionals and the pharmaceutical industry for secondary gain

Knowledge sharing versus the protection of intellectual property (both academia and the pharmaceutical industry)

Alternatives to the current academia–pharmaceutical industry structure may not be feasible

Some companies are interested in orphan diseases that may not generate blockbuster profits or significant shareholder value either as part of their overall mission (typical of the larger pharmaceutical industry) or because even a modest revenue is sufficient for their business model (smaller, biotech companies)

medicine (bench-to-bedside and bedside-to-bench) and to provide (directly and through regulatory agencies and other governance bodies) information sharing on marketed products. Indeed, the pharmaceutical industry has clearly been the leader both in the public and professional education of AD (and most other diseases), raising awareness and allowing therapies to reach many more individuals than would otherwise have been possible. Thus, to a certain degree, it is this bidirectional flow of information that helps to mitigate idiosyncratic physician practice patterns and that facilitates physician knowledge and competency which serves as the foundation of the physician's role in the care of the patient.

42.1.3   Particular issues in dealing with people with dementia – challenges for both clinicians and researchers

There are a number of issues in the treatment of dementia that, if not unique, are certainly more prominent and they add additional complexity to the relationship of health-care professionals and the pharmaceutical industry. The most obvious of these is the disease itself. With varying degrees of dementia, the patient may have limited or no capacity to understand the nature of the research and its risks and benefits. This results in family members and/or caregivers serving as both the patient proxy for consent, as well as being involved in judging the efficacy of a potential new medicine. Does the relationship between patient and caregiver alter the way that the physician provides information in seeking informed consent? If the trial is targeting challenging behaviours associated with dementia, this may be particularly problematic. Similar issues are faced by clinicians treating people with dementia and challenging behaviours. Whose symptoms are we managing and how valid is this?

The role of the physician and also of the family/caregiver to act on behalf of the patient can be biased by the type of medical facility which chooses to be involved in clinical trials. Is it the physician or is it the site which is interested in participating in clinical trials? Are the therapies studied at a particular site those showing greatest promise or those of most interest to a particular physician (the two are not mutually exclusive)? Many of the potential disease-modifying therapies now in clinical development must be administered parenterally. If a hospital or clinic is not equipped to support this paradigm, clinical trial options for their patients to consider will be much more limited.

The pharmaceutical industry must also struggle with major pragmatic issues. One of these is the cost of clinical trials for dementia. For drugs which may be potentially disease modifying, late-stage clinical trials are long (at least 18–24 months), expensive and carry a very high risk of failure due to their unprecedented nature. Of course, the risk is not only to the pharmaceutical industry, but also to patients, where the true risk of participating in the clinical trial is never certain and the benefit from an AD disease-modifying agent is unclear. The analogous experience with acute stroke is edifying, where the great risk and clinical trial expense are contributing factors to the current paucity of neuroprotective trials. The 1990s were heralded as the decade of the brain in the United States and the approval of t-PA in 1995 provided great promise. Nearly 15 years later, not a single neuroprotective therapy has been approved for stroke. It remains to be seen if dementia will follow a similar path.

There is also the issue of when is the most favourable time to treat patients with cognitive impairment. Traditionally, clinical trials target patients who are in the mild–moderate stage of the disease. This is, in part, a carry-over of the clinical development for symptomatic therapies such as ChEIs inhibitors where there was concern that patients at the severe end of the spectrum may fail to benefit from therapy due to the widespread and prolonged nature of their disease.

However, the question regarding the timing and duration of therapy remains not only about late stage disease but about earlier treatment. Most clinicians would hope that patients could be diagnosed with AD well before they reach the stage of dementia. The terminology of mild cognitive impairment (MCI) or, more recently 'early' AD (especially germane for those with 'amnestic' MCI) seeks to characterize those with objective memory impairment who are likely to develop dementia ('convert') within a relatively brief period of several years. As the scientific community better understands the disease's progression, there have been suggestions of an even earlier stage of AD called 'very early' AD. However, while some feel that there is clear merit in the treatment of AD at earlier stages before there is significant loss of brain function (much like treating patients with heart disease before there is significant heart failure), others feel that this is an industry-led example of 'disease mongering', an attempt to increase the commercial market and hence drug sales (Doran and Henry, 2008). There are a number of examples where either the criteria for diagnosing disease have been redefined or where distinct 'new' diseases have been introduced (e.g. fibromyalgia) followed by the introduction of a medicine to treat it. Federal regulators, third party payers and the public must carefully review the data to determine the societal benefit and risk, both in the short and long term, when approving and paying for these new medicines. Critical participants in this debate are the academic health-care investigators. Their influence is considerable and speaks to the need for collaboration of academia and the pharmaceutical industry, from defining the pathophysiology of disease to the education of society. Not only will the academic health-care investigators continue to be recognized as the spokesperson for the patient and other clinicians (and, by extension, for society), but will also have an important role in the creation, validation and societal uptake for the various tests and scales that will be used to both assess AD patients during the various stages of their dementia and to judge the efficacy of potential new medicines for the treatment thereof.

42.2   FUTURE DIRECTIONS

We have discussed the historical perspective of the relationship between academia and the pharmaceutical industry. This relationship has evolved over the past several decades to create a significant degree of interdependency, despite the fact that at least some of their goals are neither mutual nor similarly prioritized. This has the potential to create an inefficient and ineffective system filled with conflict.

In looking ahead, there is a need to better understand how clinicians, academic health-care investigators and the pharmaceutical industry can all benefit without issues of conflict of interest overwhelming these relationships. This chapter has cited the development of ChEIs as a successful, albeit opportunistic collaboration between the pharmaceutical industry and academic health-care investigators. In the future, a more proactive strategic alignment will assist in ensuring the timely and efficient development of improved models of health care and new medicines for patients.

42.2.1   Are there problems that need to be fixed?

As can be seen, the relationship between prescribers, other health professionals, academia and the pharmaceutical industry is complex and multi-layered. Despite this, there are substantial benefits to be obtained for patients if this collaboration can be managed successfully. A complex relationship can still be very functional. Is there evidence that these evolving inter-relationships have become dysfunctional? If so, how can these difficulties be solved proactively? Below are some examples where there have been issues of conflict and potential solutions.

42.2.2   Incomplete reporting of trial evidence

There are many people who benefit from the performance of well-conducted scientific studies. Academics receive accolades and promotion by the conduct of major studies, particularly if the reports are published in prestigious journals. Companies may make substantial profits if a new class of drugs is shown to be therapeutic, resulting in blockbuster status for these drugs. Future generations of patients will benefit from efficacious treatments to help prevent and alleviate their symptoms. The people who bear the most risk from studies and have the least likelihood of benefits are the subjects of these studies. These people consent to randomization to either ineffective treatments (placebo) or drugs that potentially may yield no benefits and may have unknown side effects. This group of people participate for many reasons but for most it is not just the desperation of seeking effective treatment. Many are driven by an altruistic desire to benefit not just themselves, but future generations. The gift of participation that these individuals give to all those who benefit from the study places an obligation on all the organizations and study investigators – that the participation of these subjects should first be reported, and the report should be an accurate and true record of the subjects' participation.

For this reason it is most important that every subject in a randomized controlled trial (RCT) (i.e. trials which are hypothesis generating) should have their data incorporated into the results of that trial and that all these trials should be reported. Unfortunately, whenever this was reviewed, the conclusion was that negative trials are much less likely to be reported than positive studies. For example, in the early trials of rivastigmine, of four pivotal phase three studies, only two were reported, and the two reported studies showed a greater response than the two unreported studies (Birks et al., 2009). It is not just the pharmaceutical industry who finds it difficult to report negative or similar results. It is difficult to convince journals to publish such studies, especially if there have been other studies which have yielded positive results. However, one of the stated purposes of Cochrane is that all RCTs will be placed in a repository and then subsequently incorporated into at least one systematic review. This approach has heightened the imperative to report all RCTs and fulfil the obligation that all parties have to the patients who participated in these trials.

42.2.2.1 SOLUTION

These concerns have resulted in the creation of trial registries, and the adoption of the position by many journals that trials will not be published unless they have been prospectively registered. The problem is that there is no compulsion that the now known studies' data should be widely available. One solution would be that repositories for unpublished trials should become widely available and should be subject to a requirement from institutional ethics committees that simple tables of the results of the primary efficacy variables be placed in such repositories within five years of the study's completion. The responsibility for completion of this requirement will need to be shared between the academic researcher and the sponsoring company.

42.2.3 Deliberate manufacture or concealment of patient data

For some years concerns have been raised regarding the deliberate manufacture of patient results. The situation is almost certainly very uncommon but the question of how often it occurs, as opposed to its detection, remains unresolved. An example of this practice was discovered in the Second European Stroke Prevention Study (ESPS 2), a major clinical trial to prevent repeat strokes. It was found, rather inadvertently, that one of the investigators fabricated data on subjects where there was no evidence that they existed. This occurred without the trial sponsor's knowledge (Enserink, 1996).

The lure of benefits has not just affected those researchers involved in pharmaceutical studies. Some academics have also fabricated patient data so as to increase their importance in the field overall (e.g. Hagmann, 2000). Fortunately, because this study's results conflicted dramatically with other investigators' work, the fabrication was detected early and did not result in the inappropriate management of patients being widely adopted. One of the difficulties with studies that arise from academia is that because of their limited budgets such studies do not have the extensive auditing procedures that are used in pharmaceutical studies. Eternal vigilance is required to ensure that such fraud does not become more common place. The propensity to fraud will always exist when there are perverse incentives for the dishonest researcher who is willing to cut corners and bow to the increasing pressure to maintain 'productivity'.

The issues become even more complex with pharmaceutical studies. Not only is there the perverse incentive of academic advancement, but there is also the added impetus of monetary gain for the investigators for recruitment of subjects and also the requirement for all pharmaceutical companies to maximize the return to shareholders. The recent inexplicable failure to report deaths in a large study of rofecoxib may point to bias by the pharmaceutical industry to suppress negative findings (Krumholz et al., 2007). Such shortcomings have severe consequences for both the general public and the company itself if these shortcomings are exposed.

42.2.3.1 SOLUTION

The perverse incentives in academia need to be addressed to discourage output for its own sake. Such pressure has been found to underlie many cases of scientific fraud. This is an issue for academic departments whose oversight of individual academic's practices often ranges from cursory to non-existent. It is not the responsibility of the institutional ethics committee to police such practices, as in some instances the ethics committee may not even be aware that fraudulent 'trials' are even taking place (Hagmann, 2000). The benefits of scientific publication and grants are usually shared by the academic investigator's institution, but these benefits should be tied to the responsibility of ensuring proper academic conduct.

The controversy surrounding rofecoxib has caused greater scrutiny on the relationship between academic researchers and the pharmaceutical industry. Late stage clinical studies in particular may require additional safeguards. These could include storage of data independently to the sponsor and analysis by independent investigators. Independent data and safety monitoring boards need not be under the control of the sponsor, and could be under the direct control of an independent academic institution. The practices of 'ghostwriting' and false claims of full access to all relevant data should be eliminated (Krumholz et al., 2007). It is in the interests of the pharmaceutical industry to lead such change as the risk for maintaining the status quo may be large.

Additionally, the FDA has recently implemented additional actions to ensure that investigators who are noncompliant with the FDA's statutes and regulations intended to protect study subjects or who knowingly reporting inaccurate study findings are not allowed to continue to participate in clinical trials. These additional actions are aimed in to expedite the review process, as well as to ensure that those engaged in misconduct are readily identified to sponsors of drug or device trials; see www.fda.gov/NewsEvents/Newsroom/PressAnnouncements/ucm176043.htm.

42.2.4 Education of clinicians

The pharmaceutical industry not only has a legitimate right to educate doctors and the general public about the advances in treatment that have been achieved, but a responsibility. It is the methods that are employed which have raised concerns.

42.2.4.1 TREATMENT GUIDED BY EVIDENCE OR TRUSTED AUTHORITIES?

Both physicians and the general public believe that evidence should guide rational prescribing. Unfortunately, when doctors are 'shadowed' this is not the mechanism by which doctors seek solutions to clinical problems. Doctors seek solutions from other doctors and due to the hierarchical relationship of this transfer of information, a relatively small number of opinion leaders guide national and international prescribing patterns. The pharmaceutical industry has a societal responsibility to contract such opinion leaders to educate them about their products and to seek their advice as to how to further investigate the benefit–risk ratio for a particular medicine. One problem has been that historically these contractual relationships are covert and unregulated and this has led to questions such as 'when does reimbursement for services rendered become coercion'? More recently, hospitals and medical centres have begun to mandate reporting of any conflict of interest, a policy that will improve transparency and the perception of the relationship between the pharmaceutical industry and healthcare professionals.

42.2.4.2   SOLUTION

There is a need for greater transparency in the relationships between opinion leaders and industry. Learned colleges and medical associations have argued for such transparency but these organizations have not indicated how compliance with these guidelines will be monitored or what would be the consequences of non-compliance to the practitioner, the industry and the colleges themselves. The level of transparency required has to be sufficient so that those people reliant on information can judge whether any reimbursement may have influenced the opinion leader and by how much. There should be limits placed on the compensation provided for different tasks, e.g. speaking at a meeting. Unfortunately, there is no evidence that such disclosure has any influence on the prescribing habits of those who have been influenced by individual opinion leaders. The provision of excessive gifts or travel grants to non-speaking participants at international conferences would appear to be frank coercion and these practices should cease.

42.3   CONCLUSIONS

In general, the relationships between clinicians, academic researchers and the pharmaceutical industry have been healthy and conducive to the best interests of patients. They have produced results for patients which would have been unachievable by the individual parties. There are particular issues regarding people with dementia that may make these relationships even more complex. There have been some recent incidents which have resulted in some tensions to appear in these relationships, which may impair the essential trust on which these relationships are founded. An ongoing dialogue between pharma and health-care professionals is critical for both understanding the issues and finding constructive solutions. Several changes are suggested which will allow greater transparency for all the parties concerned.

REFERENCES

Ames DJ, Bhathal PS, Davies BM *et al.* (1990) Heterogeneity of adverse hepatic reactions to tetrahydroaminoacridine. *Australian and New Zealand Journal of Medicine* 20: 193–5.

Birks J, Grimley Evans J, Iakovidou V, Tsolaki M. (2009) Rivastigmine for Alzheimer's disease. *Cochrane Database of Systematic Reviews* (2): CD001191.

Davies P, Maloney AJF. (1976) Selective loss of cholinergic neurons in Alzheimer's disease. *Lancet* 2: 1403.

Davies P, Verth AH. (1977) Regional distribution of muscarinic acetylcholine receptor in normal and Alzheimer-type dementia brains. *Brain Research* 138: 385–92.

Davis KL, Thal LJ, Gamzu ER *et al.* (1992) A double-blind, placebo-controlled multicenter study of tacrine for Alzheimer's disease. The Tacrine Collaborative Study Group. *New England Journal of Medicine* 327: 1253–9.

Doogan D. (2009) In support of industry-sponsored clinical research. In: Snyder PJ, Mayes LC, Spencer D (eds). *Delgado's brave bulls: The complex relationship between science and the media.* New York: Elsevier.

Doran E, Henry D. (2008) Disease mongering: expanding the boundaries of treatable disease. *Internal Medicine Journal* 38: 858–61.

Enserink M. (1996) Fraud and ethics charges hit stroke drug trial. *Science* 274: 2004–5.

Hagmann M. (2000) Scientific misconduct. Cancer researcher sacked for alleged fraud. *Science* 287: 1901–2.

Kassirer JP. (2009) Medicine's obsession with disclosure of financial conflicts: fixing the wrong problem. In: Snyder PJ, Mayes LC, Spencer D (eds). *Delgado's brave bulls: The complex relationship between science and the media.* New York: Elsevier.

Krumholz HM, Ross JS, Presler AH, Egilman DS. (2007) What have we learnt from Vioxx? *British Medical Journal* 334: 120–3.

Leber P. (1990) *Draft guidelines for the clinical evaluation of antidementia drugs.* Washington DC: Food and Drug Administration. (FDA publication no. F91-19331.)

Summers WK, Majovski LV, Marsh GM *et al.* (1986) Oral tetrahydroaminoacridine in long-term treatment of senile dementia, Alzheimer type. *New England Journal of Medicine* 315: 1241–5.

PART II

MILD COGNITIVE IMPAIRMENT

Mild cognitive impairment: a historical perspective

KAREN RITCHIE AND SYLVAINE ARTERO

43.1 COGNITIVE IMPAIRMENT AS A FEATURE OF NORMAL AGEING

Alterations in cognitive functioning in the absence of dementia have long been considered a normal aspect of ageing-related brain changes. Affecting principally episodic verbal memory, such changes are generally distinguished from neurodegenerative disorders by their far slower progression, their lesser impact on ability to perform activities of daily living, and the relative sparing of linguistic and visuospatial functions. Increased interest in the nature and long-term prognosis of ageing-related modifications in cognitive performance has now led us to question to what extent they may be considered 'normal'. The past 50 years have seen numerous attempts to define these subclinical alterations in cognitive functioning and to establish their aetiology with greater precision than the general notion of 'ageing brain changes' to which they have formerly been attributed.

One of the earliest attempts to clinically characterize normal ageing-related cognitive change as opposed to dementia (dotage) is Gulliver's description of the eternal elderly of Luggnagg. '*In talking they forget the common appellation of things, and the names of persons, even of those who are their nearest friends and relatives …. The least miserable among them appear to be those who entirely lose their memories and turn to dotage; these meet with more pity and assistance*' (Swift, 1726). Two centuries later, Kral's notion of benign senescent forgetfulness (BSF; Kral, 1962) provides further clinical precision to Swift's observation, describing normal cognitive ageing as patient complaints of a persistent difficulty in recalling detail, commonly featuring depressive symptoms. While Kral initially considered such complaints to characterize a depressive state

which he referred to as 'depressive pseudo-dementia', long-term follow up of some of these patients showed that a significant proportion went on to develop vascular dementia. BSF was diagnosed by Kral by an open psychiatric interview and no formal algorithm was proposed. Formal diagnostic criteria for non-dementia cognitive impairment were first proposed by Crook *et al.* (1986) for the National Institute of Mental Health. Referring to 'age-associated memory impairment' (AAMI), they defined these changes as subjective complaints of memory loss in elderly persons verified by a decrement of at least one standard deviation on a formal memory test in comparison with means established for young adults. Blackford and La Rue (1989) later suggested suitable tests of non-verbal and verbal secondary memory tests, proposing that AAMI be defined as performance at least one standard deviation below the mean for young adults on one or more of these tests. They also differentiate AAMI from the more severe state of 'late-life forgetfulness' (LLF), defined as performance between 1 and 2 standard deviations below the mean on at least 50 per cent of a battery of at least four tests.

Levy (1994) argued that there is little reason a priori that cognitive decline in normal old age should be confined to memory functions exclusively, and in collaboration with the International Psychogeriatric Association and the World Health Organization proposed an alternative concept of ageing-associated cognitive decline (AACD). The criteria for AACD not only admit to the possibility of a wider range of cognitive functions being affected (attention, memory, learning, thinking, language, visuospatial function), but also stipulate that the deficit should be defined in reference to norms for elderly and not young adults to avoid confounding of decline with age cohort effects. This refinement takes into account the early observations of researchers such as Schaie and Willis (1991) who have demonstrated that much of the difference in cognitive performance observed between young and elderly cohorts is attributable to generation differences (notably in education and health care) rather than to ageing-related brain changes. A comparison of the performance of AACD and AAMI criteria in the general practice setting concluded that they do not identify the same individuals within general population studies, AACD targeting a more severe state of impairment within a larger AAMI group (Richards et al., 1999).

Recognition by the major international classifications of disease of subclinical cognitive deterioration linked to the normal ageing process began with the appearance in DSM-IV (American Psychiatric Association, 1994) of the concept of age-related cognitive decline (ARCD). Like AACD it refers to an objective decline in cognitive functioning due to the physiological process of ageing, however, no operational criteria or cognitive testing procedures are specified. It is rather loosely defined as a complaint of difficulties in recalling names, appointments or in problem-solving, which cannot be related to a specific mental problem or a neurological disorder. The concepts of ARCD and AACD, while clinically meaningful, are now rarely used in research principally because of the difficulty in proving that such changes are 'normal' and not part of an as yet unidentified subclinical pathology. Many early studies employing these categories found them to subsequently be associated with underlying vascular pathology and high rates of evolution towards dementia on follow up (Celsis et al., 1997; Di Carlo et al., 2000; Ritchie et al., 2001).

43.2   DISEASE MODELS OF SUBCLINICAL COGNITIVE IMPAIRMENT

The early conceptualizations of age-related cognitive loss described above had in common the theoretical assumption that such changes are distinct from dementia and other pathologies, being the consequence of inevitable, thus normal, ageing-related cerebral changes such as atrophy and vascular fragility. As parallel research into the causes of dementia and cerebrovascular disease has now led to a clearer understanding of their aetiology, it has also been shown that many of the physiological abnormalities seen in these disorders are also present to a lesser extent in subjects identified as AAMI, ARCD and AACD. Consequently, elderly persons with subclinical cognitive deficits have become the subject of neurological as well as psychogeriatric research, the underlying question being whether cognitive deficits of this type may be due to underlying brain pathology which might be potentially treatable. Alternative concepts have subsequently appeared in the literature linking cognitive disorder to various forms of underlying pathology. The tenth revision of the International Classification of Diseases (World Health Organization, 1993), described for example 'mild cognitive disorder' (MCD), which refers to disorders of memory, learning and concentration, often accompanied by mental fatigue, which must be demonstrated by formal

neuropsychological testing and attributable to cerebral disease or damage, or systemic physical disease known to cause dysfunction. MCD is secondary to physical illness or impairment, excluding dementia, amnesic syndrome, concussion, or post-encephalitic syndrome. The concept of MCD, which was principally developed to describe the cognitive consequences of auto-immune deficiency syndrome, but then expanded to include other disorders in which cognitive change is secondary to another disease process, is applicable to all ages, not just the elderly. Attempts to apply MCD criteria to population studies of elderly persons suggest it to be of limited value in this context, casting doubt on its validity as a nosological entity (Christensen et al., 1995) for this age group. DSM-IV (American Psychiatric Association, 1994) proposed a similar entity, mild neurocognitive disorder (MNCD), which encompasses not only memory and learning difficulties, but also perceptual-motor, linguistic and central executive functions. While the concepts proposed by the two international classifications, MCD and MNCD, do not constitute adequate algorithms for application in a research context, they do provide formal recognition of subclinical cognitive disorder as a pathological state requiring treatment and as a source of handicap, and are thus likely to be important within a legal context.

A similar concept of cognitive change secondary to multiple underlying disease processes, but in this case referring to elderly populations, is that of cognitive impairment no dementia (CIND). The concept was developed within the context of the Canadian Study of Health and Aging and is defined by reference to neuropsychological testing and clinical examination (Graham et al., 1997). Persons with CIND, like MCD and MNCD, are considered to have cognitive impairment attributable to an underlying physical disorder, but may also have a 'circumscribed memory impairment' which is a modified form of AAMI. CIND encompasses a wider range of underlying pathologies (and therefore has higher prevalence rates) than MCD and MNCD, including disorders such as delirium, substance abuse and psychiatric illness, which are excluded from the ICD and DSM categories.

43.3   MILD COGNITIVE IMPAIRMENT – SUBCLINICAL COGNITIVE CHANGE AS PRODROMAL DEMENTIA

MCD, MNCD and CIND are constructs which have been developed principally for research purposes and consider cognitive disorder in the elderly to be heterogeneous, not necessarily progressive, with treatment being determined by the nature of the underlying primary systemic disease. On the other hand, many clinical observations of the long-term outcome of cognitive complaints, particularly those presenting to memory clinics and neurology departments, led to the general conclusion by many neurologists that subclinical cognitive disorder in the elderly is in fact principally, if not exclusively, early-stage dementia. Thus, whereas dementia was considered by many in the early 1990s to be an upward extension of a 'normal' process of progressive ageing-related cognitive deterioration, by the end of the decade subclinical cognitive deficit began to be perceived as a downward extension of a neurodegenerative process. In 1997, Petersen *et al.* (1997) proposed diagnostic criteria for the concept of mild cognitive impairment (MCI), initially defined as complaints of defective memory and demonstration of abnormal memory functioning for age, with normal general cognitive functioning and conserved ability to perform activities of daily living, was considered to be a prodrome of Alzheimer's disease (AD). MCI criteria proved difficult to apply as they referred to poor cognitive functioning as assessed at one point in time, thus precluding appreciation of decline over time, and difficult to differentiate from cohort effects, low IQ and education. A later definition refined the initial concept by referring to memory impairment beyond that expected for both age and education level (Petersen *et al.*, 1999). An alternative approach has been to define it in terms of early-stage dementia. For example, Krasuki *et al.* (1998) refer to cognitive impairment with a score of 20 or more on the Mini-Mental State Examination (MMSE) and Zaudig (1992) defines MCI as a score of more than 22 on MMSE or 34–47 on the SIDAM dementia scale. Others have referred to criteria based on the Clinical Dementia Rating Scale or Global Deterioration Scale scores (Flicker *et al.*, 1991; Kluger *et al.*, 1997). The concept of MCI subsequently moved from being a non-benign, non-specific form of memory impairment to a dementia prodrome. As such it became the focus of considerable interest as it opened up the possibility of widescale treatment of a subclinical state by the new anticholinergic therapies being developed at this time for AD.

43.4   OPERATIONALIZING MCI CRITERIA

Subsequent studies using MCI criteria encountered numerous difficulties. These were principally due first to a lack of consensus as to whether the concept referred to memory loss due to any cause, to dementia or specifically to AD; and second to the lack of a working definition of memory loss. The result has been that population prevalence, the clinical features of subjects identified with MCI and their clinical outcomes vary widely between studies and even within studies where there has been longitudinal follow up. A consensus conference held in Chicago in 1999 confronted the many difficulties facing the MCI concept (Petersen *et al.*, 2001), notably its two underlying assumptions that it should be confined exclusively to isolated memory impairment and whether it should refer exclusively to a prodrome of AD, or alternatively a more clinically heterogeneous group at increased risk of dementia due to any cause. While there is some limited evidence that a purely mnesic syndrome may exist (Richards *et al.*, 1999), this category appears to represent only a very small proportion (6 per cent) of elderly persons with cognitive deficit when the full range of cognitive functions are examined. Higher rates of 'circumscribed memory deficit' (31.7 per cent of CIND cases) are observed within the Canadian Longitudinal Study (Graham *et al.*, 1997), but only subjects with a score below cut-off on the MMSE are examined, and the test battery itself consists

predominantly of memory tasks. Memory tests also involve cognitive capacities other than memory, notably attentional and linguistic capacities, so that it is difficult in the absence of a detailed neuropsychological examination to conclude that an individual has an isolated mnesic impairment. Many of the studies which observe principally memory deficits in MCI have used, almost exclusively, memory tests in their diagnostic examination; a self-fulfilling prophecy.

The Chicago consensus group concluded that subjects with MCI have a condition which is different from normal ageing and are likely to progress to AD at an accelerated rate, however, they may also progress to another form of dementia or improve. This group thus proposed subtypes of MCI according to type of cognitive deficit and clinical outcome distinguishing MCI-Amnestic (MCI with pronounced memory impairment progressing to AD), MCI Multiple Domain (slight impairment across several cognitive domains leading to Alzheimer's disease, vascular dementia or stabilizing in the case of normal brain ageing changes), and MCI Single Non-Memory Domain (significant impairment in a cognitive domain other than memory leading to AD or another form of dementia). It has subsequently been suggested that MCI be further subdivided according to the suspected aetiology of the cognitive impairment, in keeping with international classifications of dementing disorders: for example MCI-AD, MCI-LBD, MCI-FTD and so on; however, clinical studies have been unable to provide consistent empirical evidence for these subdivisions. On the basis of evidence from population studies presented at this conference, it was also accepted that MCI subjects could have difficulties in everyday functioning. A recent study has confirmed functional loss to be a characteristic of all MCI subtypes (Aretouli and Brandt, 2010), and application of the revised criteria to a general population cohort has been shown to greatly increase the ability of the algorithms to differentiate a pre-dementia syndrome (Artero *et al.*, 2006).

43.5   THE FUTURE OF MCI

A number of concepts now exist to describe subclinical cognitive disorder in the elderly. Application of these concepts in general population studies gives quite different prevalence rates, both between concepts and even between studies using the same concept (**Table 43.1**).

Clearly, such deficits have multiple causes. Longitudinal population studies of subclinical cognitive deficits have demonstrated multiple patterns of cognitive change with variable clinical outcomes including dementia, depression, cardiovascular and respiratory disorders (Ritchie *et al.*, 1996; Lopez *et al.*, 2003; Palmer *et al.*, 2003; Matthews *et al.*, 2008). However, it is the identification of those cases likely to evolve towards dementia which has been given priority, especially given the development of treatments which may delay dementia onset. The potential treatment window for dementia is large, with twin studies indicating that insidious changes in cognitive performance may occur up to 20 years before disease onset (La Rue and Jarvik, 1987). For this reason, at a conceptual level MCI has been the principal focus

Table 43.1   Characteristics and estimated prevalence rates (where available) of nosological entities defining cognitive impairment in elderly persons without dementia.

Concept	Criteria		Population prevalence %
BSF	Kral (1962)	Memory complaints, forgetting details. Depression	
AAMI	Crook et al. (1986)	Memory impairment with decrement on formal cognitive test compared to young adults	7–38
LLF	Blackford and LaRue (1989)	AAMI with greater decrement on 50% of a test battery	–
AACD	Levy (1994)	Impairment on any formal cognitive test compared to peers	21–27
ARCD	DSM IV	Objective decline in cognitive functioning due to old age	8
MCD	ICD-10	Disorders of memory learning and concentration demonstrated by testing. Due to disease	4
MNCD	DSM IV	Difficulties in memory, learning, perceptual-motor, linguistic and central executive functioning. Due to disease	–
CIND	Graham et al. (1997)	Circumscribed memory impairment and low MMSE score due to disease or age	11–80
MCI	Petersen et al. (1997)	Complaints of defective memory, demonstrated by deficit on cognitive tests with normal general intellectual functioning compared to peers. Due to dementia	3–15

AACD, ageing-associated cognitive decline; AAMI, age-associated memory impairment; ARCD, age-related cognitive decline; BSF, benign senescent forgetfulness; CIND, cognitive impairment no dementia; LLF, late-life forgetfulness; MCD, mild cognitive disorder; MCI, mild cognitive impairment; MNCD, mild neurocognitive disorder.

of interest as longitudinal studies confirm the high risk rates of MCI for dementia, with conversion estimates ranging from 10 to 15 per cent per year (Petersen et al., 1997), 40 per cent over two years (Johnson et al., 1998), 20 per cent over three years (Wolf et al., 1998), 30 per cent over three years (Black, 1999), 53 per cent over three years (McKelvey et al., 1999), to 100 per cent over 4.5 years (Krasuki et al., 1998). Population studies show, however, lower dementia conversion rates 2–8 per cent per annum (Tierney et al., 1996; Johanssen et al., 1997; Kluger et al., 1999; Hogan and Ebly, 2000; Morris et al., 2001; Artero et al., 2001) than those observed in clinical studies (12–31 per cent; Flicker et al., 1991; Bowen et al., 1997; Devanand et al., 1997; Bozoki et al., 2001; Huang et al., 2000; Stephan et al., 2008) as they include a wider range of cognitive impairments which are probably also less severe than those presenting in clinical settings. Population studies further indicate that current criteria have poor specificity in the general population setting, and also miss many people who will develop dementia within a few years, but that age-adjusted cognitive measures in conjunction with measures of disability, depression and anatomical changes on cerebral imaging (volume loss in hippocampal and entorhinal cortex) may ultimately provide better dementia prediction (Tierney et al., 1996; Touchon and Ritchie, 1999; Artero et al., 2001; Ritchie et al., 2001; Visser et al., 2002; Artero et al., 2003; Palmer et al., 2003). More recently, attention has also turned towards the potential utility of biomarkers, notably amyloid β protein and tau ratios in cerebrospinal fluid as a means of identifying MCI cases most likely to develop dementia (Frankfort et al., 2008). Finally it has been suggested that both risk factors and clinical presentation of MCI may be different for men and women, such that greater specificity in detection may be achieved if sex-specific diagnostic algorithms are proposed (Artero et al., 2008; Ritchie et al., 2010).

While the recognition of MCI as a potentially pathological entity marks an early step towards the recognition of non-dementia cognitive disorder as an important clinical problem with a potential treatment, it does not meet the necessary validation criteria for a formal nosological entity (Ritchie et al., 2001). The feasibility of wide-scale treatment will very much depend on the development of more precise diagnostic criteria. Premature application of MCI criteria for the identification of subjects for clinical trials is likely to lead to either the inclusion of high numbers of non-cases (yielding high failure rates and subsequent discreditation of a treatment which may have been successful on sample subgroups) or alternatively by restriction to subjects in reality already manifesting early dementia, in which case it may be too late to demonstrate potential preventive/delaying effects. The future of MCI development will depend very much on close collaboration between specialist clinical units refining clinical criteria and epidemiologists monitoring screening efficiency within the general population where MCI will principally be detected.

REFERENCES

American Psychiatric Association. (1994) *Diagnostic and statistical manual. IV.* Washington: American Psychiatric Association.

Artero S, Touchon J, Ritchie K. (2001) Disability and mild cognitive impairment: a longitudinal population-based study. *International Journal of Geriatric Psychiatry* **16**: 1092–7.

Artero S, Tierney MC, Touchon J, Ritchie K. (2003) Prediction of transition from cognitive impairment to senile dementia: a prospective longitudinal study. *Acta Psychiatrica Scandanavica* **107**: 390–3.

Artero S, Petersen R, Touchon J, Ritchie K. (2006) Reviseed criteria for mild cognitive impairment: validation within a longitudinal population study. *Dementia and Geriatric Cognitive Disorders* 21: 198–204.

Artero S, Ancelin ML, Portet F *et al.* (2008) Risk profiles for mild cognitive impairment and progression to dementia are gender specific. *Journal of Neurology Neurosurgery and Psychiatry* 79: 979–84.

Aretouli E, Brandt J. (2010) Everyday functioning in mild cognitive impairment and its relationship with executive cognition. *International Journal of Geriatric Psychiatry* 25: 224–33.

Black SE. (1999) Can SPECT predict the future for mild cognitive impairment? *Canadian Journal of Neurological Sciences* 26: 4–6.

Blackford RC, La Rue A. (1989) Criteria for diagnosing age associated memory impairment: proposed improvements from the field. *Developmental Neuropsychology* 5: 295–306.

Bowen J, Teri L, Kukull W *et al.* (1997) Progression to dementia in patients with isolated memory loss. *Lancet* 349: 763 5.

Bozoki A, Giordani B, Heidebrink JL *et al.* (2001) Mild cognitive impairments predict dementia in nondemented elderly patients with memory loss. *Archives of Neurology* 58: 411–16.

Celsis P, Agniel A, Cardebat D *et al.* (1997) Age-related cognitive decline: a clinical entity? A longitudinal study of cerebral blood flow and memory performance. *Journal of Neurology Neurosurgery and Psychiatry* 62: 601–8.

Christensen H, Henderson AS, Jorm AF *et al.* (1995) ICD-10 mild cognitive disorder: epidemiological evidence on its validity. *Psychological Medicine* 25: 105–20.

Crook T, Bartus RT, Ferris SH *et al.* (1986) Age associated memory impairment: proposed diagnostic criteria and measures of clinical change – Report of a National Institute of Mental Health Work Group. *Developmental Neuropsychology* 2: 261–76.

Devanand DP, Folz M, Gorlyn M *et al.* (1997) Questionable dementia: clinical course and predictors of outcome. *Journal of the Americal Geriatrics Society* 45: 321–8.

DiCarlo A, Baldereschi M, Amaducci L *et al.* (2000) Cognitive impairment without dementia in older people: prevalence, vascular risk factors, impact on disability. *Journal of the American Geriatrics Society* 48: 775–82.

Flicker C, Ferris FH, Reisberg B. (1991) Mild cognitive impairment in the elderly: predictors of dementia. *Neurology* 41: 1006–9.

Frankfort SV, Tulner LR, van Campen JP *et al.* (2008) Amyloid beta protein and tau in cerebrospinal fluid and plasma as biomarkers for dementia: a review of recent literature. *Current Clinical Pharmacology* 3: 123–31.

Graham JE, Rockwood K, Beattie EL *et al.* (1997) Prevalence and severity of cognitive impairment with and without dementia in an elderly populaiton. *Lancet* 349: 1793–6.

Hogan DB, Ebly EM. (2000) Predicting who will develop dementia in a cohort of Canadian seniors. *Canadian Journal of Neurological Sciences* 27: 18–24.

Huang C, Wahlund LO, Dierks T *et al.* (2000) Discrimination of Alzheimer's disease and mild cognitive impairment by equivalent EEG sources: a cross-sectional and longitudinal study. *Clinical Neurophysiology* 111: 1961–7.

Johanssen B, Zarit SH. (1997) Early cognitive markers of the incidence of dementia and mortality: a longitudinal population-based study of the oldest old. *International Journal of Geriatric Psychiatry* 12: 53–9.

Johnson KA, Jones K, Holman BL. (1998) Preclinical prediction of Alzheimer's disease using SPECT. *Neurology* 50: 1563–72.

Kluger A, Gianutsos JG, Golomb J *et al.* (1997) Motor/psychomotor dysfunction in normal aging, mild cognitive decline, and early Alzheimer's disease: diagnostic and differential diagnostic features. *International Psychogeriatrics* 9: 307–16.

Kluger A, Ferris SH, Golomb J *et al.* (1999) Neuropsychological prediction of decline to dementia in nondemented elderly. *Journal of Geriatric Psychiatry and Neurology* 12: 168–79.

Kral VA. (1962) Senescent forgetfulness: benign and malignant. *Canadian Medical Association Journal* 86: 257–60.

Krasuki JS, Alexander GE, Horwitz B *et al.* (1998) Volumes of medial temporal lobe structures in patients with Alzheimer's disease and mild cognitive impairment (and in healthy controls). *Biological Psychiatry* 43: 60–68.

La Rue A, Jarvik LF. (1987) Cognitive function and prediction of dementia in old age. *International Journal of Aging and Human Development* 25: 79–89.

Levy R. (1994) On behalf of the Aging-Associated Cognitive Decline Working Party. Aging-associated cognitive decline. *International Psychogeriatrics* 6: 63–8.

Lopez OL, Jagust WJ, Dulberg C *et al.* (2003) Risk factors for mild cognitive impairment in the Cardiovascular Health Study Cognition Study: Part 2. *Archives of Neurology* 60: 1394–9.

McKelvey R, Bergman H, Stern J *et al.* (1999) Lack of prognostic significance of SPECT abnormalities in elderly subjects with mild memory loss. *Canadian Journal of Neurological Sciences* 26: 23–8.

Matthews FE, Stephan BC, McKeith IG *et al.* (2008) Two-year progression from mild cognitive impairment to dementia: to what extent do different definitions agree? *Journal of the American Geriatrics Society* 56: 1424–33.

Morris JC, Storandt M, Miller JP *et al.* (2001) Mild cognitive impairment represents early-stage Alzheimer disease. *Archives of Neurology* 58: 397–405.

Palmer K, Fratiglioni L, Winblad B. (2003) What is Mild Cognitive Impairment? Variations in definitions and evolution of nondemented persons with cognitive impairment. *Acta Neurologica Scandanavica* 179: 14–20.

Petersen R, Doody R, Kurz A *et al.* (2001) Current concepts in mild cognitive impairment. *Archives of Neurology* 58: 1985–92.

Petersen RC, Smith GE, Waring SC *et al.* (1997) Aging, memory and mild cognitive impairment. *International Psychogeriatrics* 9: 65–9.

Petersen RC, Smith GE, Waring SC *et al.* (1999) Mild cognitive impairment: clinical characterization and outcome. *Archives of Neurology* 56: 303–8.

Richards M, Touchon J, Ledésert B, Ritchie K. (1999) Cognitive decline in ageing: are AAMI and AACD distinct entities? *International Journal of Geriatric Psychiatry* 14: 534–40.

Ritchie K, Leibovici D, Ledésert B, Touchon J. (1996) A typology of sub-clinical senescent cognitive disorder. *British Journal of Psychiatry* 168: 470–6.

Ritchie K, Artero S, Touchon J. (2001) Classification criteria for mild cognitive impairment: a population-based validation study. *Neurology* 56: 37–42.

Ritchie K, Ancelin ML, Portet F *et al.* (2010) Retrospective identification and characterization of Mild Cognitive Impairment from a prospective population cohort. *American Journal of Geriatric Psychiatry* (in press).

Schaie KW, Willis SL. (1991) Adult personality and psychomotor performance: cross-sectional and longitudinal analyses. *Journals of Gerontology* 46: 275–84.

Stephan BC, Brayne C, McKeith IG. (2008) Mild cognitive impairment in the older population: who is missed and does it matter? *International Journal of Geriatric Psychiatry* 23: 863–71.

Swift J. (1726) *Gulliver's Travels.* London: Benjamin Motte, 223.

Tierney MC, Szalai JP, Snow WG *et al.* (1996) Prediction of probable Alzheimer's disease in memory-impaired patients: a prospective longitudinal study. *Neurology* 46: 661–5.

Touchon J, Ritchie K. (1999) Prodromal cognitive disorder in Alzheimer's disease. *International Journal of Geriatric Psychiatry* 14: 556–63.

Visser PJ, Verhey FR, Hofman PA *et al.* (2002) Medial temporal atrophy predicts Alzheimer's disease in patients with minor cognitive impairment. *Journal of Neurology Neurosurgery and Psychiatry* 72: 491–7.

Wolf H, Grunwald M, Ecke GM *et al.* (1998) The prognosis of mild cognitive impairment in the elderly. *Journal of Neural Transmission* 54: 31–50.

World Health Organization. (1993) *The ICD-10 Classification of Mental and Behavioural Disorders. Diagnostic Criteria for Research.* Geneva: World Health Organisation.

Zaudig M. (1992) A new systematic method of measurement and diagnosis of 'Mild Cognitive Impairment' and dementia according to ICD-10 and DSM III-R criteria. *International Psychogeriatrics* 4: 203–19.

Clinical characteristics of mild cognitive impairment

TARYN C SILBER, YONAS ENDALE GEDA AND RONALD C PETERSEN

44.1 INTRODUCTION

The promotion of health and prevention of disease is a time honoured axiomatic truth (Geda *et al.*, 2006b). This is particularly true of Alzheimer's disease (AD), the most common cause of dementia (Chong and Sahadevan, 2005). By the year 2050, AD is projected to afflict as many as 106.2 million people worldwide (Brookmeyer *et al.*, 2007).

For compelling reasons (see Chapter 2, The lived experience of dementia, Chapter 3, Prevalence and incidence of dementia, Chapter 8, Neuropsychiatric aspects of dementia and Chapter 15, Family carers of people with dementia) it is crucial to delay the onset of dementia. The global prevalence of AD would decrease by 22.8 million cases if it were possible to delay the onset of dementia by about two years. Effective prevention, as well as intervention, could dramatically reduce disease onset and progression (Brookmeyer *et al.*, 2007). The identification of mild cognitive impairment (MCI) contributes to the early detection and prevention effort (Petersen *et al.*, 1999).

MCI refers to an intermediate state between the cognitive changes of normal ageing and very early dementia (Petersen *et al.*, 2005; **Figure 44.1**). Individuals with MCI show cognitive impairment greater than expected for their age, but otherwise function independently and do not meet the commonly accepted criteria for dementia (Petersen *et al.*, 1999).

44.2 THE HISTORICAL GENESIS OF MCI

Reisberg and colleagues were perhaps the first to coin the term MCI (Reisberg *et al.*, 1982; Flicker *et al.*, 1991; Reisberg *et al.*, 2008). They used the Global Deterioration Scale (GDS)

to define MCI. The GDS is an ordinal scale of 1 to 7 with 1 being normal and 7 signifying severe dementia. A GDS score of 3 is defined as MCI. In 1962, VA Kral used the term 'senescent forgetfulness' as the first attempt to characterize memory concerns with ageing. This was followed by a pioneering initiative of the National Institute of Mental Health that came up with the term 'age-associated memory impairment' (AAMI; Crook *et al.*, 1986). The concept of AAMI further accelerated the research work in the grey zone between ageing and dementia. However, AAMI was noted to have its limitations, such as restriction of impairment to memory domain only and comparison of memory function in older adults with that of young adults (at least 1 standard deviation below the mean for young adults). These limitations led some to remark that, depending on the memory test selected, up to 90 per cent of those older than 50 would be labelled as impaired (Smith *et al.*, 1991).

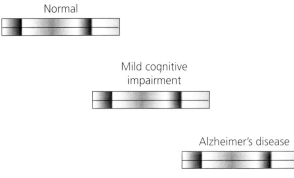

Figure 44.1 Conceptual model of mild cognitive impairment.

To address the weaknesses of AAMI, the International Psychogeriatric Association defined the term 'age associated cognitive decline' (AACD; Levy, 1994). The operational criteria for AACD referenced a variety of cognitive domains presumed to decline in normal ageing, and included age- and education-adjusted normative values as well. In addition to AAMI and AACD there are several other terms suggested (Blackford and LaRue, 1989, Graham et al., 1997) including 'questionable dementia' (Devanand et al., 1997), defined using the Clinical Dementia Rating Scale (CDR; Morris, 1993). This severity scale designates individuals with a CDR of 0.5 to have 'questionable dementia'. While both GDS and CDR are reliable scales when rating severity of MCI along the continuum of cognitive impairment, they do not necessarily coincide with various stages of impairment. Actually, patients with a GDS of 3 or CDR of 0.5 may in fact meet criteria for mild dementia or AD.

The current widely used criteria for amnestic MCI were empirically validated in a prospective study conducted in Rochester, Minnesota (Petersen et al., 1999). Since then there has been an exponential growth in the number of publications on MCI. The Mayo Clinic criteria were also endorsed by the American Academy of Neurology (AAN) that stated that the MCI construct is worthy of attention since patients with MCI develop dementia at a much higher rate of 10–15 per cent per year as compared to the general population of 1–2 per cent per year (Petersen et al., 2001).

44.3 CLINICAL FEATURES

Physicians often encounter a clinical scenario in which an elderly person presents with memory concerns. Such a patient is often interested in finding out whether the memory concerns are indicative of AD. While such concerns could represent other states such as late-life depression or the patient being in the so-called 'worried well' state, they could also be suggestive of an evolving AD. Consider, for example, a typical clinical scenario described below.

44.3.1 The case record of patient A

A 68-year-old right-handed male patient presented with forgetfulness for recent events and future engagements. Family members and close friends noticed these changes as well. The patient had difficulty identifying the onset of these symptoms but felt that they had started insidiously and progressed gradually over a period of two to three years. Otherwise, he was living independently and had no difficulty carrying out activities of daily living, such as handling his own finances, cooking and driving. He denied depression, stress or other complicating medical issues. He requested an appointment with a physician in order to determine if this memory problem should be pursued further. The clinical evaluation, i.e. meticulous history and physical examination including bedside cognitive screening using the short test of mental status, was suggestive of cognitive impairment but not severe enough to warrant the diagnosis of dementia, hence a clinical diagnosis of MCI was made. Investigations including

psychometric testing and magnetic resonance imaging (MRI) were ordered. The neuropsychological testing confirmed the clinical diagnosis. It revealed memory impairment, particularly on measures of learning and delayed recall beyond what was felt to be normal for age; but other cognitive domains such as language and visuospatial skills were relatively intact. An MRI of the head revealed mild hippocampal atrophy.

44.3.2 Comment

This patient probably has amnestic MCI. He is becoming slightly more forgetful, and this is noticeable to his family and friends. The most salient feature of the history concerns forgetfulness of insidious onset that gradually progressed over a year or so. All other cognitive domains, i.e. language, comportment-executive function, visuospatial skills, were intact. The individual did not have a decline in function. This likely represented an early disease process involving the medial temporal lobe since meaningful information could no longer be stored in an efficient manner, nor is it recalled well.

44.3.3 Diagnostic algorithm for MCI subtypes

The diagnosis of MCI is anchored upon clinical data, i.e. a detailed history, thorough physical examination and bedside cognitive screening, for example Mini-Mental State Examination (MMSE; Folstein et al., 1975) or equivalent scales (Kokmen et al., 1987) are all utilized. The original Mayo criteria for amnestic MCI included: (1) a memory complaint, preferably substantiated by an informant; (2) psychometric testing revealing memory impairment for age and education; (3) normal general cognitive function; (4) intact activities of daily living; (5) not demented (Petersen et al., 2001). Even though amnestic MCI is the most widely studied and empirically validated construct, three additional subtypes are also the subject of intense investigation (Winblad et al., 2004). **Figure 44.2** depicts the diagnostic algorithm used to identify a particular subtype of MCI. The algorithm is initiated when a patient or informant reports cognitive complaints, such as forgetfulness for recent events and future engagements. The clinician should then determine that the patient is neither demented nor normal for age. Once this is established, the next step is to make sure that there is no substantial functional decline. If it is determined that the decline in function is not of sufficient magnitude as to warrant the diagnosis of a very mild dementia, then the clinician further assumes the diagnosis of MCI and proceeds to identify the number and types of cognitive domains impaired. A diagnosis of amnestic MCI-single domain is assumed if the impairment involves only memory domain, whereas amnestic MCI-multiple domain pertains to impairments in the memory domain plus at least one other cognitive domain, such as language, executive function or visuospatial skills. Likewise, a diagnosis of non-amnestic MCI-single domain is assumed if there is impairment in a single non-memory domain, whereas non-amnestic MCI-multiple domain refers to impairments in multiple non-memory domains.

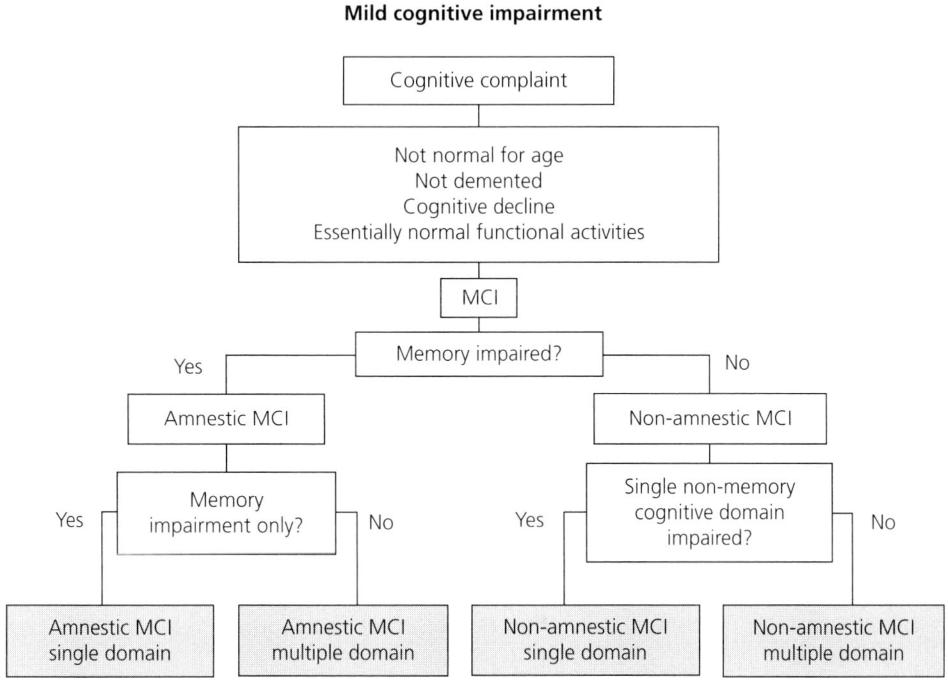

Mild cognitive impairment

Figure 44.2 Flow chart of decision process for making diagnosis of subtypes of mild cognitive impairment.

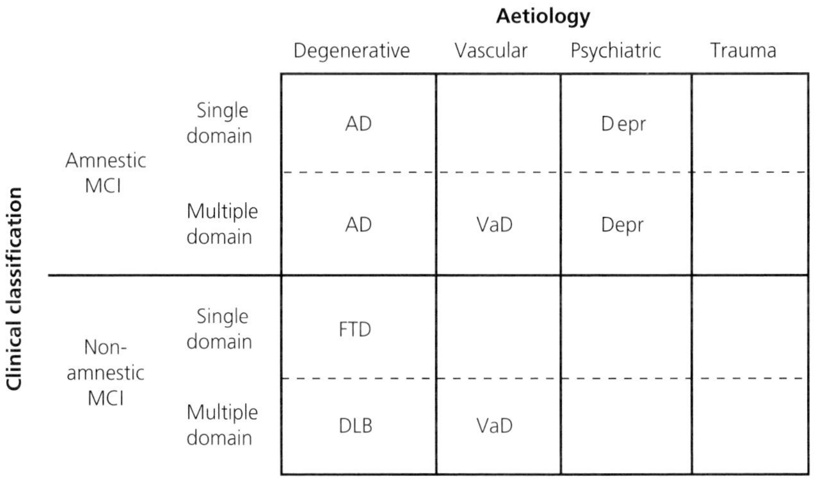

Figure 44.3 Classification of clinical subtypes of mild cognitive impairment with presumed aetiology.

The diagnostic algorithm helps to describe MCI and its subtypes. The next step is to clarify potential aetiologies of MCI. **Figure 44.3** depicts the presumed aetiologies along with clinical subtypes of MCI. The single- and multiple-domain amnestic MCI subtypes with presumed degenerative aetiology likely represent a prodromal form of AD (Winblad *et al.*, 2004). The non-amnestic subtypes that emphasize impairments in the non-memory domains may have a higher likelihood of progressing to a non-AD dementia, such as dementia with Lewy bodies (Winblad *et al.*, 2004).

44.4   THE EPIDEMIOLOGY OF MCI

The main focus of this section is the three epidemiological indices derived from descriptive studies: the prevalence of

MCI, the incidence of MCI and the conversion rate of MCI to dementia.

The incidence of MCI ranges from 1 to 6 per cent per year while prevalence estimates range from 3 to 22 per cent per year (Bennett, 2003; Hanninen *et al.*, 2002; Larrieu *et al.*, 2002; DeCarli, 2003; Lopez *et al.*, 2003; Ganguli *et al.*, 2004). This variability can in part be explained by sampling and measurement biases (Sackett, 1979). Sampling methods that may have yielded variability include using advertisements to recruit research participants (introducing a non-respondent/volunteer bias) (Sackett, 1979). Measurement bias may be introduced when retrofitting MCI criteria into a cohort assembled for non-MCI study. A population-based study utilizing the operational criteria of MCI in the elderly is likely to minimize sampling and measurement bias, thus leading to more precise estimates of prevalence and incidence rates. One such example is the population-based Mayo Clinic Study of

Aging launched in Olmsted County, Minnesota on the pre-valence date of October 1, 2004. The study is funded by the National Institute on Aging. The aim of the study is to examine the prevalence, incidence and risk factors for MCI. The study has conducted a face to face evaluation of 2050 people in person and 669 people by telephone. These assessments led to diagnostic classifications of normal cognition, MCI or dementia using specific published criteria (Roberts *et al.*, 2008). The prevalence of MCI from this study is estimated at approximately 15 per cent in the non-demented population, with a 2:1 ratio of aMCI to naMCI (Petersen *et al.*, 2009).

The Cardiovascular Health Study (CHS) was perhaps the first population-based study to estimate the prevalence of MCI subtypes. The study was originally designed to examine cardiovascular risk factors (Fried *et al.*, 1991). The CHS reported an overall prevalence of MCI to be 22 per cent with amnestic MCI accounting for 6 per cent and multi-domain MCI representing 16 per cent (Lopez *et al.*, 2003).

Researchers in Japan used the MCI criteria in a cohort of over 65-year-olds and estimated the prevalence of MCI to be in the range of 1.7–16.6 per cent (Sasaki *et al.*, 2009). An Australian research group found the prevalence of MCI to be 3.8 per cent and AACD to be 3.1 per cent in subjects 60–64 years old (Kumar *et al.*, 2005). Although the Australian study design was optimal, the cohort involved a younger age group, thus the prevalence rate was understandably low. Retrofitting the MCI criteria might have introduced measurement bias in the Japanese study.

Several studies have estimated the progression rate of MCI to dementia (Flicker *et al.*, 1991; Tierney *et al.*, 1996; Petersen *et al.*, 1999; Daly *et al.*, 2000; Petersen *et al.*, 2005; Fischer *et al.*, 2007). Their findings vary depending upon the study design and measurement instrument used (Dawe *et al.*, 1992). Researchers from Harvard University recruited study participants via advertisement. They then prospectively followed a cohort of subjects with MCI and reported a conversion rate of 6 per cent per year (Daly *et al.*, 2000) whereas a recent multi-centre randomized, double blind, placebo controlled clinical trial reported a conversion rate of 16 per cent per year (Petersen *et al.*, 2005). Another community-based birth cohort study examining progression rates between amnestic and non-amnestic subtypes of MCI to AD showed the annual rate of conversion to AD for amnestic MCI to be 19 per cent, compared to almost 11 per cent for non-amnestic MCI subjects (Fischer *et al.*, 2007). Prior to that study, Mayo Clinic and other researchers have reported a conversion rate in the range of 10–15 per cent. Hence, the rather small rate reported by the Harvard group could be attributed to non-respondent/volunteer bias (Sackett, 1979). The higher percentages from the community-based cohort study may be due to prevalence/incidence bias wherein MCI subjects with advanced cognitive impairment (prevalent MCI) may have higher conversion rates to dementia (Fischer *et al.*, 2007; Mitchell and Shiri-Feshki, 2008). The common theme in all the studies is that MCI constitutes a high risk group for dementia.

There is an ongoing controversy regarding the 'instability' of the MCI construct (Ritchie *et al.*, 2001; Larrieu *et al.*, 2002). Larrieu and colleagues from France reported a reversion rate (i.e. from MCI back to normal cognitive ageing) to

be as high as 40 per cent over a 2–3 year follow up. However, one major limitation of their study was how they defined MCI, based on only one single memory measurement, the Benton Visual Retention Test (Benton *et al.*, 1983). The international consensus panel on MCI did emphasize the importance of a progressive decline, rather than entirely relying on poor performance at any one given point in time. The broader approach of the international panel may help minimize the instability of the MCI construct (Winblad *et al.*, 2004).

44.5 NEUROIMAGING AND BIOMARKERS

Magnetic resonance imaging (MRI) of the brain has been widely investigated in the context of MCI (Jack *et al.*, 2003; Jack *et al.*, 2008). These data on quantitative MRI have been instrumental in defining the role of MRI in ageing and dementia and have contributed greatly to the development of the multi-centre AD Neuroimaging Initiative (ADNI; Petersen *et al.*, 2009).

44.5.1 Molecular imaging

An important contribution to the study of ageing is the development of amyloid-imaging positron emission tomography (PET) tracer known as Pittsburgh Compound B (PiB; Klunk *et al.*, 2004; see Chapter 13, Molecular brain imaging in dementia). This tracer labels fibrillar amyloid and allows for the assessment of cerebral amyloid burden in living people and has great potential for assessing the role of amyloid in ageing, MCI and dementia. A few studies have begun looking at the serial properties of PiB over time (Klunk *et al.*, 2005; Klunk *et al.*, 2006; see Chapter 13, Molecular brain imaging in dementia). Current data suggest that 20–30 per cent of cognitively normal subjects have positive PiB scans while about 60 per cent of MCI subjects have positive scans (Lopresti *et al.*, 2005).

44.5.2 Biomarkers

Cerebrospinal fluid (CSF) derived biomarkers, such as Amyloid-β 1 to 42 peptide ($A\beta_{1-42}$), total tau (t-tau), and tau phosphorylated at threonine 181 (p-tau) predict MCI and AD progression (Shaw *et al.*, 2009). An Italian memory clinic tested each biomarker and observed that the biomarkers had a greater sensitivity for AD (at 65–87 per cent) than MCI (at 18–50 per cent; Frisoni *et al.*, 2009).

Therefore, molecular imaging of amyloid, as well as FDG PET scans and CSF derived biomarkers add additional information on progression in the spectrum of aging, MCI and dementia (Petersen *et al.*, 2009).

44.6 NEUROPSYCHIATRIC FEATURES

Although the neurological, psychometric and neuroimaging aspects of MCI have been researched (Petersen *et al.*, 1999;

Jack *et al.*, 2000; Jak *et al.*, 2009), there has been little investigation in the neuropsychiatric aspect of MCI. It is reasonable to address this issue because the medial temporal lobe and its connections with the prefrontal cortex and other structures not only play a critical role in cognitive function but are also involved in emotional behaviour (Mesulam, 1998). The first population-based investigation of neuropsychiatric symptoms of MCI was reported in 2002 (Lyketsos *et al.*, 2002). Since then, there have been similar studies on these features involving samples from primary or tertiary care settings (Feldman *et al.*, 2004; Geda *et al.*, 2004; Hwang *et al.*, 2004; Beaulieu-Bonneau and Hudon, 2009; Edwards *et al.*, 2009).

Geda and colleagues from the Mayo Clinic Study of Aging recently reported the population-based prevalence of neuropsychiatric symptoms in normal ageing and MCI. They observed that the three most common neuropsychiatric symptoms in MCI were depression (27 per cent), apathy (18.5 per cent) and irritability (19.4 per cent; Geda *et al.*, 2008). Lyketsos and colleagues (2002) reported similar but slightly smaller frequencies of depression (20 per cent), apathy (15 per cent) and irritability (15 per cent) in the CHS. The CHS group suggested that selection bias might have led to an underestimation of their prevalence estimates. This bias may account for the differences in crude frequency rates across the two studies. The CHS did not have cognitively normal participants. The Cache County population-based study reported prevalence figures for depression (7.2 per cent), apathy (3.2 per cent), and irritability of (4.6 per cent) in cognitively normal persons (Lyketsos *et al.*, 2000). The Mayo Clinic group did observe slightly higher figures for depression (11.5 per cent), apathy (4.8 per cent) and irritability (7.6 per cent) in normal ageing (Geda *et al.*, 2008).

A previous study from the Mayo Clinic prospectively followed a cohort of 840 elderly individuals, with neither depression nor cognitive impairment at baseline, for a median period of 3.5 (1–15) years (Geda *et al.*, 2006a), to the outcome of incident MCI. Depression, as measured by the short version of GDS (Yesavage, 1988), more than doubled the risk of transition from normal ageing to incident MCI. They also observed a synergistic interaction between depression and apolipoprotein E (ApoE) genotype. They proposed four hypotheses to explain the association between depression and incident MCI (**Figure 44.4**). The first is the aetiologic pathway, where depression is hypothesized to be in the chain of causality leading to MCI by virtue of its effect on a neurobiological pathway such as the neuroendocrine axis. This hypothesis assumes causality whereby depression causes an increased secretion of corticosteroids or other 'neurotoxic' biological factor that, in turn, lead to brain parenchymal damage. The second hypothesis pertains to shared risk factor or confounding, where depression is non-causally associated with a confounder (Szklo and Nieto, 2000). The confounder at the same time is an independent risk factor for the outcome (incident MCI). The confounder could be genetic, environmental, or both. This hypothesis points to a susceptibility gene variant or another non-genetic risk factor that increases the risk of depression and MCI independently. The third hypothesis pertains to a reverse causality. Under

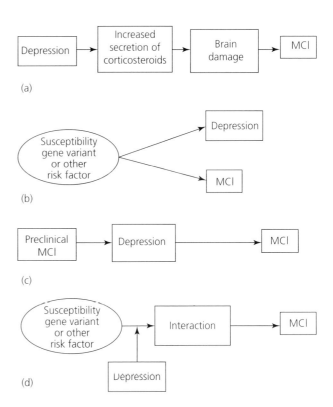

Figure 44.4 Four hypotheses of the possible mechanisms linking depression to MCI. Reproduced with permission of *Archives of Neurology* 2006; **63**: 435–40, © 2006 American Medical Association. All rights reserved.

this scenario, a person who is experiencing some degree of cognitive decline may first develop depression as a primary reaction to the symptoms. The depressive symptoms may then become an early non-cognitive manifestation of dementia, which may 'unmask' clinical MCI in individuals with limited cognitive reserve. As such, depression is an early manifestation of preclinical MCI or is a reaction to the initial symptoms of MCI. The last hypothesis suggests an interaction, where a synergistic interaction between depression and a biological variable such as a susceptibility gene variant or another non-genetic risk factor. Indeed Mayo Clinic researchers have demonstrated a synergistic interaction between depression and ApoE ε4. These four mechanisms (and other possible mechanisms; Geda *et al.*, 2006b; Butters *et al.*, 2008) are not mutually exclusive and may indeed work in tandem.

Recently an entity known as mild behavioural impairment (MBI) was reported by investigators from Argentina. They defined MBI as a late-life syndrome with prominent psychiatric and related behavioural symptoms in the absence of prominent cognitive symptoms that may also be a dementia prodrome. The investigators followed 358 elderly persons (239 with MCI and 119 with MBI) for up to five years, to the outcome of dementia. They concluded that MBI is a transitional state between normal ageing and dementia (Taragano *et al.*, 2009). However, this construct may be a new term for an old concept as the field of old age psychiatry has been investigating late life behavioural and psychological problems for several years.

Kokmen E, Naessens J, Offord K. (1987) A short test of mental status: Descripton and preliminary results. *Mayo Clinic Proceedings* 62: 281–8.

Kumar R, Dear KB, Christensen H *et al.* (2005) Prevalence of mild cognitive impairment in 60- to 64-year-old community-dwelling individuals: The Personality and Total Health through Life 60+ Study. *Dementia and Geriatric Cognitive Disorders* 19: 67–74.

Larrieu S, Letenneur L, Orgogozo JM *et al.* (2002) Incidence and outcome of mild cognitive impairment in a population-based prospective cohort. *Neurology* 59: 1594–9.

Lautenschlager NT, Cox KL, Flicker L *et al.* (2008) Effect of physical activity on cognitive function in older adults at risk for Alzheimer disease: a randomized trial. *Journal of the American Medical Association* 300: 1027–37.

Levy R. (1994) Aging-associated cognitive decline. *International Psychogeriatrics* 6: 63–8.

Lopez OL, Jagust WJ, Dekosky ST *et al.* (2003) Prevalence and classification of mild cognitive impairment in the Cardiovascular Health Study Cognition Study: part 1. *Archives of Neurology* 60: 1385–9.

Lopresti BJ, Klunk WE, Mathis CA *et al.* (2005) Simplified quantification of Pittsburgh Compound B amyloid imaging PET studies: a comparative analysis. *Journal of Nuclear Medicine* 46: 1959–72.

Lu PH, Edland SD, Teng E *et al.* (2009) Donepezil delays progression to AD in MCI subjects with depressive symptoms. *Neurology* 72: 2115–21.

Lyketsos CG, Steinberg M, Tschantz J *et al.* (2000) Mental and neuropsychiatric symptoms in dementia: findings from the Cache County Study on Memory in Aging. *American Journal of Psychiatry* 157: 708–14.

Lyketsos CG, Lopez O, Jones B *et al.* (2002) Prevalence of neuropsychiatric symptoms in dementia and mild cognitive impairment: results from the cardiovascular health study. *Journal of the American Medical Association* 288: 1475–83.

Mesulam M-M. (1998) From sensation to cognition. *Brain* 121: 1013–52.

Mitchell AJ, Shiri-Feshki M. (2008) Temporal trends in the long term risk of progression of mild cognitive impairment: a pooled analysis. *Journal of Neurology, Neurosurgery and Psychiatry* 79: 1386–91.

Morris J. (1993) The Clinical Dementia Rating (CDR): current version and scoring rules. *Neurology* 43: 2412–4.

Petersen RC. (2007) Mild cognitive impairment: current research and clinical implications. *Seminars in Neurology* 27: 22–31.

Petersen RC, Smith GE, Waring SC *et al.* (1999) Mild cognitive impairment: clinical characterization and outcome [published erratum appears in *Archives of Neurology* 1999; 56: 760]. *Archives of Neurology* 56: 303–8.

Petersen RC, Stevens JC, Ganguli M *et al.* (2001) Practice parameter: early detection of dementia: mild cognitive impairment (an evidence-based review). Report of the Quality Standards Subcommittee of the American Academy of Neurology. *Neurology* 56: 1133–42.

Petersen RC, Doody R, Kurz A *et al.* (2001) Current concepts in mild cognitive impairment. *Archives of Neurology* 58: 1985–92.

Petersen RC, Roberts RO, Knopman DS *et al.* (2009) Mild cognitive impairment: ten years later. *Archives of Neurology* 66: 1447–55.

Petersen RC, Thomas RG, Grundman M *et al.* (2005) Vitamin E and donepezil for the treatment of mild cognitive impairment. *New England Journal of Medicine* 352: 2379–88.

Petrella JR, Prince SE, Krishnan S *et al.* (2009) Effects of donepezil on cortical activation in mild cognitive impairment: a pilot double-blind placebo-controlled trial using functional MR imaging. *American Journal of Neuroradiology* 30: 411–16.

Reisberg B, Ferris SH, de Leon MJ, Crook T. (1982) The Global Deterioration Scale for assessment of primary degenerative dementia. *American Journal of Psychiatry* 139: 1136–9.

Reisberg B, Ferris SH, Kluger A *et al.* (2008) Mild cognitive impairment (MCI): a historical perspective. *International Psychogeriatrics* 20: 18–31.

Ritchie K, Artero S, Touchon J. (2001) Classification criteria for mild cognitive impairment: a population-based validation study. *Neurology* 56: 37–42.

Roberts RO, Geda YE, Knopman DS *et al.* (2008) The Mayo Clinic Study of Aging: design and sampling, participation, baseline measures and sample characteristics. *Neuroepidemiology* 30: 58–69.

Sackett DL. (1979) Bias in analytic research. *Journal of Chronic Diseases* 32: 51–63.

Sasaki M, Kodama C, Hidaka S *et al.* (2009) Prevalence of four subtypes of mild cognitive impairment and APOE in a Japanese community. *International Journal of Geriatric Psychiatry* 24: 1119–26.

Shaw LM, Vanderstichele H, Knapik-Czajka M *et al.* (2009) Cerebrospinal fluid biomarker signature in Alzheimer's disease neuroimaging initiative subjects. *Annals of Neurology* 65: 403–13.

Smith G, Ivnik RJ, Petersen RC *et al.* (1991) Age-associated memory impairment diagnoses: Problems of reliability and concerns for terminology. *Psychology and Aging* 6: 551–8.

Szklo M, Nieto FJ. (2000) *Epidemiology: beyond the basics.* Gaithersburg, MD: Aspen Publishers.

Taragano FE, Allegri RF, Krupitzki H *et al.* (2009) Mild behavioral impairment and risk of dementia: a prospective cohort study of 358 patients. *Journal of Clinical Psychiatry* 70: 584–92.

Tierney MC, Szalai JP, Snow WG *et al.* (1996) Prediction of probable Alzheimer's disease in memory-impaired patients: A prospective longitudinal study. *Neurology* 46: 661–5.

Verghese J, Lipton RB, Katz MJ *et al.* (2003) Leisure activities and the risk of dementia in the elderly. *New England Journal of Medicine* 348: 2508–16.

Verghese J, LeValley A, Derby C *et al.* (2006) Leisure activities and the risk of amnestic mild cognitive impairment in the elderly. *Neurology* 66: 821–7.

Verghese J, Cuiling W, Katz MJ *et al.* (2009) Leisure activities and risk of vascular cognitive impairment in older adults. *Journal of Geriatric Psychiatry and Neurology* 22: 110–18.

Winblad B, Palmer K, Kivipelto M *et al.* (2004) Mild cognitive impairment – beyond controversies, towards a consensus: report of the International Working Group on Mild Cognitive Impairment. *Journal of Internal Medicine* 256: 240–6.

Yesavage JA. (1988) Geriatric Depression Scale. *Psychopharmacology Bulletin* 24: 709–11.

45

Managing the patient with mild cognitive impairment

NICOLA T LAUTENSCHLAGER AND ALEXANDER F KURZ

45.1 INTRODUCTION

There has been a steadily increasing number of publications concerning mild cognitive impairment (MCI) in recent years. The majority of these papers focus on diagnostic issues and prediction of risk for future cognitive decline. More recently, the topic of prevention of dementia has taken centre stage in the MCI literature. In addition to pharmacological trials, non-pharmacological approaches investigating the role of environmental factors are being trialled in MCI. However, publications discussing how to best manage the patient with MCI outside research studies are rather sparse. With increasing awareness and knowledge in the population in relation to Alzheimer's disease (AD), specialists and memory clinics receive more and more referrals of younger patients, who, often still in the workforce, worry about their cognitive function. Managing adults with subjective memory complaints and MCI requires flexibility and spans patients from midlife to very old age. This chapter focuses on the current practical issues of managing the patient with MCI.

45.2 DISCLOSURE AND THE IMPACT OF DIAGNOSIS

The process from first raising concerns in a clinical setting regarding the cognitive performance of a person later diagnosed with MCI, to giving information on the diagnostic process and outcome, management options and regular follow-up appointments, is a journey which can last several years and often ultimately results in a dementia diagnosis. Usually the diagnostic 'label' of MCI is given by a specialist such as a neurologist, geriatrician or psychiatrist (e.g. in a memory clinic setting) to whom the family doctor had referred the patient. While initially the term MCI was very much restricted to research studies, it is now used more frequently in clinical settings (Petersen, 2007). However, since internationally accepted diagnostic criteria for MCI are not available, the criteria used for diagnosing MCI can vary widely. However, the consensus criteria of the International Working Group on MCI in 2004 represented a promising step in the right direction (Winblad et al., 2004). Various subtypes of MCI have been described, including or excluding an amnestic syndrome, which highlights the clinical heterogeneity of this diagnostic group (Petersen, 2007). There are ongoing discussions about whether MCI should be included in international classification systems (e.g. whether the amnestic subtype should be listed in DSM-V as a precursor for AD; Petersen and O'Brien, 2006). A diagnosis of MCI is a statistical risk factor for developing a dementia syndrome later on; however, due to the aetiological heterogeneity of the condition, the clinical outcomes over time vary considerably from recovering to a normal cognitive state, to maintaining a stable presentation, to progression to a dementia syndrome (Gauthier et al., 2006). In cases where MCI progressed to dementia, various pathologies have been reported in autopsy studies (Bennett et al., 2005).

Obviously, the individual clinical presentation, medical history and available evidence on the underlying cause will determine how the diagnosis should be disclosed to the patient and family and what prognostic advice is given. MCI as a diagnosis will have a different meaning for a patient from a family with familial AD as compared to someone who has no family history of cognitive impairment. Many specialists inform the patient and next of kin about the many unknowns surrounding the MCI 'label' and the fact that research in this area is a work in progress (Petersen, 2007) and this openness is usually appreciated. Where available and appropriate, the question of prognosis might make it relevant to educate patients and family members about biological markers which can help with estimating the risk of conversion to dementia. Structural changes on magnetic resonance imaging (MRI) show less predictive value (DeCarli *et al.*, 2007) than functional imaging with 2-[F]fluoro-2-deoxy-D-glucose positron emission tomography (FDG-PET; Mosconi, 2005). PIB-PET has promising potential (Okello *et al.*, 2009; see Chapter 13, Molecular brain imaging in dementia) as does elevation of tau cerebrospinal fluid (CSF; Hansson *et al.*, 2006; Mitchell, 2009; and see Chapter 53, Blood and cerebrospinal fluid biological markers for Alzheimer's disease).

Educating the patient and family in detail about the relevance of clinical symptoms, assessment process and results of tests, for example showing and explaining the relevant imaging scans, is usually helpful since it validates the concerns of the patient and family and puts the symptoms of MCI in a medical context. This should include the explanation that a thorough search for 'reversible' causes of the symptoms was part of the investigations and did not reveal any relevant potential causes. All this should help family members to accept the medical diagnosis and therefore alleviate anger, denial and guilt (Austrom and Lu, 2009). This is especially crucial in patients where the observed impairment fluctuates and the next of kin wonders whether the patient is 'putting the symptoms on'. In patients where the clinical findings strongly suggest a predementia syndrome, the possible emergence of psychological stress and depression should not only be raised with the patient, but also with the next of kin who might have already gradually moved into a carer role without necessarily having processed this consciously. It has been shown that family members of patients with MCI already experience feelings of loss and carer burden typically observed in carers of people with AD (Artero *et al.*, 2001; Garand *et al.*, 2005; Lu and Haase, 2009) and twice the general population risk for depression (Guerriero *et al.*, 2004). However, it is important to point out that the term 'carer' should be avoided when communicating with MCI patients and their families. Since the essence of the diagnostic category of MCI is that the level of independence of the patient does not justify a diagnosis of dementia the term 'carer' would contradict the diagnosis. A more neutral term like 'family member' or 'friend' is preferable (Austrom and Lu, 2009). This does not contradict recent findings showing that patients with MCI do experience some impairment in very complex activities of daily living (ADLs; Perneczky *et al.*, 2006) with family members needing to provide 'caregiving' for more complex ADLs (McIlvane *et al.*, 2008).

Ethical concerns have been raised about disclosing the 'label' MCI to patients and family members. These concerns include opening the door to distress, helplessness and hopelessness, with potential catastrophic outcomes such as suicide (Werner and Korczyn, 2008), in light of the

unavailability of effective treatment and looming AD. There is controversy about whether patients with MCI already experience limited awareness of their symptoms, but overall lack of insight is considered less common than in AD (Vogel *et al.*, 2004; Kalbe *et al.*, 2005). However, in the majority of cases the patient and family member already know that something is wrong and therefore the diagnosis does not surprise them with 'bad news' but confirms symptoms observed, often for many months. In this context, the term 'mild' in MCI might be seen as trivializing symptoms which cause great concern. It is helpful to prevent this sentiment by explaining that 'mild' is used in comparison to more severe cognitive impairment such as dementia, but not in relation to the individual, often upsetting, experience. Some clinicians therefore prefer to describe the specific clinical findings without using the tem MCI. On the other hand, similar to the disclosure process of a dementia diagnosis, it should not be overlooked that patients also have the right 'not to know' and therefore it is important to adjust the level of detail of information given accordingly.

45.3 PHARMACOLOGICAL APPROACHES

No pharmacological approaches have yet shown significant improvement of symptoms or delay of progression in MCI. Randomized controlled trials (RCTs) with negative results for the primary outcome have been conducted with cholinesterase inhibitors, vitamin E, piracetam, rofecoxib and ginkgo biloba (Salloway *et al.*, 2004; Petersen *et al.*, 2005; Thal *et al.*, 2005; Jelic *et al.*, 2006; Feldman *et al.*, 2007; DeKosky *et al.*, 2008; Winblad *et al.*, 2008). However, there is some debate about whether the RCT with donepezil and vitamin E showed some promising results by demonstrating a reduced risk for the first 12 months in the donepezil group which grew even to 24 months for apolipoprotein E (ApoE) ε4 positive patients (Petersen *et al.*, 2005). The authors of this trial reported that because of these findings donepezil could not be recommended for the treatment of MCI per se, but discussions on a one-to-one basis whether it might be appropriate in patients who seem to suffer from predementia AD would be appropriate. This off-label use of cholinesterase inhibitors continues to be discussed in the literature (Diniz *et al.*, 2009) and often in combination with memantine seems to be used by many clinicians. A recent survey in the United States showed that one quarter of patients with MCI received anti-AD medications (Weinstein *et al.*, 2009). A more recent 48-week RCT with donepezil in MCI showed small but significant changes on the Alzheimer's Disease Assessment Scale (ADAS-cog), but no significant changes on the primary outcome measure of global function (Doody *et al.*, 2009). RCTs with galantamine were overall negative, but again showed interesting results, with a non-significant reduction of progression rates and a reduced rate of progression of brain atrophy in the galantamine group. However, the same trial also showed an increased mortality in galantamine treated participants (Gold *et al.*, 2004). An RCT with rivastigmine, which showed an unexpected slow progression rate overall, was equally negative (Feldman *et al.*, 2007). A small trial with memantine in patients with age-associated memory impairment was negative in relation to measures of memory performance (Ferris et al., 2007). Trial experience to date highlights challenges in choosing the most appropriate methodology and diagnostic criteria for MCI and will be of relevance when planning future RCTs with potentially disease-modifying compounds (Knopman, 2009).

Other biological strategies to reduce cognitive decline in older adults at risk for dementia include trials with statins, B vitamins and antihypertensive therapy. Published results have been mixed (Forette et al., 2002; Heart Protection Study Collaborative Group, 2002; Lithell et al., 2003; Muldoon et al., 2004; McMahon et al., 2006; Durga et al., 2007; Fillit et al., 2008; see Chapter 58, Prevention of Alzheimer's disease).

Vascular risk factors have been clearly identified as contributing risk factors to cognitive decline, including patients with MCI. They include diabetes, hypertension, high serum levels of cholesterol and low-density lipoproteins, high levels of inflammation, obesity and smoking (Middleton and Yaffe, 2009; see Chapter 60, Vascular factors and Alzheimer's disease).

45.4   NON-PHARMACOLOGICAL APPROACHES

In the context of the prevention of dementia, potentially modifiable environmental factors such as cognitive, physical and social activities (Fratiglioni et al., 2004; Fratiglioni and Wang, 2007) have received increasing interest as part of an effective management approach for MCI (Ellison, 2008).

Several theories have been put forward to explain how cognitive activity could benefit cognition in old age and therefore potentially help patients with MCI to improve cognition or delay progression to dementia. These theories include 'use it or lose it', 'environmental enrichment', 'the cognitive reserve hypothesis' and the 'scaffolding theory of cognitive aging' approach (Fratiglioni et al., 2004; Salthouse, 2006; Stern, 2006; Park and Reuter-Lorenz, 2009). A number of trials have demonstrated that older adults without cognitive impairment can benefit from cognitive activity in that they improve their performance in the trained task (e.g. memory, problem solving, reasoning, information processing speed, attention, etc.) after completion of training (Angevaren et al., 2008; Valenzuela and Sachdev, 2009). A small number of RCTs of cognitive training in MCI have shown that improvement in areas such as memory, attention, mood and quality of life can be achieved (Belleville et al., 2006; Cipriani et al., 2006; Rozzini et al., 2006, Talassi et al., 2007). However, it is unclear how long these effects might last and whether they are meaningful in the everyday context or indeed help to delay the onset of dementia. Londos et al. (2008) were able to demonstrate in an open-label MCI study that an 8-week rehabilitation programme focusing on practical strategies to cope with memory problems improved self-rated daily function and quality of life. Another recent study exposed patients with MCI to a multi-component cognitive rehabilitation programme and compared their results to a waitlist

control group (Kurz et al., 2009). Eighteen patients with MCI participated in a 4-week cognitive rehabilitation programme in a day clinic setting. The intervention lasted for 22 hours per week and was offered in a group setting, focusing on activity planning, self-assertiveness training, relaxation techniques, stress management, use of external memory aids, memory training and motor exercise. After completion of the intervention, participants showed a significant improvement on verbal and non-verbal episodic memory, mood and activities of daily living. A waitlist control group experienced a significant practice effect on verbal episodic memory when retested, but did not show improvements for informant-rated ADLs and mood. The improvement in ADLs was independent of the reduction of depression scores on the Beck Depression Inventory. The same intervention was offered to ten patients with mild AD who failed to show any significant changes. These findings are promising, but need to be confirmed in larger RCTs. A major challenge will be to identify pragmatic and meaningful cognitive training strategies which translate into everyday life and are affordable. The exploration of whether technical support approaches might be relevant to MCI is only at the beginning (Bharucha et al., 2009).

As with cognitive activity, there are promising findings from exposing older adults to regularly physical activity. A recent meta-analysis reported a relative combined effect size of 0.32 (Colcombe and Kramer, 2003) when comparing between intervention and control groups with healthy older adults across publications. As with cognitive activity, RCTs in MCI are sparse, but a recent RCT with 170 subjective memory complainers and MCI patients aged 50 and older found significant differences between the intervention and control groups (Lautenschlager et al., 2008; Lautenschlager et al., 2009). The 24-week intervention was individually tailored and home-based, focusing on walking, but allowing combinations with other forms of physical activity depending on preference and medical history. Participants in the intervention group were asked to exercise for at least 150 minutes per week. To enhance adherence a modified behavioural intervention based on social cognitive theory (Cox et al., 2003) was implemented via a workshop, manual, newsletters and regular phone calls. Participants were re-assessed after 24 weeks, 12 and 18 months and the primary outcome measure, the ADAS-cog showed significant differences between the groups at all three time points. While this encouraging finding needs to be confirmed in larger RCTs, it demonstrates that patients with MCI can be motivated to participate in a physical activity programme and cognitively benefit from it. Currently several international groups are trying to combine potentially successful interventions in very large multi-centre trials with individuals at risk for dementia, aiming to maximize the protective effect.

Social activities are receiving increasing interest as another important environmental factor and often they are inherently part of cognitive and physical strategies (Karp et al., 2006).

A healthy, or more specifically a 'Mediterranean' diet has been suggested as another potential protective factor for healthy cognitive ageing (Bhat, 2009). This seems logical since a healthy diet positively affects the vascular risk factors mentioned above. Nutrients such as fruit, vegetables, fish, nuts, cereals and olive oil have been identified as potentially lowering the risk of dementia (Scarmeas *et al.*, 2006; Gillette-Guyonnet *et al.*, 2007). The effect of these nutrients is largely attributed to antioxidants and polyunsaturated fatty acids, however convincing evidence from RCTs is still lacking (Bhat, 2009; Fotuhi *et al.*, 2009).

A recent assessment of recently diagnosed MCI patients and their family members in the United States revealed that the majority were aware and supportive of health promotion approaches, such as mental and physical activity and diet, although the evidence is still limited (McIlvane *et al.*, 2008).

45.5 PRACTICAL CONSIDERATIONS AND CONCLUSIONS

The above findings and clinical experience suggest that after disclosure of the diagnosis of MCI to the patient and family, potential management strategies should be discussed. **Box 19.1** gives an overview of relevant topics which should be covered.

An increasing body of evidence emphasizes neuropsychiatric symptoms (Feldman *et al.*, 2004; Geda *et al.*, 2006; Simard *et al.*, 2009) as well as sleep disturbance in MCI (Beaulieu-Bonneau and Hudon, 2009). Between 35 and 75 per cent of patients with MCI experience neuropsychiatric symptoms with the most common being depression, apathy, anxiety and irritability. These patients have been reported to have a higher risk of progression to AD than those without these symptoms (Apostolova and Cummings, 2008; Edwards *et al.*, 2009). Patients with MCI report a range of emotional symptoms such as irritability, sadness and anxiety (Joosten-Weyn Banningh *et al.*, 2008). Probably the most prominent symptom in this context is depression. This is due to the ongoing discussion whether depression should be seen as a risk factor in its own right for future cognitive decline, especially if symptoms of depression have not been experienced prior to old age. Another practical question is whether MCI should be diagnosed in patients who do show symptoms of depression, or rather delayed until antidepressant treatment is successfully implemented. Usually, research studies with MCI exclude patients with clinically relevant symptoms of depression and there are findings which demonstrate that the profile of cognitive impairment differs in patients with amnestic MCI with or without additional symptoms of depression (Hudon *et al.*, 2008). However, depression can also arise as a reaction to experiencing cognitive impairment. It is safe to say that patients with MCI should be screened for symptoms of depression and treated if pharmacological treatment is indicated. Due to the cognitive impairment, the antidepressant should be chosen carefully, avoiding anticholinergic medication. An ongoing discussion is whether antidepressants could positively affect cognition directly (Doraiswamy *et al.*, 2003; Mowla *et al.*, 2007). Another common and often debilitating neuropsychiatric symptom in MCI is anxiety (Palmer *et al.*, 1997; Rozzini *et al.*, 2007); patients with MCI and anxiety experience more impairment in executive functions (Rozzini *et al.*, 2009). The clinician should screen for and treat neuropsychiatric symptoms in patients with MCI and using standard instruments, like the Neuropsychiatric Inventory, can be useful.

After considering pharmacological and non-pharmacological strategies, regular follow-up visits using standardized instruments is the best approach for identifying cognitive decline as early as possible. This approach can help to reassure patients and families member that while there is limited effective treatment for MCI, significant progression of symptoms will not be overlooked and therefore anti-dementia treatment can be started as soon as it has been proven to be helpful. Furthermore, management of potential impairment of complex ADLs should be discussed, covering important areas such as work, finances, caring for significant others, driving, etc. Recent findings demonstrate that patients with MCI perform worse on driving tests than cognitively healthy older adults (Frittelli *et al.*, 2009; Wadley *et al.*, 2009) and deteriorated in their financial skills when progressing to dementia (Triebel *et al.*, 2009). Also, medical decision-making capacity can deteriorate with progression of symptoms (Okonkwo *et al.*, 2008). Additional individual counselling for patient and family might be helpful (Ellison, 2008) if high levels of distress are detected.

In summary, the best possible management of patients with MCI is of increasing importance in light of the rising uptake of the diagnosis in clinical settings. The management approach needs to be individualized depending on the medical history, results of assessments and investigations and the personal situation of the patient and family. If available, a multidisciplinary team approach might be best to address the complex needs of the patient and family (Ellison, 2008). The approach should not be nihilistic. A proactive management plan with regular follow-up visits is crucial to help patients and family members cope in a difficult period of uncertainty.

Box 45.1 Important topics to consider in the management of MCI

Disclosure of diagnosis
Information on assessment results
Individualized information on prognosis
Pharmacological management options
Non-phamarmacological approaches
Information on research trials in the area
Monitoring health and vascular risk factors
Neuropsychiatric symptoms
Discuss ADLs (including driving)
Planning the future (e.g. finances, travelling, etc.)
Information on AD treatment in case of progression
'Carer' burden
Information on useful contacts (e.g. Alzheimer Association)
Regular follow-up appointments

REFERENCES

Angevaren M, Aufdemkampe G, Ver Haar HJ *et al.* (2008) Physical activity and enhanced fitness to improve cognitive function in older people without known cognitive impairment (update of: *Cochrane Database of Systematic Reviews*. (2: CF005381). *Cochrane Database of Systematic Reviews* 3: CD005381.

Apostolova LG, Cummings JL. (2008) Neuropsychiatric manifestations in mild cognitive impairment: a systematic review of the literature. *Dementia and Geriatric Cognitive Disorders* 25: 115–26.

Artero S, Touchon J, Ritchie K. (2001) Disability and mild cognitive impairment: a longitudinal population-based study. *International Journal of Geriatric Psychiatry* 16: 1092–7.

Austrom MG, Lu Y. (2009) Long term caregiving: helping families of persons with mild cognitive impairment cope. *Current Alzheimer Research* 6: 392–8.

Beaulieu-Bonneau S, Hudon C. (2009) Sleep disturbances in older adults with mild cognitive impairment. *International Psychogeriatrics* 21: 654–66.

Belleville S, Gilbert B, Fontaine F et al. (2006) Improvement of episodic memory in persons with mild cognitive impairment and healthy older adults: evidence from a cognitive intervention program. *Dementia and Geriatric Cognitive Disorders* 22: 486–99.

Bharucha AJ, Anand V, Forlizzi J et al. (2009) Intelligent assistive technology to dementia care: current capabilities, limitations, and future challenges. *American Journal of Geriatric Psychiatry* 17: 88–104.

Bennett DA, Schneider JA, Bienias JL et al. (2005) Mild cognitive impairment is related to Alzheimer disease pathology and cerebral infractions. *Neurology* 64: 834–41.

Bhat RS. (2009) You are what you eat: of fish, fat and folate in late-life psychiatric disorders. *Current Opinion in Psychiatry* 22: 541–5.

Cipriani G, Bianchetti A, Trabucchi M. (2006) Outcomes of a computer-based cognitive rehabilitation program on Alzheimer's disease patients compared with those on patients affected by mild cognitive impairment. *Archives of Gerontology and Geriatrics* 43: 327–35.

Colcombe S, Kramer S. (2003) Fitness effects on the cognitive function of older adults: a meta-analytic study. *Psychological Science* 14: 125–30.

Cox KL, Burke V, Gorely TJ et al. (2003) Controlled comparison of retention and adherence in home versus center-initiated exercise interventions in women age 40-65 years: the S.W.E.A.T. Study. *Preventive Medicine* 36: 17–29.

DeCarli C, Frisoni GB, Clark CM et al. (2007) Qualitative estimates of medical temporal atrophy as a predictor of progression from Mild Cognitive Impairment to dementia. *Archives of Neurology* 64: 108–15.

DeKosky ST, Williamson JD, Fitzpatrick AL et al. (2008) Ginkgo biloba for prevention of dementia: a randomized controlled trial. *Journal of the American Medical Association* 300: 2253–62.

Diniz BS, Pinto Jr JA, Gongaza MLC et al. (2009) To treat or not to treat? a meta-analysis of the use of cholinesterase inhibitors in mild cognitive impairment for delaying progression to Alzheimer's disease. *European Achives of Psychiatry and Clinical Neuroscience* 259: 248–56.

Doody RS, Ferris SH, Salloway S et al. (2009) Donepezil treatment of patients with MCI: a 48-week randomized, placebo-controlled trial. *Neurology* 72: 1555–61.

Doraiswamy PLM, Krishnan KR, Oxman T et al. (2003) Does antidepressant therapy improve cognition in elderly depressed patients? *The Journals of gerontology. Series A, Biological Sciences and Medical Sciences* 58: M1137–44.

Durga J, Van Boxtel MPJ, Schouten EG et al. (2007) Effect of 3-year folic acid supplementation on cognitive function in older adults in the FACIT trial: a randomised, double-blind controlled trial. *Lancet* 369: 208–16.

Edwards ER, Spira AP, Barnes DE, Yaffe E. (2009) Neuropsychiatric symptoms in mild cognitive impairment: differences by subtype and progression to dementia. *International Journal of Geriatric Psychiatry* 24: 716–22.

Ellison JM. (2008) A 60-year-old woman with mild memory impairment: review of mild cognitive impairment. *Journal of the American Medical Association* 300: 1566–74.

Feldman H, Scheltens P, Scarpini E et al. (2004) Behavioral symptoms in mild cognitive impairment. *Neurology* 62: 1199–201.

Feldman HH, Ferris S, Winblad B et al. (2007) Effect of rivastigmine on delay to diagnosis of Alzheimer's disease from mild cognitive impairment: the InDDEx study. *Lancet Neurology* 6: 501–12.

Ferris S, Schneider L, Farmer M et al. (2007) A double-blind, placebo-controlled trial of memantine in age-associated memory impairment (memantine in AAMI). *International Journal of Geriatric Psychiatry* 22: 448–55.

Fillit H, Nash DT, Rundek T, Zuckerman A. (2008) Cardiovascular risk factors and dementia. *American Journal of Geriatric Pharmacotherapy* 6: 100–18.

Forette F, Seux M, Staessen JA et al. (2002) The prevention of dementia with antihypertensive treatment: new evidence from the Systolic Hypertension in Europe (Syst-Eur) Study. *Archives of Internal Medicine* 162: 2046–52.

Fotuhi M, Mohassel P, Yaffe K. (2009) Fish consumption, long-chain omega-3 fatty acids and risk of cognitive decline or Alzheimer disease: a complex association. *Nature Clinic Practice. Neurology* 5: 140–52.

Fratiglioni L, Wang HX. (2007) Brain reserve hypothesis in dementia. *Journal of Alzheimers Disease* 12: 11–22.

Fratiglioni L, Paillard-Borg S, Winblad B. (2004) An active and socially integrated lifestyle in late life might protect against dementia. *Lancet Neurology* 3: 343–53.

Frittelli C, Borghetti D, Iudice G et al. (2009) Effects of Alzheimer's disease and mild cognitive impairment on driving ability: a controlled clinical study by simulated driving test. *International Journal of Geriatric Psychiatry* 24: 232–8.

Garand L, Dew MA, Eazo LR et al. (2005) Caregiving burden and psychiatric morbidity in spouses of persons with mild cognitive impairment. *International Journal of Geriatric Psychiatry* 20: 512–22.

Gauthier S, Reisberg B, Zaudig M et al. (2006) Mild cognitive impairment. *Lancet* 367: 1262–70.

Geda YE, Knopman DS, Mrazek DA et al. (2006) Depression, apolipoprotein E genotype, and the incidence of mild cognitive impairment: a prospective cohort study. *Archives of Neurology* 63: 435–40.

Gillette-Guyonnet S, Andrieu S, Dantoine T et al. (2009) Commentary on 'A roadmap for the prevention of dementia II.

Leon Thal Symposium 2008'. The Multidomain Alzheimer Preventive Trial (MAPT): a new approach to the prevention of Alzheimer's disease. MAPT Study Group. *Alzheimer's and Dementia* 5: 114–21.

Gold M, Francke S, Nye JS *et al.* (2004) Impact of APOE genotype on the efficacy of galantamine for the treatment of mild cognitive impairment. *Neurobiology of Ageing* 25: S521.

Guerriero AM, Damush TM, Hartwell CW *et al.* (2004) The development and implementation of non-pharmacological protocols for the management of patients with Alzheimer disease and their families in a multi-racial primary care setting. *Gerontologist* 44: 548–53.

Hansson O, Zetterberg H, Buchhave P *et al.* (2006) Association between CSF biomarkers and incipient Alzheimer's disease in patients with mild cognitive impairment: a follow-up study. *Lancet Neurology* 5: 228–34.

Heart Protection Study Collaborative Group. (2002) MRC/BRF heart protection study of cholesterol lowering with simvastatin in 20536 high-risk individuals: a randomised placebo-controlled trial. *Lancet* 360: 7–22.

Hudon C, Belleville S, Gauthier S. (2008) The association between depressive and cognitive symptoms in amnestic mild cognitive impairment. *International Psychogeriatrics* 20: 710–23.

Jelic V, Kivipelto M, Wilblad B. (2006) Clinical trials in mild cognitive impairment: lessons for the future. *Journal of Neurology, Neurosurgery and Psychiatry* 77: 429–38.

Joosten-Weyn Banningh L, Vernooij-Dassen M, Rikkert MO, Teunisse JP. (2008) Mild cognitive impairment: coping with an uncertain label. *International Journal of Geriatric Psychiatry* 23: 148–54.

Kalbe E, Salmon E, Perani D *et al.* (2005) Anosognosia in very mild Alzheimer's disease but not in mild cognitive impairment. *Dementia and Geriatric Cognitive Disorders* 19: 349–56.

Karp A, Paillard-Borg S, Wang HX *et al.* (2006) Mental, physical and social components in leisure activities equally contribute to decrease dementia risk. *Dementia and Geriatric Cognitive Disorders* 21: 65–73.

Knopman DS. (2009) Cracking the therapeutic nut in mild cognitive impairment: better nuts and better nutcrackers. *Neurology* 72: 1542–3.

Kurz A, Pohl C, Ramsenthaler M, Sorg C. (2009) Cognitive rehabilitation in patients with mild cognitive impairment. *International Journal of Geriatric Psychiatry* 24: 163–8.

Lautenschlager NT, Cox KL, Flicker L *et al.* (2008) Effect of physical activity on cognitive function in older adults at risk for Alzheimer disease: a randomized trial. *Journal of the American Medical Association* 300: 1027–37.

Lautenschlager NT, Xiao J, Almedia OP. (2009) Physical activity and cognitive function in Alzheimer disease (reply). *Journal of the American Medical Association* 301: 273–4.

Lithell H, Hansson L, Skoog I *et al.* (2003) The study of cognition and prognosis in the elderly (SCLOPE): principle results of a randomized double-blind intervention trial. *Hypertension* 21: 875–86.

Londos E, Boschian K, Linden A *et al.* (2008) Effects of a goal-oriented rehabilitation program in mild cognitive impairment: a pilot study. *Journal of Alzheimers Disease and Other Dementias* 23: 177–83.

Lu Y-FY, Haase JE. (2009) Experience and perspectives of caregivers of spouse with mild cognitive impairment. *Current Alzheimer Research* 6: 384–91.

McIlvane JM, Popa MA, Robinson B *et al.* (2008) Perceptions of illness, coping, and well-being in persons with mild cognitive impairment and their care partners. *Alzheimer Disease and Associated Disorders* 22: 284–92.

McMahon JA, Green TK, Skeaff CM *et al.* (2006) A controlled trial of homocysteine lowering and cognitive performance. *New England Journal of Medicine* 354: 2764–72.

Middleton LE, Yaffe K. (2009) Promising strategies for the prevention of dementia. *Archives of Neurology* 66: 1210–15.

Mitchell AJ. (2009) CSF phosphorylated tau in the diagnosis and prognosis of mild cognitive impairment and Alzheimer's disease: a meta-analysis of 51 studies. *Journal of Neurology, Neurosurgery and Psychiatry* 80: 966–75.

Mosconi L. (2005) Brain glucose metabolism in the early and specific diagnosis of Alzheimer's disease. *European Journal of Nuclear Medicine and Molecular Imaging* 32: 486–510.

Mowla A, Mosavinasab M, Pani A. (2007) Does fluoxetine have any effect on cognition of patients with mild cognitive impairment? A double-blind, placebo-controlled clinical trial. *Journal of Clinical Psychopharmacology* 27: 67–70.

Muldoon MF, Ryan CM, Sereika SM *et al.* (2004) Randomized trial of the effects of simvastatin on cognitive functioning in hypercholesterolemic adults. *American Journal of Medicine* 117: 823–9.

Okello A, Koivunen J, Edison P *et al.* (2009) Conversion of amyloid positive and negative MCI to AD over 3 years: An 11C-PIB PET study. *Neurology* 73: 754–60.

Okonkwo OC, Griffith HR, Copeland K *et al.* (2008) Medical decision-making capacity in mild cognitive impairment: a 3-year longitudinal study. *Neurology* 71: 1474–80.

Palmer BW, Jeste DV, Sheikh JI. (1997) Anxiety disorders in the elderly: DSM-IV and other barriers to diagnosis and treatment. *Journal of Affective Disorders* 46: 183–90.

Park DC, Reuter-Lorenz P. (2009) The adaptive brain: aging and neurocognitive scaffolding. *Annual Review of Psychology* 60: 173–96.

Perneczky R, Pohl C, Sorg C *et al.* (2006) Complex activities of daily living in MCI: conceptual and diagnostic issues. *Age and Ageing* 35: 240–5.

Petersen RC. (2007) Mild cognitive impairment: current research and clinical implications. *Seminars in Neurology* 27: 22–31.

Petersen RC, O'Brien J. (2006) Mild cognitive impairment should be considered for DSM-V. *Journal of Geriatric Psychiatry and Neurology* 19: 147–54.

Petersen RC, Thomas RG, Grundman M *et al.* (2005) Vitamin E and donepezil for the treatment of mild cognitive impairment. *New England Journal of Medicine* 352: 2379–88.

Rozzini L, Costardi D, Vicini-Chilovi B *et al.* (2006) Efficacy of cognitive rehabilitation in patients with mild cognitive impairment treated with cholinesterase inhibitors. *International Journal of Geriatric Psychiatry* 22: 356–60.

Rozzini L, Vicini CB, Conti M *et al.* (2007) Conversion of amnestic mild cognitive impairment to dementia of Alzheimer type is independent to memory deterioration. *International Journal of Geriatric Psychiatry* **22**: 1217–22.

Rozzini L, Chilovi BV, Peli M *et al.* (2009) Anxiety symptoms in mild cognitive impairment. *International Journal of Geriatric Psychiatry* **24**: 300–5.

Salloway S, Ferris S, Kluger A *et al.* (2004) Efficacy of donepezil in mild cognitive impairment: a randomized placebo-controlled trial. *Neurology* **63**: 651–7.

Salthouse TA. (2006) Mental exercise and mental aging: evaluating the validity of the "Use it or lose it" hypothesis. *Perspectives on Psychological Science* **1**: 68–87.

Scarmeas N, Stern Y, Tang M *et al.* (2006) Mediterranean diet and risk for Alzheimer disease. *Archives of Neurology* **63**: 1709–17.

Simard M, Hudon C, Van Reekum R. (2009) Psychological distress and risk for dementia. *Current Psychiatry Reports* **11**: 41–7.

Stern Y. (2006) Cognitive reserve and Alzheimer disease. *Alzheimer Disease and Associated Disorders* **20** (suppl 2): S69–74.

Talassi E, Guerreschi M, Feriani M *et al.* (2007) Effectiveness of a cognitive rehabilitation probram in mild dementia (MD) and mild cognitive impairment (MCI): a case control study. *Archives of Gerontology and Geriatrics* **44** (Suppl 1): 391–9.

Thal LJ, Ferris SH, Kirby L *et al.* (2005) A randomized, double-blind, study of Rofecoxib inpatients with mild cognitive impairment. *Neuropsychopharmacology* **30**: 1204–15.

Triebel KL, Martin R, Griffith HR *et al.* (2009) Declining financial capacity in mild cognitive impairment: a 1-year longitudinal study. *Neurology* **73**: 928–34.

Valenzuela M, Sachdev P. (2009) Can cognitive exercise prevent the onset of dementia? Systematic review of randomized clinical trials with longitudinal follow-up. *American Journal of Geriatric Psychiatry* **17**: 179–87.

Vogel A, Stockholm J, Gade A *et al.* (2004) Awareness of deficits in mild cognitive impairment in Alzheimer disease: do persons with MCI have impaired insight? *Dementia and Geriatric Cognitive Disorders* **17**: 181–7.

Wadley VG, Okonkwo O, Crowe M *et al.* (2009) Mild cognitive impairment and everyday function: an investigation of driving performance. *Journal of Geriatric Psychiatry and Neurology* **22**: 87–94.

Weinstein AM, Barton C, Ross L *et al.* (2009) Treatment practices of mild cognitive impairment in California Alzheimer's Disease Centers. *Journal of the American Geriatric Society* **57**: 686–90.

Werner P, Korczyn AD. (2008) Mild cognitive impairment: conceptual, assessment, ethical, and social issues. *Clinical Interventions in Aging* **3**: 413–20.

Winblad B, Palmer K, Kivipelto M *et al.* (2004) Mild cognitive impairment – beyond controversies, towards a consensus: report of the International Working Group on Mild Cognitive Impairment. *Journal of Internal Medicine* **256**: 240–6.

Winblad B, Gauthier S, Scinto L *et al.* (2008) Safety and efficacy of galantamine in subjects with mild cognitive impairment. *Neurology* **70**: 2024–35.

PART III

ALZHEIMER'S DISEASE

cognitive problems. There is an obvious, decisive and unresolved difficulty regarding the measurement of intellectual and behavioural disturbances, which usually develop over long periods and on the basis of rather variable levels of pre-morbid functioning. Erkinjuntti *et al.* (1997) demonstrated that different diagnostic criteria yield highly inconsistent results in the definition of the dementia syndrome in elderly individuals. These differences cannot be explained exclusively by different sensitivities of the examined criteria. This general difficulty is particularly pertinent in AD where the major defining criterion is the dementia syndrome. The criteria suggested by McKhann *et al.* (1984), the ICD-10 (World Health Organization, 1993) and the DSM-IV criteria (American Psychiatric Association, 1994) are given in **Boxes 46.1** and **46.2**. The daily use of such criteria and diagnostic categories misleads us to believe that they stand for natural facts, for nosological entities. However, the authors of these operational guidelines clearly stated that they are tentative and in need of further revisions. Their major drawback is a focus on the dementia syndrome instead of the underlying neurobiological disease process. Their advantage is that they state exactly what I have to describe in this chapter.

46.2.2   Clinical symptoms

Alzheimer's disease frequently follows a typical clinical course which reflects the underlying neuropathology. The length of the predementia phase cannot be reliably established with current clinical research tools. Theoretical considerations based on neuropathological and molecular biological findings suggest that this subclinical stage of illness extends over several decades. The clinical stages outlined in the present chapter overlap, and patients gradually progress from the mildest to the most severe manifestations of illness.

46.2.3   The predementia stages/mild cognitive impairment

Meticulous neuropsychological investigation may reveal mild cognitive impairment five years before the clinical diagnosis of a dementia syndrome can be established according to contemporary diagnostic standards. The pattern of the sub-diagnostic difficulties includes mild impairment in acquiring new information. Other demanding cognitive tasks, including the ability to plan or to access the semantic memory store, can also be compromised causing similar cognitive problems. The differentiation between incipient AD and a reversible condition (e.g. dementia syndrome of depression) or benign, non-progressive memory impairment is unreliable. At the predementia stage of AD, patients do not show a significant deterioration in ADL. At this stage, individuals may take advantage of memory aids and of other supportive strategies to overcome or compensate for their cognitive deficits. The performance of complex work tasks may be reduced. Patients tend to avoid difficult challenges and downplay or dissimulate their problems. In addition, non-cognitive alterations of behaviour, including social withdrawal and depressive dysphoria, may be present five years

---

Box 46.1 Diagnostic criteria for research (DCR-10) for dementia in Alzheimer's disease (ICD-10: WHO, 1993)

A. The general criteria (G1–G4) must be met.

B. There is no evidence from the history, physical examination or special investigations for any other possible cause of dementia (e.g. cerebrovascular disease, HIV disease, Parkinson's disease, Huntington's disease, normal pressure hydrocephalus), a systemic disorder (e.g. hypothyroidism, vitamin B_{12} or folic acid deficiency, hypercalcaemia), or alcohol or drug abuse.

F00.0 Dementia in Alzheimer's disease with early onset (G30.0)

1. The criteria for dementia in Alzheimer's disease (F00) must be met, and the age at onset must be below 65 years.

2. In addition, at least one of the following requirements must be met:

   (a) evidence of a relatively rapid onset and progression;

   (b) in addition to memory impairment, there must be aphasia (amnestic or sensory), agraphia, alexia, acalculia or apraxia (indicating the presence of temporal, parietal and/or frontal lobe involvement).

F00.1 Dementia in Alzheimer's disease with late onset (G30.1)

1. The criteria for dementia in Alzheimer's disease (F00) must be met and the age at onset must be 65 years or more.

2. In addition, at least one of the following requirements must be met:

   (a) evidence of a very slow, gradual onset and progression (the rate of the latter may be known only retrospectively after a course of three years or more);

   (b) predominance of memory impairment.

G1 (1) over intellectual impairment

G1 (2) (see general criteria for dementia)

F00.2 Dementia in Alzheimer's disease, atypical or mixed type (G30.8)[a]

F00.9 Dementia in Alzheimer's disease, unspecified (G30.9)

[a]Atypical dementia, Alzheimer's type. This term and code should be used for dementias that have important atypical features or that fulfil criteria for both early- and late-onset types of Alzheimer's disease. Mixed Alzheimer's and vascular dementia is also included here.

Box 46.2 DSM–IV criteria for dementia of the Alzheimer's type (American Psychiatric Association, 1994)

A. The development of multiple cognitive deficits manifested by both:
  (1) memory impairment (impaired ability to learn new information or to recall previously learned information);
  (2) one (or more) of the following cognitive disturbances:
    (a) aphasia (language disturbance);
    (b) apraxia (impaired ability to carry out motor activities despite intact motor function);
    (c) agnosia (failure to recognize or identify objects despite intact sensory function);
    (d) disturbance in executive functioning (i.e. planning, organizing, sequencing, abstracting).
B. The cognitive deficits in criteria A1 and A2 each cause significant impairment in social or occupational functioning and represent a significant decline from a previous level of functioning.
C. The course is characterized by gradual onset and continuing cognitive decline.
D. The cognitive deficits in criteria A1 and A2 are not due to any of the following:
  (1) other central nervous system conditions that cause progressive deficits in memory and cognition (e.g. cerebrovascular disease, Parkinson's disease, Huntington's disease, subdural haematoma, normal pressure hydrocephalus, brain tumour);
  (2) systemic conditions that are known to cause dementia (e.g. hypothyroidism, vitamin B_{12} or folic acid deficiency, niacin deficiency, hypercalcaemia, neurosyphilis, HIV infection);
  (3) substance-induced conditions.
E. The deficits do not occur exclusively during the course of a delirium.
F. The disturbance is not better accounted for by another Axis I disorder (e.g. major depressive disorder, schizophrenia).
With early onset: at age 65 or below
290.11 With delirium: if delirium is superimposed on the dementia.
290.12 With delusions: if delusions are the predominant feature.
290.13 With depressed mood: if depressed mood (including presentations that meet full symptom criteria for a major depressive episode) is the predominant feature. A separate diagnosis of mood disorder due to a general medical condition is not given.
290.10 Uncomplicated: if none of the above predominates in the current clinical presentation.
With late onset: after age of 65 years
290.3 With delirium: if delirium is superimposed on the dementia.
290.20 With delusions: if delusions are the predominant feature.
290.21 With depressed mood: if depressed mood (including presentations that meet full symptom criteria for a major depressive episode) is the predominant feature. A separate diagnosis of mood disorder due to a general medical condition is not given.
290.0 Uncomplicated: if none of the above predominates in the current clinical presentation.

---

before a clinical diagnosis is made. Patients with more severe alterations of cerebrospinal fluid tau- and βA_4-concentration and those developing more extensive functional brain changes will convert to dementia (Riemenschneider *et al.*, 2002; Drzezga *et al.*, 2003).

46.2.4 Mild dementia stage

In most patients, a significant impairment of learning and memory is the outstanding clinical feature. In some individuals, however, aphasic or visuoconstructional deficits may prevail. Working memory, old declarative memories from the patient's earlier years and implicit memory are affected to a much lesser degree than the declarative recent memory. Memory impairment usually interferes with various cognitive domains and usually plays a key role in the patient's difficulties with ADL. The patient's reduced ability to plan, judge and organize may not only show in complex tasks, but also in more difficult household chores (e.g. managing bank account, preparing meals). Communication may begin to suffer from shrinking vocabulary, decreasing word fluency

and less precise expressive language, even though a patient may still appear eloquent, 'fluent' and even verbose on casual inspection. An impairment of object naming and semantic difficulties with word generation can be demonstrated by means of neuropsychological tests. Constructional apraxia can be revealed on drawing tasks. Spatial disorientation frequently causes major problems in driving, as patients are less capable of estimating distances and speed. Because they have an increased risk of accidents, patients with a diagnosis of AD should be carefully assessed for driving ability, regulations for which vary between countries. At the mild stage of AD, patients may still be able to live independently for most of the time, but owing to the significant cognitive difficulties in several domains, they will need support with a variety of organizational matters. If a patient wishes to remain at home, arrangements for a support system should be made at this stage before a more intensive or permanent supervision is necessary.

Non-cognitive disturbances in AD are more frequent than previously thought. Symptoms of depression may prevail in the early stage of illness (Burns *et al.*, 1990). These emotional disturbances are typically mild and fluctuating, but also full-blown depressive episodes can occur. They may partly represent understandable emotional reactions to reduced cognitive and ADL skills or to reduced social contacts while the patient's insight is, at least, partly retained. Patients with severe depressive disturbances may show reduced cell counts in the locus caeruleus and other aminergic brainstem nuclei (Zubenko et al., 1989; Förstl et al., 1992). A reduced dorsofrontal blood flow has been demonstrated in patients with severe apathy. Subtle impairment of complex motor tasks may remain unnoticed on standard neurological examination.

46.2.5   Moderate dementia stage

Due to the severe impairment of recent memory, patients may appear to 'live in the past'. Logical reasoning, planning and organizing significantly deteriorate at this stage. Language difficulties become more obvious as word finding difficulties, paraphasia and circumstanciality increase. Reading skills deteriorate and the comprehension of texts can be incomplete. Writing becomes increasingly insecure with an increasing number of mistakes and omissions. Patients become distractible and gradually lose insight into their condition. Longer (ideomotor) sequences of action can no longer be organized, until finally the skills of using household appliances, dressing and eating are lost. The patient's spatial disorientation increases. Cortical visual agnosia is often present and can include the inability to recognize familiar faces (prosopagnosia). One-third of patients with AD at this stage develop illusionary misidentifications and other delusional symptoms, which are triggered by their cognitive deficits but also by the underlying disease process (Reisberg et al., 1996). Up to 20 per cent of the patients develop hallucinations, mostly of visual quality, which may be associated with a particularly severe cholinergic deficit (Lauter, 1968; Perry et al., 1990). At this stage, anosognosia prevails, but residues of insight may contribute to 'catastrophic reactions' following minor distress. Patients often lose emotional control and develop temper tantrums, which may be accompanied by physical or verbal aggression. Aimless and restless activities like wandering or hoarding are common (Devanand et al., 1997).

Patients in this moderate state of illness cannot survive in the community without close supervision. They are incapable of managing financial or legal matters. Household gas or electrical appliances are a constant source of danger to patients and also their carers. Hospital or nursing home admission may be delayed or even avoided, if a closely knit support system is in place. During this phase, there is a maximum strain on partners and other carers because of the patient's non-cognitive behavioural problems and somatic symptoms. Restlessness, aggression, disorientation and incontinence are the most frequent factors that precipitate the breakdown of family support. Sphincter control is insufficient and can be aggravated by 'pseudo-incontinence' as a consequence of spatial disorientation and clumsy handling of clothes. Many patients are at an increased risk of falls provoked by a hesitant, festinating gait and a stooped posture (Förstl et al., 1992).

46.2.6   Severe dementia stage

Specific modular cognitive deficits cannot be teased apart at that late stage of illness, when almost all cognitive functions are severely impaired. Even early biographical memories can be lost. Language is reduced to simple phrases or even single words. Patients are increasingly unable to articulate the simplest of needs. However, many patients can receive and return emotional signals long after the loss of language skills. This emotional receptiveness has to be remembered while the patient is completely dependent on comprehensive nursing care.

Patients often misunderstand and misinterpret nursing interventions, and this may lead to aggressive reactions. Subgroups of patients may develop stereotyped motor programmes as yelling or wandering. Restlessness and aggression may also be an expression of pain or the consequence of a profoundly disturbed circadian rhythm. A large proportion of patients show extreme apathy and exhaustion. Patients need support while eating, and even the most basic motor functions (chewing and swallowing) may be impaired as an expression of extreme apraxia. Double incontinence is frequent. Other motor disturbances (e.g. rigidity and primitive reflexes) may interfere with provision of nursing support. Extrapyramidal motor symptoms are usually due to a comorbidity with Parkinson's disease. Snouting and grasping reactions are the most frequent primitive reflexes and are associated with frontal lobe atrophy. Myoclonus and epileptic seizures can be observed in a smaller proportion of patients with severe AD, but are more frequent as compared with the general elderly population. Many bedridden patients develop decubitus ulcerations, contractions and infections. Pneumonia followed by myocardial infarction and septicaemia are the most frequent causes of death in AD.

46.3   BASIC DEFINITION OF AD

46.3.1   Neurophysiology and neuroimaging

Neither cranial computed tomography (CT) nor magnetic resonance tomography (MRT) or single photon emission computed tomography (SPECT), nor positron emission tomography (PET), not even electroencephalography (EEG) and quantitative electroencephalography analysis (qEEG) are appropriate tools for diagnosing AD. Each of these methods can, however, contribute to a clinical diagnosis:

- by excluding other specific causes of dementia that are incompatible with AD, and
- by documenting functional and morphological changes that are characteristic of AD.

46.3.1.1   EEG

Hans Berger's original observation of a slowed background activity in the EEG of demented patients was repeatedly confirmed with modern quantitative methods. This slowing exceeds the changes observed in elderly individuals without cognitive changes, but is significantly less severe than in patients with reversible confusional states or other types of brain changes underlying cognitive impairment. The decrease of α power and the increase of slow θ and δ activity are correlated with the severity of illness. The dimensional complexity and the synchronicity (coherence) of the EEG signals are significantly reduced in clinically manifest AD. A statistical discrimination of patients from elderly controls can be achieved in more than 80 per cent (Besthorn et al., 1997).

46.3.1.2   SPECT AND PET

Numerous SPECT studies have demonstrated a typical asymmetric temporoparietal hypoperfusion in a large proportion of patients with AD. A decrease of temporoparietal perfusion is an important sign of AD and this typical perfusion pattern represents a valuable aid for the differentiation of AD from forms of dementia with a strong vascular component and from frontal or frontotemporal brain degenerations. PET methods are possibly more sensitive for the early observation of characteristic functional changes. The correlations between reduced perfusion or reduced metabolism with cognitive deficits, stage or duration of illness are statistically significant (Bartenstein et al., 1997). Similar to qEEG, SPECT and PET allow a statistical discrimination of patients with AD from elderly controls in more than 80 per cent.

46.3.1.3   CT/MRT

The intracranial cerebrospinal fluid spaces show an age-related increase. A significant AD-associated atrophy is superimposed on this age-related effect. The corresponding decrease of brain volume is significantly correlated with the decrease of cognitive performance. As the hippocampus is an early target for neurofibrillary tangles, neuronal and gross volume loss, it should be visualized accurately at the first occasion for a thorough clinical and neuroradiological examination. The demonstration of an increasing volume loss in the mediotemporal cortex is of diagnostic importance. Similar to qEEG, SPECT and PET, planimetric and volumetric estimates of brain atrophy permit a statistical discrimination between patients with AD and elderly controls in more than 80 per cent – which is not necessarily of great clinical importance.

46.3.2   Neuropathology

Some authors have argued that plaques and neurofibrillary tangles could also be found in the brains of non-demented persons who appeared clinically intact until their death and that their pathophysiological significance was, therefore, doubtful (e.g. Rothschild, 1937). Blessed et al. (1968) established a statistical correlation between the severity of cortical plaque depositions and the ADL and also of cognitive performance. This approach reintroduced reason, or at

least common sense, into the scientific investigation of the mind–brain relationship of dementing patients. Brun and Gustafson (1976) pointed out the typical distribution of cerebral degeneration in AD, which is usually most pronounced in the mediotemporal limbic area, the posterior inferior temporal areas, adjoining parieto-occipital lobes and posterior cingulate gyrus. The frontal lobes are less severely involved. The primary sensory projection areas are frequently spared in typical AD. Braak and Braak (1991) elaborated a topographic distribution of neurofibrillary tangles, neuritic plaques and neuropil threads, including non-demented individuals in their studies. In stages I and II, the trans-entorhinal cortex is affected; the neurofibrillary tangles extend into the entorhinal cortex in stages III and IV; the hemispheral isocortex shows neurofibrillary and plaque depositions in stages V and VI, when patients usually develop clinical deficits. The clinical validity of Braak and Braak's staging has been confirmed in several studies (e.g. Delacourte et al., 1998a).

46.3.3   Diagnostic confirmation

According to the clinicopathological paradigm, a histopathological confirmation of clinically suspected AD is still considered the gold standard. The clinical diagnosis of AD can be confirmed by the neuropathological work up in 80 per cent of the cases or more, similar to qEEG, SPECT, PET, CT and MRI studies. This high percentage is often mistaken as a proof of our clinical skills and may mislead to undue complacency. It must not be forgotten that the *a priori* probability of choosing the right diagnosis is higher than 60 per cent, simply because of the high prevalence of AD. The probability that a patient who satisfies clinical diagnostic criteria for AD will also satisfy neuropathological criteria for AD is – according to Bayes' theory – directly proportional to the prevalence of AD (i.e. critical levels of plaques and neurofibrillary tangles according to standard neuropathological criteria) in the study population. In dealing with prevalent brain changes, highly sensitive – and highly unspecific – diagnostic criteria will inevitably lead to a frequent diagnostic confirmation. Numerous selection mechanisms lead to strongly biased patient samples in memory clinics and in scientific long-term studies that lead to these high, impressive validation rates. The patients have usually undergone repeated examinations, many reached a severe stage of illness before death, and cases difficult to examine and with evidence of mixed pathology had been eliminated from these studies at an earlier stage. Such samples have little to do with the normal clinical situation and the diagnostic difficulties at early and mild stages of illness when diagnostic certainty is much lower. Recent studies, using operational, clinical and neuropathological criteria, have shown that the presence of Alzheimer-type changes in the brains of demented patients can be predicted with a rather high reliability (owing to their prevalence), but that the admixture of other pathologies is not infrequent (Bowler et al., 1998; Holmes et al., 1998). Modern neuropathological criteria (Hyman and Trojanowski, 1997) do not offer a categorical 'yes-or-no' decision for the verification of

AD, but yield an estimate for the likelihood that the observed plaque – and tangle counts and their distribution – explain the clinical deficits (**Box 46.3**).

It remains questionable whether it is appropriate for clinicians to speculate about the exclusive presence of Alzheimer-type plaques and tangles in their patients' brains, or whether it would be more adequate to aim at identifying as many treatable pathogenic cofactors as possible.

46.4   THE FUNCTIONAL NEUROANATOMY OF AD

46.4.1   Corticocortical disconnection

Blessed *et al.* (1968) confirmed a relationship between the isocortical plaque density and the clinical deficits. This is illustrated by the severity and extension of primarily temporoparietal hypoperfusion and hypometabolism in SPECT and PET studies. Brun and Gustafson (1976) pronounced the plausible correlation between the pattern of neuropsychological deficits and the topographical pattern of the brain changes. Delacourte *et al.* (1998b) observed that cognitive deficits are inevitably associated with neurofibrillary changes in the polymodal isocortical association areas. Neurofibrillary and plaque depositions in the isocortical layers III and V are associated with a degeneration of glutamatergic pyramidal cells responsible for corticocortical and corticosubcortical projections (Pearson *et al.*, 1985; Arendt, 1999). Up to 50 per cent of the neocortical neurones can be lost (Gomez-Isla *et al.*, 1997). This leads to a functional impairment of feed-forward loops from the lower to the higher association areas, and of feedback systems from higher to lower association areas. Its cognitive consequence is an increased noise from disturbed amplification and filtering of information. A decreased EEG coherence can be considered as a neurophysiological result of this disconnection. A callosal atrophy is evidence for corticocortical axons. The cortical localization of the process can be associated with the clinical symptoms: a disruption of cortical pathways mediating visuospatial cognition is associated with constructional apraxia; damage of high order visual association areas with apperceptive agnosia.

46.4.2   Hippocampal de-afferentiation and de-efferentiation

Hyman *et al.* (1984) demonstrated an isolation of the hippocampal formation due to a cell-specific pathology in layers II and IV of entorhinal cortex and the subiculum, normally responsible for the connection with basal forebrain, thalamus, hypothalamus and association cortices. This leads to a perforant pathway destruction with consecutive glutamate depletion in the dentate gyrus (Hyman *et al.*, 1987). It is now well known that the transentorhinal followed by the entorhinal regions are early targets of neurofibrillary tangle formation and neuronal degeneration in AD (Braak and Braak, 1991; Delacourte *et al.*, 1998a). Intact hippocampal pyramidal cells ('index neurones') are part of extensive hippocampal-neocortical neuronal networks and represent essential prerequisites for the storage and retrieval of declarative memories in adult individuals. Deficits of recent episodic memory are frequent presenting symptoms in AD. According to Ribot's law, recent declarative memory functions are more severely impaired than older episodic and semantic memories, which are affected in the course of illness. The volume of the amygdala–hippocampus complex is positively correlated with the performance on memory tasks and inversely correlated with the severity of dementia (Fama *et al.*, 1997; Pantel *et al.*, 1997). There is a close association between the severity of mediotemporal lobe atrophy and hypoperfusion or hypometabolism of the temporoparietal neocortex (Lavenu *et al.*, 1997; Yamaguchi *et al.*, 1997). The severity of mediotemporal degeneration increases while the disease process extends over the isocortex. The individual contribution of the archicortical and isocortical changes to the clinical deficits are, therefore, difficult to disentangle. The situation is further complicated by severe alterations in the upper brainstem.

46.4.3   Cholinergic denervation

As explained in other chapters of this volume, the basal nucleus of Meynert and other cholinergic nuclei in the basal forebrain are the only sources of acetylcholine for the isocortex and the hippocampus. Acetylcholine in the neocortex reduces the potassium resting potential, thereby increasing neuronal excitability, and also stimulates the activity of GABAergic interneurones allowing a focused cortical excitation. In addition, acetylcholine reduces the activity of thalamic pacemaker neurones. This is how acetylcholine increases attention and allows the organized processing of information in the neocortex and limbic system (Arendt, 2002). In summary, acetylcholine reduces the resistance in hippocampo-neocortical oscillating circuits responsible for the formation and retrieval of memories. Acetylcholinesterase inhibitors temporarily reduce the resistance in these circuits.

46.4.4   Heterogeneity

There are presenile and senile, sporadic and familial forms of AD. The patients are examined at different stages of illness;

and the topographic patterns – reflected by the clinical symptoms – may show some heterogeneity and deviate from the standard course of illness described above. Most of these heterogeneous patterns are not sufficiently distinctive and stable over time to warrant the definition of meaningful subtypes of AD. Few patients have been described in whom an atypical pattern of deficit, related to plaque and tangle pathology, persisted over a longer period of time, e.g. in progressive biparietal atrophy. As mentioned above, Alzheimer pathology does not protect against other forms of neuropathological change. In old age, the admixture of other pathologies, e.g. of vascular changes, Lewy bodies, etc., is not infrequent. Some neuropathological changes would be extremely difficult to detect under the cover of plaques and tangles, e.g. brain degenerations with focal cortical onset, lacking distinctive histopathology.

46.5   DIFFERENTIAL DIAGNOSES

46.5.1   What is (probably) not AD

Alzheimer's disease should not be considered as a synonym for normal ageing. Also, AD is not a synonym for dementia; this is often forgotten, even in diagnostic guidelines. AD is not just the clinical Alzheimer dementia syndrome, but the underlying neurodegenerative process together with its typical clinical manifestation. AD is not (only) a presenile, but also a senile form of degenerative dementia. AD is more severe than age-associated memory impairment, benign senescent forgetfulness and the like. AD is more than an amnestic syndrome, even if deficits of episodic memory may frequently represent the core symptom of AD. AD is not a confusional state, but a confusional state may represent a first transient manifestation of a subclinical cholinergic deficit and the threshold for confusional states is reduced in patients who are cholinergically challenged due to Lewy body and/or plaque and tangle pathology in the basal forebrain nuclei.

Alzheimer's disease is different from other forms of dementia with specific features that satisfy standard clinical and neuropathological criteria, e.g. so-called vascular dementia, dementia with Lewy bodies, Pick-complex diseases and other brain degenerations with focal cortical onset and characteristic histopathological hallmarks, Creutzfeldt–Jakob disease, AIDS-related complex, Huntington's disease, alcohol-related cognitive impairment, cognitive impairment and schizophrenia, the dementia syndrome of depression or other uncommon forms of dementia.

46.5.2   What may be(come) AD

As mentioned earlier, patients satisfying clinical criteria for the diseases listed above may still have critical numbers of plaques and neurofibrillary tangles, and a cholinergic deficit, and may, therefore, benefit from cholinergic and other anti-dementia treatment with efficacy demonstrated for typical AD. To date, there is no method for ruling out significant numbers of plaques and neurofibrillary tangles in the

patients' brains with sufficient certainty during their lifetime, but there may be features that make the presence of significant Alzheimer pathology, or comorbidity, more likely, for example,

- a slow onset of cognitive impairment before a stroke;
- a continuous progression of dementia after treatment for normal pressure hydrocephalus;
- hippocampal atrophy;
- temporoparietal and more extensive hypoperfusion and hypometabolism (Drzezga *et al.*, 2003);
- a family history of AD;
- a molecular-genetic risk or diagnostic factor; or
- increased tau and decreased βA4 in the cerebrospinal fluid (Riemenschneider *et al.*, 2002).

Double pathology decreases the threshold for the manifestation of deficits. Less severe vascular changes would be required for the manifestation of dementia, if a moderate amount of plaques and neurofibrillary tangles is already present. This appears to be confirmed by observations from pivotal landmark studies (Snowdon *et al.*, 1997; MRC-CFAS 2001). Therefore a clinical deficit unexplained by the severity and extension of a single type of specific brain changes suggests the presence of cerebral multimorbidity.

Clinically, any mild cognitive impairment, amnestic syndrome, confusional state, depression, etc. may represent an early preclinical stage of AD. Pathophysiologically, a low α power, a discrete temporoparietal hypoperfusion or hypometabolism, early molecular cerebrospinal fluid alterations may herald incipient AD. Morphologically, anyone with mild brain atrophy, any person with subthreshold counts of plaques and neurofibrillary tangles would be a candidate for AD. Genetically, asymptomatic carriers of dominant mutations or risk factors are disposed to developing AD.

46.5.3   Alzheimer–Plus

There is nearly no senile dementia without relevant Alzheimer pathology (MRC-CFAS 2001). Cognition (C) should therefore be considered as the difference between initial intellectual capability (I) and the cumulative effects of the severity (S) and extension (e) of different types of brain changes, neurofibrillary tangles (NFT), plaques (PL), Lewy bodies (LB), frontotemporal (Pi), microangiopathic (MIC), macroangiopathic (MAC), etc.:

$$C = I - (S_{NFT} \times e_{NFT} + S_{PL} \times e_{PL}$$
$$+ S_{LB} \times e_{LB} + S_{Pi} \times e_{Pi}$$
$$+ S_{mic} \times e_{mic} + S_{MAC} \times e_{MAC}+)$$

The correlations between individual morphological features and specific symptoms are not as clear cut as in other neuropsychiatric syndromes observed in younger patients. The relationship between neuropathological changes and clinical deficits appears more fuzzy due to the variabilities of severity, extensions and admixtures (NFT – learning, declarative recent memory, hippocampal atrophy, increased tau concentrations; plaques – 'higher' neocortical neuropsychological

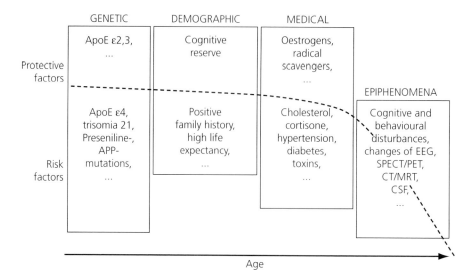

Figure 46.1 Risk model of cognitive deterioration.

deficits, neocortical atrophy, decreased βA_4-concentration; LB – motivational, affective and extrapyramidal motor symptoms, pigmented nuclei pathology; Pick-complex – behavioural and language deficits, frontotemporal atrophy, tau mutations; microangiopathy – slowing, gait apraxia, leukoaraiosis; macroangiopathy – see localization and extension of lesion).

46.5.4 Future diagnostic approaches

We are, presently, concentrating our diagnostic and therapeutic efforts on the epiphenomena of AD. It is now known that the disease process develops over many decades before it becomes clinically evident. It is hardly a rewarding exercise for patient and physician to establish the diagnosis of AD, once significant and irreversible brain changes have accrued. However, this will be the case as long as a diagnosis relies on the manifestation of a clinical dementia syndrome and does not aim at pathophysiological factors that could represent the targets of an early intervention. Cumulative incidence and morbidity suggest that everyone runs a remarkable risk of developing the symptoms of AD in old age. Therefore, risk or chance models should help to plan the timing and intensity of early interventions. Such models will include genetic, sociodemographic, somatic and environmental protective and risk factors together with the 'early' psychological and biological epiphenomena of illness (**Figure 46.1**). Most of these factors are discussed elsewhere in this volume. Genetic factors are currently frequently discussed. Several sociodemographic factors are of self-explanatory importance (age, life expectancy, cognitive reserve). The influence of somatic and environmental cofactors is usually disregarded because they are not considered part of the Alzheimer pathophysiology. Some of them are now receiving increasing attention (oestrogen, cholesterol, cortisone; non-steroidal anti-inflammatory agents, homocysteine, vascular comorbidity). Subclinical changes that can occur in the course of the biological disease process and be discovered with special laboratory methods before the patient develops clinical

symptoms can be considered as 'early epiphenomena'. These can be discrete cognitive, predominantly amnestic deficits, associated functional brain changes (Desgranges *et al.*, 1998), discrete morphological alterations in the mediotemporal lobe (Reiman *et al.*, 1998) and early alterations of cerebrospinal fluid. The gaps in **Figure 46.1** need to be filled in the years to come in order to develop individualized risk profiles for early interventions preceding the medical manifestation of epiphenomena.

REFERENCES

Albert E. (1963) Senile Demenz und Alzheimer – die gleiche Krankheit? *Zentralblatt für die Gesamte Neurologie und Psychiatrie* **172**: 164.

Alzheimer A. (1898) Neure Arbeiten über die Dementia senilis und die auf atherot matöser Gefässerkrankung basierenden Gehirnkrankheiten. *Monatsschrift für Psychiatrie und Neurologie* **3**: 101–15.

American Psychiatric Association. (1994) *Desk Reference to the Diagnostic Criteria from DSM-IV.* Washington DC: APA, 85.

Arendt T. (1999) Pathologische Anatomie der Alzheimer Krankheit. In: Förstl H, Bickel H, Kurz A (eds). *Alzheimer Demenz – Grundlagen, Klinik, Therapie.* Heidelberg: Springer, 87–108.

Arendt T. (2002) Neuronal pathology in Alzheimer's disease. In: Beyrenther K, Einhäupl K (eds). *Dementia.* Stuttgart: Thieme, 106–17.

Bartenstein P, Minoshima S, Hirsch C et al. (1997) Quantitative assessment of cerebral blood flow in patients with Alzheimer's disease by SPECT. *Journal of Nuclear Medicine* **38**: 1095–101.

Besthorn C, Zerfass R, Geiger-Kabisch C et al. (1997) Discrimination of Alzheimer's disease and normal aging by EEG data. *EEG and Clinical Neurophysiology* **103**: 241–8.

Blessed G, Tomlinson BE, Roth M. (1968) The association between quantitative measures of dementia and of senile change in the cerebral grey matter of elderly subjects. *British Journal of Psychiatry* **114**: 797–811.

Bowler JV, Munoz DG, Merskey H *et al.* (1998) Fallacies in the pathological confirmation of the diagnosis of Alzheimer's disease. *Journal of Neurology, Neurosurgery, and Psychiatry* **64**: 18–24.

Braak H, Braak E. (1991) Neuropathological staging of Alzheimer-related changes. *Acta Neuropathologica* **82**: 239–59.

Brun A, Gustafson L. (1976) Distribution of cerebral degeneration in Alzheimer's disease – a clinico-pathological study. *Archiv fur Psychiatrie und Nervenkrankheiten* **223**: 15–23.

Burns A, Jacoby R, Levy R. (1990) Psychiatric phenomena in Alzheimer's disease. III: Disorders of mood. *British Journal of Psychiatry* **157**: 81–6.

Corsellis JAN. (1969) The pathology of dementia. *British Journal of Hospital Medicine* **2**: 695–702.

Delacourte A, Buée L, David JP *et al.* (1998a) Lack of continuum between cerebral aging and Alzheimer's disease as revealed by PHF-tau and Aβ biochemistry. *Alzheimer's Reports* **1**: 101–10.

Delacourte A, Sergeant N, Wattez A *et al.* (1998b) Vulnerable neuronal subsets in Alzheimer's and Pick's disease are distinguished by their tau isoform distribution and phosphorylation. *Annals of Neurology* **43**: 193–204.

Desgranges B, Baron JC, de la Sayette V *et al.* (1998) The neural substrates of memory systems impairment in Alzheimer's disease. A PET study of resting brain glucose utilization. *Brain* **121**: 611–31.

Devanand DP, Jacobs DM, Tang MX *et al.* (1997) The course of psychopathology in mild to moderate Alzheimer's disease. *Archives of General Psychiatry* **54**: 257–63.

Drzezga A, Lautenschlager N, Siebner H *et al.* (2003) Cerebral metabolic changes accompanying conversion of mild cognitive impairment into Alzheimer's disease: a PET follow-up study. *European Journal of Nuclear Medicine and Molecular Imaging* **30**: 1104–13.

Erkinjuntti T, Ostbye T, Steenhuis R, Hachinski V. (1997) The effect of different diagnostic criteria on the prevalence of dementia. *New England Journal of Medicine* **337**: 1667–74.

Fama R, Sullivan ER, Shear PK *et al.* (1997) Selective cortical and hippocampal volume correlates of the Mattis Dementia Rating Scale in Alzheimer disease. *Archives of Neurology* **54**: 719–28.

Förstl H, Burns A, Levy R *et al.* (1992) Neurological signs in Alzheimer's disease. *Archives of Neurology* **49**: 1038–42.

Gomez-Isla T, Hollister R, West H *et al.* (1997) Neuronal loss correlates with but exceeds neurofibrillary tangles in Alzheimer's disease. *Annals of Neurology* **41**: 17–24.

Gowers WR. (1902) A lecture on abiotrophy. *Lancet* i: 1003–7.

Holmes C, Cairns N, Lantos P, Mann A. (1998) Validity of current clinical criteria for Alzheimer's disease, vascular dementia and dementia with Lewy bodies. *British Journal of Psychiatry* **174**: 45–50.

Hyman BT, Trojanowski JQ. (1997) Editorial on consensus recommendations for the postmortem diagnosis of Alzheimer disease from the National Institute on Aging and the Reagan Institute Working group on diagnostic criteria for the neuropathological assessment of Alzheimer disease. *Journal of Neuropathology and Experimental Neurology* **56**: 1095–7.

Hyman BT, Van Hoesen GW, Damasio AR, Barnes CL. (1984) Alzheimer's disease: Cell-specific pathology isolates the hippocampal formation. *Science* **225**: 1168–70.

Hyman BT, Van Hoesen GW, Damasio AR. (1987) Alzheimer's disease: Glutamate depletion in the hippocampal perforant pathway zone. *Annals of Neurology* **22**: 37–41.

Kraepelin E. (1910) *Psychiatrie. Ein Lehrbuch für Studierende und Ärzte*, 8th edn. Auflage, Bd. II, Teil 1. Leipzig: Barth, 624–32.

Lauter H. (1968) Zur Klinik und Psychopathologie der Alzheimerschen Krankheit. *Psychiatrica Clinica* **1**: 85–108.

Lauter H, Meyer JE. (1968) Clinical and nosological concepts of senile dementia. In: Müller CH, Ciompi L (eds). *Senile dementia*. Bern/Stuttgart: Hans Huber, 13–26.

Lavenu I, Pasquier F, Leber F *et al.* (1997) Association between medial temporal lobe atrophy on CT and parietotemporal uptake decrease on SPECT in Alzheimer disease. *Journal of Neurology, Neurosurgery, and Psychiatry* **63**: 441–5.

McKhann G, Drachman D, Folstein N *et al.* (1984) Clinical diagnosis of Alzheimer's disease. *Neurology* **34**: 939–44.

MRC-CFAS. (2001) Pathological correlates of late-onset dementia in a multicentre, community-based population in England and Wales. *Lancet* **357**: 169–75.

Pantel J, Schröder J, Schad LR *et al.* (1997) Quantitative magnetic resonance imaging and neurophysiological functions in dementia of the Alzheimer type. *Psychological Medicine* **27**: 221–9.

Pearson RCA, Esiri MM, Hiorns RW *et al.* (1985) Anatomical correlates of the distribution of the pathological changes in the neocortex in Alzheimer disease. *Proceedings of the National Academy of Science of the United States of America* **82**: 4531–4.

Perry EK, Kerwin J, Perry RH *et al.* (1990) Visual hallucinations and the cholinergic system in dementia. *Journal of Neurology, Neurosurgery, and Psychiatry* **53**: 88.

Reiman EM, Uecker A, Caselli RJ *et al.* (1998) Hippocampal volumes in cognitively normal persons at genetic risk for Alzheimer's disease. The nun study. *Journal of the American Medical Association* **44**: 288–91.

Reisberg B, Auer SR, Bonteiro I *et al.* (1996) Behavioral disturbances of dementia: an overview of phenomenology and methodologic concerns. *International Psychogeriatrics* **8**: 169–80.

Riemenschneider M, Lautenschlager N, Wagenpfeil S. (2002) Cerebrospinal fluid tau and beta-amyloid 42 proteins identify Alzheimer disease in subjects with mild cognitive impairment. *Archives of Neurology* **59**: 1729–34.

Rothschild D. (1937) Pathologic changes in senile psychosis and their psychobiologic significance. *American Journal of Psychiatry* **93**: 757–88.

Snowdon DA, Greiner LH, Mortimer JA *et al.* (1997) Brain infarction and the clinical expression of Alzheimer disease. The nun study. *Journal of the American Medical Association* **277**: 813–17.

World Health Organization. (1993) *The ICD-10 Classification of Mental and Behavioural Disorders: Diagnostic Criteria for Research*. Geneva: WHO.

Yamaguchi S, Meguro K, Itoh M. (1997) Decreased cortical glucose metabolism correlates with hippocampal atrophy in Alzheimer's disease as shown by MRI and PET. *Journal of Neurology, Neurosurgery, and Psychiatry* **62**: 596–600.

Zubenko GS, Moossy J, Martinez AJ *et al.* (1989) A brain regional analysis of morphologic and cholinergic abnormalities in Alzheimer's disease. *Archives of Neurology* **46**: 634–8.

Risk factors for Alzheimer's disease

PATRICIA A BOYLE AND ROBERT S WILSON

47.1 INTRODUCTION

By the time a clinical diagnosis of Alzheimer's disease (AD) can be made, widespread brain damage has already occurred and current therapies are not thought to alter disease progression. As a result, there is an urgent need for strategies to delay dementia onset. Identification of risk factors for the disease is a critical step towards that goal.

47.2 RISK FACTORS FOR AD

This chapter reviews the major factors associated with the risk of AD, with an emphasis on those supported by data from prospective studies of incident disease. Importantly, although much of the initial information regarding risk factors came from studies involving people who sought the attention of medical providers or population-based studies of people with prevalent disease, such studies are susceptible to bias because they involve only a limited, non-random fraction of people with AD. Further, because disease prevalence is highly related to survival, population-based studies of prevalent disease can lead to the identification of factors associated with survival with disease rather than actual risk of disease. Thus, population-based studies of incident disease, in which risk factors are identified prior to disease onset, are better positioned for identifying risk factors. Data from such studies have become available in recent years, and several factors, including genetic, experiential and medical risk factors for AD have been identified. Some of these are associated with an increased risk of AD, whereas others are associated with a decreased risk.

In addition to reviewing risk factors, the possible neurobiologic mechanisms by which various risk factors influence

the development of AD are discussed, with the caveat that not all risk factors have been well studied in this regard. Moreover, the relationships between risk factors, common age-related neuropathologies, such as the pathology of AD, and cognitive impairment are complex. There are three primary ways in which risk factors can be associated with AD: first, they can initiate pathological processes that lead to cognitive impairment and AD; second, they can modify or alter the relation of pathology to cognition; and third, they can be related to the clinical expression of AD but unrelated to its pathology. Although in many cases the neurobiologic basis of the association between a risk factor and AD remains unknown, we discuss neurobiologic mechanisms whenever possible because an understanding of how risk factors lead to AD may suggest novel strategies for delaying dementia onset. Thus, we present findings from clinicopathological studies and focus in particular on the role of AD pathologic hallmarks (i.e. amyloid plaques and neurofibrillary tangles) and cerebral infarction, the most common causes of cognitive impairment in old age.

47.3 GENETIC RISK FACTORS

47.3.1 Amyloid precursor protein, the presenilins and apolipoprotein E

Several studies have examined the role of genetic factors as determinants of AD, and mutations in three genes are known to cause AD (i.e. amyloid precursor protein (APP), presenilin 1 and presenilin 2). Notably, however, these mutations account for only about 1 per cent of AD cases, those that are early onset. In contrast to mutations, several polymorphisms have been reported to be associated with an increased risk of AD, but the apolipoprotein E (ApoE) gene is the only consistently replicated risk factor for the most common expression of AD, that which begins after 65 years of age. People with one or more copies of the ε4 allele have about a two- to three-fold greater risk of developing AD compared to those without the ε4 allele (Evans *et al.*, 1997a; Jellinger, 2006; Murrell *et al.*, 2006), and some data suggest that this association may be stronger among whites than African Americans. The mechanism underlying the association of the ε4 allele with AD risk has not yet been fully elucidated, but AD pathology appears to have an important role. The ε4 allele has been associated with the burden of AD pathology in clinicopathological studies, and findings suggest that the ε4 allele works through amyloid deposition and subsequent tangle formation to cause cognitive impairment (Bennett *et al.*, 2003; Bennett *et al.*, 2005a). Finally, the ε4 allele also increases the likelihood of cerebral infarcts, which also increase the likelihood of AD (Schneider *et al.*, 2005). Taken together, these findings suggest that the ε4 allele leads to the accumulation of AD pathology but also interacts with other risk factors to cause cognitive impairment and AD.

47.3.2   ApoE ε2 allele status

In contrast to the ε4 allele, which increases the risk of AD, the presence of the ε2 allele is associated with a reduced risk of AD (Wilson *et al.*, 2002c; Jellinger, 2006). Although the data are limited, because the ε2 allele is not very common, a meta-analysis reported that people with an ε2 allele have about a 40 per cent lower risk of AD compared to those without the allele (Farrer *et al.*, 1997). Although various mechanisms have been proposed, clinicopathological findings suggest that the ApoE genotype affects the risk of AD primarily by affecting the accumulation of AD pathology (Bennett *et al.*, 2003; Bennett *et al.*, 2005a).

47.4   EXPERIENTIAL FACTORS

47.4.1   Age

Old age is often touted as the strongest risk factor for AD. Indeed, the occurrence of AD is strongly related to age; AD is fairly rare among younger people, but the risk of AD increases dramatically after age 65, with one in ten individuals over 65 and nearly half of those over 85 affected. Importantly, however, although age is commonly viewed as a risk factor, it is unlikely that age actually causes AD. Age is more likely a proxy for other as yet unknown disease processes that are associated with the development of AD.

47.4.2   Female sex

Female sex is often considered a risk factor for AD, as the disease is more common among women than men, particularly over the age of 80. However, this sex difference appears to be due in large part to increased longevity among women.

Overall, studies of people under 85 years of age do not suggest strong sex differences in AD incidence. The situation after age 85 is uncertain because of the paucity of men in this age group. It has been hypothesized that women may be more vulnerable to AD due to hormonal changes that follow menopause, but we are not aware of data showing the mechanistic role of hormones. One clinicopathological study suggested that AD pathology was more likely to be expressed as a clinical dementia syndrome in women than in men (Barnes *et al.*, 2005), and some animal data suggest possible sex differences in APP processing (Maynard *et al.*, 2006). Overall, however, current data do not suggest strong sex differences in risk of AD.

47.4.3   Education

Many studies have shown reduced AD risk among people with higher levels of education (Evans *et al.*, 1997b; Karp *et al.*, 2004; Caamano-Isorna *et al.*, 2006). Notably, however, a recent review of published studies (Wilson *et al.*, 2009b) concluded that education is not related to the rate of cognitive decline, the primary clinical manifestation of AD. This suggests that the association of education with AD is largely due to its robust association with the level of cognitive function (which holds at all ages). Nevertheless, it has been hypothesized that education contributes to neural reserve by somehow reducing the adverse clinical impact of mild to moderate pathologic burden. Towards this end, clinicopathological studies have shown that education reduces the association of AD pathologic burden, particularly amyloid, with the level of cognition proximate to death (Bennett *et al.*, 2005b).

47.4.4   Race/ethnicity

There are relatively scant data on race/ethnicity, but some studies have reported that African Americans and Hispanics are more likely than non-Hispanic whites to develop AD (Tang *et al.*, 2001; Evans *et al.*, 2003). These findings are difficult to interpret, because race and ethnicity are entangled with socioeconomic and cultural variables that strongly influence cognitive test performance. Statistical adjustment for variables such as education and income does not account for all of the potentially confounding effects of race. Thus, data on the association of race/ethnicity and AD should be interpreted with great caution.

47.4.5   Depressive symptoms and loneliness

Data from several large prospective studies support an association between depressive symptoms and the risk of AD (Wilson *et al.*, 2002a; Wilson *et al.*, 2003b; Andersen *et al.*, 2005; see Chapter 74, Depression with cognitive impairment), with one prospective study reporting that the risk of developing AD increased by about 20 per cent for each depressive symptom endorsed (Wilson *et al.*, 2002a). In addition, a related psychological construct referred to as loneliness (i.e. the subjective sense of connectedness to

because motor dysfunction is an early clinical sign of a pathologic process rather than a true risk factor.

47.5.6   Olfactory dysfunction

Prospective studies have shown that olfactory impairment (e.g. difficulty identifying familiar odours) predicts cognitive decline and the development of AD and its precursor, mild cognitive impairment (Wilson *et al.*, 2007b; Wilson *et al.*, 2007e; Wilson *et al.*, 2009a). Clinicopathological studies show that impaired odour recognition is robustly related to level of AD pathologic changes in the brain, particularly density of neurofibrillary tangles in central olfactory regions (Wilson *et al.*, 2007b) and this association is seen even in older people without apparent cognitive dysfunction (Wilson *et al.*, 2009a).

47.5.7   Inflammatory markers

Increasing evidence suggests that inflammation may play an important role in the pathogenesis of AD, and findings from some prospective studies suggest that the level of systemic markers of inflammation, particularly C-reactive protein and interleukin-6, are associated with an increased risk of AD (Schmidt *et al.*, 2002; Ravaglia *et al.*, 2007). In particular, one large study reported a three-fold increase in the risk of AD among men with high levels of C-reactive protein. Several potential mechanisms underlie the association between inflammation and AD. Inflammation can occur as a consequence of neurodegeneration or, alternatively, it may be a causal part of a cascade of events that lead to the accumulation of AD pathology, particularly amyloid deposition. Inflammation is also associated with vascular disease and may be related to dementia via cerebrovascular disease. Additional research is needed to further clarify the role of inflammation in the development of AD and the basis of this association.

47.5.8   Medications

Several medications, including oestrogen, non-steroidal anti-inflammatory drugs (NSAIDs) and statins have been examined for their potential to protect against dementia (Honig *et al.*, 2003). Oestrogen has been associated with a reduced risk of AD in several observational studies, with some evidence of a dose–response relationship, whereby longer duration of oestrogen therapy was associated with greater protection. Similar findings have been reported for NSAIDs, with some studies reporting a reduced risk of dementia among users (particularly those using for more than two years), although findings are inconsistent. Finally, some cross-sectional or case-control studies have shown a protective effect for statins, but prospective cohort studies generally have not replicated those findings. Clinical trials examining the potential for oestrogen and NSAIDs to prevent or delay the onset of dementia have failed because hormone replacement and NSAIDs are associated with serious adverse health outcomes. Therefore, such trials have been discontinued, but trials of statins are ongoing (see Chapter 55, Drug treatments in development for Alzheimer's disease).

47.6   CONCLUSION

Using data from prospective studies of incident disease, several factors associated with the risk of AD have been identified, including genetic, experiential and medical factors. Whereas some of these are probably true risk factors and causative of AD, others probaby reflect the earliest manifestations of the pathology of AD or another ongoing disease process. Further, the relationships between risk factors, common age-related neuropathologies and AD are complex and in many cases unclear. Whereas some risk factors work directly via their influence on the accumulation of AD and other common age-related pathologies (e.g. infarcts), others appear to modify the association of cognition with pathology, such that they provide benefit in the face of accumulating neuropathology. Finally, many risk factors also likely interact with each other. Additional research from prospective studies of incident disease is needed to clarify the true risk factors for AD and to establish the neurobiologic basis of the link between various risk factors and AD, an understanding that is essential to the goal of preventing or delaying the onset of dementia in old age.

REFERENCES

Andersen K, Lolk A, Kragh-Sorensen P *et al.* (2005) Depression and the risk of Alzheimer disease. *Epidemiology* **16**: 233–8.

Arvanitakis Z, Schneider JA, Wilson RS *et al.* (2006) Diabetes is related to cerebral infarction but not to AD pathology in older persons. *Neurology* **67**: 1960–5.

Barnes LL, Mendes de Leon CF, Wilson RS *et al.* (2004) Social resources and cognitive decline in a population of older African Americans and whites. *Neurology* **63**: 2322–6.

Barnes LL, Wilson RS, Bienias JL *et al.* (2005) Sex differences in the clinical manifestations of Alzheimer disease pathology. *Archives of General Psychiatry* **62**: 685–91.

Bassuk SS, Glass TA, Berkman LF. (1999) Social disengagement and incident cognitive decline in community-dwelling elderly persons. *Annals of Internal Medicine* **131**: 165–73.

Bennett DA, Schneider JA, Wilson RS *et al.* (2005a) Amyloid mediates the association of apolipoprotein E e4 allele to cognitive function in older people. *Journal of Neurology, Neurosurgery, and Psychiatry* **76**: 1194–9.

Bennett DA, Schneider JA, Wilson RS *et al.* (2005b) Education modifies the association of amyloid but not tangles with cognitive function. *Neurology* **65**: 953–5.

Bennett DA, Schneider JA, Tang Y *et al.* (2006) The effect of social networks on the relation between AD pathology and level of cognitive function in old people: A longitudinal cohort study. *Lancet Neurology* **5**: 406–12.

Bennett DA, Wilson RS, Schneider JA *et al.* (2003) Apolipoprotein E ε4 allele, AD pathology, and the clinical expression of AD. *Neurology* 60: 246–55.

Boyle PA, Buchman AS, Barnes LL, Bennett DA. (2009a) Purpose in life is associated with a reduced risk of Alzheimer's disease and Mild Cognitive Impairment among community based older persons. *Archives of General Psychiatry* 71: 574–9.

Boyle PA, Buchman AS, Wilson RS *et al.* (2009b) Association of muscle strength with the risk of Alzheimer disease and the rate of cognitive decline in community-dwelling older persons. *Archives of Neurology* 66: 1339–44.

Buchman AS, Wilson RS, Bienias JL *et al.* (2005) Change in body mass index and risk of incident Alzheimer disease. *Neurology* 65: 892–7.

Buchman AS, Wilson RS, Schneider JA *et al.* (2006) Body mass index in older persons is associated with AD pathology. *Neurology* 67: 1949–54.

Buchman AS, Boyle PA, Wilson RS *et al.* (2007) Frailty is associated with incident Alzheimer's disease and cognitive decline in the elderly. *Psychosomatic Medicine* 69: 483–9.

Caamano-Isorna F, Corral M, Montes-Martinez A *et al.* (2006) Education and dementia: A meta-analytic study. *Neuroepidemiology* 26: 226–32.

Evans D, Beckett L, Field T *et al.* (1997a) Apolipoprotein E e4 and incidence of Alzheimer's disease in a community population of older persons. *JAMA* 277: 822–4.

Evans D, Hebert L, Beckett L *et al.* (1997b) Education and other measures of socioeconomic status and risk of incident Alzheimer disease in a population of older persons. *Archives of Neurology* 54: 1399–05.

Evans DA, Bennett DA, Wilson RS *et al.* (2003) Incidence of Alzheimer disease in a biracial urban community: Relation to apolipoprotein E allele status. *Archives of Neurology* 60: 185–9.

Farrer LA, Cupples LA, Haines JL *et al.* (1997) Effects of age, sex, and ethnicity on the association between apolipoprotein E genotype and Alzheimer disease. A meta-analysis. APOE and Alzheimer Disease Meta Analysis Consortium. *Journal of the American Medical Association* 278: 1349–56.

Fratiglioni L, Wang HX, Ericsson K *et al.* (2000) Influence of social network on occurrence of dementia: A community-based longitudinal study. *Lancet* 355: 1315–19.

Hall KS, Gao S, Unverzagt FW *et al.* (2000) Low education and childhood rural residence: Risk for AD in African Americans. *Neurology* 54: 95–9.

Honig LS, Tang MX, Albert S *et al.* (2003) Stroke and the risk of Alzheimer disease. *Archives of Neurology* 60: 1707–12.

Jellinger KA. (2006) Alzheimer 100 – highlights in the history of Alzheimer research. *Journal of Neural Transmission* 113: 1603–23.

Karp A, Kareholt I, Oui C. (2004) Relation of education and occupation-based socioeconomic status to incident AD. *American Journal of Epidemiology* 159: 175–83.

Kawas CH. (2006) Medications and diet: protective factors for AD? *Alzheimer Disease and Associated Disorders* 20 (Suppl 2): S89–96.

Kivipelto M, Ngandu T, Fratiglioni L *et al.* (2005) Obesity and vascular risk factors at midlife and the risk of dementia and Alzheimer disease. *Archives of Neurology* 62: 1556–60.

Maynard CJ, Cappai R, Volitakis I *et al.* (2006) Gender and genetic background effects on brain metal levels in APP transgenic and normal mice: Implications for Alzheimer beta-amyloid pathology. *Journal of Inorganic Biochemistry* 100: 952–62.

Morris MC. (2009) The role of nutrition in Alzheimer's disease: Epidemiological evidence. *European Journal of Neurology* 16 (Suppl 1): 1–7.

Murrell JR, Price B, Lane KA *et al.* (2006) Association of apolipoprotein E genotyoe and Alzheimer disease in African Americans. *Archives of Neurology* 63: 431–4.

Podewils LJ, Guallar E, Kuller LH *et al.* (2005) Physical activity, APOE genotype, and dementia risk: Findings from the Cardiovascular Health Cognition Study. *American Journal of Epidemiology* 161: 639–51.

Ravaglia G, Forti P, Maioli F *et al.* (2007) Blood inflammatory markers and risk of dementia: The Conselice Study of Brain Aging. *Neurobiology of Aging* 28: 1810–20.

Scarmeas N, Luchsinger JA, Schupf N *et al.* (2009) Physical activity, diet, and risk of Alzheimer disease. *Journal of the American Medical Association* 302: 627–37.

Schmidt R, Schmidt H, Curb JD *et al.* (2002) Early inflammation and dementia: A 25-year follow-up of the Honolulu-Asia Aging Study. *Annals of Neurology* 52: 168–74.

Schneider JA, Bienias JL, Wilson RS *et al.* (2005) The apolipoprotein E ε4 allele increases the odds of chronic cerebral infarction detected at autopsy in older persons. *Stroke* 36: 954–9.

Soetanto A, Wilson RS, Talbot K *et al.* (2010) Association of anxiety and depression with microtubule-associated protein 2- and synaptopodin-immunolabeled dendrite and spine densities in hippocampal CA3 of older humans. *Archives of General Psychiatry* 67: 448–57.

Sturman MT, Morris MC, Mendes de Leon CF *et al.* (2005) Physical activity, cognitive activity, and cognitive decline in a biracial community population. *Archives of Neurology* 62: 1750–4.

Tang MX, Cross P, Andrews H *et al.* (2001) Incidence of AD in African-Americans, Caribbean Hispanics, and Caucasians in northern Manhattan. *Neurology* 56: 49–56.

Wilson RS, Barnes LL, Mendes de Leon CF *et al.* (2002a) Depressive symptoms, cognitive decline, and risk of AD in older persons. *Neurology* 59: 364–70.

Wilson RS, Bennett DA, Bienias JL *et al.* (2002b) Cognitive activity and incident AD in a population-based sample of older persons. *Neurology* 59: 1910–14.

Wilson RS, Bienias JL, Berry-Kravis E *et al.* (2002c) The apolipoprotein E epsilon 2 allele and decline in episodic memory. *Journal of Neurology, Neurosurgery, and Psychiatry* 73: 672–7.

Wilson RS, Mendes De Leon CF, Barnes LL *et al.* (2002d) Participation in cognitively stimulating activities and risk of incident Alzheimer disease. *Journal of the American Medical Association* 287: 742–8.

Wilson RS, Bennett DA, Bienias JL *et al.* (2003a) Cognitive activity and cognitive decline in a biracial community population. *Neurology* 61: 812–16.

Wilson RS, Schneider JA, Bienias JL et al. (2003b) Depressive symptoms, clinical AD, and cortical plaques and tangles in older persons. *Neurology* **61**: 1102–7.

Wilson RS, Arnold SE, Schneider JA et al. (2006) Chronic psychological distress and risk of AD in old age. *Neuroepidemiology* **27**: 143–53.

Wilson RS, Arnold SE, Schneider JA et al. (2007a) Chronic distress, age-related neuropathology, and late-life dementia. *Psychosomatic Medicine* **69**: 47–53.

Wilson RS, Arnold SE, Schneider JA et al. (2007b) The relation between cerebral Alzheimer's disease pathology and odour identification in old age. *Journal of Neurology, Neurosurgery, and Psychiatry* **78**: 30–5.

Wilson RS, Krueger KR, Arnold SE et al. (2007c) Loneliness and risk of AD. *Archives of General Psychiatry* **64**: 234–40.

Wilson RS, Schneider JA, Arnold SE et al. (2007d) Conscientiousness and the incidence of Alzheimer disease and mild cognitive impairment. *Archives of General Psychiatry* **64**: 1204–8.

Wilson RS, Schneider JA, Arnold SE et al. (2007e) Olfactory identification and incidence of mild cognitive impairment in older age. *Archives of General Psychiatry* **64**: 802–8.

Wilson RS, Scherr PA, Schneider JA et al. (2007f) Relation of cognitive activity to risk of developing Alzheimer disease. *Neurology* **69**: 1911–20.

Wilson RS, Arnold SE, Beck TL et al. (2008) Change in depressive symptoms during the prodromal phase of Alzheimer disease. *Archives of General Psychiatry* **65**: 439–45.

Wilson RS, Arnold SE, Schneider JA et al. (2009a) Olfactory impairment in presymptomatic Alzheimer's disease. *Annals of the New York Academy of Sciences* **1170**: 730–5.

Wilson RS, Hebert LE, Scherr PA et al. (2009b) Educational attainment and cognitive decline in old age. *Neurology* **72**: 460–5.

Yaffe K, Kanaya A, Lindquist K et al. (2004) The metabolic syndrome, inflammation, and risk of cognitive decline. *Journal of the American Medical Association* **292**: 2237–42.

The natural history of Alzheimer's disease

ADAM S FLEISHER AND JODY COREY-BLOOM

48.1 CLINICAL FEATURES

The diverse spectrum of symptoms of Alzheimer's disease (AD) reflects dysfunction of widespread regions of the cerebral cortex. Symptoms begin insidiously, making it difficult to date the onset of cognitive and functional decline precisely. Progression is generally gradual, yet can be interleaved with occasional plateaus; however, reliable measurement of disease progression is difficult because of variability between and within subjects.

Memory loss is the cardinal and commonest presenting complaint in AD. Initially, the patient has difficulty recalling new information such as names or details of conversation, while remote memories are relatively preserved. With progression, the memory loss worsens to include remote memory (Wilson et al., 1983; Sullivan et al., 1986; Cummings and Cole, 2002). Early in AD, judgement and abstraction are often impaired, suggesting involvement of the frontal lobes. Social comportment and interpersonal skills are often strikingly preserved, and may remain relatively intact long after memory and insight have been lost.

Language is frequently normal early in AD, although reduced conversational output may be noted. As dementia progresses, many patients become more recognizably aphasic. Initially, this manifests as dysnomia and mild loss of fluency, with paraphasic errors and relative preservation of repetition, a pattern resembling transcortical sensory aphasia (Cummings et al., 1985; Cummings and Cole, 2002). At a later stage, language is obviously dysfluent and repetition impaired; terminally, a state of near-mutism may occur (Murdoch et al., 1987).

Visuospatial impairment in AD results in symptoms such as misplacing objects or getting lost, and difficulty with tasks such as recognizing and drawing complex figures (Brouwers et al., 1984; Kavcic and Duffy, 2003). Calculation difficulty (affecting skills such as handling money), apraxia and agnosia are further problems that develop in AD. Apraxia may impair activities such as operating appliances or dressing; as might be expected, more complex skills tend to break down first, while highly over-learned motor tasks (e.g. playing a musical instrument, using tools) may be retained until relatively late in the course (Rapcsak et al., 1989; Helmes and Ostbye, 2002). Agnosia develops in middle to late stages of AD, and includes features such as failing to recognize family members or spouses.

Behavioural or psychiatric symptoms occur frequently in AD (see Chapter 8, Neuropsychiatric aspects of dementia and Chapter 9, Measurement of behaviour disturbance, non-cognitive symptoms and quality of life). Over and above a general decline of activity and interest in virtually all AD patients, depressive symptoms occur in about 25 per cent, although severe depression is uncommon (Cummings et al., 1987; Rapcsak et al., 1989; Rosen and Zubenko, 1991; Becker et al., 1994; Cummings and Cole, 2002; Helmes and Ostbye, 2002; Starkstein et al., 2008). The frequency of significantly depressed mood in patients with AD ranged from 0 to 87 per cent in 30 studies reviewed by Wragg and Jeste (1989) with higher rates reported from acute care facilities than in series from outpatient research sites. While many AD patients have depressive symptoms, most do not display enough features to meet DSM-IV criteria for major depressive disorders. The fact that vegetative symptoms such as sleep disturbance, weight gain, loss of libido, lack of interest and reduced motor activity are common to both AD and depression may account for the high rate of 'depression' found in some studies (Lazarus et al., 1987; Becker et al., 1994; Jost and Grossberg,

1996). In patients with severe dementia, there is an apparent paucity of depressive symptoms. A likely explanation is that certain features of depression (guilt, hopelessness, anxiety) are less discernible in subjects with severe dementia. But, symptoms such as crying and diminished sleep can be expressed even at late stages of AD.

Delusions are common in AD, although they are rarely as systematized as in schizophrenia. They often have a paranoid flavour, with fears of personal harm, theft of personal property and marital infidelity. Misidentification syndromes also occur; whether these represent true delusions is unclear. The prevalence of psychotic symptoms in AD, the relationship of hallucinations and delusions to the severity of cognitive impairment, and the influence of psychosis on the rate of cognitive decline are controversial. Estimates of the prevalence of psychotic symptoms in AD range from 10 to 73 per cent, with most in the range of 28–38 per cent (Wragg and Jeste, 1989; Mega et al., 1999). Delusions have been reported in 13–75 per cent of AD patients, and hallucinations, more commonly visual than auditory, in 3–50 per cent (Mayeux et al., 1985; Cummings et al., 1987; Reisberg et al., 1987; Drevets and Rubin, 1989; Reisberg et al., 1989; Becker et al., 1994; Jost and Grossberg, 1996; Cook et al., 2003). This substantial variation in frequencies is probably due to different methodologic approaches, especially in defining delusions and hallucinations, and to differences in the range of severity of AD in each series. Although psychotic symptoms may occur throughout the course of AD, they have their highest frequency at a moderate level of dementia (Drevets and Rubin, 1989).

In addition to depression and psychotic symptoms, AD patients show a wide range of behavioural abnormalities including agitation, wandering, sleep disturbances and disinhibition (Becker et al., 1994; Jost and Grossberg, 1996; Lyketsos et al., 2002). In contrast to psychotic symptoms, behavioural disturbances are more clearly associated with the degree of dementia. A study of 127 AD patients found that the overall number of behavioural problems increased significantly with worsening cognitive function (Teri et al., 1988). Agitation includes physical aggression, verbal aggression, and non-aggressive behaviours. Physically non-aggressive behaviours, such as motor restlessness and pacing, are the most common forms of agitation in outpatients with AD. However, physical aggression is the most distressing behaviour to custodians, and occurs in about 20 per cent of patients (Reisberg et al., 1987; Burns et al., 1990; Hooker et al., 2002). Various factors appear to be important predictors of aggressive behaviour, including pre-morbid history of aggression, a troubled pre-morbid relationship between the caregiver and patient, and a greater number of social and medical problems. Wandering behaviour affects 3–26 per cent of AD outpatients. Insomnia and sleep disturbances are inconstant features of AD, and sexual disinhibition has been reported in less than 10 per cent of patients (Burns et al., 1990; Becker et al., 1994). Thus, behavioural symptoms are a pervasive and poorly understood concomitant symptom of cognitive deterioration in AD.

Excluding mental status testing, the neurologic examination is usually normal in AD, and the presence of significant or lateralizing abnormalities often suggests other diagnoses.

However, primitive reflexes (snout, glabellar, grasp), impaired graphesthesia, and an abnormal response to double simultaneous stimulation (face–hand test) are frequently encountered in AD (Galasko et al., 1990; Becker et al., 1994). Variable features, including extrapyramidal signs (rigidity and bradykinesia), gait disturbances, and myoclonus may occasionally be seen early in the course of AD, and increase in prevalence with the severity of AD (Stern et al., 1987). The frequency of extrapyramidal signs in patients with AD was as low as 12–14 per cent in some series (Galasko et al., 1990; Burns et al., 1991; Becker et al., 1994), and as high as 28–92 per cent in others (Mayeux et al., 1985; Molsa et al., 1986; Bakchine et al., 1989; Lopez et al., 2000), depending on the severity of dementia in patients studied. In intermediate or advanced stages of dementia, patients often develop nonspecific impairment of gait and balance, leading to an increased risk of falls. Myoclonus develops late in the course of AD and longitudinal studies report an increase in its frequency during follow up (Mayeux et al., 1985; Tschampa et al., 2001). Its prevalence in AD has varied widely from 0 to 68 per cent, although the usual reported rate is about 10 per cent (Hauser et al., 1986).

As neuronal degeneration progresses in AD, all of the above symptoms worsen, and eventually patients become uncommunicative, and unable to care for themselves, walk or maintain continence. They require total care, including feeding, and are often institutionalized. In end-stage AD, death usually results from the complications of being bedbound, such as aspiration pneumonia, urinary tract infections, sepsis or pulmonary embolism (Molsa et al., 1986).

48.2   CLINICAL UTILITY OF ASSESSING CHANGE

The course of AD and the combination of symptoms that manifest in each patient are markedly heterogeneous; however, there are several direct clinical applications of tracking change. First, in early cases of AD, where impairment is mild, documenting progression helps to confirm or establish the diagnosis of dementia. Clearly, progressive cognitive deterioration is incompatible with normal ageing, depression, delirium or a static encephalopathy. The clinical follow up of patients who are initially classified as having AD greatly increases the accuracy of the diagnosis.

Second, progression to a greater degree than expected may prompt the physician to look for a superimposed factor that may be treatable, such as hypothyroidism, intercurrent infection, medication toxicity or depression. Improvement or stabilization of psychometric scores indicates a favourable response to treating a remediable factor contributing to dementia.

Third, defining the anticipated course of AD in detail enables clinicians to provide patients and families with realistic expectations regarding the disease, and aids in making decisions for day care or institutionalization.

Longitudinal cognitive change may be fruitfully applied to several problems in clinical research. Change over time on mental status scores may be used to construct models of the clinical course of 'typical' AD. This methodologic approach has ramifications, such as testing whether genetic/environmental factors or experimental treatment influence the rate of progression of dementia.

Attempts to refine the natural history of AD have utilized two basic methods: global staging systems and serial changes on psychometric test scores.

48.2.1 Measuring change with global staging systems

Staging systems for AD comprise information on intellectual, social and community functioning obtained by history rather than formal rating scales. Two widely used schemes are the Washington University Clinical Dementia Rating (CDR) (Hughes et al., 1982; Morris, 1997) and the Global Deterioration Scale (GDS) (Reisberg et al., 1982; Reisberg et al., 1986), which divide AD into a succession of stages. These scales reflect an overall, indirect evaluation of cognition, primarily obtained from caregivers, rather than a direct assessment of the patient but are able to assess the influence of cognitive loss on the ability to conduct everyday activities. They provide information about clinically meaningful function and behaviour and are less affected by the 'floor' and 'ceiling' effects commonly associated with psychometric tests.

The CDR incorporates information from patients and informants concerning six areas of mental function: memory, orientation, judgement and problem solving, community affairs, home and hobbies, and personal care. Each area is scored as 0 = normal, 0.5 = questionable, 1 = mild, 2 = moderate, or 3 = severe impairment, and integrated to obtain an overall stage of dementia, using similar definitions of 0, 0.5 and 1 to 3. Inter-rater reliability is high, with a correlation of 0.91, and the CDR has been standardized for multi-centre use (Morris et al., 1997). Since the CDR includes cognitive items and activities of daily living (ADL), it is not surprising that it correlates well with the cognitive Blessed Information-Memory-Concentration (BIMC) scale ($r = 0.55$) and with the ADL-based Blessed Dementia Scale (BDS) ($r = 0.53$) (Berg et al., 1988). Putting the CDR into practice, these authors followed a cohort of 43 initially mild AD patients (CDR 1) for 90 months. Over 67 per cent of patients progressed to CDR 3 (severe dementia) by 50 months, and over 80 per cent by 66 months. Many patients in this CDR 1 group reached end points: 50 per cent of patients were institutionalized by 40 months, and 80 per cent by 60 months. Thirty per cent of patients died by 40 months, and 40 per cent by 72 months. Although the CDR is clearly a useful staging instrument and has become widely accepted in the clinical setting as a reliable and valid global assessment measure for AD, it is not as sensitive a measure of annual or short-term rate of change, as movement from one stage to the next may take several years (Storandt et al., 2002).

The GDS divides AD into a succession of seven major, clinically distinguishable stages (further subdivided into 16) ranging from normal cognition (GDS 1) to severe dementia (GDS 7) (Reisberg et al., 1982). Criteria for many of the stages combine history (initially of memory decline, later of functional impairment, progressing to loss of self-care,

language and gait), and mental status examination. Stages defined by this integration of history, ADL and cognition should show high correlations with mental state screening tests: indeed, the GDS correlates well with the Mini-Mental State Examination (MMSE) ($r = 0.9$, $p < 0.001$) and the BIMC ($r = 0.8$, $p < 0.001$) (Reisberg et al., 1989). GDS stages 1 and 2 correspond to CDR 0, representing normal ageing, and GDS 3 is equivalent to CDR 0.5. In a longitudinal study, only 5 per cent of GDS 2 subjects became demented over three to four years, whereas 15 per cent of GDS 3 subjects progressed to more advanced stages of dementia (Reisberg et al., 1986).

The GDS has similar virtues and drawbacks to the CDR, namely difficulty in defining a natural history over periods shorter than a year or two. The primary use of these staging systems may be in research settings and in following patients longitudinally over extended periods, since the transitions from one stage to the next occur over relatively long intervals.

48.2.2 Measuring change by rate of decline on cognitive tests

As a more flexible longitudinal index of brain function, some studies have measured the annual rate of change (ARC) of mental status test scores in AD. Longitudinal data exist for ARC on five mental status tests in common use: the BIMC test, the MMSE, the Dementia Rating Scale (DRS), the Cambridge Cognitive Examination (CAMCOG) (Roth et al., 1986) and the Alzheimer's Disease Assessment Scale (ADAS) (Rosen et al., 1984). Unfortunately, although these rates of decline are available, their generalizability is uncertain.

Katzman et al. (1988) compared four groups of subjects with AD on the BIMC, with follow up over one year (Reisberg et al., 1989). These cohorts differed substantially with regard to age, education, sex, severity of dementia and place of residence, and included community-dwelling and institutionalized subjects seen in private practice or public hospital settings. The mean rate of change on the BIMC did not differ significantly among the four groups for subjects who initially made 24 or fewer errors (out of a possible 33). In those patients, the ARC on the BIMC was 4.4 errors per year, and did not vary with age, education or place of residence. Among demented subjects with an initial BIMC score of more than 24 errors, the rate of change was lower, presumably because the test had reached a floor. A similar overall rate of progression for the BIMC was found in a group of outpatients with AD (Ortof and Crystal, 1989). Subjects lost an average of 4.1 points per year, regardless of age of onset, duration of illness or family history of dementia. Two further studies observed a comparable ARC in community-dwelling AD patients (Thal et al., 1988; Salmon et al., 1990). In all of these studies, the standard deviation was slightly less than the mean ARC over one year and the range of ARC varied widely. Significant variation in the mean ARC on the BIMC has been observed however by other investigators. For example, Lucca et al. (1993) noted a change of only 2.6 (± 4.9) points on the BIMC over one year in a group of 56 patients with AD comprising out-patients and in-patients at geriatric institutions. Using data from the California Alzheimer's Disease Diagnostic and

Treatment Centers, we observed an annual rate of change of 2.8 points on the BIMC (Corey-Bloom *et al.*, 1993).

For the MMSE, a number of studies have reported a mean ARC in AD ranging from 1.8 to 4.2 points. Of these studies, the one with the lowest ARC entered patients at a very mild stage of AD (Becker *et al.*, 1988). Studies with the highest ARC had more severely impaired subjects at entry (Yesavage *et al.*, 1988; Burns *et al.*, 1991), while the remaining studies showed an intermediate ARC (about 2.5 points per year) in patients with an intermediate initial level of impairment (Salmon *et al.*, 1990; Teri *et al.*, 1990; Corey-Bloom *et al.*, 1993; Aguero-Torres *et al.*, 1998; Swanwick *et al.*, 1998; Thal *et al.*, 2000; Winblad *et al.*, 2001). This illustrates that rate of change of the MMSE is affected by the severity of cognitive impairment even before the test reaches a floor. The MMSE tests a wide range of cognitive skills, and individuals may be expected to decline at varying rates and over different cognitive tasks during the progression of AD. For example, patients lose points on the orientation, recall and construction items before language or praxis become abnormal. The degree of variability of ARC for the BIMC (reflected by the standard deviations in ARC studies) is significantly smaller than that of the MMSE (Schneider, 1992), suggesting that the BIMC has less noise and may be more reliable as a change measure.

Few studies of longitudinal cognitive change in AD have used extended follow-up periods. In a study distinguished by seven years of follow up, Aguero-Torres *et al.* (1998) found a mean ARC of 2.8 points on the MMSE during their first period of evaluation (entry–three years) and 3.0 points thereafter (three–seven years). Salmon *et al.* (1990) compared the BIMC, MMSE and DRS in 55 community-dwelling patients with AD over two years. Each subject's scores on the three tests were highly correlated at entry and after one and two years. Over the study period, patients lost a mean of 3.2 points on the BIMC, 2.8 points on the MMSE and 11.4 points on the DRS per year. In general, the group declined to a greater degree on all three scales in the second year than in the first, but this was statistically significant only for the DRS. For individuals, however, the ARC of mental status scores in the first year did not predict the next year's rate of decline. Unlike the BIMC and the MMSE, the ARC of the DRS did not decrease with more advanced dementia, indicating that the DRS has a wider range for detecting change than these other tests.

Two longer instruments, similar to the DRS, have been used for serial assessment: the CAMCOG and the ADAS. The CAMCOG is the cognitive component of the Cambridge Mental Disorders of the Elderly Examination (CAMDEX), an instrument designed for assessing dementia. It has sections testing memory, language, praxis, orientation, attention, calculation, abstraction and perception, with a maximum total score of 107. In a survey of 110 patients spanning a wide spectrum of severity of AD, Burns *et al.* (1991) found a significant decline over one year in the overall score (12.3 points), and in virtually every abstraction were close to 'floor' on initial evaluation, and declined further over one year. The initial mean MMSE for this group was 10 (± 5.9), lower than in studies cited above, and changed by an average of 3.5 points (Burns *et al.*, 1991). In a study of 95 less demented

subjects (mean MMSE of 19.6 ± 3.8), Swanwick *et al.* (1998) reported an annual decline on the CAMCOG of 9.42 points (± 9.52). However, as reflected by the large standard deviation, the ARC was normally distributed with a high degree of individual variability. Additionally, the rate of decline in the first year did not predict subsequent ARC.

The ADAS includes a cognitive portion, with a maximum of 70 points, and a non-cognitive subscale scored out of 40. Kramer-Ginsberg *et al.* (1988); R Mohs (personal communication) found an average ARC on the ADAS of 9.3 points in 60 AD patients. Yesavage *et al.* (1988) reported a similar ARC on the ADAS of 8.3 points in 30 patients with AD, and additionally noted a high correlation between selected subscales of the ADAS and the MMSE. In a larger group of 102 AD patients participating in the ALCAR clinical trial, Thal *et al.* (2000) reported an ARC of 7.5 points. The ADAS-Cog is the most common cognitive outcome measure used in randomized clinical treatment trials for AD (Wolfson *et al.*, 2002; Jones *et al.*, 2009). It should be noted that rates of decline in clinical trials may be less than those seen in natural history studies because of inherent selection biases. Clinical trial volunteers tend to have better overall health care, are selected to reduce co-morbidities, and typically have more involved carers.

Unfortunately, while mean ARC for each of these cognitive scales was reasonably consistent between studies, the standard deviations were fairly large, roughly equal to the means, indicating substantial individual variability. Some patients' scores did not decline, and even improved over one to two years of follow up. This variability has several possible explanations. First, AD may not progress uniformly, since patients with early dementia may enter a 'plateau' phase with relatively slow deterioration. Second, performance on these cognitive tests probably does not decline in a linear fashion. Third, test–retest variability is influenced by patients' mood, attention and motivation and many other factors which have an impact on day-to-day mental performance, adding a further element of uncertainty to ARC calculations. A fourth possibility is that a number of biological and clinical factors may modify the rate of progression of AD. These include demographic factors such as age of onset, gender and education; co-morbid disease such as cerebrovascular disease, diabetes and hypertension; historical features such as lipid-lowering agents, vitamin and non-steroidal anti-inflammatory drug use; genetic factors such as apolipoprotein E status; and clinical features such as psychosis and extrapyramidal signs.

48.3   CLINICAL PREDICTORS OF RATE OF PROGRESSION

As noted, a number of factors appear to affect the rate of decline in AD; however, this is a thorny issue since variables thought to have independent prognostic significance may simply be markers of the level of disease severity (Drachman *et al.*, 1990).

For example, using a large well-characterized sample of Consortium to Establish a Registry for Alzheimer's Disease

(CERAD) subjects, Morris *et al.* (1993) found that dementia progression may be non-linear, that rate-of-change determinations were less reliable when the observation period was one year or less, and that rate of progression in AD was determined by the severity of cognitive impairment: the less severe the dementia, the slower the rate of decline. Similarly, Teri *et al.* (1995), using a community-based sample of 156 patients diagnosed with probable AD followed for up to five years, found that average rate of decline in cognitive function, as measured by the MMSE and Mattis DRS, becomes more rapid as the disease progresses. This has been confirmed by a more recent study by Storandt *et al.* (2002). Using a large cohort of mildly demented subjects, they found that initial dementia severity was the most significant predictor of annual rate of progression on composite psychometric testing, with increasingly steeper slopes as severity increased. In addition, these authors found that the rates of decline were highly variable from person to person and between groups as well. There was limited evidence for any systematic predictors of cognitive decline, including combined psychometric measures.

Several studies investigating age at onset as a predictor of deterioration have reported a significant association between earlier age at onset and greater rate of cognitive or functional worsening (Lucca *et al.*, 1993; Jacobs *et al.*, 1994; Teri *et al.*, 1995; Mungas *et al.*, 2001; Backman *et al.*, 2003). This is not supported, however, by one study of 95 subjects with AD attending a memory clinic (Swanwick *et al.*, 1998).

Gender was not seen to influence cognitive decline in several studies of AD (Reisberg *et al.*, 1986; Drachman *et al.*, 1990; Burns *et al.*, 1991; Mortimer *et al.*, 1992; Jacobs *et al.*, 1994; Swanwick *et al.*, 1998; Storandt *et al.*, 2002). However, this was not the case for others who reported slower (Heston *et al.*, 1981; Lucca *et al.*, 1993; Aguero-Torres *et al.*, 1998) and faster (Swanwick *et al.*, 1998) rates of progression in men as compared to women.

Level of education has been examined as a predictor of decline in several studies (Heston *et al.*, 1981; Filley *et al.*, 1985; Berg *et al.*, 1988; Katzman *et al.*, 1988; Drachman *et al.*, 1990; Lucca *et al.*, 1993; Teri *et al.*, 1995; Storandt *et al.*, 2002). A recent study of 154 persons with a mean education of 8 years (± 4.4) with mild to moderate AD demonstrated that more educated individuals were more likely to have faster cognitive progression (Musicco *et al.*, 2009).

The apolipoprotein E (ApoE) ε4 allele is associated with both a high likelihood of developing AD and an earlier age of onset; nonetheless, there have been conflicting results with regard to the influence of ApoE genotype on the course of cognitive decline in AD. Gomez-Isla *et al.* (1996), in a prospective longitudinal study of 359 AD patients, found that the ApoE ε4 allele was not associated with any change in rate of progression of dementia. Likewise, Growdon *et al.* (1996) reported that rate of decline did not vary significantly across ApoE genotype on any neuropsychological test administered to 66 probable AD patients over a span of up to 5.5 years and Kurz *et al.* (1996) noted no association between ε4 status and rate of cognitive decline over three years on the CAMCOG and MMSE in 64 subjects with clinically diagnosed AD. Furthermore, Frisoni *et al.* (1995) reported a slower rate of progression with increasing ε4 gene dose in a retrospective

examination of 62 sporadic AD patients. These latter findings were similar to those of Stern *et al.* (1997) who noted a slower rate of decline on the modified MMSE among patients with ApoE ε4 alleles compared to patients with other genotypes. This is not supported, however, by Craft *et al.* (1998) who reported an accelerated rate of decline on the DRS in ApoE ε4 homozygotes with probable AD, and Hirono *et al.* (2003) who reported a similar accelerated rate of decline on the ADAS-Cog, even after controlling for age, gender, education, test interval and baseline scores.

Concomitant cerebrovascular disease has not been shown to significantly increase rate of cognitive decline in AD (Lee *et al.*, 2000; Storandt *et al.*, 2002). However, one longitudinal study with autopsy follow up of 50 patients with AD and strokes, compared to 218 AD patients without strokes, showed a slight increase in rate of decline on MMSE scores in the co-morbid stroke group for subjects over the age of 80 (Mungas *et al.*, 2001).

Although it has been suggested that patients who develop extrapyramidal symptoms (EPSs) such as tremor, bradykinesia, rigid tone or masked facial features, have a faster rate of decline, many earlier studies probably included patients on neuroleptics and those with Lewy body variant and diffuse Lewy body (DLB) disease (Miller *et al.*, 1991; Mortimer *et al.*, 1992; Chui *et al.* 1994; Stern *et al.*, 1994). Furthermore, it is now clear that there is a pathological subset of AD patients with alpha-synuclein-positive cortical Lewy bodies in addition to typical AD pathology (Fleisher and Olichney, 2005; Weisman *et al.*, 2007). A retrospective study by Lopez *et al.* (2000) compared clinical characteristics of 185 autopsy-proven AD and 60 autopsy-proven AD plus Lewy bodies (DLB) subjects. These authors found no differences in rate of cognitive decline between the two, although DLB subjects developed EPS earlier. However, in a more recent study of 56 patients with DLB compared to 111 AD patients, who were examined for up to five years on end points of hospitalization, institutionalization and death (Hanyu *et al.*, 2009), DLB patients had a significantly shorter time to clinical end points than those with AD (median time; 40 versus 52 months, $p < 0.0001$). The proportion of hospitalizations (and death) was significantly higher in DLB than in AD patients (30 versus 14 per cent, $p < 0.05$), but differences with regard to nursing home placement did not reach statistical significance (25 versus 17 per cent). Rates of decline on the MMSE were equivalent for both patient groups. Although there is strong evidence that the addition of Lewy bodies to AD pathology expedites clinical decline, it is not clear that the EPS of typical AD, free from Lewy body pathology, predicts more rapid decline.

Whether neuropsychiatric symptoms superimposed on AD influence cognitive deterioration has been examined by several authors. Initial reports suggested that AD patients reached end points on a modified MMSE or BDS score more rapidly when psychotic symptoms were present (Mayeux *et al.*, 1985; Drevets and Rubin, 1989; Stern *et al.*, 1990). However, these investigations did not match patients for their level of dementia. Controlling for severity of AD, other studies were unable to replicate these findings (Reisberg *et al.*, 1986; Chen *et al.*, 1991), although two more have confirmed psychosis as a robust predictor of cognitive decline (Chui *et al.*, 1994; Stern *et al.*, 1994). Lopez *et al.* (1999) examined the effect of psychiatric symptoms and medications on progression in 179 mild to moderate probable AD patients, followed for a mean of 49.5 ± 27.4 months. These authors found that the presence of psychiatric symptoms and the use of psychiatric medications were associated with increased rate of functional (BDRS) but not cognitive (MMSE) decline. One cross-sectional study reported that AD patients with depression had more ADL impairment than those without (Pearson *et al.*, 1989), however, other longitudinal studies found no effect of depression on rate of decline (Lopez *et al.*, 1990; Storandt *et al.*, 2002).

Whether vitamin use, oestrogen, lipid-lowering agents or non-steroidal anti-inflammatory drugs (NSAIDs) affect progression of AD has been investigated. High-dose vitamin E appeared to slow disease progression in a double-blind, placebo-controlled trial in patients with AD of moderate severity (Sano *et al.*, 1997). Reduction of serum homocysteine with folate, B_6 and B_{12} has shown no benefit in slowing the progression of AD (Aisen *et al.*, 2008). An omega-3 fatty acid, docosohexanoic acid, was recently shown in a large placebo-controlled, randomized, clinical trial to not be effective in slowing cognitive decline in AD (Quinn *et al.*, 2009). Although several observational studies have suggested that oestrogen replacement therapy may have a beneficial effect on cognitive performance in women with AD, many have substantial methodologic problems (Haskell *et al.*, 1997; Yaffe *et al.*, 1998). Furthermore, a study of the association between serum oestradiol and oestrone levels in 120 hysterectomized women taking replacement found no significant association between hormone levels and cognitive functioning after either two or twelve months of treatment (Thal *et al.*, 2003). Additional evidence that oestrogen may not be beneficial in AD comes from the Women's Health Initiative Memory Study, a randomized, double-blind, placebo-controlled clinical trial of 4532 post-menopausal women, comparing oestrogen and progesterone versus placebo effects on incidence of dementia over four years. The authors found that oestrogen plus progestin therapy increased the risk of probable dementia in post-menopausal women aged 65 years or older (Shumaker *et al.*, 2003). Several large cohort analyses have demonstrated decreased prevalence of AD with use of various lipid-lowering agents (Rockwood *et al.*, 2002). Although a large multi-centre placebo-controlled trial investigating the effect of simvastatin on progression of cognitive decline in AD recently concluded, results of this trial have not yet been published. Analysis of longitudinal changes over one year revealed less decline among NSAID patients than among non-NSAID patients on measures of verbal fluency, spatial recognition and orientation, in a study of 210 patients with AD (Rich *et al.*, 1995). On the other hand, a randomized, placebo-controlled trial of naproxen and rofecoxib showed no effect on cognitive decline in 351 patients with mild to moderate AD (Aisen *et al.*, 2003).

48.4   PREDICTING NURSING HOME PLACEMENT IN AD

Most patients with AD reside in nursing homes or related institutions late in the course of the illness. The interval between the diagnosis of AD and the need for institutional placement has much practical and clinical importance, but is not easy to predict. Behavioural symptoms such as agitation, wandering or aggression may pre-empt nursing home placement, regardless of the level of cognitive impairment. Other variables that greatly influence the decision for institutional placement of a demented patient may include social support and caregiver burden. Many studies have evaluated such predictors of nursing home placement. In a systematic review of the literature, Gaugler *et al.* (2009) reviewed 782 studies on nursing home placement of dementia patients, performing analysis on the 80 most relevant and high quality studies. They found that the most consistent predictors of nursing home admission in dementia patients included severity of cognitive impairment, basic activity of daily living dependencies, behavioural symptoms and depression. Caregivers who reported greater emotional stress also increased risk for placement. Demographic variables, incontinence and use of available services did not predict nursing home placement.

A large population-based historical cohort study suggests, not surprisingly, that the mere presence of dementia increases the overall risk of nursing home admission (Eaker *et al.*, 2002). In their study, the adjusted hazard ratio for institutionalization, compared to non-demented controls, was 5.44 (95% confidence interval, CI: 3.68, 8.05) for AD cases and 5.08 (95% CI: 3.38, 7.63) for non-AD dementia cases, independent of co-morbid conditions.

As noted, several studies have examined predictors of institutionalization in AD. As expected, the predictive factors are complex and vary greatly among studies. One investigation of 14 married men with AD found that urinary or faecal incontinence, inability to speak coherently and loss of skills needed for bathing and grooming were major determinants of institutionalization (Hutton *et al.*, 1985). In a five-year study of 92 patients who developed AD before the age of 70, lower mental status scores or aphasia were more common in those who were institutionalized (Hutton *et al.*, 1985; Heyman *et al.*, 1987). In most instances, nursing home placement occurred because the patients had become almost completely helpless and required 24-hour supervision; for ten patients the decision was prompted by death or serious illness of their caregivers.

A prospective study of 101 initially community-dwelling AD patients found that 12 per cent with 'mild AD' were in nursing homes after one year, and 35 per cent after two years (Knopman *et al.*, 1988). For 'advanced AD', the figures were 39 per cent at one year and 62 per cent at two years. Total ADL scores were significantly related to institutionalization, while incontinence, irritability, inability to walk, wandering, hyperactivity and nocturnal behavioural problems were the leading reasons for placement cited by caregivers.

A CERAD analysis, comprising 20 university medical centres, found that the median time from enrolment to nursing home placement was 3.1 years, with significantly reduced times (2.1 years) for males who were unmarried (Heyman *et al.*, 1997). The major predictors of time to admission were measures of dementia severity upon entry into the study, including the degree of cognitive impairment, functional disability and overall stage. Age at entry and marital status (men only) also predicted time to nursing home admission. Similar findings with regard to marital status have been reported by others (Haupt and Kurz, 1993).

Finally, a large multi-regional, prospective study distinguished by an extremely large number of patients ($n = 3944$), found that specific caregiver traits (including age ≥ 80, low income, poor health and high perceived burden as a result of caregiving) predicted earlier placement for care recipients (Gaugler *et al.*, 2003).

48.5   SURVIVAL IN AD

Length of survival in AD is highly variable although an excess mortality has consistently been reported (Katzman, 1976; Jorm *et al.*, 1987; Aevarsson *et al.*, 1998). Although mean survival after symptom onset may range from two to over 16 years, the observed survival rate among AD populations is generally significantly less than the expected rate, based on life expectancy tables (Walsh *et al.*, 1990). Depending on the study, survival at five years ranges from 10 to 40 per cent in different AD populations. Of course, the most favourable survival rates are seen in mild cohorts followed up in outpatient settings, with lowest survival rates reported in relatively severely demented subjects from hospital series. The median duration of survival among CERAD patients from time of study entry was 5.9 years (Heyman *et al.*, 1996), which compares favourably to the 5.3 years reported by Walsh *et al.* (1990), the 5.7 years noted by Molsa *et al.* (1986) and the 5.8 years described by Jost and Grossberg (1995). Three other studies found shorter median periods of survival of 3.4 years (Schoenberg *et al.*, 1987), 3.5 years (Barclay *et al.*, 1985) and 4.3 years (Claus *et al.*, 1998), possibly due to inclusion of more severe subjects.

The shortened survival of AD patients results from complications due to severe mental decline. Malnutrition, dehydration, pneumonia and other infections occur frequently in the terminal stages when patients are bed-bound, incontinent and unable to communicate or feed themselves. Compared to other elderly individuals, AD patients are not especially predisposed to cancer, cerebrovascular or cardiovascular disease (Molsa *et al.*, 1986).

Unremarkably, the most consistent predictors of mortality in AD patients are age, gender and dementia severity. Age was significantly associated with survival time in a large sample of patients with AD, drawn from throughout the state of California (Moritz *et al.*, 1997). Increasing age has also been related to shorter survival in several additional studies (Hier *et al.*, 1989; Walsh *et al.*, 1990; van Dijk *et al.*, 1991; Heyman *et al.*, 1996; Reisberg *et al.*, 1996; Aguero-Torres *et al.*, 1998; Claus *et al.*, 1998; Gambassi *et al.*, 1999; Ueki *et al.*, 2001). Although two reports have indicated that survival rates of patients with early-onset AD are considerably less than those of late-onset AD (Heyman *et al.*, 1987; McGonigal *et al.*, 1992), this finding has not been confirmed by others (Walsh *et al.*, 1990; Bracco *et al.*, 1994; Corder *et al.*, 1995; Bowen *et al.*, 1996; Heyman *et al.*, 1996).

Most investigators have reported shorter survival times for men than women (Schoenberg *et al.*, 1987; Berg *et al.*, 1988; Burns *et al.*, 1991; van Dijk *et al.*, 1991; Corder *et al.*, 1995; Jagger *et al.*, 1995; Molsa *et al.*, 1995; Stern *et al.*, 1995; Bowen *et al.*, 1996; Heyman *et al.*, 1996; Reisberg *et al.*, 1996; Moritz *et al.*, 1997; Claus *et al.*, 1998; Gambassi *et al.*, 1999; Lapane *et al.*, 2001; Ueki *et al.*, 2001), although this has not been the case for all studies (Hier *et al.*, 1989; Walsh *et al.*, 1990; Becker *et al.*, 1994). Furthermore, it has been suggested by some that predictors may differ by gender. Moritz *et al.* (1997) found that among men, but not women, survival

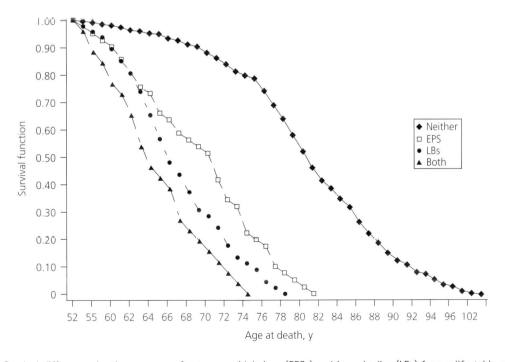

Figure 48.1   Survival differences by the presence of extrapyramidal signs (EPSs) and Lewy bodies (LBs) from a life-table analysis. Reproduced with permission (Haan *et al.*, 2002).

times were negatively associated with selected neurological symptoms, particularly aphasia and apraxia. Among women, but not men, a history of cardiovascular conditions was associated with poorer survival. Lapane *et al.* (2001), on the other hand, found that the most important predictors of mortality for men were severity of dementia and the occurrence of delirium. For women, death was associated with impairment of ADL, presence of pressure sores, malnutrition and co-morbidity.

Patients with more severe dementia at study entry have shorter durations of survival (Walsh *et al.*, 1990; Burns *et al.*, 1991; Evans *et al.*, 1991; Jagger *et al.*, 1995; Heyman *et al.*, 1996; Moritz *et al.*, 1997; Claus *et al.*, 1998; Ueki *et al.*, 2001; Storandt *et al.*, 2002). In addition, functional disability has been shown to decrease survival time in AD (Martin *et al.*, 1987; Bianchetti *et al.*, 1995; Heyman *et al.*, 1996; Ueki *et al.*, 2001).

Additional variables that may influence survival time in patients with AD have not been well established, including level of education (Becker *et al.*, 1994; Stern *et al.*, 1995; Geerlings *et al.*, 1997), medical co-morbidity (Moritz *et al.*, 1997; Aguero-Torres *et al.*, 1998) and psychiatric or behavioural symptoms (Barclay *et al.*, 1985; Molsa *et al.*, 1986; Walsh *et al.*, 1990; Stern *et al.*, 1994; Samson *et al.*, 1996), among others.

Survival in AD appeared to be unrelated to ApoE ε4 gene dose in one study (Corder *et al.*, 1995). However, Tilvis *et al.* (1998) noted increased mortality in elderly demented patients with the ε4 allele, a finding supported, at least for men, in a recent study of 92 autopsy-confirmed AD cases (Dal Forno *et al.*, 2002). On the other hand, Stern *et al.* (1997) found that the presence of at least one ε4 allele was associated with a less aggressive form of AD and a decreased risk of mortality in 99 patients with probable AD followed for up to six years.

Extrapyramidal symptoms appeared to be an important predictor of mortality in a population-based study of 198 patients with probable early-onset AD (Samson *et al.*, 1996). EPS at entry were also associated with a higher relative risk of death in 236 patients with mild AD followed semi-annually (Stern *et al.*, 1994). A study of 379 AD patients found similar heightened mortality for EPS and demonstrated that individuals with EPS were three times more likely to have Lewy bodies at autopsy (Haan *et al.*, 2002) (**Figure 48.1**). Both EPS and LBs were associated with earlier age at death. This was not the case for a study by Lopez *et al.* (2000) who reported no differences between AD and AD+LB with regard to survival.

48.6   CONCLUSIONS

Despite an abundance of observations about the natural history of AD, the variability of its clinical features and rate of progression has not been explained, and the validity of 'subtypes' of AD has not been proven. The most consistent predictor of more rapid deterioration and death in AD appears to be the degree of cognitive and functional disability. Because of the relatively low prevalence of clinical features such as EPS, depression and psychosis at early stages

of the disease, larger studies, carefully controlling for the potential confounding effect of dementia severity, are needed to clarify their effect on prognosis.

REFERENCES

Aevarsson O, Svanborg A, Skoog I. (1998) Seven-year survival rate after age 85 years: relation to Alzheimer disease and vascular dementia. *Archives of Neurology* **55**: 1226–32.

Aguero-Torres H, Fratiglioni L, Guo Z *et al.* (1998) Prognostic factors in very old demented adults: A seven-year follow-up from a population-based survey in Stockholm. *Journal of the American Geriatrics Society* **46**: 444–52.

Aisen PS, Schafer K, Grundman M *et al.* (2003) Results of a multicenter trial of rofecoxib and naproxen in Alzheimer's disease. *Journal of the American Medical Association* **289**: 2819–26.

Aisen PS, Schneider LS, Sano M *et al.* (2008) High-dose B vitamin supplementation and cognitive decline in Alzheimer disease: a randomized controlled trial. *Journal of the American Medical Association* **300**: 1774–83.

Backman L, Jones S, Small BJ *et al.* (2003) Rate of cognitive decline in preclinical Alzheimer's disease: The role of comorbidity. *Journals of Gerontology. Series B Psychological Sciences and Social Sciences* **58**: P228–36.

Bakchine S, Lacomblez L, Palisson E *et al.* (1989) Relationship between primitive reflexes, extra-pyramidal signs, reflective apraxia and severity of cognitive impairment in dementia of the Alzheimer type. *Acta Neurologica Scandinavica* **79**: 38–46.

Barclay LL, Zemcov A, Blass JP, McDowell FH. (1985) Factors associated with duration of survival in Alzheimer's disease. *Biological Psychiatry* **20**: 86–93.

Becker JT, Boller F, Lopez OL *et al.* (1994) The natural history of Alzheimer's disease. Description of study cohort and accuracy of diagnosis. *Archives of Neurology* **51**: 585–94.

Becker JT, Huff FJ, Nebes RD *et al.* (1988) Neuropsychological function in Alzheimer's disease. Pattern of impairment and rates of progression. *Archives of Neurology* **45**: 263–8.

Berg L, Miller JP, Storandt M *et al.* (1988) Mild senile dementia of the Alzheimer type: 2. Longitudinal assessment. *Annals of Neurology* **23**: 477–84.

Bianchetti A, Scuratti A, Zanetti O *et al.* (1995) Predictors of mortality and institutionalization in Alzheimer disease patients 1 year after discharge from an Alzheimer dementia unit. *Dementia* **6**: 108–12.

Bowen JD, Malter AD, Sheppard L *et al.* (1996) Predictors of mortality in patients diagnosed with probable Alzheimer's disease. *Neurology* **47**: 433–9.

Bracco L, Gallato R, Grigoletto F *et al.* (1994) Factors affecting course and survival in Alzheimer's disease. A 9-year longitudinal study. *Archives of Neurology* **51**: 1213–19.

Brouwers P, Cox C, Martin A *et al.* (1984) Differential perceptual-spatial impairment in Huntington's and Alzheimer's dementias. *Archives of Neurology* **41**: 1073–6.

Burns A, Jacoby R, Levy R. (1990) Psychiatric phenomena in Alzheimer's disease. IV: Disorders of behaviour. *British Journal of Psychiatry* **157**: 86–94.

Burns A, Jacoby R, Levy R. (1991) Progression of cognitive impairment in Alzheimer's disease. *Journal of the American Geriatrics Society* **39**: 39–45.

Burns A, Lewis G, Jacoby R, Levy R. (1991) Factors affecting survival in Alzheimer's disease. *Psychological Medicine* **21**: 363–70.

Chen JY, Stern Y, Sano M, Mayeux R. (1991) Cumulative risks of developing extrapyramidal signs, psychosis, or myoclonus in the course of Alzheimer's disease. *Archives of Neurology* **48**: 1141–3.

Chui HC, Lyness SA, Sobel E, Schneider LS. (1994) Extrapyramidal signs and psychiatric symptoms predict faster cognitive decline in Alzheimer's disease. *Archives of Neurology* **51**: 676–81.

Claus JJ, van Gool WA, Teunisse S *et al.* (1998) Predicting survival in patients with early Alzheimer's disease. *Dementia and Geriatric Cognitive Disorders* **9**: 284–93.

Cook SE, Miyahara S, Bacanu SA *et al.* (2003) Psychotic symptoms in Alzheimer disease: Evidence for subtypes. *American Journal of Geriatric Psychiatry* **11**: 406–13.

Corder EH, Saunders AM, Strittmatter WJ *et al.* (1995) Apolipoprotein E, survival in Alzheimer's disease patients, and the competing risks of death and Alzheimer's disease. *Neurology* **45**: 1323–8.

Corey-Bloom J, Galasko D, Hofstetter CR *et al.* (1993) Clinical features distinguishing large cohorts with possible AD, probable AD, and mixed dementia. *Journal of the American Geriatrics Society* **41**: 31–7.

Craft S, Teri L, Edland SD *et al.* (1998) Accelerated decline in apolipoprotein E-epsilon4 homozygotes with Alzheimer's disease. *Neurology* **51**: 149–53.

Cummings JL, Benson F, Hill MA, Read S. (1985) Aphasia in dementia of the Alzheimer type. *Neurology* **35**: 394–7.

Cummings JL, Miller B, Hill MA, Neshkes R. (1987) Neuropsychiatric aspects of multi-infarct dementia and dementia of the Alzheimer type. *Archives of Neurology* **44**: 389–93.

Cummings JL, Cole G. (2002) Alzheimer disease. *Journal of the American Medical Association* **287**: 2335–8.

Dal Forno G, Carson KA, Brookmeyer R *et al.* (2002) APOE genotype and survival in men and women with Alzheimer's disease. *Neurology* **58**: 1045–50.

Drachman DA, O'Donnell BF, Lew RA, Swearer JM. (1990) The prognosis in Alzheimer's disease. 'How far' rather than 'how fast' best predicts the course. *Archives of Neurology* **47**: 851–6.

Drevets WC, Rubin EH. (1989) Psychotic symptoms and the longitudinal course of senile dementia of the Alzheimer type. *Biological Psychiatry* **25**: 39–48.

Eaker ED, Vierkant RA, Mickel SF. (2002) Predictors of nursing home admission and/or death in incident Alzheimer's disease and other dementia cases compared to controls: A population-based study. *Journal of Clinical Epidemiology* **55**: 462–8.

Evans DA, Smith LA, Scherr PA *et al.* (1991) Risk of death from Alzheimer's disease in a community population of older persons. *American Journal of Epidemiology* **134**: 403–12.

Filley CM, Brownell HH, Albert ML. (1985) Education provides no protection against Alzheimer's disease. *Neurology* **35**: 1781–4.

Fleisher AS, Olichney JM. (2005) Neurodegenerative disorders with diffuse cortical Lewy bodies. *Advances in Neurology* **96**: 148–65.

Frisoni GB, Govoni S, Geroldi C *et al.* (1995) Gene dose of the epsilon 4 allele of apolipoprotein E and disease progression in sporadic late-onset Alzheimer's disease. *Annals of Neurology* **37**: 596–604.

Galasko D, Kwo-on-Yuen PF, Klauber MR, Thal LJ. (1990) Neurological findings in Alzheimer's disease and normal aging. *Archives of Neurology* **47**: 625–7.

Gambassi G, Landi F, Lapane KL *et al.* (1999) Predictors of mortality in patients with Alzheimer's disease living in nursing homes. *Journal of Neurology, Neurosurgery, and Psychiatry* **67**: 59–65.

Gaugler JE, Kane RL, Kane RA *et al.* (2003) Caregiving and institutionalization of cognitively impaired older people: Utilizing dynamic predictors of change. *Gerontologist* **43**: 219–29.

Gaugler JE, Yu F, Krichbaum K, Wyman JF. (2009) Predictors of nursing home admission for persons with dementia. *Medical Care* **47**: 191–8.

Geerlings MI, Deeg DJ, Schmand B *et al.* (1997) Increased risk of mortality in Alzheimer's disease patients with higher education? A replication study. *Neurology* **49**: 798–802.

Gomez-Isla T, West HL, Rebeck GW *et al.* (1996) Clinical and pathological correlates of apolipoprotein E epsilon 4 in Alzheimer's disease. *Annals of Neurology* **39**: 62–70.

Growdon JH, Locascio JJ, Corkin S *et al.* (1996) Apolipoprotein E genotype does not influence rates of cognitive decline in Alzheimer's disease. *Neurology* **47**: 444–8.

Haan MN, Jagust WJ, Galasko D, Kaye J. (2002) Effect of extrapyramidal signs and Lewy bodies on survival in patients with Alzheimer disease. *Archives of Neurology* **59**: 588–93.

Hanyu H, Sato T, Hirao K *et al.* (2009) Differences in clinical course between dementia with Lewy bodies and Alzheimer's disease. *European Journal of Neurology* **16**: 212–17.

Haskell SG, Richardson ED, Horwitz RI. (1997) The effect of estrogen replacement therapy on cognitive function in women: A critical review of the literature. *Journal of Clinical Epidemiology* **50**: 1249–64.

Haupt M, Kurz A. (1993) Predictors of nursing home placement in patients with Alzheimer's disease. *Internation Journal of Geriatric Psychiatry* **8**: 741–6.

Hauser WA, Morris ML, Heston LL, Anderson VE. (1986) Seizures and myoclonus in patients with Alzheimer's disease. *Neurology* **36**: 1226–30.

Helmes E, Ostbye T. (2002) Beyond memory impairment: Cognitive changes in Alzheimer's disease. *Archives of Clinical Neuropsychology* **17**: 179–93.

Heston LL, Mastri AR, Anderson VE, White J. (1981) Dementia of the Alzheimer type. Clinical genetics, natural history, and associated conditions. *Archives of General Psychiatry* **38**: 1085–90.

Heyman A, Wilkinson WE, Hurwitz BJ *et al.* (1987) Early-onset Alzheimer's disease: Clinical predictors of institutionalization and death. *Neurology* **37**: 980–4.

Heyman A, Peterson B, Fillenbaum G, Pieper C. (1996) The consortium to establish a registry for Alzheimer's disease

(CERAD). Part XIV: Demographic and clinical predictors of survival in patients with Alzheimer's disease. *Neurology* **46**: 656–60.

Heyman A, Peterson B, Fillenbaum G, Pieper C. (1997) Predictors of time to institutionalization of patients with Alzheimer's disease: The CERAD experience, part XVII. *Neurology* **48**: 1304–9.

Hier DB, Warach JD, Gorelick PB, Thomas J. (1989) Predictors of survival in clinically diagnosed Alzheimer's disease and multi-infarct dementia. *Archives of Neurology* **46**: 1213–16.

Hirono N, Hashimoto M, Yasuda M et al. (2003) Accelerated memory decline in Alzheimer's disease with apolipoprotein epsilon4 allele. *Journal of Neuropsychiatry and Clinical Neurosciences* **15**: 354–8.

Hooker K, Bowman SR, Coehlo DP et al. (2002) Behavioral change in persons with dementia: Relationships with mental and physical health of caregivers. *Journals of Gerontology. Series B Psychological Sciences and Social Sciences* **57**: P453–60.

Hughes CP, Berg L, Danziger WL et al. (1982) A new clinical scale for the staging of dementia. *British Journal of Psychiatry* **140**: 566–72.

Hutton JT, Dippel RL, Loewenson RB et al. (1985) Predictors of nursing home placement of patients with Alzheimer's disease. *Texas Medicine* **81**: 40–3.

Jacobs D, Sano M, Marder K et al. (1994) Age at onset of Alzheimer's disease: Relation to pattern of cognitive dysfunction and rate of decline. *Neurology* **44**: 1215–20.

Jagger C, Clarke M, Stone A. (1995) Predictors of survival with Alzheimer's disease: A community-based study. *Psychological Medicine* **25**: 171–7.

Jones RW, Schwam E, Wilkinson D et al. (2009) Rates of cognitive change in Alzheimer disease: Observations across a decade of placebo-controlled clinical trials with donepezil. *Alzheimer Disease and Associated Disorders* **23**: 357–64.

Jorm AF, Korten AE, Henderson AS. (1987) The prevalence of dementia: A quantitative integration of the literature. *Acta Psychiatrica Scandinavica* **76**: 465–79.

Jost BC, Grossberg GT. (1995) The natural history of Alzheimer's disease: A brain bank study. *Journal of the American Geriatrics Society* **43**: 1248–55.

Jost BC, Grossberg GT. (1996) The evolution of psychiatric symptoms in Alzheimer's disease: A natural history study. *Journal of the American Geriatrics Society* **44**: 1078–81.

Katzman R. (1976) Editorial: The prevalence and malignancy of Alzheimer disease. A major killer. *Archives of Neurology* **33**: 217–18.

Katzman R, Brown T, Thal LJ et al. (1988) Comparison of rate of annual change of mental status score in four independent studies of patients with Alzheimer's disease. *Annals of Neurology* **24**: 384–9.

Kavcic V, Duffy CJ. (2003) Attentional dynamics and visual perception: Mechanisms of spatial disorientation in Alzheimer's disease. *Brain* **126**: 1173–81.

Knopman DS, Kitto J, Deinard S, Heiring J. (1988) Longitudinal study of death and institutionalization in patients with primary degenerative dementia. *Journal of the American Geriatrics Society* **36**: 108–12.

Kramer-Ginsberg E, Mohs RC, Aryan M et al. (1988) Clinical predictors of course for Alzheimer patients in a longitudinal study: A preliminary report. *Psychopharmacology Bulletin* **24**: 458–62.

Kurz A, Egensperger R, Haupt M et al. (1996) Apolipoprotein E epsilon 4 allele, cognitive decline, and deterioration of everyday performance in Alzheimer's disease. *Neurology* **47**: 440–3.

Lapane KL, Gambassi G, Landi F et al. (2001) Gender differences in predictors of mortality in nursing home residents with AD. *Neurology* **56**: 650–4.

Lazarus LW, Newton N, Cohler B et al. (1987) Frequency and presentation of depressive symptoms in patients with primary degenerative dementia. *American Journal of Psychiatry* **144**: 41–5.

Lee JH, Olichney JM, Hansen LA et al. (2000) Small concomitant vascular lesions do not influence rates of cognitive decline in patients with Alzheimer disease. *Archives of Neurology* **57**: 1474–9.

Lopez OL, Boller F, Becker JT et al. (1990) Alzheimer's disease and depression: Neuropsychological impairment and progression of the illness. *American Journal of Psychiatry* **147**: 855–60.

Lopez OL, Wisniewski SR, Becker JT et al. (1999) Psychiatric medication and abnormal behavior as predictors of progression in probable Alzheimer disease. *Archives of Neurology* **56**: 1266–72.

Lopez OL, Wisniewski S, Hamilton RL et al. (2000) Predictors of progression in patients with AD and Lewy bodies. *Neurology* **54**: 1774–9.

Lucca U, Comelli M, Tettamanti M et al. (1993) Rate of progression and prognostic factors in Alzheimer's disease: A prospective study. *Journal of the American Geriatrics Society* **41**: 45–9.

Lyketsos CG, Lopez O, Jones B et al. (2002) Prevalence of neuropsychiatric symptoms in dementia and mild cognitive impairment: Results from the cardiovascular health study. *Journal of the American Medical Association* **288**: 1475–83.

Martin DC, Miller JK, Kapoor W et al. (1987) A controlled study of survival with dementia. *Archives of Neurology* **44**: 1122–6.

Mayeux R, Stern Y, Spanton S. (1985) Heterogeneity in dementia of the Alzheimer type: Evidence of subgroups. *Neurology* **35**: 453–61.

McGonigal G, McQuade CA, Thomas BM, Whalley LJ. (1992) Survival in presenile Alzheimer's and multi-infarct dementias. *Neuroepidemiology* **11**: 121–6.

Mega MS, Masterman DM, O'Connor SM et al. (1999) The spectrum of behavioral responses to cholinesterase inhibitor therapy in Alzheimer disease. *Archives of Neurology* **56**: 1388–93.

Miller TP, Tinklenberg JR, Brooks III JO, Yesavage JA. (1991) Cognitive decline in patients with Alzheimer disease: Differences in patients with and without extrapyramidal signs. *Alzheimer Disease and Associated Disorders* **5**: 251–6.

Molsa PK, Marttila RJ, Rinne UK. (1986) Survival and cause of death in Alzheimer's disease and multi-infarct dementia. *Acta Neurologica Scandinavica* **74**: 103–7.

Molsa PK, Marttila RJ, Rinne UK. (1995) Long-term survival and predictors of mortality in Alzheimer's disease and multi-infarct dementia. *Acta Neurologica Scandinavica* **91**: 159–64.

Moritz DJ, Fox PJ, Luscombe FA, Kraemer HC. (1997) Neurological and psychiatric predictors of mortality in patients with Alzheimer disease in California. *Archives of Neurology* 54: 878–85.

Morris JC. (1997) Clinical dementia rating: A reliable and valid diagnostic and staging measure for dementia of the Alzheimer type. *International Psychogeriatrics* 9: 173–6.

Morris JC, Edland S, Clark C et al. (1993) The consortium to establish a registry for Alzheimer's disease (CERAD). Part IV. Rates of cognitive change in the longitudinal assessment of probable Alzheimer's disease. *Neurology* 43: 2457–65.

Morris JC, Ernesto C, Schafer K et al. (1997) Clinical dementia rating training and reliability in multicenter studies: The Alzheimer's Disease Cooperative Study experience. *Neurology* 48: 1508–10.

Mortimer JA, Ebbitt B, Jun SP, Finch MD. (1992) Predictors of cognitive and functional progression in patients with probable Alzheimer's disease. *Neurology* 42: 1689–96.

Mungas D, Reed BR, Ellis WG, Jagust WJ. (2001) The effects of age on rate of progression of Alzheimer disease and dementia with associated cerebrovascular disease. *Archives of Neurology* 58: 1243–7.

Murdoch BE, Chenery HJ, Wilks V, Boyle RS. (1987) Language disorders in dementia of the Alzheimer type. *Brain and Language* 31: 122–37.

Musicco M, Palmer K, Salamone G et al. (2009) Predictors of progression of cognitive decline in Alzheimer's disease: The role of vascular and sociodemographic factors. *Journal of Neurology* 256: 1288–95.

Ortof E, Crystal HA. (1989) Rate of progression of Alzheimer's disease. *Journal of the American Geriatrics Society* 37: 511–14.

Pearson JL, Teri L, Reifler BV, Raskind MA. (1989) Functional status and cognitive impairment in Alzheimer's patients with and without depression. *Journal of the American Geriatrics Society* 37: 1117–21.

Quinn JF, Raman R, Thomas RG et al. (2009) A clinical trial of docosohexanoic acid (DHA) for the treatment of Alzheimer's disease. Paper presented at the International Conference on Alzheimer's Disease, Vienna, July 2009.

Rapcsak SZ, Croswell SC, Rubens AB. (1989) Apraxia in Alzheimer's disease. *Neurology* 39: 664–8.

Reisberg B, Ferris SH, de Leon MJ, Crook T. (1982) The Global Deterioration Scale for assessment of primary degenerative dementia. *American Journal of Psychiatry* 139: 1136–9.

Reisberg B, Ferris SH, Shulman E et al. (1986) Longitudinal course of normal aging and progressive dementia of the Alzheimer's type: A prospective study of 106 subjects over a 3.6 year mean interval. *Progress in Neuropsychopharmacology and Biological Psychiatry* 10: 571–8.

Reisberg B, Borenstein J, Salob SP et al. (1987) Behavioral symptoms in Alzheimer's disease: phenomenology and treatment. *Journal of Clinical Psychiatry* 48 (Suppl): 9–15.

Reisberg B, Ferris SH, de Leon MJ et al. (1989) The stage specific temporal course of Alzheimer's disease: Functional and behavioral concomitants based upon cross-sectional and longitudinal observation. *Progress in Clinical Biological Research* 317: 23–41.

Reisberg B, Ferris SH, Franssen EH et al. (1996) Mortality and temporal course of probable Alzheimer's disease: A 5-year prospective study. *International Psychogeriatrics* 8: 291–311.

Rich JB, Rasmusson DX, Folstein MF et al. (1995) Nonsteroidal anti-inflammatory drugs in Alzheimer's disease. *Neurology* 45: 51–5.

Rockwood K, Kirkland S, Hogan DB et al. (2002) Use of lipid-lowering agents, indication bias, and the risk of dementia in community-dwelling elderly people. *Archives of Neurology* 59: 223–7.

Rosen J, Zubenko GS. (1991) Emergence of psychosis and depression in the longitudinal evaluation of Alzheimer's disease. *Biological Psychiatry* 29: 224–32.

Rosen WG, Mohs RC, Davis KL. (1984) A new rating scale for Alzheimer's disease. *American Journal of Psychiatry* 141: 1356–64.

Roth M, Tym E, Mountjoy CQ et al. (1986) CAMDEX. A standardised instrument for the diagnosis of mental disorder in the elderly with special reference to the early detection of dementia. *British Journal of Psychiatry* 149: 698–709.

Salmon DP, Thal LJ, Butters N, Heindel WC. (1990) Longitudinal evaluation of dementia of the Alzheimer type: A comparison of 3 standardized mental status examinations. *Neurology* 40: 1225–30.

Samson WN, van Duijn CM, Hop WC, Hofman A. (1996) Clinical features and mortality in patients with early-onset Alzheimer's disease. *European Neurology* 36: 103–6.

Sano M, Ernesto C, Thomas RG et al. (1997) A controlled trial of selegiline, alpha-tocopherol, or both as treatment for Alzheimer's disease. The Alzheimer's Disease Cooperative Study. *New England Journal of Medicine* 336: 1216–22.

Schneider LS. (1992) Tracking dementia by the IMC and the MMSE. *Journal of the American Geriatrics Society* 40: 537–8.

Schoenberg BS, Kokmen E, Okazaki H. (1987) Alzheimer's disease and other dementing illnesses in a defined United States population: Incidence rates and clinical features. *Annals of Neurology* 22: 724–9.

Shumaker SA, Legault C, Rapp SR et al. (2003) Estrogen plus progestin and the incidence of dementia and mild cognitive impairment in postmenopausal women: The Women's Health Initiative Memory Study: A randomized controlled trial. *Journal of the American Medical Association* 289: 2651–62.

Starkstein SE, Mizrahi R, Power BD. (2008) Depression in Alzheimer's disease: Phenomenology, clinical correlates and treatment. *International Review of Psychiatry* 20: 382–8.

Stern Y, Mayeux R, Sano M et al. (1987) Predictors of disease course in patients with probable Alzheimer's disease. *Neurology* 37: 1649–53.

Stern Y, Hesdorffer D, Sano M, Mayeux R. (1990) Measurement and prediction of functional capacity in Alzheimer's disease. *Neurology* 40: 8–14.

Stern Y, Albert M, Brandt J et al. (1994) Utility of extrapyramidal signs and psychosis as predictors of cognitive and functional decline, nursing home admission, and death in Alzheimer's disease: prospective analyses from the Predictors Study. *Neurology* 44: 2300–7.

Stern Y, Tang MX, Denaro J, Mayeux R. (1995) Increased risk of mortality in Alzheimer's disease patients with more advanced educational and occupational attainment. *Annals of Neurology* **37**: 590–5.

Stern Y, Brandt J, Albert M *et al.* (1997) The absence of an apolipoprotein ε4 allele is associated with a more aggressive form of Alzheimer's disease. *Annals of Neurology* **41**: 615–20.

Storandt M, Grant EA, Miller JP, Morris JC. (2002) Rates of progression in mild cognitive impairment and early Alzheimer's disease. *Neurology* **59**: 1034–41.

Sullivan EV, Corkin S, Growdon JH. (1986) Verbal and nonverbal short-term memory in patients with Alzheimer's disease and in healthy elderly subjects. *Developmental Neuropsychology* **2**: 387–400.

Swanwick GR, Coen RF, Coakley D, Lawlor BA. (1998) Assessment of progression and prognosis in 'possible' and 'probable' Alzheimer's disease. *International Journal of Geriatric Psychiatry* **13**: 331–5.

Teri L, Larson EB, Reifler BV. (1988) Behavioral disturbance in dementia of the Alzheimer's type. *Journal of the American Geriatrics Society* **36**: 1–6.

Teri L, Hughes JP, Larson EB. (1990) Cognitive deterioration in Alzheimer's disease: Behavioral and health factors. *Journal of Gerontology* **45**: P58–63.

Teri L, McCurry SM, Edland SD *et al.* (1995) Cognitive decline in Alzheimer's disease: A longitudinal investigation of risk factors for accelerated decline. *Journals of Gerontology. Series A, Biological Sciences and Medical Sciences* **50A**: M49–55.

Thal LJ, Grundman M, Klauber MR. (1988) Dementia: Characteristics of a referral population and factors associated with progression. *Neurology* **38**: 1083–90.

Thal LJ, Calvani M, Amato A, Carta A. (2000) A 1-year controlled trial of acetyl-l-carnitine in early-onset AD. *Neurology* **55**: 805–10.

Thal LJ, Thomas RG, Mulnard R *et al.* (2003) Estrogen levels do not correlate with improvement in cognition. *Archives of Neurology* **60**: 209–12.

Tilvis RS, Strandberg TE, Juva K. (1998) Apolipoprotein E phenotypes, dementia and mortality in a prospective population sample. *Journal of the American Geriatrics Society* **46**: 712–15.

Tschampa HJ, Neumann M, Zerr I *et al.* (2001) Patients with Alzheimer's disease and dementia with Lewy bodies mistaken for Creutzfeldt–Jakob disease. *Journal of Neurology, Neurosurgery, and Psychiatry* **71**: 33–9.

Ueki A, Shinjo H, Shimode H *et al.* (2001) Factors associated with mortality in patients with early-onset Alzheimer's disease: A five-year longitudinal study. *International Journal of Geriatric Psychiatry* **16**: 810–5.

van Dijk PT, Dippel DW, Habbema JD. (1991) Survival of patients with dementia. *Journal of the American Geriatrics Society* **39**: 603–10.

Walsh JS, Welch HG, Larson EB. (1990) Survival of outpatients with Alzheimer-type dementia. *Annals of Internal Medicine* **113**: 429–34.

Weisman D, Cho M, Taylor C *et al.* (2007) In dementia with Lewy bodies, Braak stage determines phenotype, not Lewy body distribution. *Neurology* **69**: 356–9.

Wilson RS, Bacon LD, Fox JH, Kaszniak AW. (1983) Primary memory and secondary memory in dementia of the Alzheimer type. *Journal of Clinical Neuropsychology* **5**: 337–44.

Winblad B, Engedal K, Soininen H *et al.* (2001) A 1-year, randomized, placebo-controlled study of donepezil in patients with mild to moderate AD. *Neurology* **57**: 489–95.

Wolfson C, Oremus M, Shukla V *et al.* (2002) Donepezil and rivastigmine in the treatment of Alzheimer's disease: A best-evidence synthesis of the published data on their efficacy and cost-effectiveness. *Clinical Therapeutics* **24**: 862–6.

Wragg RE, Jeste DV. (1989) Overview of depression and psychosis in Alzheimer's disease. *American Journal of Psychiatry* **146**: 577–87.

Yaffe K, Grady D, Pressman A, Cummings S. (1998) Serum estrogen levels, cognitive performance, and risk of cognitive decline in older community women. *Journal of the American Geriatrics Society* **46**: 816–21.

Yesavage JA, Poulsen SL, Sheikh J, Tanke E. (1988) Rates of change of common measures of impairment in senile dementia of the Alzheimer's type. *Psychopharmacology Bulletin* **24**: 531–4.

49

The neuropathology of Alzheimer's disease

COLIN L MASTERS

49.1 INTRODUCTION

Although Alzheimer (1907) highlighted the two key histological lesions, amyloid plaques and neurofibrillary tangles (NFTs) more than 100 years ago, recent developments in molecular biology, molecular genetics, immunohistochemistry, image analysis and protein chemistry have transformed our understanding of the pathogenesis of Alzheimer's disease (AD). For practising neuropathologists, immunohistochemistry in particular has become an essential part of the diagnostic armoury to complement the neurohistology of the common neurodegenerative conditions.

49.2 PATHOLOGIC CHANGES OUTSIDE THE CENTRAL NERVOUS SYSTEM

General post-mortem examination does not reveal any specific abnormalities outside the central nervous system (CNS). Patients with AD usually die from terminal respiratory illness, and bronchopneumonia is most often the cause of death. Ongoing investigations have, however, revealed that subtle biochemical abnormalities may not be restricted to the brain. AD may, like a systemic illness, cause secondary changes in the cerebrospinal fluid (CSF) and peripheral blood which reflect neuronal metabolism of the amyloid beta (Aβ) amyloid and tau proteins. As the disease progresses, the total metabolic pools of Aβ and tau increase within the brain, CSF and blood, even though the Aβ levels in CSF and blood decrease as the disease develops (Ritchie *et al.*, 2003; Bates *et al.*, 2009; Craig-Shapiro *et al.*, 2009; Fagan *et al.*, 2009).

That sensory outposts associated with the brain undergo degeneration has been suspected for some time. The optic nerve (Hinton *et al.*, 1986) and retinal ganglion cells (Blanks *et al.*, 1989) show degenerative changes and the anterior olfactory nucleus develops NFTs (Esiri and Wilcock, 1984). In addition, abnormalities in the processes of olfactory neurones in the nasal mucosa have been reported (Talamo *et al.*, 1989) and tau-reactive filaments, absent from controls, have been described in the olfactory mucosa in biopsy specimens of patients with probable AD (Tabaton *et al.*, 1991a). Deposition of Aβ in the periphery of the lens may also be linked to AD, although more studies are required to confirm this association (Goldstein *et al*, 2003).

49.3 MACROSCOPIC NEUROPATHOLOGIC CHANGES

The naked eye appearances of the brain range from unremarkable to grossly abnormal. The leptomeninges may be thickened, particularly over the convexity, and may show orange-brown areas of various sizes, indicating old, circumscribed subarachnoid haemorrhages, which most often result from amyloid (congophilic) angiopathy (ACA). The cranial nerves are normal and the large cerebral vessels in uncomplicated cases of AD have not been damaged more by atherosclerosis than expected for the patient's age. Brain weight is quite often reduced, sometimes below 1000 g. Since brain weight normally depends on the patient's age, sex and constitution, the degree of atrophy should be considered in the light of these factors. A discrepancy between the findings of neuroimaging and neuropathology is not unusual: cerebral atrophy reported on computed tomography scans or magnetic resonance imaging may not always be confirmed at post-mortem examination. Agonal changes of haemodynamics, post-mortem delay, and the effects of fixation on the brain may be partly responsible for this discrepancy. The normal ratio of 8:1 of total brain weight to that of the brainstem and cerebellum may decrease, indicating loss of tissue from the cerebral hemispheres. The atrophy is usually diffuse and symmetrical, although the frontoparietal region and the temporal lobes may be more severely affected than the rest of the brain (**Figure 49.1**). Moderate-to-severe atrophy is easy to discern: the sulci are widened and the gyri narrowed both on the outside and on coronal slices. These latter also reveal enlarged lateral ventricles with rounded angles and additional space between the hippocampi and the wall of the temporal horns. Decrease in the thickness of neocortical ribbon, apart from extreme cases of atrophy, is difficult, and may prove deceptive, to assess on naked-eye appearances. A quantitative study, however, revealed a decrease of neocortical areas of all lobes in AD, whereas in patients over the age of 80, only the temporal cortex was atrophied (Hubbard and Anderson, 1981; Hubbard and Anderson, 1985). Reduction in cortical area may result from a decrease in the length rather than in the width of cortex, indicating loss of columns of cells and fibres perpendicular to the pial surface. A correlation appears to exist between the length, but not the thickness, of the cortical ribbon and dementia score (Duyckaerts *et al.*, 1985). Apart from

occasional small, orange-coloured old haemorrhages in the cortex, suggestive of ACA, uncomplicated AD usually is not associated with any other focal lesions. There is a growing awareness that the topographic dispersion of the lesions of AD are related to an underlying functional property of the higher nervous system. The brain's 'default network' may explain why certain areas are more affected by atrophy and amyloid deposition (Buckner *et al.*, 2009; Dickerson *et al.*, 2009). In turn, the evolution of amyloid deposition at the macroscopic scale is now able to be visualized by positron emission tomography (PET)-amyloid tracers as the disease begins and progresses (Rowe *et al*, 2007; Jack *et al*, 2009; see Chapter 13, Molecular brain imaging in dementia).

49.4   HISTOLOGY, ULTRASTRUCTURE, IMMUNOCYTOCHEMISTRY AND MORPHOMETRY

The neurohistological features of AD are complex and variable. The two hallmark lesions, amyloid plaques and NFTs (**Figure 49.2**) are complemented by granulovacuolar degeneration, Hirano bodies, neuronal and synaptic loss, abnormalities of neuronal processes and synapses, astrocytic and microglial response, and vascular changes. The white matter may also be affected (Esiri *et al.*, 1997).

49.4.1   Amyloid plaques

The amyloid or neuritic plaque ('senile' plaque) is one of the major lesions found in the AD brain, first described by Blocq and Marinesco in 1892 (Blocq and Marinesco, 1892). These structures, ranging in size from 50 to 200 μm (Terry, 1985), can be readily demonstrated in frozen and paraffin-embedded sections by silver impregnation methods (**Figure 49.3**) and immunocytochemistry. The lesion consists of an Aβ amyloid core with a corona of argyrophilic axonal and dendritic processes, Aβ amyloid fibrils, glial cell processes and microglial cells. Neuritic processes in the periphery of the plaque are frequently dystrophic and contain paired helical

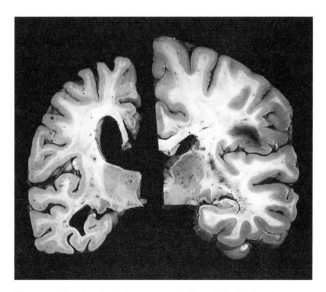

Figure 49.1   On the left, a coronal slice of the brain of a patient with severe Alzheimer's disease showing atrophy: the lateral ventricle is enlarged with rounding of its angle and there is additional space between the hippocampus and the inferior horn of the lateral ventricle. Several gyri are narrowed and the lateral fissure is widened. On the right, a slice of the right hemibrain of a normal subject.

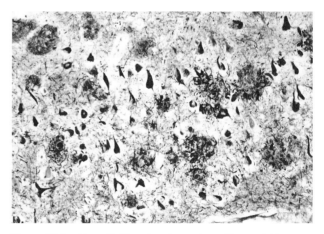

Figure 49.2   Neurofibrillary tangles and neuritic amyloid plaques in the neocortex. Modified Bielschowsky silver impregnation.

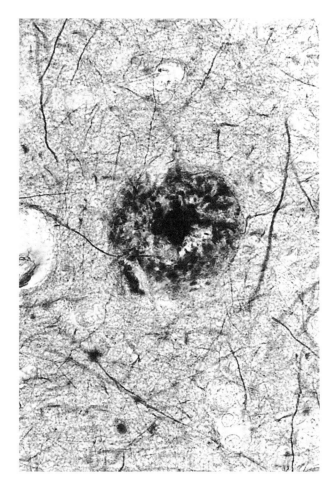

Figure 49.3 An argyrophilic amyloid plaque in the neocortex showing a neuritic ring with an amyloid core formation. Modified Bielschowsky silver impregnation.

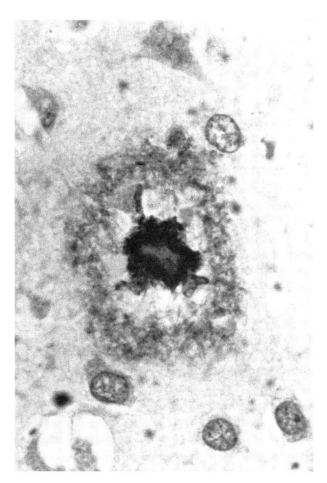

Figure 49.4 An amyloid plaque with a dense core and corona. Aβ-amyloid immunohistochemistry.

filaments, which are composed largely of ubiquinated and phosphorylated tau protein (Gonatas *et al.*, 1967; Hanger *et al.*, 1991). In 1927, Divry (Divry, 1927) demonstrated that the core of the AD plaque contained a congophilic amyloid substance which gave an apple green colour under polarized light. The plaque amyloid is composed of 5–10 nm filaments made up of a 38–43 amino acid (4 kDa) peptide (Masters *et al.*, 1985), now referred to as Aβ peptide, derived from neurones by proteolytic cleavage of the amyloid precursor protein (APP) (Kang *et al.*, 1987).

Three types of plaque have been identified in conventional silver staining preparations: 'primitive' or 'early', 'classical' or 'mature', and 'burnt-out' or 'compact'. On the basis of light and electron microscopic studies, a three-stage evolution of the plaque has been proposed. The first stage is the 'primitive' plaque, composed of a small number of distorted neurites, largely presynaptic in origin with few amyloid fibres, astrocytic processes and the occasional microglial cell. The second stage is the 'classical' or 'mature' plaque with a dense amyloid core with a halo of dystrophic neurites, astrocytic processes and cell bodies and the occasional microglial cell. The final stage in this sequence is the 'burnt-out' plaque consisting of a dense core of amyloid (Terry *et al.*, 1981; Esiri and Morris, 1997). The relationship between dystrophic neurites,

neurofibrillary degeneration and Aβ amyloid deposition is not fully understood (Adalbert *et al.*, 2009), but the neurites and tangles appear to be downstream of Aβ accumulation. These three stages of plaque development have not been confirmed in experimental transgenic mice and therefore the temporal relationships suggested above remain speculative: it may yet transpire that the three types of plaques are independent of each other.

Studies using antibodies raised against Aβ peptide reveal a much more widespread deposition of amyloid than is visualized by traditional staining methods (Majocha *et al.*, 1988; Gentleman *et al.*, 1989; Armstrong *et al.*, 1996; **Figures 49.4, 49.5, 49.6, 49.7 and 49.8**). Aβ immunoreactivity has been detected throughout the CNS including the neocortex, hippocampus, thalamus, amygdala, caudate nucleus, putamen, nucleus basalis of Meynert, midbrain, pons, medulla oblongata, the cerebellar cortex and spinal cord (Joachim *et al.*, 1989; Ogomori *et al.*, 1989). These deposits take a variety of forms and include subpial, vascular, dyshoric, punctate or granular, diffuse, stellar, ring-with-core and compact deposits (Ogomori *et al.*, 1989). A laminar pattern of Aβ deposits in the neocortex has been described with concentrations in layers II, III and V (Majocha *et al.*, 1988).

As noted, the Aβ peptide is a 38–43 residue cleavage product of a larger precursor protein, the APP (Kang *et al.*,

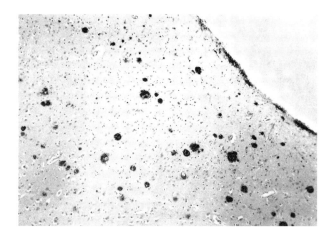

Figure 49.5 Aβ-amyloid protein deposits in the temporal lobe of a patient with Alzheimer's disease. Several deposit morphologies can be seen. Aβ-amyloid immunohistochemistry.

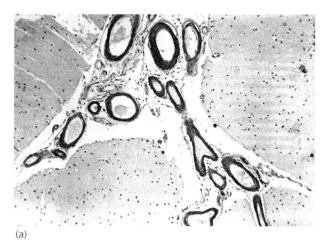

(a)

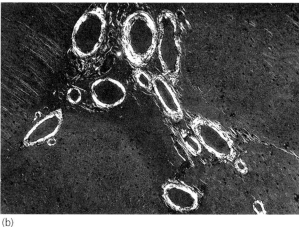

(b)

Figure 49.7 Congophilic angiopathy. Blood vessels stained with Congo red showing birefringence under polarized light (a) and β-amyloid immunohistochemistry (b).

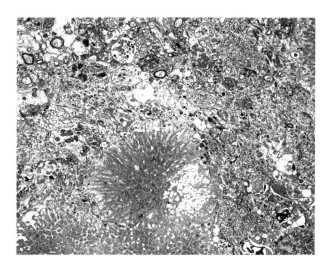

Figure 49.6 A high-power electron micrograph revealing Aβ-amyloid fibrils (A) of a plaque. (Courtesy Dr I Janota, Institute of Psychiatry, London.)

1987). Although most cells have the potential to produce APP, neurones and platelets express APP to high levels. Moreover, neurones process APP with β-secretase (BACE) to a greater extent than most other cell types, which in turn leads to the formation of full Aβ sequences. The theory that Aβ deposition is an early event in AD pathogenesis has been given support by the presence of extracellular Aβ in diffuse plaques not associated with any neuritic change, or astrocytic involvement (Yamaguchi *et al.*, 1991). More condensed Aβ is, however, associated with a neuritic change, reactive astrocytosis and microglial infiltration and phagocytosis. Most species of Aβ have been detected by immunohistochemistry using antibodies that recognize epitopes within the full-length $Aβ_{(1-42)}$ or a truncated $Aβ_{(1-40)}$. The predominant species in sporadic AD is $Aβ_{42(43)}$ and this is found in plaques of all morphological types. Diffuse plaques contain mainly $Aβ_{42(43)}$ (Mann *et al.*, 1996a; Mann *et al.*, 1996b).

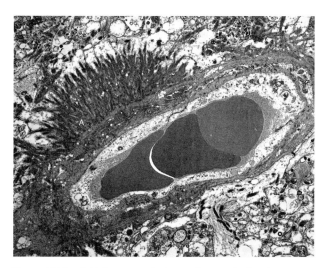

Figure 49.8 A high-power electron micrograph showing β-amyloid fibrils (A) surrounding a blood vessel: dyshoric angiopathy. (Courtesy Dr I Janota, Institute of Psychiatry, London.)

A number of other proteins co-localize with Aβ including apolipoprotein E (ApoE), a widely distributed protein involved in the transport of cholesterol. There are three common isoforms of ApoE which are encoded by three alleles, ε2, ε3 and ε4, and there is a strong association between the presence of the ε4 allele and the age of onset of AD. ApoE has been shown to bind to Aβ and a high proportion of Aβ and ApoE deposits tend to be co-localized. Thus, both diffuse and compact Aβ plaques may be immunolabelled by anti-Aβ and anti-ApoE antibodies (Cairns et al., 1997b; Armstrong et al., 1998). The presence of one or more ε4 alleles leads to both an earlier onset and a more severe Aβ amyloidosis (Roses, 1994; Agosta et al, 2009). The relationship between Aβ and ApoE is still imperfectly understood, as ApoE knock-out mice have an increased amount of Aβ deposition on a transgenic APP background.

The plaques are also immunohistochemically positive for a number of neuroactive substances. Acetylcholinesterase, a marker of the cholinergic system, can be demonstrated within and around the neuritic elements of the corona. Many of these elements derive from cholinergic neurones in the basal forebrain, particularly the nucleus basalis of Meynert, the diagonal band of Broca and the medial septal nuclei. Several other neurotransmitters have been demonstrated in the plaque. These include substance P, neuropeptide Y, neurotensin, cholecystokinin, 5-hydroxytryptamine and catecholamine (Walker et al., 1988; Hauw et al., 1991). Ubiquitin, a protein acting as a signal for degradation of abnormal proteins, is also present in intracellular neurites and NFTs (Perry et al., 1987). The protease inhibitor α1-antichymotrypsin has been localized to the plaque using immunohistochemical methods (Walker et al., 1988). Serum amyloid P component is a glycoprotein complex produced in the liver, distributed in serum, and has been detected in diffuse and consolidated Aβ deposits, NFTs and neuritic degeneration.

The plaques are more numerous in associative regions of neocortex than in sensory areas and are also largest in those laminae characterized by large pyramidal neurones (Rogers and Morrison, 1985). Accumulations of Aβ peptide are found in the neocortex of non-demented elderly individuals without any neurofibrillary change, suggesting that Aβ deposition precedes neurofibrillary changes. However, NFT formation has been reported in areas devoid of Aβ (Braak et al., 1986; Duyckaerts et al., 1988; Delaère et al., 1990; Armstrong et al., 1993), indicating that factors in addition to Aβ may be required to cause aggregation of tau. Tangle-bearing neurones generally project into areas with Aβ deposition, suggesting some form of retrograde transport of the toxic elements which are associated with Aβ.

49.4.2 NFTs

The second histological hallmark of AD is the NFT. These are not specific to AD, since they occur in other neurodegenerative disorders, including Down's syndrome, post-encephalitic parkinsonism, dementia pugilistica, amyotrophic lateral sclerosis–parkinsonism–dementia complex of Guam, subacute sclerosing panencephalitis, dementia with tangles with and without calcification, and in myotonic dystrophy

(Kiuchi et al., 1991). Globose NFTs also develop in progressive supranuclear palsy and sporadic motor neurone disease, but their morphology and ultrastructure differ from those seen in AD.

In AD, NFTs are common in the medial temporal structures, in the hippocampus, amygdala and parahippocampal gyrus, and also occur throughout the neocortex and the deep grey matter including the lentiform nucleus, the nucleus basalis of Meynert, the thalamus, the mamillary bodies, substantia nigra, locus caeruleus, periaqueductal grey matter, the raphé nuclei of the brainstem and the pedunculopontine nucleus.

Neurofibrillary tangles are intracellular inclusions composed of ubiquinated and phosphorylated tau. Their configuration is determined in part by the shape of neurones in which they develop. NFTs are flame-shaped in pyramidal neurones, while in the neurones of the brainstem they assume more complex, globose forms. They can be easily discerned in histological sections stained with haematoxylin and eosin, silver impregnation techniques or with Congo red, which renders them birefringent under polarized light. They can be best demonstrated by immunocytochemistry using antibodies against tau and ubiquitin (**Figure 49.9**).

Electron microscopy reveals the fine structural details (**Figure 49.10**). NFTs are mainly composed of paired helical filaments (Kidd, 1963), which in turn are formed by two filaments wound around each other. Each filament has a diameter of 10 nm with crossover points every 80 nm, resulting in the typical periodicity of a double helix. A negative staining technique has demonstrated that each filament is composed of four protofilaments with a diameter of 3–5 nm (Wisniewski et al., 1984). NFTs also contain straight filaments with an average diameter of 15 nm. These straight and the paired helical filaments may form hybrid filaments, displaying both morphologies, share surface epitopes and have identically shaped structural units. These common features indicate that paired helical and straight filaments are related and they represent only somewhat different assemblies of the same basic molecular unit (Crowther, 1991).

A major component of the NFT is a microtubule-associated protein called tau, which is involved in microtubule assembly and stabilization. In the adult human

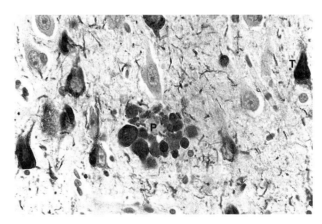

Figure 49.9 A neuritic plaque (P) and neurofibrillary tangles (T) demonstrated by anti-tau immunohistochemistry.

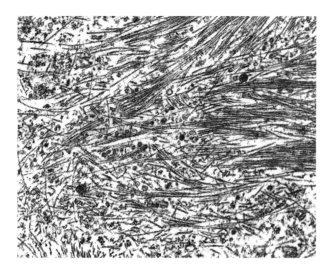

Figure 49.10 A high-power electron micrograph revealing paired helical filaments of a neurofibrillary tangle. (Courtesy of the late Professor LW Duchen, Institute of Psychiatry, London.)

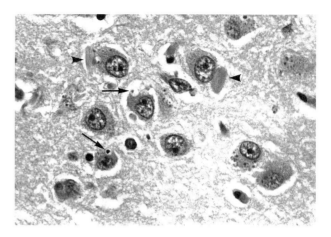

Figure 49.11 Granulovacuolar degeneration (arrows) and Hirano bodies (arrowheads) in the pyramidal cell layer of the hippocampus. Haematoxylin and eosin.

NFTs may be enveloped by glial processes and eventually be internalized as part of their degradative cycle.

49.4.3 Granulovacuolar degeneration

Granulovacuolar degeneration was first described by Simchowicz (1911) in the hippocampal neurones of senile dementia patients (**Figure 49.11**). Granulovacuoles are abnormal cytoplasmic structures: one or more vacuoles of 3.5 mm in diameter each contain a single granule. The electron microscope shows a dense granular core, embedded in a translucent matrix. This granular component gives a positive reaction with antibodies to tubulin (Price *et al.*, 1985), to phosphorylated epitopes of the heavy neurofilament peptide (Kahn *et al.*, 1985), to tau (Dickson *et al.*, 1987) and, in some neurones, to ubiquitin (Leigh *et al.*, 1989). A detailed immunocytochemical study has demonstrated that most epitopes of the tau molecule are sequestered in granulo-vacuoles and this tau protein is antigenically similar to that found in paired helical filaments. Granulovacuoles are now considered to be special autophagosomes that are formed by the sequestration of electron-dense material by a two-layered membrane. Granulovacuoles are virtually restricted to the pyramidal neurones of the hippocampus and in severe AD cases the neuronal cytoplasm is replete with these abnormal structures. They also occur, much less often, in a variety of diseases, including progressive supranuclear palsy, amyotrophic lateral sclerosis–parkinsonism–dementia complex of Guam and tuberous sclerosis.

49.4.4 Hirano bodies

These abnormal structures were first described by Hirano (1965). They are most commonly seen in and among the pyramidal cells of the hippocampus. Hirano bodies occur in normal subjects and their frequency increases with age. However, AD patients have significantly more Hirano bodies than age-matched controls. They also occur in various neurological diseases, including Pick's disease, motor neurone

brain, there are six isoforms of tau and all of these are hyperphosphorylated in AD (Hanger *et al.*, 1991; Goedert *et al.*, 1992). Antibodies that recognize specific phosphorylation-dependent epitopes may be used to identify the three sites of tau aggregation: the NFT, dystrophic neurites of plaques and neuropil threads. Phosphorylation-dependent antibodies may also be used to distinguish the tauopathy in AD from other neurological disorders (Cairns *et al.*, 1997a). Other neuronal inclusions which have confused neuropathologists until recently have been elucidated as containing the TDP-43 protein (Arai *et al.*, 2009). This type of neuronal inclusion is prominent in the frontotemporal lobar atrophies of the non-Pick type, ALS, and also in selected areas of the AD-affected brain. Its significance in AD is the subject of intense scrutiny.

Biochemically, NFTs are composed of phosphorylated isoforms of tau (Goedert *et al.*, 1988), and monoclonal antibodies can be used to quantify NFTs (Harrington *et al.*, 1991). They also contain ubiquitin, and anti-ubiquitin antibodies give strongly positive reaction with NFTs (Mori *et al.*, 1987; Perry *et al.*, 1987).

While NFTs are intracytoplasmic neuronal inclusions, they may become extracellular after the neurone that contained them has vanished. These extraneuronal NFTs are most often seen in the hippocampus and entorhinal cortex in advanced disease, and both their antigenic properties and ultrastructural features differ from their intraneuronal counterparts (Tabaton *et al.*, 1991b). They are chiefly composed of straight, not paired, helical filaments and react differently with antibodies to tau and ubiquitin. A small subset of extraneuronal tangles gives positive reactions with antibodies to both tau and Aβ protein. The degradation of the NFT (the transition from intracellular to extracellular form) is a series of distinct stages involving complex molecular events that alter both the antigenicity and configuration of the tangle (Bondareff *et al.*, 1990). It is the insolubility of NFTs that is most likely to be responsible for the occurrence of extraneuronal forms (Terry, 1990). The extraneuronal disease and kuru, and in animals infected with kuru and scrapie (Gibson and Tomlinson, 1977). Hirano bodies stand out in sections stained with haematoxylin and eosin as bright pink, homogeneous structures which are circular in cross section with a diameter up to 25 μm, and rectangular or spindle-shaped up to 30 μm in length in longitudinal sections. Ultrastructurally, they are composed of a complex, crystalline array of interlacing filaments forming a lattice-like or 'herring-bone' configuration (Tomonaga, 1974). They stain positively with antibodies to actin (Goldman, 1983) and immunostaining for tau has been reported (Galloway et al., 1987).

49.4.5 Neuronal loss

Neuronal loss is far more difficult to assess than the histological abnormalities previously described, although the decrease of particular neuronal populations is more readily accepted than in normal ageing (Terry, 1990). While well-defined, neuronal groups, like the locus ceruleus, are easier to count, the cerebral cortex presents considerable technical problems. Nevertheless, it has been established that there is a significant decrease of 36–46 per cent in the concentration of large neurones, particularly from layers III and V of the neocortex (Terry et al., 1981). The loss of the large cortical neurones is age-dependent: the column of these cells is reduced in patients under 80 years of age, but appears to be normal for age in older subjects (Hubbard and Anderson, 1985). This neuronal loss, however, does not affect the neocortex evenly; it appears to be restricted to the frontal and temporal lobes, whereas the parietal and occipital regions are less involved (Mountjoy et al., 1983). The hippocampus is even more severely affected: neuronal fall-out reaches an average of 47 per cent (Ball, 1977) and the number of pyramidal neurones is reduced by 40 per cent in area H1 (Mann et al., 1985). This loss appears to correlate with the number of tangle-bearing cells, while the end plate and area H2 are less affected. There is also a substantial decrease of neurones in the cholinergic nucleus basalis of Meynert (Whitehouse et al., 1981), in the cholinergic pedunculopontine nucleus (Jellinger, 1988), in the noradrenergic locus ceruleus (Tomlinson et al., 1981; Marcyniuk et al., 1986) and in the serotonergic raphé nuclei in the brainstem (Yamamoto and Hirano, 1985).

49.4.6 Abnormalities of neuronal processes and synapses

Neuropil threads or 'curly' fibres and dystrophic neurites have been well documented in silver impregnated preparations developed by Gallyas (1971), but they attracted attention when it was realized that their occurrence was associated with the severity of dementia (Braak et al., 1986). Neuropil threads or curly fibres are slender, short structures found in the neuropil of the cortex. Dystrophic neurites, some of which contribute to the formation of plaques, also appear as somewhat contorted, thread-like structures in these preparations. These abnormal neurites are likely to be a heterogeneous population of dendrites and axons (Tourtellotte and

Van Hoesen, 1991). Their ultrastructural and immunocytochemical features are strikingly similar to those of NFTs, indicating that they also originate from the altered neuronal cytoskeleton. Neuropil threads immunostain with antibodies to tau (Kowall and Kosik, 1987; Probst et al., 1989) and to ubiquitin (Joachim et al., 1987). Electron microscopy has revealed that they are often in dendrites and contain straight filaments of 14–16 nm in diameter in addition to paired helical filaments (Tabaton et al., 1989; Yamaguchi et al., 1990b). Moreover, they are often in the dendrites of those nerve cells that contain NFTs in their cell body (Braak and Braak, 1988). There is increasing evidence that their distribution is more closely associated with NFTs than with plaques. Considerable decrease of synapses also occurs and this loss is likely to contribute to the development of the disease (Davis et al., 1987). Moreover, immunocytochemical quantification of synaptophysin, a protein localized in pre-synaptic terminals, revealed an average decrease of 50 per cent in the density of the granular neuropil immunoreaction in the parietal, temporal and midfrontal cortex (Masliah et al., 1989). In the electron microscope, some presynaptic terminals were distended and contained altered synaptic organelles, including swollen vesicles and dense bodies, similar to those seen in dystrophic neurites. These latter structures gave positive staining with antibodies to synaptophysin and immunoreactivity was mainly localized to the outer membranes of synaptic vesicles and dense bodies. This finding lends further support to the view that progressive synaptic derangements occur in the neocortex of AD (Masliah et al., 1991).

49.4.7 Glial changes

Astrocytes can be readily observed immunohistochemically by using an antibody to glial fibrillary acidic protein (see **Figure 49.12**). Both NFTs and plaques are more prevalent in the pyramidal cell-rich layers II, III and V than in other laminae (Mann et al., 1985; Majocha et al., 1988; Braak et al., 1989) and both have been associated with patterns of gliosis in AD (Itagakai et al., 1989; Cairns et al., 1992) where perivascular gliosis is prominent throughout the cerebrum. In AD extensive gliosis has a laminar pattern in the neocortex, but there does not appear to be an AD-specific pattern of subcortical gliosis. In addition to NFTs, plaques and dystrophic neurites, reactive astrocytosis is associated with degenerating neurones in AD. In the pathogenesis of the plaque it appears that Aβ deposition is an early event preceding gliosis (Yamaguchi et al., 1990a).

The presence of major histocompatibility complex class II antigens on reactive microglia in association with plaques in AD is indicative of an immune response, although the significance of such expression on the cell surfaces of reactive microglial cells is uncertain. Reactive microglial cells have been found in association with diffuse Aβ deposits and, more frequently, with compact cores of plaques (Itagakai et al., 1989). Leukocyte common antigen and complement receptors, including the cell adhesion molecules, the β-2 integrins, have been localized on microglial cells around plaques. These data are consistent with a phagocytic role for microglia and

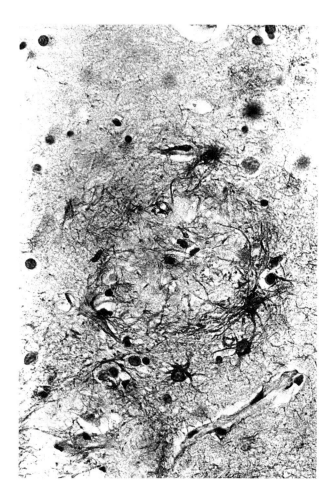

Figure 49.12 Astrocyte cell bodies and processes encircling a plaque. Glial fibrillary acidic protein immunohistochemistry.

provide evidence for an inflammatory response of brain tissue in AD.

49.4.8   Vascular abnormalities

When stained with the dye Congo red, cerebral blood vessels containing amyloid appear apple green under polarized light. Pantelakis (1954) called this deposition congophilic angiopathy (see **Figure 49.7**). These changes affect leptomeningeal and cortical arterioles, and occasionally intracortical capillaries and venules. The parieto-occipital cortex is usually more affected than that in the frontal and temporal lobes and the change is most easily identified in the striate cortex in the occipital lobe. The brainstem and cerebellar cortex are less frequently affected. The occurrence of ACA in conjunction with AD is quite common (Keage *et al.*, 2009).

Vascular amyloid is the same protein as the Aβ amyloid found in plaques. Although vascular amyloid is frequently present in AD, it may be absent even when there are abundant plaques and parenchymal deposits. Occasionally, Aβ appears to extend from the vessel wall into the surrounding cerebral tissue; this is referred to as dyshoric angiopathy (or the *drusige Entartung* of Scholz). This is commonly seen in lamina III of the striate cortex and adjacent occipital cortex, occasionally in Ammon's horn and in the cerebellum (Hauw *et al.*, 1991).

At least three forms of autosomal dominant familial cerebral amyloid angiopathy have been identified at the molecular level. In the Dutch (Levy *et al.*, 1990) and Icelandic forms, patients suffer from recurrent cerebral haemorrhages that lead to an early death (before 40 years of age in Icelandic patients, and between 50 and 60 years in Dutch patients). The amyloid fibrils in patients with the Icelandic type are made up of cystatin C, a degradation product of a larger protease inhibitor. In the Dutch patients, the amyloid fibrils are composed of the same Aβ protein found in amyloid angiopathy in AD, Down's syndrome, and sporadic amyloid angiopathy. In British and Danish pedigrees, another form of diffuse cerebrovascular amyloidosis has elucidated the Worster-Drought syndrome (Masters and Beyreuther, 2001) in which another novel amyloidogenic peptide aggregates in the brain.

49.4.9   White matter changes

Although the degenerative process in AD primarily affects the grey matter, the white matter may not be spared. Computed tomography scans may show areas of hypodensity. The precise pathological substrate remains controversial. Since amyloid angiopathy is often part of AD, it is possible that the white matter changes result mainly from vascular causes. Symmetrical, incomplete infarctions of the white matter histologically correspond to partial loss of myelin sheaths, axons and oligodendrocytes. These changes are accompanied by mild astrocytosis and macrophage response, while there is hyaline fibrosis of small vessels. Cavitating infarctions do not develop and this white matter damage, which occurs in the absence of hypertensive vascular degeneration, is thought to be caused by hypoperfusion (Brun and England, 1986). However, severe loss of cortical neurones may also contribute to fibre loss and consequent pallor of white matter.

49.5   FAMILIAL AD

Alzheimer's disease is a disease primarily of old age and it is difficult to determine the proportion of genetic cases as many family members will die before expressing the disease. Familial forms of AD with multiple affected individuals are rare and account for probably fewer than 5 per cent of AD cases. Mutations in the APP gene and two related genes, presenilin-1 (PS1) and presenilin-2 (PS2), account for the majority of early-onset autosomal dominant cases of familial AD (Lamb, 1997; see Chapter 52, Genetics of Alzheimer's disease). Although clinical features may differ between families, the neuropathological features are not markedly different familial AD and early-onset sporadic cases. However, prominent cerebellar plaques and Aβ deposition have been reported in familial cases (Iseki *et al.*, 1990; Struble *et al.*, 1991; Fukutani *et al.*, 1996; Fukutani *et al.*, 1997). Computerized methods of image analysis have been used to more accurately define the pathological phenotype of AD. Using these techniques, differences in Aβ load have been reported. Mann *et al.* (Mann *et al.*, 1996a; Mann *et al.*, 1996b) have shown that both APP and PS mutations lead to

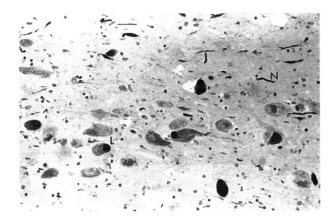

Figure 49.13 Lewy bodies (L) and dystrophic neurites (N) in the midbrain of a patient who died with familial Alzheimer's disease with the amyloid precursor protein 717valine-isoleucine mutation. α-Synuclein immunohistochemistry.

measurable increases in Aβ load. More recent studies using PET-amyloid ligands show a very distinctive accentuation of Aβ amyloid in the striatum (Villemagne *et al.*, 2009).

In those cases with an early onset, below 65 years of age, the duration of illness tends to be shorter, and the density of NFTs and plaques is often greater than in sporadic, late-onset patients. Cortical and brainstem Lewy bodies may coexist with AD in APP (Lantos *et al.*, 1992) and PS mutation patients (**Figure 49.13**). It is now known that the Lewy body and dystrophic neurites of Parkinson's disease and dementia with Lewy bodies contain the protein α-synuclein (Spillantini *et al.*, 1997). Familial and sporadic forms of AD may also be found in combination with cerebrovascular disease. Rare sporadic cases of AD have been found in combination with other neurodegenerative disorders including Pick's disease, Creutzfeldt–Jakob disease, motor neurone disease and progressive supranuclear palsy.

49.6 PATHOGENESIS

While the cause of AD is now clearly defined as the cerebral deposition of Aβ amyloid, the pathogenesis of AD is not fully understood. Although many risk factors have been proposed, the evidence for most of these is weak except for age, family history and ApoE genotype (Alafuzoff *et al.*, 2009; Chen *et al.*, 2009). A genetic contribution to the aetiology of AD has received strong support in recent years and it is likely that more genes (such as LRP, α_2M and IDE) will be associated with the disease. In the more common non-familial, sporadic cases, and in discordant monozygotic twins, environmental factors may be important in the aetiology.

The discovery of mutations in the APP and PS genes, all of which lead to overproduction of Aβ or preferential production of a long 42-amino acid form of Aβ, has confirmed the central role of APP and Aβ deposition in the pathogenesis of AD (Lamb, 1997). Deposition of Aβ appears to be an early event in both AD and Down's syndrome and precedes the development of plaques, NFTs, microgliosis and astrocytosis (Rozemuller *et al.*, 1989; Woltjer *et al.*, 2009). The amyloid

deposits characteristic of AD, 42–43 amino acid Aβ fragments, are the abnormal proteolytic cleavage products of APP. It is known that Aβ has both toxic (Yanker *et al.*, 1989) and trophic effects on neurones in culture, which may relate to plaque and NFT formation.

Metal ions such as aluminium, iron, copper and zinc have been implicated as an environmental toxic agent in the pathogenesis of AD. Accumulations of aluminosilicates and iron in the central region of the core of plaques and within neurones containing NFTs have been reported (Candy *et al.*, 1986). Another environmental factor implicated in Aβ deposition is head trauma. Although Roberts *et al.* (1991) showed that in a series of patients suffering sustained head injury, there were extensive deposits of Aβ in the neocortex, longer term follow-up studies have failed to confirm any association (Chen *et al.*, 2009).

Although varying amounts of Aβ with a range of morphologies may be found in cognitively normal elderly individuals, it is quantitatively much more severe and cytoarchitectonically defined in AD (Majocha *et al.*, 1988; Cairns *et al.*, 1991). The importance of overexpression of APP and its abnormal cleavage product, Aβ, in the pathogenesis of AD has been demonstrated by transgenic mouse models (Borchelt *et al.*, 1998). Transgenic mice expressing the full-length human APP develop Aβ deposits similar in morphology to those found in AD, but as noted above, differing somewhat in their human 'subtype' counterparts. These animal models will be useful for testing anti-amyloid drugs (Morrissette *et al.*, 2009).

49.7 NEUROPATHOLOGY AND CLINICAL FINDINGS

Alzheimer first suggested a correlation between the presence of NFTs, plaques and dementia in 1906. Roth *et al.* (1966) and Wilcock and Esiri (1982) demonstrated that elderly patients' mental test scores correlated with the neuropathological lesions characteristic of AD. Many other neuropathological (Nelson *et al.*, 2009) and neurochemical changes (Zubenko *et al.*, 1991) have been associated with AD and the accuracy of clinical diagnosis ranges from 43 to 87 per cent (Boller *et al.*, 1989; Jellinger *et al.*, 1990) and, in one sample of 26 cases, 100 per cent (Morris *et al.*, 1988). Conversely, inaccuracy in the ante-mortem diagnosis of AD is common, and for this reason, post-mortem examination remains an essential component of AD research. An accurate differential diagnosis is made difficult by the problems of distinguishing between mild dementia and the cognitive changes of 'normal ageing'. Mild cognitive impairment is the earliest clinically recognizable form of AD, which is now being evaluated with *in vivo* neuroimaging of Aβ load using PET radioliogands (Rowe *et al.*, 2008).

Although not all studies have produced positive findings, there is general agreement that cases with earlier onset, shorter duration of illness and greater cognitive impairment have more cortical plaques, whereas late-onset cases which take a milder course tend to show less cortical change (Bowen *et al.*, 1979; Hansen *et al.*, 1988). High correlations were observed between cognitive performance and plaque counts in brain biopsies from dementing patients examined earlier in the course of illness (Mann *et al.*, 1986; Neary *et al.*, 1986; Mann *et al.*, 1988). Plaques and NFTs were detected in 38 (75 per cent) of 51 unselected non-demented patients who died between the ages of 55 and 64 years (Ulrich, 1985). These lesions were consistently found in the entorhinal cortex, the hippocampus, or both, suggesting that this region is a site of origin of the lesions. A morphometric analysis of cerebral slices by de la Monte (1989) showed that patients with 'preclinical' AD had shrinkage of white matter comparable to that found in AD, yet the cortical areas were normal, suggesting that white matter degeneration is an intrinsic component of AD. In clinical AD, there was global cerebral atrophy of both cortex and white matter. Neuronal death in patients with AD is closely associated with extensive synapse loss in the neocortex and this has been correlated with cognitive impairment (Terry *et al.*, 1991). Measures of the morphological substrates of brain function frequently show an overlap between AD and control groups (Coleman and Flood, 1987). There does not appear to be a consistent relationship between the pattern of vascular amyloid and the distribution of plaques. Neither is there a correlation between vascular amyloid and dementia (Mountjoy *et al.*, 1982). More recent studies have confirmed that the Aβ amyloid per se is probably not the best indicator of severity of disease – rather, the soluble Aβ which are a prelude to plaque formation show a closer correlation with the degree of neurodegeneration (McLean *et al.*, 1999). With the advent of molecular imaging probes for Aβ, many of the above issues will be resolved (Jack *et al.*, 2009).

49.8 DIAGNOSTIC PROBLEMS AND CRITERIA

Despite the fact that the neurohistological abnormalities of AD have been established, the neuropathological diagnosis is not always straightforward (Cruz-Sanchez *et al.*, 1995). There are several reasons to explain this problem. First, the histopathology of AD is complex and the various abnormalities, previously described, when severe and extensive enable a diagnosis to be made. However, there are considerable differences from case to case and this histological heterogeneity of disease presents the most formidable difficulties for the neuropathologist. The severity and distribution of any of the histological lesions may considerably vary and are influenced by the age and genetic background of the patient, among other factors. Quantitative morphometry and neurochemistry have supported the view that AD is not a uniformly diffuse disorder: morphological abnormalities and neurochemical deficits tend to be more severe and more extensive in younger patients. There may be subtle differences in the pathology of familial and sporadic cases, and atypical cases exist both in the familial and sporadic forms. Second, although there are several histological abnormalities in AD, only Aβ deposition approaches a level of specificity, since many of these lesions occur in normal ageing and in other diseases of the nervous system. Third, AD may concurrently occur with other diseases, most commonly with vascular

disease and more rarely with other neurodegenerative disorders.

For these reasons, it is important to establish a set of neuropathological or neurochemical criteria. Although several attempts have been made, no universally accepted criteria exist for the neuropathological diagnosis of AD. An attempt has been made to define AD in terms of hippocampal pathology. Based on quantitative morphometry, it was suggested that more than 20 tangle-bearing neurones per mm³ and fewer than 5600 neurones per mm³ should be diagnostic (Ball *et al.*, 1985). This threshold, however, has proven too low and would include 30 per cent of mentally normal elderly people (Anderson and Hubbard, 1985). A North American panel of neuropathologists has recommended age-adjusted plaque and tangle counts. In patients under 50, plaques and tangles in excess of 2–5 per mm² in the neocortex should secure the diagnosis of AD. Between 60 and 65 years, there should be more than 8 plaques per mm², between 66 and 75 years more than 10 and over the age of 75, more than 15. In the first two age groups, some NFTs may be found, but in the last group these may not be necessary for diagnosis (Khachaturian, 1985). The value of these criteria has, however, been diminished by the statement that these figures can be revised downwards by as much as 50 per cent in the presence of positive clinical history of AD. A survey of the practical application of these criteria has revealed considerable variations in the use of criteria and the methods of examination (Wisniewski *et al.*, 1989). A European Multicentre Study found that subjective assessment currently was more reliable to compare cases from different laboratories, since quantitative values are greatly influenced by the neurohistological technique employed (Duyckaerts *et al.*, 1990).

The most widely used protocol for neuropathological assessment is that developed by the Task Force of the Consortium to Establish a Registry for AD (CERAD). This takes clinical findings into consideration, and neuropathological criteria for 'definite', 'probable' and 'possible' AD are proposed (Mirra *et al.*, 1991). This system is based on a semiquantitative assessment of plaque scores. The presence or absence of tangles does not enter into the formal assessment. The more recent National Institute on Aging and Reagan Institute (NIA-RI) criteria require both semi-quantitative measures of plaque and tangle distribution and additional sampling (Geddes *et al.*, 1997; Hyman and Trojanowski, 1997). A change from previous criteria is the opinion that any Alzheimer lesions should be considered as pathological even when they appear to be incidental. By acknowledging that a spectrum of changes exists within AD, these criteria may prove more successful than previous ones (Geddes *et al.*, 1997; Hyman and Trojanowski, 1997).

In the final analysis, it is likely that a combination of morphologic and biochemical assays will yield a set of criteria through which a secure diagnosis of AD will be made. Current indications are that blood, CSF and brain tissue levels of Aβ (soluble, insoluble), tau, ApoE and BACE may provide a more practical method for the diagnosis and therapeutic monitoring of AD (McLean *et al.*, 1999; Holsinger *et al.*, 2002; Holsinger *et al.*, 2004; Bates *et al.*, 2009; Craig-Shapiro *et al.*, 2009; Fagan *et al.*, 2009; Woltjer *et al.*, 2009).

REFERENCES

Adalbert R, Nogradi A, Babetto E *et al.* (2009) Severely dystrophic axons at amyloid plaques remain continuous and connected to viable cell bodies. *Brain* 132: 402–16.

Agosta F, Vossel KA, Miller BL *et al.* (2009) Apolipoprotein E ε4 is associated with disease-specific effects on brain atrophy in Alzheimer's disease and frontotemporal dementia. *Proceedings of the National Academy of Sciences of the United States of America* 106: 2018–22.

Alafuzoff I, Aho L, Helisalmi S *et al.* (2009) β-Amyloid deposition in brains of subjects with diabetes. *Neuropathology and Applied Neurobiology* 35: 60–8.

Alzheimer A. (1907) Über eine eigenartige Erkrankung der Hirnrinde. *Allgemeine Zeitschrift für Psychiatrie* 64: 146–8.

Anderson JM, Hubbard BM. (1985) Definition of Alzheimer's disease. *Lancet* 1: 408.

Arai T, Mackenzie IRA, Hasegawa M *et al.* (2009) Phosphorylated TDP-43 in Alzheimer's disease and dementia with Lewy bodies. *Acta Neuropathologica* 117: 125–36.

Armstrong RA, Myers D, Smith CUM. (1993) The spatial patterns of β/4 deposit subtypes in Alzheimer's disease. *Acta Neuropathologica* 86: 36–41.

Armstrong RA, Cairns NJ, Lantos PL. (1998) The spatial pattern of β-amyloid (Ab) deposits in Alzheimer's disease patients is related to apolipoprotein genotype. *Neuroscience Research Communications* 22: 99–106.

Armstrong RA, Cairns NJ, Myers D *et al.* (1996) A comparison of β-amyloid deposition in the medial temporal lobe in sporadic Alzheimer's disease, Down's syndrome and normal elderly brains. *Neurodegeneration* 5: 35–41.

Ball MJ. (1977) Neuronal loss, neurofibrillary tangles and granulovacuolar degeneration in the hippocampus with ageing brain and senile dementia: A quantitative study. *Acta Neuropathologica* 37: 111–18.

Ball MJ, Fisman M, Hachinski V *et al.* (1985) A new definition of Alzheimer's disease: A hippocampal dementia. *Lancet* 1: 14–16.

Bates KA, Verdile G, Li Q-X *et al.* (2009) Clearance mechanisms of Alzheimer's amyloid-β peptide: Implications for therapeutic design and diagnostic tests. *Molecular Psychiatry* 14: 469–86.

Blanks JC, Hinton DR, Sadun AA, Miller CA. (1989) Retinal ganglion cell degeneration in Alzheimer's disease. *Brain Research* 501: 364–72.

Blocq P, Marinesco G. (1892) Sur les lesions et la pathogénie de l'epilepsie dite essentielle. *Semaine Medicale* 12: 445–6.

Boller F, Lopez OL, Moossy J. (1989) Diagnosis of dementia: Clinicopathologic correlations. *Neurology* 39: 76–9.

Bondareff E, Wischik CM, Novak M *et al.* (1990) Molecular analysis of neurofibrillary degeneration in Alzheimer's disease. *American Journal of Pathology* 137: 711–23.

Borchelt DR, Woing PC, Sisodia SS, Price DL. (1998) Transgenic mouse models of Alzheimer's disease and amyotrophic lateral sclerosis. *Brain Pathology* 8: 735–57.

Bowen DM, Spillane JA, Curzon G *et al.* (1979) Accelerated ageing or selective neuronal loss as an important cause of dementia? *Lancet* 1: 11–14.

Braak H, Braak E. (1988) Neuropil threads occur in dendrites of tangle-bearing nerve cells. *Neuropathology and Applied Neurobiology* 14: 39–44.

Braak H, Braak E, Grundke-Iqbal I, Iqbal K. (1986) Occurrence of neuropil thread, in the senile human brain and in Alzheimer's disease: A third location of paired helical filaments outside of neurofibrillary tangles and neuritic plaques. *Neuroscience Letters* 65: 351–5.

Braak H, Braak E, Kalus P. (1989) Alzheimer's disease areal and laminar pathology in the occipital isocortex. *Acta Neuropathologica* 77: 494–506.

Brun A, Englund E. (1986) A white matter disorder in dementia of the Alzheimer type: A pathoanatomical study. *Annals of Neurology* 19: 253–62.

Buckner RL, Sepulcre J, Talukdar T *et al.* (2009) Cortical hubs revealed by intrinsic functional connectivity: mapping, assessment of stability and relation to Alzheimer's disease. *Journal of Neuroscience* 29: 1860–73.

Cairns NJ, Chadwick A, Luthert PJ, Lantos PL. (1991) β-Amyloid protein load is relatively uniform throughout neocortex and hippocampus in elderly Alzheimer's disease patients. *Neuroscience Letters* 129: 115–18.

Cairns NJ, Chadwick A, Luthert PJ, Lantos PL. (1992) Astrocytosis, βA4-protein deposition and paired helical filament formation in Alzheimer's disease. *Journal of the Neurological Sciences* 112: 68–75.

Cairns NJ, Atkinson PF, Hanger DP *et al.* (1997a) Tau protein in the glial cytoplasmic inclusions of multiple system atrophy can be distinguished from abnormal tau in Alzheimer's disease. *Neuroscience Letters* 230: 49–52.

Cairns NJ, Fukutani Y, Chadwick A *et al.* (1997b) Apolipoprotein E, β-amyloid (Aβ), phosphorylated tau and apolipoprotein E genotype in Alzheimer's disease. *Alzheimer Research* 3: 109–14.

Candy JM, Oakley AE, Klinowski J *et al.* (1986) Aluminoscilicates and senile plaque formation in Alzheimer's disease. *Lancet* 1: 354–7.

Chen X-H, Johnson VE, Uryu K *et al.* (2009) A lack of amyloid β plaques despite persistent accumulation of amyloid β in axons of long-term survivors of traumatic brain injury. *Brain Pathology* 19: 214–23.

Coleman PD, Flood DG. (1987) Neuron numbers and dendritic extent in normal aging and Alzheimer's disease. *Neurobiology of Aging* 8: 521–45.

Craig-Shapiro R, Fagan AM, Holtzman DM. (2009) Biomarkers of Alzheimer's disease. *Neurobiology of Disease* 35: 128–40.

Crowther RA. (1991) Straight and paired helical filaments in Alzheimer's have a common structural unit. *Proceedings of the National Academy of Sciences of the United States of America* 88: 2288–92.

Cruz-Sánchez FF, Ravid R, Cuzner ML. (eds) (1995) *Neuropathological diagnostic criteria for brain banking.* Oxford: IOS Press.

Davis CA, Mann DMA, Sumpter PQ, Yates PO. (1987) A quantitative morphometric analysis of the neuronal and synaptic content of the frontal and temporal cortex in patients with Alzheimer's disease. *Journal of the Neurological Sciences* 78: 151–64.

Delaère P, Duyckaerts C, Masters C et al. (1990) Large amounts of neocortical βA4 deposits without neuritic plaques nor tangles in a psychometrically assessed, non-demented person. Neuroscience Letters 116: 87–93.

de la Monte SM. (1989) Quantitation of cerebral atrophy in preclinical and end-stage Alzheimer's disease. Annals of Neurology 25: 450–9.

Dickerson BC, Bakkour A, Salat DH et al. (2009) The cortical signature of Alzheimer's disease: Regionally specific cortical thinning relates to symptom severity in very mild to mild AD dementia and is detectable in asymptomatic amyloid-positive individuals. Cerebral Cortex 19: 497–510.

Dickson DW, Ksiezak-Reding H, Davies P, Yen SH. (1987) A monoclonal antibody that recognises a phosphorylated epitope in Alzheimer neurofibrillary tangles, neurofilaments and tau proteins immunostains granulovacuolar degeneration. Acta Neuropathologica 73: 254–8.

Divry P. (1927) Etude histo-chimique des plaques séniles. Journal Belge de Neurologie et de Psychiatrie 27: 643–57.

Duyckaerts C, Hauw J-J, Piette F et al. (1985) Cortical atrophy in senile dementia of the Alzheimer type is mainly due to a decrease in cortical length. Acta Neuropathologica 66: 72–4.

Duyckaerts C, Delaère P, Poulain V et al. (1988) Does amyloid precede paired helical filaments in the senile plaques? A study of 15 cases with graded intellectual status in aging and Alzheimer's disease. Neuroscience Letters 91: 354–9.

Duyckaerts C, Delaère P, Hauw J-J et al. (1990) Rating of the lesions in senile dementia of the Alzheimer type: A concordance between laboratories. A European multicenter study under the auspices of EURAGE. Journal of the Neurological Sciences 7: 295–323.

Esiri MM, Wilcock GK. (1984) The olfactory bulbs in Alzheimer's disease. Journal of Neurology, Neurosurgery, and Psychiatry 47: 56–60.

Esiri MM, Morris JH. (1997) The neuropathology of dementia. Cambridge: Cambridge University Press.

Esiri MM, Hyman BT, Beyreuther K, Masters CL. (1997) Ageing and dementia. In: Graham DI, Lantos PL (eds). Greenfield's Neuropathology, 6th edn. Vol. II. London: Arnold, 153–233.

Fagan AM, Head D, Shah AR et al. (2009) Decreased cerebrospinal fluid Aβ$_{42}$ correlates with brain atrophy in cognitively normal elderly. Annals of Neurology 65: 176–83.

Fukutani Y, Cairns NJ, Rossor MN, Lantos PL. (1996) Purkinje cell loss and astrocytosis in the cerebellum in familial and sporadic Alzheimer's disease. Neuroscience Letters 214: 33–6.

Fukutani Y, Cairns NJ, Rossor MN, Lantos PL. (1997) Cerebellar pathology in sporadic and familial Alzheimer's disease including APP 717(val-ile) mutation cases: A morphometric investigation. Journal of the Neurological Sciences 149: 177–84.

Galloway PG, Perry G, Kosik KS, Gambetti P. (1987) Hirano bodies contain tau protein. Brain Research 403: 337–40.

Gallyas F. (1971) Silver staining of Alzheimer's neurofibrillary changes by means of physical development. Acta Morphologica Academiae Scientifica Hungarica 19: 1–8.

Geddes JW, Tekirian TL, Soultanian NS et al. (1997) Comparison of neuropathologic criteria for the diagnosis of Alzheimer's disease. Neurobiology of Aging 18 (4 Suppl.): S99–105.

Gentleman SM, Bruton C, Allsop D et al. (1989) A demonstration of the advantages of immunostaining in the quantification of amyloid plaque deposits. Histochemistry 92: 355–8.

Gibson PH, Tomlinson BE. (1977) Numbers of Hirano bodies in the hippocampus of normal and demented people with Alzheimer's disease. Journal of the Neurological Sciences 33: 199–206.

Goedert M, Wischik CM, Crowther RA et al. (1988) Cloning and sequencing of the cDNA encoding a core protein of the paired helical filament of Alzheimer's disease: Identification as the microtubule-associated protein tau. Proceedings of the National Academy of Sciences of the United States of America 85: 4051–5.

Goedert M, Spillantini MG, Cairns NJ, Crowther RA. (1992) Tau proteins of Alzheimer paired helical filaments; abnormal phosphorylation of all six isoforms. Neuron 8: 159–68.

Goldman JE. (1983) The association of actin with Hirano bodies. Journal of Neuropathology and Experimental Neurology 42: 146–52.

Goldstein LE, Muffat JA, Cherny RA et al. (2003) Cystolic beta-amyloid deposition and supranuclear cataracts in lenses from people with Alzheimer's disease. Lancet 361: 1258–65.

Gonatas NK, Anderson A, Vongelista I. (1967) The contribution of altered synapses in the senile plaque: An electronmicroscopic study in Alzheimer's dementia. Journal of Neuropathology and Experimental Neurology 26: 25–39.

Hanger DP, Brion J-P, Gallo J-M et al. (1991) Tau in Alzheimer's disease and Down's syndrome is insoluble and abnormally phosphorylated. Biochemical Journal 275: 99–104.

Hansen LA, De Teresa R, Davies P, Terry RD. (1988) Neocortical morphometry, lesion counts, and choline acetyltransferase levels in the age spectrum of Alzheimer's disease. Neurology 38: 48–55.

Harrington CR, Mukaetova-Ladinska EB, Hills R et al. (1991) Measurement of distinct immunochemical presentations of tau protein in Alzheimer's disease. Proceedings of the National Academy of Sciences of the United States of America 88: 5842–6.

Hauw J-J, Duyckaerts C, Delaere P. (1991) Alzheimer's disease. In: Duckett S (ed). The pathology of the aging nervous system. London: Lea and Febiger, 113–47.

Hinton DR, Sadun AA, Blanks JC, Miller CA. (1986) Optic nerve degeneration in Alzheimer's disease. New England Journal of Medicine 315: 485–7.

Hirano A. (1965) Pathology of amyotrophic lateral sclerosis. In: Gajdusek DC, Gibbs Jr CJ, Alpers M (eds). Slow, latent and temperate virus infections. Washington DC: US Government Printing Office, 23–6.

Holsinger RMD, McLean CA, Beyreuther K et al. (2002) Increased expression of the amyloid precursor β-secretase in Alzheimer's disease. Annals of Neurology 51: 783–6.

Holsinger RMD, Mclean CA, Collins SJ et al. (2004) Increased β-secretase activity in cerebrospinal fluid of Alzheimer's disease subjects. Annals of Neurology 55: 898–9.

Hubbard BM, Anderson JM. (1981) A quantitative study of cerebral atrophy in old age and senile dementia. Journal of the Neurological Sciences 50: 135–45.

Hubbard BM, Anderson JM. (1985) Age-related variations in the neuron content of the cerebral cortex in senile dementia of Alzheimer type. *Neuropathology and Applied Neurobiology* **11**: 369–82.

Hyman BT, Trojanowski JQ. (1997). Editorial on consensus recommendations for the postmortem diagnosis of Alzheimer disease from the National Institute on Aging and the Reagan Institute Working Group on diagnostic criteria for the neuropathological assessment of Alzheimer's disease. *Journal of Neuropathology and Experimental Neurology* **56**: 1095–7.

Iseki E, Matsushita M, Kosaka K *et al*. (1990) Morphological characteristics of senile plaques in familial Alzheimer's disease. *Acta Neuropathologica* **80**: 227–32.

Itagakai S, McGeer PL, Akiyama H *et al*. (1989) Relationship of microglia and astrocytes to amyloid deposits of Alzheimer's disease. *Journal of Neuroimmunology* **24**: 173–82.

Jack CR, Lowe VJ, Weigand SD *et al*. (2009) and the Alzheimer's Disease Neuroimaging Initiative. Serial PIB and MRI in normal, mild cognitive impairment and Alzheimer's disease: Implications for sequence of pathological events in Alzheimer's disease. *Brain* **132**: 1355–65.

Jellinger K. (1988) The pedunculopontine nucleus in Parkinson's disease, progressive supranuclear palsy and Alzheimer's disease. *Journal of Neurology, Neurosurgery, and Psychiatry* **51**: 540–3.

Jellinger K, Danielczyk W, Fischer P, Gabriel E. (1990) Clinicopathological analysis of dementia disorders in the elderly. *Journal of the Neurological Sciences* **95**: 239–58.

Joachim CL, Morris JH, Selkoe DJ, Kosik KS. (1987) Tau epitopes are incorporated into a wide range of lesions in Alzheimer's disease. *Journal of Neuropathology and Experimental Neurology* **46**: 611–22.

Joachim CL, Morris JH, Selkoe DJ. (1989) Diffuse senile plaques occur commonly in the cerebellum in Alzheimer's disease. *American Journal of Pathology* **135**: 309–19.

Kahn J, Anderton BH, Probert A *et al*. (1985) Immunohistological study of granulovacuolar degeneration using monoclonal antibodies to neurofilaments. *Journal of Neurology, Neurosurgery, and Psychiatry* **48**: 924–6.

Kang J, Lemaire HG, Unterbeck A *et al*. (1987) The precursor of Alzheimer's disease amyloid A4 protein resembles a cell-surface receptor. *Nature* **325**: 733–6.

Keage HAD, Carare RO, Friedland RP *et al*. (2009) Population studies of sporadic cerebral amyloid angiopathy and dementia: A systematic review. *BMC Neurology* **9**: 3.

Khachaturian ZS. (1985) Diagnosis of Alzheimer's disease. *Archives of Neurology* **42**: 1097–104.

Kidd M. (1963) Paired helical filaments in electron microscopy of Alzheimer's disease. *Nature* **197**: 192–3.

Kiuchi A, Utsuka N, Namba Y *et al*. (1991) Presenile appearance of abundant neurofibrillary tangles without senile plaques in the brain in myotonic dystrophy. *Acta Neuropathologica* **82**: 1–5.

Kowall NW, Kosik KS. (1987) Axonal disruption and aberrant localization of tau protein characterize the neuropil pathology of Alzheimer's disease. *Annals of Neurology* **22**: 639–43.

Lamb BT. (1997) Presenilins, amyloid-β and Alzheimer's disease. *Nature Medicine* **3**: 28–9.

Lantos PL, Luthert PJ, Hanger D *et al*. (1992) Familial Alzheimer's disease with the amyloid precursor protein position 717 mutation and sporadic Alzheimer's disease have the same cytoskeletal pathology. *Neuroscience Letters* **137**: 221–4.

Leigh PN, Probst A, Dale GE *et al*. (1989) New aspects of the pathology of neurodegenerative disorders as revealed by ubiquitin antibodies. *Acta Neuropathologica* **79**: 61–72.

Levy E, Carman MD, Fernandez-Madrid IJ *et al*. (1990) Mutation of the Alzheimer's disease amyloid gene in hereditary cerebral hemorrhage, Dutch type. *Science* **248**: 1124–6.

Majocha RE, Benes FM, Reifel JL *et al*. (1988) Laminar-specific distribution and infrastructural detail of amyloid in the Alzheimer's disease cortex visualized by computer-enhanced imaging of epitopes recognized by monoclonal antibodies. *Proceedings of the National Academy of Sciences of the United States of America* **85**: 6182–6.

Mann DMA, Yates PO, Marcynink B. (1985) Some morphometric observations in the cerebral cortex and hippocampus in presenile Alzheimer's disease, senile dementia of Alzheimer type and Down's syndrome in middle age. *Journal of the Neurological Sciences* **69**: 139–59.

Mann DMA, Yates PO, Marcyniuk B. (1986) A comparison of nerve cell loss in cortical and subcortical structures in Alzheimer's disease. *Journal of Neurology, Neurosurgery, and Psychiatry* **49**: 310–12.

Mann DMA, Yates PO, Marcyniuk B *et al*. (1988) The progression of the pathological changes of Alzheimer's disease in frontal and temporal neocortex examined both at biopsy and at autopsy. *Neuropathology and Applied Neurobiology* **14**: 177–95.

Mann DMA, Iwatsubo T, Cairns NJ *et al*. (1996a) Amyloid β protein (Aβ) deposition in chromosome 14-linked Alzheimer's disease: Predominance of Aβ$_{42(43)}$. *Annals of Neurology* **40**: 149–56.

Mann DMA, Iwatsubo T, Ihara Y *et al*. (1996b) Predominant deposition of amyloid-β$_{42(43)}$ in plaques in cases of Alzheimer's disease and hereditary cerebral hemorrhage associated with mutations in the amyloid precursor protein gene. *American Journal of Pathology* **148**: 1257–66.

Marcyniuk B, Mann DMA, Yates PO. (1986) The topography of cell loss from locus ceruleus in Alzheimer's disease. *Journal of the Neurological Sciences* **76**: 335–45.

Masliah E, Terry RD, DeTeresa RM, Hansen LA. (1989) Immunohistochemical quantification of the synapse-related protein synaptophysin in Alzheimer disease. *Neuroscience Letters* **103**: 234–9.

Masliah E, Hansen L, Albright T *et al*. (1991) Immunoelectron microscopic study of synaptic pathology in Alzheimer's disease. *Acta Neuropathologica* **81**: 428–33.

Masters CL, Beyreuther K. (2001) The Worster-Drought syndrome and other syndromes of dementia with spastic paraparesis: The paradox of molecular pathology. *Journal of Neuropathology and Experimental Neurology* **60**: 317–19.

Masters CL, Simms G, Weinman NA *et al*. (1985) Amyloid plaque core protein in Alzheimer disease and Down syndrome. *Proceedings of the National Academy of Sciences of the United States of America* **82**: 4245–9.

McLean CA, Cherny RA, Fraser FW et al. (1999) Soluble pool of Aβ as a determinant of severity of neurodegeration in Alzheimer's disease. *Annals of Neurology* **46**: 860–6.

Mirra SS, Heyman A, McKeel D et al. (1991) The consortium to establish a registry for Alzheimer's disease (CERAD). Part II. Standardization of the neuropathologic assessment of Alzheimer's disease. *Neurology* **41**: 479–86.

Mori H, Kondo J, Ihara Y. (1987) Ubiquitin is a component of paired helical filaments in Alzheimer's disease. *Science* **235**: 1641–4.

Morris JC, McKeel DW, Fulling K et al. (1988) Validation of clinical diagnostic criteria for Alzheimer's disease. *Annals of Neurology* **24**: 17–22.

Morrissette DA, Parachikova A, Green KN, LaFerla FM. (2009) Relevance of transgenic mouse models to human Alzheimer disease. *Journal of Biological Chemistry* **284**: 6033–7.

Mountjoy CQ, Thomlinson BE, Gibson PH. (1982) Amyloid senile plaques and cerebral blood vessels. A semi-quantitative investigation of a possible relationship. *Journal of the Neurological Sciences* **57**: 89–103.

Mountjoy CQ, Roth M, Evans NJR, Evans HM. (1983) Cortical neuronal counts in normal elderly controls and demented patients. *Neurobiology of Aging* **4**: 1–11.

Neary D, Snowden JS, Bowen DM et al. (1986) Neuropsychological syndromes in presenile dementia due to cerebral atrophy. *Journal of Neurology, Neurosurgery, and Psychiatry* **49**: 163–74.

Nelson PT, Braak H, Markesbery WR. (2009) Neuropathology and cognitive impairment in Alzheimer disease: A complex but coherent relationship. *Journal of Neuropathology and Experimental Neurology* **68**: 1–14.

Ogomori K, Kitamoto T, Tateishi J et al. (1989) β-Protein amyloid is widely distributed in the central nervous system of patients with Alzheimer's disease. *American Journal of Pathology* **134**: 243–51.

Pantelakis S. (1954) Un type particulier d'angiopathie sénile du système nervaux central: l'angiopathie congophile. Topographie et fréquence. *Monatsschrift für Psychiatrie und Neurologie* **128**: 219–56.

Perry G, Friedman R, Shaw G, Chau V. (1987) Ubiquitin is detected in neurofibrillary tangles and senile plaque neurites of Alzheimer's disease brains. *Proceedings of the National Academy of Sciences of the United States of America* **84**: 3033–6.

Price DL, Stuble RG, Altschuler RJ et al. (1985) Aggregation of tubulin in neurons in Alzheimer's disease. *Journal of Neuropathology and Experimental Neurology* **44**: 366.

Probst A, Anderton BH, Brion J-P, Ulrich J. (1989) Senile plaque neurites fail to demonstrate anti-paired helical filament and anti-microtubule associated protein-tau immunoreactive proteins in the absence of neurofibrillary tangles in the neocortex. *Acta Neuropathologica* **77**: 430–6.

Ritchie CW, Bush AI, Mackinnon A et al. (2003) Metal-protein attenuation with iodochlorhydroxyquin (clioquinol) targeting Aβ amyloid deposition and toxicity in Alzheimer disease: A pilot phase 2 clinical trial. *Archives of Neurology* **60**: 1678–91.

Roberts GW, Gentleman SM, Lynch A, Graham DI. (1991) βA4 amyloid protein deposition in brain after head trauma. *Lancet* **338**: 1422–3.

Rogers J, Morrison JH. (1985) Quantitative morphology and laminar distribution of senile plaques in Alzheimer's disease. *Journal of Neuroscience* **5**: 2801–8.

Roses AD. (1994) Apolipoprotein E affects the rate of Alzheimer's disease expression: β amyloid burden is a secondary consequence dependent on *APOE* genotype and duration of disease. *Journal of Neuropathology and Experimental Neurology* **53**: 429–37.

Roth M, Tomlinson BE, Blessed G. (1966) Correlations between scores for dementia and counts of 'senile plaques' in cerebral grey matter of elderly subjects. *Nature* **209**: 109–10.

Rowe CC, Ng S, Ackermann U et al. (2007) Imaging β-amyloid burden in aging and dementia. *Neurology* **68**: 1718–25.

Rowe CC, Ackerman U, Browne W et al. (2008) Imaging of amyloid β in Alzheimer's disease with 18F-BAY94-9172, a novel PET tracer: proof of mechanism. *Lancet Neurology* **7**: 129–35.

Rozemuller JM, Eikelenboom P, Stam FC et al. (1989) A4 protein in Alzheimer's disease: Primary and secondary cellular events in extracellular amyloid deposition. *Journal of Neuropathology and Experimental Neurology* **48**: 674–91.

Simchowicz T. (1911) Histologische Studien über die senile Demenz. *Histologische und Histopathologische Arbeiten* **4**: 267–444.

Spillantini MG, Schmidt ML, Lee VM et al. (1997) α-Synuclein in Lewy bodies. *Nature* **388**: 839–40.

Struble RG, Polinsky RJ, Hedreen JC et al. (1991) Hippocampal lesions in dominantly inherited Alzheimer's disease. *Journal of Neuropathology and Experimental Neurology* **50**: 82–94.

Tabaton M, Mandybur TI, Perry G et al. (1989) The widespread alteration of neurites in Alzheimer's disease may be unrelated to amyloid deposition. *Annals of Neurology* **26**: 771–8.

Tabaton M, Cammarata S, Mancardi GL et al. (1991a) Abnormal tau-reactive filaments in olfactory mucosa in biopsy specimens of patients with probable Alzheimer's disease. *Neurology* **41**: 391–4.

Tabaton M, Cammarata S, Mancardi G et al. (1991b) Ultrastructural localization of β-amyloid, tau, and ubiquitin epitopes in extracellular neurofibrillary tangles. *Proceedings of the National Academy of Sciences of the United States of America* **88**: 2098–102.

Talamo BR, Ruder RA, Kosik KS et al. (1989) Pathological changes in olfactory neurons in patients with Alzheimer's disease. *Nature* **337**: 736–9.

Terry RD. (1985) Alzheimer's disease. In: Davis RL, Robertson DM (eds). *Textbook of neuropathology*. Baltimore: Williams & Wilkins, 824–41.

Terry RD. (1990) Normal aging and Alzheimer's disease: growing problems. In: Cancilla PA, Vogel FS, Kaufman N (eds). *Neuropathology. International Academy of Pathology Monograph*. Baltimore: Williams & Wilkins, 41–54.

Terry RD, Peck A, DeTeresa R et al. (1981) Some morphometric aspects of the brain in senile dementia of the Alzheimer type. *Annals of Neurology* **10**: 184–92.

Terry RD, Masliah E, Salmon DP et al. (1991) Physical basis of cognitive alterations in Alzheimer's disease: Synapse loss is the major correlate of cognitive impairment. *Annals of Neurology* **30**: 572–80.

Tomlinson BE, Irving D, Blessed G. (1981) Cell loss in the locus ceruleus in senile dementia of Alzheimer type. *Journal of the Neurological Sciences* **49**: 419–28.

Tomonaga M. (1974) Ultrastructure of Hirano bodies. *Acta Neuropathologica* **28**: 365–6.

Tourtellotte WG, Van Hoesen GW. (1991) The axonal origin of a subpopulation of dystrophic neurites in Alzheimer's disease. *Neuroscience Letters* **129**: 11–16.

Ulrich J. (1985) Alzheimer changes in nondemented patients younger than sixty-five: Possible early stages of Alzheimer's disease and senile dementia of the Alzheimer type. *Annals of Neurology* **17**: 273–7.

Villemagne VL, Ataka S, Mizuno T et al. (2009) High striatal amyloid beta-peptide deposition across different autosomal Alzheimer disease mutation types. *Archives of Neurology* **66**: 1537–44.

Walker LC, Kitt CA, Cork LC et al. (1988) Multiple transmitter systems contribute neurites to individual senile plaques. *Journal of Neuropathology and Experimental Neurology* **47**: 138–44.

Whitehouse PJ, Price DL, Clark AW et al. (1981) Alzheimer's disease: Evidence for selective loss of cholinergic neurons in the nucleus basalis. *Annals of Neurology* **10**: 122–6.

Wilcock GK, Esiri MM. (1982) Plaques, tangles and dementia. *Journal of the Neurological Sciences* **56**: 343–56.

Wisniewski HM, Merz PA, Iqbal K. (1984) Ultrastructure of paired helical filaments of Alzheimer's neurofibrillary tangle. *Journal of Neuropathology and Experimental Neurology* **43**: 643–56.

Wisniewski HM, Rabe A, Zigman W, Silverman W. (1989) Neuropathological diagnosis of Alzheimer's disease. *Journal of Neuropathology and Experimental Neurology* **48**: 606–9.

Woltjer RL, Sonnen JA et al. (2009) Quantitation and mapping of cerebral detergent-insoluble proteins in the elderly. *Brain Pathology* **19**: 365–74.

Yamaguchi H, Nakazato Y, Hirai S, Shoji M. (1990a) Immunoelectron microscopic localization of amyloid β protein in the diffuse plaques of Alzheimer-type dementia. *Brain Research* **508**: 320–4.

Yamaguchi H, Nakazato Y, Shoji M et al. (1990b) Ultrastructure of the neuropil threads in the Alzheimer brain: Their dendritic origin and accumulation in the senile plaques. *Acta Neuropathologica* **80**: 368–74.

Yamaguchi H, Nakazato Y, Shoji M et al. (1991) Ultrastructure of diffuse plaques in senile dementia of the Alzheimer type: Comparison with primitive plaques. *Acta Neuropathologica* **82**: 13–20.

Yamamoto T, Hirano A. (1985) Nucleus raphe dorsalis in Alzheimer's disease: Neurofibrillary tangles and loss of large neurons. *Annals of Neurology* **17**: 573–7.

Yanker BA, Dawes LR, Fisher S et al. (1989) Neurotoxicity of a fragment of the amyloid precursor associated with Alzheimer's disease. *Science* **245**: 417–20.

Zubenko GS, Moossy J, Martinez J et al. (1991) Neuropathologic and neurochemical correlates of psychosis in primary dementia. *Archives of Neurology* **48**: 619–24.

Neurochemistry of Alzheimer's disease

PAUL T FRANCIS

50.1   INTRODUCTION

The demonstration of deficits in choline acetyltransferase (ChAT) activity in patients dying with Alzheimer's disease (AD) (Bowen *et al.*, 1976; Davies and Maloney, 1976), together with human anticholinergic drug studies (Drachman and Leavitt, 1974), led to the eventual development of cholinesterase inhibitors (ChEIs) for the symptomatic treatment of AD. Present neurochemical investigations of this system attempt to understand how early the cholinergic deficit develops and the extent to which it occurs in mild cognitive impairment (MCI). In addition, recognition of the role of the glutamatergic system in learning and memory has prompted study of biochemical markers of the major excitatory neurotransmitter system. Anatomical studies suggest interconnectivity between glutamatergic and cholinergic systems but their exact role in AD still requires further elucidation. Just as cholinergic and glutamatergic disruption may be additive in contributing to cognitive and behavioural symptoms of dementia, so pharmacological replacement therapy may be synergistic (Francis *et al.*, 1993; Francis 2005).

The amyloid cascade hypothesis has undergone many revisions but still provides a framework in which to understand disease progression in AD (Hardy, 2006; see Chapter 51, The central role of Aβ amyloid in the pathogenesis of Alzheimer's disease). It is widely accepted that neurotransmitter deficits, neuronal and synapse loss and subsequent decline, are final consequences of this cascade, however many studies suggest that modulation of neurotransmitter activity and synaptic function may have the potential to influence disease progression.

50.2   NEUROCHEMISTRY

From a neurochemical standpoint acetylcholine (ACh), glutamate, serotonin and noradrenaline are the major transmitter systems affected in AD with relative sparing of dopamine, GABA and most peptides (Francis *et al.*, 1993). This chapter examines both cognitive and non-cognitive (behavioural) correlates of neurotransmitter dysfunction, the latter also being considered to relate to structural and functional alterations in the central nervous system. Such changes are important, in part because carers find behavioural disturbances difficult to cope with and the presence of such behaviours in AD patients often leads to institutionalization. The chapter focuses on cholinergic and glutamatergic systems; for a comprehensive review of neurotransmission in AD see Lai *et al.* (2007).

50.2.1   Acetylcholine

Neuropathologically, loss of neurones from the nucleus of Meynert (CH 4 cholinergic nucleus) is well documented in AD, although the extent of the loss reported varies from moderate to severe, and it has been suggested that in AD cholinergic dysfunction exceeds neuronal degeneration (Perry *et al.*, 1982). This is consistent with studies of cholinergic markers in biopsy samples from patients who had AD for approximately three years, where reduction in functional cholinergic measures, ACh synthesis and choline uptake exceeded the reduction in ChAT activity (Francis *et al.*, 1985).

On the basis of the above evidence, neocortical cholinergic innervation appears to be lost at an early stage of the disease. Beach *et al.* (2000) reported neurofibrillary tangles (NFTs) in entorhinal cortex and a 20–30 per cent loss of ChAT activity in brains from patients at the earliest stages of AD, namely Braak stages I and II, and tangle formation in the main cholinergic nucleus is present in MCI (Mesulam *et al.*, 2004). However, another study using the Clinical Dementia Rating scale (CDR) suggests that the greatest reduction in markers of the cholinergic system occurs between moderate (CDR 2.0) and severe (CDR 5.0) disease with little change between the non-demented and mild stages (CDR 0-2) (Davis *et al.*, 1999). In contrast, a study of MCI, the suggested AD prodrome, reported an increase in ChAT activity in some cortical regions (DeKosky *et al.*, 2002). The acknowledged problems of these latter studies is that ChAT activity is not the rate-limiting step of ACh synthesis and hence there could be cholinergic dysfunction before structural loss, possibly linked to aberrant sprouting. Changes in cholinergic neurones appear to relate to aspects of cognitive function (Francis *et al.*, 1985) as well as non-cognitive behaviour (Minger *et al.*, 2000; Gauthier *et al.*, 2002). It has also been suggested that ACh is centrally involved in the process of conscious awareness (Perry *et al.*, 1999), and that the variety of clinical symptoms associated with cholinergic dysfunction in AD and related disorders reflects disturbances in the conscious processing of information. There is evidence that implicit memory for example (which does not involve conscious awareness) is relatively intact in AD (Postle *et al.*, 1996).

Nicotinic and muscarinic (M2) ACh receptors, most of which are considered to be located on cholinergic terminals, are reduced in AD (Court *et al.*, 2001; Lai *et al.*, 2001). Reductions in nicotinic receptors are confined to the $\alpha_4\beta_2$ subtype. The postsynaptic cholinergic system (usually present upon glutamatergic neurones) appears to be less affected, which is hopeful for therapeutic intervention. Postsynaptic muscarinic M1 receptors (Perry *et al.*, 1990) are relatively preserved although there may be a degree of functional uncoupling (Tsang *et al.*, 2006). The enzyme responsible for the breakdown of ACh, acetylcholinesterase, is reduced, perhaps in part due to a loss of cholinergic terminals, while butyrylcholinesterase activity (the function of which is not yet fully understood and which is present in extrasynaptic areas and plaques) increases (Perry *et al.*, 1978).

50.2.2   Acetylcholine and cognition

A prediction of the cholinergic hypothesis is that drugs likely to potentiate this function should improve cognition in AD patients. There are a number of treatment approaches to the amelioration of the cholinergic deficit, however the use of ChEIs is the most well-developed approach to date (Francis *et al.*, 1999).

During the late 1980s and early 1990s, the first cholinomimetic compound, tacrine, underwent large-scale clinical studies and established the benefits of ChEI treatment in patients with probable AD. A so-called second generation of ChEIs has been developed including donepezil, rivastigmine, metrifonate and galantamine (Francis *et al.*, 1999; Wilkinson *et al.*, 2004). Such compounds demonstrate a clinical effect and magnitude of benefit of at least that reported for tacrine, but with a more favourable clinical profile. Evidence has emerged from clinical trials of ChEIs that such drugs may improve the behavioural symptoms of AD. Physostigmine, tacrine, rivastigmine and metrifonate have variously been reported in placebo controlled trials to decrease psychotic symptoms, agitation, apathy, anxiety, disinhibition, pacing, aberrant motor behaviour and lack of cooperation (Cummings and Kaufer, 1996). In one study muscarinic M2 receptor density was increased in the frontal cortex of AD

patients with delusions and in the temporal cortex of those with hallucinations, compared to patients without psychotic symptoms. This suggests a role for M2 receptors in the psychosis of AD and may provide the rationale for treatment of behaviourally disturbed AD patients with M2 antagonists (Lai *et al.*, 2001).

Possibly related to these findings in AD, a study of rivastigmine in patients with Parkinson's disease dementia showed a positive outcome (Emre *et al.*, 2004); such patients have a greater cholinergic deficit than AD (Perry *et al.*, 1994).

50.2.3   The cholinergic system and AD pathology

Many preclinical studies indicate that activation of cholinergic receptors influence the metabolism of one of the two key proteins involved in AD, APP, diverting metabolism away from the formation of amyloid (Aβ) (Nitsch, 1996; Francis *et al.*, 1999). In support of this hypothesis two clinical studies show that muscarinic M1 agonists are able to reduce cerebrospinal fluid (CSF) concentrations of Aβ (Hock *et al.*, 2000; Nitsch *et al.*, 2000). Finally, an M1 agonist reversed Aβ accumulation in a triple transgenic model of AD (Caccamo *et al.*, 2006). Furthermore, nicotinic receptor stimulation is associated with reduced plaque densities in human brain (Court *et al.*, 1998) and transgenic mice (Hellstrom-Lindahl *et al.*, 2004). These results suggest that compounds being developed for symptomatic treatment may have a serendipitous effect on the continuing emergence of pathology, by reducing the production of Aβ. There is also evidence for a possible beneficial role of cholinergic neurotransmission by modulation in the generation of NFTs via reduced phosphorylation of tau protein. One of the primary intracellular enzymes responsible, glycogen synthase kinase-3 can be regulated by muscarinic activation (Sadot *et al.*, 1996) and tau phosphorylation was reduced by an M1 agonist (Caccamo *et al.*, 2006). Cholinergic neurotransmission may also be a specific target for Aβ, since it has been shown to reduce both choline uptake and ACh release *in vitro* (Auld *et al.*, 1998). Furthermore, Aβ is reported to bind with high affinity to the α7 subtype of the nicotinic receptor, suggesting that cholinergic function through this receptor may be compromised because of high levels of (soluble) peptide in AD brains (Wang *et al.*, 2000; Abbott *et al.*, 2008).

50.2.4   Glutamate

Glutamate is the principal excitatory neurotransmitter of the brain, being used at approximately two-thirds of synapses and, as a consequence, the majority of neurones and glia have receptors for glutamate. An integral part of protein, energy and ammonia metabolism of all cells, with a high intracellular concentration, it has been difficult to distinguish the presynaptic transmitter pool of glutamate from the metabolic pool (Francis *et al.*, 1993). Considered to be the main neurotransmitter of neocortical and hippocampal pyramidal neurones, glutamate is thus involved in higher mental functions such as cognition and memory (Francis *et al.*, 1993). An important mechanism by which glutamate may contribute to learning and memory functions is via long-term potentiation (LTP) at pyramidal neurone synapses (Baudry and Lynch, 2001). LTP is a form of synaptic strengthening following brief, high frequency, stimulation.

Histological AD studies indicate loss of pyramidal neurones and their synapses together with surrounding neuropil (Esiri, 1991). Corticocortical and corticofugal-projecting pyramidal neurones are lost together with those of the entorhinal and hippocampal CA1 region. Remaining neurones are subject to NFT formation. Uptake of D–aspartate, a putative marker of glutamatergic nerve endings, is reduced in many cortical areas in AD brains (Procter et al., 1988).

Biochemical evidence suggests a presynaptic 'double blow' as the activity of glutamatergic neurones is heavily influenced by the cholinergic system, also dysfunctional in AD. The clinical relevance of these changes is emphasized because glutamatergic and cholinergic dysfunction are both strong correlates of cognitive decline in AD. Glutamatergic (and cholinergic) cells die over a period of years and in a very specific regional and neurochemically selective pattern (Francis et al., 1993). The selectivity is intriguing, because cholinergic neurones of the basal forebrain die while those of the pons are spared; glutamatergic neurones of the frontal, temporal and parietal cortex are lost while apparently similar neurones in the motor and sensory cortex are unaffected. Factors that may lead to necrosis or apoptosis in selected groups of neurones in AD may include tangles, Aβ toxicity, microglia, free radical generation, excitotoxicity (too much and too little glutamatergic neurotransmission) and withdrawal of trophic factors. The strongest evidence suggests that most of glutamatergic pyramidal neurones die as a consequence of the presence of NFT within the cytoplasm (Kowall and Beal, 1991). However, this may only account for up to 50 per cent of such cells.

Glutamate is synthesized in nerve terminals by one of several possible enzymes. First, glutamine can be converted to glutamate by the action of the mitochondrial enzyme glutaminase (Procter et al., 1988); alternatively, glutamate can be produced by transamination from aspartate in the cytosol. Direct measurement of glutaminase activity was unaffected in AD (Procter et al., 1988). By contrast, glutaminase-positive neurones were reduced in number and subject to tangle formation (Kowall and Beal, 1991). Several groups have shown reductions in the concentration of glutamate in AD tissue and lumbar CSF (Lowe et al., 1990). Although glutamate neurotransmission failure was not extensive in these studies, glutamate concentration was reduced by 14 per cent in temporal lobe biopsy samples and by 86 per cent in the terminal zone of the perforant pathway at autopsy of AD patients (Hyman et al., 1987).

We have recently begun to investigate the status of the vesicular glutamate transporters (VGLUT), VGLUT1 and VGLUT2 (Bellocchio et al., 2000). These proteins are only present in the glutamatergic neurone terminals and therefore represent a useful marker of their number. Studies indicate that there is a reduction in VGLUT1 (but not VGLUT2) in parietal and occipital cortex in AD but not in temporal cortex (Kirvell et al., 2006). Other studies link this reduction to cognitive impairment (Kashani et al., 2008).

Upon release into the synapse, approximately 95 per cent of glutamate is removed by glutamate transporter proteins present upon glial cells named GLT, GLAST and EAAC (Danbolt, 2001). Reductions in glutamate uptake in AD cases have been reported in fresh (unfrozen) post-mortem brains (Procter et al., 1994). Antibodies directed against the individual glutamate transporters reveal conflicting data. Reduced levels of GLT protein (but not its mRNA), with normal levels of both GLAST and EAAC have been reported (Danbolt, 2001). Even assuming there was no reduction of transporter protein, there is considerable evidence for oxidative damage of proteins such as these glutamate transporters (Keller et al., 1997; Begni et al., 2004). This might explain the functional deficit in glutamate uptake, identified above, and is likely to lead to elevations in synaptic concentrations of glutamate (Parsons et al., 2007; Francis, 2009).

50.2.5 Glutamate and cognition

A role for glutamate and glutamate receptors in learning and memory is widely recognized. For example, NMDA antagonists impair learning and memory, while NMDA agonists and facilitators improve memory (Francis et al., 1993). Likewise, AMPAkines (positive modulators of AMPA receptor function) facilitate learning and memory (Lynch, 1998). Circumstantial evidence of the involvement of glutamatergic pathways includes the well-established role of structures such as the hippocampus in learning and memory. More specifically, lesions of certain glutamatergic pathways impair learning and memory. In addition, glutamate and glutamate receptors are involved in mechanisms of synaptic plasticity (LTP and long-term depression of the synapse) which are considered to underlie learning and memory (Baudry and Lynch, 2001). Loss of synapses and pyramidal cell perikarya from the neocortex of AD patients correlates with measures of cognitive decline and is considered to be the best evidence for a functional role of glutamatergic involvement in cognitive dysfunction in AD (Francis et al., 1993).

50.2.6 The glutamatergic system and AD pathology

Excitotoxic cell death involves excess activation of receptors, leading to raised intracellular Ca^{2+} and consequent activation of a cascade of enzymes, resulting in cell death by necrosis or apoptosis (Lipton, 1999). During the 1980s it was also suggested that endogenous glutamate could accumulate and become excitotoxic, perhaps as a result of impaired clearance (as a consequence of disrupted transporter function or indirectly in conditions of reduced energy availability). There is some evidence that energy levels may be reduced in AD due to perturbed mitochondrial function (Francis et al., 1993) and considerable evidence for oxidative damage of proteins including the glutamate transporter (Keller et al., 1997). Others have cautioned that there is no simple relationship between raised extracellular glutamate concentrations and cell death in vivo. It remains possible that changes in numbers of glutamate receptors or changes in ion selectivity may lead over time to cell death. For instance the large numbers of calcium-permeable AMPA receptors present on basal forebrain cholinergic neurones may be linked to their loss in AD (Ikonomovic and Armstrong, 1996).

The glutamatergic system is a significant target for AD-related pathology in that tangles occur principally in glutamatergic pyramidal neurones; these cells are lost and much of the observed synaptic pathology will involve these cells. Tangles and cell and synapse loss are the strongest correlates of cognitive impairment in AD (Neary et al., 1986; Terry et al., 1991). There is also an emerging role for tangle formation within pyramidal neurones of specific brain regions as a causative mechanism of agitation and aggression in AD (Tekin et al., 2001; Francis, 2009).

50.2.7 Interactions between cholinergic and glutamatergic systems

It is important to remember that glutamatergic neurones of the neocortex and hippocampus are influenced by acetylcholine through nicotinic and muscarinic receptors (Chessell and Humphrey, 1995; Dijk et al., 1995). Terminals of cholinergic neurones are found in all layers of the neocortex, synapsing with pyramidal neurones in layers II/III and V (Turrini et al., 2001). Both muscarinic and nicotinic receptors activate pyramidal neurones and hence facilitate glutamate release in a rat model (Chessell and Humphrey, 1995; Dijk et al., 1995). Thus underactivity of the cholinergic system is likely to have effects on the activity of the glutamatergic system and conversely, it therefore follows that treatment of patients with cholinomimetics is likely to increase glutamatergic function.

50.2.8 Treatment strategies based on facilitating glutamatergic neurotransmission

Cholinergic stimulation is one pathway to enhance glutamatergic function. Other treatment strategies that more directly increase the activity of remaining glutamatergic neurones, without causing excitotoxicity, represent an important target for the symptomatic treatment of AD, and may have a disease-modifying effect. Several approaches have been tried including positive modulation of both AMPA and NMDA receptors. AMPAkines, which are considered to work by increasing the sensitivity of these receptors, have been in clinical trial for MCI but with modest success (Johnson and Simmon, 2002). Modulation of the NMDA receptor has been attempted via the glycine co-agonist site with clear indication in preclinical studies that the partial agonist D-cycloserine improved learning and memory (Myhrer and Paulsen, 1997). Clinical studies have suggested some benefit but full-scale trials have not been initiated (Schwartz et al., 1996). There is no evidence that these drugs enhance excitotoxicity.

Perhaps the most surprising development is the success of the uncompetitive NMDA antagonist memantine in clinical trials in moderate and severe AD (Reisberg et al., 2003). One would normally consider that such an approach – blockade of a receptor that would normally be activated in learning

and memory – would be counter-intuitive. However there is evidence that this molecule acts like the endogenous NMDA antagonist, magnesium ions, able to prevent background activation of the NMDA receptor ('noise'), while allowing activation of this receptor for LTP formation (Francis, 2003; Parsons et al., 2007). The observed effects of memantine on agitation and aggression may be explained by this mechanism, however there is preclinical evidence to suggest that this drug is capable of altering the phosphorylation state of tau, the precursor to tangle formation (Francis, 2009). There is also evidence of a benefit of the addition of memantine to established treatment with a ChEI in AD patients (Tariot et al., 2004). Since ChEIs are likely to act in part by increasing glutamate release ('signal') (Dijk et al., 1995; Francis et al., 1999) the benefit may be hypothesized to come from the combination of a reduction in glutamate 'noise' (by memantine) and an increase in discrete glutamate signals (donepezil) (Francis, 2003).

50.3   CONCLUSION

The changes in cholinergic neurotransmission seen in the brains of patients dying with AD provided the rationale for the development of compounds aimed at symptomatic relief. Treatment of AD patients with ChEIs has confirmed the relevance of this finding. However it has long been recognized that the major changes in AD are likely to involve the more abundant cortical glutamatergic pyramidal neurones. Hence there is a need for this change to be addressed. Since increasing cholinergic function will also increase glutamatergic activity, there may be synergistic benefit from co-administration of drugs that target both the cholinergic system (ChEIs) and glutamatergic systems (memantine). As disease-modifying treatments become available it is likely that symptomatic therapy will continue to be required, and indeed there is evidence that such treatments may also slow disease progression.

REFERENCES

Abbott JJ, Howlett DR, Francis PT, Williams RJ. (2008) Aß$_{1-42}$ modulation of Akt phosphorylation via a7 nAChR and NMDA receptors. *Neurobiology of Aging* 29: 992–1001.

Auld DS, Kar S, Quirion R. (1998) Beta-amyloid peptides as direct cholinergic neuromodulators: A missing link? *Trends in Neuroscience* 21: 43–9.

Baudry M, Lynch G. (2001) Remembrance of arguments past: How well is the glutamate receptor hypothesis of LTP holding up after 20 years? *Neurobiology of Learning and Memory* 76: 284–97.

Beach TG, Kuo YM, Spiegel K et al. (2000) The cholinergic deficit coincides with A beta deposition at the earliest histopathologic stages of Alzheimer disease. *Journal of Neuropathology and Experimental Neurology* 59: 308–13.

Begni B, Brighina L, Sirtori E et al. (2004) Oxidative stress impairs glutamate uptake in fibroblasts from patients with Alzheimer's disease. *Free Radical Biology and Medicine* 37: 892–901.

Bellocchio EE, Reimer RJ, Fremeau Jr RT, Edwards RH. (2000) Uptake of glutamate into synaptic vesicles by an inorganic phosphate transporter. *Science* 289: 957–60.

Bowen DM, Smith CB, White P, Davison AN. (1976) Neurotransmitter-related enzymes and indices of hypoxia in senile dementia and other abiotrophies. *Brain* 99: 459–96.

Caccamo A, Oddo S, Billings LM *et al.* (2006) M1 receptors play a central role in modulating AD-like pathology in transgenic mice. *Neuron* 49: 671–82.

Chessell IP, Humphrey PPA. (1995) Nicotinic and muscarinic receptor-evoked depolarisations recorded from a novel cortical brain slice preparation. *Neuropharmacology* 34: 1289–96.

Court JA, Lloyd S, Thomas N *et al.* (1998) Dopamine and nicotinic receptor binding and the levels of dopamine and homovanillic acid in human brain related to tobacco use. *Neuroscience* 87: 63–78.

Court J, Martin-Ruiz C, Piggott M *et al.* (2001) Nicotinic receptor abnormalities in Alzheimer's disease. *Biological Psychiatry* 49: 175–84.

Cummings JL, Kaufer DI. (1996) Neuropsychiatric aspects of Alzheimer's disease: The cholinergic hypothesis revisited. *Neurology* 47: 876–83.

Danbolt NC. (2001) Glutamate uptake. *Progress in Neurobiology* 65: 1–105.

Davies P, Maloney AJF. (1976) Selective loss of central cholinergic neurones in Alzheimer's disease. *Lancet* ii: 1403.

Davis KL, Mohs RC, Marin D *et al.* (1999) Cholinergic markers in elderly patients with early signs of Alzheimer disease. *Journal of the American Medical Association* 281: 1401–6.

DeKosky ST, Ikonomovic MD, Styren SD *et al.* (2002) Upregulation of choline acetyltransferase activity in hippocampus and frontal cortex of elderly subjects with mild cognitive impairment. *Annals of Neurology* 51: 145–55.

Dijk SN, Francis PT, Stratmann GC, Bowen DM. (1995) Cholinomimetics increase glutamate outflow by an action on the corticostriatal pathway: Implications for Alzheimer's disease. *Journal of Neurochemistry* 65: 2165–9.

Drachman DA, Leavitt J. (1974) Human memory and the cholinergic system. *Archives of Neurology* 30: 113–21.

Emre M, Aarsland D, Albanese A *et al.* (2004) Rivastigmine for dementia associated with Parkinson's disease. *New England Journal of Medicine* 351: 2509–18.

Esiri M. (1991) Neuropathology. In: Jacoby R, Oppenheimer C (eds). *Psychiatry in the elderly.* Oxford: Oxford University Press, 113–47.

Francis PT. (2003) Glutamatergic systems in Alzheimer's disease. *International Journal of Geriatric Psychiatry* 18 (Suppl 1): S15–21.

Francis PT. (2005) The interplay of neurotransmitters in Alzheimer's disease. *CNS Spectrums* 10 (Suppl 18): 6–9.

Francis PT. (2009) Altered glutamate neurotransmission and behaviour in dementia: Evidence from studies of memantine. *Current Molecular Pharmacology* 2: 77–82.

Francis PT, Palmer AM, Sims NR *et al.* (1985) Neurochemical studies of early-onset Alzheimer's disease. Possible influence on treatment. *New England Journal of Medicine* 313: 7–11.

Francis PT, Sims NR, Procter AW, Bowen DM. (1993) Cortical pyramidal neurone loss may cause glutamatergic hypoactivity and cognitive impairment in Alzheimer's disease: Investigative and therapeutic perspectives. *Journal of Neurochemistry* 60: 1589–604.

Francis PT, Palmer AM, Snape M, Wilcock GK. (1999) The cholinergic hypothesis of Alzheimer's disease: A review of progress. *Journal of Neurology, Neurosurgery, and Psychiatry* 66: 137–47.

Gauthier S, Feldman H, Hecker J *et al.* (2002) Efficacy of donepezil on behavioral symptoms in patients with moderate to severe Alzheimer's disease. *International Psychogeriatrics* 14: 389–404.

Hardy J. (2006) A hundred years of Alzheimer's disease research. *Neuron* 52: 3–13.

Hellstrom-Lindahl E, Court J, Keverne J *et al.* (2004) Nicotine reduces A beta in the brain and cerebral vessels of APPsw mice. *European Journal of Neuroscience* 19: 2703–10.

Hock C, Maddalena A, Heuser I *et al.* (2000) Treatment with the selective muscarinic agonist talsaclidine decreases cerebrospinal fluid levels of total amyloid beta-peptide in patients with Alzheimer's disease. *Annals of the New York Academy of Sciences* 920: 285–91.

Hyman BT, Van Hoesen GW, Damasio AR. (1987) Alzheimer's disease: Glutamate depletion in the hippocampal perforant pathway zone. *Annals of Neurology* 22: 37–40.

Ikonomovic MD, Armstrong DM. (1996) Distribution of AMPA receptor subunits in the nucleus basalis of Meynert in aged humans: Implications for selective neuronal degeneration. *Brain Research* 716: 229–32.

Johnson SA, Simmon VF. (2002) Randomized, double-blind, placebo-controlled international clinical trial of the Ampakine CX516 in elderly participants with mild cognitive impairment: A progress report. *Journal of Molecular Neuroscience* 19: 197–200.

Kashani A, Lepicard E, Poirel O *et al.* (2008) Loss of VGLUT1 and VGLUT2 in the prefrontal cortex is correlated with cognitive decline in Alzheimer disease. *Neurobiology of Aging* 29: 1619–30.

Keller JN, Mark RJ, Bruce AJ *et al.* (1997) 4-hydroxynonenal, an aldehydic product of membrane lipid peroxidation, impairs glutamate transport and mitochondrial function in synaptosomes. *Neuroscience* 80: 685–96.

Kirvell SL, Esiri MM, Francis PT. (2006) Down regulation of vesicular glutamate transporters precede cell loss and pathology in Alzheimer's disease. *Journal of Neurochemistry* 98: 939–50.

Kowall NW, Beal MF. (1991) Glutamate-, glutaminase-, and taurine-immunoreactive neurones develop neurofibrillary tangles in Alzheimer's disease. *Annals of Neurology* 29: 162–7.

Lai MK, Lai OF, Keene J *et al.* (2001) Psychosis of Alzheimer's disease is associated with elevated muscarinic M2 binding in the cortex. *Neurology* 57: 805–11.

Lai MKP, Ramirez MJ, Tsang SW, Francis PT. (2007) Alzheimer's disease as a neurotransmitter disease. In: Dawbarn D, Allen SJ (eds). *Neurobiology of Alzheimer's disease*, 3rd edn. Oxford: Oxford University Press, 245–82.

Lipton P. (1999) Ischemic cell death in brain neurons. *Physiological Reviews* 79: 1431–568.

Lowe SL, Bowen DM, Francis PT, Neary D. (1990) Ante mortem cerebral amino acid concentrations indicate selective degeneration of glutamate-enriched neurons in Alzheimer's disease. *Neuroscience* 38: 571–7.

Lynch G. (1998) Memory and the brain: Unexpected chemistries and a new pharmacology. *Neurobiology of Learning and Memory* 70: 82–100.

Mesulam M, Shaw P, Mash D, Weintraub S. (2004) Cholinergic nucleus basalis tauopathy emerges early in the aging-MCI-AD continuum. *Annals of Neurology* 55: 815–28.

Minger SL, Esiri MM, McDonald B *et al.* (2000) Cholinergic deficits contribute to behavioural disturbance in patients with dementia. *Neurology* 55: 1460–7.

Myhrer T, Paulsen RE. (1997) Infusion of D-cycloserine into temporal-hippocampal areas and restoration of mnemonic function in rats with disrupted glutamatergic temporal systems. *European Journal of Pharmacology* 328: 1–7.

Neary D, Snowden JS, Mann DM *et al.* (1986) Alzheimer's disease: A correlative study. *Journal of Neurology, Neurosurgery, and Psychiatry* 49: 229–37.

Nitsch RM. (1996) From acetylcholine to amyloid: Neurotransmitters and the pathology of Alzheimer's disease. *Neurodegeneration* 5: 477–82.

Nitsch RM, Deng M, Tennis M *et al.* (2000) The selective muscarinic M1 agonist AF102B decreases levels of total Abeta in cerebrospinal fluid of patients with Alzheimer's disease. *Annals of Neurology* 48: 913–8.

Parsons CG, Stoffler A, Danysz W. (2007) Memantine: A NMDA receptor antagonist that improves memory by restoration of homeostasis in the glutamatergic system – too little activation is bad, too much is even worse. *Neuropharmacology* 53: 699–723.

Perry EK, Perry RH, Blessed G, Tomlinson BE. (1978) Changes in brain cholinesterases in senile dementia of Alzheimer type. *Neuropathology and Applied Neurobiology* 4: 273–7.

Perry RH, Candy JM, Perry EK *et al.* (1982) Extensive loss of choline acetyltransferase activity is not reflected by neuronal loss in the nucleus of Meynert in Alzheimer's disease. *Neuroscience Letters* 33: 311–5.

Perry EK, Smith CJ, Court JA, Perry RH. (1990) Cholinergic nictotinic and muscarinic receptors in dementia of Alzheimer, Parkinson and Lewy body types. *Journal of Neural Transmission. Parkinson's Disease and Dementia section* 2: 149–58.

Perry EK, Haroutunian V, Davis KL *et al.* (1994) Neocortical cholinergic activities differentiate Lewy body dementia from classical Alzheimer's disease. *NeuroReport* 5: 747–9.

Perry EK, Walker M, Grace J, Perry RH. (1999) Acetylcholine in mind: A neurotransmitter correlate of consciousness? *Trends in Neuroscience* 22: 273–80.

Postle BR, Corkin S, Growdon JH. (1996) Intact implicit memory for novel patterns in Alzheimer's disease. *Learning and Memory* 3: 305–12.

Procter AW, Palmer AM, Francis PT *et al.* (1988) Evidence of glutamatergic denervation and possible abnormal metabolism in Alzheimer's disease. *Journal of Neurochemistry* 50: 790–802.

Procter AW, Francis PT, Holmes C *et al.* (1994) APP isoforms show correlations with neurones but not with glia in brains of demented subjects. *Acta Neuropathologica* 88: 545–52.

Reisberg B, Doody R, Stoffler A *et al.* (2003) Memantine in moderate-to-severe Alzheimer's disease. *New England Journal of Medicine* 348: 1333–41.

Sadot E, Gurwitz D, Barg J *et al.* (1996) Activation of m_1 muscarinic acetylcholine receptor regulates τ phosphorylation in transfected PC12 cells. *Journal of Neurochemistry* 66: 877–80.

Schwartz BL, Hashtroudi S, Herting RL *et al.* (1996) D-cycloserine enhances implicit memory in Alzheimer patients. *Neurology* 46: 420–4.

Tariot PN, Farlow MR, Grossberg GT *et al.* (2004) Memantine treatment in patients with moderate to severe Alzheimer disease already receiving donepezil: A randomized controlled trial. *JAMA* 291: 317–24.

Tekin S, Mega MS, Masterman DM *et al.* (2001) Orbitofrontal and anterior cingulate cortex neurofibrillary tangle burden is associated with agitation in Alzheimer disease. *Annals of Neurology* 49: 355–61.

Terry RD, Masliah E, Salmon DP *et al.* (1991) Physical basis of cognitive alterations in Alzheimer's disease: Synapse loss is the major correlate of cognitive impairment. *Annals of Neurology* 30: 572–80.

Tsang SW, Lai MK, Kirvell S *et al.* (2006) Impaired coupling of muscarinic M(1) receptors to G-proteins in the neocortex is associated with severity of dementia in Alzheimer's disease. *Neurobiology of Aging* 27: 1216–23.

Turrini P, Casu MA, Wong TP *et al.* (2001) Cholinergic nerve terminals establish classical synapses in the rat cerebral cortex: Synaptic pattern and age-related atrophy. *Neuroscience* 105: 277–85.

Wang HY, Lee DHS, Dandrea MR *et al.* (2000) Beta-amyloid(1-42) binds to alpha 7 nicotinic acetylcholine receptor with high affinity – implications for Alzheimer's disease pathology. *Journal of Biological Chemistry* 275: 5626–32.

Wilkinson DG, Francis PT, Schwam E, Payne-Parrish J. (2004) Cholinesterase inhibitors used in the treatment of Alzheimer's disease: The relationship between pharmacological effects and clinical efficacy. *Drugs and Aging* 21: 453–78.

The central role of Aβ amyloid in the pathogenesis of Alzheimer's disease

CRAIG RITCHIE, CATRIONA MCLEAN, KONRAD BEYREUTHER AND COLIN L MASTERS

51.1 INTRODUCTION

The details of the molecular neuropathology of Alzheimer's disease (AD), from the amyloid precursor protein (APP) through to the production of amyloid Aβ, plaque formation, neurodegeneration and to final neuronal death are discussed in this chapter. This process, like Alexander's Gordian knot, has been scrutinized over the last three decades with the ongoing hope that a decisive therapeutic incision is not too distant. Points in the biochemical pathway that may be amenable to therapeutic intervention are highlighted.

The theory that Aβ amyloid underlies the neurodegenerative changes in AD remains pre-eminent (**Figure 51.1**) despite the emergence in recent years of alternative disease pathways. It is clear that there are both proven and hypothetical links between the alternate pathways (mitochondrial dysfunction, neuroinflammation, elevation of cortisol and the destabilization of tubulin) and Aβ protein. Integral to the pivotal role of Aβ and AD is the presumed neurotoxicity of Aβ, especially in its oligomeric form, whilst the monomeric form may have important physiological properties.

This peptide is the main constituent of the amyloid plaque, one of the characteristic pathological features of AD. It is also found in vessel walls as a congophilic amyloid angiopathy (Glenner and Wong, 1984; Masters et al., 1985).

Neurofibrillary changes are also major features in the brains of patients with AD. Tau protein, a microtubule-associated protein, is ubiquinated, phosphorylated and accumulates as neurofibrillary tangles (NFT) forming dystrophic neurites (Kosik et al., 1986; Wood et al., 1986). The actual link between Aβ accumulation and tau-associated NFT remains unknown, although NFT appear to be downstream of the events which surround Aβ accumulation in the AD brain. The hyperphosphorylation of tau protein may result within energy deficient neuronal cells that achieve this state through mitochondrial dysfunction. It has been demonstrated that mitochondria are susceptible to damage arising from internalized Aβ binding to the mitochondrial membrane. This observation would place intracellular Aβ accumulation at an upstream point in the genesis of two subsequent intracellular pathological processes seen in AD, namely mitochondrial dysfunction and tau hyperphosphorylation.

The biogenesis of Aβ from APP and putative mechanisms for its neurotoxicity, together with genetic risk factors such as apolipoprotein E (ApoE) that may interact with Aβ and affect its clearance from the brain, is the focus of this chapter. More detailed reviews on these subjects can be found elsewhere (Blacker and Tanzi, 1998; Hardy et al., 1998; Multhaup et al., 1998; Price et al., 1998; Lansbury, 1999; Scheper et al., 1999; Butterfield, 2002; Citron, 2002; Lahiri et al., 2002; Suh and

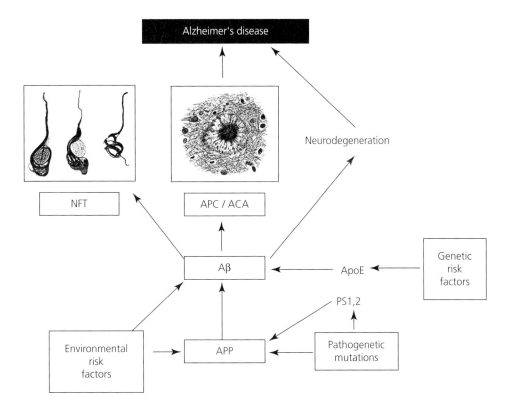

Figure 51.1   The amyloidocentric pathway that leads to Alzheimer's disease proceeds from the proteolytic processing of the amyloid β precursor protein (APP) into the Aβ amyloid. The amyloid forms visible plaques (amyloid plaque cores, APC; amyloid congophilic angiopathy, ACA). The relationship between Aβ and neurofibrillary tangle (NFT) formation remains unclear. The mechanisms that underly the basic neurodegenerative changes in Alzheimer's disease are also uncertain. This pathway is subject to modulation by environmental and genetic factors at various points.

Checler, 2002; Walsh *et al.*, 2002; Atwood *et al.*, 2003; Butterfield, 2003; Bertram and Tanzi, 2004).

51.2   Aβ AMYLOID ACCUMULATION AND PLAQUE DEVELOPMENT

One of the two characteristic microscopic features of AD is the accumulation of Aβ amyloid in plaques of varying morphology. These are extracellular or perivascular congophilic deposits of aggregated Aβ with a high content of β-pleated sheet secondary structure. The amyloid plaque itself is the end result of a process of Aβ oligomerization, fibril formation, aggregation and precipitation occurring in several stages, with each stage potentially having a different impact on surrounding neurones. Initially it was postulated that a soluble species of Aβ forms oligomers. Over time there has developed a consensus that it is the oligomeric form of Aβ that is the most synaptotoxic (Naylor *et al.*, 2008; Shankar and Walsh, 2009) and neurotoxic (Mclean *et al.*, 1999). Oligomers are formed from monomeric Aβ through the formation of covalent di-tyrosine bonds that are relatively resistant to catabolism (Naylor *et al.*, 2008). The formation of oligomers is dependent upon the presence of metal ions (in particular copper and zinc) and generates free radicals as these metal ions are reduced (Smith *et al.*, 2007). These oligomers may then aggregate into protofibrillar structures,

which may first be seen as precipitates in diffuse amyloid plaques; this progresses with dystrophic neurite formation both within the neuropil and around dense crystalloid precipitates of amyloid cores. Following this, an intermediate stage is reached where the plaque increases in complexity before a final stage of a non-neuritic 'burned out' or 'end-stage plaque' is reached. The genesis of plaques may well represent a physiological response to neutralize the toxicity of the Aβ oligomers.

In AD, processing of APP creates a high ratio of $A\beta_{42}$ ('long' Aβ of 42 amino acids) to $A\beta_{40}$ ('short' Aβ of 40 amino acids). The more insoluble long Aβ is the primary constituent of the amyloid plaque. However, immunocytochemical techniques have demonstrated that diffuse plaques contain not only $A\beta_{42}$ but also $A\beta_{40}$ and, in a small proportion of plaques (most of which have a dense amyloid core), $A\beta_{(16-40/42)}$ (the p3 fragment) (Dickson, 1997). Perivascular amyloid identified in the congophilic angiopathies predominantly consists of $A\beta_{40}$ (Suzuki *et al.*, 1994; Barelli *et al.*, 1997).

Plaque morphology also varies as a function of topographic location. Smaller granular deposits are seen in the deep grey matter nuclei, and linear streaks occur in the molecular layer of the cerebellum. The morphology of the amyloid plaque therefore varies depending upon both location and stage of development.

The number of amyloid plaques at post-mortem does not correlate well with the severity of clinical disease (McKee et al., 1991; Morris et al., 1991; Terry et al., 1991; Berg et al., 1998). However, plaque formation may correlate with the degree of neuronal injury as identified by the cellular pro-apoptotic response as measured by the TUNEL technique (Sheng et al., 1998). The poor correlation may also be explained in part by a process of growth and resolution of plaques with the establishment of a plateau phase for plaque production (Hyman and Tanzi, 1992). In concert with traditional explanations of the disconnect between plaque number and disease severity, there is now a gathering consensus that the soluble $A\beta_{42}$ load may be more closely related to clinical severity (McLean et al., 1999), whether or not the $A\beta_{42}$ exists as an oligomer or complexed to other proteins (Lorenzo and Yanker, 1994; Howlett et al., 1995). A major argument raised by opponents of the amyloid theory is that individuals can have numerous plaques but no clinical cognitive impairment. This may be countered by the observation, as will be elaborated below, that Aβ, while being the crucial factor in triggering the neuronal compromise resulting in neurodegeneration in AD, will only act upon compromised cells, such compromise appearing, for example, in the form of age-related oxidative stress (Lockhart et al., 1994). Moreover, Aβ may mediate clinical symptomatology predominantly through synaptotoxicity and neurotoxicity which precedes frank neurodegeneration. Finally, Aβ and the plaque are components within a very complex biological system that relies on numerous other pathological processes before AD develops clinically. These processes are mediated by other biological, genetic and environmental risk factors. It may be that to trigger AD from the physiological production of monomeric Aβ requires the 'perfect storm' combining several biological (e.g. neuro-inflammation, mitochondrial dysfunction and genentic vulnerability) and environmental (e.g. cerebrovascular pathology, elevated levels of cerebral trace metals or stress) factors – all of which are more likely to accumulate and co-occur with advancing age.

51.3   GENETIC EVIDENCE FOR THE ROLE OF Aβ IN AD

The most convincing support for the central role of Aβ and APP in the pathogenesis of AD is that all of the known fully penetrant autosomal dominant gene mutations that cause early onset AD lead to an increase of $A\beta_{42}$ production (**Table 51.1**). Mutations in the APP gene itself lead to the development of aberrant APP that is preferentially processed to produce an increase in the $A\beta_{42:40}$ ratio. All causative APP mutations identified to date occur in proximity to the Aβ domain of the protein. Similarly, multiple mutations in the two presenilin genes have a dramatic effect on the $A\beta_{42:40}$ ratio.

51.4   AMYLOID PRECURSOR PROTEIN

The APP is a transmembrane protein that is found in most cell types including neuronal and glial cells (**Figure 51.2**). It is especially enriched in the alpha-granule of platelets. The APP gene is located on chromosome 21 (Kang et al., 1987). The pathogenic APP mutations account for less than 5 per cent of all cases of AD inherited in an autosomal dominant manner.

The precise physiological function of APP is unknown, though no doubt it is complex and possibly related to synaptic plasticity, repair and regeneration. The structural domains suggest that it may have a role in cell–cell (synapse) or cell–matrix interactions (neurite stabilization). In the platelet, APP has been shown to be involved in inhibition of platelet aggregation via an effect on arachidonic acid metabolism (Henry et al., 1998). There is also evidence to suggest that APP is affected by metal ion binding, calcium levels and heparin binding. APP has also been associated with cell proliferation and neurite outgrowth in response to nerve growth factor (Milward et al., 1992; Small et al., 1994; Yankner, 1996). Other

Table 51.1   Pathogenic mutations that cause Alzheimer's disease.

Mutations	Mechanism of action	Effect
APPgene dosage or aberrant regulation		
Down's syndrome (trisomy 21)	Upregulation of APP gene promotor up to 5- to 6-fold	Increased total Aβ
Pathogenic APP gene mutations		
APP codons:		
670/671 (Swedish)	Increase β-secretase cleavage	Excess total Aβ production
692 and 693 (Dutch and Flemish)	Decrease α-secretase activity?	Resultant increase in β- and γ-activity with consequent increased total Aβ
715 (French)	Affects γ-secretase activity	Increased amounts of Aβ p3 fragment
717 (London)	Altered γ-secretase activity	Increased ratio of $A\beta_{42:40}$
723 (Australian)	Affects γ-secretase activity	Increased ratio of $A\beta_{42:40}$
Pathogenic PS1, 2 gene mutations		
More than 70 point or missense mutations and exon deletion mutations	Direct or indirect alteration of γ-secretase	Increased ratio of $A\beta_{42:40}$

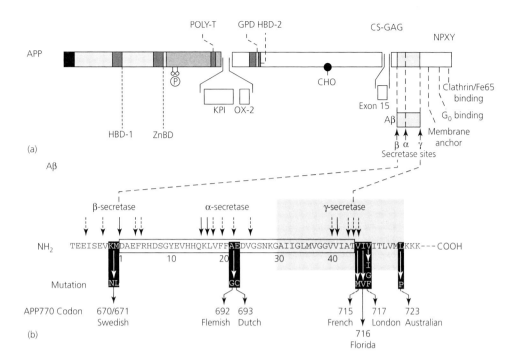

Figure 51.2   The structural domains of APP are schematically shown. Within the large extracellular ectodomain there are heparin-binding sites (HBD-1,2), metal-binding sites (ZnBD), growth-promoting domains (GPD), carbohydrate-attachment sites (CHO; CS-GAG) and alternatively spliced exons (KPI, OX2, exon 15). The shorter cytoplasmic domain has interacting motifs for G_0 protein, clathrin (NPXY) and the Fe65 family of proteins. The Aβ (juxtatransmembrane and transmembrane) domains are shown in more detail. The β-, α- and γ-secretase sites are shown, with the major cleavage sites indicated by unbroken arrows. The critical pathogenic mutations are shown to be clustered near the secretase sites (see also **Table 51.1**).

in vitro experiments have suggested that a deficiency of APP renders cells more susceptible to a variety of neurotoxic insults.

51.5   APP PROCESSING BY α-, β- AND γ-SECRETASES

APP exists in three major isoforms of 695, 751 and 770 amino acids. The 695 amino acid isoform (APP695) is predominantly expressed in neurones (Kang *et al.*, 1987; Tanzi *et al.*, 1987). The APP751 and APP770 isoforms are predominantly expressed in peripheral tissues and astrocytes (Golde *et al.*, 1990; Kang and Müller-Hill, 1990). APP is synthesized in the endoplasmic reticulum and is then transported through the Golgi apparatus to the cell surface. In its transmembrane orientation (as shown in **Figure 51.2**) it undergoes proteolytic cleavage to produce Aβ. The half-life of APP is short and is processed by at least two pathways (α- and β-/γ-secretase activities). In peripheral cells, α-secretase activity predominates, cleaving the Aβ domain of APP at position 16/17. This leads to the production of soluble ectodomain protein sAPPα (Evin *et al.*, 1994). The soluble ectodomains of APP (both sAPPα and sAPPβ) do not aggregate and do not participate in plaque formation. α-Secretase activity leaves in the membrane a small carboxyl-terminal fragment which undergoes further processing. The α-secretase activity may be sequence non-specific and act on several other transmembrane proteins. Furthermore, recent work has identified a disintegrin and metalloprotease

(ADAM), as being a potent effector of α-secretase activity (Lammich *et al.*, 1999). Increase of ADAM-10 expression and activity may theoretically be effective as a treatment for AD.

Aβ therefore exists in several forms depending on the site of cleavage by as yet largely undefined α-, β- or γ-secretases. The length of the Aβ fragment varies depending on the site of cleavage leading to a product between 39 and 43 amino acids in length. The N-terminal 28 residues are from the extracellular portion of APP, and the 11–15 C-terminal residues are derived from the transmembrane domain. It is the $Aβ_{42}$ which is considered to be the more insoluble and toxic moiety and is a product of γ-secretase cleavage of the APP molecule. β- and γ-secretase activity involves cleavage of APP at sites corresponding to positions 1 (β-secretase) and 40 or 42 (γ-secretase) of the Aβ fragment, releasing the insoluble amyloidogenic peptide $Aβ_{(1-40/42)}$ commonly referred to as $Aβ_{42}$. It is intriguing to note that in animal models, elevated levels of cortisol are associated with preferential activity of the β-secretase pathway (Green *et al.*, 2006) as well as hippocampal atrophy and increased amyloid plaque development (Butters *et al.*, 2008) in patients with depression. These biological observations provide a basis for the described epidemiological and clinical link between depression/stress and AD (Jorm, 2001; Huang *et al.*, 2009).

Determination of the identity of γ-secretase could have important therapeutic implications. Recent evidence suggests an intimate relationship between presenilin (PS)1 and γ-secretase, and there is increasing evidence that the active site of γ-secretase lies within the transmembrane domains of the

PS molecule (De Strooper *et al.*, 1999; Struhl and Greenwald, 1999; Wolfe *et al.*, 1999; Ye *et al.*, 1999). The macromolecular complex which constitutes γ-secretase activity is presently discerned as >400 kDa in mass, and contains at least three other molecules: Aph1, Pen2 and nicastrin (Iwatsubo, 2004). Active development of inhibitors of γ-secretase has progressed at a radical pace, and the results of clinical trials are expected soon.

51.6   APP MUTATIONS AND Aβ PRODUCTION

The various APP mutations inevitably produce increased ratios of Aβ42 through a variety of mechanisms (**Table 51.1**). The mutations at codons 670/671 (the 'Swedish' mutation), increase β-secretase cleavage and lead to an overall excess amyloid production (Cai *et al.*, 1993). Mutations at codon 717 (the 'London' mutation), 715 (the 'French' mutation), 716 (the 'Florida' mutation) and 723 (the 'Australian' mutation) act at the γ-secretase site, increasing the ratio of Aβ42:40 (Suzuki *et al.*, 1994; Brooks *et al.*, 1995; Eckman *et al.*, 1997; Ancolio *et al.*, 1999; Kwok *et al.*, 2000). Mutations at 692 and 693 (the 'Dutch' and 'Flemish' mutations) are either associated with α-secretase activity, presumably leading to a decrease in this pathway with a resultant increase in β- and γ-activity (Haass *et al.*, 1994) or yield a mutant Aβ peptide with enhanced toxicity or propensity to aggregation. In Down's syndrome (trisomy 21), where there is an extra copy of the APP gene, there is a similar increase in the overall levels of Aβ42 (Teller *et al.*, 1996).

It is necessary to elucidate the mechanisms that regulate the activity of the secretase enzymes involved in APP metabolism, as a greater understanding of these processes will aid the development of therapeutic interventions. One factor that may predict which form of cleavage is utilized is cell type, with glial cells and neurones (both differentiated and undifferentiated) producing different isoforms of APP (Haass *et al.*, 1991; Baskin *et al.*, 1992; Hung *et al.*, 1992). Another factor that influences the cleavage pathway may be the release of APP by protein kinase C (PKC) which leads to a predominance of the α-secretase pathway (Caporaso *et al.*, 1992; Gillespie *et al.*, 1992; Sinha and Lieberburg, 1992). Of interest, PKC-mediated α-secretase activity may be induced by neurotransmitters and other first messenger ligands (Buxbaum *et al.*, 1992; Lahiri *et al.*, 1992; Nitsch *et al.*, 1992). If these first and second messenger pathways prove to directly influence the production of Aβ42, then these systems could provide another target for pharmacological intervention.

51.7   PRESENILINS 1 AND 2

The PS1 gene is located on chromosome 14 and PS2 on chromosome 1. In the brain, PS1 is found in both neurones and glia. It has a multi-pass transmembrane orientation (**Figure 51.3**). PS2 expression in the pancreas and muscle exceeds other sites including the brain (Rogaev, 1998). The presenilin molecules undergo cleavage by unidentified mechanisms to yield N- and C-terminal fragments. The functions of PS1 and PS2 are unknown, though it has been proposed that they may have a role in signalling pathways from plasma membranes to the cell nucleus during cell differentiation, or they may play a role in receptor trafficking and protein recycling.

A link between PS mutations and Aβ production has been confirmed as an increased ratio of Aβ42:40 is noted in

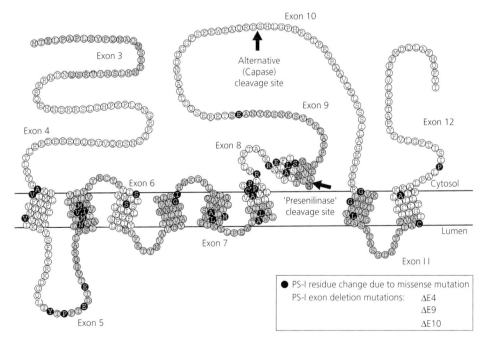

Figure 51.3   A model of the presenilin 1 molecule. The multiple mutations that cause early-onset Alzheimer's disease are seen to cluster in the transmembrane domains and in proximity to the normal 'presenilinase' cleavage site. The cytosolic loop between transmembrane domains 6 and 7 may play a critical role in γ-secretase activity.

transfected cell lines and transgenic mice expressing mutant forms of PS1 (Borchelt *et al.*, 1996; Citron *et al.*, 1996; Duff *et al.*, 1996; Lemere *et al.*, 1996). Knock-out PS1 cells lose γ-secretase activity, consistent with the concept of PS harbouring the active γ-secretase site (De Strooper *et al.*, 1998). Furthermore, patients and at-risk individuals with PS mutations have increased ratios of Aβ$_{42:40}$ (Scheuner *et al.*, 1996). PS1 may have an anti-apoptotic activity (Roperch *et al.*, 1998) and mutations in PS1 may sensitize neuronal cells to apoptosis by disruption of intracellular calcium levels (Keller *et al.*, 1998).

In summary, all the identified genotypes in autosomal dominant AD have, as their common denominator, an increase in the production of Aβ$_{42}$. This observation suggests a direct causal relationship between Aβ$_{42}$ and the development of AD.

51.8   Aβ AND NEUROTOXICITY

Despite evidence that an increase in the proportion of Aβ$_{42}$ is a common end point for all the autosomal dominant mutations that lead to AD, the exact mechanism of underlying Aβ$_{42}$ and neuronal degeneration remains unclear (**Table 51.2**).

Aβ has been shown to be directly neurotoxic to hippocampal neurones that are particularly sensitive to oxidative stress and are affected first in the spread of AD throughout the cerebral cortex. While some authors have been unable to demonstrate neurotoxicity of Aβ when it exists in an immature, non-fibrillar, amorphous aggregate (Lorenzo and Yanker, 1994), there is now an emerging consensus that the smaller oligomeric aggregates of Aβ, in association with factors such as metal ions, constitute the principal forms of the toxic Aβ species. Aβ can potentiate the neuronal insult of excitatory amino acids (Koh *et al.*, 1990), oxidative stress (Lockhart *et al.*, 1994) and glucose deprivation (Copani *et al.*, 1991). This may explain why the cumulative exposure of the ageing brain to other risk factors renders it more vulnerable to the toxic effects of Aβ. Aβ has also been shown *in vitro* to cause plasma membrane lipid peroxidation, impairment of ion motive ATPases, glutamate uptake and uncoupling of γ-protein linked receptors (Behl *et al.*, 1994; Butterfield *et al.*, 1994; Hensley *et al.*, 1994; Mark *et al.*, 1996). These pathological processes may contribute to a loss of intracellular calcium homeostasis that has been reported in cultured neurones (Mattson *et al.*, 1993). Aβ, when introduced into neuronal cultures, leads to a gradual increase in intracellular calcium, though this activity is not affected by the addition of either calcium channel blockers or chelating agents (Lorenzo and Yanker, 1994; Whitson and Appel, 1995). Aβ may also impair redox activity in mitochondria, leading to the

Table 51.2 Aβ toxicity-proposed mechanisms.

Generation of reactive oxygen species, metal mediated
Physical disruption of cellular membrane
Receptor-mediated uptake and apoptotic signalling
Disturbance of intracellular calcium homeostasis

production of free radicals (Shearman *et al.*, 1994). Cellular damage mediated by Aβ is inhibited by vitamin E (Behl *et al.*, 1992). This supports the above observation that a free radical-based process, mediated by Aβ, leads to neuronal damage and that this process, *in vitro*, can be inhibited by antioxidants. The use of antioxidants in the treatment of AD has been investigated clinically in recent years and some clinical efficacy has been shown with vitamin E (Sano *et al.*, 1997) though a summation of the evidence to date has concluded that this intervention may well be too late in advanced disease or early dementia (Ames and Ritchie, 2007). Moreover, preliminary trials with compounds which target the redox-active metal binding sites on Aβ have yielded encouraging results (Ritchie *et al.*, 2003; Lannfelt *et al.*, 2008).

51.9   Aβ INTERACTION WITH APOE AND OTHER RISK FACTOR GENES

51.9.1   ApoE

Apolipoprotein E isoforms represent a major genetic susceptibility factor for sporadic AD, affecting all people aged over 60 years. It is the first of what may prove to be a multiple set of genetic risk factors that have the potential to modify any putative environmental risk factor.

The ApoE gene, located on chromosome 19, was the first polymorphic gene to be associated with a complex disease using positional cloning strategies. The ApoE gene products vary depending upon the inherited pair of polymorphic alleles. There are three allelic varieties: ε2, ε3 and ε4. ApoE is a glycoprotein of 299 amino acids that is a normal constituent of plasma and cerebrospinal fluid lipoprotein particles. The physiological function of the protein is to mediate cholesterol uptake, storage, transport and metabolism. There is a binding site for Aβ present near the C-terminus of the ApoE molecule (Wisniewski *et al.*, 1993). ApoE is a component of the very low-density lipoprotein (VLDL) and high-density lipoprotein complexes involved in cellular uptake and metabolism of cholesterol (Mahley, 1988). ApoE is normally upregulated and released from astrocytes following neuronal injury and not only affects lipid metabolism following this trauma, but may also complex with VLDL to increase neurite outgrowth and synaptogenesis. However, the different ApoE genotypes differentially affect this process. Individuals carrying the ε4 allele have a decreased capacity for compensatory neurite outgrowth and synaptogenesis following neuronal injury (Poirier, 1994).

It has also been demonstrated that individuals with at least one ε4 allele develop greater numbers of neuritic plaques (Olichney *et al.*, 1996) irrespective of whether or not they have clinical AD (Rebeck *et al.*, 1993; Schmechel *et al.*, 1993; Polvikoski *et al.*, 1995). ApoE ε4 also complexes with Aβ, whereas ApoE ε3 does not have the same affinity, thus promoting protofibril formation, which, as has been alluded to already, may be the immediate neurotoxic product in AD. A model therefore exists that outlines the interaction between Aβ and ApoE which explains why the latter exists as one of many contributing genetic risk factors to the development of

AD. At the very least, it links the metabolism of cholesterol into the Aβ-mediated pathway of AD causation.

Not only is the genotype that an individual carries relevant as a risk factor for AD, but variations in ApoE levels may also be an important factor in predicting disease onset. The promoter of ApoE that regulates the synthesis of the lipoprotein is polymorphic. The allelic variants at −491 (Bullido et al., 1998), −427 (Artiga et al., 1998) and −219 (Lambert et al., 1998) of the ApoE promoter region, when homozygous, may be associated with increased risk of AD, and a combination of the adverse alleles of the promoter and coding regions confer even greater risk of developing AD (Artiga et al., 1998).

Clinically, possession of the ε4 allele increases the risk of developing AD at any particular age. In individuals who are ε4 heterozygotes, there is an approximate doubling of risk and for those that are homozygous for ε4 the risk is increased by a factor of between 6 and 8 (National Institute on Aging/Alzheimer's Association Working Group, 1996). Possession of an ε4 allele may lead to an earlier age of onset (Blacker et al., 1997; Burlinson et al., 1998) and there may be an even greater risk of developing AD in females who carry the ε4 allele (Poirier et al., 1993; Payami et al., 1994; Duara et al., 1996). There are, however, conflicting reports regarding the rate of decline associated with different genotypes. The ApoE ε2 allele may confer protection against the development of AD (Corder et al., 1994; Myers et al., 1996).

The ε4 allele also confers additional risk of developing AD in those patients who have suffered strokes (Slooter et al., 1997), though other authors, in smaller studies, have failed to replicate this finding (Burlinson et al., 1998). Other cerebral insults such as head injuries have been associated with increased Aβ deposition in patients who carry an ε4 allele (Nicoll et al., 1995). Determining the ApoE status of a patient may be of value in aiding the diagnosis of AD where there is already a high clinical suspicion of the condition. However, there may only be a marginal increase in diagnostic accuracy (American College of Medical Genetics/American Society of Human Genetics Working Group on Apo E and Alzheimer's disease, 1995; National Institute on Aging/Alzheimer's Association Working Group, 1996). In isolation, knowledge of the ApoE genotype of any given individual lacks the sensitivity, specificity or positive predictive value to be useful as a screening tool.

51.9.2 α2-Macroglobulin, low–density lipoprotein receptor–related protein 1 and insulin degrading enzyme

While the ApoE gene was the first polymorphic marker to be identified as a genetic modifier of risk for AD, other candidate genetic loci are being investigated, including α2-macroglobulin (α2M), a protease inhibitor found in association with amyloid plaques in AD. The gene for α2M is located on chromosome 12, binds Aβ with high affinity, and may influence fibril formation and the toxicity of Aβ *in vitro* (Hughes et al., 1998). The activity of α2M has also been associated with low-density lipoprotein receptor-related protein 1 (LRP1). Both α2M and LRP1 are upregulated

following neuronal injury (Lopes et al., 1994). Furthermore, α2M is thought to mediate Aβ degradation via endocytosis through LRP1 (Narita et al., 1997). As ApoE and APP are also ligands of LRP1, it is postulated that different isoforms of ApoE and α2M may interact differentially and competitively for this system, affecting the clearance of Aβ.

Several investigators have now shown that, like ApoE, different LRP1 genotypes are associated with the development of AD (Kang et al., 1997; Hollenbach et al., 1998), mediated possibly through an increase in Aβ burden. α2M genotypes, unlike ApoE genotypes, have seemingly no affect on the age of onset in AD (Liao et al., 1998). The odds ratio for AD associated with the γ/γ α2M genotype was shown to be 1.77 (1.16–2.70, $p < 0.01$) and in combination with ApoE ε4 was 9.68 (3.91–24.0, $p < 0.001$). In the same study, there was no increased risk of AD demonstrated in heterozygotic individuals with γ/γ genotype, and stratification of the sample based on the presence or absence of the ApoE ε4 allele demonstrated a similar overrepresentation of the γ/γ genotype in both strata (Liao et al., 1998). This finding was demonstrated in a population-based study. This initial work suggests that the α2M γ/γ genotype may increase the risk of developing AD, that this risk is independent of the effects of ApoE ε4, and that the risks are additive and substantial. The studies to date require further replication and the effect requires demonstration in different populations in a similar manner to studies defining the risks associated with ApoE ε4. If future studies do conclude that α2M is an independent risk factor for AD, then predictive testing considering both genes (and also including genotyping of the ApoE promoter regions) could be developed with much higher positive predictive values than those demonstrated with ApoE testing alone. Whole genome search strategies (Blacker et al., 2003; Ertekin-Taner et al., 2004) have yielded other 'hot spots' of interest, the most intriguing of which is that on chromosome 10, close to the insulin degrading enzyme (IDE) locus. Attempts to identify IDE as a risk factor have so far failed, but it remains an attractive candidate for its demonstrated role in promoting the clearance of Aβ from the brain (Farris et al., 2004).

51.9.3 Translocase of mitochondrial membrane 40

Translocase of mitochondrial membrane 40 (TOMM40) is an enzyme that assists in moving proteins into mitochondria. (The acronym TOMM40 has also been used to describe the same protein called 'the outer mitochondrial membrane translocase' by other authors.) Recently it has been shown that C-trunctated APP may show arrested passage across TOMM40 in the mitochondria of patients with AD leading to dysfunction (Devi et al., 2006). The propensity for TOMM40 to arrest such movement may be influenced by genetic variability of this protein's constitution predicting both the risk of disease and age of onset (Roses et al., 2009). The gene encoding TOMM40 is closely adjacent to the ApoE gene on chromosome 19 and in linkage disequilibrium with both ApoE and APOC1. Within intron 6 of the TOMM40 gene, the variable length deoxythymidine homopolymer (poly-T) is associated with the risk and age of onset of AD. The implications are that the risk of developing AD is closely associated with the interplay of an individual's TOMM40, ApoE and APOOC1 status which can all be determined at a predisease stage. Ongoing work is developing this hypothesis and whether this risk is modifiable through intervention.

51.10   LINKING Aβ PRODUCTION AND AGGREGATION TO OTHER OBSERVED PATHOLOGIES IN AD

51.10.1   Aβ and tau hyperphosphorylation

The two most well-defined pathological processes in AD are the hyperphosphorylation of tau protein and subsequent destabilization of the cytoskeletal protein tubulin and the aggregation of Aβ to form amyloid plaques. While there has been debate about which process is upstream from the other and hence more 'important', less prosaic thinking would lead one to develop hypotheses about how these two important lesions are linked. One such hypothesis recognizes the importance of the pivotal role of the protein glycogen synthase kinase 3 (GSK3) in the pathological events observed in AD (Hooper et al., 2008).

GSK3 has a multiplicity of functions including roles in maintaining microtubule stability, apoptosis and gene transcription. Upregulation of the protein is associated with induction of tau hyperphosphorylation (Lovestone et al., 1994), an effect inhibited by insulin (Lesort et al., 1999). The role of insulin not only to inhibit GSK3 but also promote the expression of insulin degrading enzyme which is an Aβ protease as well as a promoter of APP processing through the α-secretase pathway has led to the proposition that AD could be labelled 'type 3 diabetes' (de la Monte and Wands, 2008).

Moreover, the GSK3α isoform has been shown to regulate APP processing leading to increased Aβ production (Phiel et al., 2003) which, in turn, has been shown in neurones to further increase GSK3β expression. Both the GSK3 isoforms are associated with tau hyperphosphorylation.

Although there are other theories associating tau and Aβ protein in the genesis of the disease, GSK3 overexpression and its interaction with insulin would appear probable linking processes with much consistent evidence supporting this theory.

51.10.2   Aβ and mitochondrial dysfunction

Mitochondria are the energy source of the cell and any disruption of mitochondrial function will necessarily lead to impaired neuronal function, defences, repair and integrity. Again, the question arises as to whether Aβ overproduction leads to mitochondrial damage or whether the latter precedes the former.

An energy-deficient neurone will tend to favour less energy-dependent processes where an alternative exists. In this regard it has been demonstrated that β-secretase increases in function in energy-deprived neurones (Vassar et al., 2009).

Therefore, upstream mitochondrial damage may lead to increased Aβ42 production. Downstream from this though, mitochondrial membranes and multiple mitochondrial processes are damaged by intracellular Aβ (Reddy and Beal, 2008) and the C-truncated fragment of APP can lead to further mitochondrial dysfunction through disruption of TOMM40. It is also worth noting that the hyperphosphorylation of tau protein is more likely to occur in energy-deficient cells (Rhein and Eckert, 2007).

51.10.3   Aβ and neuroinflammation

There has been a long-held hypothesis that glial activation is central to the pathology seen in AD (Meda et al., 2001). Glial cells activate in response to inflammatory signalling from both peripheral and central sources (including the amyloid plaque). The response of glia to systemic inflammation may explain the genesis of delirium in patients with systemic infections and the apparent acceleration of decline in AD as a result of delirium (Fong et al., 2009). When activated, glial cells overproduce the excitotoxic neurotransmitter glutamate and proinflammatory cytokines also influence concentrations of zinc (Vasto et al., 2007). Whilst the glutamate is directly neurotoxic through the NMDA receptor, the heightened levels of zinc may drive the oligomerization of Aβ leading to both acute (synaptotoxic) delirium generating events as well as – over time – neurotoxicity and neurodegeneration leading to more entrenched and irreversible symptoms. This observation may explain why PBT2 was shown to have an acute effect in phase II trials despite being developed predominantly as a disease-modifying agent (Lannfelt et al., 2008).

51.11   A PHYSIOLOGICAL ROLE FOR Aβ

It is highly unlikely that there is an invariably toxic protein or single process which explains the pathology of AD – rather it is the interaction of many (normally) physiological processes whose interactions associated with genetic and environmental risks associated with ageing become pathological. In this light Aβ may well perform an important physiological role to act as an antioxidant and to chaperone elevating metals towards biological inactivity embedded within the β-pleated sheet of the plaque. When the system is in homeostatic equilibrium between trace metal elevation, Aβ genesis and aggregation, there is little if any synaptotoxicity, but when multiple systems start to fail under the influence of genetic vulnerability and in the context of ageing mediating accumulation of risks, the normally benign systems tip into a pathological, malignant cascade that evolution has not found a way (or a need) to switch off.

Accordingly, to intervene beyond what is possible from a preventative perspective, one must not throw the baby out with the bathwater; interventions will need to be subtle and no doubt used in combinations with other interventions affecting other parts of the process.

51.12   INTERVENTIONS

Being able to determine the risk that a given individual has of developing AD late in life has important clinical implications, as risk modification strategies are most likely to be of greatest benefit when disease processes are nascent or indolent. As proven disease-modifying treatments for AD do not exist, another benefit of defining a population with AD but without dementia is to be able to define a cohort for clinical trials of drugs or biological agents with a postulated preventative or significant disease-modifying action.

Current therapeutic interventions for AD operate far downstream from the postulated initial toxicity of $A\beta_{42}$. Their efficacy is dependent upon augmenting the activity of surviving cholinergic neurones; the cholinesterase inhibitors (donepezil, galantamine and rivastigmine) have shown only modest effect on clinical progression of AD and have no demonstrable disease-modifying effect (Ritchie *et al.*, 2004). To prevent neuronal damage and clinical impairment, effective therapies must either affect the pathological levels of production of $A\beta_{42}$ from APP or mediate its toxicity or clearance. Therapeutic paradigms may therefore (and this list is not exhaustive) target inhibition of γ-secretase, or β-secretase or upregulate the α-secretase pathway; influence the phosphorylation state of the APP molecule; inderdict metal ions' interaction with Aβ and hence prevent oligomerization; scavenge free radicals; affect the postulated overactivation of microglial cells in response to amyloid deposition and systemic inflammatory signals; inhibit GSK3; stabilize or protect TOMM40; improve insulin sensitivity; protect α7 nicotinic receptors and do so as a combination of these approaches.

These actions may, if the amyloid theory is correct, decrease $A\beta_{42}$'s oligomerization and downstream toxic effects thereby protecting both the synapse at the early stage of disease and latterly the neurone itself.

51.13   CONCLUSIONS

This chapter highlights the complexity and intricacies of the various systems that tie Aβ to the neuronal degeneration of AD. One sword blow upon the Gordian Knot will not work, rather the interventions and untying should represent a thoughtful, careful unpicking. Intensive investigation of these biochemical systems has elucidated several potential targets for rational therapeutic intervention. The test of the amyloid theory will be in the examination of interventions that modulate the production and accumulation of Aβ42, initially in mice before human trials take place. In preparation for these trials, defining a high-risk population based on genetic risk factors and the observation of biological changes in patients pre-cognitive decline will continue with the hope that more effective disease-modifying drugs will be available for trial in the not too distant future.

REFERENCES

American College of Medical Genetics/American Society of Human Genetics Working Group on ApoE and Alzheimer disease. (1995) Statement on use of apolipoprotein E testing for Alzheimer's disease. *Journal of the American Medical Association* **274**: 1627–9.

Ames D, Ritchie C. (2007) Antioxidants and Alzheimer's disease: Time to stop feeding vitamin E to dementia patients? *International Psychogeriatrics* **19**: 1–8.

Ancolio K, Dumanchin C, Barelli H *et al.* (1999) Unusual phenotypic alteration of β-amyloid precursor protein maturation (βAPP) by a new Val-715 to met βAPP-770 mutation responsible for probable early-onset Alzheimer's disease. *Proceedings of the National Academy of Sciences of the United States of America* **96**: 4119–24.

Artiga MJ, Bullido MJ, Frank A *et al.* (1998) Risk for Alzheimer's disease correlates with transcriptional activity of the ApoE gene. *Human Molecular Genetics* **7**: 1887–92.

Atwood CS, Obrenovich ME, Liu TB *et al.* (2003) Amyloid-β: A chameleon walking in two worlds: a review of the trophic and toxic properties of amyloid-β. *Brain Research Reviews* **43**: 1–16.

Barelli H, Lebeau A, Vizzavona J *et al.* (1997) Characterization of new polyclonal antibodies specific for 40 and 42 amino acid-long amyloid β peptides: Their use to examine the cell biology of presenilins and the immunohistochemistry of sporadic Alzheimer's disease and cerebral amyloid angiopathy cases. *Molecular Medicine* **3**: 695–707.

Baskin F, Rosenberg R, Davis RM. (1992) Morphological differentiation and proteoglycan synthesis regulate Alzheimer amyloid precursor protein processing in PC-12 and human astrocyte cultures. *Journal of Neuroscience Research* **32**: 274–9.

Behl C, Davis J, Cole GM, Schubert D. (1992) Vitamin E protects nerve cells from amyloid β protein toxicity. *Biochemical and Biophysical Research Communications* **186**: 944–50.

Behl C, Davis JB, Lesley R, Schubert D. (1994) Hydrogen peroxide mediates amyloid beta protein toxicity. *Cell* **77**: 817–27.

Berg L, McKeel DW, Miller P *et al.* (1998) Clinicopathologic studies in cognitively healthy aging and Alzheimer disease. Relation of histologic markers to dementia severity, age, sex, and apolipoprotein E genotype. *Archives of Neurology* **55**: 326–35.

Bertram L, Tanzi RE. (2004) Alzheimer's disease: One disorder, too many genes? *Human Molecular Genetics* **13**: R135–41.

Blacker D, Haines JL, Rodes L *et al.* (1997) ApoE4 and age at onset of Alzheimer's disease: The NIMH genetics initiative. *Neurology* **48**: 139–47.

Blacker D, Tanzi RE. (1998) The genetics of Alzheimer's disease. Current status and future prospects. *Archives of Neurology* **55**: 294–6.

Blacker D, Bertram L, Saunders AJ *et al.* (2003) Results of a high-resolution genome screen of 437 Alzheimer's disease families. *Human Molecular Genetics* **12**: 23–32.

Borchelt DR, Thinakaran G, Eckman CB *et al.* (1996) Familial Alzheimer's disease-linked presenilin 1 variants elevate Aβ-1-42/1-40 ratio *in vitro* and *in vivo*. *Neuron* **17**: 1005–13.

Brooks WS, Martins RN, Devoecht J *et al.* (1995) A mutation in codon 717 of the amyloid precursor protein gene in an Australian family with Alzheimer's disease. *Neuroscience Letters* **199**: 183–6.

Bullido MJ, Artiga MJ, Recuero M *et al.* (1998) A polymorphism in the regulatory region of ApoE associated with risk of Alzheimer's dementia. *Nature Genetics* **18**: 69–71.

Burlinson S, Burns A, Mann D *et al.* (1998) Effect of apolipoprotein E status on clinical features of dementia. *International Journal of Geriatric Psychology* **13**: 177–85.

Butterfield DA, Hensley K, Harris M *et al.* (1994) β-Amyloid peptide free radical fragments initiate synaptosomal lipoperoxidation in a sequence-specific fashion: Implications to Alzheimer's disease. *Biochemical and Biophysical Research Communications* **200**: 710–15.

Butterfield DA. (2002) Amyloid β-peptide (1–42)-induced oxidative stress and neurotoxicity: Implications for neurodegeneration in Alzheimer's disease brain. A review. *Free Radical Research* **36**: 1307–13.

Butterfield DA. (2003) Amyloid β-peptide 1–42-associated free radical-induced oxidative stress and neurodegeneration in Alzheimer's disease brain: Mechanisms and consequences. *Current Medicinal Chemistry* **10**: 2651–9.

Butters MA, Young JB, Lopez O. (2008) Pathways linking late-life depression to persistent cognitive impairment and dementia. *Dialogues in Clinical Neuroscience* **10**: 345–57.

Buxbaum JD, Oishi M, Chen HI *et al.* (1992) Cholinergic agonists and interleukin 1 regulate processing and secretion of the Alzheimer β/A4 amyloid protein precursor. *Proceedings of the National Academy of Sciences of the United States of America* **89**: 10075–8.

Cai XD, Golde TE, Younkin SG. (1993) Release of excess amyloid beta protein from a mutant amyloid beta protein precursor. *Science* **259**: 514–16.

Caporaso GL, Gandy SE, Buxbaum JD. (1992) Protein phosphorylation regulates secretion of Alzheimer β/A4 amyloid precursor protein. *Proceedings of the National Academy of Sciences of the United States of America* **89**: 3055–9.

Citron M, Diehl TS, Gordon G *et al.* (1996) Evidence that the 42- and 40-amino acid forms of amyloid β protein are generated from the β-amyloid precursor protein by different protease activities. *Proceedings of the National Academy of Sciences of the United States of America* **93**: 13170–5.

Citron M. (2002) Alzheimer's disease: Treatments in discovery and development. *Nature Neuroscience* **5**: 1055–7.

Copani A, Koh J, Cotman CW. (1991) β-Amyloid increases neuronal susceptibility to injury by glucose deprivation. *Neuropharmacology and Neurotoxicology* **2**: 763–5.

Corder EH, Saunders AM, Risch NJ *et al.* (1994) Protective effect of apolipoprotein E type 2 allele for late onset Alzheimer's disease. *Nature Genetics* **7**: 180–4.

de la Monte SM, Wands JR. (2008) Alzheimer's disease is type 3 diabetes – evidence reviewed. *Journal of Diabetes Science and Technology* **2**: 1101–13.

De Strooper B, Saftig P, Craessaerts K *et al.* (1998) Deficiency of presenilin-1 inhibits the normal cleavage of amyloid precursor protein. *Nature* **391**: 387–90.

De Strooper B, Annaert W, Cupers P *et al.* (1999) A presenilin-1-dependent γ-secretase-like protease mediates release of Notch intracellular domain. *Nature* **398**: 518–22.

Devi L, Prabhu B, Galati DF *et al.* (2006) Accumulation of amyloid precursor protein in the mitochondrial import channels of human Alzheimer's disease brain is associated with mitochondrial dysfunction. *Journal of Neuroscience* **26**: 9057–68.

Dickson DW. (1997) The pathogenesis of senile plaques. *Journal of Neuropathology and Experimental Neurology* **56**: 321–39.

Duara R, Barker WW, Lopez-Alberola R *et al.* (1996) Alzheimer's disease: Interaction of apolipoprotein E genotype, family history of dementia, gender, education, ethnicity and age of onset. *Neurology* **46**: 1575–9.

Duff K, Eckman C, Zehr C *et al.* (1996) Increased amyloid-β42(43) in brains of mice expressing mutant presenilin 1. *Nature* **383**: 710–13.

Eckman CB, Mehta ND, Crook R *et al.* (1997) A new pathogenic mutation in the APP gene (I716V) increases the relative proportion of Aβ 42(43). *Human Molecular Genetics* **6**: 2087–9.

Ertekin-Taner N, Allen M, Fadale D *et al.* (2004) Genetic variants in haplotype block spanning IDE are signficantly associated with plasma Aβ42 levels and risk for Alzheimer disease. *Human Mutation* **23**: 334–42.

Evin G, Beyreuther K, Masters CL. (1994) Alzheimer's disease amyloid precursor protein (APP): Proteolytic processing, secretases and βA4 amyloid production. *Amyloid: International Journal of Experimental and Clinical Investigation* **1**: 263–80.

Farris W, Mansourian S, Leissring MA *et al.* (2004) Partial loss-of-function mutations in insulin-degrading enzyme that induce diabetes also impair degradation of amyloid β–protein. *American Journal of Pathology* **164**: 1425–34.

Fong TG, Jones RN, Shi P *et al.* (2009) Delirium accelerates cognitive decline in Alzheimer disease. *Neurology* **72**: 1570–5.

Gillespie SL, Golde TE, Younkin SG. (1992) Secretory processing of the Alzheimer amyloid β/A4 protein precursor is increased by protein phosphorylation. *Biochemical and Biophysical Research Communications* **187**: 1285–90.

Glenner GG, Wong CW. (1984) Alzheimer's disease: Initial report of the purification and characterization of a novel cerebrovascular amyloid protein. *Biochemical and Biophysical Research Communications* **120**: 885–90.

Golde TE, Estus S, Usiak M *et al.* (1990) Expression of β amyloid protein precursor mRNAs: Recognition of a novel alternatively spliced form and quantitation in Alzheimer's disease using PCR. *Neuron* **4**: 253–67.

Green KN, Billings LM, Roozendaal B *et al.* (2006) Glucocorticoids increase amyloid-beta and tau pathology in a mouse model of Alzheimer's disease. *Journal of Neuroscience* **26**: 9047–56.

Haass C, Hung AY, Selkoe DJ. (1991) Processing of β-amyloid precursor protein in microglia and astrocytes favors an internal localization over constitutive secretion. *Journal of Neuroscience* **11**: 3783–93.

Haass C, Hung AY, Selkoe DJ, Teplow DB. (1994) Mutations associated with a locus for familial Alzheimer's disease result in alternative processing of amyloid β protein precursor. *Journal of Biological Chemistry* **269**: 17741–8.

Hardy J, Duff K, Gwinn Hardy K *et al.* (1998) Genetic dissection of Alzheimer's disease and related dementias: Amyloid and its relationship to tau. *Nature Neuroscience* **1**: 355–8.

Henry A, Li QX, Galatis D et al. (1998) Inhibition of platelet activation by the Alzheimer's disease amyloid precursor protein. British Journal of Haematology 103: 402–15.

Hensley K, Carney JM, Mattson MP et al. (1994) A model for β-amyloid aggregation and neurotoxicity based on free radical generation by the peptide: Relevance to Alzheimer disease. Proceedings of the National Academy of Sciences of the United States of America 91: 3270–4.

Hollenbach E, Ackerman S, Hyman BT, Rebeck GW. (1998) Confirmation of an association between a polymorphism in exon 3 of the low-density lipoprotein receptor-related protein gene and Alzheimer's disease. Neurology 50: 1905–7.

Hooper C, Killick R, Lovestone S. (2008) The GSK3 hypothesis of Alzheimer's disease. Journal of Neurochemistry 104: 1433–9.

Howlett DR, Jennings KH, Lee DC et al. (1995) Aggregation state and neurotoxic properties of Alzheimer beta-amyloid peptide. Neurodegeneration 4: 23–32.

Huang CW, Lui CC, Chang WN et al. (2009) Elevated basal cortisol level predicts lower hippocampal volume and cognitive decline in Alzheimer's disease. Journal of Clinical Neuroscience 16: 1283–6.

Hughes SR, Khorkova O, Goyal S et al. (1998) α2-Macroglobulin associates with β-amyloid peptide and prevents fibril formation. Proceedings of the National Academy of Sciences of the United States of America 95: 3275–80.

Hung AY, Koo EH, Haass C, Selkoe DJ. (1992) Increased expression of β-amyloid precursor protein during neuronal differentiation is not accompanied by secretory cleavage. Journal of Biological Chemistry 268: 22959–62.

Hyman BT, Tanzi RE. (1992) Amyloid, dementia and Alzheimer's disease. Current Opinion in Neurology and Neurosurgery 5: 88–93.

Iwatsubo T. (2004) The γ-secretase complex: machinery for intramembrane proteolysis. Current Opinion in Neurobiology 14: 379–83.

Jorm AF. (2001) History of depression as a risk factor for dementia: An updated review. Australian and New Zealand Journal of Psychiatry 35: 776–81.

Kang DE, Saitoh T, Chen X et al. (1997) Genetic association of the low-density lipoprotein receptor-related protein gene (LRP), an apolipoprotein E receptor, with late onset Alzheimer's disease. Neurology 49: 56–61.

Kang J, Lemaire H, Unterbeck A et al. (1987) The precursor of Alzheimer's disease amyloid A4 protein resembles a cell-surface receptor. Nature 325: 733–6.

Kang J, Müller-Hill B. (1990) Differential splicing of Alzheimer's disease amyloid A4 precursor RNA in rat tissues: PreA4695 mRNA is predominantly produced in rat and human brain. Biochemical and Biophysical Research Communications 166: 1192–200.

Keller JN, Guo Q, Holtsberg FW et al. (1998) Increased sensitivity to mitochondrial toxin-induced apoptosis in neural cells expressing mutant presenilin-1 is linked to perturbed calcium homeostasis and enhanced oxyradical production. Journal of Neuroscience 18: 4439–50.

Koh J, Yang LL, Cotman CW. (1990) β-Amyloid protein increases the vulnerability of cultured cortical neurons to excitotoxic damage. Brain Research 533: 315–20.

Kosik KS, Joachim CL, Selkoe DJ. (1986) Microtubule-associated protein tau (tau) is a major antigenic component of paired helical filaments in Alzheimer disease. Proceedings of the National Academy of Sciences of the United States of America 83: 4044–8.

Kwok JBJ, Li Q-X, Hallup M et al. (2000) Novel Leu 723 pro amyloid precursor protein mutation increases amyloid β42 (43) peptide levels and induces apoptosis. Annals of Neurology 47: 249–53.

Lahiri DK, Nall C, Farlow M. (1992) The cholinergic agonist carbachol reduces intracellular β-amyloid precursor protein in PC 12 and C6 cells. Biochemistry International 28: 853–60.

Lahiri DK, Farlow MR, Greig NH, Sambamurti K. (2002) Current drug targets for Alzheimer's disease treatment. Drug Development Research 56: 267–81.

Lambert JC, Pasquier F, Cottel D et al. (1998) A new polymorphism in the ApoE promoter associated with risk of developing Alzheimer's dementia. Human Molecular Genetics 7: 533–40.

Lammich S, Kojro E, Postina R et al. (1999) Constitutive and regulated α-secretase cleavage of Alzheimer's amyloid precursor protein by a disintegrin metalloprotease. Proceedings of the National Academy of Sciences of the United States of America 96: 3922–7.

Lannfelt L, Blennow K, Zetterberg H et al. (2008) Safety, efficacy, and biomarker findings of PBT2 in targeting Abeta as a modifying therapy for Alzheimer's disease: A phase IIa, double-blind, randomised, placebo-controlled trial. Lancet Neurology 7: 779–86.

Lansbury Jr PT. (1999) Evolution of amyloid: What normal protein folding may tell us about fibrillogenesis and disease. Proceedings of the National Academy of Sciences of the United States of America 96: 3342–4.

Lemere CA, Lopera F, Kosik KS et al. (1996) The E280A presenilin 1 Alzheimer mutation produces increased Aβ42 deposition and severe cerebellar pathology. Nature Medicine 2: 1146–50.

Lesort M, Jope R, Johnson GV et al. (1999) Insulin transiently increases tau phosphorylation: Involvement in glycogen synthase kinase-3 and Fyn tyrosine kinase. Journal of Neurochemistry 72: 576–84.

Liao A, Nitsch RM, Greenberg SM et al. (1998) Genetic association of an α2-macroglobulin (Val 1000 Ile) polymorphism and Alzheimer's disease. Human Molecular Genetics 7: 1953–6.

Lockhart BP, Benicourt C, Junien JL, Privat A. (1994) Inhibitors of free radical formation fail to attenuate direct β-amyloid(25–35) peptide-mediated neurotoxicity in rat hippocampal cultures. Journal of Neuroscience Research 39: 494–505.

Lopes MB, Bogaev CA, Gonias SL, Vandenberg SR. (1994) Expression of α2-macroglobulin receptor/low density lipoprotein receptor-related protein is increased in reactive and neoplastic glial cells. FEBS Letters 338: 301–5.

Lorenzo A, Yanker BA. (1994) β-Amyloid neurotoxicity requires fibril formation and is inhibited by Congo red. Proceedings of the National Academy of Sciences of the United States of America 91: 12243–7.

Lovestone S, Reynolds C, Latimer D et al. (1994) Alzheimer's disease-like phosphorylation of the microtubule-associated protein tau by glycogen synthase kinase-3 in transfected mammalian cells. Current Biology 4: 10.

McKee AC, Kosik KS, Kowall NW. (1991) Neuritic pathology and dementia in Alzheimer's disease. *Annals of Neurology* **30**: 156–65.

McLean CA, Cherney RA, Fraser FW *et al.* (1999) Soluble pool of Aβ as a determinant of severity of neurodegeneration in Alzheimer's disease. *Annals of Neurology* **46**: 860–6.

Mahley RW. (1988) Apoliprotein E: Cholesterol transport protein with expanding role in cell biology. *Science* **240**: 622–30.

Mark RJ, Blanc EM, Mattson MP. (1996) Amyloid β-peptide and oxidative cellular injury in Alzheimer's disease. *Molecular Neurobiology* **12**: 211–24.

Masters CL, Simms G, Weinman NA *et al.* (1985) Amyloid plaque core protein in Alzheimer disease and Down syndrome. *Proceedings of the National Academy of Sciences of the United States of America* **82**: 4245–9.

Mattson MP, Cheng B, Culwell AR *et al.* (1993) Evidence for excitoprotective and intraneuronal calcium-regulating roles for secreted forms of the β-amyloid precursor protein. *Neuron* **10**: 243–54.

Meda L, Baron P, Scarlato G *et al.* (2001) Glial activation in Alzheimer's disease: The role of Abeta and its associated proteins. *Neurobiology of Aging* **22**: 885–93.

Milward E, Papadopoulos R, Fuller SJ *et al.* (1992) The amyloid protein precursor of Alzheimer's disease is a mediator of the effects of nerve growth factor on neurite outgrowth. *Neuron* **9**: 129–37.

Morris JC, McKeel DW, Storandt M *et al.* (1991) Very mild Alzheimer's disease: Informant-based clinical psychometric and pathologic distinction from normal aging. *Neurology* **41**: 469–78.

Multhaup G, Masters CL, Beyreuther K. (1998) Oxidative stress in Alzheimer's disease. *Alzheimer's Reports* **1**: 147–54.

Myers R, Schaeter EJ, Wilson PW *et al.* (1996) Apolipoprotein E4 association with dementia in a population based study: The Framingham study. *Neurology* **46**: 673–7.

Narita M, Holtzman DM, Schwartz AL, Bu GJ. (1997) α2-Macroglobulin complexes with and mediates the endocytosis of β-amyloid peptide via cell surface low-density lipoprotein receptor-related protein. *Journal of Neurochemistry* **69**: 1904–11.

National Institute on Aging/Alzheimer's Association Working Group. (1996) Apolipoprotein E genotyping in Alzheimer's disease. *Lancet* **347**: 1091–5.

Naylor R, Hill AF, Barnham K. (2008) Is covalently crosslinked Abeta responsible for synaptotoxicity in Alzheimer's disease? *Current Alzheimer Research* **5**: 533–9.

Nicoll J, Roberts GW, Graham D. (1995) Apolipoprotein E ε4 allele is associated with deposition of amyloid following head injury. *Nature Medicine* **1**: 135–7.

Nitsch RM, Slack BE, Wurtman RJ, Growdon JH. (1992) Release of Alzheimer amyloid precursor derivatives stimulated by activation of muscarinic acetylcholine receptors. *Science* **258**: 304–7.

Olichney JM, Hansen LA, Galasko D *et al.* (1996) The apolipoprotein E ε4 allele is associated with increased neuritic plaques and cerebral amyloid angiopathy in Alzheimer's disease and Lewy body variant. *Neurology* **47**: 190–6.

Payami H, Montee KR, Kaye JA *et al.* (1994) Alzheimer's disease, apolipoprotein ε4, and gender. *Journal of the American Medical Association* **271**: 1316–17.

Phiel CJ, Wilson CA, Lee VM, Klein PS. (2003) GSK-3alpha regulates production of Alzheimer's disease amyloid-beta peptides. *Nature* **423**: 435–9.

Poirier J, Davignon J, Bouthillier D *et al.* (1993) Apolipoprotein E polymorphism and Alzheimer's disease. *Lancet* **342**: 697–9.

Poirier J. (1994) Apolipoprotein E in CNS models of CNS injury and in Alzheimer's disease. *Trends in Neuroscience* **17**: 525–30.

Polvikoski T, Sulkava R, Haltia M *et al.* (1995) Apolipoprotein E, dementia and cortical deposition of β-amyloid protein. *New England Journal of Medicine* **333**: 1242–7.

Price DL, Sisodia SS, Borchelt DR. (1998) Genetic neurodegenerative diseases: The human illness and transgenic models. *Science* **282**: 1079–83.

Rebeck GW, Reiter JS, Strickland DK, Hyman BT. (1993) Apolipoprotein E in sporadic Alzheimer's disease: Allelic variation and receptor interactions. *Neuron* **11**: 575–80.

Reddy PH, Beal MF. (2008) Amyloid beta, mitochondrial dysfunction and synaptic damage: Implications for cognitive decline in aging and Alzheimer's disease. *Trends in Molecular Medicine* **14**: 45–53.

Rhein V, Eckert A. (2007) Effects of Alzheimer's amyloid-beta and tau protein on mitochondrial function – role of glucose metabolism and insulin signalling. *Archives of Physiology and Biochemistry* **113**: 131–41.

Ritchie CW, Bush AI, Mackinnon A *et al.* (2003) Metal-protein attenuation with iodochlorhydroxyquin (clioquinol) targeting A beta amyloid deposition and toxicity in Alzheimer disease – a pilot phase 2 clinical trial. *Archives of Neurology* **60**: 1685–91.

Ritchie CW, Ames D, Clayton T, Lai R. (2004) Metaanalysis of randomized trials of the efficacy and safety of donepezil, galantamine, and rivastigmine for the treatment of Alzheimer disease. *American Journal of Geriatric Psychiatry* **12**: 358–69.

Rogaev EI. (1998) Presenilins – discovery and characterization of the genes of Alzheimer's disease. *Molecular Biology* **32**: 58–69.

Roperch JP, Alvaro V, Pricur S *et al.* (1998) Inhibition of presenilin 1 expression is promoted by p53 and p21waf-1 and results in apoptosis and tumor suppression. *Nature Medicine* **4**: 835–8.

Roses A, Lutz M, Amrine-Madsen H *et al.* (2009) A TOMM 40 variable length polymorphism determines the age of late-onset Alzheimer's disease. *Pharmacogenomics Journal*. Available from: www.nature.com/tpj/journal/vaop/ncurrent/full/tpj200969a.html.

Sano M, Ernesto C, Thomas RG *et al.* (1997) A controlled trial of selegiline, alpha-tocopherol, or both as treatment for Alzheimer's disease. *New England Journal of Medicine* **336**: 1216–22.

Scheper W, Annaert W, Cupers P *et al.* (1999) Function and dysfunction of the presenilins. *Alzheimer's Reports* **2**: 73–81.

Scheuner D, Eckman C, Jensen M *et al.* (1996) Secreted amyloid β-protein similar to that in the senile plaques of Alzheimer's disease is increased *in vivo* by the presenilin 1 and 2 and APP mutations linked to familial Alzheimer's disease. *Nature Medicine* **2**: 864–70.

Schmechel DE, Saunders AM, Strittmatter WJ et al. (1993) Increased amyloid β-peptide deposition in cerebral cortex as a consequence of apolipoprotein E genotype in late-onset Alzheimer's disease. *Proceedings of the National Academy of Sciences of the United States of America* **90**: 9649–53.

Shearman MS, Ragan CI, Iversen LL. (1994) Inhibition of PC12 cell redox activity is a specific, early indicator of the mechanism of β-amyloid-mediated cell death. *Proceedings of the National Academy of Sciences of the United States of America* **91**: 1470–4.

Sheng JG, Zhou XQ, Mrak RE, Griffin WS. (1998) Progressive neuronal injury associated with amyloid plaque formation in Alzheimer's disease. *Journal of Neuropathology and Experimental Neurology* **57**: 714–17.

Sinha S, Lieberburg I. (1992) Normal metabolism of the amyloid precursor protein (APP). *Neurodegeneration* **1**: 169–75.

Slooter AJC, Tang MX, van Duijn CM et al. (1997) Apolipoprotein E ε4 and the risk of dementia with stroke (a population based investigation). *Journal of the American Medical Association* **277**: 818–21.

Small DH, Nurcombe V, Reed G et al. (1994) A heparin-binding domain in the amyloid protein precursor of Alzheimer's disease is involved in the regulation of neurite outgrowth. *Journal of Neuroscience* **14**: 2117–27.

Smith DG, Cappai R, Barnham KJ et al. (2007) The redox chemistry of the Alzheimer's disease amyloid beta peptide. *Biochimica et Biophysica Acta* **1768**: 1976–90.

Struhl G, Greenwald I. (1999) Presenilin is required for activity and nuclear access of notch in Drosophila. *Nature* **398**: 522–4.

Suh YH, Checler F. (2002) Amyloid precursor protein, presenilins, and α-synuclein: Molecular pathogenesis and pharmacological applications in Alzheimer's disease. *Pharmacological Reviews* **54**: 469–525.

Suzuki N, Iwatsubo T, Odaka A et al. (1994) High tissue content of soluble beta 1–40 is linked to cerebral amyloid angiopathy. *American Journal of Pathology* **145**: 452–60.

Tanzi RE, Gusella JF, Watkins PC et al. (1987) Amyloid β protein gene: cDNA, mRNA distribution and genetic linkage near the Alzheimer locus. *Science* **235**: 880–4.

Teller JK, Russo C, DeBusk LM et al. (1996) Presence of soluble amyloid β-peptide precedes amyloid plaque formation in Down's syndrome. *Nature Medicine* **2**: 93–5.

Terry RD, Masliah E, Salmon DP et al. (1991) Physical basis of cognitive alterations in Alzheimer's disease: Synapse loss is the major correlate of cognitive impairment. *Annals of Neurology* **30**: 572–80.

Vassar R, Kovacs DM, Yan R, Wong PC. (2009) The beta-secretase enzyme BACE in health and Alzheimer's disease: Regulation, cell biology, function, and therapeutic potential. *Journal of Neuroscience* **29**: 12787–94.

Vasto S, Mocchegiani E, Malavolta M. (2007) Zinc and inflammatory/immune response in aging. *Annals of the New York Academy of Sciences* **1100**: 111–22.

Walsh DM, Klyubin I, Fadeeva JV et al. (2002) Amyloid-beta oligomers: Their production, toxicity and therapeutic inhibition. *Biochemical Society Transactions* **30**: 552–7.

Whitson JS, Appel SH. (1995) Neurotoxicity of Aβ amyloid protein in vitro is not altered by calcium channel blockade. *Neurobiology of Aging* **16**: 5–10.

Wisniewski T, Golabek A, Matsubara E et al. (1993) Apolipoprotein E: Binding to soluble Alzheimer's β-amyloid. *Biochemical and Biophysical Research Communications* **192**: 359–65.

Wolfe MS, Xia W, Ostaszewski BL et al. (1999) Two transmembrane aspartates in presenilin-1 required for presenilin endoproteolysis and γ-secretase activity. *Nature* **398**: 513–17.

Wood JG, Mirra SS, Pollock NJ, Binder LI. (1986) Neurofibrillary tangles of Alzheimer disease share antigenic determinants with the axonal microtubule associated protein tau. *Proceedings of the National Academy of Sciences of the United States of America* **83**: 4040–3.

Yankner BA. (1996) Mechanisms of neuronal degeneration in Alzheimer's disease. *Neurology* **16**: 921–32.

Ye Y, Lukinova N, Fortini ME. (1999) Neurogenic phenotypes and altered Notch processing in Drosophila presenilin mutants. *Nature* **398**: 525–9.

Genetics of Alzheimer's disease

MARGIE SMITH

52.1 INTRODUCTION

The genetic architecture of Alzheimer's disease (AD) remains elusive despite the success in identifying patients with rare autosomal dominant early-onset Alzheimer's disease (EOAD). Mutations in three genes, the amyloid protein precursor (APP) and the presenilin genes (PS1 and PS2) located on chromosomes 21, 14 and 1, respectively, exert their effect in a fully penetrant manner. The gene that encodes apolipoprotein E (ApoE) is the only genetic variant which consistently influences disease risk. Contrastingly, susceptibility for late-onset Alzheimer's disease (LOAD) shows a less obvious familial aggregation and is therefore likely to be governed by a number of risk alleles located on a number of different genes. Continued research in this complex area of the genes and proteins involved in AD will help establish a logical basis for therapeutics and management.

52.2 MOLECULAR GENETICS OF EOAD

Mutations in three genes, APP, PS1 and PS2 genes, alter production of the amyloid-β (Aβ) peptide, the principle component of senile plaques (Tanzi and Bertram, 2005). In the 20 years since the discovery of the APP gene, it has only been relatively recently that the interaction with the PS1 and PS2 genes has been elucidated. Aβ is generated from APP by sequential cleavage of two enzymes: β-secretase and γ-secretase. All of the pathogenic mutations that are currently known to cause autosomal dominant EOAD are located either in the APP gene itself or in genes that encode the proteins that are located in the catalytic centre of the γ-secretase complex.

Unique pathologies not seen in the 'sporadic' or LOAD have been reported when these genes are mutated. The historical review of each gene gives a perspective into the understanding of EOAD, the phenotypes and the early understanding of the biochemical pathways involved. The molgen website has a catalogue of all of the reported mutations in the APP, PS1 and PS2 genes (www.molgen.ua.ac.be/AD).

52.2.1 Mutations in the APP gene

The APP gene was implicated as a potential locus for AD mutations based on four main intersecting lines of evidence. First, it is well known that individuals with Downs's syndrome (trisomy 21) develop the pathological lesions of AD by the fourth decade. This evidence implied a relationship between chromosome 21 and AD pathology (Mann et al., 1984; Mann et al., 1989). Second, a 40–42 amino acid proteolytic peptide (Aβ) of the full-length APP is a major constituent of senile plaques (Masters et al., 1985; Goldgaber et al., 1987; Kang et al., 1987). Genetic linkage studies have shown an additional line of evidence for linkage to a locus associated with EOAD in the region of chromosome 21 containing the APP gene (St George-Hyslop et al., 1987; Goate et al., 1989). Finally, a missense mutation (APP E693Q) was identified in the Aβ region of the APP gene characterized by hereditary cerebral haemorrhage with amyloidosis of the Dutch type (HCHWA-D) (Levy et al., 1990; Kamino et al., 1992). This is a rare disorder caused by severe βA4 amyloid deposition in meningeal and cerebral microvessels (Levy et al., 1990; Van Broeckhoven et al., 1990). It was then shown that E693G mutation causes AD by increasing amyloid β-protofibril formation and decreasing amyloid β levels in plasma and conditioned media (Nilsberth et al., 2000). Three different mutations were reported at codon 693: the 'Dutch' mutation (Glu22Gln), the Arctic Glu22Gly mutation and 'Italian' mutation (Glu22Lys). Peptides of the wild-type 'Dutch' and 'Italian' variants were made and their cytotoxic effects were evaluated in human cerebral endothelial cells in culture. The effect of each mutation was different under these conditions, the E22Q peptide exhibiting the highest content of beta-sheet formation and aggregation properties. In contrast the 'Dutch' variant peptide induced apoptosis of cerebral endothelial cells. These results indicated that a change in amino acid at position 22 confers distinct structural properties on the peptides that affect the onset of the inexorable disease process (Miravalle et al., 2000). After the initial finding of the E693Q mutation, a sequence variation affecting the valine at codon 717 (position 46 relative to the βA4 sequence) was found to be associated with the EOAD phenotype. At least 13 families worldwide were identified with a V717I mutation, conferring an age of onset for AD in the mid-fifties (Goate et al., 1991; Hardy et al., 1991; Naruse et al., 1991; Fidani et al., 1992; Sorbi et al., 1993; Brooks et al., 1995; Sorbi et al., 1995; Campion et al., 1996; Matsumura et al., 1996; Campion et al., 1999; Finckh et al., 2000). A 'mixed' phenotype of AD and/or severe cerebral amyloid angiopathy is caused by a mutation (A692G) at the βA4 residue 21 adjacent to the E693Q HCHWA-D (Hendriks et al., 1992). This finding provided supporting evidence for the hypothesis that HCHWA-D and AD are pathological variants of the same disease, being associated with a phenotype of AD or other βA4 amyloidosis-related disorders. A double mutation (K670N and M671L) in a large Swedish EOAD kindred with a mean age of onset of 55 years was identified (Mullan et al., 1992). More recently, four other APP mutations have been identified, the Austrian (Thr714Ile) (De Jonghe et al., 2000), Florida (Ile716Val) (Eckman et al., 1997), French (Val715Met) (Ancolio et al., 1999) and the Australian (Leu723Pro) (Kwok et al., 2000a).

The Swedish double mutation was the first APP mutation for which a direct effect on βA4 processing could be demonstrated (Mullan et al., 1992). This double point mutation (the 'Swedish' mutation) Lys670Met and Asp671Leu is upstream of the β-secretase cleavage site and results in a five- to eight-fold increase in the formation of both $A\beta_{40}$ and $A\beta_{42}$ (Citron et al., 1992). Two single point mutations at amino acid 717 (the 'London' mutation Val717Ile and the 'Indiana' mutation Val717Phe) are adjacent to the γ-secretase site and specifically increase the production of $A\beta_{42}$ (Suzuki et al., 1994), which is known to form insoluble amyloid fibrils (Selkoe, 1994). Synthetic peptides containing the HCHWA mutation show accelerated fibril formation (Wisniewski et al., 1991). The majority of APP mutations' molecular effect is to increase $A\beta_{42}$ production (Hardy, 1997); however, overexpression of the Val715Met mutation in human HEK293 cells and murine neurones reduces the total Aβ production and increases the recovery of the physiologically secreted product, APPα. It was initially thought that some cases of familial AD were associated with a reduction in the overall production of Aβ, however it was shown to be caused by an increased production of truncated forms of Aβ ending at the 42 position (Ancolio et al., 1999).

To date, there have been 32 APP mutations identified in 86 kindreds. These mutations exert their effect by increasing Aβ production or $A\beta_{42}:A\beta_{40}$ ratio. The mutations are located in the Aβ coding region or close to the β and γ-secretase sites of APP (Hardy, 1997). Recently, three groups have reported a chromosome 21 genomic duplication of unknown size. The phenotype is variable with congophillic amyloid angiopathy and Lewy body dementia being described (Rovelet-Lecrux et al., 2006; Sleegers et al., 2006; Rovelet-Lecrux et al., 2007). The duplications are of unknown size and include not only the APP gene but NCAM2, NMRPL39, JAM2, ATPJ, GABPA, CYYR1 ADAMTS1 and ADAMTS5 genes or APP, MRPL39, JAM2, ATP5J, GABPA, CYYR1, ADAMTS1, ADAMTS5, ZNF294, USP16, CCT8 AND BACH1 genes (Rovelet-Lecrux et al., 2006). The age onset and duration of the early-onset disease are variable across the eight kindreds reported.

52.2.2   Mutations in the PS1 gene

After the initial finding of an EOAD locus on chromosome 21 it became apparent that the majority of EOAD kindreds did not show linkage to chromosome 21 (Tanzi et al., 1987; Van Broeckhoven et al., 1987; Schellenberg et al., 1988; St George-Hyslop et al., 1990). The PS1 gene was identified in 1995 through positional cloning strategies. Five mutations were identified in eight of 14 pedigrees analysed (Sherrington et al., 1995). All the mutations occurred within highly conserved domains of the PS1 protein as shown by comparison to the murine homologue that provides supporting evidence that these mutations are indeed pathogenic. Not all mutations occur at residues that are conserved between PS1 and PS2. The PS1 gene was previously denoted as the S182 or AD3 locus; to date, 177 mutations have been detected in 392 kindreds in the PS1 gene.

The age of onset of AD due to PS1 mutations is accelerated, however, variability in age onset is observed. The M139V and M146V mutations have an age onset around 40 years (Clark et al., 1995; Van Broeckhoven, 1995), whereas for kindreds identified with the E280 and C410Y mutations the age of onset is between 45 and 50 (Clark et al., 1995; Sherrington et al., 1995); the Ala409Thr mutation has an onset of 85 years (Aldudo et al., 1999). EOAD linked to chromosome 14 is estimated to account for 70 per cent of all EOAD pedigrees (St George-Hyslop et al., 1992; Van Broeckhoven et al., 1992).

The phenotype of PS1 mutations is heterogeneous. It was initially thought that the only difference between AD and EOAD was the earlier age of onset (Sherrington et al., 1995); however, there are five reports of AD associated with spastic paraparesis (SP) of the lower limbs. The brain pathology in one kindred was described as unique with large plaques lacking the classical core of amyloid fibrils. The term 'cotton wool' was coined by virtue of their size and appearance (Crook et al., 1998). PS1 mutations associated with SP include a small deletion in exon 4 (DeltaI83/M84) (Steiner et al., 2001), an insertion of six nucleotides in the coding region of exon 5 (from TAC to TTTATATAC) between amino acids K155 and Y156, point mutations in the coding region of exon 8 (Val261Phe) (Farlow et al., 2000) and (Arg278Thr) (Kwok et al., 1997), a point mutation in the splice acceptor consensus of intron 8 resulting in in-frame skipping of exon 9 and an amino acid change at the splice junction of exon 8 and exon 10 (g.58304G > A, c.869–955del) (Sato *et al.*, 1998; Kwok *et al.*, 2000b), (g.58304G > T, c.869–955del) (Perez-Tur *et al.*, 1995; Hutton *et al.*, 1996; Kwok *et al.*, 1997; Kwok *et al.*, 2000b) and large genomic deletions (g.56305–62162del) (Kwok *et al.*, 1997; Smith *et al.*, 2001) identified in an Australian kindred and (g.56681–61235) the Delta9Finn kindred (Crook *et al.*, 1998). Interestingly, a point mutation in the splice donor consensus site of intron 4 resulting in three different transcripts with a single codon insertion, partial and complete deletion of exon 4, respectively, the latter two resulting in a frameshift and premature stop codon (g.23024delG, c.338–339insTAC, c.170–338del, c.88–338del) (Tysoe *et al.*, 1998) is not associated with spastic paraparesis. It was hypothesized that this mutation leads to AD through haploinsufficiency of full-length PS1. This is in direct contrast to other PS1 mutations, which are thought to confer a 'toxic' gain of function in which Aβ_{42} secretion is selectively increased (Tysoe *et al.*, 1998). Other phenotypes associated with EOAD are frontotemporal features (Raux *et al.*, 2000), myoclonic seizures (Ezquerra *et al.*, 1999) and a psychiatric disorder (Tedde *et al.*, 2000).

Mutations are located throughout the PS1 protein; however, their distribution may not be random. Mutations tend to occur at residues conserved between PS1 and PS2 and, as such, the majority are in transmembrane domains. Specifically the cluster of mutations in transmembrane 1, 2, 3, 4 and 6 line up on one side of the α-helix. This helical face may be important for the interaction with other transmembrane proteins (Clark *et al.*, 1995). It was suggested that disruption of the helical faces impairs presenilin function so that more Aβ_{42} is produced (Hardy and Crook, 2001). The majority of PS1 mutations cluster in exon 8, which is close to the cleavage site. If this is a functional domain then disruption of its function may be critical to pathogenicity. The clustering of APP mutations around the α-, β- and γ-secretase sites leads to different molecular mechanisms however the outcome is the same.

The normal biological and pathological functions of PS1 were at that time poorly understood; however, there was ample evidence for a role of PS1 in the proteolytic processing of APP and in Notch processing (Wolfe *et al.*, 1999). PS1 is endoproteolytically cleaved between amino acids 291 and 299 resulting in an N-terminal fragment of 30 kDa and a C-terminal fragment of 18 kDa (Thinakaran *et al.*, 1996). The proteolytic cleavage site is located in that part of PS1 encoded by exon 9; therefore the delta 9 mutant does not undergo cleavage and accumulates as full-length PS1 (Thinakaran *et al.*, 1996). Conversely, the efficiency of processing was shown not to be affected by missense mutations in AD brains (Hendriks *et al.*, 1997), in brains of transgenic mice (Duff *et al.*, 1996) and in transfected cells (Borchelt *et al.*, 1996). Cells transfected with PS1 mutants (M146V, A246G, A260V, G384A, C410T) have impaired proteolysis (Mercken *et al.*, 1996) and in lymphocytes of mutation carriers (Takahashi *et al.*, 1999). There is no correlation between different PS1 mutations, age onset and A$\beta_{42(43)}$ production in transfected embryonic kidney cells (Mehta *et al.*, 1998).

Overall, PS1 mutations increase the Aβ_{42}:Aβ_{40} ratio, the mutations are located throughout the protein and it has been shown to have an enzymatic role in the γ-secretase complex. To date, 177 PS1 mutations have been identified in 392 kindreds (www.molgen.ua.ac.be/AD).

52.2.3   Mutations in the PS2 gene

Directly after the identification of the PS1 cDNA sequence, 'expressed sequence tags' were described with considerable homology to two different segments within the PS1 open reading frame (T03796). Cloning of the full-length cDNA of this corresponding gene, mapped to chromosome 1, enabled the identification of missense mutations in cDNAs in affected Volga-German subjects (Levy-Lahad *et al.*, 1995). Evidence of the physical genome mapping of PS2 on chromosome 1q42.1 was performed using fluorescence *in situ* hybridization (Tokano *et al.*, 1997). The majority of kindreds analysed exhibited the N141I missense mutation thereby identifying a founder effect. EOAD onset in these kindreds generally occurs later than in EOAD kindreds linked to chromosome 14 but with a broader range of age at onset from 54.8 ± 8.4 years. The mean duration of disease is 11.3 ± 4.6 years and mean age at death approximately 66 years. Clinically, kindreds with PS1 mutations have a more aggressive disease than those with PS2 mutations (Lampe *et al.*, 1994). The wide variation in age of onset indicates that other genetic and/or environmental factors influence the age of onset. Non-penetrance over the age of 80 years has also been observed (Sherrington *et al.*, 1996). The penetrance is over 95 per cent for PS2 kindreds; however, presymptomatic individuals harbouring the mutation over the age of 80 may escape disease.

The exon 5 T122P mutation was found to be highly penetrant unlike the previously reported PS2 mutations N141I and M239V (Levy-Lehad *et al.*, 1995). Consistent with the variable penetrance of the N141I and M239V mutations, the M239I mutation has associated phenotypic variability with some affected individuals having an earlier onset and more severe course than the index case (Finckh *et al.*, 2000).

Fourteen mutations have been identified in 23 kindreds (www.molgen.ua.ac.be/AD). The majority of these mutations are localized to exons 3, 5, 6, 7, 10 and 12 of the PS2 gene.

52.3   APPROACHES TO IDENTIFYING NEW AD GENES

52.3.1   Genome–wide association analysis

Generally, a handful of markers are selected for each genetic association study. The choice of markers is based on a prior hypothesis that has implicated these genes in AD; hence the term 'candidate genes'. Such selection does not allow for conclusions that lie beyond the scope of the hypothesis, such as the elucidation of pathogenetic pathways beyond those that initially drove the selection of the tested candidate genes to be reached. In contrast, genome-wide association studies (GWAS) test several hundreds of thousands of markers in an unbiased or hypothesis-free fashion. Recently, there have been three large GWAS studies in AD spanning 17 343 to

502 627 single nucleotide polymorphisms (SNPs) (Coon *et al.*, 2007; Grupe *et al.*, 2007; Reiman *et al.*, 2007; Li *et al.*, 2008). The GWAS conducted by Grupe *et al.* (2007) was the first study of its type in which putative functional variants in or near coding regions were analysed. Reiman *et al.* (2007) was the first high-density GWAS that reported evidence of an AD association with variants in the gene that encodes GRB2-associated binding protein 2, GAB2 that is located on chromosome 11q14. This association only became evident when AD cases and controls were divided into carrier and non-carriers of the e4 allele of ApoE. Finally, Li *et al.* (2008) reported an association with variants in the Golgi membrane protein 1 (GOLM1) located on chromosome 9q22 and two currently uncharacterized loci on chromosomes 9p and 15q.

The results of the most powerful GWAS of AD involving over 16 000 individuals from Europe observed genome-wide significant association with SNPs and three loci not previously associated with disease, CLU (also known as APOJ), PICALM and CR1 (Harold *et al.*, 2009; Lambert *et al.*, 2009). The combined data from these two groups suggest that certain variations of the three genes could increase the risk of having late-onset dementia by up to 20 per cent.

A more recent addition to GWAS markers are probes that allow the systematic assessment of copy-number variants. Such variants represent deletion or multiplications of certain chromosomal segments. However, some arrays only assay SNPs that are located in known or predicted coding regions (cSNPs). While this approach leads to enrichment of potentially functionally relevant variants, it is at the expense of overall genome-wide coverage.

52.3.2   Systematic meta-analysis

One of the major problems in genetics today is one of sorting through the large data outputs of the many reported risk factors; which ones are real and which are statistical artefacts. A publicly available database, AlzGene, which systematically collects, summarizes and meta-analyses all AD genetic association studies has recently become available (Bertram *et al.*, 2007). The AlzGene group searches literature and databases for genetic-association studies in AD samples. The results are included if the publication is peer reviewed and written in English. All entries into the database are double-checked and the allelic random effects are calculated if genotype data are available from at least four independent case–control samples. The data and results are then made available online (www.alzgene.org). In the previous month, the AlzGene database included 1236 studies, 598 genes and 2335 polymorphisms.

This is a valuable resource that should be consulted for up to date summaries and rankings. Below is a discussion of a handful of the candidate genes selected from the current list.

52.4   CANDIDATE GENES

The identification of genes and SNPs must be further evaluated in the context of potential functional genomic consequences and more specifically how these variants contribute

to neurodegeneration and dementia. Six of the top ten genes listed in the AlzGene resource are discussed more fully in relation to how their contribution may affect AD.

52.4.1   ApoE as a risk factor

Analysis has shown that that the ApoE locus located on chromosome 19 cannot account for all the genetic risk associated with sporadic early- and late-onset forms of AD (Templeton, 1995). The association of ApoE with LOAD has been studied extensively (Saunders, 2000). Polymorphisms within the ApoE promoter region correlate with increased transcriptional activity of the ApoE gene *in vitro*. Association studies of ApoE polymorphisms suggest that the −491 A/T genotype, the −491 AA genotype, the −219 T/G, the −427 C/T genotype and the Th1/E47cs genotype increase the risk of developing AD. Not surprisingly, results from other groups show positive and partial association of ApoE polymorphisms and increased risk of developing AD (Bullido *et al.*, 1998). The AlzGene resource has over 40 ApoE association studies documented in which a positive association has been reported (Bertram *et al.*, 2007). To date, this gene is the only confirmed susceptibility locus for LOAD, with ε4 allele homozygotes representing the greatest AD risk.

52.4.2   Angiotensin I-converting enzyme

Angiotensin I-converting enzyme (ACE) located on chromosome 17 encodes angiotensin I-converting enzyme 1 (ACE1), a ubiquitously expressed zinc metalloprotease that is involved in regulating blood pressure. Three polymorphisms have shown significant odds ratios in AlzGene. The relevance of ACE in AD is the observation that ACE1 can degrade naturally secreted Aβ *in vitro* (Hu *et al.* 2001; Hemming and Selkoe, 2005). However, two reports did not show supporting evidence *in vitro* (Eckman *et al.*, 2006; Hemming and Selkoe, 2007). ACE1 in the pathogenesis of AD may contribute via its role in blood pressure regulation since individuals with high mid-life blood pressure have shown an increased risk (Takeda *et al.*, 2008). Edwards *et al.* (2009) reported a putative multilocus association between ACE, A2M and LRRTM3. These three genes are related to Aβ clearance and their combined effects may contribute susceptibility to LOAD. Finally, the D allele variant of ACE is associated with a number of diseases, including atherosclerosis, diabetic nephropathy, stroke and coronary heart disease (Sayed-Tabatabaei *et al.*, 2006).

52.4.3   CST3

Cystatin C (CysC) located on chromosome 20 encoded by CST3 is an abundant ubiquitously expressed extracellular inhibitor of cysteine proteases. CST3 is upregulated following injury and is found in high levels in most body fluids including cerebrospinal fluid. Two CST3 SNPs analysed in AlzGene show significant association with AD with the most pronounced effects observed in the homozygous carriers of the Thr25 allele (Balbin and Abrahamson, 1991). CysC binds

Aβ (Vinters *et al.*, 1990) and inhibits Aβ-fibril formation in a concentration-dependent manner *in vitro* (Sastre *et al.*, 2004) and *in vivo* (Kaeser *et al.*, 2007) therefore; it is of potential relevance in AD. In addition, CysC is also involved in the development of C amyloid angiopathy (HCCAA) caused by a mutation at codon 68 (Leu68Gln). CAA lesions composed of Aβ bound to CysC are observed in AD brains (Levy *et al.*, 2006).

52.4.4   CLU, PICALM and CR1

CLU (ApoJ/clusterin) located on chromosome 8, PICALM (phosphatidylinositol-binding clathrin assembly protein) located on chromosome 11 and CR1 (complement component 3b/4b receptor) located on chromosome 1 sequence variants have recently been found to have association with AD (Harold *et al.*, 2009; Lambert *et al.*, 2009). It has been postulated that genetic variations in these three genes could account for more than one in five cases of AD. However, another 13 gene variants were also identified that warrant further investigation.

While more studies are required to determine the biological significance of the genetic contribution of these genes, the researchers have noted that CLU levels are often elevated when brain tissue is injured or inflamed. Increased levels of CLU and CR1 are found in brains and cerebrospinal fluids of Alzheimer's patients. PICALM may play a role in synaptic health and it may affect the levels of Aβ deposits in the brain.

The reader is encouraged to use the AlzGene resource to follow these recently identified genes and their likely biological contribution to LOAD.

52.5   DIAGNOSTIC GENETIC TESTING FOR AD

The identification of three genes causative for EOAD, APP and recently PS1 and PS2 raises the question of the role for genetic testing in AD. A consensus statement discussing the ethical aspects of the clinical introduction of genetic testing for AD concluded, 'except for autosomal dominant early-onset families, genetic testing in asymptomatic individuals is unwarranted'. Predictive testing for EOAD was offered in research settings following the identification of APP mutations on chromosome 21 using established Huntington's disease guidelines (Lennox *et al.*, 1994). The experience of three individuals belonging to a Swedish kindred with early-onset autosomal dominant AD was documented. Only three members of this large kindred proceeded with predictive testing, indicating a low demand for testing. One individual who was found to harbour the mutation reacted with depressive and suicidal feelings while the other two subjects expressed relief (Lannfelt *et al.*, 1995).

The ApoE gene, which confers some susceptibility to LOAD, has high commercial potential but the sensitivity and specificity of the test is low. An asymptomatic individual with an ε4 allele will not necessarily develop AD. However, testing for ApoE ε4 may be useful as an aid for the diagnosis of individuals presenting with AD. Use of ApoE genetic testing as a diagnostic adjunct in patients already presenting with dementia may prove useful, but it remains under investigation. The premature introduction of genetic testing and possible adverse consequences 'are to be avoided' (Post *et al.*, 1997). Athena Neurosciences (South San Francisco, CA, USA) in 1996 introduced the Admark ApoE Genetic Test 'for greater certainty in differential diagnosis of AD'. The requesting physician must sign a consent stating that the individual has dementia prior to ApoE genotyping being performed.

Predictive testing is performed when a known family mutation has been identified in at least one other affected family member. Pretest assessment and counselling involves obtaining an accurate pedigree, neurological examination (not compulsory) and psychological appraisal. This is critical to understanding the individual's ability to cope with the results of the test. EOAD contributes less than 5 per cent of all AD cases; therefore, there is no logical reason to perform genetic testing beyond this small cohort.

52.6   CONCLUSION

Genetic studies of EOAD have had a significant impact on our understanding of the pathogenesis of AD that, in turn, has led to research into diagnostic and therapeutic strategies and the availability of predictive testing of EOAD families. However, as people with EOAD represent only 5 per cent of all those with AD, some of the focus of genetic research has now shifted towards LOAD. Currently in LOAD, there appears to be a complex interplay of many risk factors, much as is seen in other pathogenic processes such as atherosclerosis. The current complexity of this area undermines the role for risk factor testing in LOAD. Understanding this genetic interplay is pivotal and likely to be the focus of genetic research in the next decade.

REFERENCES

Aldudo J, Bullido MJ, Valdivieso F. (1999) DGGE method for the mutational analysis of the coding and proximal promoter regions of the Alzheimer's disease presenilin-1 gene: Two novel mutations. *Human Mutation* 14: 433–9.

Ancolio K, Dumanchin C, Barelli H *et al.* (1999) Unusual phenotypic alteration of beta amyloid precursor protein (betaAPP) maturation by a new Val-715 > Met betaAPP-770 mutation responsible for probable early-onset Alzheimer's disease. *Proceedings of the National Academy of Science of the United States of America* 96: 4119–24.

Balbin M, Abrahamson M. (1991) SstII polymorphic sites in the promoter region of the human cystatin C gene. *Human Genetics* 87: 751–2.

Bertram L, McQueen MB, Mullin K *et al.* (2007) Systematic meta-analysis of Alzheimer disease genetic association studies: The AlzGene database. *Nature Genetics* 39: 17–23.

Borchelt DR, Thinakaran G, Eckman CB *et al.* (1996) Familial Alzheimer's disease-linked presenilin 1 variants elevate Ab1–42/1–40 ratio *in vitro* and *in vivo*. *Neuron* 17: 1005–13.

Brooks WS, Martins RN, De Voecht J et al. (1995) A mutation in codon 717 of the amyloid precursor protein in an Australian family with Alzheimer's disease. Neuroscience Letters 199: 183–6.

Bullido MJ, Artiga MJ, Recuero M et al. (1998) A polymorphism in the regulatory region of APoE associated with risk for Alzheimer's dementia. Nature Genetics 18: 69–71.

Campion D, Brice A, Hannequin D et al. (1996) No founder effect in three novel Alzheimer's disease families with APP 717 Val->Ile mutation. Journal of Medical Genetics 33: 661–4.

Campion D, Dumanchin C, Hannequin D et al. (1999) Early-onset autosomal dominant Alzheimer's disease: Prevalence, genetic heterogeneity, and mutation spectrum. American Journal of Human Genetics 65: 664–70.

Citron M, Oltersdorf T, Haass C et al. (1992) Mutation of the beta-amyloid precursor protein in familial Alzheimer's disease increases b-protein production. Nature 360: 672–4.

Clark RF, Hutton M, Fuldner RA et al. (1995) The structure of the presenilin 1 gene and identification of six novel mutations in early onset AD families. Nature Genetics 11: 219–22.

Coon KD, Myers AJ, Craig DW et al. (2007) A high-density whole genome association study reveals that APOE is the major susceptibility gene for sporadic late-onset Alzheimer disease. Journal of Clinical Psychiatry 68: 611–12.

Crook R, Verkkoniemi A, Perez-Tur J et al. (1998) A variant of Alzheimer's disease with spastic paraparesis and unusual plaques due to deletion of exon 9 of presenilin. Nature Medicine 4: 452–5.

De Jonghe C, Kumar-Singh S, Cruts M et al. (2000) Unusual Ab amyloid in Alzheimer's disease due to an APP T7141 mutation at the g42-secretase site. Neurobiology of Aging ; (Suppl. 1): S200.

Duff K, Eckman C, Zehr C et al. (1996) Increased amyloid-beta42(43) in brains of mice expressing mutant presenilin 1. Nature 383: 710–13.

Eckman CB, Mehta ND, Crook R et al. (1997) A new pathogenic mutation in the APP gene (I716V) increases the relative proportion of A beta 42(43). Human Molecular Genetics 6: 2087–9.

Eckman EA, Adams SK, Troendle FJ et al. (2006) Regulation of steady-state beta-amyloid levels in the brain by neprilysin and endothelin-converting enzyme but not angiotensin-converting enzyme. Journal of Biological Chemistry 281: 30471–8.

Edwards TL, Pericak-Vance M, Gilbert JR et al. (2009) An association analysis of Alzheimer disease candidate genes detects an ancestral risk haplotype clade in ACE and putative multilocus association between ACE, A2M, and LRRTM3. American Journal of Medical Genetics Part B: Neuropsychiatric Genetics 150B: 721–35.

Ezquerra M, Carnero C, Blesa R et al. (1999) A presenilin 1 mutation (Ser169Pro) associated with early-onset AD and myoclonic seizures. Neurology 52: 566–70.

Farlow MR, Murrell JR, Hulette CM et al. (2000) Hereditary lateral sclerosis and Alzheimer disease associated with mutation at codon 261 of the presenilin 1 (PS1) gene. Neurobiology of Aging 21 (Suppl.): S62.

Fidani L, Rooke K, Chartier-Harlin M et al. (1992) Screening for mutations in the open reading frame and promoter of the b-amyloid precursor protein in familial Alzheimer's disease: Identification of a further family with APP Val->Ile. Human Molecular Genetics 1: 165–8.

Finckh U, Muller-Thomsen T, Mann U et al. (2000) High prevalence of pathogenic mutations in patients with early-onset dementia detected by sequence analyses of four different genes. American Journal of Human Genetics 66: 110–17.

Goate A, Haynes AR, Owen MJ et al. (1989) Predisposing locus for Alzheimer disease on chromosome 21. Lancet 1: 352–5.

Goate A, Chartier HM, Mullan M et al. (1991) Segregation of a missense mutation in the amyloid precursor protein gene with familial Alzheimer's disease. Nature 349: 704–6.

Goldgaber D, Lerman MI, McBride OW. (1987) Characterisation and chromosomal localization of a cDNA encoding brain amyloid of Alzheimer disease on chromosome 21. Science 235: 877–80.

Grupe A, Abraham R, Li Y et al. (2007) Evidence for novel susceptibility genes for late-onset Alzheimer's disease from a genome-wide association study of putative functional variants. Human Molecular Genetics 16: 865–73.

Hardy J. (1997) Amyloid, the presenilins and Alzheimer's disease. Trends in Neuroscience 20: 154–9.

Hardy J, Crook R. (2001) Presenilin mutations line up along transmembrane a-helices. Neuroscience Letters 306: 203–5.

Hardy J, Mullan M, Chartier-Harlin MC et al. (1991) Molecular classification of Alzheimer's disease. Lancet 337: 1342–3.

Harold D, Abraham R, Hollingworth P et al. (2009) Genome-wide association study identifies variants at CLU and PICALM associated with Alzheimer's disease. Nature Genetics 41: 1088–93.

Hemming ML, Selkoe DJ. (2005) Amyloid β-protein is degraded by cellular angiotensin-converting enzyme (ACE) and elevated by an ACE inhibitor. Journal of Biological Chemistry 280: 37644–50.

Hemming ML, Selkoe DJ. (2007) Effects of prolonged angiotensin-converting enzyme inhibitor treatment on amyloid β-protein metabolism in mouse models of Alzheimer's disease. Neurobiology of Disease 26: 273–81.

Hendriks L, van Duijn C, Cras P et al. (1992) Presenilin dementia and cerebral haemorrhage linked to a mutation at condon 692 of the B-amyloid precursor protein gene. Nature Genetics 1: 218–21.

Hendriks L, Thinakaran G, Harris CL et al. (1997) Processing of presenilin 1 in brains of patients with Alzheimer's disease and controls. NeuroReport 8: 1717–21.

Hu J, Igarashi A, Kamata M et al. (2001) Angiotensin-converting enzyme degrades Alzheimer amyloid β-peptide (AB); retards Aβ aggregation, deposition, fibril formation; and inhibits cytotoxicity. Journal of Biological Chemistry 276: 47863–8.

Hutton M, Busfield F, Wragg M et al. (1996) Complete analysis of the presenilin 1 gene in early onset Alzheimer's disease. NeuroReport 7: 801–5.

Kaeser SA, Herzig MC, Coomaraswammy J, Kilger E. (2007) Cystatin C modulates cerebral beta-amyloidosis. Nature Genetics 39: 1437–9.

Kamino K, Orr HT, Payami H et al. (1992) Linkage and mutational analysis of familial Alzheimer disease kindreds for the APP gene region. American Journal of Human Genetics 51: 998–1014.

Kang J, Lemaire HG, Unterbeck A. (1987) The precursor of Alzheimer disease amyloid A4 protein resembles a cell surface receptor. *Nature* **325**: 733–6.

Kwok JB, Taddei K, Hallupp M *et al.* (1997) Two novel (M233T and R278T) presenilin-1 mutations in early-onset Alzheimer's disease pedigrees and preliminary evidence for association of presenilin-1 mutations with a novel phenotype. *NeuroReport* **8**: 1537–42.

Kwok JBJ, Li Q-X, Hallup M *et al.* (2000a) Novel Leu723Pro amyloid precursor protein mutation increases amyloid beta42(43) peptide levels and induces apoptosis. *Annals of Neurology* **47**: 249–53.

Kwok JBJ, Smith MJ, Brooks WS *et al.* (2000b) Variable presentation of Alzheimer's disease and/or spastic paraparesis phenotypes in pedigrees with a novel PS-1 exon 9 deletion or exon 9 splice acceptor mutations. *Neurobiology of Aging* **21** (Suppl.): S25.

Lambert J-C, Health S, Even G *et al.* (2009) Genome-wide association study identifies variants at CLU and CR1 associated with Alzheimer's disease. *Nature Genetics* **41**: 1094–9.

Lampe TH, Bird TD, Nochlin D *et al.* (1994) Phenotype of chromosome 14-linked familial Alzheimer's disease in a large kindred. *Annals of Neurology* **36**: 368–78.

Lannfelt H, Axelman K, Lilius L, Basun H. (1995) Genetic counseling of a Swedish Alzheimer family with amyloid precursor protein mutation. *American Journal of Human Genetics* **56**: 332–5.

Lennox A, Karlinsky H, Meschino W *et al.* (1994) Molecular genetic predictive testing for Alzheimer disease: Deliberations and preliminary recommendations. *Alzheimer Disease and Associated Disorders* **8**: 126–47.

Levy E, Carman MD, Fernandez-Madrid IJ *et al.* (1990) Mutation of the Alzheimer's disease amyloid gene in hereditary cerebral hemorrhage, Dutch type. *Science* **248**: 1124–6.

Levy-Lahad E, Wijsman EM, Nemens E *et al.* (1995) A familial Alzheimer's disease locus on chromosome 1. *Science* **269**: 970–3.

Levy E, Jaskolski M, Grubb A. (2006) The role of cystatin C in cerebral amyloid angiopathy and stroke: Cell biology and animal models. *Brain Pathology* **16**: 60–70.

Li H, Wetten S, Li L *et al.* (2008) Candidate single-nucleotide polymorphisms from a genomewide association study of Alzheimer disease. *Archives of Neurology* **65**: 45–53.

Mann DMA, Yates PO, Marcyniuk B. (1984) Alzheimer's presenile dementia, senile dementia, of the Alzheimer type, and Down's syndrome in middle age form a continuum of pathologic changes. *Neuropathology and Applied Neurobiology* **10**: 185–207.

Mann DM, Brown A, Prinja D *et al.* (1989) An analysis of the morphology of senile plaques in Down's syndrome patients of different ages using immunocytochemical and lectin histochemical techniques. *Neuropathology and Applied Neurobiology* **15**: 317–29.

Masters CL, Simms G, Weinman NA *et al.* (1985) Amyloid plaque core protein in Alzheimer disease and Down syndrome. *Proceedings of the National Academy of Sciences of the United States of America* **82**: 4245–9.

Matsumura Y, Kitamura E, Miyoshi K *et al.* (1996) Japanese siblings with missense mutation (717Val->Ile) in amyloid precursor protein of early-onset Alzheimer's disease. *Neurology* **46**: 1721–3.

Mehta ND, Refolo LM, Eckman C *et al.* (1998) Increased Abeta42(43) from cell lines expressing presenilin 1 mutations. *Annals of Neurology* **43**: 256–8.

Mercken M, Takahashi H, Honda T *et al.* (1996) Characterisation of human presenilin 1 using *N*-terminal specific monoclonal antibodies: Evidence that Alzheimer mutations affect proteolytic processing. *FEBS Letters* **389**: 297–303.

Miravalle H, Tokuda T, Chiarle R *et al.* (2000) Substitutions at codon 22 of Alzheimer's A-beta peptide induce diverse conformational changes and apoptotic effects in human cerebral endothelial cells. *Journal of Biological Chemistry* **275**: 27110–16.

Mullan M, Crawford F, Axelman K *et al.* (1992) A pathogenic mutation for probable Alzheimer's disease in the APP gene at the *N*-terminus of b-amyloid. *Nature Genetics* **1**: 345–7.

Naruse S, Igarashi S, Aoki K *et al.* (1991) Mis-sense mutation Val to ILE in exon 17 of amyloid precursor protein in Japanese familial Alzheimer's disease. *Lancet* **337**: 978–9.

Nilsberth C, Westlind-Danielsson A, Eckman CB *et al.* (2000) The Arctic mutation (E693G) causes Alzheimer's disease through a novel mechanism: Increased amyloid b protofibril formation and decreased amyloid b levels in plasma and conditioned media. *Neurobiology of Aging* **21**(Suppl. 1): S58.

Perez-Tur J, Froelich S, Prihar G *et al.* (1995) A mutation in Alzheimer's disease destroying a splice acceptor site in the presenilin-1 gene. *NeuroReport* **7**: 297–301.

Post SG, Whitehouse PJ, Binstock RH *et al.* (1997) The clinical introduction of genetic testing for Alzheimer disease. *Journal of the American Medical Association* **277**: 832–6.

Raux G, Gantier R, Thomas-Anterion C *et al.* (2000) Dementia with prominent frontotemporal features associated with L113P presenilin 1 mutation. *Neurology* **55**: 1577–9.

Reiman EM, Webster JA, Myers AJ *et al.* (2007) GAB2 alleles modify Alzheimer's risk in APOE epsilon4 carriers. *Neuron* **54**: 713–20.

Rovelet-Lecrux A, Hannequin D, Raux G *et al.* (2006) APP locus duplication causes autosomal dominant early-onset Alzheimer disease with cerebral amyloid angiopathy. *Nature Genetics* **38**: 24–6.

Rovelet-Lecrux A, Frebourg T, Tuominen H *et al.* (2007) APP locus duplication in a Finnish family with dementia and intracerebral haemorrhage. *Journal of Neurology, Neurosurgery, and Psychiatry* **78**: 1158–9.

St George-Hyslop PH, Tanzi RE, Polinsky RJ *et al.* (1987) The genetic defect causing familial Alzheimer disease maps on chromosome 21. *Science* **235**: 885–9.

St George-Hyslop PH, Haines JL, Farrer LA *et al.* (1990) Genetic linkage studies suggest that Alzheimer's disease is not a single homogenous disorder. *Nature* **347**: 194–7.

St George-Hyslop PH, Haines J, Rogaev E *et al.* (1992) Genetic evidence for a novel familial Alzheimer's disease locus on chromosome 14. *Nature Genetics* **2**: 330–4.

Sato S, Kamino K, Miki T *et al.* (1998) Splicing mutation of presenilin-1 gene for early-onset familial Alzheimer's disease. *Human Mutation* (Suppl. 1): S91–4.

Sastre M, Calero M, Pawlik M *et al.* (2004) Binding of cystatin C to Alzheimer's amyloid b I inhibits in vitro amylid fibril formation. *Neurobiology of Ageing* 25: 1033–43.

Saunders AM. (2000) Apolipoprotein E and Alzheimer's disease: An update on genetic and functional analyses. *Journal of Neuropathology and Experimental Neurology* 59: 751–8.

Sayed-Tabatabaei FA, Oostra BA, Isaacs A *et al.* (2006) ACE polymorphisms. *Circulation Research* 98: 1123–33.

Schellenberg GD, Bird TD, Wijsman EM *et al.* (1988) Absence of linkage of chromosome 21q21 markers to familial Alzheimer's disease. *Science* 241: 1507–10.

Selkoe D. (1994) Cell biology of the amyloid beta-protein precursor and the mechanism of Alzheimer's disease. *Annual Review of Cell Biology* 10: 373–403.

Sherrington R, Rogaev EI, Liang Y *et al.* (1995) Cloning a gene bearing missense mutations in early-onset familial Alzheimer's disease. *Nature* 375: 754–60.

Sherrington R, Froelich S, Sorbi S *et al.* (1996) Alzheimer's disease associated with mutations in presenilin 2 is rare and variably penetrant. *Human Molecular Genetics* 5: 985–8.

Sleegers K, Brouwers N, Gijselinck I *et al.* (2006) APP duplication is sufficient to cause early onset Alzheimer's dementia with cerebral amyloid angiopathy. *Brain* 129: 2977–83.

Smith MJ, Kwok JBJ, McLean CA *et al.* (2001) Variable phenotype of Alzheimer's disease with spastic paraparesis. *Annals of Neurology* 49: 125–9.

Sorbi S, Nacmias B, Forleo P *et al.* (1993) APP717 and Alzheimer's disease in Italy. *Nature Genetics* 4: 10.

Sorbi S, Nacmiass B, Forleo P *et al.* (1995) Epistatic effect of APP717 mutation and apolipoprotein E genotype in familial Alzheimer's disease. *Annals of Neurology* 38: 124–7.

Steiner H, Revesz T, Neumann M *et al.* (2001) A pathogenic presenilin-1 deletion causes aberrant Ab42 production in the absence of congophilic amyloid plaques. *Journal of Biological Chemistry* 276: 7233–9.

Suzuki N, Cheung TT, Cai XD *et al.* (1994) An increased percentage of long amyloid beta protein secreted by familial amyloid beta protein precursor (beta APP717) mutants. *Science* 264: 1336–40.

Takahashi H, Mercken M, Honda T *et al.* (1999) Impaired proteolytic processing of presenilin-1 in chromosome 14-linked familial Alzheimer's disease patient lymphocytes. *Neuroscience Letters* 260: 121–4.

Takeda S, Sato N, Ogihara T *et al.* (2008) The rennin-angiotensin system, hypertension and cognitive dysfunction in Alzheimer's disease: New therapeutic potential. *Frontiers of Bioscience* 13: 2253–65.

Tanzi RE, St George-Hyslop PH, Haines JL *et al.* (1987) The genetic defect in familial Alzheimer's disease is not tightly linked to the amyloid b-protein gene. *Nature* 329: 156–7.

Tanzi RE, Bertram L. (2005) Twenty years of the Alzheimer's disease amyloid hypothesis: A genetic perspective. *Cell* 120: 545–55.

Tedde A, Forleo P, Nacmias B *et al.* (2000) A presenilin 1 mutation (Leu392Pro) in a familial AD kindred with psychiatric symptoms at onset. *Neurology* 55: 1590–1.

Templeton AR. (1995) A cladistic analysis of phenotypic associations with haplotypes inferred from restriction endonucleases mapping or DNA sequencing. V. Analysis of case/control sampling designs: Alzheimer's disease and apolipoprotein E locus. *Genetics* 140: 403–9.

Thinakaran G, Borchelt DR, Lee MK *et al.* (1996) Endoproteolysis of presenilin 1 and accumulation of processed derivatives in vivo. *Neuron* 17: 181–90.

Tokano T, Sahara N, Yamanouchi Y, Mori H. (1997) Assignment of Alzheimer's presenilin-2 (PS-2) gene to 1q42.1 by fluorescence in situ hybridisation. *Neuroscience Letters* 221: 205–7.

Tysoe C, Whittaker J, Xuereb J *et al.* (1998) A Presenilin-1 truncating mutation is present in two cases with autopsy-confirmed early-onset Alzheimer disease. *American Journal of Human Genetics* 62: 70–6.

Van Broeckhoven C. (1995) Presenilins and Alzheimer's disease. *Nature Genetics* 11: 230–2.

Van Broeckhoven C, Genthe AM, Vandenberghe A *et al.* (1987) Failure of familial Alzheimer's disease to segregate with the A4-amyloid gene in several European families. *Nature* 329: 153–5.

Van Broeckhoven C, Hann J, Bakker E *et al.* (1990) Amyloid beta protein precursor gene and hereditary cerebral hemorrhage with amyloidosis (Dutch). *Science* 248: 1120–2.

Van Broeckhoven C, Backhovens H, Cruts M *et al.* (1992) Mapping of a gene predisposing to early-onset Alzheimer's disease to chromosome 14q24.3. *Nature Genetics* 2: 335–9.

Vinters HV, Nishimura GS, Secor DL. (1990) Immunoreactive A4 and gamma trace peptide colocalization in amyloidotic arteriolar lesions in brains of patients with Alzheimer's disease. *American Journal of Pathology* 137: 233–40.

Wisniewski T, Ghiso J, Frangione B. (1991) Peptides homologous to the amyloid protein of Alzheimer's disease containing a glutamine for glutamic acid substitution have accelerated amyloid fibril formation. *Biochemical and Biophysical Research Communications* 179: 1247–54.

Wolfe MS, Xia W, Moore CL *et al.* (1999) Peptidomimetic probes and molecular modeling suggest Alzheimer's g-secretases are intramembrane-cleaving aspartyl proteases. *Biochemistry* 38: 4720–7.

Blood and cerebrospinal fluid biological markers for Alzheimer's disease

JOHANNES PANTEL AND HARALD HAMPEL

53.1 FUNCTION AND PURPOSE OF BIOMARKERS IN THE DIAGNOSIS AND TREATMENT OF ALZHEIMER'S DISEASE

In general, a biomarker defines a disease characteristic that is objectively measured and evaluated as an indicator of normal biological processes, pathogenic processes or pharmacological responses to a therapeutic intervention (Shaw *et al.*, 2007). The Working Group on Molecular and Biochemical Markers of Alzheimer's disease (AD) aimed to stipulate the relevance of the single biomarkers and therefore proposed guidelines to achieve this goal (Consensus Report, 1998). Accordingly, the ideal biomarker for AD should detect a fundamental feature of neuropathology and be validated in neuropathologically confirmed cases. With respect to the diagnosis and treatment of a given disease, biomarkers may subserve certain functions (Kroll, 2008). These include:

- **Diagnostic function**: Diagnostic markers assist in the clinical diagnosis and in the differential diagnosis. In the context of a dementia diagnosis these markers might facilitate the differentiation of dementia from non-dementing cognitive disorders in the elderly (e.g. geriatric depression), or enable the differentiation of AD from non-AD dementias. A diagnostic biomarker should have a sensitivity for detecting AD of at least 85 per cent and its specificity in differentiating AD patients from

age-matched control subjects and from patients with other forms of dementia should reach at least 75 per cent (Consensus Report, 1998). In clinically diagnosed populations a higher level of specificity for biomarkers probably will not be achieved for methodological reasons, as even the gold standard, the clinical diagnostic criteria, cannot be absolutely specific. The same applies to controls of the same age, as some of them might have presymptomatic AD (Morris and Price, 2001). In large groups, this fact will inevitably affect the specificity of the results of even the best biomarker.

- **Screening function**: Screening markers discriminate the 'healthy' state from an early disease state, preferably in the asymptomatic phase (e.g. predementia stage of AD). They might subserve early (preclinical) diagnosis of AD and thus enable early intervention. Targets for the screening approach can be an entire population or subpopulations at risk (e.g. mild cognitive impairment (MCI)).

- **Prognostic function**: Prognostic markers can predict the likely course of the disease. They are associated with outcome regardless of treatment used.

- **Predictive function**: Prediction or stratifications markers are associated with outcome from a specific therapy. They predict the likely response to a drug (e.g. an acetylcholin inhibitor or an anti-amyloid substance) before starting treatment. These markers classify individuals as 'responders' as compared with likely 'non-responders'.

- **Monitoring function**: A monitoring marker can be used to monitor efficacy of a drug treatment once the responder status is established. Within the setting of a clinical drug trial a monitoring marker may also serve as a 'surrogate marker' if it is closely linked to a clinically meaningful treatment outcome (e.g cognition, functional abilities, quality of life). In that sense, a useful monitoring marker can be used as an outcome parameter under a particular treatment.

The same marker can subserve different listed functions, e.g. it can be both predictive and prognostic, or it might be diagnostic and also be a useful screening tool.

53.2 BIOMARKER DEVELOPMENT

Ideally, a biomarker should be reliable, reproducible, non-invasive, simple to perform and inexpensive. Positive predictive value should approach 90 per cent. Recommended steps to establish a biomarker include confirmation by at least two independent studies conducted by qualified investigators with the results published in peer-reviewed journals (Consensus Report, 1998).

Although a large number of AD biomarker studies have been published, the clinical relevance and feasibility of the investigated biomarkers are not completely elucidated (Buerger and Hampel, 2009). A number of steps are required before a biomarker becomes a reliable and precise asset to clinicians. First, the technical feasibility of the new marker has to be established, including the availability of a validated assay with high precision and reliability of measurement and well-described reagents and standards. A large number of potential markers have successfully passed this first step. Second, the possible marker has to be evaluated in a relatively pure sample of diseased and comparison groups. This is similar to the phase 2 trial in therapeutics, but the goal here is to make an initial assessment of its sensitivity and specificity. Only few potential markers have passed this step. In the next step, the new marker has to be studied in a more representative population-based sample, providing an assessment of its true diagnostic properties and thus demonstrating its clinical usefulness. Large-scale, controlled multicentre biomarker trials are currently being conducted in the US, Japanese, Australian and European Alzheimer networks in an attempt to systematically develop and validate core feasible candidate biomarkers in research areas such as neurochemistry and structural and functional imaging (Hampel et al., 2009).

Two different approaches exist for the identification of cerebrospinal fluid (CSF) biomarkers: the hypothesis driven candidate biomarker approach and the exploratory proteome approach. The candidate biomarker approach tries to identify a protein or molecule reflecting neurochemical changes underlying central mechanistic molecular and pathogenic processes leading to neurodegeneration. In AD biomarker research, the candidate approach should, that is, reflect neuronal and synaptic degeneration, mismetabolism of amyloid precursor protein (APP) and/or aggregation of amyloid-β (Aβ) with subsequent deposition in plaques, and/or hyperphosphorylation of tau with subsequent formation of paired helical filaments and tangles. The proteome approach uses unbiased hypothesis independent proteomic methods that try to identify biomarkers that can differentiate affected cases from healthy controls and other comparisons, such as various brain disorders, regardless of whether the biomarkers may be directly known as linked to molecular or pathogenetic processes (Zetzsche et al., 2010). Exploratory proteome-based methods include 2D electrophoresis (2DE), protein chips or liquid chromatography, combined with mass spectrometry (Blennow, 2005).

53.3 DIAGNOSTIC BIOMARKERS FOR AD

Biomarker research in AD is most advanced in the field of diagnosis. In their position paper on the revision of research criteria for the diagnosis of AD, Dubois et al. (2007) list characteristic pathological signatures of 'abnormal cerebrospinal fluid biomarkers' (including low Aβ_{42} concentrations or increased total tau or phospho-tau concentrations) as a major supportive feature for the diagnosis of probable AD. Currently the most promising diagnostic biomarker candidates originate from CSF (Buerger and Hampel, 2009). Therefore, this chapter will focus on current 'gold standard' diagnostic 'core feasible' (as defined by the NIA Biological Marker Working Group (Frank et al., 2003)) CSF markers. Other applications in blood, serum or plasma and additional candidate markers will be reviewed below, however, results are still experimental and preliminary (Blennow et al., 2010; Hampel et al., 2010).

Diagnostic biomarkers should improve early (termed 'diagnosis' in symptomatic or 'detection' in studies on pre-symptomatic cases) and differential diagnosis ('classification'), particularly when symptoms are absent, vague or unspecific. Nonetheless, diagnostic biomarkers should best be used and interpreted in combination with clinical examination and other investigations such as blood tests, structural imaging and neuropsychological testing.

53.3.1 Aβ in blood plasma

Efforts to discover and develop diagnostic biomarkers for AD in peripheral blood, plasma or serum is still experimental and at phase 1–2 of diagnostic validation; there are few candidates in pilot and first single-centre studies that seem to perform close to the diagnostic accuracy range achieved by established core feasible CSF biomarkers (see below). The best-studied candidate biomarker in plasma so far is Aβ, but the findings are contradictory. Some groups have reported high concentrations in plasma of either Aβ_{42} or Aβ_{40} in AD with a broad overlap between cases and controls, whereas most groups find no change (Irizarry, 2004). Some studies have also reported high plasma Aβ_{42} (but not Aβ_{40}) in non-demented elderly people who later developed either progressive cognitive decline or AD (Mayeux et al., 2003; Pomara et al., 2005). In contrast, van Oijen and colleagues recently reported an association between high $A\beta_{40}$, low $A\beta_{42}$, and risk of dementia (van Oijen *et al.*, 2006). This result is in general agreement with the findings of Graff-Radford *et al.* (2007), who observed a weak association between low plasma $A\beta_{42}:A\beta_{40}$ ratio and risk of future MCI or AD in a healthy elderly population. Similar findings were reported by Lewczuk *et al.* (2009). Apart from disease-related factors, the opposing results may be due to the fact that $A\beta_{42}$ is difficult to measure in plasma. Moreover, it is still unclear what effect $A\beta$ oligomerization has on $A\beta$ concentrations in plasma measured by immunoassays. This possible confounder might differ between different methods, which could explain some of the contradictory results in the literature. It is still unclear whether the disturbed metabolism of $A\beta_{42}$ in the AD brain is reflected by changes in the levels of $A\beta$ markers in plasma. In fact, $A\beta$ is produced by many different bodily cells and there seems to be no correlation between the levels of $A\beta_{42}$ in plasma and CSF (Vanderstichele *et al.*, 2000; Mehta *et al.*, 2001). Similarly, other investigations have shown that plasma $A\beta_{42}$ and $A\beta_{40}$ do not reflect $A\beta$ accumulation in the brains of individuals with AD (Fagan *et al.*, 2006; Freeman *et al.*, 2007).

53.3.2 $A\beta$ in CSF

As all currently known genetic causes of familial AD are linked to increased deposition of $A\beta$, it seems very likely that $A\beta$ could be a useful marker for the disease (Consensus Report, 1998). The soluble $A\beta$ peptide is a component of normal cell metabolism that, if abnormally proteolysed, becomes insoluble and aggregates in the brain (Mehta *et al.*, 1991). Unfortunately, total $A\beta$ level shows no clear diagnostic utility (Motter *et al.*, 1995). The 42-amino acid $A\beta$ deposits more rapidly than 40-amino acid $A\beta$ protein (Iwatsubo *et al.*, 1994; Wisniewski and Wegiel, 1995). Thus, CSF $A\beta_{42}$ seems to be the initial form of extracellular aggregation and studies have focused on this peptide. About 20 studies have been conducted on 2000 patients and controls, showing a reduction of $A\beta_{42}$ by about 50 per cent in AD patients compared with non-demented controls of the same age; the diagnostic sensitivity and specificity levels range between 80 and 90 per cent (Blennow and Hampel, 2003). A non-age-dependent cut-off level of 500 pg/mL was found between AD patients and healthy controls (Sjoegren *et al.*, 2001). The sensitivity was higher for patients with the apolipoprotein E (ApoE) ε4 allele (83.6 per cent) than for patients without one (54.2 per cent) (Tapiola *et al.*, 2000). Decreased $A\beta_{42}$ levels were also found in patients with vascular dementia (Hulstaert *et al.*, 1999). Many studies have found decreased CSF $A\beta_{42}$ in patients with MCI as compared with controls (Andreasen *et al.*, 1999), but one study found increased levels in patients with MCI. Since disorders not related to $A\beta$ plaques, such as amyotrophic lateral sclerosis and multiple system atrophy, are also associated with reduced $A\beta_{42}$ level (Sjoegren *et al.*, 2002; Holmberg *et al.*, 2003), it is not clear if the decreased level of CSF $A\beta_{42}$ reflects the deposition of $A\beta_{42}$ in plaques or if other processes such as decreased $A\beta$ production or increased $A\beta$ clearance or proteolysis are involved.

In distinguishing AD from other types of dementia the specificity level achieves unsatisfactory results; as a mean only approximately 60 per cent (Hulstaert *et al.*, 1999). An autopsy study demonstrated an inverse correlation between $A\beta_{42}$ levels in the CSF and the number of plaques (Strozyk *et al.*, 2003), and it has been shown that subjects with evidence of amyloid plaque accumulation in the brain using positron emission tomography studies with Pittsburgh Compound B (PIB; see below and Chapter 13, Molecular brain imaging in dementia) had the lowest CSF $A\beta_{42}$ concentrations (Fagan *et al.*, 2006), however future studies need to take account of the considerable diurnal fluctuations in CSF $A\beta$ levels (Bateman *et al.*, 2007).

Data on CSF $A\beta_{40}$ are less clear. Several studies showed similar levels in AD patients and controls (Mecocci *et al.*, 1995; Tamaoka *et al.*, 1997). Only one study (Jensen *et al.*, 1999) showed lower $A\beta_{40}$ levels in patients with AD with a considerable overlap between patients and controls.

In addition to $A\beta_{42}$ and $A\beta_{40}$ in CSF alone, the ratio of $A\beta_{42}$ to $A\beta_{40}$ has been investigated. The $A\beta_{42}:A\beta_{40}$ ratio is reduced in CSF (or, conversely, $A\beta_{40}:A\beta_{42}$ ratio is increased). The reduction of CSF $A\beta_{42}:A\beta_{40}$ ratio seems to be more marked than the reduction of CSF $A\beta_{42}$ alone (Fukuyama *et al.*, 2000; Lewczuk *et al.*, 2004). Further studies are needed to determine if the CSF $A\beta_{42}:A\beta_{40}$ ratio has a higher diagnostic potential than CSF $A\beta_{42}$ alone (Lewczuk *et al.*, 2004), especially in cases of MCI and early AD.

Thus, $A\beta_{42}$ comes close to fulfilling the criteria for a useful diagnostic test for AD (Consensus Report, 1998), but is of limited value in differentiating AD from other primary dementias.

53.3.3   Total tau protein in CSF

The main component relating to intraneuronal changes in AD patients is the microtubule-associated tau protein. Abnormal aggregates can only be formed if the tau protein is released from its sites of binding (Spillantini *et al.*, 1990). In AD patients, tau protein is present in a pathological, hyperphosphorylated form. Tau pathology can also be observed in other neurodegenerative diseases, but differs from tau pathology in AD patients at the molecular level (Hasegawa, 2006). Tau protein was quantified in the CSF under the hypothesis that it is released extracellularly as a result of the neurodegenerative process. The methods initially available analysed all forms of tau regardless of their phosphorylation status at specific epitopes, i.e. total tau protein (t-tau).

More than 50 studies have been conducted with some 5000 cases and controls and all have demonstrated an increase in the concentration of t-tau in AD patients by approximately 300 per cent compared with non-demented elderly subjects, and a systematic increase in the concentration with age was observed in the control groups (Buerger née Buch *et al.*, 1999; Wahlund *et al.*, 2001). The sensitivity and specificity levels were between 80 and 90 per cent for t-tau (Blennow and Hampel, 2003). In subjects younger than 50 years, the concentrations in the CSF are usually lower than 300 pg/mL, in subjects younger than 70 years lower than 450 pg/mL, and in the over seventies lower than 500 pg/mL (Sjoegren *et al.*, 2001). Both t-tau and $A\beta_{42}$ were already significantly altered in MCI subjects who are at increased risk of AD (Hampel *et al.*, 2004d). Although the AD group could be differentiated from healthy controls of the same age using a combination of the two markers (sensitivity = 85 per cent, specificity = 86 per cent), the differential diagnosis (classification) between AD and other primary degenerative dementias was unsatisfactory (sensitivity = 85 per cent, specificity = 58 per cent) (Hulstaert *et al.*, 1999). Therefore, more specific biomarkers were sought.

53.3.4   Hxyperphosphorylated tau protein in CSF

Approximately 30 phosphorylation epitopes have been detected in AD. Around 1999 the first methods were published and demonstrated concentrations of hyperphosphorylated tau protein (p-tau) in the CSF. Most of these studies have investigated tau protein hyperphosphorylated at threonine 231 (p-tau$_{231P}$) and at threonine 181 (p-tau$_{181P}$), and a few results have been obtained for serine 199 (p-tau$_{199P}$). A correlation with neurofibrillary neocortical pathology was demonstrated for p-tau$_{231P}$ in the CSF (Buerger *et al.*, 2006), but not for p-tau$_{181P}$ (Buerger *et al.*, 2007). Single studies are available on other epitopes as well.

An increase in p-tau has consistently been found in the CSF of AD patients compared with controls. Around 20 studies have been conducted on 2000 patients and controls with sensitivity and specificity levels of between 80 and 90 per cent. Differences have certainly been observed between the individual p-tau subtypes in distinguishing between the groups. P-tau$_{231P}$ and p-tau$_{181P}$ show better results than p-tau$_{199P}$ in distinguishing AD from control groups and even from other types of dementia (Hampel *et al.*, 2004a). These and other studies suggest that p-tau is promising in distinguishing AD from frontotemporal dementia (FTD), with sensitivity and specificity rates of 85–90 per cent (Buerger *et al.*, 2002c; Hampel *et al.*, 2004b). A combination of various p-tau subtypes did not provide improved results in distinguishing between the groups due to ceiling effects. P-tau may also be useful in distinguishing AD from idiopathic normal pressure hydrocephalus. A study found similarly altered concentrations of t-tau and Aβ$_{42}$ in both groups compared with controls, while p-tau$_{181P}$ was considerably higher in the AD group only (Kapaki *et al.*, 2007). The sensitivity and specificity rates were higher than 85 per cent. A systematic review discusses what clinical benefit p-tau might offer. The high negative predictive value of p-tau of approximately 90 per cent appears to be particularly significant. Normal values rule out the presence of AD with almost 90 per cent probability (Mitchell and Brindle, 2003).

53.3.5   CSF Aβ and tau protein in the distinction of AD from other forms of dementia

There have been several studies of the potential of CSF Aβ$_{42}$ to differentiate AD from other neurodegenerative disorders. Compared to control subjects with other neurological conditions, a slight decrease has been described in non-AD dementias (Galasko, 1998). Low levels of Aβ$_{42}$ protein have

been detected in dementia with Lewy bodies (DLB); the range of Aβ$_{42}$ protein concentrations overlaps with Aβ$_{42}$ concentrations found in AD patients (Andreasen *et al.*, 1999; Kanemaru *et al.*, 2000; Parnetti *et al.*, 2001; Vanmechelen *et al.*, 2001; Mollenhauer *et al.*, 2005), but part of the overlap may be due to concomitant AD pathology. There is also marked reduction in CSF Aβ$_{42}$ in disorders without β-amyloid plaques, such as Creutzfeldt–Jakob disease (CJD) (Otto *et al.*, 2000), frontotemporal dementia and vascular dementia (VaD) (Hulstaert *et al.*, 1999; Sjoegren *et al.*, 2000).

An increase of CSF t-tau has been found in a proportion of cases with other dementia disorders, including VaD, FTD and DLB (Blennow and Hampel, 2003). Other studies, however, found normal levels in these disorders (Blennow and Hampel, 2003). The potential of t-tau is limited in its ability to discriminate AD from other relevant dementia disorders. At a sensitivity level of 81 per cent, CSF t-tau reached a specificity of only 57 per cent in distinguishing AD from other dementias (Hulstaert *et al.*, 1999; Parnetti *et al.*, 2000). Therefore, t-tau seems an unlikely candidate as a marker for the differential diagnosis of AD.

The supposition that t-tau reflects non-specific processes of axonal damage and neuronal degeneration is further supported by increased CSF t-tau in disorders with extensive and/or rapid neuronal degeneration such as CJD (Otto *et al.*, 2002). A highly significant increase of 580 per cent was documented in CJD compared to AD patients. At a cut-off level of 2130 pg/mL t-tau yielded a sensitivity of 93 per cent and a specificity of 100 per cent between AD and CJD (Kapaki *et al.*, 2001).

For differentiating between AD and FTD, p-tau$_{231}$ showed a sensitivity of 90.2 per cent and a specificity of 92.3 per cent (Buerger *et al.*, 2002b). In the differentiation from geriatric major depression p-tau$_{231}$ showed good results and a higher discriminative power than t-tau (Buerger *et al.*, 2003). P-tau$_{181}$ has been proposed as a potential marker for differentiating AD from DLB (Mollenhauer *et al.*, 2005) or VaD (Schoenknecht *et al.*, 2003). In differentiating between AD and DLB, specificity at a given sensitivity level was improved by p-tau$_{181}$ compared to t-tau (Parnetti *et al.*, 2001; Vanmechelen *et al.*, 2001). Despite a very marked increase in t-tau in CJD, there is only a slight elevation of p-tau$_{181}$ (Buerger *et al.*, 2006). This suggests that CSF p-tau is not simply a mechanistic marker for neuronal damage, like CSF t-tau, but might specifically reflect the phosphorylation state of tau, and thus possibly the formation of tangles in AD.

53.3.6   Aβ and tau protein in combination

It would seem obvious to combine a specific set of different neurochemical markers to achieve more accurate early and differential diagnosis and to compare the validity of the individual methods. In agreement with this view, combined measurements have higher predictive power than either diagnostic approach alone in MCI settings. The combination of different CSF biomarkers has been evaluated by several studies which used different algorithms/methods: discrimination lines, classification trees, quadrants with cut-off points and ratios.

The most investigated combination utilizes CSF t-tau and $A\beta_{42}$, but other combinations like CSF p-tau$_{181}$ and $A\beta_{42}$ have shown good results. The combination of biomarkers has slightly higher sensitivity and specificity than for a single biomarker. The combined use of CSF-tau and CSF-$A\beta_{42}$ markers seems to allow differentiation between AD and normal ageing or other disorders such as depression (Andreasen et al., 2001; Sunderland et al., 2003). Several studies suggest that concomitant measurement of CSF-tau and CSF-$A\beta_{42}$ increases the diagnostic precision for AD. Fagan et al. (2007) showed that CSF-tau/$A\beta_{42}$ and p-tau$_{181}$:$A\beta_{42}$ ratio significantly predicted conversion from cognitively normal subjects to subjects with very mild or mild AD and proposed CSF-tau:$A\beta_{42}$ ratios as promising antecedent biomarkers predicting future dementia in cognitively normal older adults. Other studies with MCI subjects confirm these results (Herukka et al., 2007). Hansson et al. (2006) found a slightly higher specificity using the combination of t-tau and the $A\beta_{42}$:p-tau$_{181}$ ratio than with the combination of CSF t-tau and $A\beta_{42}$ in the detection of incipient AD in MCI subjects.

53.3.7   Other biomarkers and new approaches

As mentioned above, the most promising candidate biomarkers for diagnostic purposes are amyloid β peptides (Aβ) and tau proteins. However there are other potential AD biomarkers (Frank et al., 2003), such as isoprostanes, sulphatides and homocysteine, PP, ApoE, 8-hydroxy-2DD'-deoxyguanosine, α1-antichymotrypsin (ACT), interleukin-6 (IL-6), IL-6 receptor complex proteins, C-reactive protein and C1q protein (see **Table 53.1**) (Blennow and Hampel, 2003; Blennow et al., 2006; Blennow et al., 2010; Hampel et al., 2010).

A particularly promising new approach focuses on CSF β-secretase (BACE-1), one of the key enzymes responsible for the pathological cleavage of the APP (for review see Hampel and Shen, 2008; Zhao et al., 2007). A significant increase was found in BACE-1 concentration and activity in the CSF of MCI subjects compared with healthy controls. Patients with the ApoE ε4 risk allele were found to have the highest concentrations. BACE-1 may have value in early detection, prediction and biological activity of AD (Zhong et al., 2007).

Isoprostanes are also being studied as markers of lipid peroxidation. An increase was found in the CSF of MCI subjects compared with controls, and levels also increased over time. With regard to their diagnostic precision, the CSF markers isoprostanes and p-tau performed better than memory tests (de Leon et al., 2006). However, due to the very demanding analysis method, isoprostanes should still be regarded as a merely scientific approach. This also holds true for markers of apoptosis, oxidative stress, and mitochondrial dysfunction measured in lymphocytes which are currently under investigation as potential prognostic AD biomarkers (Leuner et al., 2007).

Other biomarker candidates for AD include ApoE in CSF, antichymotrypsin, soluble IL-6, IL-6R, gp130, C-reactive protein; C1q; homocysteine; oxysterols and cholesterol metabolites, 3-nitrotyrosine, which are currently under

Table 53.1 Candidate AD biomarkers (modified after Shaw et al., 2007).

Analyte	Biofluid
Aβ antibodies	Serum, plasma, CSF
A-antichymotrypsin	Blood, CSF
APP	CSF
APP isoform ratio in platelets	Platelets
BACE	Platelets, CSF, blood
CD59	Serum, plasma, CSF
C-reactive protein	Serum, plasma, CSF
C1q	Serum, plasma, CSF
8-hydroxy-deoxyguanine	Urine, plasma, CSF
Glutamine synthetase	Serum, CSF
GFAP and antibodies to GFAP	CSF
Interleukin-6-receptor complex	Serum, CSF
Isoprostanes	CSF
Kallikrein	Plasma, CSF
Melanotransferrin	Serum, CSF
Microvascular marker (VCAM-1, ICAM-1, ET-1, ADM, ANP)	Blood
Neurofilament proteins	CSF
Nitrotyrosine	CSF
Oxysterols	Plasma, CSF
Sulphatides	CSF
Synaptic markers	CSF
S100β	Blood, CSF

Aβ, amyloid-β; ADM, adrenomedulline; ANP, atrial natriuretic peptide; APP, amyloid precursor protein; BACE, beta-secretase; CSF, cerebrospinal fluid; ET-1, endotheline; GFAP, glial fibrillary acidic protein; ICAM-1, intercellular adhesion molecule-1; VCAM-1, vascular cell adhesion molecule-1.

investigation. They are discussed in detail in Buerger and Hampel (2009).

There is also emerging clinical diagnostic evidence for blood-based microvascular biomarkers in AD (Ewers et al., 2010). These candidates include blood concentration of vascular cell adhesion molecule-1 (VCAM-1) and intercellular adhesion molecule-1 (ICAM-1) which are increased in AD. Measures of endothelial vasodilatory function including blood levels of endotheline (ET-1), adrenomedulline (ADM) and atrial natriuretic peptide (ANP), as well as sphingolipids are significantly altered early during the predementia stage of MCI, suggesting sensitivity of these biomarkers for early detection and diagnosis; however, this requires validation in phase II and III diagnostic studies. Moreover, it is still unclear how the detected systemic microvascular alterations relate to cerebrovascular and neuronal pathologies in the AD brain.

Recent analysis of plasma suggests that a panel of 18 exploratory markers derived from proteome analysis can distinguish AD patients from non-demented controls and predicts conversion to AD for 20 of 22 MCI subjects (Carrillo *et al.*, 2009). This was also shown using a hypothesis-based combination of established blood-based markers indicative for microvascular changes in AD patients compared to control subjects (Scheltens *et al.*, 2002; Ewers *et al.*, 2010). Another study showed decreased serum levels of abeta autoantibodies in AD compared to controls (Brettschneider *et al.*, 2005; Buerger *et al.*, 2009). Further validation of these approaches is needed, but first data suggest that a plasma-based assay might be achievable (Ray *et al.*, 2007).

53.4   SCREENING AND PROGNOSTIC BIOMARKERS FOR AD

53.4.1   Genetic testing

Genetic polymorphisms can be detected by simple blood testing. Some are associated with an increased risk for the progression of dementia in preclinical or prodromal AD (Myers and Goate, 2001). This qualifies the well-known genetic risk genes for AD as screening and/or prognostic biomarkers. In addition to the three genes that are associated with inherited, early-onset AD, there are also genetic risk factors for late-onset AD. ApoE is the best known, but there are likely to be others that have a relatively smaller role.

Of course, finding risk genes for AD raises the issue of genetic testing (Risner *et al.*, 2006; Sonnen *et al.*, 2009). The ApoE ε4 risk allele has been known for decades and five consensus conferences have concluded that ApoE status should not be revealed to unaffected individuals since there is no treatment available to slow the progression of the disease. In a recent perspective paper published by the Alzheimer's Association the problem of genetic testing was discussed in the light of findings from the REVEAL study (Watson *et al.*, 2006), which assessed this issue in a clinical trial-like setting. It found that there is a 'wish to know' ApoE status among first-degree adult children of AD patients. Reasons given included a desire to arrange personal affairs and long-term care, to prepare their family or because of simple curiosity. The trial divided 162 people into two arms. Each was tested, but only one group was given the result, which was presented with a detailed explanation of how ApoE status affects AD risk (Reger *et al.*, 2008). Surprisingly, in 6-week, 6-month and 12-month follow ups, it was found that those volunteers who were ApoE ε4-positive exhibited no increased anxiety or stress compared to baseline measurements. Those who found they were ApoE ε4-negative, on the other hand, exhibited reduced stress and anxiety. It seems that people generally expect the worst and when they get it, it has little effect on them, but when they get good news it comes as a relief.

A second phase of the study, using a condensed protocol with no genetic counselling and just a mailed brochure, found much the same effect, though there was initially, at 6 weeks, slightly increased stress among those with ApoE ε4 alleles. This became insignificant at 6 and 12 months. The findings suggest that taking the time and money for counselling makes a difference, but only early on. Overall, the studies suggest that when presented in context and with

sufficient explanation to preclude misinterpretation, personal genetic testing may reasonably safely fulfil people's desire to know their own genetic predispositions. Additionally, since ApoE ε4 carriers in the REVEAL study did begin to take steps (such as exercise and vitamin E) to prevent AD, it suggests a willingness among the public to take necessary interventions that might be proven beneficial (Silverman *et al.*, 2000).

53.4.2   Early diagnostic and prognostic value of CSF Aβ and tau in MCI

The diagnosis of MCI is generally applied to elderly individuals who experience cognitive decline but do not meet the clinical criteria for dementia. Many studies have shown that subjects with MCI have an increased risk for dementia. Ten to 15 per cent of subjects with MCI convert to AD in a year (Petersen *et al.*, 1999). In MCI subjects who converted to AD during follow up, elevated t-tau levels at baseline were found in a relatively high number of individuals (Arai *et al.*, 1997b; Andreasen *et al.*, 1999). Memory-impaired subjects who later developed AD could be discriminated by high CSF t-tau with 90 per cent sensitivity and 100 per cent specificity from those who did not progress (Arai *et al.*, 1997a). Longitudinally, elevated CSF levels of t-tau in MCI subjects were found and still remained elevated after conversion to clinical AD. Another study showed that 88 per cent of subjects with MCI had elevated t-tau concentrations and/or low CSF $A\beta_{42}$ levels at baseline (Andreasen *et al.*, 2001). Thus, elevated CSF t-tau in MCI may have the potential to predict AD, a finding that was supported by Hampel *et al.* (2004c). CSF t-tau remained elevated for up to two years in mild to moderate AD. Initial and follow-up levels of t-tau correlated strongly, suggesting a stable rate of neurodegeneration during this time period. It is possible that CSF t-tau will decrease over time if there is effective disease modification and neuroprotection in AD patients (Galasko, 2001). CSF $p\text{-}tau_{231}$ shows promise in predicting cognitive decline and conversion to AD from MCI (de Leon *et al.*, 2002; Ewers *et al.*, 2007). High CSF $p\text{-}tau_{231}$ concentration significantly correlated with subsequent cognitive decline and conversion to AD. Thus, high $p\text{-}tau_{231}$ may be a predictor variable for progressive cognitive decline in MCI subjects, but in addition to $p\text{-}tau_{231}$, old age and ApoE ε4 carrier status independently predicted cognitive decline (Buerger *et al.*, 2002a). In a study performed by Schoenknecht *et al.* (2007) CSF levels of t-tau and $p\text{-}tau_{181}$ were determined in 80 subjects with MCI, 54 patients with geriatric major depression and 24 age-matched controls. Patients were reassessed after at least 12 months. During follow up 29 per cent of the MCI subjects but only one patient with geriatric depression converted to AD. Already at baseline converters to AD were characterized by significantly higher t-tau and p-tau levels compared to MCI non-converters and depressed patients. With respect to conversion to AD the negative predictive value of t-tau (p-tau) was 90 per cent (87 per cent), while the positive predictive value was relatively low at 53 per cent (40 per cent). These findings show that a low level of CSF tau can assist in the identification of prodromal AD in subjects at risk (MCI), and might also be of value in the differentiation of geriatric depression from incipient dementia.

A recently published multicentre study including data on 750 subjects with MCI, 529 patients with AD and 304 non-demented control subjects found that CSF $A\beta_{42}$, t-tau and p-tau identify incipient AD (in subjects with MCI) with good accuracy, but less accurately than reported from single centre-studies (Mattsson *et al.*, 2009). In this study, inter-site assay variability highlighted a need for standardization of analytical techniques and clinical procedures.

53.5   PREDICTIVE BIOMARKERS FOR AD

53.5.1   Pharmacogenomic markers of drug response

Predictive biomarkers are used to predict the likely response to a drug (e.g. a cholinesterase inhibitor or an anti-amyloid substance) before the treatment is initiated. It is estimated that genes account for 20–95 per cent of variability in drug disposition and pharmacodynamics (Cacabelos, 2008). Recent studies indicate that the therapeutic response in AD is genotype-specific depending upon genes associated with AD pathogenesis and/or genes responsible for drug metabolism (CYPs). Several studies indicate that the presence of the ApoE ε4 allele differentially affects the quality and size of drug response in AD patients treated with cholinesterase inhibitors. For example, the presence of this allele predicts a less favourable outcome in patients treated with tacrine, while it seems to have a neutral effect in galantamine (Suh *et al.*, 2006), and a positive influence in donepezil (Petersen *et al.*, 2005; Choi *et al.*, 2008). In monogenic-related studies of responsiveness to a combination therapy, ApoE ε4/4 carriers are the worst responders (Cacabelos, 2008). In trigenic (ApoE-PS1-PS2 clusters)-related studies the best responders are those patients carrying the 331222–, 341122–, 341222– and 441112– genomic profiles. The worst responders in all genomic clusters are patients with the 441122+ genotype, indicating the powerful, deleterious effect of the ApoE ε4/4 genotype on therapeutics in networking activity with other AD-related genes. Taken together, pharmacogenomic data on drug response in available drugs for the treatment of AD are still preliminary and no definite clinical recommendations can be drawn from the evidence. Longer prospective studies with larger patient populations are necessary to confirm and enhance previous findings. This holds particularly true for the influence of genetic polymorphism on the efficacy of novel disease-modifying substances.

53.5.2   Predictive CSF biomarkers in AD

Only a little is known about using CSF-derived biomarkers as predictors of AD treatment response. In a study by Wallin *et al.* (2009) including 191 patients with AD treated in a routine setting, a fast pre-treatment progression was the most consistent predictor of response to a treatment with cholinestrase inhibitors. However, fast progression did not correlate with CSF biomarkers and the baseline levels of CSF biomarkers including $A\beta_{42}$, t-tau and p-tau did not predict treatment response. As pointed out above, the CSF biomarkers are useful state markers for AD and it is likely that they are stable even over a six-month treatment period with cholinesterase inhibitors (Blennow *et al.*, 2007). Since available antidementia drugs primarily modulate neural transmission, but do not directly affect the molecular pathology of AD, one would not expect a predictive value of $A\beta$ and tau concentrations with respect to treatment with these substances. In might be speculated that CSF levels of $A\beta$ and tau are more meaningful in the prediction of treatment effects induced by disease-modifying anti-amyloid substances.

53.6   BLOOD AND CSF BIOMARKERS FOR THE MONITORING OF TREATMENT EFFECTS IN AD

To date, the monitoring of the efficacy of drug treatments for AD is based on solely clinical and/or psychometric assessment. There are currently no blood- or CSF-derived biomarkers which can be used or recommended as valid outcome parameters or surrogates for a particular treatment. However, there is emerging evidence that blood- and CSF-derived biomarkers can help to determine whether certain types of targeted AD treatments are hitting drug targets in the brain and are even linked to a meaningful clinical outcome (Siemers *et al.*, 2007; Galasko, 2009; Siemers, 2009). This is being investigated in the context of clinical drug trials (see also 53.7 The role of blood and CSF biomarkers in drug development). To select, apply and interpret blood and CSF biomarkers in clinical trials, one needs to understand (1) the events and neurobiological processes that CSF biomarkers can measure, (2) the targets of the drug(s) and the effect of successful targeting on the (concentration of) biomarkers and (3) the time point of intervention during the disease process (e.g. treatment versus prevention). To date, no disease-modifying drug for AD has convincingly demonstrated success in phase II or phase III studies. However, CSF biomarker analyses performed in current drug trials suggest that it is possible to lower production of, or improve clearance of $A\beta$, and possibly to decrease oxidative stress. In contrast, downstream markers (e.g. of neuronal damage) have not shown convincing improvement in studies as yet (Galasko, 2009). If and when a disease-modifying drug has proven efficacy, the dynamics of the investigated biomarker should be analysed with respect to its validity as a surrogate for clinical outcome. This could lead to the use of the relevant plasma or CSF biomarkers as outcome measures or surrogates in the clinical routine setting.

53.7   THE ROLE OF BLOOD AND CSF BIOMARKERS IN DRUG DEVELOPMENT

53.7.1   Biomarkers as end points in AD clinical drug trials

Several new therapeutic substances aiming at 'disease modification' in AD are currently under clinical investigation (Hampel *et al.*, 2009). These novel therapeutic approaches require novel biomarkers to ensure objectivity and efficiency in drug development as well as relating to the initiation and monitoring of drug treatment once the drug has been approved. Blood and CSF biomarkers can provide useful information for all phases of AD clinical trials (Siemers *et al.*, 2007; Hampel *et al.*, 2009; Siemers, 2009). For example, various biomarkers were used in the development of a γ-secretase inhibitor (semagacestat), and a monoclonal antibody that binds to the mid-domain of $A\beta$ (solanezumab). These include CSF and plasma $A\beta_{42}$ and $A\beta_{40}$, CSF t-tau and P-tau$_{181}$, pyro-Glu 3-42 $A\beta$ (N3pGluAβ) in plasma, and an N-terminal truncated form of $A\beta$, known as 'fragment 2' (plasma and CSF). Biomarkers were assessed during all three stages of drug development (Siemers, 2009). Among other findings, the dynamics of biomarker concentration indicated an effect of the drugs on core pathologic features of AD. Furthermore, determination of biomarkers in phase 1 studies provided mechanistic information that could be used to determine appropriate drug dosing for phases 2 and 3. In order to qualify as a surrogate marker which might serve as an objectively measurable primary end point in clinical studies, a biomarker should be closely linked to a clinically meaningful treatment outcome (e.g. cognition, functional abilities, quality of life). None of the biomarker candidates has yet fulfilled these requirements. Internal biomarker qualification programmes through all preclinical and clinical trial stages closely linked to specific drug development programmes are highly recommended for pharmaceutical companies in order to generate biomarkers for various necessary roles and for qualification processes conducted in close interaction with regulatory authorities. There is a lively ongoing debate between academic researchers, industry and regulatory authorities on how biomarkers can best be qualified and validated for use in trials. Several large-scale international controlled multicentre trials should provide further diagnostic validation, which is besides real biomarker qualification only one specific side of the coin, of selected 'core feasible' biomarker candidates which could serve as candidate outcome measures for enrichment, stratification, proof-of-concept and potential use in phase III confirmatory efficacy trials.

53.7.2 'Enrichment' of patient samples for clinical drug trials

The diagnostic accuracy of clinical MCI criteria for predementia or prodromal AD is low to moderate (Visser *et al.*, 2005). Their use may lead to inclusion of many patients who do not have predementia AD or to exclusion of many who do. This might partly explain the failure of many of the previous drug trials in MCI populations (Jelic *et al.*, 2006). In future trials CSF-derived biomarkers (e.g. different species of $A\beta$ and tau protein) can serve as early diagnostic indicators in order to enrich the number of 'true' cases among subjects selected primarily on clinical criteria (Hampel and Broich, 2009). This approach could considerably increase the statistical power and, in turn, decrease sample size and trial costs. Core feasible CSF biomarker candidates, in addition to ApoE genotyping, are currently recommended to be introduced for meaningful enrichment in MCI populations to decrease inhomogeneity of study population, data variance and enhance rate of cognitive decline and progression as well as time to conversion to AD, particularly in proof-of-concept studies.

53.7.3 Regulatory aspects

New guideline documents of regulatory authorities, such as the Food and Drug Administration (FDA) and the European Medicines Agency (EMEA), will most likely strongly recommend thorough validation of biological as well as imaging candidate markers as primary and secondary end points in upcoming phase II and III treatment trials of compounds claiming disease-modifying properties. Currently the FDA would not likely grant approval based on a change in a biomarker (surrogate) alone, because it is yet not clear what such a change would mean clinically (Carrillo *et al.*, 2009). Though that is an important goal, it comes back to the problem of the 'unvalidated surrogate'. Development of surrogate markers is of utmost importance for trial programmes and to substantiate claims for disease modification, however, the problem seems far from resolved by academic and industry stakeholders. The EMEA, the European Medicines Agency, released new guidelines in July 2008. They seem more positive about using biomarkers as surrogate markers' outcome markers, but still want to see a clinical effect. Biomarker data may be seen as supportive, especially for any claims of disease modification. Generally, they recognize the urgency of treating as early as possible. For disease-modifying agents the situation is slightly different, since it is unchartered territory. The EMEA may recognize a disease-modifying effect if there is a measurable delay in underlying pathological/pathophysiological disease process and this is accompanied by clinical improvement. They will allow a limited claim of disease modification if there is delayed disease progression based on clinical signs, and a full claim if that effect is supported by biomarker (biological or imaging data).

In the wake of numerous therapeutic trials for disease modification in AD, there is an urgent need for paralleled drug and biomarker development programmes, efforts to qualify and validate markers for specific functions and roles, as well as a strong interaction between academic researchers, industry and regulatory authorities. Future questions will elucidate whether compounds should treat clinical symptoms or syndromes or rather pathology and specific molecular mechanisms. This would be a 'paradigm shift' in the treatment of neurodegenerative disorders, such as AD and biological markers would gain centre stage in this process. Moreover, biomarkers will provide the only means to identify mechanisms, disease or pathology at potentially reversible presymptomatic stages at which subjects at risk for AD may be treated most effectively in the future of individualized disease prevention. Currently underrated blood marker candidates may one day become essential primary tools for screening larger at-risk populations to channel subjects into more costly, sensitive and specific diagnostic programmes before initiating therapy. A 'diagnostic flow model' for AD is as yet under development and proposed by consensus groups (Hampel *et al.*, personal communication).

REFERENCES

Consensus Report of the Working Group on: "Molecular and Biochemical Markers of Alzheimer's Disease". (1998) The Ronald and Nancy Reagan Research Institute of the Alzheimer's Association and the National Institute on Aging Working Group. *Neurobiology of Aging* **19**: 109–16.

Andreasen N, Minthon L, Vanmechelen E *et al.* (1999) Cerebrospinal fluid tau and Abeta42 as predictors of development of Alzheimer's disease in patients with mild cognitive impairment. *Neuroscience Letters* **273**: 5–8.

Andreasen N, Minthon L, Davidsson P *et al.* (2001) Evaluation of CSF-tau and CSF-Abeta42 as diagnostic markers for Alzheimer disease in clinical practice. *Archives of Neurology* **58**: 373–9.

Arai H, Morikawa Y, Higuchi M *et al.* (1997a) Cerebrospinal fluid tau levels in neurodegenerative diseases with distinct tau-related pathology. *Biochemical and Biophysical Research Commununications* **236**: 262–4.

Arai H, Nakagawa T, Kosaka Y *et al.* (1997b) Elevated cerebrospinal fluid tau protein levels as a predictor of dementia in memory-impaired individuals. *Alzheimer Disease and Associated Disorders* **3**: 211–13.

Bateman RJ, Wen G, Morris JC *et al.* (2007) Fluctuations of CSF amyloid-beta levels: implications for a diagnostic and therapeutic biomarker. *Neurology* **68**: 666–9.

Blennow K, Hampel H. (2003) CSF markers for incipient Alzheimer's disease. *Lancet Neurology* **2**: 605–13.

Blennow K. (2005) CSF biomarkers for Alzheimer's disease: use in early diagnosis and evaluation of drug treatment. *Expert Review of Molecular Diagnostics* **5**: 661–72.

Blennow K, de Leon MJ, Zetterberg H. (2006) Alzheimer's disease. *Lancet* **368**: 387–403.

Blennow K, Zetterberg H, Minthon L *et al.* (2007) Longitudinal stability of CSF biomarkers in Alzheimer's disease. *Neuroscience Letters* **419**: 18–22.

Blennow K, Hampel H, Weiner M, Zetterberg H. (2010) Cerebrospinal fluid and plasma biomarkers in Alzheimer's disease. *Nature Reviews Neurology* **6**: 131–44.

Brettschneider S, Morgenthaler NG, Teipel SJ *et al.* (2005) Decreased serum amyloid beta(1-42) autoantibody levels in Alzheimer's disease, determined by a newly developed immuno-precipitation assay with radiolabeled amyloid beta(1-42) peptide. *Biological Psychiatry* **57**: 813–6.

Buerger K, Teipel SJ, Zinkowski R *et al.* (2002a) CSF tau protein phosphorylated at threonine 231 correlates with cognitive decline in MCI subjects. *Neurology* **59**: 627–9.

Buerger K, Zinkowski R, Teipel SJ *et al.* (2002b) Differential diagnosis of Alzheimer disease with cerebrospinal fluid levels of tau protein phosphorylated at threonine 231. *Archives of Neurology* **59**: 1267–72.

Buerger K, Zinkowski R, Teipel SJ *et al.* (2002c) Differential diagnosis of Alzheimer disease with cerebrospinal fluid levels of tau protein phosphorylated at threonine 231. *Archives of Neurology* **59**: 1267–72.

Buerger K, Zinkowski R, Teipel SJ *et al.* (2003) Differentiation of geriatric major depression from Alzheimer's disease with CSF tau protein phosphorylated at threonine 231. *American Journal of Psychiatry* **160**: 376–9.

Buerger K, Ewers M, Pirttila T *et al.* (2006) CSF phosphorylated tau protein correlates with neocortical neurofibrillary pathology in Alzheimer's disease. *Brain* **129**: 3035–41.

Buerger K, Alafuzoff I, Ewers M *et al.* (2007) No correlation between CSF tau protein phosphorylated at threonine 181 with neocortical neurofibrillary pathology in Alzheimer's disease. *Brain* **130**: e82.

Buerger K, Ernst A, Ewers M *et al.* (2009) Blood-based microcirculation markers in Alzheimer's disease-diagnostic value of midregional pro-atrial natriuretic peptide/C-terminal endothelin-1 precursor fragment ratio. *Biological Psychiatry* **65**: 979–84.

Buerger K, Hampel H. (2009) Biomarkers for the dementias. In: Weiner MF, Lipton AM (eds). *The American Psychiatric Publishing textbook of Alzheimer disease and other dementias.* Arlington, VA: American Psychiatric Publishing, 407–21.

Buerger née Buch K, Padberg F, Nolde T *et al.* (1999) Cerebrospinal fluid tau protein shows a better discrimination in young old (<70 years) than in old patients with Alzheimer's disease compared with controls. *Neuroscience Letters* **277**: 21–24.

Cacabelos R. (2008) Pharmacogenomics and therapeutic prospects in dementia. *European Archives of Psychiatry and Clinical Neuroscience* **258** (Suppl. 1): 28–47.

Carrillo MC, Blackwell A, Hampel H *et al.* (2009) Early risk assessment for Alzheimer's disease. *Alzheimer's and Dementia* **5**: 182–96.

Choi SH, Kim SY, Na HR *et al.* (2008) Effect of ApoE genotype on response to donepezil in patients with Alzheimer's disease. *Dementia and Geriatric Cognitive Disorders* **25**: 445–50.

de Leon MJ, Segal S, Tarshish CY *et al.* (2002) Longitudinal cerebrospinal fluid tau load increases in mild cognitive impairment. *Neuroscience Letters* **333**: 183–6.

de Leon MJ, DeSanti S, Zinkowski R *et al.* (2006) Longitudinal CSF and MRI biomarkers improve the diagnosis of mild cognitive impairment. *Neurobiology of Aging* **27**: 394–401.

Dubois B, Feldman HH, Jacova C *et al.* (2007) Research criteria for the diagnosis of Alzheimer's disease: revising the NINCDS-ADRDA criteria. *Lancet. Neurology* **6**: 734–46.

Ewers M, Buerger K, Teipel SJ *et al.* (2007) Multicenter assessment of CSF-phosphorylated tau for the prediction of conversion of MCI. *Neurology* **69**: 2205–12.

Ewers M, Mielke MM, Hampel H. (2010) Blood-based biological markers of microvascular pathology in Alzheimer's disease. *Experimental Gerontology* **45**: 75–9.

Fagan AM, Mintun MA, Mach RH *et al.* (2006) Inverse relation between in vivo amyloid imaging load and cerebrospinal fluid Abeta42 in humans. *Annals of Neurology* **59**: 512–9.

Fagan AM, Roe CM, Xiong C *et al.* (2007) Cerebrospinal fluid tau/beta-amyloid(42) ratio as a prediction of cognitive decline in nondemented older adults. *Archives of Neurology* **64**: 343–9.

Frank RA, Galasko D, Hampel H *et al.* (2003) Biological markers for therapeutic trials in Alzheimer's disease. Proceedings of the biological markers working group; NIA initiative on neuroimaging in Alzheimer's disease. *Neurobiology of Aging* **24**: 521–36.

Freeman SH, Raju S, Hyman BT *et al.* (2007) Plasma Abeta levels do not reflect brain Abeta levels. *Journal of Neuropathology and Experimental Neurology* **66**: 264–71.

Fukuyama R, Mizuno T, Mori S *et al.* (2000) Age-dependent change in the levels of Abeta40 and Abeta42 in cerebrospinal fluid from control subjects, and a decrease in the ratio of Abeta42 to Abeta40 level in cerebrospinal fluid from Alzheimer's disease patients. *European Neurology* **43**: 155–60.

Galasko D. (1998) Cerebrospinal fluid levels of A beta 42 and tau: potential markers of Alzheimer's disease. *Journal of Neural Transmission. Supplementum* **53**: 209–21.

Galasko D. (2001) Lewy bodies and dementia. *Current Neurology and Neuroscience Reports* **1**: 435–41.

Galasko D. (2009) CSF biomarkers as outcome measures in clinical trials. *Alzheimer's and Dementia* **5** (Suppl. 1): 95.

Graff-Radford NR, Crook JE, Lucas J *et al.* (2007) Association of low plasma Abeta42/Abeta40 ratios with increased imminent risk for mild cognitive impairment and Alzheimer disease. *Archives of Neurology* **64**: 354–62.

Hampel H, Buerger K, Zinkowski R *et al.* (2004a) Measurement of phosphorylated tau epitopes in the differential diagnosis of Alzheimer disease: a comparative cerebrospinal fluid study. *Archives of General Psychiatry* **61**: 95–102.

Hampel H, Buerger K, Zinkowski R *et al.* (2004b) Measurement of phosphorylated tau epitopes in the differential diagnosis of Alzheimer disease: a comparative cerebrospinal fluid study. *Archives of General Psychiatry* **61**: 95–102.

Hampel H, Mitchell A, Blennow K *et al.* (2004c) Core biological marker candidates of Alzheimer's disease – perspectives for diagnosis, prediction of outcome and reflection of biological activity. *Journal of Neural Transmission. Supplementum* **111**: 247–72.

Hampel H, Teipel SJ, Fuchsberger T *et al.* (2004d) Value of CSF beta-amyloid1-42 and tau as predictors of Alzheimer's disease in patients with mild cognitive impairment. *Molecular Psychiatry* **9**: 705–10.

Hampel H, Shen Y. (2008) Beta-site amyloid precursor protein cleaving enzyme 1 (BACE1) as a biological candidate marker of Alzheimer's disease. *Scandinavian Journal of Clinical and Laboratory Investigations* **69**: 8–12.

Hampel H, Broich K. (2009) Enrichment of MCI and early Alzheimer's disease treatment trials using neurochemical and imaging candidate biomarkers. *The Journal of Nutrition, Health and Aging* **13**: 373–5.

Hampel H, Broich K, Hoessler Y *et al.* (2009) Biological markers for early detection and pharmacological treatment of Alzheimer's disease. *Dialogues in Clinical Neuroscience* **11**: 141–57.

Hampel H, Frank R Broich K *et al.* (2010) Biomarkers for diagnosis and as endpoints for clinical trials in Alzheimer's disease. *Nature Reviews Drug Discovery* **9**: 560–74.

Hansson O, Zetterberg H, Buchhave P *et al.* (2006) Association between CSF biomarkers and incipient Alzheimer's disease in patients with mild cognitive impairment: a follow-up study. *Lancet. Neurology* **5**: 228–34.

Hasegawa M. (2006) Biochemistry and molecular biology of tauopathies. *Neuropathology* **26**: 484–90.

Herukka SK, Helisalmi S, Hallikainen M *et al.* (2007) CSF Abeta42, Tau and phosphorylated Tau, APOE epsilon4 allele and MCI type in progressive MCI. *Neurobiology of Aging* **28**: 507–14.

Holmberg B, Johnels B, Blennow K *et al.* (2003) Cerebrospinal fluid Abeta42 is reduced in multiple system atrophy but normal in Parkinson's disease and progressive supranuclear palsy. *Movement Disorders* **18**: 186–90.

Hulstaert F, Blennow K, Ivanoiu A *et al.* (1999) Improved discrimination of AD patients using beta-amyloid(1-42) and tau levels in CSF. *Neurology* **52**: 1555–62.

Irizarry MC. (2004) Biomarkers of Alzheimer disease in plasma. *NeuroRx* **1**: 226–34.

Iwatsubo T, Odaka A, Suzuki N *et al.* (1994) Visualization of A beta 42(43) and A beta 40 in senile plaques with end-specific A beta monoclonals: evidence that an initially deposited species is A beta 42(43). *Neuron* **13**: 45–53.

Jelic V, Kivipelto M, Winblad B. (2006) Clinical trials in mild cognitive impairment: lessons for the future. *Journal of Neurology, Neurosurgery, and Psychiatry* **77**: 429–38.

Jensen M, Schroeder J, Blomberg M *et al.* (1999) Cerebrospinal fluid A beta42 is increased early in sporadic Alzheimer's disease and declines with disease progression. *Annals of Neurology* **45**: 504–11.

Kanemaru K, Kameda N, Yamanouchi H. (2000) Decreased CSF amyloid beta42 and normal tau levels in dementia with Lewy bodies. *Neurology* **54**: 1875–6.

Kapaki E, Kilidireas K, Paraskevas GP *et al.* (2001) Highly increased CSF tau protein and decreased beta-amyloid (1-42) in sporadic CJD: a discrimination from Alzheimer's disease? *Journal of Neurology, Neurosurgery, and Psychiatry* **71**: 401–3.

Kapaki EN, Paraskevas GP, Tzerakis NG *et al.* (2007) Cerebrospinal fluid tau, phospho-tau181 and beta-amyloid1-42 in idiopathic normal pressure hydrocephalus: a discrimination from Alzheimer's disease. *European Journal of Neurology* **14**: 168–73.

Kroll W. (2008) Biomarkers – predictors, surrogate parameters – a concept definition. In: Schmitz G, Endres S, Götte D (eds). *Biomarker*. Stuttgart: Schattauer, 1–14.

Leuner K, Pantel J, Frey C *et al.* (2007) Enhanced apoptosis, oxidative stress and mitochondrial dysfunction in lymphocytes as potential biomarkers for Alzheimer's disease. *Journal of Neural Transmission. Supplementum* **72**: 207–15.

Lewczuk P, Esselmann H, Otto M *et al.* (2004) Neurochemical diagnosis of Alzheimer's dementia by CSF Abeta42, Abeta42/Abeta40 ratio and total tau. *Neurobiology of Aging* **25**: 273–81.

Lewczuk P, Kornhuber J, Vanmechelen E *et al.* (2009) Amyloid beta peptides in plasma in early diagnosis of Alzheimer's disease: a multicenter study with multiplexing. *Experimental Neurology.* cited 5 August 2009. Available from: www.ncbi.nlm.nih.gov/pubmed/19664622.

Mattsson N, Zetterberg H, Hansson O *et al.* (2009) CSF biomarkers and incipient Alzheimer disease in patients with mild cognitive impairment. *Journal of the American Medical Association* **302**: 385–93.

Mayeux R, Honig LS, Tang MX *et al.* (2003) Plasma A[beta]40 and A[beta]42 and Alzheimer's disease: relation to age, mortality, and risk. *Neurology* **61**: 1185–90.

Mecocci P, Parnetti L, Romano G et al. (1995) Serum anti-GFAP and anti-S100 autoantibodies in brain aging, Alzheimer's disease and vascular dementia. Journal of Neuroimmunology 57: 165–70.

Mehta PD, Kim KS, Wisniewski HM. (1991) ELISA as a laboratory test to aid the diagnosis of Alzheimer's disease. In: Bullock GR, van Velzen D, Warhol MJ, Herbrink P (eds). Techniques in diagnostic pathology, vol. 2. San Diego, CA: Academic Press, 99–112.

Mehta PD, Pirttila T, Patrick BA et al. (2001) Amyloid beta protein 1-40 and 1-42 levels in matched cerebrospinal fluid and plasma from patients with Alzheimer disease. Neuroscience Letters 304: 102–6.

Mitchell A, Brindle N. (2003) CSF phosphorylated tau – does it constitute an accurate biological test for Alzheimer's disease? International Journal of Geriatric Psychiatry 18: 407–11.

Mollenhauer B, Cepek L, Bibl M et al. (2005) Tau protein, Abeta42 and S-100B protein in cerebrospinal fluid of patients with dementia with Lewy bodies. Dementia and Geriatric Cognitive Disorders 19: 164–70.

Morris JC, Price AL. (2001) Pathologic correlates of nondemented aging, mild cognitive impairment, and early-stage Alzheimer's disease. Journal of Molecular Neuroscience 17: 101–18.

Motter R, Vigo-Pelfrey C, Kholodenko D et al. (1995) Reduction of beta-amyloid peptide42 in the cerebrospinal fluid of patients with Alzheimer's disease. Annals of Neurology 38: 643–8.

Myers AJ, Goate AM. (2001) The genetics of late-onset Alzheimer's disease. Current Opinion in Neurology 14: 433–40.

Otto M, Esselmann H, Schulz-Shaeffer W et al. (2000) Decreased beta-amyloid1-42 in cerebrospinal fluid of patients with Creutzfeldt–Jakob disease. Neurology 54: 1099–102.

Otto M, Wiltfang J, Cepek L et al. (2002) Tau protein and 14-3-3 protein in the differential diagnosis of Creutzfeldt–Jakob disease. Neurology 58: 192–7.

Parnetti L, Reboldi GP, Gallai V. (2000) Cerebrospinal fluid pyruvate levels in Alzheimer's disease and vascular dementia. Neurology 54: 735–7.

Parnetti L, Lanari A, Amici S et al. (2001) CSF phosphorylated tau is a possible marker for discriminating Alzheimer's disease from dementia with Lewy bodies. Phospho-Tau International Study Group. Neurological Sciences 22: 77–8.

Petersen RC, Smith GE, Waring SC et al. (1999) Mild cognitive impairment: clinical characterization and outcome. Archives of Neurology 56: 303–8.

Petersen RC, Thomas RG, Grundman M et al. (2005) Vitamin E and donepezil for the treatment of mild cognitive impairment. New England Journal of Medicine 352: 2379–88.

Pomara N, Willoughby LM, Sidtis JJ et al. (2005) Selective reductions in plasma Abeta 1-42 in healthy elderly subjects during longitudinal follow-up: a preliminary report. American Journal of Geriatric Psychiatry 13: 914–17.

Ray S, Britschgi M, Herbert C et al. (2007) Classification and prediction of clinical Alzheimer's diagnosis based on plasma signaling proteins. Nature Medicine 13: 1359–62.

Reger MA, Watson GS, Green PS et al. (2008) Intranasal insulin administration dose-dependently modulates verbal memory and plasma amyloid-beta in memory-impaired older adults. Journal of Alzheimer's Disease 13: 323–31.

Risner ME, Saunders AM, Altman JF et al. (2006) Efficacy of rosiglitazone in a genetically defined population with mild-to-moderate Alzheimer's disease. Pharmacogenomics Journal 6: 246–54.

Scheltens P, Fox N, Barkhof F et al. (2002) Structural magnetic resonance imaging in the practical assessment of dementia: beyond exclusion. Lancet Neurology 1: 13–21.

Schoenknecht P, Pantel J, Hartmann T et al. (2003) Cerebrospinal fluid tau levels in Alzheimer's disease are elevated when compared with vascular dementia but do not correlate with measures of cerebral atrophy. Psychiatry Research 120: 231–8.

Schoenknecht P, Pantel J, Kaiser E et al. (2007) Increased tau protein differentiates mild cognitive impairment from geriatric depression and predicts conversion to dementia. Neuroscience Letters 416: 39–42.

Shaw LM, Korecka M, Clark CM et al. (2007) Biomarkers of neurodegeneration for diagnosis and monitoring therapeutics. Nature Reviews in Drug Discovery 6: 295–303.

Siemers E. (2009) Biochemical markers as endpoint in clinical trials: applications in phase 1, 2 and 3 studies. Alzheimer's and Dementia 5 (Suppl. 1); P95.

Siemers ER, Dean RA, Friedrich S et al. (2007) Safety, tolerability, and effects on plasma and cerebrospinal fluid amyloid-beta after inhibition of gamma-secretase. Clinical Neuropharmacology 30: 317–25.

Silverman JM, Smith CM, Marin DB et al. (2000) Has familial aggregation in Alzheimer's disease been overestimated? International Journal of Geriatric Psychiatry 15: 631–7.

Sjoegren M, Minthon L, Davidsson P et al. (2000) CSF levels of tau, beta-amyloid(1-42) and GAP-43 in frontotemporal dementia, other types of dementia and normal aging. Journal of Neural Transmission. Supplementum 107: 563–79.

Sjoegren M, Vanderstichele H, Agren H et al. (2001) Tau and Abeta42 in cerebrospinal fluid from healthy adults 21–93 years of age: establishment of reference values. Clinical Chemistry 47: 1776–81.

Sjoegren M, Davidsson P, Wallin A et al. (2002) Decreased CSF-beta-amyloid 42 in Alzheimer's disease and amyotrophic lateral sclerosis may reflect mismetabolism of beta-amyloid induced by disparate mechanisms. Dementia and Geriatric Cognitive Disorders 13: 112–18.

Sonnen JA, Larson EB, Brickell K et al. (2009) Different patterns of cerebral injury in dementia with or without diabetes. Archives of Neurology 66: 315–22.

Spillantini MG, Goedert M, Jakes R et al. (1990) Topographical relationship between beta-amyloid and tau protein epitopes in tangle-bearing cells in Alzheimer disease. Proceedings of the National Academy of Sciences of the United States of America 87: 3952–6.

Strozyk D, Blennow K, White LR et al. (2003) CSF Abeta 42 levels correlate with amyloid-neuropathology in a population-based autopsy study. Neurology 60: 652–6.

Suh GH, Jung HY, Lee CU et al. (2006) Effect of the apolipoprotein E epsilon4 allele on the efficacy and tolerability of galantamine in the treatment of Alzheimer's disease. Dementia and Geriatric Cognitive Disorders 21: 33–9.

Sunderland T, Linker G, Mirza N et al. (2003) Decreased beta-amyloid1-42 and increased tau levels in cerebrospinal fluid of patients with Alzheimer disease. *Journal of the American Medical Association* **289**: 2094–103.

Tamaoka A, Sawamura N, Fukushima T et al. (1997) Amyloid beta protein 42(43) in cerebrospinal fluid of patients with Alzheimer's disease. *Journal of the Neurological Sciences* **148**: 41–5.

Tapiola T, Pirttila T, Mehta PD et al. (2000) Relationship between apoE genotype and CSF beta-amyloid (1-42) and tau in patients with probable and definite Alzheimer's disease. *Neurobiology of Aging* **21**: 735–40.

van Oijen M, Hofman A, Soares HD et al. (2006) Plasma Abeta(1-40) and Abeta(1-42) and the risk of dementia: a prospective case-cohort study. *Lancet Neurology* **5**: 655–60.

Vanderstichele H, Van Kerschaver E, Hesse C et al. (2000) Standardization of measurement of beta-amyloid(1-42) in cerebrospinal fluid and plasma. *Amyloid* **7**: 245–58.

Vanmechelen E, Vanderstichele H, Hulstaert F et al. (2001) Cerebrospinal fluid tau and beta-amyloid(1-42) in dementia disorders. *Mechanisms of Ageing and Development* **122**: 2005–11.

Visser PJ, Scheltens P, Verhey FR. (2005) Do MCI criteria in drug trials accurately identify subjects with predementia Alzheimer's disease? *Journal of Neurology, Neurosurgery, and Psychiatry* **76**: 1348–54.

Wahlund LO, Barkhof F, Fazekas F et al. (2001) A new rating scale for age-related white matter changes applicable to MRI and CT. *Stroke* **32**: 1318–22.

Wallin AK, Hansson O, Blennow K et al. (2009) Can CSF biomarkers or pre-treatment progression rate predict response to cholinesterase inhibitor treatment in Alzheimer's disease? *International Journal of Geriatric Psychiatry* **24**: 638–47.

Watson GS, Reger MA, Baker LD et al. (2006) Effects of exercise and nutrition on memory in Japanese Americans with impaired glucose tolerance. *Diabetes Care* **29**: 135–6.

Wisniewski HM, Wegiel J. (1995) The neuropathology of Alzheimer's disease. *Neuroimaging Clinics of North America* **5**: 45–57.

Zetzsche T, Rujescu D, Hardy J, Hample H. (2010) Advances and perspectives from genetic research: development of biological markers in Alzheimer's disease. *Expert Review of Molecular Diagnostics* **10**: 667–90.

Zhao J, Fu Y, Yasvoina M et al. (2007) Beta-site amyloid precursor protein cleaving enzyme 1 levels become elevated in neurons around amyloid plaques: implications for Alzheimer's disease pathogenesis. *Journal of Neuroscience* **27**: 3639–49.

Zhong Z, Ewers M, Teipel S et al. (2007) Levels of beta-secretase (BACE1) in cerebrospinal fluid as a predictor of risk in mild cognitive impairment. *Archives of General Psychiatry* **64**: 718–26.

Established treatments for Alzheimer's disease: cholinesterase inhibitors and memantine

ALEXANDER F KURZ AND NICOLA T LAUTENSCHLAGER

54.1 INTRODUCTION

Approved treatments for Alzheimer's disease (AD) target biochemical abnormalities which occur as a consequence of nerve cell loss in forebrain nuclei and in the cerebral cortex. This mode of action addresses the final stretch of a complex pathological cascade (Hardy, 2009) and does not interfere with the mechanisms that induce neuronal degeneration. Cholinesterase inhibitors (ChEIs) partially restore the deficit in acetylcholine which arises from a significant deficit of neurones in the nucleus basalis of Meynert and in the central septal area which project to many cortical regions (Bartus et al., 1982). Memantine attenuates the toxic effects of glutamate which is released in excess from degenerating cortical neurones, but preserves physiological glutamate-mediated signalling (Greenamyre et al., 1988). Whether these therapies confer additional neuroprotective potential in addition to purely symptomatic effects has been widely debated, but never demonstrated in human studies (Lleó et al., 2006). Cholinesterase inhibitors and memantine may only be used for the treatment of patients with AD diagnosed with dementia. In subjects with subdiagnostic cognitive impairment, ChEIs did not achieve a clinically meaningful delay of progression to dementia (Raschetti et al., 2007). There are no published studies with memantine in this patient population.

54.2 CLINICAL EFFICACY

The clinical efficacy of antidementia treatments has been evaluated in double-blind, randomized controlled clinical trials (RCTs). These studies are usually designed to meet the requirements for approval by regulatory authorities. Current criteria for efficacy require demonstration of statistically significant differences between patients receiving active treatment and patients receiving placebo on two or more relevant domains. The US Food and Drug Administration (FDA) applies a dual outcome, which includes cognition, to document the specificity of the effect and a global assessment of overall functioning to ensure that the effect is clinically meaningful (Ad Hoc FDA Dementia Assessment Task Force, 1991). The European regulatory authority (EMEA) favours a triple outcome including global impression, cognition and functional ability (Broich, 2007; Katona et al., 2007). Treatment differences on these domains are assessed using standardized, validated psychometric instruments. Some frequently used clinical scales are listed in **Table 54.1**. Since AD is a progressive disorder, deterioration will occur in the placebo group over time. Hence, a difference between active treatment and placebo does not necessarily imply improvement from baseline, but often indicates less worsening in actively treated patients. Participants in clinical drug trials, particularly in studies commissioned by manufacturers, are usually selected in terms of high treatment expectations, low co-morbidity, restricted concomitant medications and few behavioural disturbances. Therefore, these populations are often not representative of patients seen in primary or secondary care settings. Industry-sponsored trials typically apply strict inclusion and exclusion criteria which exclude the majority of outpatients with AD (Gill et al., 2004). Treatment duration is usually short, not exceeding 12–24 weeks. There are only three studies of antidementia drugs which provide

Table 54.1   Frequently used assessment instruments in clinical antidementia trials.

Domain	Instrument	Score range	Polarity	Reference
Global assessment	CIBIC, CIBIC-plus	1–7	≤3 better, 4 no change, ≥5 worse	Schneider, 1997
	GBS	0–162	Lower better	Gottfries et al., 1982
	CDR-SB	0–18	Lower better	Morris, 1993
Cognition	MMSE	0–30	Higher better	Folstein et al., 1975
	ADAS-Cog	0–70	Lower better	Rosen et al., 1984
	SIB	0–100	Higher better	Schmitt et al., 1997
Activities of daily living	ADCS-ADL	0–110	Higher better	Galasko et al., 1997
	ADCS-ADL sev	0–54	Higher better	Galasko et al., 2005
	PDS	0–100	Higher better	De Jong et al., 1989
	DAD	0–40	Higher better	Gélinas et al., 1995
Behavioural disturbance	NPI	0–144	Lower better	Cummings, 1997

ADAS-Cog, Alzheimer's Disease Assessment Scale, cognitive part; ADCS-ADL, Alzheimer's Disease Cooperative Study Activities of Daily Living Scale; ADCS-ADL sev, Alzheimer's Disease Cooperative Study Activities of Daily Living Scale (for patients with moderate to severe dementia); CDR-SB, Clinical Dementia Rating Sum of Boxes; CIBIC, Clinician-Based Impression of Change; CIBIC-plus, Clinician-Based Impression of Change (plus caregiver input); DAD, Disability Assessment in Dementia; GBS, Gottfries–Bråne–Steen Scale; MMSE, Mini-Mental State Examination; NPI, Neuropsychiatric Inventory; PDS, Progressive Deterioration Scale; SIB, Severe Impairment Battery.

placebo-controlled data beyond six months. For these reasons, clinical trials purvey an incomplete and biased perspective on the efficacy and tolerability of antidementia treatments. Many important questions regarding generalizability of effects to less selected patient populations, optimal duration of treatment, impact on neuropsychiatric symptoms of dementia, and relevance for patient or caregiver quality of life remain largely unanswered. This chapter draws primarily on meta-analyses. Individual studies are referenced with regard to patient subgroups not covered by these analyses, and in consideration of less frequently used outcomes, treatment combinations and comparisons between drugs. Data are presented on intent-to-treat populations if available.

54.2.1   Tacrine

Tacrine (tetrahydroaminoacridine, THA) is a non-competitive, reversible, ChEI with a higher affinity for butyryl cholinesterase (BChE) than acetylcholinesterase (AChE). In addition to its effects on cholinesterases, tacrine inhibits monoamine oxidase activity, affects noradrenaline, dopamine and serotonin uptake and release, increases histamine levels, stimulates insulin secretion and increases glucose metabolism (Wagstaff and McTavish, 1994). Tacrine is metabolized in the liver. The plasma elimination half-life is 3–4 hours with repeated oral doses. Tacrine was the first ChEI approved for use in mild to moderate AD in 1993. Dosing is titrated according to tolerability, starting with 10 mg four times daily, increasing up 40 mg four times daily, with increases at 4–6 week intervals. Weekly monitoring of serum transaminase levels is recommended for the first 18 weeks of therapy and for the 6 weeks following each further increase in dosage. Monitoring should be carried out every three months after this. The clinical efficacy of tacrine was initially evaluated in crossover studies on small patient samples which yielded mixed results. These studies were followed by larger trials which shaped the current methodology of antidementia drug

evaluation (Wagstaff and McTavish, 1994). In a meta-analysis data were summarized from 12 studies on a total of 1984 patients. Six studies had a crossover design of which four involved exposure to tacrine prior to randomization (enrichment), another six had a parallel-group design of which three employed an enrichment strategy (Qizilbash et al., 1998). Outcome measures varied greatly across these studies.

In these studies, which had durations of 12–30 weeks, significant advantages were found favouring tacrine on global assessment and cognition, but not on activities of daily living (ADL). The difference from placebo was two points on the ADAS-Cog at 12 weeks and 1.4 units on the Mini-Mental State Examination (MMSE) at 24 weeks (**Table 54.2**).

The major side effect of tacrine is liver toxicity which manifests as serum transaminase elevation (Watkins et al., 1994). An increase above the upper limit of the norm occurs in 36–66 per cent of patients, an increase more than three times the upper limit of the norm is observed in 13–50 per cent of treated individuals (Wagstaff and McTavish, 1994). Most instances of liver toxicity are asymptomatic and reverse within 4 weeks. Changes in liver function are rare. Tacrine treatment is also associated with dose-dependent cholinergic adverse events including nausea, vomiting, diarrhoea, dyspepsia and anorexia. Reported incidence rates are 14–35 per cent for nausea and 4–18 per cent for diarrhoea (Raina et al., 2008). In non-enriched studies the likelihood of withdrawal was significantly greater for tacrine as compared with placebo. The most frequent reason for premature termination was transaminase elevation.

54.2.2   Donepezil

Donepezil is a piperidine-based, non-competitive, reversible ChEI which shows much greater selectivity for AChE than for BChE. It has a half-life of approximately 70 hours which allows once daily administration. Absorption of donepezil is

Table 54.2   Summary of clinical trials with tacrine.

Domain	Instrument	Duration (weeks)	Treatment difference	Statistical significance
Global assessment	CIBIC	12–30	OR 1.58	0.002
Cognition	ADAS-Cog	12	2.07	<0.001
	MMSE	24	1.41	0.001
Activities of daily living	PDS	6	0.75	n.s.
Tolerability	Withdrawals	12–30	OR 3.68	<0.001

ADAS-Cog, Alzheimer's Disease Assessment Scale, cognitive part; CIBIC, Clinician-Based Impression of Change; MMSE, Mini-Mental State Examination; n.s., not significant; PDS, Progressive Deterioration Scale.

Table 54.3   Summary of clinical trials with donepezil.

Domain	Instrument	Dose (mg/day)	Duration (weeks)	Treatment difference	Statistical significance
Global assessment	CIBIC-plus, % improved	5	24	15%	<0.0001
		10		11%	<0.0001
	GBS	10	52	6.01	0.05
	CDR-SB	5	24	0.51	<0.0001
		10		0.53	<0.0001
Cognition	ADAS-Cog	5	24	2.02	<0.0001
		10		2.81	<0.0001
	MMSE	5	24	1.44	0.0004
		10		1.34	<0.0001
		10	52	1.84	0.006
	SIB	10	24	5.55	<0.0001
Activities of daily living	DAD	10	24	8.00	0.0004
	ADCS-ADL	10		1.60	0.02
	PDS	10	52	3.80	0.0004
Behavioural disturbance	NPI	10	24	2.62	0.02
Tolerability	Withdrawals due to adverse event	10	24	5%	0.003
	Patients with at least one adverse event	5	24	7%	0.03
		10		5%	0.008

ADAS-Cog, Alzheimer's Disease Assessment Scale, cognitive part; ADCS-ADL; Alzheimer's Disease Cooperative Study Activities of Daily Living Scale; CDR-SB, Clinical Dementia Rating Sum of Boxes; CIBIC-plus, Clinician-Based Impression of Change (plus caregiver input); DAD, Disability Assessment in Dementia; MMSE, Mini-Mental State Examination; NPI, Neuropsychiatric Inventory; PDS, Progressive Deterioration Scale; SIB, Severe Impairment Battery.

complete and uninfluenced by food or time of administration. The drug is available in 5 and 10 mg preparations, the lower dose often being prescribed in the initial 4 weeks of treatment. Donepezil is metabolized via the hepatic route and eliminated primarily through the kidneys (Wilkinson, 1999). It received FDA approval for the treatment of mild to moderate dementia in AD in 1996, which was expanded to the treatment of severe dementia in AD in 2006. The evidence that accrued from 15 clinical trials including 4406 participants was summarized in a meta-analysis by Birks and Harvey (2006) (**Table 54.3**).

Global assessment scales revealed significant advantages favouring donepezil at both the 5 and 10 mg daily doses after 24 and 52 weeks of treatment. The proportion of patients rated as improved on the Clinician-Based Impression of Change (plus caregiver input) (CIBIC-plus) was 10–15 per cent larger in actively treated patients than in patients receiving placebo. On cognitive scales, there were significant treatment differences on the ADAS-Cog of 2.0 and 2.8 points

for the 5 and 10 mg doses, respectively, on the MMSE of 1.4 points at 24 weeks independently of the dose and 1.8 points for the high dose at 52 weeks, and on the Severe Impairment Battery (SIB) of 5.5 points for the high dose at 24 weeks. Donepezil significantly improved ADL and behavioural disturbances relative to placebo levels. Withdrawals due to adverse events and patients suffering at least one adverse event were significantly more frequent in the donepezil than in the placebo groups. Adverse events seen more frequently in the donepezil groups than in the placebo groups were cholinergic in nature and included nausea, vomiting and diarrhoea.

In one study on patients with very mild dementia a significant improvement of approximately two points above baseline was observed in the donepezil group on the ADAS-Cog after 24 weeks of treatment, whereas little decline was noted in the placebo group (Seltzer et al., 2004). No significant group difference was found in this trial regarding global assessment. In patients with moderate to severe dementia (MMSE baseline score 5–17) statistically significant advantages of donepezil relative to placebo were observed at 24 weeks on global assessment, cognitive ability, ADL and behavioural disturbances of similar magnitude as seen in the mild to moderate subgroup (Feldman *et al.*, 2001). In one study on patients with severe dementia (baseline MMSE score ≤10) a statistically significant improvement of cognitive ability over baseline was observed in conjunction with less decline on ADL (Winblad *et al.*, 2006). In a second, independent study on patients with severe dementia (baseline MMSE score ≤12) subjects receiving donepezil showed a significant advantage of cognitive ability relative to placebo-treated patients at 24 weeks which was mainly due to deterioration in the placebo group. There was also a significant advantage on global assessment but no treatment difference on ADL in this study (Black *et al.*, 2007). No effect of donepezil on behavioural disturbances was seen in studies involving patients with more severe dementia.

Donepezil is the only antidementia medication for which placebo-controlled data are available beyond treatment durations of six months. Information on 12 months was obtained from a trial on 286 patients with mild to moderate dementia (MMSE scores 10–26). On a global assessment scale (Gottfries–Bråne–Steen scale (GBS)) patients receiving donepezil had declined by week 52, as had placebo-treated subjects, but there was a statistically significant advantage for active treatment. Regarding cognitive ability, patients treated with donepezil showed little deterioration on the MMSE at study end point relative to baseline, whereas worsening by 2.2 points had occurred in patients receiving placebo. This indicates that donepezil offsets cognitive decline in this patient group by almost one year. No statistically significant effects on behavioural disturbances were observed (Winblad *et al.*, 2001). Another 12-month study on 531 patients with moderate dementia (MMSE score 10–20) used predefined clinically evident decline in function as the primary outcome. Significantly more patients in the placebo group than in the donepezil group reached this end point. Survival analysis revealed that the mean time to clinically evident functional decline was five months longer in the actively treated patients (Mohs *et al.*, 2001).

The only study which provided randomized and placebo-controlled evidence on the efficacy of donepezil beyond one year was carried out in a primary care setting independently of the manufacturer. Small but statistically significant treatment differences on cognitive ability and ADL were maintained for two years. However, no significant effect of donepezil was detected on nursing home admissions and progression of disability which had been defined as primary outcomes in this study (Courtney *et al.*, 2004). Due to methodological problems including lack of statistical power, high dropout rate and unusual treatment schemes, this trial probably underestimated the true drug effects (Black and Szalai, 2004).

54.2.3   Rivastigmine

Rivastigmine is a slowly reversible, non-competitive inhibitor of AChE and BChE and has a phenylcarbamate structure.

Since the activity of AChE declines, whereas the activity of BChE remains unchanged, or even increases as AD progresses (Perry *et al.*, 1978), the dual enzyme inhibition holds particular promise for patients with moderate and severe dementia. The metabolism of rivastigmine is largely independent of the cytochrome P450 (CYP) liver enzyme system, and the risk of interactions with other drugs is low. After binding to its target enzyme, the carbamate portion of rivastigmine is slowly hydrolysed and excreted. Rivastigmine has a half-life of 2 hours, so requires at least twice daily dosing, initially starting with 3 mg/day, increasing to between 6 and 12 mg/day according to individual tolerability (Polinsky, 1998). Rivastigmine was approved for the treatment of mild to moderate dementia in AD in 2000. A meta-analysis summarized the results of 13 RCTs which included a total of 5121 participants with mild to severe dementia in AD (baseline MMSE 10–26) who were treated for up to 12 months (Birks *et al.*, 2009) (**Table 54.4**).

After 24–26 weeks of treatment, rivastigmine at a dose of 6–12 mg/day was associated with significant advantages relative to placebo on global assessment, cognitive ability and ADL. The treatment differences were 2 ADAS-Cog points, 0.8 MMSE points and 4.5 points on the SIB. No significant effect on behavioural disturbances was found. The lower dose of 1–4 mg/day was associated with significant treatment differences on global assessment and cognition, but not on ADL. The incidence of withdrawals due to adverse events and the proportion of patients suffering at least one adverse event were significantly higher in patients treated with 6–12 mg/day rivastigmine than in patients receiving placebo. The most frequent adverse events seen in these patients were vomiting, diarrhoea, anorexia, headache, syncope, abdominal pain and dizziness.

In 2007 a transdermal formulation of rivastigmine became available which delivers 9.8 mg over 24 hours. The efficacy of the rivastigmine patch is equivalent to the capsule at a dose of 12 mg/day, but tolerability is better. The number of patients experiencing at least one adverse event was 51 per cent in patients using the patch as compared with 63 per cent in patients treated with capsules ($p = 0.02$). The incidence of gastrointestinal side effects including nausea, vomiting and weight loss is particularly reduced. The dermatological tolerability of the patch is acceptable. Mild skin irritation appears common in clinical practice, and 7–8 per cent of patients experience moderate to severe erythema or pruritus (Cummings *et al.*, 2010).

In one study on patients with severe dementia in AD (MMSE score 5–12) there were statistically significant advantages of rivastigmine relative to placebo on global assessment and cognitive ability but not on ADL or behavioural disturbance at 26 weeks (López-Pousa *et al.*, 2004). The treatment difference was four points on the SIB.

There is only one small placebo-controlled RCT on rivastigmine over 12 months (Karaman *et al.*, 2005). Patients were included with 'advanced moderate' dementia in AD (MMSE score ≤14). At study end point statistically significant treatment differences favouring rivastigmine were observed of 0.4 units on the Alzheimer's Disease Cooperative Study (ADCS)-Clinical Global Impression of Change (CGIC), of 5.3 points on the ADAS-Cog and of 4.3 units on

Table 54.4 Summary of clinical trials with rivastigmine.

Domain	Instrument	Dose (mg/day)	Duration (weeks)	Treatment difference	Statistical significance
Global assessment	CIBIC-plus, improved	1–4	26	6%	0.01
		6–12	26	7%	<0.0001
Cognition	ADAS-Cog	1–4	26	0.84	0.01
		6–12	26	1.99	<0.0001
	ADAS-Cog, ≥4 units	1–4	26	2%	n.s.
		6–12	26	6%	<0.01
	MMSE	1–4	26	0.43	0.02
		6–12	26	0.83	<0.0001
	SIB	6–12	26	4.53	0.03
Activities of daily living	PDS	1–4	26	0.4	n.s.
		6–12	26	2.15	<0.0001
	ADCS-ADL	6–12	24	1.80	0.03
Behavioural disturbance	NPI	3–12	24	2.20	n.s.
Tolerability	Withdrawals due to adverse event	1–4	26	0%	n.s.
		6–12	26	15%	<0.01
	Patients with at least one adverse event	1–4	26	1%	n.s.
		6–12	26	12%	<0.01

ADAS-Cog, Alzheimer's Disease Assessment Scale, cognitive part; ADCS-ADL, Alzheimer's Disease Cooperative Study Activities of Daily Living Scale; CIBIC-plus, Clinician-Based Impression of Change (plus caregiver input); MMSE, Mini-Mental State Examination; NPI, Neuropsychiatric Inventory; PDS, Progressive Deterioration Scale; SIB, Severe Impairment Battery.

the Progressive Deterioration Scale (PDS). Patients treated with 6–12 mg/day showed greater benefit than patients treated with a lower dose.

54.2.4   Galantamine

Galantamine is a tertiary alkaloid which was first isolated from the bulbs of snowdrop and narcissus but is now produced synthetically. It is a competitive, reversible inhibitor of AChE with very little BChE activity (Harvey, 1995). In addition, galantamine is an allosteric potentiatior of the action of AChE on nicotinic receptors (Maelicke, 2000). It has a half-life of approximately 6 hours. The recommended maintenance dose is 16–24 mg/day taken in two daily doses. Galantamine was approved by the FDA for the treatment of mild to moderate dementia in AD in 2001. A meta-analysis summarized the data from ten clinical trials on a total of 6805 patients with mild to moderate dementia (Loy and Schneider, 2004) (**Table 54.5**).

In six-month studies, galantamine treatment was associated with significant advantages relative to placebo on global assessment, cognitive ability, ADL and behavioural disturbance at the 16 mg/day dose. For the 8 mg/day dose the only significant treatment difference was observed on measures of cognition. The 24 mg/day dose was not superior to the 16 mg/day dose. The treatment difference on the ADAS-Cog was three points at six months. At a dose of 24 mg/day, but not at a dose of 16 mg/day, the incidence of withdrawals due to adverse events was higher in patients treated with galantamine than in patients receiving placebo. Adverse events that were more frequently seen in patients on active treatment with 16 mg/day galantamine included nausea, vomiting and diarrhoea. At the higher dose galantamine treatment was associated with an increased incidence of nausea, vomiting, dizziness, weight loss, anorexia, tremor and headache.

In nursing home residents with severe dementia ($n = 407$) galantamine titrated up to a maximum dose of 24 mg/day over six months was associated with a significant advantage over placebo on cognitive ability but not on ADL (Burns et al., 2009). Since 2005 galantamine has been available as a prolonged release once daily dosage formulation (8, 16 and 24 mg) which shows similar efficacy and tolerability to immediate release galantamine at comparable doses (Brodaty et al., 2005).

54.2.5   Memantine

Memantine is a non-competitive modulator of the NMDA receptor and works by normalizing glutamatergic neurotransmission. It prevents excitatory amino acid neurotoxicity, but does not interfere with the physiological function of glutamate for learning and memory (Butterfield and Pocernich, 2003). Memantine reaches maximal plasma concentrations 3–8 hours after oral administration, is eliminated renally, has no inhibitory effect on the CYP system, and does not inhibit cholinesterase inhibitors (Jarvis and Figgitt, 2003). It is administered twice daily up to a maximum dose of 20 mg/day. Memantine was approved by the FDA in 2003 for use in moderate to severe dementia in AD. A meta-analysis summarized the data from three clinical trials on 1291 patients with moderate to severe dementia (baseline MMSE 3–14) and from three unpublished studies in 997 patients with mild to moderate dementia in AD, all over six-month periods (McShane et al., 2009) (**Table 54.6**).

In patients with mild to moderate dementia, memantine treatment is associated with significant benefits relative to

Table 54.5 Summary of clinical trials with galantamine.

Domain	Instrument	Dose (mg/day)	Duration (months)	Treatment difference	Statistical significance
Global assessment	CIBIC-plus, no change or improved	8	6	4%	n.s.
		16		17%	<0.0001
		24		16%	<0.0001
Cognition	ADAS-Cog	8	6	1.30	<0.05
		16		3.10	<0.0001
		24		3.13	<0.0001
Activities of daily living	ADCS-ADL	8	6	0.60	n.s.
		16		3.10	<0.0001
		24		2.30	<0.01
	DAD	24	6	3.66	<0.01
Behavioural disturbance	NPI	8	6	0.30	n.s.
		16		2.10	0.034
		24		1.49	n.s.
Tolerability	Withdrawals due to adverse event	8	6	1%	n.s.
		16		0%	n.s.
		24		7%	<0.001

ADAS-Cog, Alzheimer's Disease Assessment Scale, cognitive part; ADCS-ADL, Alzheimer's Disease Cooperative Study Activities of Daily Living Scale; CIBIC-plus, Clinician-Based Impression of Change (plus caregiver input); DAD, Disability Assessment in Dementia; NPI, Neuropsychiatric Inventory.

Table 54.6 Summary of clinical trials with memantine.

Domain	Instrument	Severity	Duration (months)	Treatment difference	Statistical significance
Global impression	CIBIC-plus	Mild to moderate	6	0.13	0.03
		Moderate to severe	6	0.28	<0.0001
Cognition	ADAS-Cog	Mild to moderate	6	0.99	0.001
	SIB	Moderate to severe	6	2.97	0.0001
Activities of daily living	ADCS-ADL	Mild to moderate	6	0.20	n.s.
	ADCS-ADL sev	Moderate to severe	6	1.27	0.003
Behavioural disturbance	NPI	Mild to moderate	6	0.25	n.s.
		Moderate to severe	6	2.76	0.004
Tolerability	Withdrawals before end	Mild to moderate	6	1.4%	n.s.
		Moderate to severe	6	7.6%[a]	0.005
	Patients with at least one adverse event	Mild to moderate	6	3%	n.s.
		Moderate to severe	6	2%	n.s.

[a] In favour of memantine.
ADAS-Cog, Alzheimer's Disease Assessment Scale, cognitive part; ADCS-ADL; Alzheimer's Disease Cooperative Study Activities of Daily Living Scale; ADCS-ADL sev, Alzheimer's Disease Cooperative Study Activities of Daily Living Scale (for patients with moderate to severe dementia); CIBIC-plus, Clinician-Based Impression of Change (plus caregiver input); NPI, Neuropsychiatric Inventory; SIB, Severe Impairment Battery.

placebo on global assessment and cognition, but not on ADL or behavioural disturbance. In patients with moderate to severe dementia, on the other hand, memantine provides significant advantages over placebo on all four outcome domains (Jarvis and Figgitt, 2003). Another large RCT in patients with moderate to severe dementia in AD, however, failed to demonstrate statistically significant advantages for memantine over placebo on any outcome domain after 24 weeks of treatment (van Dyck et al., 2007). The tolerability of memantine does not differ from placebo (Farlow and Pejovic, 2008). There are no controlled data on the efficacy of memantine beyond six months.

54.2.6   Comparisons between treatments

Donepezil was directly compared with rivastigmine in one 12-week trial and one two-year study. The short-term trial was sponsored by the makers of donepezil and included 111 subjects with mild to moderate dementia. The study was not blinded since dosing scheme and number of study visits were different. Mean changes from baseline were similar in both groups, with treatment differences of 0.16 points on the ADAS-Cog and 0.49 points on the MMSE. ADL and behavioural disturbance were not assessed in this study. The proportion of study completers was significantly greater in the donepezil group (89 per cent) than in the rivastigmine group (60 per cent), whereas the frequency of adverse events resulting in premature discontinuation was higher in the rivastigmine group (22 per cent) than in the donepezil group (11 per cent) (Wilkinson *et al.*, 2002). The two-year study was sponsored by the manufacturer of rivastigmine. It included 998 individuals with moderate dementia and preserved blinding by employing a double-dummy design and identical visit schedules in both groups. There was an almost identical decline of cognitive ability from baseline in both groups at end point. On ADL, however, patients treated with donepezil showed significantly greater deterioration than patients receiving rivastigmine. The treatment difference was two units on the Alzheimer's Disease Cooperative Study Activities of Daily Living Scale (ADCS-ADL) scale. No statistically significant difference was detected between the two groups on behavioural disturbance. During the 16 week dose titration period of the study more gastrointestinal adverse events and more premature discontinuations were recorded in the rivastigmine group than in the donepezil group. During the maintenance period, however, the incidence of gastrointestinal adverse events and the number of withdrawals before the end of study was similar in both groups (Bullock *et al.*, 2005).

There are also two studies comparing donepezil with galantamine. A 12-week study sponsored by the makers of donepezil which included 120 subjects with mild to moderate dementia showed significantly greater improvements from baseline on cognitive ability and ADL in the donepezil group as compared with the galantamine group. Treatment differences were 2.5 points on the ADAS-Cog, 1 point on the MMSE and 2.1 units on the Disability Assessment in Dementia (DAD) (Jones *et al.*, 2004). In contrast, a 52-week head-to-head trial including 182 patients with moderate dementia sponsored by the manufacturer of galantamine did not demonstrate statistically significant differences between the two treatments on cognition (ADAS-Cog, MMSE), ADL (Bristol Activities of Daily Living Scale) and behavioural disturbance (Neuropsychiatric Inventory (NPI)). Rates of gastrointestinal adverse events were similar in both groups (Wilcock *et al.*, 2003).

The only study to directly compare donepezil with memantine was conducted in China, where 100 patients with mild to moderate dementia were randomized to receive either donepezil at 5 mg/day, or memantine, titrated up to 20 mg/day, throughout the trial. At the 16-month end point there were no statistically significant differences between the two groups regarding cognitive ability (MMSE) or ADL (Blessed scale) (Hu *et al.*, 2006). Results are questionable because donepezil was administered at a low dose and the instrument used for assessing everyday activities probably lacked sensitivity to change.

54.2.7   Treatment combinations

The additional effect of memantine in patients who declined despite continuing donepezil treatment was evaluated in an RCT involving 404 patients with moderate to severe dementia in AD (MMSE 5–14). Participants were randomized to

receive memantine (titrated up to 20 mg/day) or placebo in addition to the ChEI for 24 weeks. Statistically significant advantages were observed at study end point on global assessment, cognitive ability, ADL and behavioural disturbance (Tariot *et al.*, 2004). Another RCT examined the additional effect of memantine in 433 patients with mild to moderate AD (MMSE score 10–22) already receiving stable treatment with a ChEI (donepezil, rivastigmine or galantamine). At 24 weeks there were no statistically significant differences between patient groups who received memantine or placebo in addition to cholinergic treatment with regard to global assessment, cognitive ability, ADL or behavioural disturbance (Porsteinsson *et al.*, 2008). A third study showed additional benefit effects of memantine in patients with moderate to severe dementia (MMSE <18) who did not respond satisfactorily to rivastigmine after switching from donepezil (Dantoine *et al.*, 2006). Combinations of memantine and ChEIs were well tolerated. A large trial evaluating the combination of donepezil and memantine in patients with moderate to severe AD is ongoing (Jones *et al.*, 2009).

54.3   CLINICAL IMPORTANCE

The advantages provided by the active treatments relative to placebo are small in comparison to the range of the assessment instruments used for measurement. The average treatment differences of ChEIs are 3–4 per cent on the ADAS-Cog (range 0–70), 3–7 per cent on the MMSE (range 0–30), 1–2 per cent on the ADCS-ADL (range 0–110) and 1–2 per cent on the NPI (range 0–144). For memantine, the average treatment differences are less than 2 per cent on the ADAS-Cog, less than 1 per cent on the ADCS-ADL and 1–2 per cent on the NPI. Even if treatment gains of this magnitude attain statistical significance in sufficiently large patient samples, whether they are clinically meaningful is questionable (Molnar *et al.*, 2009). In the absence of a general consensus, several criteria have been proposed for the evaluation of treatment effects in the real-world context. These include improvement on global assessment, slowing of cognitive deterioration, delay in reaching significant clinical end points, reduction of behavioural disturbance, attainment of individual patient and caregiver goals, and lowering the incidence of nursing home admissions (Chin, 2008; Qaseem *et al.*, 2008; Molnar *et al.*, 2009).

54.3.1   Improvement on global rating

A one unit change on a seven-stage global assessment instrument such as the CIBIC would probably qualify as clinically meaningful. However, the average advantage of antidementia treatments relative to placebo is less than 0.5 units. In a pooled analysis of clinical trials with ChEIs the proportion of patients on active treatment who were rated as improved on a global scale varied between 18 and 35 per cent, as compared with 11–28 per cent in patients receiving placebo. This means that less than 10 per cent more patients improve with treatment than without (Lanctôt *et al.*, 2003).

54.3.2 Slowing of cognitive deterioration

According to the FDA, compensating the natural history of cognitive decline by at least six months is clinically relevant. This equates to a four point or greater difference on the ADAS-Cog (Kramer-Ginsberg *et al.*, 1988). None of the approved AD treatments has achieved an average effect of this magnitude. However, in a one-year study donepezil delayed the decline of cognitive ability by almost one year (Winblad *et al.*, 2001).

54.3.3 Delay in reaching significant clinical end points

Progression to disability is a robust criterion for the clinical relevance of treatment effects. This outcome was addressed in two double-blind, placebo-controlled studies with donepezil. A one-year study showed that donepezil treatment extended the time to loss of critical ADL by five months (Mohs *et al.*, 2001). On the other hand, a longer-term study conducted independently of the pharmaceutical industry in a primary care setting failed to demonstrate a delay in the progression of disability and in reaching the threshold of severe cognitive impairment, probably due to methodological problems (Courtney *et al.*, 2004).

54.3.4 Reduction of behavioural disturbance

Clinical trials of antidementia drugs usually were not designed to evaluate their effects on behavioural disturbance associated with dementia, but measures of neuropsychiatric symptoms were often used as secondary outcomes. Two independent meta-analyses evaluating the behavioural effects of ChEIs concluded that active treatment was associated with an advantage relative to placebo of less than two units on the NPI. Even smaller effects were seen in patients with moderate to severe dementia where neuropsychiatric symptoms are particularly prevalent and effective treatment is most needed (Trinh *et al.*, 2003; Campbell *et al.*, 2008). A systematic review concluded that ChEIs have a weak impact on behavioural disturbance of doubtful clinical importance (Grimmer and Kurz, 2006). The only RCT examining the effects of a ChEI on acute neuropsychiatric symptoms in patients with severe dementia was negative (Holmes *et al.*, 2007). According to a review of three double-blind, placebo-controlled trials with memantine in patients with moderate to severe dementia in AD, two studies found no statistically significant difference between memantine and placebo. One study detected a significant advantage favouring memantine of 3.84 units on the NPI which was due to worsening in the placebo group (Grossberg *et al.*, 2009).

54.3.5 Attainment of individual patient and caregiver goals

In a 24-week study with galantamine, 12 weeks of which were double-blind and placebo-controlled, patients on active treatment showed statistically significant advantages relative to placebo of two points on the ADAS-Cog and 0.4 units on the CIBIC-plus. These treatment gains were entirely consistent with the results of the meta-analyses reviewed above. The attainment of individual goals, however, as defined by patients and caregivers, was not different between the two groups (Rockwood *et al.*, 2006). Few trials included caregiver burden or time spent on caregiving as an outcome and showed small overall effects (Lingler *et al.*, 2005).

54.3.6 Lowering the incidence of nursing home admissions

As a criterion for the clinical relevance of antidementia drug effects, the incidence of nursing home admissions is problematic. Institutionalization is not exclusively determined by factors that are modifiable through medications such as cognitive impairment, limitation of everyday activities or behavioural disturbance. It is also triggered by factors which are intangible to antidementia drugs including patient and caregiver physical health, and availability of community resources (Gaugel *et al.*, 2009). Depending on individual circumstances, nursing home care may be a better alternative for patients with dementia than remaining in the community. For ChEIs, uncontrolled studies have demonstrated that higher dosage and longer duration of treatment were associated with reduced incidence (Knopman *et al.*, 1996; Beusterien *et al.*, 2004) or delay (Lopez *et al.*, 2002; Geldmacher *et al.*, 2003; Feldman *et al.*, 2009) of nursing home admissions. The risk of institutionalization was further reduced by combining ChEI treatment with memantine (Lopez *et al.*, 2009). These investigations are flawed, however, because patients were not randomly allocated to dosage and duration of drug exposure (Karlawish, 2004; Schneider and Qizilbash, 2004). The only long-term placebo-controlled RCT which incorporated nursing home admission as a primary outcome criterion failed to show an impact of donepezil on the rate of institutionalization (Courtney *et al.*, 2004). Economic analyses suggest that the cost savings associated with reducing the time spent in full-time care do not offset the cost of treatment (Loveman *et al.*, 2006).

54.4 PRACTICAL CONSIDERATIONS

The pharmacological effects of current AD treatments are not large. Among the various outcomes examined, the delay of cognitive and functional decline can be considered as clinically meaningful, whereas the impact on behavioural disturbance and caregiver burden is probably insignificant. Even modest clinical benefits, however, are highly desirable in a disease which deprives affected individuals of their intellectual capacity, undermines personal autonomy and heavily burdens family carers (Burns and O'Brien, 2006). Against this background, opportunities for better quality of life, more activity and increased participation must not be missed, while avoiding treatment which lacks practical utility. Achievement of these goals requires timely initiation of treatment, careful monitoring of individual response, attention to safety issues, skilful use of switching and combination strategies, and long-term continuation.

54.4.1 Treatment initiation

To take full advantage of the symptom-delaying effect of current medications, treatment should be initiated early, as soon as the clinical diagnosis can be established with confidence. Due to ceiling effects of the most common assessment instruments (MMSE, ADAS-Cog), this rational strategy collides with treatment guidelines requiring improvement rather than maintenance of cognition as a criterion of efficacy. The role of early treatment is to preserve a maximum of cognitive ability and functional independence for as long as possible. In patients with mild dementia a ChEI should be used, in patients with moderate dementia either a ChEI or memantine may be prescribed. Treatment expectations of patients and carers should be focused on delaying decline and extending patient independence, rather than on overall and durable improvement of symptoms (Farlow and Pejovic, 2008).

54.4.2 Safety issues

The only contraindication to the use of antidementia medications is known hypersensitiviy to a specific drug or its derivatives. ChEIs should be used with caution in patients who have a previous history of severe liver disease, pre-existing bradycardia, peptic ulcer disease, current alcoholism, asthma or chronic obstructive pulmonary disease (Bonner and Peskind, 2002). Memantine should be used at a lower dose than usual in patients with severe renal impairment. Possible interactions with drugs which inhibit the CYP pathways can be observed for tacrine, donepezil and galantamine, but are uncommon with rivastigmine (Standridge, 2004). No metabolic interactions with other drugs have been observed with memantine (Farlow and Pejovic, 2008).

54.4.3 Monitoring treatment response

Evaluating whether and to what extent an individual patient has responded to the treatment provided is a difficult task in a gradually progressive disease such as AD.

The rate of clinical worsening varies widely across patients, is unforeseeable, and previous deterioration is not helpful for predicting further decline (Swanwick et al., 1998). Response to treatment is also highly variable, with only a minority of patients showing true pharmacological improvement. On the other hand, placebo effects are large. For these reasons, the paradigm of treatment decisions guided by the patient's feeling or doing better is inappropriate to AD (Swanwick and Lawlor, 1999). In particular, lack of improvement does not provide an indication for stopping treatment. No change in the patient's condition is the most likely outcome after three to six months' treatment with an antidementia agent. Moreover, a true pharmacological gain may be masked by a dip in the natural progression.

Therefore, the only rational grounds for discontinuation are poor tolerance, low compliance, dramatic decline following the initiation of treatment and absence of deterioration after a drug-free period of 6 weeks (Swanwick and Lawlor, 1999).

54.4.4 Switching drugs

The ChEIs share one basic mode of action but differ with regard to other pharmacological properties. In case of poor tolerance or rapid deterioration despite treatment, switching to another drug within the same class is a viable therapeutic option (Gauthier et al., 2003). Several open-label studies have demonstrated that up to 50 per cent of patients who experienced lack of efficacy or poor tolerability with the initial drug responded favourably to subsequent treatment with another ChEI. In patients with moderate to severe dementia, switching to memantine is another possibility. Open-label studies have demonstrated that many patients experience improvement or stabilization after previously unsatisfactory treatment response and that tolerability is good (Waldemar et al., 2008). Conversely, improvement has been reported in patients with moderate to severe dementia who were switched to donepezil who experienced lack of efficacy from previous treatment with memantine (Sakka et al., 2007).

54.4.5 Treatment combinations

Patients with moderate to severe AD who show tolerability problems or marked deterioration despite stable treatment with a ChEI may respond favourably to combination treatment with memantine (Farlow and Pejovic, 2008). Another important way to optimize the management of dementia is to combine pharmacological treatment with non-pharmacological interventions. An enhancement of clinical efficacy over standard antidementia drugs has been demonstrated for cognitive rehabilitation in patients with mild dementia (Bottino et al., 2005) and for reality orientation in subjects with mild to moderate dementia (Onder et al., 2005).

54.4.6 Discontinuation

There is no evidence from RCTs on the efficacy of current treatments beyond 12 months. After this duration of treatment, patients receiving donepezil do significantly better in terms of cognitive performance and functional ability than patients on placebo. Several open-label extension studies have suggested that treatment gains are maintained for significantly longer periods, although both the actively treated group and the placebo group will continue to decline. These results must be interpreted with caution, however, because patients remaining in treatment were positively selected in terms of treatment response and drug tolerability, and because placebo data were generated by statistical extrapolation (Rodda and Walker, 2009). It is highly probable that the trajectories of treated groups and placebo groups will meet, but it is not clear when this will occur. As noted, gradual deterioration despite treatment is not a criterion for withdrawing treatment, because the natural course of symptoms in an individual patient is unknown. A drug-free interval of several weeks is one way to determine whether a patient still benefits from treatment. On the other hand, drug withdrawal carries a risk of rapid deterioration which cannot be fully compensated by reinitiating treatment. At present, it appears to be a rational strategy to continue treatment as long as neither tolerability problems nor rapid worsening occur, and as long as the patient's condition can be maintained at a stage where the pharmacological properties of the present treatment still have a chance of being beneficial.

54.5 CONCLUSION

We concur with other comparative reviews in concluding that the clinical effects of the currently approved AD treatments are modest (Harry and Zakzanis, 2005; Birks, 2006; Hansen et al., 2007; Shah et al., 2008; Rodda and Walker, 2009). The most salient outcome is a temporary delay of cognitive performance and functional ability by up to 12 months. The effect size is dose-related for donepezil and rivastigmine (Ritchie et al., 2004). Impacts on behavioural disturbances have also been demonstrated but are probably not clinically meaningful (Campbell et al., 2008; Cummings et al., 2008). Clinically detectable improvement only occurs in a minority of patients. The ChEIs do not show clinically relevant differences regarding efficacy and are therefore interchangeable. Advantages for the dual enzyme inhibition of rivastigmine or for the nicotinic receptor enhancement of galantamine are not clinically apparent. Most likely, ChEIs achieve similar clinical benefits in patients with mild dementia and in individuals with severe dementia as in the mild-to-moderate subgroup (Birks, 2006). Memantine is probably less efficacious than a cholinesterase inhibitor in patients with mild dementia, and has not been approved for this population. In patients with moderate to severe dementia, data on clinical efficacy are less consistent for memantine than for cholinesterase inhibitors. Premature withdrawals are more frequent in patients treated with ChEIs as compared with patients receiving placebo. The most common adverse events are nausea, vomiting, diarrhoea, dizziness and weight loss. Differences between drugs regarding the frequency of these adverse events (Lanctôt et al., 2003) have become negligible with the introduction of a transdermal formulation for rivastigmine. A high incidence of liver enzyme elevations in conjunction with a four times daily dosing scheme significantly limits the usability of tacrine. Memantine has an excellent tolerability, with rates of adverse events being no different from placebo. Reliable placebo-controlled data are only available for treatment with cholinesterase inhibitors up to one year. At that point patients on active treatment do better in terms of global assessment, cognitive ability and ADL than patients receiving placebo. It is likely that treatment differences are maintained beyond 12 months, although gradual decline will invariably occur. How long ChEI treatment can maintain patients above placebo levels is unclear. To provide meaningful benefits to patients with AD and their

family carers, the modest effects of currently approved treatments must be applied within a skillful management strategy. It includes early treatment initiation, observation of safety issues and monitoring of individual treatment response on the grounds of appropriate criteria. Physicians must be aware of existing alternatives in case of tolerability problems or marked deterioration, and they should not give up treatment too early. The currently approved symptomatic treatments for AD will remain the standard of care until novel disease-modifying therapies are determined to be safe and efficacious (Shah et al., 2008). They will continue to be an important part of the management of dementia once the new pharmacological strategies become available.

REFERENCES

Ad Hoc FDA Dementia Assessment Task Force. (1991) Antidementia drug assessment symposium. *Neurobiology of Aging* 12: 379–82.

Bartus RT, Dean RL, Beer B, Lippa AS. (1982) The cholinergic hypothesis of geriatric memory dysfunction. *Science* 217: 408–17.

Beusterien KM, Thomas SK, Gause D et al. (2004) Impact of rivastigmine use on the risk of nursing home placement in a US sample. *CNS Drugs* 18: 1143–8.

Birks J. (2006) Cholinesterase inhibitors for Alzheimer's disease. *Cochrane Database of Systematic Reviews* (1): CD005593.

Birks J, Harvey RJ. (2006) Donepezil for dementia due to Alzheimer's disease (review). *Cochrane Database of Systematic Reviews* (1): CD001190.

Birks J, Grimley-Evans J, Iakovidou V et al. (2009) Rivastigmine for Alzheimer's disease. *Cochrane Database of Systematic Reviews* (2): CD001191.

Black SE, Szalai JP. (2004) Are there long-term benefits of donepezil in Alzheimer's disease? *Canadian Medical Association Journal* 171: 1174–5.

Black SE, Li RD, McRae T et al. (2007) Donepezil preserves cognition and global function in patients with severe Alzheimer disease. *Neurology* 69: 459–69.

Bonner LT, Peskind ER. (2002) Pharmacologic treatments of dementia. *Medical Clinics of North America* 86: 657–74.

Bottino CMC, Carvalho IAM, Alvarez AMMA et al. (2005) Cognitive rehabilitation combined with drug treatment in Alzheimer's disease patients: A pilot study. *Clinical Rehabilitation* 19: 861–9.

Brodaty H, Corey-Bloom J, Potocnik FCV et al. (2005) Galantamine prolonged-release formulation in the treatment of mild to moderate Alzheimer's disease. *Dementia and Geriatric Cognitive Disorders* 20: 120–32.

Broich K. (2007) Outcome measures in clinical trials on medicinal products for the tretment of dementia: A European regulatory perspective. *International Psychogeriatrics* 19: 509–24.

Bullock R, Touchon J, Bergman H et al. (2005) Rivastigmine and donepezil treatment in moderate to moderately-severe Alzheimer's disease over a 2-year period. *Current Medical Research and Opinion* 21: 1317–27.

Burns A, O'Brien J. (2006) Clinical practice with anti-dementia drugs: A consensus statement of the British Association for Psychopharmacology. *Journal of Psychopharmacology* **20**: 732–55.

Burns A, Bernabei R, Bullock R *et al.* (2009) Safety and efficacy of galantamine (Reminyl) in severe Alzheimer's disease (the SERAD study): A randomised, placebo-controlled, double blind trial. *Lancet Neurology* **8**: 39–47.

Butterfield DA, Pocernich CB. (2003) The glutamatergic system and Alzheimer's disease. Therapeutic implications. *CNS Drugs* **17**: 641–52.

Campbell N, Ayub A, Boustani MA *et al.* (2008) Impact of cholinesterase inhibitors on behavioral and psychological symptoms of Alzheimer's disease. A meta-analysis. *Clinical Interventions in Aging* **3**: 719–28.

Chin JJ. (2008) Alzheimer's disease – towards more patient-centred and meaningful clinical outcomes. *Annals of the Academy of Medicine, Singapore* **37**: 535–7.

Courtney C, Farrell D, Gray R *et al.* (2004) Long-term donepezil treatment in 656 patients with Alzheimer's disease (AD2000): Randomised double-blind trial. *Lancet* **363**: 2105–15.

Cummings JL. (1997) The Neuropsychiatric Inventory. Assessing psychopathology in dementia patients. *Neurology* **48** (Suppl. 6): 10S–16S.

Cummings JL, Mackell J, Kaufer D. (2008) Behavioral effects of current Alzheimer's disease treatments: A descriptive review. *Alzheimer's and Dementia* **4**: 49–60.

Cummings JL, Farlow MR, Meng X *et al.* (2010) Rivastigmine transdermal patch skin tolerability. Results of a 1-year clinical trial in patients with mild-to-moderate Alzheimer's disease. *Clinical Drug Investigation* **30**: 41–9.

Dantoine T, Auriacombe S, Sarazin M *et al.* (2006) Rivastigmine monotherapy and combination therapy with memantine in patients with moderately severe Alzheimer's disease who failed to benefit from previous cholinesterase inhibitor treatment. *International Journal of Clinical Practice* **60**: 110–18.

De Jong R, Ostersund OW, Roy GW. (1989) Measurement of quality-of-life changes in patients with Alzheimer's disease. *Clinical Therapeutics* **11**: 545–54.

Farlow MR, Pejovic MLMV. (2008) Treatment options in Alzheimer's disease: Maximizing benefit, managing expectations. *Dementia and Geriatric Cognitive Disorders* **25**: 408–22.

Feldman H, Gauthier S, Hecker J *et al.* (2001) A 24-week, randomized, double-blind study of donepezil in moderate to severe Alzheimer's disease. *Neurology* **57**: 613–20.

Feldman H, Pirttila T, Dartigues JF *et al.* (2009) Treatment with galantamine and time to nursing home placement in Alzheimer's disease patients with and without cerebrovascular disease. *International Journal of Geriatric Psychiatry* **24**: 479–88.

Folstein MF, Folstein SE, McHugh PR. (1975) 'Mini Mental State'. A practical method for grading the cognitive state of patients for the clinician. *Journal of Psychiatric Research* **12**: 189–98.

Galasko D, Bennett D, Sano M *et al.* (1997) An inventory to assess activities of daily living for clinical trials in patients with Alzheimer's disase. *Alzheimer Disease and Associated Disorders* **11** (Suppl. 2): S33–9.

Galasko D, Schmitt F, Thomas R *et al.* (2005) Detailed assessment of activities of daily living in moderate to severe Alzheimer's disease. *Journal of the International Neuropsychological Society* **11**: 446–53.

Gaugel JE, Yu F, Krichbaum K, Wyman JF. (2009) Predictors of nursing home admission for persons with dementia. *Medical Care* **47**: 191–8.

Gauthier S, Emre M, Farlow MR *et al.* (2003) Strategies for continued successful treatment of Alzheimer's disease: Switching cholinesterase inhibitors. *Current Medical Research and Opinion* **19**: 707–14.

Geldmacher DS, Provenzano G, McRae T *et al.* (2003) Donepezil is associated with delayed nursing home placement in patients with Alzheimer's disease. *Journal of the American Geriatrics Society* **51**: 937–44.

Gélinas I, Gauthier L, McIntyre M *et al.* (1999) Development of a functional measure for persons with Alzheimer's disease: the disability assessment for dementia. *American Journal of Occupational Therapy* **53**: 471–81.

Gill SS, Bronskill SE, Mamdani M *et al.* (2004) Representation of patients with dementia in clinical trials of donepezil. *Canadian Journal of Clinical Pharmacology* **11**: e274–85.

Gottfries CG, Brane G, Gullberg B, Steen G. (1982) A new rating scale for dementia syndromes. *Archives of Gerontology and Geriatrics* **1**: 311–30.

Greenamyre JT, Maragos EF, Albin RL *et al.* (1988) Glutamate transmission and toxicity in Alzheimer's disease. *Progress in Neuropsychopharmacology and Biological Psychiatry* **12**: 421–30.

Grimmer T, Kurz A. (2006) Effects of cholinesterase inhibitors on behavioural disturbances in Alzheimer's disease. A systematic review. *Drugs and Aging* **23**: 957–67.

Grossberg GT, Pejovic V, Miller ML, Graham SM. (2009) Mementine therapy of behavioral symptoms in community-dwelling patients with moderate to severe Alzheimer's disease. *Dementia and Geriatric Cognitive Disorders* **27**: 164–72.

Hansen RA, Garlehner G, Lohr KN, Kauffer DI. (2007) Functional outcomes of drug treatment in Alzheimer's disease. A systematic review and meta-analysis. *Drugs and Aging* **24**: 155–67.

Hardy J. (2009) The amyloid hypothesis for Alzheimer's disease: A critical reappraisal. *Journal of Neurochemistry* **110**: 1129–34.

Harry RDJ, Zakzanis KK. (2005) A comparison of donepezil and galantamine in the treatment of cognitive symptoms of Alzheimer's disease: A meta-analysis. *Human Psychopharmacology* **20**: 183–7.

Harvey AL. (1995) The pharmacology of galanthamine and its analogues. *Pharmacological Therapeutics* **68**: 113–28.

Holmes C, Wilkinson D, Dean C *et al.* (2007) Risperidone and rivastigmine and agitated bahviour in severe Alzheimer's disease: A randomised double blind placebo controlled study. *International Journal of Geriatric Psychiatry* **22**: 380–1.

Hu HT, Zhang ZX, Yao JL *et al.* (2006) Clinical efficacy and safety of akatinol memantine in treatment of mild to moderate Alzheimer disease. A donepezil-controlled, randomized trial. *Zhonghua Nei Ke Za Zhi* **45**: 277–80.

Jarvis B, Figgitt DP. (2003) Memantine. *Drugs and Aging* 20: 465–76.

Jones RW, Soininen H, Hager K *et al.* (2004) A multinational, randomised, 12-week study comparing the effects of donepezil and galantamine in patients with mild to moderate Alzheimer's disease. *International Journal of Geriatric Psychiatry* 19: 58–67.

Jones R, Sheehan B, Phillips P *et al.* (2009) DOMINO-AD protocol: Donepezil and memantine in moderate to severe Alzheimer's disease – a multicentre RCT. *Trials* 10: 57.

Karaman V, Edrogan F, Köseoglu E, Turan T, Özdemir-Ersoy A. (2005) A 12-month study of the efficacy of rivastigmine in patients with advanced moderate Alzheimer's disease. *Dementia and Geriatric Cognitive Disorders* 19: 51–6.

Karlawish JHT. (2004) Donepezil delay to nursing home placement study is flawed. *Journal of the American Geriatrics Society* 52: 845.

Katona C, Livingston G, Cooper C *et al.* (2007) International Psychogeriatric Association consensus statement on defining and measuring treatment benefits in dementia. *International Psychogeriatrics* 19: 345–54.

Knopman D, Schneider L, Davis K *et al.* (1996) Long-term tacrine (Cognex) treatment: Effects on nursing home placement and mortality. *Neurology* 47: 166–77.

Kramer-Ginsberg E, Mohs RC, Aryan M *et al.* (1988) Clinical predictors of course for Alzheimer patients in a longitudinal study: A preliminary report. *Psychopharmacology Bulletin* 24: 458–62.

Lanctôt KL, Herrmann N, Yau KK *et al.* (2003) Efficacy and safety of cholinesterase inhibitors in Alzheimer's disease: A meta-analysis. *Canadian Medical Association Journal* 169: 557–63.

Lingler JH, Martire LM, Sshulz R. (2005) Caregiver-specific outcomes in antidementia clinical drug trials: A systematic review and meta-analysis. *Journal of the American Geriatrics Society* 53: 983–90.

Lleó A, Greenberg SM, Growdon JH. (2006) Current pharmacotherapy for Alzheimer's disease. *Annual Review of Medicine* 57: 513–33.

Lopez OL, Becker JT, Wisniewski S *et al.* (2002) Cholinesterase inhibitor treatment alters the natural history of Alzheimer's disease. *Journal of Neurology, Neurosurgery, and Psychiatry* 2: 310–4.

Lopez OL, Becker JT, Wahed AS *et al.* (2009) Long-term effects of the concomitant use of memantine with cholinesterase inhibition in Alzheimer disease. *Journal of Neurology, Neurosurgery, and Psychiatry* 80: 600–7.

López-Pousa S, Hernandez B, Rapatz G. (2004) Efficacy of rivastigmine in patients with severe Alzheimer's disease: A double-blind, randomized pilot study. *Brain Aging* 4: 26–34.

Loveman E, Green C, Kirby J *et al.* (2006) The clinical and cost-effectiveness of donepezil, rivastigmine, galantamine, and memantine for Alzheimer's disease. *Health Technology Assessment* 10: 1.

Loy C, Schneider L. (2004) Galantamine for Alzheimer's disease. *Cochrane Database of Systematic Reviews* (4): CD001747.

McShane R, Areosa-Satre A, Minikaran N. (2009) Memantine for dementia. *Cochrane Database of Systematic Reviews* (2): CD003154.

Maelicke A. (2000) Allosteric modulation of nicotinic receptors as a treatment strategy for Alzheimer's disease. *Dementia and Geriatric Cognitive Disorders* 11: 11–18.

Mohs RC, Doody RS, Morris JC *et al.* (2001) A 1-year, placebo-controlled preservation of function survival study of donepezil in AD patients. *Neurology* 57: 481–8.

Molnar FJ, Man-Son-Hing M, Fergusson D. (2009) Systematic review of measures of clinical significance employed in randomized controlled trials of drugs for dementia. *Journal of the American Geriatrics Society* 57: 536–46.

Morris JC. (1993) The Clinical Dementia Rating (CDR): Current version and scoring rules. *Neurology* 43: 2412–14.

Onder G, Zanetti O, Giacobini E *et al.* (2005) Reality orientation therapy combined with cholinesterase inhibitors in Alzheimer's disease: Randomised controlled trial. *British Journal of Psychiatry* 187: 450–5.

Perry EK, Perry RH, Blessed G, Tomlinson BE. (1978) Changes in brain cholinesterases in senile dementia of Alzheimer type. *Neuropathology and Applied Neurobiology* 4: 273–7.

Polinsky RN. (1998) Clinical pharmacology of rivastigmine: A new-generation acetylcholinesterase inhibitor for the treatment of Alzheimer's disease. *Clinical Therapeutics* 20: 634–47.

Porsteinsson AP, Grossberg GT, Mintzer J, Olin JT. (2008) Memantine treatment in patients with mild to moderate Alzheimer's disease already receiving a cholinesterase inhibitor: A randomized, double-blind, placebo-controlled trial. *Current Alzheimer Research* 5: 83–9.

Qaseem A, Snow V, Cross JT *et al.* (2008) Current pharmacologic treatment of dementia: A clinical practice guideline from the American College of Physicians and the American Academy of Family Physicians. *Annals of Internal Medicine* 148: 370–8.

Qizilbash N, Whitehead A, Higgins J *et al.* (1998) Cholinesterase inhibition for Alzheimer disease. A meta-analysis of the tacrine trials. *Journal of the American Medical Association* 281: 2287–8.

Raina P, Santaguida P, Ismaila A *et al.* (2008) Effectiveness of cholinesterase inhibitors and memantine for treatment of dementia: Evidence review for a clinical practice guideline. *Annals of Internal Medicine* 148: 379–97.

Raschetti R, Albanese E, Vanacore N, Maggini M. (2007) Cholinesterase inhibitors in mild cognitive impairment: A systematic review of randomised trials. *PLoS Medicine* 4: 1818–28.

Ritchie CW, Ames D, Clayton T, Lai R. (2004) Metaanalysis of randomized trials of the efficacy and safety of donepezil, galantamine, and rivastigmine for the treatment of Alzheimer disease. *American Journal of Geriatric Psychiatry* 12: 358–69.

Rockwood K, Fay S, Song X *et al.* (2006) Attainment of goals by people with Alzheimer's disease receiving galantamine: A randomized controlled trial. *Canadian Medical Association Journal* 174: 1099–105.

Rodda J, Walker Z. (2009) Ten years of cholinesterase inhibitors. *International Journal of Geriatric Psychiatry* 24: 437–42.

Rosen WG, Mohs R, Davis KL. (1984) A new rating scale for Alzheimer's disease. *American Journal of Psychiatry* 11: 1356–64.

Sakka P, Tsolake M, Hort J *et al.* (2007) Effectiveness of open-label donepezil treatment in patients with Alzheimer's disease discontinuing memantine monotherapy. *Current Medical Research and Opinion* **23**: 3153–65.

Schmitt FA, Ashford W, Ernesto W *et al.* (1997) The Severe Impairment Battery: Concurrent validity and the assessment of longitudinal change in Alzheimer's disease. *Alzheimer Disease and Associated Disorders* **11** (Suppl. 2): S51–6.

Schneider LS. (1997) Validity and reliability of the Alzheimer's Disease Study – Clinical Global Impression of Change (ADCS-CGIC). *Alzheimer Disease and Associated Disorders* **11**: 13–23.

Schneider LS, Qizilbash N. (2004) Delay in nursing home placement with donepezil. *Journal of the American Geriatrics Society* **52**: 1024–926.

Seltzer B, Zolnouni P, Nunez M *et al.* (2004) Efficacy of donepezil in early-stage Alzheimer disease. A randomized placebo-controlled trial. *Archives of Neurology* **61**: 1852–6.

Shah RS, Lee HG, Xiongwei Z *et al.* (2008) Current approaches in the treatment of Alzheimer's disease. *Biomedicine and Pharmacotherapy* **62**: 199–207.

Standridge JB. (2004) Pharmacotherapeutic approaches to the treatment of Alzheimer's disease. *Clinical Therapeutics* **26**: 615–30.

Swanwick GRJ, Coen RF, Coakley D, Lawlor BA. (1998) Assessment of progression and prognosis in 'possible' and 'probable' Alzheimer's disease. *International Journal of Geriatric Psychiatry* **13**: 331–5.

Swanwick GRJ, Lawlor BA. (1999) Initiating and monitoring cholinesterase inhibitor treatment for Alzheimer's disease. *International Journal of Geriatric Psychiatry* **14**: 244–8.

Tariot PN, Farlow MR, Grossberg GT *et al.* (2004) Memantine treatment in patients with moderate to severe Alzheimer disease already receiving donepezil. A randomized controlled trial. *Journal of the American Medical Association* **291**: 317–24.

Trinh NH, Hoblyn J, Mohanty S, Yaffe K. (2003) Efficacy of cholinesterase inhibitors in the treatment of neuropsychiatric symptoms and functional impairment in Alzheimer disease. A meta-analysis. *Journal of the American Medical Association* **289**: 210–16.

Van Dyck CH, Tariot PN, Myers B, Resnick EM. (2007) A 24-week randomized, controlled trial of memantine in patients with moderate-to-severe Alzheimer disease. *Alzheimer Disease and Associated Disorders* **21**: 136–43.

Wagstaff AJ, McTavish D. (1994) Tacrine. A review of its pharmacodynamic and pharmacokinetic properties, and therapeutic efficacy in Alzheimer's disease. *Drugs and Aging* **4**: 510–40.

Waldemar G, Hyvärinen M, Krog-Josiassen M *et al.* (2008) Tolerability of switching from donepezil to memantine treatment in patients with moderate to severe Alzheimer's disease. *International Journal of Geriatric Psychiatry* **23**: 979–81.

Watkins PB, Zimmerman HJ, Knapp MG *et al.* (1994) Hepatotoxic effects of tacrine administration in patients with Alzheimer's disease. *Journal of the American Medical Association* **271**: 992–8.

Wilcock G, Howe I, Coles H *et al.* (2003) A long-term comparison of galanamine and donepezil in the treatment of Alzheimer's disease. *Drugs and Aging* **20**: 777–89.

Wilkinson DG. (1999) The pharmacology of donepezil: A new treatment for Alzheimer's disease. *Expert Opinion on Pharmacotherapy* **1**: 121–35.

Wilkinson D, Passmore AP, Bullock R *et al.* (2002) A multinational, randomised, 12-week, comparative study of donepezil and rivastigmine in patients with mild to moderate Alzheimer's disease. *International Journal of Clinical Practice* **56**: 441–6.

Winblad B, Engedal K, Soininen H *et al.* (2001) A 1-year, randomized, placebo-conrolled study of donepezil in patients with mild to moderate AD. *Neurology* **57**: 489–95.

Winblad B, Kilander L, Eriksson S *et al.* (2006) Donepezil in patients with severe Alzheimer's disease: Double-blind, parallel-group, placebo-controlled study. *Lancet* **367**: 1057–65.

55

Drug treatments in development for Alzheimer's disease

MICHAEL WOODWARD

55.1 INTRODUCTION

It is unfortunate that 24 years after initial descriptions of the therapeutic benefits of tacrine (Summers *et al.*, 1986) we still only have symptomatic therapies for Alzheimer's disease (AD) and no therapies for the other dementias. Only four drugs are regularly used for AD (donepezil, galantamine, rivastigmine and memantine) and no new drug has been marketed for almost 15 years. We desperately need disease-modifying therapies as well as new symptomatic therapies for AD.

In many respects the course of developing therapies for AD has resembled that of developing cancer drugs. There were initially only symptomatic therapies, then, as the molecular basis of cancer was better understood, an enthusiasm that a single magic bullet would be developed that would cure and indeed prevent all cancer. It is likely that the future course of AD drug development will also track that of cancer drugs, with therapies that have modest effects on the disease process often used sequentially or in combination, along with symptomatic therapies, without a sudden major development that cures all. As with some cancer therapies, there are likely to be some drugs that dramatically alter the course of some types of dementia (e.g. TDP-43 related frontotemporal lobar degeneration) rather than being effective for all dementias. Over decades, we may achieve a situation where most people with dementia treated with the new therapies can look forward to another 15–20 years of productive life, rather than the current average of five to ten years. Unlike cancer, most people with dementia are already of advanced age and even without dementia their life expectancy is limited.

The holy grail of dementia therapies is primary prevention – identifying those at increased risk of developing a form of dementia then treating them with a therapy that prevents dementia developing. Such a therapy would need to be very safe, as many people who would never develop dementia will be given it. These therapeutic agents would probably, but not necessarily, be effective in treating established dementia too. Conversely, a drug that fails in dementia therapeutic trials may however be effective as a preventative agent. The non-steroidal anti-inflammatory drugs (NSAIDs) could fall into this class – all therapeutic trials for AD were negative but they still may have a preventative role. Indeed, this hypothesis was to be tested in the ADAPT trial of the AD Cooperative Studies group (Martin *et al.*, 2008) but unfortunately the trial was terminated early due to concerns about toxicity of the agent (celecoxib) in a large healthy population. Chapter 58, Prevention of Alzheimer's disease, addresses prevention of AD in detail.

We stand on an exciting threshold with more dementia therapeutic trials than at any time – aimed at developing both disease-modifying and symptomatic therapies. It is quite likely that within two to three years a disease-modifying agent will be marketed. This will be the first major development in over 25 years of dementia therapies.

55.2 TARGETS OF DEMENTIA THERAPIES

An increase in understanding of the genetic, cellular and molecular basis of dementia has led to a wide range of

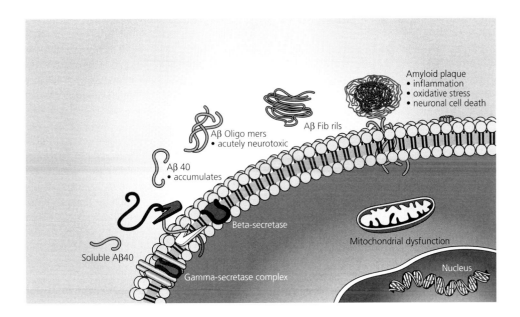

Figure 55.1   Potential molecular targets for AD therapies.

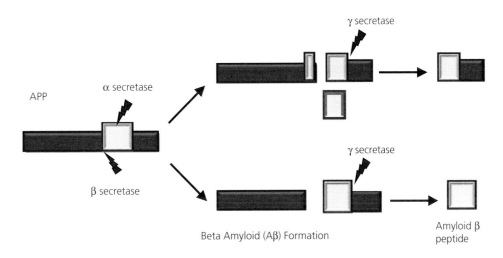

Figure 55.2   Beta amyloid (Aβ) formation.

potential therapeutic targets. Only those targets with current therapeutic trials are described in this chapter, but it is highly likely that many more molecules and disease processes will be targeted in future (**Figure 55.1**).

55.2.1   Amyloid

The amyloid precursor protein (APP) is a transmembrane protein that is cleaved by enzymes called secretases (see also Chapter 51, The central role of Aβ amyloid in the pathogenesis of Alzheimer's disease). The amyloidogenic beta amyloid (Aβ) fragment is cleaved at either end by γ and β secretases, but can also be cleaved in the middle by α secretase, making harmless fragments (**Figure 55.2**). The Aβ then forms oligomers before eventually aggregating as amyloid (Aβ) plaques. The Aβ peptide is also taken up from the periphery by the receptor for advanced glycation end

products (RAGE) (**Figure 55.3**). Thus, potential anti-amyloid approaches include inhibitors of α and β secretase, enhancers of α secretase, inhibitors of Aβ aggregation, drugs that de-aggregate amyloid, inhibitors of RAGE and antibodies directed against Aβ.

55.2.2   Tau

Tau is a protein that stabilizes microtubules, allowing transport of vesicles and other products of neuronal cell bodies down the axon to the synapse. In AD, tau becomes hyperphosphorylated and this disrupts the microtubules, with the tau eventually aggregating to create neurofibrillary tangles. Several mechanisms can be targeted therapeutically, including hyperphosphorylation and tau aggregation. Such approaches may also work in some of the non-AD dementias such as some types of frontotemporal lobar degeneration.

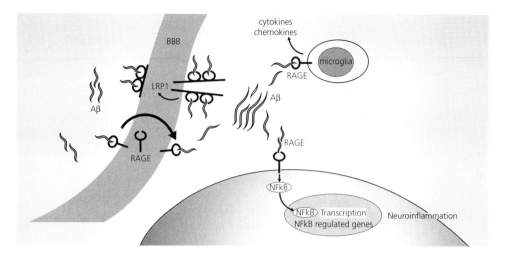

Figure 55.3　Receptor for advanced glycation end products.

55.2.3　Neurones and synapses

Neural regeneration and replacement is being attempted with stem cell transplants/infusions (see Chapter 56, Stem cell therapies for Alzheimer's disease and other dementias) and the delivery of nerve growth factors and other neurotrophic agents. It is reassuring that in regions of most intense neural response to dementia pathology (e.g. around amyloid plaques) there are often neurones that can be revived and any cell death is more from apoptosis than necrosis, meaning damage to other cells is limited. However, the brain is the most complex organ with respect to cellular structure so neural regeneration or replacement may never be fully possible.

55.2.4　Inflammation

There is an inflammatory response around amyloid plaques in AD, and inflammation may occur with other dementias. This presents potential targets, using anti-inflammatory agents to limit cell damage and modify the clinical course of dementia.

55.2.5　Mitochondria

These organelles generate the energy required for cellular processes and damage to mitochondria has been implicated as one of the primary causes of cell damage in dementia. Mitochondria have their own genes and are the site of numerous metabolic pathways, many of which present potential targets for dementia therapies.

55.2.6　Oxidative processes

Closely linked with mitochondrial function, all cells generate damaging oxidative species and have regulatory antioxidant mechanisms. AD therapies that enhance this antioxidant response may protect cells from damage and alter the course of the dementia.

55.2.7　Neurotransmitters and receptors

Symptomatic AD therapies to date have targeted a small number of neurotransmitters and their receptors, and other neurotransmitter symptoms are potential targets for new symptomatic therapies. These include the various histaminergic, 5-hydroxytryptamine (5-HT) and glutamatergic neurotransmitters and receptors.

55.2.8　Other mechanisms

The cholesterol-lowering statins have been examined as potential disease-modifying agents following epidemiological evidence that their use may be associated with a lower risk of developing dementia. There are several potential mechanisms by which they may attenuate AD pathology, including interaction with APP processing and cerebrovascular effects.

Other potentially disease-modifying agents target the perioxisome proliferator-activated receptor-γ (PPAR-γ) receptor or have multiple modes of action and will be described below.

55.3　THERAPEUTIC TRIALS

The numerous potential targets described above have led to a plethora of well-constructed trials of new dementia therapies. This chapter concentrates on therapeutic areas where trials have been conducted and results presented. However, it is likely that many new targets and agents are being developed and may soon have sufficient data to review.

55.3.1　Amyloid

55.3.1.1　ACTIVE IMMUNIZATION

Antibodies against Aβ can be induced by injecting Aβ and these antibodies may modify the amyloid cascade, preventing AD progression (Schenk et al., 1999). The first trial of the

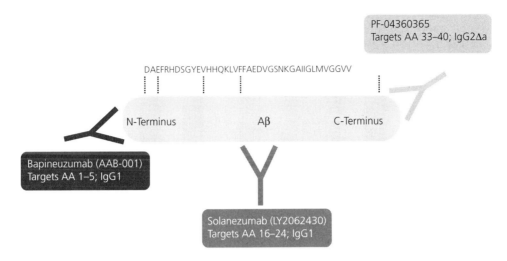

DAEFRHDSGYEVHHQKLVFFAEDVGSNKGAIIGLMVGGVV

PF-04360365
Targets AA 33–40; IgG2Δa

N-Terminus   Aβ   C-Terminus

Bapineuzumab (AAB-001)
Targets AA 1–5; IgG1

Solanezumab (LY2062430)
Targets AA 16–24; IgG1

Figure 55.4 Examples of anti-Aβ monoclonal antibodies epitopes.

active immunization against Aβ began after transgenic animal studies showed that such an approach prevented deposition of amyloid (if used early), and reduced amyloid load (if used later), leading to clinical benefits including prevention of memory loss (Morgan *et al.*, 2000). A phase I clinical trial of immunotherapy of patients with AD, using Aβ$_{42}$ as the antigen, showed a highly variable development of antibodies (Bayer *et al.*, 2005) but no significant clinical benefits (though the trial was not powered for clinical end points). A subsequent phase IIa study was halted when 6 per cent of the patients developed a sterile meningoencephalitis (Orgogozo *et al.*, 2003), but showed no major differences in cognitive outcomes when antibody responders were compared with the placebo group after one year, despite evidence of high serum antibodies to Aβ$_{42}$ in a group who received active treatment (Hock *et al.*, 2003). More recently, neuropathological examination of eight patients who had received active immunization revealed removal of amyloid plaque proportional to the antibody response, but no survival advantage in time to severe dementia, with all reaching severe AD before death (Holmes *et al.*, 2008).

The finding that plaque removal is not enough to halt progressive neurodegeneration in AD poses challenges to the amyloid hypothesis. It is possible that amyloid (Aβ) plaques may be needed to initiate but not to maintain progressive neurodegeneration. It is also hypothesized that it is oligomeric Aβ, rather than the fibrillar Aβ in plaques, that is responsible for most neurodegeneration in AD and that as immunization fails to reduce oligomeric Aβ (or indeed increases this as Aβ in plaques is mobilized) this approach may be ineffective clinically. Additionally, full-length Aβ immunization may be overactivating the immune system, causing the meningoencephalitis seen (Orgogozo *et al.*, 2003) and compromising potential clinical improvements from plaque removal. Thus, more recent active immunization approaches have utilized Aβ fragments that are less likely to activate unwanted immune responses. These trials are in progress but may be the last throw of the dice for active immunization. Novartis has evaluated Aβ fragments inserted into a biosphere, to increase immunogenicity. In two small cohorts, each subject received three injections of 50 and 180 μg doses, and 18 of 22 actively treated subjects developed detectable antibodies. Cognitive end points were negative but there were no serious adverse events. Wyeth/Elan are also continuing to pursue an active immunization approach with their antigen ACC-001.

55.3.1.2 PASSIVE IMMUNIZATION

An approach that bypasses the need to respond to an antigen and, variably, produce antibodies is to inject the antibodies themselves. This can be done by using pooled immunoglobulin, which contain anti-Aβ antibodies, or developing monoclonal antibodies (mAbs) against Aβ (**Figure 55.4**). These monoclonal antibodies, usually produced from animal immunoglobulin, can be humanized and modified in other ways that can impact on efficacy and reduce unwanted immune/inflammatory effects.

Currently mAbs in clinical trials are directed against either the C or N-terminus of Aβ, or the mid-portion of the Aβ peptide. The most advanced mAb, in clinical trials, is bapineuzumab, which is directed against the N-terminus. Phase II results from a trial in 234 subjects with six infusions 13 weeks apart have been published. The primary end points Alzheimer's Disease Assessment Scale-cognitive subscale (ADAS-Cog) and Disability Assessment for Dementia did not significantly improve in the overall group but did improve significantly in the 79 subjects who were apolipoprotein E (ApoE) ε4 non-carriers (**Figure 55.5**). There was also a suggestion of reduced loss of whole brain volume over 71 weeks, assessed by magnetic resonance imaging (MRI), in the ApoE ε4 non-carriers (**Figure 55.6**) (Salloway *et al.*, 2009). Cerebrospinal fluid (CSF) Aβ and phospho-tau levels were insignificantly different in the treated and untreated groups.

Adverse effects have however been quite significant, with vasogenic oedema (VE) occurring in about 10 per cent of actively treated subjects, compared to none of the controls. Most occurred in ApoE ε4 carriers and most were asymptomatic, but at least one required steroids for lethargy and confusion. Cases occurred after the first or second dose but none have recurred after rechallenging. Microhaemorrhages

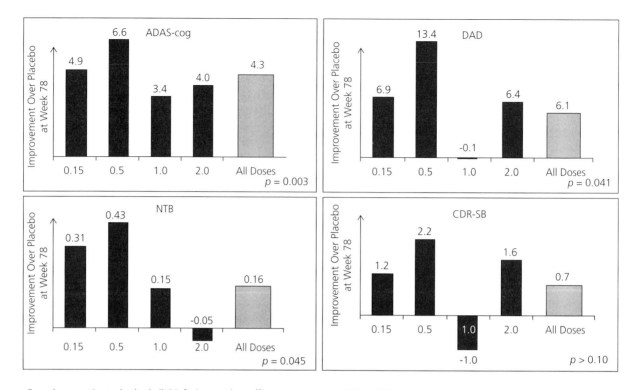

Completer: patient who had all 6 infusions and an efficacy assessment at Week 78
Bars above zero indicated improvement relative to placebo
Patient populations for "all doses" comparisons: bapineuzumab, N = 78; placebo, N =78

Figure 55.5   Clinical efficacy end points: total population (completer). Bapineuzumab-ApoE4 non-carrier results.

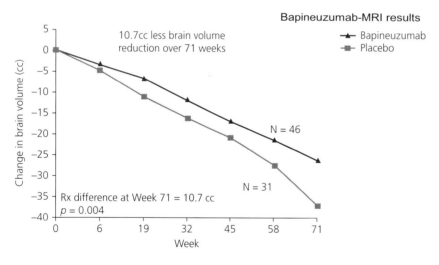

*Brain volume as measured by brain boundary shift integral (BBSI)
MITT analyses using RM model without assumption of linearity, adjusted for whole brain volume at baseline, MMSE at baseline and ApoE4 status

Figure 55.6   Change in MRI brain volume*: ApoE4 non-carrier population (MITT).

were seen and it has been postulated that removal of amyloid from blood vessels may cause these microhaemorrhages and the subsequent VE. The highest rate has been seen in those treated with the higher doses of bapineuzumab and this, along with the possible differential ApoE ε4 response effects, has been factored into a huge phase III trial programme now in progress. Lower doses are being used and there is intensive MRI monitoring for microhaemorrhages and VE.

The phase III programme consists of two parallel trials – one in those who are ApoE ε4 carriers and another in those who are ApoE ε4 negative. To date, there have been no increased safety concerns and the trials proceed, aiming to recruit nearly 4000 subjects into the two studies. Substudies will examine CSF biomarker responses, MRI brain volumetrics and positron emission tomography (PET) measurements of hypometabolism and amyloid load. The results should be available in 2011 and, if favourable, bapineuzumab is likely to be the first marketed disease-modifying AD therapy, with a possible launch date as early as 2013.

Solanezumab is a mAb directed against the mid-portion of Aβ. A study in subjects with mild to moderate AD, with infusions every 4 weeks for three months, showed no change in cognitive end points. CSF Aβ levels increased, which is probably desirable as levels are lower in AD subjects compared to controls. Total plasma Aβ levels increased in a dose-dependent manner. The drug appeared to be well tolerated (Siemers *et al.*, 2009).

Pfizer have a C-terminus mAb, PF-04360365, that has progressed through phase I and phase II trials. The antibody is an IgG2 delta A humanized mouse immunoglobin which may have less unwanted immunological effects than other mAbs. A phase I trial in 37 AD subjects showed the drug was well tolerated and the higher doses were affecting plasma Aβ levels. There have been no cases of VE or microhaemorrhages to date. The results of a phase II trial are being processed but progression to phase III trials is planned. It is likely that most effects of the mAb are in the periphery, essentially binding Aβ to produce a gradient from the central nervous system CNS ('peripheral sink'), but this remains to be established.

The Roche IgG$_1$ mAb, gantenerumab, targets fibrillar Aβ and a phase I trial has been completed, with a phase II trial in progress.

Other companies no doubt also have mAb under development, as these approaches target the core of the amyloid hypothesis. Failure would cast an even greater shadow over this anti-amyloid approach, although a role in prevention is still possible even if therapy of established AD is unsuccessful. The main concerns to date, apart from lack of unequivocal evidence of clinical efficacy, are VE and microhaemorrhages. If efficacy is established, the 'cost' (VE) will need to be carefully factored in when determining the clinical usefulness of this immunotherapy approach. VE may limit the doses that can be utilized and this may in turn impact on clinical end points.

55.3.1.3 POLYCLONAL ANTIBODIES

Human immunoglobulin contains polyclonal anti-Aβ antibodies (IgG and IgM classes) that bind to both oligomeric and fibrillar Aβ and at least three companies are trialling human immunoglobulin infusions for the treatment of AD. It is reassuring that such treatment is already utilized for a range of other immune-mediated conditions, and indeed individuals previously exposed to immunoglobulin therapy for other reasons have a reduced risk of subsequent AD (Fillit *et al.*, 2009).

Most trials have progressed to phase II (Grifols, Octapharma) but Baxter, in conjunction with the USA AD Cooperative Studies group, have progressed to a phase III (efficacy) trial. Interim analysis of a small number of subjects (eight on placebo, 16 on active immunoglobulin) showed near significant improvement of the ADAS-Cog at six months ($p = 0.054$) and a significant benefit on the ADAS-Cog at nine months ($p = 0.009$). On the global scale, the CGIC, significant benefits were seen at six and nine months ($p = 0.017$ and $p = 0.003$).

55.3.1.4 CSF DRAINAGE

It is possible that continuous CSF drainage will remove Aβ from the brain, essentially creating an Aβ gradient. A randomized controlled trial (RCT) of 215 subjects utilized a sham (occluded) shunt as the control arm. At nine months there was no significant difference in cognitive or global end points between the two groups. There was a total of 12 CNS infections. It is unlikely that this approach will be subjected to further trials (Silverberg *et al.*, 2008).

55.3.1.5 NEW MODES OF DELIVERY OF IMMUNOTHERAPY

A significant drawback of immunotherapy is the need to infuse the treatment, usually intravenously. Aβ fragments delivered mucosally (e.g. via the nose) have elicited an antibody response in mice, avoiding the need for parenteral administration. An oral Aβ vaccine is also being developed but efficacy is not yet in the public domain.

Other methods of delivery of Aβ, or (mAbs), include utilizing filamentous viral bacteriophages, and modifying an adenovirus to include a 'payload' of antigen or antibody.

55.3.1.6 OTHER IMMUNOTHERAPIES

Anti-Aβ DNA vaccination is a promising approach that is being trialled. Additionally, an antibody has been developed from a subject with the British APP mutation that interacts with various β-pleated protein sheets. This antibody potentially targets both amyloid and tau (as neurofibrillary tangles) as both are β sheets and it may thus have benefits beyond those of individual anti-amyloid or anti-tau therapies.

55.3.1.7 GAMMA SECRETASE INHIBITION/MODULATION

The β secretase releases the major portion of APP, and subsequently the γ secretase complex liberates Aβ – either Aβ$_{40}$ or the much more amyloidogenic and toxic Aβ$_{42}$. Gamma secretase is a transmembrane complex of four proteins – presenilin, nicastrin, Aph-1 and Pen-2 (Panza *et al.*, 2009). It has numerous substrates apart from APP, and some (e.g. Notch) are vital in embryogenesis and also important in adult cellular functions. Thus, blanket inhibition of γ secretase may have unwanted toxic effects, but the components of γ secretase can be differentially inhibited, potentially leading to efficacy against APP cleavage but also an acceptable adverse effect profile by sparing other functions of the complex.

The γ secretase inhibitor most advanced in therapeutic trials for AD is semagacestat (previously known as LY450139). Phase II results from a 14-week trial in 51 subjects have been published (Fleisher *et al.*, 2008). Fifteen subjects received placebo, 22 received 100 mg and 14 received 140 mg daily. Whilst not powered for clinical efficacy end points, there were no significant differences seen in the ADAS-Cog or the Alzheimer's Disease Cooperative Study-activities of daily living (ADCS-ADL) (functional) scale, but the three groups did differ in baseline Mini-Mental State Examination (MMSE) scores. A main outcome measure of the study was adverse events and the active treatment was associated with a significantly greater risk of skin rash and hair colour change which reversed when the drug was ceased. Gastrointestinal symptoms were insignificantly more frequent in those treated with semagacestat.

The trial also measured CSF Aβ levels and these were not significantly reduced in any of the three groups. Plasma Aβ_{40} concentration fell by 58.2 per cent in the 100-mg group and 64.6 per cent in the 140-mg group ($p < 0.001$ compared with baseline values); there was no reduction in the placebo group. This suggests an effect of the therapy, but the clinical significance of reduced plasma Aβ is yet to be established. Reduced CNS Aβ production, in a dose-dependent fashion, has also been shown in healthy men treated with semagacestat (Bateman et al., 2009) supporting the efficacy of the drug against APP cleavage. A large phase III trial (called 'IDENTITY') of semagacestat is in progress, with results expected in 2011.

Merk also has a γ secretase (MK-0752) in the phase II trial stage (Panza et al., 2009) after phase I data showed the compound reduced CSF Aβ_{40} level in healthy men (Rosen et al., 2006). At least four other γ secretase inhibitors have progressed to clinical trials (Panza et al., 2009). New molecules targeting γ secretase may not fully inhibit the enzyme but act more as a modulator of enzyme function, potentially reducing unwanted adverse effects while maintaining therapeutic efficacy (Kuker et al., 2008). Intriguingly, a substrate labelling technique has suggested that γ secretase modulators may also reduce Aβ aggregation as well as reducing Aβ production (Kuker et al., 2008). Eisai, Merck and Chiese are all developing γ secretase modulators and the Eisai compound (E2012) has progressed to early phase trials (Panza et al., 2009).

55.3.1.8   BETA SECRETASE INHIBITION

The β secretase (BACE) enzyme is very large and this poses difficulties in producing an inhibitor that would also cross the blood–brain barrier. The enzyme has however been crystallized and knowledge of its structure has assisted rational drug development. Small molecule inhibitors that bind to the active enzymatic site have been developed, including GRL-8234 which was discussed at ICAD 2009. It is a 660 dalton agent with 0.8 micromolar potency that demonstrates good selectivity and promising effects on both CSF and plasma Aβ levels in transgenic mice models. The mice also had improved memory seen in the Morris water maze.

A phase I study of another β secretase inhibitor, CTS-21166 (also known as ASP-1702), in 48 healthy volunteers has showed a reduction in plasma Aβ and phase II studies in AD subjects are planned (Panza et al., 2009). Other BACE inhibitors (e.g. KMI-429) are being developed but human trial results are yet to be reported.

55.3.1.9   ALPHA SECRETASE ENHANCEMENT

The α secretase processes APP in a non-amyloidogenic pathway by cleaving APP near the middle of the Aβ portion, preventing Aβ formation. Thus, a potential AD therapy is

α secretase enhancement. An α secretase activator EHT-0202, has recently commenced a three-month phase II evaluation in 35 AD subjects (Panza et al., 2009). Unfortunately, there is only a limited amount of natural α secretase so augmentation may not lead to a large reduction of Aβ. However, theoretically it is possible to introduce extra α secretase, akin to enzyme replacement therapy in deficiency disorders. Such replacement therapy could be genetically based.

55.3.1.10   RAGE ANTAGONISTS

RAGE is a multiligand receptor on cell surfaces. Ligands recognized by RAGE include Aβ which is first released from APP extracellularly, so uptake into cells may be inhibited by RAGE antagonism, reducing intracellular amyloid load and the inflammatory effects of Aβ. Pfizer have developed a RAGE antagonist, PF-04494700, that does inhibit plaque formation and improves behavioural performance in an APP transgenic mouse model. The compound is being developed both for AD and diabetic neuropathy.

55.3.1.11   AMYLOID AGGREGATION INHIBITORS

Glycosaminoglycans (GAGS) are components of proteoglycans, which are incorporated into the amyloid plaque. Tramiprosate ('Alzhemed') is a GAG-mimetic that binds to Aβ and inhibits fibril formation. In a phase II trial tramiprosate reduced brain levels of Aβ_{42} but did not improve cognition scores compared to placebo (Aisan et al., 2006). The drug proceeded to an 18-month phase III trial which was negative on primary end points so it will almost certainly not be further developed.

Curcumin is found in the spice tumeric and has antioxidant, anti-inflammatory and anti-aggregation properties. Curcumin binds Aβ and reduces amyloid plaque burden in mice (Garcia-Alloza et al., 2007). A phase II trial is ongoing and it may be a favoured therapy, if effective, as toxicity is likely to be low and it will be seen as a 'nutraceutical'.

Aβ binds copper and zinc and some metal chelating compounds affect Aβ aggregation, particularly into the most toxic oligomeric species. Original studies with clioquinol, a copper-zinc chelator, showed reduced Aβ deposition in a mouse model of AD (Cheney et al., 2001). A structural analogue, PBT-2, has completed a 12-week phase II trial in 78 subjects (placebo, 50 and 250 mg daily) (**Figure 55.7**) (Lannfelt et al., 2008). The trial was not powered for cognitive end points but did show a significant benefit of the 250-mg dose, compared to placebo, on two executive function subscales. There was also a highly significant ($p = 0.0060$) reduction in CSF Aβ_{42} with the 250-mg dose but it is unclear whether a reduction is desirable in a condition which is associated with lower CSF Aβ levels. Funding has now been nearly fully acquired for the phase III trial, which will proceed shortly.

Colostrinin is a proline-rich polypeptide found in sheep colostrum which affects amyloid aggregation. A small open-label study suggests possible clinical benefit (Leszek et al., 2002) and the peptide components of colostrinin are under investigation. Like curcumin, the agent may be favourable regarded due to its 'nutraceutical' categorization.

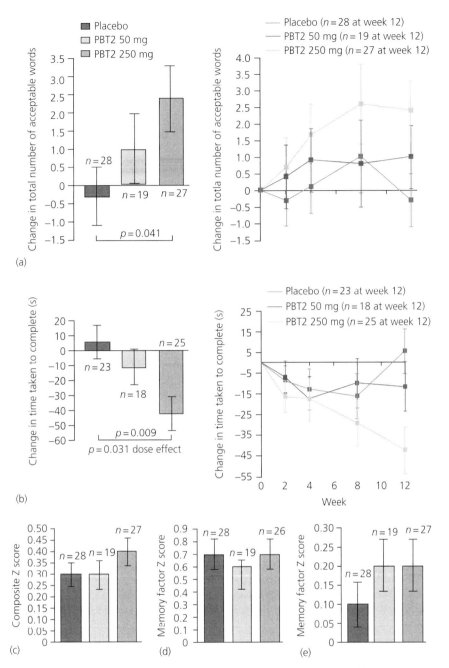

Figure 55.7 Effect of PBT2 and placebo on the change from pretreatment at 12 weeks in NTB. (a) Category fluency test, (b) trial making test part b, (c) composite factor Z-score, (d) memory factor Z-score and (e) executive factor Z-score. Executive function is not as impaired as memory, which is at floor levels, in this group of AD subjects. ADAS-cog has no tests of executive function. Lannfelt *et al.*, *Lancet Neurology* (2008).

55.3.1.12   OTHER ANTI-AMYLOID APPROACHES

Tarenflurbil (Flurizan[TM]; Myriad Genetics, Salt Lake City, UT, USA) was originally developed as an anti-inflammatory with anti-amyloid effects. In fact, it is primarily a selective amyloid-lowering agent with no anti-inflammatory effects. The anti-amyloid property is primarily through modulating γ secretase without interfering with other biological essential functions of the enzyme (Weggen *et al.*, 2003), producing shorter Aβ fragments that appear to be non-toxic. Tarenflurbil decreased brain levels of Aβ_{42} and improved spatial learning and memory performance in mouse models of AD (Eriksen *et al.*,

2003; Kukar *et al.*, 2007). In a 3-week phase I study in 48 healthy volunteers, doses up to 800 mg twice daily were as well tolerated as placebo and higher plasma drug levels were related to lower plasma Aβ_{42} levels (Galasko *et al.*, 2007). A 12-month phase II study in 210 subjects on stable doses of cholinesterase inhibitors, again using doses up to 800 mg twice daily, showed a significantly lower rate of decline in activities of daily living (ADCS-ADL) and global function (CDR-sb) compared to placebo, along with an insignificantly slower rate of cognitive decline (ADAS-Cog), in the milder AD patients (Wilcock *et al.*, 2008). In a 12-month extension all patients were treated with tarenflurbil and when those treated for the full 24 months with the agent were compared with the delayed start group, there was a significantly ($p < 0.001$) slower rate of decline on each of the primary outcome measures, suggesting a disease-modifying effect.

Unfortunately, the 18-month phase III trial results using 800 mg tarenfurbil twice daily were negative. In one of the two large studies, in 1684 randomized participants, tarenfurbil had no beneficial effect on either of the two primary outcomes: difference in change from baseline to month 18 versus placebo for the ADAS-Cog and for the ADCS-ADL (Green *et al.*, 2009). There was also no significant benefit seen in any of the secondary outcomes. The second large phase III trial was also negative. It is highly unlikely that this drug will be further developed for AD, and the negative results support those arguing against the amyloid hypothesis of AD pathogenesis.

Phenserine has both cholinesterase inhibiting and anti-amyloid effects and preclinical results were promising (Lahiri *et al.*, 2007). Subsequently a phase II trial was negative (Winblad *et al.*, 2006), perhaps due to unfavourable pharmacokinetics, but there is no indication that the drug will be further developed.

A fascinating study showed that activation of microglia by a nasally administered proteosome-based adjuvant reduced the level of fibrillar amyloid and both insoluble and soluble Aβ fragments in transgenic mice (Frenkel *et al.*, 2008). This type of approach can also be regarded as an antibody-independent immunotherapy. Human trial results are awaited.

55.3.2   Tau

55.3.2.1   IMMUNOTHERAPY

A number of potential targets exist for immunotherapy against tau. These include the microtubule binding region of tau and the pathogenic phosphorylated (as opposed to non-phosphorylated) tau. To date, tau immunotherapy has not progressed beyond animal models, but it appears promising and human trials are likely.

55.3.2.2   METHYLTHIOMINIUM CHLORIDE ('REMBER')

There has been a completed trial of the first therapeutic agent targeting tau, utilizing a drug derived from the dye used to stain neurofibrillary tangles in neuropathological studies. The agent primarily inhibits tau aggregation. The 84-week phase II study in 321 subjects showed significant benefits, compared to placebo, in the cognitive (ADAS-Cog) and global (CDR) primary end points but only for the lower doses (Wischik *et al.*, 2008). The 100-mg (high-dose) formulation may have had formulation deficiencies (cross-linking with the gelatine capsule) which have subsequently been addressed. Neuroimaging end points were also promising, including SPECT in 125 subjects (with no decline in perfusion seen with the 60-mg dose, compared to a decline in the placebo group) and FDG-PET in 19 subjects (improved metabolism in the actively treated group). The agent is poorly absorbed and diarrhoea occurred in some treated subjects. A phase III trial is soon to proceed to as formulation issues have been resolved, although unblinding remains an issue as the active agent stains urine blue.

It is noteworthy that by 2050 there will be 600 million people with significant tau pathology (BRAAK stage II or above) – not all with AD. Anti-tau therapy could thus have widespread application for those so affected, including people with AD, some frontotemporal lobar degenerations and mild cognitive impairment.

55.3.2.3   INHIBITION OF TAU HYPERPHOSPHORYLATION

Several phosphorylation inhibitors have been developed, as have agents that dephosphorylate tau. None have yet undergone extensive human testing. Selenium is an inhibitor of a tau phosphatase and has shown promising effects in mouse models. The first planned trial in AD subjects has, to date, been obstructed by a hospital ethics committee concerned about the risk of selenosis despite adequate tolerability being demonstrated in subjects treated with the same planned doses for a different condition.

55.3.3   Neurones and synapses

55.3.3.1   NERVE GROWTH FACTOR

The first trial of nerve growth factor (NGF) directly infused into the CSF was halted due to a high proportion of subjects experiencing intense axial (back) pain. This may have been due to the presence of NGF receptors in the spinal cord, but a further trial of this mode of delivery has been flagged.

A variation on this direct neurorestorative approach was examined in a phase I trial in eight patients with mild AD (Tuszynski *et al.*, 2005). Fibroblasts were extracted from their fingers, genetically modified to express human NGF then injected directly back into the cholinergic nucleus basalis of their forebrain. After a mean follow up of 22 months in six subjects, no long-term adverse effects were seen but two (non-anaesthetized) subjects moved abruptly during the procedure, causing subcortical haemorrhage. All subsequent procedures were performed under general anaesthesia. The MMSE and ADAS-Cog showed improvements in the rate of decline and serial FDG-PET scans showed significant ($p < 0.05$) widespread increases in metabolism after the procedure. Brain autopsy from one subject showed robust growth responses to the NGF expression. Unfortunately, there have been no further studies of this procedure, which is best seen as a proof of concept.

55.3.3.2   NEUROTROPHIC THERAPIES

Xaliproden is a neurotrophic factor enhancer that demonstrated neuroprotective and neurorestorative effects in preclinical studies. It proceeded to large phase III clinical trials in subjects with AD which were negative (Porzner *et al.*, 2009).

55.3.3.3   CEREBROLYSIN

The peptide mixture, extracted from pig brains, has neurotrophic activity and also reduced Aβ deposition in animal models. Human trials in AD subjects have shown that cerebrolysin infusion improves function and cognition (Alvarez et al., 2006) and is well tolerated. It is unclear why it has not yet been marketed.

55.3.3.4   PHOSPHODIESTERASE 9A INHIBITION

The Pfizer drug PF-04447943 is a high affinity inhibitor of phosphodiesterase (PDE)-9A and this action should elevate cyclic guanosine monophosphate, in turn improving synaptic function and stabilizing vulnerable synapses. To date, only preclinical data have been published. The α secretase activator EHT-0202, described above, is also a PDE inhibitor, but targets PDE-4.

55.3.4   Neurotransmitters and receptors

Most therapies directed at neurotransmitters and their receptors are symptomatic rather than disease modifying, although the distinction between these two classes of effects is less clear than originally thought. Modifying synaptic activity may have neuroprotective effects, although it has been difficult to demonstrate this with the cholinesterase inhibitors. Several new neurotransmitter approaches are being trialled and some may have to be both symptomatic and disease modifying.

55.3.4.1   HISTAMINE-3 RECEPTOR

The histamine-3 (H3) receptor is preserved even in severe AD and drugs that antagonize it increase levels of acetylcholine, noradrenaline and dopamine in the cingulate cortex and hippocampus. Two compounds are being evaluated for cognitive benefits through H3 receptor antagonism. The GSK drug (Medhurst et al., 2007) has undergone a phase I study and a Servier compound is also undergoing early phase evaluation.

55.3.4.2   5-HT6 RECEPTOR ANTAGONISM

Earlier studies with a 5-HTI$_A$ receptor antagonist, lecozatan, were negative in AD subjects, but there are numerous 5-HT receptor subtypes and antagonism of 5-HT$_6$ seems promising. This receptor is localized almost exclusively in the CNS. Antagonism enhances cholinergic and glutamatergic neurotransmission (Upton et al., 2008).

One such compound, SB-742457, is undergoing early phase trials by GSK in AD and at least five other companies have early phase trials with 5-HT$_6$ receptor antagonists. These compounds are well tolerated and cognitive benefits in AD subjects have been seen (Upton et al., 2008).

55.3.4.3   AMPA RECEPTOR MODULATION

The glutamatergic receptor AMPA is downscaled in AD and agents targeting this may improve neurotransmission in AD subjects. An initial trial of an AMPA modulator in mild cognitive impairment (MCI) cases by Servier was disastrous, with severe adverse effects, but other AMPA modulators for AD are being developed (Doraiswamy, 2002; Salloway et al., 2008).

55.3.4.4   NICOTINIC RECEPTOR AGONISTS AND MODULATORS

Galantamine, a cholinesterase inhibitor used in AD, has nicotinic receptor activity and agents that act predominantly on the α7 nicotinic receptor have been developed for AD. These agents may have other neurotransmitter benefits beyond increasing levels of acetylcholine. One agent, TC-1734 has progressed to phase II trials in MCI (Salloway et al., 2008).

55.3.4.5   MUSCARINIC RECEPTOR AGONISTS

The M1 musarinic agonist AF267B increased non-amyloidogenic APP processing and in a mouse model it has attenuated both plaque and tangle formation (Salloway et al., 2008).

Earlier trials with direct muscarinic receptor agonists were abandoned largely due to unacceptable adverse effects (these drugs included milameline, xanomeline and talsaclidine). There are several muscarinic receptor subtypes and it is possible that an effective therapy with an acceptable adverse effects profile will emerge.

55.3.5   Anti-inflammatory therapies

55.3.5.1   NSAIDS

Alzheimer recognized the presence of activated microglia cells around plaques and tangles and many other markers of inflammation have been documented. Large epidemiological studies have demonstrated a lower prevalence of AD in long-term users of NSAIDs and this led to a large number of therapeutic trials of these agents in AD, from 1993 to 2004 (Woodward, 2007). All were negative and it is unlikely that any further development of existing agents (including steroids, NSAIDs and hydroxychloroquine) will occur.

55.3.5.2   ETANERCEPT

Involvement of the proinflammatory cytokine tumour necrosis factor-α (TNF-α) in the pathogenesis of AD has long been suspected. Etanercept is a biological antagonist of TNF-α and when delivered by perispinal administration it improved cognitive function in a small number of cases from a single centre (Tobinick and Gross, 2008) but larger multicentre RCTs are needed.

55.3.6   Mitochondrial agents

55.3.6.1   LATREPIRDINE (DIMEBON)

Latrepirdine was developed as an antihistamine but has several modes of action relevant to AD. It is a weak

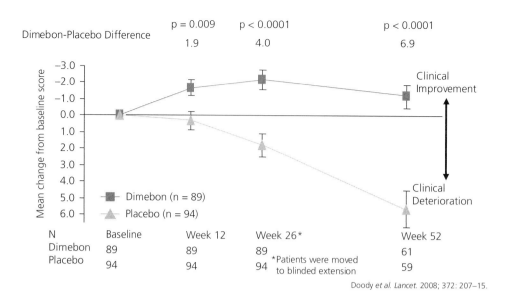

Doody *et al. Lancet.* 2008; 372: 207–15.

Figure 55.8 Dimebon – effect on cognition. Scale used is ADAS-Cog.

cholinesterase inhibitor and a weak NMDA antagonist. There are deteriorations of mitochondrial functions in AD and latrepirdine appears to enhance some of these functions. A double-blind placebo-controlled RCT in 193 subjects with AD, conducted at 11 sites in Russia, was positive for the primary and all secondary end points at six months, and also after an additional six-month blinded extension (Doody *et al.*, 2008). The primary outcome, the ADAS-Cog, improved by six to nine points over placebo at 12 months ($p < 0.001$) (see **Figure 55.8**) and similar very significant benefits over placebo were seen for the MMSE, ADCS-ADL and the NPI. The agent was well tolerated. Two large 26-week multi-centre RCTs have been conducted ('Connection' in those not on a cholinesterase inhibitor for which trial results were negative, and 'Concert' for those on such an agent – this trial is still proceeding as of July 2010). Results should be available in 2011/2012.

55.3.7 Antioxidants

Following encouraging results from a trial of the antioxidant vitamin E in patients with moderate to severe AD (Sano *et al.*, 1997) there was a negative trial of vitamin E in subjects with MCI – the therapy did not delay progression to AD over three years (Petersen *et al.*, 2005). Concerns about the cardiovascular risk of vitamin E at high doses are likely to prevent further studies of this antioxidant as an AD therapy but other agents may be examined (Frank and Gupta, 2005; see also Chapter 57, Vitamins and complementary therapies used to treat Alzheimer's disease).

55.3.8 Other agents

55.3.8.1 STATINS

A large reduced risk of AD in those using statins (3-hydroxy-3-methylglutaryl coenzyme A reductase inhibitors) has been found in most epidemiological studies, irrespective of cholesterol levels. Statins affect APP processing by γ secretase so any efficacy in AD could be due to decreased Aβ production. A small study of atorvastatin in 63 individuals showed some promising results (Sparks *et al.*, 2005) but a large phase III trial of the same agent for those with AD (Jones *et al.*, 2008) was negative. Statins may yet have a role as add-on therapy, but only positive trial results could support this usage.

55.3.8.2 PPAR-γ AGONISTS

Insulin abnormalities and insulin resistance could contribute to the neuropathology and clinical features of AD (Craft, 2005). Rosiglitazone is a PPAR-γ agonist that increases peripheral insulin sensitivity. In transgenic mice it attenuates reductions in insulin-degrading enzyme (IDE) and decreases Aβ$_{42}$ levels. Perhaps reduced insulin 'frees up' IDE to metabolize Aβ.

Trials of rosiglitazone in AD subjects showed better cognitive measures in those lacking the ApoE ε4 allele but there was no change in the plasma Aβ levels, compared with baseline (Watson *et al.*, 2005). A recent large phase III trial of rosiglitazone had negative results. This, combined with concerns about side effects, including cardiac failure, almost certainly means the end of the use of this PPAR-γ agonist in AD, but pioglitzone, potentially a safer PPAR-γ agonist, has also been trialled in AD.

55.3.8.3 HORMONE THERAPY

Driven by observational evidence in population studies (females) and studies of treatments for prostate cancer (males), the potential therapeutic role for hormones in those with AD has led to several trials. Hormone replacement therapy has not been effective for the treatment of AD in females and most recently the 'CO-STAR' study of tamoxifen/raloxifen was negative. Leuprolide, which affects levels of luteinizing hormone (Casadeus *et al.*, 2004) was ineffective in two large 52-week phase III trials conducted by Voyager Pharmaceuticals despite earlier promising phase II results.

Dehydroepiandrosterone dione has also been trialled in AD subjects, and again results were negative. It appears very unlikely that any hormonal therapy for AD will be available within the next decade.

55.3.8.4   HOMOCYSTEINE LOWERING THERAPIES

Homocysteine levels are higher in AD patients than in age-matched controls (Seshadri et al., 2002) and this may relate to reduced DNA repair or cerebrovascular effects of homocysteine, but trials of the homocysteine-lowering agent folate and vitamins B_{12} and B_6 in AD have been negative.

55.3.8.5   APOE ε4 MODULATION

The association between ApoE ε4 and AD risk has led to early phase trials of agents that modulate or reduce ε4 expression or activity (Mahley et al., 2006). One group of agents that inhibit ApoE ε4 domain interactions looks promising, but large human trials are awaited.

55.4   THE NEAR FUTURE: NEW THERAPIES LIKELY TO BE USED IN DEMENTIA

The most promising new therapies are bapineuzumab and semagacestat, although latrepirdine may also be marketed soon. It is likely that AD therapy will be used similarly to therapies for other chronic diseases – a mixture of disease-modifying and symptomatic therapies used both in combination and sequentially. Affordability is sure to be a limiting factor in uptake of new therapies.

A likely scenario is:

1. begin a cholinesterase inhibitor;
2. at the same time, use a disease-modifying drug such as bapineuzumab (monthly infusions);
3. change to another disease-modifying agent (e.g. semagacestat) as/if the disease progresses;
4. consider changing to or adding another symptomatic drug such as a $5-HT_6$ or H3 receptor modulator.

At any time, a person with AD may be on two to six different therapies, with adverse effects and affordability being the main limiting factors. One thing is certain, after 24 years of waiting we will soon have several more therapies available to fight AD.

REFERENCES

Alvarez XA, Cacabelos R, Laredo M *et al*. (2006) A 24-week, double-blind, placebo-controlled study of three doses of Cerebrolysin in patients with mild to moderate Alzheimer's disease. *European Journal of Neurology* 13: 43–54.

Aisan PS, Saumier D, Briand R *et al*. (2006) A phase I study targeting amyloid- beta with 3APS in mild-to-moderate Alzheimer disease. *Neurology* 67: 1757–63.

Bateman RJ, Siemers ER, Mawuenyega KG *et al*. (2009) A γ-secretase inhibitor decreases amyloid-β production in the central nervous system. *Annals of Neurology* 66: 48–54.

Bayer AJ, Bullock R, Jones RW *et al*. (2005) Evaluation of the safety and immunogenicity of synthetic Abeta42 (AN1792) in patients with AD. *Neurology* 64: 94–101.

Casadeus G, Zhu X, Atwood CS *et al*. (2004) Beyond oestrogen: targeting gonadotropin hormones in the treatment of Alzheimer's disease. *Current Drug Targets–CNS and Neurological Disorders* 3: 281–5.

Cheney RA, Atwood CS, Xilmas E *et al*. (2001) Treatment with a copper-zinc chelator markedly and rapidly inhibits beta-amyloid accumulation in Alzheimer's disease transgenic mice. *Neurone* 30: 655–76.

Craft S. (2005) Insulin resistance syndrome and Alzheimer's disease: age and obesity-related effects on memory, amyloid and inflammation. *Neurobiology of Aging* 26 (Suppl. 1): 65–9.

Doody R, Gavrilova S, Sano M *et al*. (2008) Effect of dimebon on cognition, activities of daily living, behaviour, and global function in patients with mild-to-moderate Alzheimer's disease: a randomised, double-blind, placebo-controlled study. *Lancet* 372: 207–15.

Doraiswamy PM. (2002) Non-cholinergic strategies for treating and preventing Alzheimer's disease. *CNS Drugs* 16: 811–24.

Eriksen JL, Sagi SA, Smith TE *et al*. (2003) NSAIDs and enantiomers of flurbiprofen target γ-secretase and lower Aβ42 *in vivo*. *Journal of Clinical Investigation* 112: 440–9.

Fillit H, Hess G, Hill J *et al*. (2009) IV immunoglobulin is associated with a reduced risk of Alzheimer disease and related disorders. *Neurology* 73: 180–5.

Frank B, Gupta S. (2005) A review of antioxidants and Alzheimer's disease. *Annals of Clinical Psychiatry* 17: 269–86.

Frenkel D, Puckett L, Petrovic S *et al*. (2008) A nasal proteosome adjuvant activates microglia and prevents amyloid deposition. *Annals of Neurology* 63: 591–601.

Fleisher AS, Raman R, Siemers ER *et al*. (2008) Phase 2 safety trial targeting amyloid β production with a γ-secretase inhibitor in Alzheimer disease. *Archives of Neurology* 65: 1031–8.

Galasko DR, Graff-Radford N, May S *et al*. (2007) Safety, tolerability, pharmacokinetics, and Abeta levels after short-term administration of R-flurbiprofen in healthy elderly individuals. *Alzheimer's Disease and Associated Disorders* 21: 292–9.

Garcia-Alloza M, Borrelli LA, Rozkaine A *et al*. (2007) Curcumin labels amyloid pathology *in vivo*, disrupts existing plaques, and partially restores neurites in an Alzheimer mouse model. *Journal of Neurochemistry* 102: 1095–104.

Green RC, Schneider LS, Amato DA *et al*. (2009) Effect of tarenflurbil on cognitive decline and activities of daily living in patients with mild Alzheimer Disease. A randomised controlled trial. *Journal of the American Medical Association* 302: 2557–64.

Hock C, Konietzko U, Steffer JR *et al*. (2003) Antibodies against beta-amyloid slow cognitive decline in Alzheimer's disease. *Nature* 38: 547–54.

Holmes C, Boche D, Wilkinson D et al. (2008) Long-term effects of Aβ42 immunisation in Alzheimer's disease: follow-up of a randomised, placebo-controlled phase I trial. Lancet 372: 216–23.

Jones R, Kivipelto M, Feldman H et al. (2008) The atorvastatin/donepezil in Alzheimer's disease srudy (LEADe): design and baseline characteristics. Alzheimer's and Dementia 4: 145–53.

Kukar T, Prescott S, Eriksen JL et al. (2007) Chronic administration of R-flurbiprofen attenuates learning impairments in transgenic amyloid precursor protein mice. BMC Neuroscience 8: 54.

Kuker TL, Ladd TB, Bann MA et al. (2008) Substrate-targeting gamma-secretase modulators. Nature 453: 925–9.

Lannfelt L, Blennow K, Zetterberg H et al. (2008) Safety, efficacy, and biomarker findings of PBT2 in targeting Aβ as a modifying therapy for Alzheimer's disease: a phase IIa, double-blind, randomised, placebo-controlled trial. Lancet Neurology 7: 779–86.

Lahiri DK, Chen D, Maloney B et al. (2007) The experimental Alzheimer's disease drug posiphen [(+)-phenserine] lowers amyloid-β peptide levels in cell culture and mice. Journal of Pharmacology and Experimental Therapeutics 320: 386–96.

Leszek J, Inglot AD, Janusz M et al. (2002) Colostrinin proline-rich polypeptide complex from ovine colostrum – a long-term study of its efficacy in Alzheimer's disease. Medical Science Monitor 8: P193–6.

Mahley RW, Weisgraber KH, Huang Y. (2006) Apolipoprotein E4: a causative factor and therapeutic target in neuropathology, including Alzheimer's disease. Proceedings of the National Academy of Science of the United States of America 103: 5644–51.

Martin BK, Szekely C, Brandt J et al. (2008) Cognitive function over time in the Alzheimer's Disease Anti-inflammatory Prevention Trial (ADAPT): results of a randomized, controlled trial of naproxen and celecoxib. Archives of Neurology 65: 896–905.

Medhurst AD, Atkins AR, Beresford IJ et al. (2007) GSK189254, a novel receptor antagonist that binds to histamine H3 receptors in Alzheimer's disease brain and improves cognitive performance in preclinical models. Journal of Pharmacology and Experimental Therapeutics 321: 1032–45.

Morgan D, Diamond DM, Gottschall PE et al. (2000) A beta peptide vaccination prevents memory loss in an animal model of Alzheimer's disease. Nature 408: 982–5.

Orgogozo J-M, Gilman S, Dartigues J-F et al. (2003) Subacute meningoencephalitis in a subset of patients with AD after Abeta42 immunization. Neurology 61: 46–51.

Panza F, Solfrizzi V, Frisardi V et al. (2009) Disease-modifying approach to the treatment of Alzheimer's disease. From α-secretase activators to γ-secretase inhibitors and modulators. Drugs and Aging 26: 537–55.

Petersen RC, Thomas RG, Grundman M et al. (2005) Vitamin E and donepezil for the treatment of mild cognitive impairment. New England Journal of Medicine 352: 2379–88.

Porzner M, Müller T, Seufferlein T et al. (2009) SR 7746A/xaliproden, a non-peptide neurotrophic compound: prospects and constraints for the treatment of nervous system diseases. Expert Opinion on Investigational Drugs 18: 1765–72.

Rosen LB, Stone JA, Plump A et al. (2006) The β secretase inhibitor MK-0752 acutely and significantly reduces CSF Aβ concentrations in humans. Alzheimer's and Dementia 2 (Suppl. 1): S79. (Abstr. O4-03-02)

Salloway S, Mintzer J, Weiner MF, Cummings JL. (2008) Disease-modifying therapies in Alzheimer's disease. Alzheimer's and Dementia 4: 65–79.

Salloway S, Sperling R, Gilman S et al. (2009) A phase 2 multiple ascending dose trial of bapineuzumab in mild to moderate Alzheimer disease. Neurology 73: 2061–70.

Sano M, Ernesto C, Thomas RG et al. (1997) A controlled trial of selegiline, alpha-tocopherol, or both as treatment for Alzheimer's disease. New England Journal of Medicine 336: 1216–22.

Seshadri S, Beiser A, Selhub J et al. (2002) Plasma homocysteine as a risk factor for dementia and Alzheimer's disease. New England Journal of Medicine 346: 476–83.

Schenk D, Barbour R, Dunn W et al. (1999) Immunization with amyloid-beta attenuates Alzheimer-disease-like-pathology in PDAPP mouse. Nature 400: 173–7.

Siemers E, Dean R, Lachno D et al. (2009) Measurement of cerebrospinal fluid total tau and phospho-tau in phase 2 trials of therapies targeting Aβ. Alzheimer and Dementia 5: 258–8.

Silverberg GD, Mayo M, Saul T et al. (2008) Continuous CSF drainage in AD: results of a double-blind, randomised, placebo-controlled study. Neurology 71: 202–9.

Sparks DL, Sabbagh MN, Connor DJ et al. (2005) Atorvastatin for the treatment of mild to moderate Alzheimer's disease: preliminary results. Archives of Neurology 62: 753–7.

Summers WK, Majovski IV, Marsh GM et al. (1986) Oral tetrahydroaminoacridine in long-term treatment of senile dementia, Alzheimer type. New England Journal of Medicine 315: 1241–5.

Tobinick EL, Gross H. (2008) Rapid cognitive improvement in Alzheimer's disease following perispinal etanercept administration. Journal of Neuroinflammation 5: 2.

Tuszynski MH, Thal L, Pay M et al. (2005) A phase I clinical trial of nerve growth factor gene therapy for Alzheimer disease. Nature Medicine 11: 551–5.

Upton N, Chuang TT, Hunter AJ, Virley DJ. (2008) 5-HT6 receptor antagonists as novel cognitive enhancing agents for Alzheimer's disease. Neurotherapeutics 5: 458–69.

Watson GS, Cholerton BA, Reger MA et al. (2005) Preserved cognition in patients with early Alzheimer's disease and amnestic mild cognitive impairment after treatment with rosiglitazone; a preliminary study. American Journal of Geriatric Psychiatry 13: 950–8.

Weggen S, Eriksen JL, Sagi SA et al. (2003) Aβ42-lowering nonsteroidal anti-inflammatory drugs preserve intra-membrane cleavage of the amyloid precursor protein (APP) and ErbE-4 receptor and signalling through the APP intracellular domain. Journal of Biological Chemistry 278: 30748–54.

Wilcock G, Black S, Hendrix S et al. (2008) Efficacy and safety of tarenflurbil in mild to moderate Alzheimer's disease: a randomised phase II trial. Lancet Neurology 7: 483–93.

Winblad B, Giacobini E, Froelich L et al. (2006) Double-blind placebo-controlled evaluation of the safety and efficacy of phenserine tartrate for the treatment of mild to moderate Alzheimer disease. Paper presented at the 9th International Geneva/Springfield Symposium on Advances in Alzheimer Therapy, April 2006 (Abstr. 11A).

Wischik C, Bentham P, Wischik D *et al.* (2008) Tau aggregation inhibitor (TAI) therapy with rember[TM] arrests disease progression in mild and moderate Alzheimer's disease over 50 weeks. Paper presented at International conference on Alzheimer disease, Chicago, July 2008. Abstract in *Alzheimer's and Dementia*. 4: T167.

Woodward M. (2007) Anti-inflammatory drugs. In: Ritchie CW, Ames D, Masters CL, Cummings J (eds). *Therapeutic strategies in dementia*. Oxford: Atlas Medical Publishing, 111–19.

Stem cell therapies for Alzheimer's disease and other dementias

ANTIGONI EKONOMOU AND STEPHEN L MINGER

56.1 CELL THERAPY IN THE CENTRAL NERVOUS SYSTEM

Current dementia treatments alleviatiate symptoms but there are no therapies that are disease modifying, or that delay or reverse the symptoms of dementia. Thus, the need for novel therapeutic strategies is of paramount importance. One such novel strategy is the cell replacement of lost neurones.

The potential therapeutic efficacy of cell therapy in the central nervous system (CNS) was first demonstrated in the late 1980s and early 1990s by pioneering translational research in Sweden. Based on a series of elegant studies which demonstrated functional benefit of transplanted post-mitotic fetal dopaminergic neurones in animal models of Parkinson's disease, research quickly translated into assessing the potential of these cells in human patients. The first published reports in humans appeared in the early 1990s (Freed *et al.*, 1990; Lindvall *et al.*, 1990; Spencer *et al.*, 1992; Freeman *et al.*, 1995) where fetal dopaminergic neurones were grafted into the striatum of Parkinson's disease. These cells engrafted and released dopamine, resulting in long-term and sustained improvement in some but not all patients, with no evidence of tumour formation (Piccini *et al.*, 1997). Although the use of fetal cells for transplantation studies has generally been abandoned due to limited availability of fetal tissue, the large variability in tissue quality and gestational age and ethical issues associated with tissue procurement, these experiments were a very valuable source of information and proof-of-concept of the therapeutic potential of cellular replacement in the CNS.

Following on from the studies using post-mitotic fetal tissue, attention turned to the generation of alternative cell populations that might impart the same clinical benefit as fetal tissue, but without the continuous reliance on human fetuses as a source population. The generation of highly expandable neural stem cells from developing brain (Reynolds and Weiss, 1992; Minger *et al.*, 1996) heralded a new era in the potential for cell therapy in the CNS. Over the last 15 years, a number of studies have been performed using transplanted stem cells in a variety of animal models of human neurological conditions, many of which demonstrated significant functional improvement following implantation (Bjorklund *et al.*, 2002; Machimoto *et al.*, 2007; Van't Hof *et al.*, 2007; Muraoka *et al.*, 2008). These results have stimulated the prospects for the use of stem cells for transplantation in humans.

56.2 STEM CELLS

Within the last 30 years researchers discovered, isolated and expanded stem cells from a variety of human tissues, revealing a new scientific field with enormous therapeutic potential. Although the first human stem cells derived from the haematopoietic system were used many years ago in bone marrow transplantation in the treatment of leukaemia, there has been an explosion of research in stem cell biology and a huge increase in both public and scientific interest in this field.

Stem cells are all cells that are characterized by the ability of self-renewal and the potential to differentiate into a variety of other cell types. They can be derived from the inner cell mass of the early embryo (embryonic stem cells), from the developing fetus (fetal stem cells) and from the adult body (adult stem cells). Embryonic stem cells are considered to be pluripotent, as they can potentially differentiate into all 210 different cell types of the human body whereas fetal and adult stem cells are generally defined as multipotent and thus can only differentiate into the cell types forming the organ from where they are isolated. Some but not all stem cell populations can proliferate *in vitro* for extended periods under defined culture conditions, and can be expanded and stored without losing their potency and retaining a normal karyotype. Once they are established as cell lines, they can be 'deposited' in stem cell banks around the world and can be made available to researchers. Based on these properties, the therapeutic potential of stem cells can be easily recognized in conditions that result in loss of key functional cell groups, such as pancreatic beta cells (as in Type I diabetes), hepatic cells or dopaminergic neurones (as in the case of Parkinson's disease) by introducing stem cells or their progeny to replace the function of cells lost in these diseases.

Under a very controlled regulatory process in the UK, researchers are allowed to use human embryos that are in excess or not suitable from *in vitro* fertilization (IVF) treatment programmes for the derivation of embryonic stem cells, with parents' consent. Fetal stem cells can be obtained from human fetuses that are available as a result of surgical abortion under the Polkinghorne guidelines, again with parents' consent and appropriate ethical approval. Adult stem cells can be isolated from a variety of organs of the human body, when their location permits their derivation without serious side effects.

How feasible is it to create a specific set of cells for treatment of all diseases/injuries that result from cell loss? First, the immunocompatibility of the transplanted cells and the patient is crucial for the success of the cell replacement treatment. If that is not possible, immunosuppression of the patient or some other technique to evade immune recognition is necessary. All types of stem cells destined to be used for transplantation should be isolated and expanded under good manufacturing process conditions. Optimization of the culture techniques and protocols in order to create sufficient cell numbers for patient treatment is necessary. Modification of the current protocols for the partial or terminal differentiation of stem cells to the desired cell type in high percentages is of high importance. The manipulation of the micro-environment at the site of transplantation that will lead to the optimal survival and anatomical and functional integration of the transplanted cells is a crucial step for cell replacement therapy. Finally, each disease entity should be assessed for individual factors that may influence the optimal therapeutic efficacy of stem cell therapy. How do all of these have an effect on the use of stem cells for cell replacement in the human nervous system and, more specifically, for the treatment of dementias?

56.3 STEM CELLS TO TREAT DEMENTIA

All trials are and should be under very strict regulatory control in order to avoid any scientific misconduct and ethical implications. The first approved clinical safety trial by the Food and Drug Administration using embryonic stem cell-derived oligodendrocytes for the treatment of spinal cord injuries is underway by the biotechnology company Geron (USA) (Couzin, 2009). It is the first one involving the use of human embryonic stem cells in cell replacement therapy and, as such, has received an immense amount of media and patient attention. This potential represents a watershed moment in the evolution of cell therapy for CNS and other human degenerative and traumatic conditions. Currently, there are no such trials for cell replacement in the case of dementing illnesses. Why is that so?

Dementia describes a group of symptoms that occur after various diseases and conditions that lead to the loss of mental functions, changes in personality, mood and behaviour severe enough to interfere with a person's daily functioning (see Chapter 1, Dementia: historical overview). Certain causes of dementia can be reversed, if the underlying cause can be treated, such as alcohol-related dementia. The incurable forms of dementia include Alzheimer's disease (AD, the most common cause of dementia) (Small and Cappai, 2006), vascular dementia, dementia with Lewy bodies (DLB) and frontotemporal dementia (including Pick's disease). All these dementias are characterized by neuronal cell loss which eventually leads to disruption of neuronal circuits. Lost cells are mainly glutamatergic and cholinergic neurones located in the hippocampus, cortex and basal forebrain, areas responsible for memory, cognition, personality and emotional behaviour. Thus, the use of stem cells as a cell replacement therapy provides a very appealing option. Indeed, the following animal studies have provided very encouraging results.

First, cholinergic-rich tissue (Fine *et al.*, 1985) and peripheral cholinergic neurones (Itakura *et al.*, 1992) have been transplanted in a rat animal model of AD with lesions of nucleus basalis of Meynert. These animal trials showed a memory improvement which indicated a partial neuronal rescue in the disease model. In aged rats, transplantation of human neural stem cells differentiated into neurones and astrocytes and improved the cognitive function of the aged animals, with no signs of tumour formation, confirming a beneficial effect of the transplanted cells in the brain (Qu *et al.*, 2001). In another, more recent study, Wang *et al.*, (2006) transplanted neurospheres and human embryonic stem cells in the cortex of a mouse model of AD produced by ibotenic acid injections into nucleus basalis of Meynert. Neurosphere transplantation produced cholinergic neurones and improved the cognitive function of the lesioned animals in contrast to the embryonic stem cell transplantation that produced teratocarcinomas.

Another aspect of transplanted stem cells is their potential use as 'drug delivery vehicles'. Stem cells can be genetically modified by using plasmid-based or viral-based (using retroviruses or lentiviruses) insertion of an exogenous DNA in the stem cells. After transplantation, the genetically modified stem cells and their progeny will express the 'foreign' DNA *in situ*. The exogenous DNA may be that of a neurotrophic factor, a neuroprotective agent, an enzyme, etc. (Ourednik *et al.*, 2002; Tai and Svendsen, 2004; Ben-Dor *et al.*, 2006; Dass *et al.*, 2006; Suter *et al.*, 2006). Even better, some stem cells such as neural stem cells also express and secrete neurotrophic and neuroprotective factors. Therefore, the transplantation of stem cells at the affected area may possibly modify a 'hostile' micro-environment and promote the survival of the remaining neurones and even the rescue of the ones that are affected.

There are already some very encouraging animal studies of other neurodegenerative diseases supporting this view. One using glial-derived neurotrophic factor (GDNF)-expressing neural precursor cells showed successful integration and differentiation of these cells as well as a stable GDNF expression for up to four months after the surgery, which was also accompanied by a behavioural improvement in a rat model of Parkinson's disease (Akerud et al., 2001). Similarly, GDNF-expressing neural stem cells survived and expanded after grafting when transplanted in quinolinate-lesioned mouse striata, prevented neuronal degeneration and improved behaviour in the lesioned mice (Pineda et al., 2007). In addition, genetically engineered neural stem cells overexpressing nerve growth factor were transplanted in the cortex of an animal model of cognitive impairment, were integrated in the local neuronal circuit and improved their cognitive impairment (Wu et al., 2008).

As the neuronal cell loss in dementia is widespread and progressive, transplantation for cell replacement may be technically challenging or insufficient. Thus, an alternative therapeutic strategy would be the activation of stem cells already present in the adult brain that could potentially provide an endogenous source of replacement neurones.

Historically, the first indication of the presence of dividing cells in the brain was by Altman and Das (1965), although it took many more years for the scientific community to abolish the dogma by Santiago Ramon y Cajal that the adult brain is not capable of generating new neurones. It took a few more decades to prove the existence of adult neurogenesis, first in birds (Goldman and Nottebohm, 1983) and then in other organisms, including humans; (Eriksson et al., 1998; van Praag et al., 2002; Carleton et al., 2003; Sanai et al., 2004; Zupanc, 2006; for review see Nottebohm, 2002; Jordan et al., 2007).

It is now widely accepted there are two main neurogenic regions (niches) where multipotent neural stem cells (NSCs) and their progeny are located: the subventricular zone (SVZ), underlying the wall of the lateral ventricles, and the dentate gyrus subgranular zone in the hippocampus. NSCs can be isolated from the SVZ and the hippocampus and develop in culture with the subsequent potential to differentiate into neurones, astrocytes or oligodendrocytes, thus displaying characteristics of bona fide stem cells (Reynolds and Weiss, 1992; Palmer et al., 1997).

In the healthy adult brain, NSCs constantly replace neurones in the olfactory bulb and in the hippocampus, but not all of the newly generated neurones survive and integrate into the local neuronal circuit (Kempermann and Gage, 1999; Temple and Alvarez-Buylla, 1999; Ming and Song, 2005). Production of new neurones can be influenced by a variety of stimulatory and inhibitory factors; for example it is known that certain hormones, growth factors, antidepressants, anti-inflammatory drugs, caloric restriction, physical exercise and learning, and cholinesterase inhibitors all have a positive effect on endogenous neurogenesis. In comparison, stress, opiates, ageing and seizures have negative effects on the production of neural stem cells. These factors exert their effects selectively on proliferation, migration, differentiation and survival of NSCs and their progeny (for review see Ming and Song, 2005; Abrous et al., 2005; Goldman, 2007; Hsu et al., 2007). Thus, one can increase endogenous neurogenesis by promoting positive environmental factors or delivery of pro-neurogenic pharmacological agents and negating inhibitory influences where possible.

Certain neurological conditions have a stimulatory effect on adult neurogenesis, at least early in the course of disease or damage. Studies using animal models of neurodegenerative diseases and injuries have shown that there is an upregulation in number of NSCs (Levine and Reynolds, 1999; Arvidsson et al., 2002; Kleindienst et al., 2005) and, in some cases, subsequent migration from one of the neurogenic niches, the SVZ, to the affected areas where some of them can differentiate into neurones, replacing the ones lost due to the disease and resulting in an improved outcome (Magavi and Macklis, 2001). This has been proved also true for humans, where recent studies have provided the first evidence that regenerative mechanisms may be active in adult human brain in response to ischaemia (Jin et al., 2006; Minger et al., 2007; Mattiesen et al., 2009). This potential 'regeneration' is consistent with recent clinical findings indicating that delayed post-stroke improvement in cognition is common in older patients with mild vascular cognitive impairment (Ballard et al., 2003).

In the case of dementia, a variety of animal models have been developed, bearing the human genes that are mutated in the familial forms of the disease. Depending on the promoter used for the gene expression and the gene that is mutated, as well as if they are single, double or triple transgenics, neuropathological landmarks of the dementias start appearing at different age and endogenous neurogenesis is differently altered. None of the models though recapitulates the full neuropathological changes observed in AD patients.

Specifically, in the case of animal models of dementia, at least four different genes responsible for hereditary dementing illnesses have been introduced into mice in their mutant form: APP (amyloid precursor protein), presenilins (PS)1 and PS2 and tau. Transgenic mice carrying different PS1 P117L (Wen et al., 2002) and M146V (Wang et al., 2004) mutations exhibit reduced neurogenesis in the hippocampus compared with their non-transgenic littermates. In contrast to these findings (Chevallier et al., 2005), observed a transient, enhanced proliferation of progenitor cells in mice bearing the A246E PS1 mutation. Using two different strains of mice over overexpressing the Swedish double mutation of APP (Dong et al., 2004 and Haughey et al., 2002), demonstrated a decreased capacity for cell proliferation in the hippocampus of transgenic mice compared with their non-transgenic littermates. In contrast Jin et al. (2004a), showed increased neuronal production in the dentate gyrus and SVZ of mice with both the Swedish and Indiana mutations of APP.

The differences between these studies may be due to differences in the protocols for the creation of the transgenic mice which translate into different spatial and temporal neuropathology and cognitive performance, leading to different experimental results. Nevertheless, these models confirmed that the neurogenic potential is still present and active in the disease – alas possibly less effective – and constitute a very valuable tool for studying how manipulation of endogenous neurogenesis can be used as an endogenous cell replacement therapy.

A few experimental studies on endogenous neurogenesis have been performed using brain tissue from patients suffering from dementia. Post-mortem analysis of human brains by Jin et al. (2004b) showed increased numbers of proliferating neuronal progenitors in the hippocampus of patients with AD at all stages of the disease. Furthermore, our previous work (Ziabreva et al., 2006) revealed significant increases in nestin-positive neural stem cells and a decrease in Musashi-1-positive progenitors in the SVZ of AD patients at the latest stages of the disease, suggesting an altered turnover of neural stem cells and their progeny in AD.

Hoglinger et al. (2004) suggested a dopaminergic control on endogenous neurogenesis, as they found reduced numbers of proliferating cells in the SVZ and fewer neural precursor cells in the olfactory bulb and dentate gyrus of individuals with Parkinson's disease with and without dementia. Using autopsy tissue (Ziabreva et al., 2007), showed a significant reduction of Musashi-1-expressing neural progenitors in the SVZ of DLB patients which was also associated with the cholinergic impairment detected in these patients. These two studies also confirm a change in endogenous neurogenesis in a different form of dementia and highlight a close association between neurogenesis and neurotransmission; possibly a new potential drug target for dementia.

All the studies point to the fact of an altered endogenous neurogenic mechanism in dementia. Currently, it is not known if these alterations are a compensatory mechanism to the brain insult or a consequence of the disease. Further time-course experiments in animal models and in human autopsy tissue before any clinical changes are evident compared to later stages of disease progression are required to clarify this. It is still uncertain the extent to which endogenous neurogenic mechanism still exists in dementia, thus understanding the mechanism(s) how dementia affects or alters neurogenesis and the fate of newly generated cells will be of great importance. Furthermore, research for the discovery of new factors that can enhance all aspects of endogenous neurogenesis will be of great benefit for the potential use of endogenous neural stem cells in the treatment of dementia.

56.4 CONCLUSION

Stem cells provide a very appealing approach for the treatment of neurodegenerative diseases. There have been many groundbreaking studies highlighting their exciting therapeutic opportunity; alas there are still numerous hurdles to be overcome before they become a routine treatment. As the number of laboratories working in the field of stem cell biology is constantly increasing and exciting results add to our stem cell knowledge, our optimism remains for their use in the treatment of disorders such as dementia.

REFERENCES

Abrous DN, Koehl M, Le Moal M. (2005) Adult neurogenesis: From precursors to network and physiology. *Physiological Reviews* **85**: 523–69.

Akerud P, Canals JM, Snyder EY, Arenas E. (2001) Neuroprotection through delivery of glial cell line-derived neurotrophic factor by neural stem cells in a mouse model of Parkinson's disease. *Journal of Neuroscience* **21**: 8108–18.

Altman J, Das GD. (1965) Autoradiographic and histological evidence of postnatal hippocampal neurogenesis in rats. *Journal of Comparative Neurology* **124**: 319–35.

Arvidsson A, Collin T, Kirik D et al. (2002) Neuronal replacement from endogenous precursors in the adult brain after stroke. *Nature Medicine* **8**: 963–70.

Ballard C, Rowan E, Stephens S et al. (2003) Prospective follow-up study between 3 and 15 months after stroke: Improvements and decline in cognitive function among dementia-free stroke survivors >75 years of age. *Stroke* **34**: 2440–4.

Ben-Dor I, Itsykson P, Goldenberg D et al. (2006) Lentiviral vectors harboring a dual-gene system allow high and homogeneous transgene expression in selected polyclonal human embryonic stem cells. *Molecular Therapy* **14**: 255–67.

Bjorklund LM, Sanchez-Pernaute R, Chung S et al. (2002) Embryonic stem cells develop into functional dopaminergic neurons after transplantation in a Parkinson rat model. *Proceedings of the National Academy of Sciences of the United States of America* **99**: 2344–9.

Carleton A, Petreanu LT, Lansford R et al. (2003) Becoming a new neuron in the adult olfactory bulb. *Nature Neuroscience* **6**: 507–18.

Chevallier NL, Soriano S, Kang DE et al. (2005) Perturbed neurogenesis in the adult hippocampus associated with presenilin-1 A246E mutation. *American Journal of Pathology* **167**: 151–9.

Couzin J. (2009) Biotechnology. Celebration and concern over U.S. trial of embryonic stem cells. *Science* **323**: 568.

Dass B, Olanow CW, Kordower JH. (2006) Gene transfer of trophic factors and stem cell grafting as treatments for Parkinson's disease. *Neurology* **66**: S89–103.

Dong H, Goico B, Martin M et al. (2004) Modulation of hippocampal cell proliferation, memory, and amyloid plaque deposition in APPsw (Tg2576) mutant mice by isolation stress. *Neuroscience* **127**: 601–9.

Eriksson PS, Perfilieva E, Bjork-Eriksson T et al. (1998) Neurogenesis in the adult human hippocampus. *Nature Medicine* **4**: 1313–7.

Fine A, Dunnett SB, Bjorklund A, Iversen SD. (1985) Cholinergic ventral forebrain grafts into the neocortex improve passive avoidance memory in a rat model of Alzheimer disease. *Proceedings of the National Academy of Sciences of the United States of America* **82**: 5227–30.

Freed CR, Breeze RE, Rosenberg NL et al. (1990) Therapeutic effects of human fetal dopamine cells transplanted in a patient with Parkinson's disease. *Progress in Brain Research* **82**: 715–21.

Freeman TB, Olanow CW, Hauser RA et al. (1995) Bilateral fetal nigral transplantation into the postcommissural putamen in Parkinson's disease. Annals of Neurology 38: 379–88.

Goldman SA. (2007) Disease targets and strategies for the therapeutic modulation of endogenous neural stem and progenitor cells. Clinical Pharmacology and Therapeutics 82: 453–60.

Goldman SA, Nottebohm F. (1983) Neuronal production, migration, and differentiation in a vocal control nucleus of the adult female canary brain. Proceedings of the National Academy of the Sciences of the United States of America 80: 2390–4.

Haughey NJ, Liu D, Nath A et al. (2002) Disruption of neurogenesis in the subventricular zone of adult mice, and in human cortical neuronal precursor cells in culture, by amyloid beta-peptide: Implications for the pathogenesis of Alzheimer's disease. NeuroMolecular Medicine 1: 125–35.

Hoglinger GU, Rizk P, Muriel MP et al. (2004) Dopamine depletion impairs precursor cell proliferation in Parkinson disease. Nature Neuroscience 7: 726–35.

Hsu YC, Lee DC, Chiu IM. (2007) Neural stem cells, neural progenitors, and neurotrophic factors. Cell Transplantation 16: 133–50.

Itakura T, Umemoto M, Kamei I et al. (1992) Autotransplantation of peripheral cholinergic neurons into the brains of Alzheimer model rats. Acta Neurochirurigca (Wien) 115: 127–32.

Jin K, Galvan V, Xie L et al. (2004a) Enhanced neurogenesis in Alzheimer's disease transgenic (PDGF-APPSw,Ind) mice. Proceedings of the National Academy of Sciences of the United States of America 101: 13363–7.

Jin K, Peel AL, Mao XO et al. (2004b) Increased hippocampal neurogenesis in Alzheimer's disease. Proceedings of the National Academy of Sciences of the United States of America 101: 343–7.

Jin K, Wang X, Xie L et al. (2006) Evidence for stroke-induced neurogenesis in the human brain. Proceedings of the National Academy of Science of the United States of America 103: 13198–202.

Jordan JD, Ma DK, Ming GL, Song H. (2007) Cellular niches for endogenous neural stem cells in the adult brain. CNS and Neurological Disorders Drug Targets 6: 336–41.

Kempermann G, Gage FH. (1999) Experience-dependent regulation of adult hippocampal neurogenesis: effects of long-term stimulation and stimulus withdrawal. Hippocampus 9: 321–32.

Kleindienst A, McGinn MJ, Harvey HB et al. (2005) Enhanced hippocampal neurogenesis by intraventricular S100B infusion is associated with improved cognitive recovery after traumatic brain injury. Journal of Neurotrauma 22: 645–55.

Levine JM, Reynolds R. (1999) Activation and proliferation of endogenous oligodendrocyte precursor cells during ethidium bromide-induced demyelination. Experimental Neurology 160: 333–47.

Lindvall O, Brundin P, Widner H et al. (1990) Grafts of fetal dopamine neurons survive and improve motor function in Parkinson's disease. Science 247: 574–7.

Machimoto T, Yasuchika K, Komori J et al. (2007) Improvement of the survival rate by fetal liver cell transplantation in a mice lethal liver failure model. Transplantation 84: 1233–9.

Magavi SS, Macklis JD. (2001) Manipulation of neural precursors in situ: Induction of neurogenesis in the neocortex of adult mice. Neuropsychopharmacology 25: 816–35.

Mattiesen WR, Tauber SC, Gerber J et al. (2009) Increased neurogenesis after hypoxic-ischemic encephalopathy in humans is age related. Acta Neuropathologica 117: 525–34.

Ming GL, Song H. (2005) Adult neurogenesis in the mammalian central nervous system. Annual Review of Neuroscience 28: 223–50.

Minger SL, Fisher LJ, Ray J, Gage FH. (1996) Long-term survival of transplanted basal forebrain cells following in vitro propagation with fibroblast growth factor-2. Experimental Neurology 141: 12–24.

Minger SL, Ekonomou A, Carta EM et al. (2007) Endogenous neurogenesis in the human brain following cerebral infarction. Regenerative Medicine 2: 69–74.

Muraoka K, Shingo T, Yasuhara T et al. (2008) Comparison of the therapeutic potential of adult and embryonic neural precursor cells in a rat model of Parkinson disease. Journal of Neurosurgery 108: 149–59.

Nottebohm F. (2002) Why are some neurons replaced in adult brain? Journal of Neuroscience 22: 624–8.

Ourednik J, Ourednik V, Lynch WP et al. (2002) Neural stem cells display an inherent mechanism for rescuing dysfunctional neurons. Nature Biotechnology 20: 1103–10.

Palmer TD, Takahashi J, Gage FH. (1997) The adult rat hippocampus contains primordial neural stem cells. Molecular and Cellular Neuroscience 8: 389–404.

Piccini P, Morrish PK, Turjanski N et al. (1997) Dopaminergic function in familial Parkinson's disease: A clinical and 18F-dopa positron emission tomography study. Annals of Neurology 41: 222–9.

Pineda JR, Rubio N, Akerud P et al. (2007) Neuroprotection by GDNF-secreting stem cells in a Huntington's disease model: Optical neuroimage tracking of brain-grafted cells. Gene Therapy 14: 118–28.

Qu T, Brannen CL, Kim HM, Sugaya K. (2001) Human neural stem cells improve cognitive function of aged brain. Neuroreport 12: 1127–32.

Reynolds BA, Weiss S. (1992) Generation of neurons and astrocytes from isolated cells of the adult mammalian central nervous system. Science 255: 1707–10.

Sanai N, Tramontin AD, Quinones-Hinojosa A et al. (2004) Unique astrocyte ribbon in adult human brain contains neural stem cells but lacks chain migration. Nature 427: 740–4.

Small DH, Cappai R. (2006) Alois Alzheimer and Alzheimer's disease: A centennial perspective. Journal of Neurochemistry 99: 708–10.

Spencer DD, Robbins RJ, Naftolin F et al. (1992) Unilateral transplantation of human fetal mesencephalic tissue into the caudate nucleus of patients with Parkinson's disease. New England Journal of Medicine 327: 1541–8.

Suter DM, Cartier L, Bettiol E et al. (2006) Rapid generation of stable transgenic embryonic stem cell lines using modular lentivectors. Stem Cells 24: 615–23.

Tai YT, Svendsen CN. (2004) Stem cells as a potential treatment of neurological disorders. *Current Opinion in Pharmacology* **4**: 98–104.

Temple S, Alvarez-Buylla A. (1999) Stem cells in the adult mammalian central nervous system. *Current Opinion in Neurobiology* **9**: 135–41.

van Praag H, Schinder AF, Christie BR *et al.* (2002) Functional neurogenesis in the adult hippocampus. *Nature* **415**: 1030–4.

Van't Hof W, Mal N, Huang Y *et al.* (2007) Direct delivery of syngeneic and allogeneic large-scale expanded multipotent adult progenitor cells improves cardiac function after myocardial infarct. *Cytotherapy* **9**: 477–87.

Wang R, Dineley KT, Sweatt JD, Zheng H. (2004) Presenilin 1 familial Alzheimer's disease mutation leads to defective associative learning and impaired adult neurogenesis. *Neuroscience* **126**: 305–12.

Wang TT, Jing AH, Luo XY *et al.* (2006) Neural stem cells: Isolation and differentiation into cholinergic neurons. *Neuroreport* **17**: 1433–6.

Wen PH, Shao X, Shao Z *et al.* (2002) Overexpression of wild type but not an FAD mutant presenilin-1 promotes neurogenesis in the hippocampus of adult mice. *Neurobiology of Disease* **10**: 8–19.

Wu S, Sasaki A, Yoshimoto R *et al.* (2008) Neural stem cells improve learning and memory in rats with Alzheimer's disease. *Pathobiology* **75**: 186–94.

Ziabreva I, Perry E, Perry R *et al.* (2006) Altered neurogenesis in Alzheimer's disease. *Journal of Psychosomatic Research* **61**: 311–6.

Ziabreva I, Ballard C, Johnson M *et al.* (2007) Loss of Musashi1 in Lewy body dementia associated with cholinergic deficit. *Neuropathology and Applied Neurobiology* **33**: 586–90.

Zupanc GK. (2006) Neurogenesis and neuronal regeneration in the adult fish brain. *Journal of Comparative Physiology. A, Neuroethology, Sensory, Neural, and Behavioral Physiology* **192**: 649–70.

57

Vitamins and complementary therapies used to treat Alzheimer's disease

DENNIS CHANG, DILIP GHOSH AND ALAN BENSOUSSAN

57.1 INTRODUCTION

The current conventional treatment of Alzheimer's disease (AD) offers only modest symptomatic relief, which is not satisfactory considering the magnitude of the disease burden on patients and community as a whole. Several classes of pharmaceutical agents are currently used for the management of AD, among which cholinesterase inhibitors and glutamate receptor antagonists are suggested to produce the best clinical outcomes (Farlow *et al.*, 2008).

Complementary and alternative medicine (CAM) has an extensive history of use worldwide and several interventions have been explored as therapeutic options for the management or prevention of AD. According to a recent US national survey conducted by the National Center for Complementary and Alternative Medicine, approximately 38 per cent of US adults and approximately 12 per cent of children use some form of CAM (Barnes *et al.*, 2008). The World Health Organization (WHO) estimates that almost 75 per cent of the world's population has therapeutic experience with herbal remedies (Dubey *et al.*, 2004).

The use of CAM for treatment of ageing-related disorders dates to 5000 years ago in ancient China where herbal remedies were used to boost memory function and increase longevity. The common forms of CAM currently used in the management of AD include herbal medicine (including Western herbal medicine, Chinese herbal medicine, Ayurvedic medicine), vitamins and dietary supplements (e.g. fish oil), acupuncture, aromatherapy, mind-body therapy (e.g.

medication, qigong exercise), physical therapies (e.g. chiropractic, reflexology, remedial massage, therapeutic touch), music therapy and melatonin and light therapy (**Table 57.1**).

This chapter focuses in particular on the scientific evidence in support of the use of herbal medicine, vitamins and fish oil in the management of AD.

57.2 HERBAL MEDICINE FOR AD

Herbal medicines have been used in many cultures over thousands of years to boost memory function and manage behavioural and psychological symptoms. Specific herbs which have attracted most attention include *Ginkgo biloba*, *Bacopa monniera*, *Huperzia serrata*, *Panax ginseng*, *Curcuma longa* and *Melissa officinalis*. Tea, especially green tea (*Camellia sinensis*) is also considered beneficial for cognitive function owing to its antioxidant effects. The mechanisms of action, adverse effects and herb–drug interactions of these herbal medicines for AD are summarized in **Table 57.2**.

Unlike pharmaceutical agents, herbal medicines often contain multiple bioactive components which can affect different therapeutic targets of diseases with multifactorial/multisystem pathophysiological components such as dementia. In addition, evidence suggests that the complex chemical mixtures of herbal medicines enhance therapeutic efficacy by facilitating synergistic action via various mechanisms; for example, constituents of herbal extracts

Table 57.1 Overview of common vitamins and complementary therapies for the treatment of Alzheimer's disease.

Common vitamins and complementary therapies	
Herbal medicine	*Ginkgo biloba*
	Huperzia serrata (Huperzine A)
	Bacopa monniera
	Curcuma longa
	Panax ginseng
	Melissa officinalis
	Camellia sinensis (tea)
Vitamins and dietary supplements	Vitamins C and E
	Vitamin B and folic acid
	Vitamin D
	Fish oil
Other complementary therapies	Acupuncture
	Aromatherapy
	Physical therapy (such as chiropractic, reflexology, remedial massage, therapeutic touch)
	Mind-body therapy (meditation, qigong exercise)
	Music therapy
	Melatonin and light therapy

interacting with one another to improve their solubility and hence bioavailability (Wagner and Ulrich-Merzenich, 2009).

57.2.1   *Gingko biloba*

Ginkgo biloba leaf extract (ginkgo) is one of the most studied herbs. The principal active components in ginkgo are flavonol glycosides (e.g. quercetin and kaempferol) and terpenoids (e.g. ginkgolide and bilobalide). Preclinical studies demonstrate that gingko's neuroprotective effects derive from its ability to decrease oxygen radical discharge and pro-inflammatory functions of macrophages (antioxidant and anti-inflammatory), reduce corticosteroid production (anti-anxiety), increase glucose uptake and utilization and adenosine triphosphate production, improve blood flow by increasing red blood cell deformability, decrease red cell aggregation, induce nitric oxide production and inhibit platelet activating factor receptors (Chan *et al.*, 2007). In healthy young adults, ginkgo has been shown to improve speed of processing, working memory, executive function and cognitive function (Kennedy *et al.*, 2007). In clinical trials with dementia patients, however, the effectiveness of ginkgo for enhancing memory and cognitive function remains controversial. Several early controlled clinical studies demonstrated some improvement in memory loss, concentration, anxiety and other symptoms associated with dementia (Howes and Houghton, 2003). For example, a randomized, double-blind, placebo-controlled trial of 216 participants with AD or vascular dementia (VaD) showed significant improvement in the attention and memory function in the

EGb761 (a standard ginkgo preparation)-treated group after 24 weeks of treatment (Kanowski *et al.*, 1996). One key issue relating to some of these early studies is the use of self-assessment questionnaires which raise concerns about the reliability of the results (Howes and Houghton, 2003). Several more recent clinical trials with greater participant numbers and longer intervention periods reported no difference between ginkgo and placebo (Schneider, 2008). A recently updated Cochrane systematic review on the use of ginkgo for dementia concludes that the existing evidence remains inconsistent and unconvincing (Birks and Evans, 2009).

57.2.2   *Huperzia serrata*

Huperzine A (HupA) is an alkaloid derived from the club moss, *Huperzia serrata*. It has been used to treat dementia in China and is sold over the counter as a dietary supplement in the US for memory loss and mental impairment. Besides HupA's well-known cholinesterase inhibiting property, it has been suggested to exert other pharmacological effects including antioxidant, anti-β-amyloid peptide fragmentation, inhibition of oxygen-glucose deprivation and N-methyl-D-aspartic acid receptor antagonism (Howes and Houghton, 2003) (**Table 57.2**). Most clinical trials of HupA were conducted and published in China. A meta-analysis of HupA for the treatment of AD identified 11 studies (one open-label study, two centre reports and eight controlled clinical trials) among which four trials involving 474 patients (235 in the HupA treatment group and 239 in the control group) were included in the final analysis (Wang *et al.*, 2009). The results demonstrated that HupA (300–500 μg/day) significantly improved cognitive function (as assessed by the Mini-Mental State Examination (MMSE)) and activities of daily living (ADL). A recent Cochrane systematic review conducted in China that recruited six clinical trials with a total of 454 patients also suggest that HupA may improve general cognitive function, global clinical status, behavioural disturbance and functional performance with minimal side effects in AD patients (Li *et al.*, 2009). However, due to the limitations of these systematic reviews and meta-analyses caused by the lack of quality data, small sample sizes of individual clinical trials and short intervention periods, more rigorous randomized controlled trials with large sample sizes are needed to confirm the clinical effectiveness of HupA.

57.2.3   *Bacopa monniera*

Bacopa monniera (Brahmi) is a medicinal plant which occurs naturally in India and has been mentioned in several ancient Ayurvedic treatises including the *Caraka Samhita* (sixth century AD) and the *Bravprakash Var-Prakarana* (sixteenth century AD) for the management of a range of mental conditions including anxiety, poor cognition and lack of concentration (Russo and Borrelli, 2005). Brahmi is marketed in Western countries as a memory enhancing agent. The major constituents of Brahmi are two saponins – bacosides A and B. Animal studies have found Brahmi can enhance several aspects of mental function and learning ability (Russo and

Table 57.2 Mechanisms of action, adverse effects and herb–drug interactions of commonly used herbs for Alzheimer's disease.

Herb	Possible mechanisms of action	Adverse effects	Herb–drug interaction
Ginkgo biloba	Decrease oxygen radical discharge and proinflammatory functions of macrophages, reduce corticosteroid production, increase glucose uptake and utilization and adenosine triphosphate production; improve blood flow by increasing red blood cell deformability; decrease red cell aggregation; induce nitric oxide production; inhibit platelet activating factors	Dizziness, tinnitus, headache, nausea, vomiting, diarrhoea, headache, weakness, restless and skin rash, etc.	Possess antiplatelet activity; caution when used with anticoagulant and antiplatelet agents (such as warfarin)
Huperzia serrata (Huperzine A)	Anticholinesterase; antioxidant; anti-β-amyloic peptide fragment; inhibition of oxygen–glucose deprivation; muscaric receptor antagonism	Nausea, vomiting, anorexia, diarrhoea, hyperactivity, insomnia, indigestion and mild abdominal pain	May cause additive effects when used with other anticholinesterase agents such as donepezil
Bacopa monniera	Enhance nerve impulse transmission; improve memory and cognition	Therapeutic doses are not associated with major adverse effects	Slightly sedative effect; caution when used with other known sedatives; inhibits the effect of thyroid-suppressant drugs
Curcuma longa	Antioxidant; anti-inflammatory; cholesterol-lowering properties; block aggregation and fibril formation	No significant side effects reported	Possess anticoagulant or antiplatelet activity; caution when used with anticoagulant and antiplatelet medications
Panax ginseng	Stimulating central cholinergic and dopaminerg c receptors; stimulating hypothalamic–pituitary–adrenal axis	Insomnia, diarrhoea, headache, tremor and skin eruptions	Combination of antidepressants and ginseng may induce mania; caution when used with antidiabetic drugs as ginseng may induce fasting blood glucose levels
Melissa officinalis	Nicotinic and muscarinic binding properties; strong antioxidant effect	No significant side effects. May cause drowsiness	Caution when used together with sedatives, anti-anxiety drugs, narcotic pain relievers (e.g. codeine), antihistamines
Camellia sinensis (tea)	The phenolic compounds (especially epigallocatechin gallate) have antioxidant effect	No significant side effects; excessive caffeine may lead to agitation, tremors and insomnia	Caution when used with theophylline and ephedrine

Borrelli, 2005). The exact mechanisms for these actions remain unclear; however, it has been suggested that neuro-pharmacological/nootropic actions of Brahmi are induced by antioxidant effects via metal chelation at the initiation level and also as a lipid peroxidation chain action breaker, and modulation of cholinergic system via reversing acetyl choline (ACh) depletion, reducing choline acetylase activity and decreasing muscarinic receptor binding (Russo and Borrelli, 2005; Stough et al., 2008).

Data from human studies are consistent with results from animal studies. In a double-blind, placebo-controlled study to examine the chronic effects of a Brahmi extract (KeenMind) on memory enhancement in 46 healthy human subjects aged between 18 and 60 years, 12 weeks treatment of 300 mg KeenMind improved early information processing, verbal learning and memory consolidation (Stough et al., 2001). This study received support from another trial involving 76 older study participants (40–65 years) (Roodenrys et al., 2002). In this study, 90 days of Brahmi treatment significantly decreased the rate of forgetting newly acquired information. Two further clinical trials were recently conducted with Brahmi extract in healthy participants. Calabrese and colleagues undertook a randomized, double-blind, placebo-controlled clinical trial with a treatment period of 12 weeks to evaluate effects of a standardized dry extract of Brahmi on cognitive function and its safety and tolerability in healthy elderly participants (average age 73 years) (Calabrese et al., 2008). The results demonstrated that Brahmi has positive benefits on multiple measures of cognitive performance and affect. Stough and co-workers (2008) also provide further support for the cognitive enhancing effect of Brahmi in a randomized controlled trial of 107 healthy participants aged between 18 and 60 years. Ninety days treatment with Brahmi extract significantly improved spatial working memory accuracy and reduced false-positives recorded in rapid visual information processing tasks. Further studies are required to ascertain the effective dosage range, and the longer term effects of administration and potential therapeutic effects of Brahmi for AD will also need to be validated in AD patients.

57.2.4   Curcuma longa

The perennial herb *Curcuma longa* (turmeric) contains three structurally closely related chemical components – curcumin, demethoxycurcumin and bisdemethoxycurcumin, which together are commonly referred to as 'curcumin' or 'curcuminoids' (Goel et al., 2008). Commercially available 'curcumin' extracts are often claimed to contain either 70 or 95 per cent curcuminoids.

In folk medicine, turmeric has been applied as a therapeutic preparation over centuries in different parts of the world. In Ayurvedic medicine, turmeric is a well-documented treatment for disease conditions including asthma, bronchial hyperactivity, respiratory allergy, liver disorders, anorexia, rheumatism, diabetic wounds, runny nose, cough and sinusitis as well as for neurodegenerative disorders (Goel et al., 2008). Data from animal and *in vitro* studies suggest that curcuminoids possess antioxidant, anti-inflammatory and cholesterol lowering properties, all of which are key processes involved in pathogenesis of AD (Ringman et al., 2005). It has also been suggested that curcuminoids directly bind small β-amyloid species to block aggregation and fibril formation supporting the rationale for curcuminoids to be used therapeutically for AD (Yang et al., 2005). However, evidence from rigorous clinical trials to support this therapeutic claim is lacking. In a large, population-based study, the relation between consumption of curry (turmeric) and cognitive function was investigated in 1010 elderly non-demented Singaporeans. Consumption of turmeric containing curry was associated with a significantly better cognitive performance measured by MMSE compared to those who 'never or rarely' consumed curry (Ng et al., 2006). A randomized, double-blind, placebo-controlled trial was recently undertaken in 34 AD patients in Hong Kong to evaluate curcumin's effect on AD (Baum et al., 2008). Six months treatment with 1 or 4 grams of curcumin did not significantly change MMSE scores or other pathological parameters although there was a trend towards increase in serum $A\beta_{40}$ which may represent an increase in disaggregation of $A\beta$ deposits by curcumin treatment. This study was one of the earliest attempts to evaluate the clinical effectiveness of curcumin for AD, and several factors (small sample size, relatively short intervention period, lack of cognitive decline in the placebo group) significantly limited the generalizability of the data. Several larger-scale clinical trials are underway or soon to be completed. The upcoming results will help to determine if curcumin has therapeutic value for the treatment and prevention of dementia.

57.2.5   Panax ginseng

Panax ginseng (ginseng) root has been used for the management of AD in many Asian countries. Most of the cognitive effects of ginseng have been studied in animals and healthy individuals. The principal bioactive components of ginseng are ginsenosides which have been suggested to have antioxidant, anti-inflammatory and anti-apoptotic effects (Radad et al., 2006). A recent *in vitro* study also demonstrated that ginsenoside Rg3 promotes beta-amyloid peptide degradation via enhancing gene expression (Yang et al., 2009).

Data from human studies suggest that ginseng modestly improves thinking and secondary and working memory in healthy volunteers (Kennedy et al., 2003a; Reay et al., 2006). Two recent small open-label trials demonstrated potential therapeutic benefits of ginseng for AD (Heo et al., 2008; Lee et al., 2008). In the first study, 12-week treatment with low-dose (4.5 g per day; $n=15$) and high-dose (9 g per day; $n=15$) Korean ginseng showed significant effects on the Alzheimer's Disease Assessment Scale-cognitive subscale (ADAS-Cog) and the Clinical Dementia Rating (CDR) when compared with those in the control group ($n=31$) (Heo et al., 2008). In the second study in which 87 AD patients ($n=58$ in the ginseng group; $n=39$ in the control group) were involved, 12-week treatment with ginseng powder (4.5 g per day) was associated with significant improvements in ADAS-Cog and MMSE scores (Lee et al., 2008). Ginseng has also demonstrated clinical benefits when combined with ginkgo in improving cognitive function in humans (Wesnes *et al.*, 2000; Kennedy *et al.*, 2001). Large-scale, long-term studies using standardized extracts are required to determine the clinical efficacy of ginseng therapy in AD.

57.2.6   *Melissa officinalis*

Melissa officinalis (lemon balm) has acetylcholine receptor activity in the central nervous system with both nicotinic and muscarinic binding properties (Perry *et al.*, 1999) as well as a strong antioxidant effect (Dastmalchi *et al.*, 2008), both of which are desirable in the management of AD. Human studies have shown that the plant extract can modulate mood and cognitive performance when administered to young, healthy volunteers (Kennedy *et al.*, 2003b). In a randomized, double-blind, placebo-controlled clinical trial, four-month treatment of *Melissa* extract produced significantly improved cognitive function and reduced agitation in patients with mild to moderate AD aged between 65 and 80 years (Akhondzadeh *et al.*, 2003). The results suggest that *Melissa officinalis* may be of value in the management of mild to moderate AD.

57.2.7   *Camellia sinensis* (tea)

Data from animal and epidemiological studies suggested that drinking tea (mostly green tea) may help to protect the brain against ageing. Evidence suggests a probable inverse correlation between tea consumption and the incidence of AD and other neurodegenerative diseases (e.g. Parkinson's disease) (Sharangi, 2009). The chief bioactive components of tea are polyphenols, caffeine and amino acids, and polyphenols are responsible for its antioxidant properties (Sharangi, 2009). In particular, its main catechin polyphenol constituent, epigallocatechin gallate, has been shown to exert neuroprotective/neurorescue activities in a wide array of cellular and animal models of neurological disorders (Mandel *et al.*, 2008). In a human cross-sectional study assessing the effect of green tea on cognitive functions in elderly Japanese participants, it was reported that green tea consumption of two or more cups (100 mL/cup) per day reduced the prevalence of cognitive function impairments in the participant cohort (Kuriyama *et al.*, 2006). More recently, Nurk and colleagues (2009) examined the relationship between intake of three flavonoid-rich foods (chocolate, wine and tea) in participants aged between 70 and 74 years. Consumption of these foods (especially tea) was associated with enhanced cognitive function in a dose-dependent manner (Nurk *et al.*, 2009).

57.3   FISH OILS FOR AD

High total fat intake, in particular that of omega-6 saturated fatty acids, is associated with poor cognitive performance and higher prevalence of AD (Ortega, 2006). A higher ratio of omega-6 to polyunsaturated fatty acids (PUFAs) is also associated with decreased insulin sensitivity and type II diabetes, which is also linked to cognitive impairment and

dementia (Greenwood and Winocur, 2005). Data from animal and epidemiologic studies suggest that PUFAs, particularly long-chain omega-3 fatty acids including docosahexaenoic acid (DHA) and eicosapentaenoic acid (EPA), can provide protection against cognitive decline and hence dementia. The mechanisms underpinning the neuroprotective effects of PUFAs may include reduction of cardiovascular risk factors (e.g. triglyceridaemia), attenuation of the inflammation process and reduction of amyloid production and increased clearance (Fotuhi *et al.*, 2009).

Numerous clinical studies conducted to evaluate the effectiveness of long-chain omega-3 fatty acids in patients with impaired cognitive function and dementia have generated conflicting results. For example, in a preliminary randomized, double-blind, placebo-controlled trial, 24-week treatment with omega-3 PUFAs (1.8 g per day) in 23 patients with mild to moderate AD improved the Clinician's Interview-Based Impression of Change Scale (CIBIC-plus) but not the ADAS-Cog scores when compared with placebo (Chiu *et al.*, 2008). A randomized, double-blind trial involving 174 patients with mild to moderate AD showed that six-month treatment with a daily intake of 1.7 g DHA and 0.6 g EPA did not delay the rate of cognitive decline measured by the MMSE and ADAS-Cog, although positive effects were observed in a small subgroup with very mild AD (MMSE > 27) (Freund-Levi *et al.*, 2008). A recent systematic review concludes that the current data are insufficient to confirm the effects of PUFAs on cognitive function in patients with impaired cognitive and dementia (Fotuhi *et al.*, 2009), so it is too early to provide any definite guidelines for the use of long-chain omega-3 fatty acid supplements in the prevention or treatment of AD.

57.4   VITAMINS FOR AD

57.4.1   Vitamin E and vitamin C

Animal and human studies strongly indicate the involvement of oxygen-free radicals in the pathological process of cognitive function impairment in AD (Pratico, 2008). This oxidative stress hypothesis has led to interest in the use of antioxidant vitamins such as vitamins E and C for the treatment of AD.

Data from cross-sectional and prospective cohort epidemiological studies on the relationship between intake of antioxidant vitamins and AD are inconsistent. A study in 4000 elderly participants aged 65 years or over showed a strong link between a combination of vitamin C and E supplements (but not individually) and a lower risk of AD, but another study in 980 individuals with the same age profile over four years failed to demonstrate an association between vitamin C or E supplementation separately and incidence of AD (Luchsinger *et al.*, 2007).

A number of randomized controlled trials have been conducted to evaluate the effects of vitamin E supplementation in AD patients. In one of the earlier clinical trials in patients with moderate AD, two-year treatment with high-dose vitamin E (2000 IU per day) was associated with significant delay in time to institutionalization, loss of ability to perform basic activities and progression to severe dementia (Sano *et al.*, 1997), though post hoc statistical manipulation of the study's data was required to produce any positive result (Ames and Ritchie, 2007). This finding was not replicated in a large clinical trial with 769 patients with mild cognitive impairment (MCI) where the probability of progression to AD and change in cognitive function were investigated. Compared with a placebo group, three years of treatment with vitamin E (2000 IU per day) did not reduce the likelihood of progression to AD or improve cognitive function at all (Petersen *et al.*, 2005). In another large randomized, double-blind, placebo-controlled trial with 6377 healthy women aged 65 years or above using much lower dose vitamin E supplementation (600 IU per day on alternate days), no differences in global scores of cognitive function between the vitamin E and placebo control groups were found after 5.6 years and 9.6 years of treatment (Kang *et al.*, 2006). A Cochrane systematic review, which reviewed two studies (Sano *et al.*, 1997; Petersen *et al.*, 2005), concluded that there is no convincing evidence of efficacy of vitamin E in the prevention or treatment of people with AD (Isaac *et al.*, 2008). A slightly increased rate of death among subjects taking high-dose vitamin E for a variety of indications in a number of trials is another good reason not to advocate its use for AD (Ames and Ritchie, 2007).

57.4.2 B Vitamins and folate

Data from a retrospective case-controlled study and a number of prospective cohort studies suggest that elevated serum total homocysteine level is a potential risk factor for AD and VaD (Clark, 2008). Homocysteine can act in the brain and possibly in the AD pathway through vascular mechanisms or as a neurotoxin. Homocysteine levels in blood can be controlled by levels of vitamins B_{12}, B_6 and folate that convert homocysteine to methionine and cysteine, respectively, and hence reduce the homocysteine levels. This theory has lead to considerable interest in using B vitamins and folate for the treatment/prevention of AD (Clark, 2008).

However, this therapeutic approach has not received consistent support from clinical trials. In a small study of 30 mild to moderate dementia patients aged over 60 years with low serum B_{12}, 40-week supplementation with vitamin B_{12} did not produce significant changes in cognitive function, although a reduction in delirium associated with dementia was observed (Kwok *et al.*, 2008). Similarly, a 26-week supplementation study with multivitamins (including vitamins B_6, B_{12} and folic acid) as adjunctive treatment with a cholinesterase inhibitor in patients with AD ($n = 89$) did not show any significant beneficial effects on cognition or ADL function (Sun *et al.*, 2007). Further, in a randomized placebo-controlled trial in patients with MCI, one year supplementation with vitamins B_6, B_{12} and folic acid failed to produce significant improvement in quality of life measures (van Uffelen *et al.*, 2007). In a larger-scale multicentre, randomized, double-blind controlled trial, 409 patients with mild to moderate AD were randomly allocated to receive high-dose supplements of 5 mg/day of folate, 25 mg/day of

vitamin B_6 and 1 mg/day of vitamin B_{12} or identical placebo. The 18-month treatment did not slow cognitive decline measured by the ADAS-Cog scores (Aisen *et al.*, 2008). A recent Cochrane review concluded that the existing small number of studies did not provide consistent evidence that folic acid with or without vitamin B_{12} has a beneficial effect on the cognitive function of healthy or cognitively impaired older people (Malouf and Evans, 2008).

57.4.3 Vitamin D

Although strong biological evidence exists to suggest a close relationship of vitamin D with brain development and function, direct effects of inadequacy of vitamin D on cognition and behaviour in humans are lacking (McCann and Ames, 2008). A recent study comparing the prevalence of vitamin D insufficiency in patients with Parkinson's disease and AD failed to demonstrate a convincing correlation between vitamin D deficiency and AD (Evatt *et al.*, 2008). Despite this uncertainty, vitamin D supplementation is recommended by some authors for at-risk groups to treat cognitive or behavioural dysfunction, especially those with an extremely low 25-hydroxycholecalciferol (25OHD3) concentration (McCann and Ames, 2008).

57.5 OTHER COMPLEMENTARY THERAPIES FOR AD

Other complementary therapies have been used to treat AD or other dementias and/or alleviate associated symptoms. These interventions include, but are not limited to, acupuncture, chiropractic, reflexology, remedial massage, therapeutic touch, aromatherapy, mind-body therapy (e.g. meditation, qigong exercise), music therapy (see Chapter 29, Sexuality and dementia), and melatonin and light therapy (**Table 57.1**). Relatively low levels of evidence exist to support the use of some of these therapies. For example, acupressure and Montessori-based activities were effective in reducing agitated behaviours, aggressive behaviours, physically non-aggressive behaviours and in improving emotional expression and response (Montessori group only) in 133 institutionalized residents with dementia in Taiwan (Lin *et al.*, 2009). In a cross-over randomized trial with 70 patients with dementia, lavender inhalation significantly alleviated agitated behaviours when compared with the control group (sunflower inhalation) (Lin *et al.*, 2007). More rigorous scientific research is needed to evaluate the effectiveness of these therapies (see also Chapter 23, The role of physiotherapy in the management of dementia).

57.6 CONCLUSION

Due to the unsatisfactory effects of approved antidementia therapies (see Chapter 54, Established treatments for Alzheimer's disease: cholinesterase inhibitors and memantine), it is imperative that potentially suitable complementary medicines and therapies be thoroughly examined and validated if appropriate.

AD is complex in nature in terms of its pathogenesis. Complementary interventions such as herbal medicines and multivitamin supplementation often contain multiple components and therefore can affect different targets, which make them ideal therapies for disorders with multifactorial/multisystem pathophysiological components. This hypothesis needs to be further validated in future pharmacological studies and clinical trials.

A large proportion of the existing evidence to support the use of complementary medicine for AD comes from animal and *in vitro* studies and epidemiological data. Unfortunately, clinical trials of these interventions frequently produced disappointing and inconsistent results. The overall clinical evidence for these interventions remains thin and conflicting. Further large-scale, randomized, double-blind, placebo-controlled trials are needed to evaluate the effectiveness and safety of these interventions. Some traditional medical systems such as Chinese and Ayurvedic medicine emphasize health maintenance and disease prevention, which is currently poorly studied. Hence, research to assess the protective and preventive effects of these medicines should also be carried out.

REFERENCES

Aisen P, Scheider LS, Sano M *et al.* (2008) High-dose B vitamin supplementation and cognitive decline in Alzheimer disease: A randomized controlled trial. *Journal of American Medical Association* **300**: 1774–83.

Akhondzadeh S, Noroozian M, Mohammadi M *et al.* (2003) *Melissa officinalis* extract in the treatment of patients with mild to moderate Alzheimer's disease: A double blind, randomised, placebo controlled trial. *Journal of Neurology, Neurosurgery, and Psychiatry* **28**: 53–9.

Ames D, Ritchie C. (2007) Antioxidants and Alzheimer's disease: Time to stop feeding Vitamin E to dementia patients? *International Psychogeriatrics* **19**: 1–8.

Barnes PM, Bloom B, Nahin R. (2007) Complementary and alternative medicine use among adults and children: United States. CDC National Health Statistics Report no. 12. December 10, 2008.

Baum L, Lam CWK, Cheung SKK *et al.* (2008) Six-month randomized placebo-controlled, double-blind, pilot clinical trial of curcumin in patients with Alzheimer disease. *Journal of Clinical Psychopharmacology* **28**: 110–13.

Birks J, Evans JG. (2009) Ginkgo biloba for cognitive impairment and dementia. *Cochrane Database of Systematic Reviews* (1): CD003120.

Calabrese C, Gregory WL, Leo M *et al.* (2008) Effects of a standardized *Bacopa monnieri* extract on cognitive performance, anxiety, and depression in the elderly: A randomized, double-blind, placebo-controlled trial. *Journal of Alternative and Complementary Medicine* **14**: 707–13.

Chan P-C, Xia Q, Fu PP. (2007) *Ginkgo biloba* leave extract: biological, medicinal and toxicological effects. *Journal of Environmental Science Health Part C* **25**: 211–44.

Chiu CC, Su KP, Cheng TC *et al.* (2008) The effects of omega-3 fatty acids monotherapy in Alzheimer's disease and mild cognitive impairment: A preliminary randomized double-blind placebo-controlled study. *Progress in Neuro-Psychopharmacolgy and Biological Psychiatry* **32**: 1538–44.

Clark R. (2008) Plenary Lecture: B-vitamins and prevention of dementia. *Proceedings of the Nutrition Society* **67**: 75–81.

Dastmalchi K, Dorman HJD, Oinonen PP *et al.* (2008) Chemical composition and *in vitro* antioxidative activity of a lemon balm (*Melissa officinalis* L.) extract. *LWT Food Science and Technology* **41**: 391–400.

Dubey NK, Kumar R, Tripathi P. (2004) Global promotion of herbal medicine: India's opportunity. *Current Science* **86**: 37–41.

Evatt ML, Lelong MR, Khazai N *et al.* (2008) Prevalence of vitamin D insufficiency in patients with Parkinson disease and Alzheimer disease. *Archives of Neurology* **65**: 1348–52.

Farlow MR, Miller ML, Pejovic V. (2008) Treatment options in Alzheimer's disease: Maximizing benefit, managing expectations. *Dementia and Geriatic Cognitive Disorders* **25**: 408–22.

Fotuhi M, Mohassel P, Yaffe K. (2009) Fish consumption, long-chain omega-3 fatty acids and risk of cognitive decline or Alzheimer disease: A complex association. *Nature Clinical Practice Neurology* **5**: 140–52.

Freund-Levi Y, Basun H, Cederholm T *et al.* (2008) Omega-3 supplementation in mild to moderate Alzheimer's disease: Effects on neuropsychiatric symptoms. *International Journal of Geriatric Psychiatry* **23**: 161–9.

Goel A, Kunnumakkara AB, Aggarwal BB. (2008) Curcumin as "Curecumin": From kitchen to clinic. *Biochemical Pharmacology* **75**: 787–809.

Greenwood CE, Winocur G. (2005) High-fat diets, insulin resistance and declining cognitive function. *Neurobiology of Aging* **26**: 42–5.

Heo JH, Lee ST, Chu K *et al.* (2008) An open-label trial of Korean red ginseng as an adjuvant treatment for cognitive impairment in patients with Alzheimer's disease. *European Journal of Neurology* **15**: 865–8.

Howes M-JR, Houghton PJ. (2003) Plants used in Chinese and Indian traditional medicine for improvement of memory and cognitive function. *Pharmacology Biochemistry and Behavior* **75**: 513–27.

Isaac MGEKN, Quinn R, Tabet N. (2008) Vitamin E for Alzheimer's disease and mild cognitive impairment. *Cochrane Database of Systematic Reviews* (3): CD002854.

Kang JH, Cook N, Manson J *et al.* (2006) A randomised trial of vitamin E supplementation and cognitive function in women. *Archives of Internal Medicine* **166**: 2462–8.

Kanowski S, Herrmann WM, Stephan K *et al.* (1996) Proof of efficacy of the ginkgo biloba special extract EGb 761 in outpatients suffering from mild to moderate primary degenerative dementia of the Alzheimer type or multiinfarct dementia. *Pharmacopsychiatry* **29**: 47–56.

Kennedy DO, Scholey AB, Wesnes KA. (2001) Differential, dose dependent changes in cognitive performance following acute administration of a *Ginkgo biloba/Panax ginseng* combination to healthy young volunteers. *Nutritional Neuroscience* 4: 399–412.

Kennedy DO, Scholey AB, Drewery L et al. (2003a) Electroencephalograph (EEG) effects of single doses of *Ginkgo biloba* and *Panax ginseng* in healthy young volunteers. *Pharmacology, Biochemistry and Behavior* 75: 701 0.

Kennedy DO, Wake G, Savelev S et al. (2003b) Modulation of mood and cognitive performance following acute administration of single doses of Melissa officinalis (Lemon Balm) with human CNS nicotinic and muscarinic receptor-binding properties. *Neuropsychopharmacology* 28: 1871–81.

Kennedy DO, Jackson PA, Haskell CF, Scholey AM. (2007) Modulation of cognitive performance following single doses of 120 mg Ginkgo biloba extract administered to healthy young volunteers. *Human Psychopharmacology: Clinical and Experimental* 22: 559–66.

Kuriyama S, Hozawa A, Ohmori K et al. (2006) Green tea consumption and cognitive function: A cross-sectional study from the Tsurugaya Project. *American Journal of Clinical Nutrition* 83: 355–61.

Kwok T, Lee J, Lam L, Woo J. (2008) Vitamin B12 supplementation did not improve cognition but reduced delirium in demented patients with vitamin B12 deficiency. *Archives of Gerontology and Geriatrics* 46: 273–82.

Lee ST, Chu K, Sim JY et al. (2008) Panax ginseng enhances cognitive performance in Alzheimer disease. *Alzheimer Disease and Associated Disorders* 22: 222–6.

Li J, Wu HM, Zhou RL et al. (2009) Huperzine A for Alzheimer's disease. *Cochrane Database of Systematic Reviews* (2): CD005592.

Lin L-C, Yang M-H, Kao C-C et al. (2009) Using acupressure and Montessori-based activities to decrease agitation for residents with dementia: A cross-over trial. *Journal of the American Geriatrics Society* 57: 1022–9.

Lin P, Chan W-C, Ng F-L, Lam L. (2007) Efficacy of aromatherapy (*Lavendula angustifolia*) as an intervention for agitated behaviours in Chinese older persons with dementia: A cross-over randomized trial. *International Journal of Geriatric Psychiatry* 22: 405–10.

Luchsinger JA, Noble JM, Scarmeas N. (2007) Diet and Alzheimer's disease. *Current Neurology and Neuroscience Reports* 7: 366–72.

McCann JC, Ames BN. (2007) Is there convincing biological or behavioral evidence linking vitamin D deficiency to brain dysfunction? *The FASEB Journal* 22: 982–1001.

Malouf R, Evans JG. (2008) Folic acid with or without vitamin B12 for the prevention and treatment of healthy elderly and demented people. *Cochrane Database of Systematic Reviews* (4): CD004514.

Mandel SA, Amit T, Kalfon L et al. (2008) Targeting multiple neurodegenerative diseases etiologies with multimodal-acting green tea catechins. *Journal of Nutrition* 138: 1578S–83S.

Ng T-P, Chiam P-C, Lee T et al. (2006) Curry consumption and cognitive function in the elderly. *American Journal Epidemiologist* 164: 898–906.

Nurk E, Refsum H, Drevon CA et al. (2009) Intake of flavonoid-rich wine, tea, and chocolate by elderly men and women is associated with better cognitive test performance. *Journal of Nutrition* 139: 120–7.

Ortega RM. (2006) Importance of functional foods in the Mediterranean diet. *Public Health Nutrition* 9: 1136–40.

Perry EK, Pikering AT, Wang WW et al. (1999) Medicinal plants and Alzheimer's disease: From etnobotany to phytotherapy. *Journal of Pharmacy and Pharmacology* 51: 527–34.

Petersen RC, Thomas RG, Grundman M. (2005) Vitamin E and donepezil for the treatment of mild cognitive impairment. *New England Journal of Medicine* 352: 2379–88.

Pratico D. (2008) Evidence of oxidative stress in Alzheimer's disease brain and antioxidant therapy. *Annals of the New York Academy of Science* 1147: 70–8.

Radad K, Gille G, Liu LL, Rausch WD. (2006) Use of ginseng in medicine with emphasis on neurodegenerative disorders. *Journal of Pharmacological Science* 100: 175–86.

Reay JL, Kennedy DO, Scholey AB. (2006) Effects of *Panax ginseng*, consumed with and without glucose, on blood glucose levels and cognitive performance during sustained 'mentally demanding' tasks. *Journal of Psychopharmcology* 20: 771–81.

Ringman JM, Frautschy SA, Cole GM et al. (2005) A potential role of the curry spice in Alzheimer's disease. *Current Alzheimer Research* 2: 131–6.

Roodenrys S, Booth D, Bulzomi S et al. (2002) Chronic effects of Brahmi (Bacopa monnieri) on human memory. *Neuropsychopharmacology* 27: 279–81.

Russo A, Borrelli F. (2005) *Bacopa monniera*, a reputed nootropic plant: an overview. *Phytomedicine* 12: 305–17.

Sano M, Ernesto C, Thomas RG et al. (1997) A controlled trial of seligiline, alpha-tocopherol, or both as treatment for Alzheimer's disease. *New England Journal of Medicine* 336: 1216–22.

Schneider LS. (2008) *Ginkgo biloba* extract and preventing Alzheimer's disease. *Journal of American Medical Association* 300: 2306–8.

Sharangi AB. (2009) Medicinal and therapeutic potentialities of tea (Camellia sinensis L.) – A review. *Food Research International* 42: 529–35.

Stough C, Lloyd J, Clarke J et al. (2001) The chronic effect of *Bacopa monnieri* (Brahmi) on cognitive functions on healthy human subjects. *Psychopharmacology* 156: 481–4.

Stough C, Downey LA, Lloyd J et al. (2008) Examining the nootropic effects of a special extract of Bacopa monniera on human cognitive functioning: 90 day double-blind placebo-controlled randomized trial. *Phytotherapy Research* 22: 1629–34.

Sun Y, Lu CJ, Chien KL et al. (2007) Efficacy of multivitamin supplementation containing vitamins B6 and B12 and folic acid as adjunctive treatment with a cholinesterase inhibitor in Alzheimer's disease: A 26-week, randomized, double-blind, placebo-controlled study in Taiwanese patients. *Clinical Therapeutics* 29: 2204–14.

van Uffelen JGZ, Paw MJMCM, Hopman-Rock M, van Mechelen W. (2007) The effect of walking and vitamin B supplementation on quality of life in community-dwelling adults with mild cognitive impairment: A randomised, controlled trial. *Quality of Life Research* **16**: 1137–46.

Wagner H, Ulrich-Merzenich G. (2009) Synergy research: approaching a new generation of phytopharmaceuticals. Part 1. *Phytomedicine* **16**: 97–107.

Wang B-S, Wang H, Wei Z-H *et al.* (2009) Efficacy and safety of natural acetylcholinesterase inhibitor huperzine A in the treatment of Alzheimer's disease: An updated meta-analysis. *Journal of Neural Transmission* **116**: 457–65.

Wesnes KA, Ward T, McGinty A, Petrini O. (2000) The memory enhancing effects of a Ginkgo biloba/Panax ginseng combination in healthy middle-aged volunteers. *Psychopharmacology* **152**: 353–61.

Yang F, Lim GP, Begum AN *et al.* (2005) Curcumin inhibits formation of amyloid beta oligomers and fibrils, binds plaques, and reduces amyloid *in vivo*. *Journal of Biological Chemistry* **280**: 5892–901.

Yang L, Hao J, Zhang J *et al.* (2009) Ginsenoside Rg3 promotes beta-amyloid peptide degradation by enhancing gene expression of neprilysin. *Journal of Pharmacy and Pharmacology* **61**: 375–80.

Prevention of Alzheimer's disease

NITIN PURANDARE

58.1 INTRODUCTION

Primary prevention of Alzheimer's disease (AD) is the ultimate goal of therapeutic intervention. The prevalence of dementia would be reduced by 50 per cent if risk reduction strategies were successful in delaying the onset of dementia by five years (Jorm et al., 1987). This chapter focuses on four key areas that are particularly amenable to therapeutic intervention: control of risk factors for cerebrovascular disease, anti-inflammatory drugs, antioxidants and increasing neuronal reserve.

58.2 CONTROL OF RISK FACTORS FOR CEREBROVASCULAR DISEASE

58.2.1 Hypertension

58.2.1.1 EPIDEMIOLOGICAL EVIDENCE

Epidemiological studies have shown hypertension in midlife (systolic and diastolic) to be a risk factor for AD and vascular dementia (VaD) in later life. For example, the Honolulu Asia Aging Study (HAAS) followed over 3500 Japanese-American men for 25 years, and found hypertension to increase the risk of dementia by four- to five-fold in those who were never treated with antihypertensives. The risk was greatest in those with systolic hypertension and apolipoprotein E (ApoE) ε4 allele after controlling for other risk factors (odds ratio, OR = 13.0) (Peila et al., 2001). In HAAS the OR for dementia in patients with systolic hypertension and ApoE ε4 decreased from 13.0 to 1.9 in those receiving antihypertensives.

Hypertension was also associated with lower total brain weight, increased stratum pyramidale (SP) count and hippocampal atrophy. A coexistence of SP and lacunar infarcts further increased the risk of incident dementia (Petrovitch et al., 2005). The blood pressure (BP) drops around the time of or soon after the onset of clinical dementia and current research is trying to ascertain whether this is a risk factor or risk marker for dementia. The Kungsholmen project followed 947 people aged ≥75 years every three years for six years. BP decreased significantly over three years prior to and following diagnosis of dementia. In people with baseline systolic BP < 160 mmHg, a drop of ≥15 mmHg over the first follow up was associated with an increased risk of dementia at the second follow up (relative risk, RR = 3.1) (Qiu et al., 2004). However, another prospective study of 2356 people ≥65 years over eight years concluded that the association between BP and dementia depended on age at which BP was measured and not the time relative to the onset of dementia. In a 65–74 years age group high systolic BP and borderline-high diastolic BP was associated with an increased risk of dementia while in those ≥75 years there was a trend towards high systolic BP being associated with low risk of developing dementia (Li et al., 2007). However, the Women's Health Initiative Memory Study did not find independent association between hypertension and mild cognitive impairment (MCI) or dementia over a 4.5 years follow up of postmenopausal women with mean age of 71 years (Johnson et al., 2008).

58.2.1.2 RANDOMIZED CONTROLLED TRIALS

A number of randomized controlled trials (RCTs) of antihypertensives have been published with cognition and or dementia as one of the outcomes (see **Table 58.1**). Earlier trials using diuretics or β-blockers did not demonstrate a lower risk of incident dementia (Applegate *et al.*, 1994; Prince *et al.*, 1996). The results of more trials using calcium channel blockers (Syst-Eur trial, Forette *et al.*, 1998; Forette *et al.*, 2002) or angiotensin convering enzyme (ACE) inhibitors (HOPE trial, Bosch *et al.*, 2002; PROGRESS trial, Tzourio *et al.*, 2003) have been mixed but more encouraging. The PROGRESS trial, which included both normotensive and hypertensive patients with previous history of cerebrovascular disease, found a significant reduction in stroke-related dementia in patients treated with perindopril (ACE inhibitor) as the main antihypertensive. The SCOPE trial (Lithell *et al.*, 2003) included a much older (70–89 years) patient group and excluded those with stroke or myocardial infarction in the previous six months. Candesartan (angiotensin II type 1 (AT1) receptor blocker) did not have any positive effect on progression of cognitive impairment over 3.7 years. However, antihypertensives were used in 84 per cent of the controls.

The Syst-Eur trial included 2410 older people with isolated systolic hypertension (systolic BP 160–219 and diastolic BP < 95 mmHg). The intervention group ($n = 1238$) received nitrendipine (calcium channel blocker) and if required, enalapril and hydrochlorthiazide. Over two year follow up the intervention group had a 50 per cent reduced risk of incident dementia compared to the group receiving placebo (Forette *et al.*, 1998). The controls were given antihypertensive medications at the end of the trial and both groups followed for a further two years. Long-term treatment with nitrendipine reduced incident dementia by 55 per cent (from 7.4 to 3.3 cases per 1000 person years). Treatment of 1000 patients for five years could prevent 20 (95 per cent CI: 7, 33) cases of dementia (Forette *et al.*, 2002). The hypertension in the Very Elderly trial (HYVET, Peters *et al.*, 2008a) included patients with hypertension (systolic BP 160–200 and diastolic BP < 110 mmHg, respectively) aged 80 years or older who were followed for two years. There was no significant reduction in incident dementia between active (indapamide ± perindopril) and placebo arms. However, when the data were combined in a meta-analysis with other placebo-controlled trials the combined risk ratio favoured active treatment with antihypertensive HR 0.87 (95 per cent CI: 0.76, 1.00).

The statistical power of these studies is limited by the low incident risk of dementia in these populations because of the young age and modest study durations. In all RCTs, incident dementia has been a secondary outcome, heart disease or stroke being the primary outcomes, and generally, brief assessment instruments lacking sensitivity to subtle changes have been employed. Also, epidemiological evidence suggests that the time lapse between diagnosis of hypertension and onset of dementia can be over 15 years, and it is not known whether the protective effect of starting antihypertensives on incident dementia extends throughout this period.

The treatment issues may be slightly different in established VaD. One study has indicated that maintaining systolic BP within upper limits of normal (135–150 mmHg) was more beneficial in preserving cognitive functions than reducing systolic BP below this level (Meyer *et al.*, 1986).

Another issue which needs further clarification is whether the risk reduction is related to actual reduction in the BP and/or some other neuroprotective action of the individual hypertensive, such as calcium channel antagonists, ACE inhibitors or AT1 receptor blockers. In animal studies, angiotensin II has been shown to inhibit acetylcholine release while AT1 receptor blockers improve cognitive performance (Barnes *et al.*, 1989; Fogari *et al.*, 2003).

58.2.2 Hypercholesterolaemia

58.2.2.1 BIOLOGICAL BASIS FOR IMPORTANCE IN PREVENTION OF AD

Hypercholesterolaemia, especially increased low density lipoproteins, is a known risk factor for coronary heart disease, atherosclerosis and stroke, which are all associated with increased risk of dementia. The ApoE ε4 allele affects stabilization of membrane lipoproteins and is a risk factor for hypercholesterolaemia. Lowering of cholesterol promotes the non-amyloidogenic α-secretase pathway (Kojro *et al.*, 2001). Statins reduce cholesterol levels by inhibiting the enzyme 3-hydroxy-3-methylglutaryl coenzyme A (HMG-CoA). In addition, statins have an antioxidant action, decrease proinflammatory process and improve cerebral blood flow. Lovastatin reduced amyloid β protein 42 ($A\beta_{42}$) in cultured hippocampal neurones (Simons *et al.*, 1998) and simvastatin had a similar effect in cerebrospinal fluid and brain tissue of guinea pigs (Fassbender *et al.*, 2001).

58.2.2.2 CLINICAL EVIDENCE

A number of case–control and epidemiological studies have reported hypercholesterolaemia as a risk factor for dementia, including AD. For example, Moroney *et al.* (1999) followed over 2000 older people in New York City over two years and found those with cholesterol levels in the highest quartile to be at increased risk of dementia, especially VaD (OR = 3–4) compared to those in the lowest quartile. A similar sized study but with much longer follow up (21 years) in Eastern Finland reported that raised cholesterol in midlife (≥ 6.5 mmol/L) to more than double the risk of dementia, including AD, independently of other risk factors such as hypertension and ApoE ε4 (Kivipelto *et al.*, 2002).

There are some important inconsistencies in the epidemiological evidence. Studies have found no risk reduction (Zandi *et al.*, 2005; Arvanitakis *et al.*, 2008) or risk reduction with lipid lowering agents (LLAs) in general (Dufouil *et al.*, 2005) or with statins alone (Haag *et al.*, 2009). A meta-analysis of seven observational studies indicated risk reduction in cognitive impairment to be significant only for statins (OR = 0.43) and not other LLAs (Etminan *et al.*, 2003). However, a recent meta-analysis which included seven observational studies found that statin use did not reduce the risk of dementia or AD (Zhou *et al.*, 2007). Other inconsistencies may relate to differential effect in certain age groups (statins lower risk of AD in those younger than 80 years; Rockwood *et al.*, 2002) and specific actions of

Table 58.1 Effect of antihypertensive treatment on cognitive function and dementia.

Randomized controlled trials	Sample size	Participants (characteristics, age in years)	Duration	Treatment	Impact on dementia or cognition
Peters et al., 2008a; (HYVET-COG)	3336	>80: systolic BP 160–200 mmHg, diastolic BP <110 mmHg	2.2 years	Indapamide, perindopril	No significant effect on incidence of dementia but when data combined with previous trials in meta-analysis results favoured active treatment
Forette et al., 1998; (Syst-Eur)	2418	>60: systolic hypertension	2 years	Nitrendipine	50% reduction in the incidence of dementia (7.7–3.8 cases per 1000 patient-years, $p = 0.05$)
Forette et al., 2002; (extended follow-up of Syst-Eur)	2902	>60: systolic hypertension	3.9 years	Nitrendipine, enalapril maleate, hydrochlorothiazide	55% reduction in the risk of dementia (7.4–3.3 cases per 1000 patient-years, $p < 0.001$)
Applegate et al., 1994; (Systolic Hypertension in the Elderly)	2034	>60: systolic hypertension	5 years	Chlorthalidone	No significant impact of cognition or incident dementia
Prince et al., 1996; (MRC Older people with HT)	2584	65–74: systolic BP 160–209 mmHg	4.5 years	Atenolol, hydrochlorothiazide amiloride	No significant impact on cognition or incident dementia
Bosch et al., 2002; (HOPE)	9297	>55: left ventricular dysfunction	4.5 years	Ramipril, vitamin E	Significantly better outcome with respect to cognition and function
Tzourio et al. (2003 The PROGRESS Collaborative Group)	6105	Mean age 64: stroke or transient ischaemic attack with and without hypertension	4 years	Perindopril, indapamide	Significant reduction in cognitive decline and incident dementia associated with recurrent stroke
Lithell et al., 2003; (SCOPE)	4964	70–89: systolic and or diastolic hypertension	3.7 years	Candesartan (antihypertensive used in 84% of controls)	No difference on progression of cognitive impairment

BP, blood pressure.

individual statins. For example, simvastatin acts directly on processing of amyloid precursor protein by inhibiting both α- and β-secretase (Sjogren *et al.*, 2003).

The results of intervention trials, with cognition as one of the many secondary outcomes, have been disappointing. MRC/BHF Heart Protection Study (Heart Protection Study Collaborative Group, 2002), comparing simvastatin versus placebo, found simvastatin to reduce risk of major vascular events by one-third. The study examined potential effects on cognition by modified Telephone Interview for Cognitive Status (TICS). There was no difference between two groups in either proportion of patients scoring below the cut off of 22 out of 39 or in the mean TICS score. The PROSPER study (Shepherd *et al.*, 2002), an RCT of pravastatin ($n = 2891$) versus placebo ($n = 2913$) over three years, found pravastatin to significantly reduce mortality from coronary disease but had no effect on cognition. The statistical power of both studies was limited by the low incident dementia in study subjects (0.3 per cent in active or placebo group in the Heart Protection Study). A Cochrane review based on the above two studies concluded that statins given in late life to individuals at risk of vascular disease have no effect in preventing AD or dementia (McGuinness *et al.*, 2009).

58.2.3   Elevated homocysteine

58.2.3.1   BIOLOGICAL BASIS

Plasma or serum homocysteine, or total homocysteine (tHcy), refers to the sum of the sulfhydryl amino acid homocysteine and the homocysteinyl moieties of the disulphides homocystine and homocysteine-cysteine, whether free or bound to plasma proteins. A number of factors such as age, diet, B_{12} and folate, plasma albumin, use of diuretics and renal function influence homocysteine levels in the blood. Elevated tHcy may lead to an excessive production of homocysteic acid and cysteine sulphinic acid, which act as endogenous agonists of N-methyl-D-aspartic acid (NMDA) receptors. In addition to this excitotoxic effect, homocysteine is also known to cause damage to vascular endothelium.

58.2.3.2   CLINICAL EVIDENCE

In older people without dementia, elevated tHcy is associated with more subtle cognitive impairment. Dufouil *et al.* (2003) followed up 1241 subjects aged 61–73 years over four years and found higher concentrations of tHcy were associated with poor performance on all neuropsychological tests with the odds of cognitive decline 2.8-fold ($p < 0.05$) higher in subjects with tHcy levels above 15 μmol/L compared with those with levels below 10 μmol/L. Fasting tHcy levels predicted cognitive decline in a follow-up study of 32 healthy elderly people over five years ($p < 0.001$), especially word recall, orientation and special copying skills (McCaddon *et al.*, 2001). Case–control studies have shown elevated tHcy to be associated with AD after adjusting for age, sex, nutritional status and ApoE ε4 allele (Clarke *et al.*, 1998). A large epidemiological study in Framingham, USA, involving 1092

older residents in the community (mean age 76 years, median follow up eight years) reported that the risk of AD nearly doubled (relative risk (RR) 1.8; confidence intervals (CI) 1.3–2.5) with one standard deviation increase in tHcy levels at baseline (Seshadri *et al.*, 2002).

Intervention trials to lower homocysteine levels need to consider three things. First, whether to target people with tHcy levels in the highest quartile of local population or use an arbitrary cut off of such as > 15 μmol/L. Second, the best treatment combination to lower tHcy from various forms of B_{12} and folate needs to be determined, also considering merits of additional nutrients such as *N*-acetylcysteine. Third, a better understanding is required of factors affecting tHcy levels and their response to vitamin supplementation. Age, plasma albumin, use of diuretics and renal function are just some of them (Ventura *et al.*, 2001). The C677T mutation of methelenetetrahydrofolate reductase (MTHFR) gene, present in about one-fifth of people with AD, may be yet another important factor that may affect treatment response. MTHFR acts as a methyl donor for homocysteine methylation and hence reduces homocysteine levels. The C677T mutation is common in the Caucasian population (30 per cent), which results in lower MTHFR activity and elevated tHcy (Frosst *et al.*, 1995; Bottiglieri *et al.*, 2001).

Although elevated tHcy levels have been associated with cognitive impairment in AD, the effect of reducing tHcy on cognition is unclear. In patients with AD, two small RCTs of folic acid with or without vitamin B_{12} supplementation showed positive effect on cognitive (Nilsson *et al.*, 2001) and functional decline (Connelly *et al.*, 2008). However, another small RCT of folic acid (Sun *et al.*, 2007) and a much larger RCT of folate with B_6 and B_{12} showed only reduction in tHcy but no effect on cognitive or functional decline (Aisen *et al.*, 2008). Unlike previous studies which were of six months duration, the latter study was much longer with a total of 340/ 409 participants (202 in active treatment group and 138 in placebo) completing the 18-month follow up. Plasma levels of tHcy show significant cross-sectional correlation with $A\beta_{40}$ levels and vitamin supplementation does reduce tHcy but not necessarily $A\beta_{40}$ with two similar size studies of two years duration showing positive (Flicker *et al.*, 2008) or no effect (Viswanathan *et al.*, 2009). This raises the question of whether the elevated tHcy is a 'risk factor' or a 'risk marker' for AD (Seshadri, 2006). A Cochrane review (Malouf and Grimley Evans, 2008) did not find any evidence to support risk factor status. However, the review did include a large RCT from the Netherlands in which 818 older people (50–70 years) with raised plasma tHcy and normal serum vitamin B_{12} at screening were assigned to receive 800 μg daily oral folic acid or placebo for three years (Durga *et al.*, 2007). The intervention group did significantly better on certain cognitive domains such as memory storage and information processing speed.

58.2.4   Other cardiovascular risk factors

Diabetes, carotid atherosclerosis, heart disease and smoking are risk factors for stroke, VaD and AD. Obesity in midlife is yet another risk factor for AD in late life. It is unclear as to whether a specific combination of vascular risk factors (e.g.

metabolic syndrome; Vanhanen *et al.*, 2006) or just number of risk factors (Kivipelto *et al.*, 2006) contribute additively to the overall risk of developing AD. Their control reduces the occurrence of cerebrovascular disease and one would expect a similar risk reduction in AD, but so far there is no RCT. Nonetheless, understanding underlying pathophysiological mechanisms may open new avenues for prevention. For example, mutations in insulin degrading enzyme that induce diabetes, also impair degradation of beta amyloid (Farris *et al.*, 2004). Similarly, spontaneous cerebral microemboli (SCE), common in carotid disease but thought to be asymptomatic, have been associated with cognitive impairment following carotid and heart bypass surgery. We examined the frequency of SCE in AD and VaD by transcranial Doppler monitoring of middle cerebral arteries over 1 hour. Among 85 AD–control and 85 VaD–control pairs, we found SCE in 37–38 per cent of patients with AD or VaD compared to 13–14 per cent of their controls ($p < 0.001$; Purandare *et al.*, 2006). Those with SCE showed a more rapid decline in cognition and function over six months compared with those in whom no SCE were detected (Purandare *et al.*, 2007). SCE are potentially treatable and if they are found to be predictive of cognitive decline then they could be a target in prevention of dementia, both AD and VaD. Yet another example would be smoking. Whilst smoking overall appears to be associated with a doubling of the risk of AD (presumably because of cardiovascular factors), nicotine itself may have neuroprotective properties and possibly reduce amyloid burden (Nordberg *et al.*, 2002).

58.3 CONTROL OF SUBCLINICAL INFLAMMATORY PROCESSES

58.3.1 Biological basis

The importance of inflammatory processes in causation of dementia is established with evidence from biochemical, neuropathological and epidemiological studies. Primary inflammatory cytokines such as interleukins 1β (IL-1β), IL-6 and α2-macroglobulin are increased in brains of patients with AD. The neuropathological features of AD include accumulation of microglia and astrocytes around senile plaques. Both express human leukocyte antigens and are involved in activation of the complement cascade. These inflammatory changes are thought to lead to further amyloid deposition and neuronal damage.

Non-steroidal anti-inflammatory drugs (NSAIDs) differ in their mechanisms of action and as yet we do not know the mechanism that is most important in offering neuroprotection in AD. Traditional NSAIDs such as ibuprofen, indomethacin affect both cyclooxygenases (Cox-1 and Cox-2). Newer NSAIDs such as celecoxib and rofecoxib specifically inhibit Cox-2 and hence have less propensity to cause gastrointestinal side effects. Cox-1 is prominent in CA-1 of hippocampus and is involved in microglial activation surrounding senile plaques. Cox-2 is prominent in dendrites of pyramidal neurones and is increased in many areas of brains in AD. Cox-2 levels correlate with Aβ amyloid levels in AD brains. Cox-2 is required in neurones with NMDA receptors which are responsible for glutamate-induced excitotoxicity in AD. NSAIDs also exhibit actions other than suppression of inflammation. NSAIDs inhibit Cox in platelets (resulting in reduced platelet aggregation and reduced Aβ amyloid in blood) and in vascular endothelium (protecting the endothelium from free radicals). The importance of the non-inflammatory actions of NSAIDs is highlighted by observations that both 'low' and 'high' doses offer neuroprotection. It is also possible that some NSAIDs influence amyloid deposition by inhibiting gamma secretase, independent of Cox activity (Weggen *et al.*, 2001).

58.3.2 Clinical evidence

A number of epidemiological studies have shown long-term use of NSAIDs to be associated with a two- to four-fold reduced risk of AD, but some have been inconclusive (McGeer *et al.*, 1996). A systematic review and meta-analysis of nine observational studies concluded that NSAIDs do offer some protection against AD (Etminan *et al.*, 2003). In't Veld *et al.* (2001) suggest that the conflicting evidence may be related to inaccurate recording and reliance on patients' and/ or relatives' memory or incomplete medical records. They examined computerized pharmacy records in the follow-up study of almost 7000 residents of Rotterdam over seven years. NSAIDs were associated with a reduced risk of AD depending on the duration of use (< 1 month: RR 0.95; 1–24 months: RR 0.83; > 24 months: RR 0.20). Zandi and Breitner (2001) suggest that to be protective in AD, NSAIDs would need to be taken several years before the onset of disease, and secondary or tertiary prevention trials are unlikely to show a positive effect. This is in keeping with a very modest effect observed in RCTs of low-dose prednisone and NSAID in AD, including a trial of rofecoxib (Cox-2 inhibitor) or naproxen versus placebo with negative results (Aisen *et al.*, 2000; Aisen *et al.*, 2003). The Alzheimer's Disease Anti-inflammatory Prevention Trial (ADAPT) which aimed to examine the efficacy of celecoxib and naproxen in older people (over 70s with a family history of AD) was suspended due to the cardiovascular safety of NSAID (Meinert *et al.*, 2009) and the analysis of the longitudinal data did not find any beneficial effect of either drugs on cognition (Martin *et al.*, 2008).

58.4 CONTROL OF OXIDATIVE STRESS AND FREE RADICALS

58.4.1 Biological basis

Oxidative stress can cause lipoprotein oxidation, Aβ polymerization and generation of excessive free radicals. *In vitro* studies suggest that ApoE ε4 reduces the antioxidant capacity of neurones. Vitamins E and C along with alcohol (in moderation) scavenge these free radicals.

58.4.2 Clinical evidence

A number of epidemiological studies have found higher dietary intake of vitamins E and C, and moderate alcohol consumption to lower risk of dementia. A systematic review which included 23 studies found small amounts of alcohol to have a protective effect against dementia (random effects model, RR 0.63; 95 per cent CI 0.53–0.75) and Alzheimer's disease (RR 0.57; 95 per cent CI 0.44–0.74) (Peters *et al.*, 2008b). However, studies varied in terms of lengths of follow up, measurement of alcohol intake and assessment of potential confounders. Additional studies are needed to examine the effect of type of alcohol on risk reduction, as micronutrients in red wine, especially resveratrol, may offer specific protection against beta-amyloid toxicity, an effect also observed with green tea extracts and the curry spice, curcumin.

A study in which 341 patients with moderate to severe AD were randomized to receive selegiline (monoamine oxidase inhibitor) and vitamin E (either alone or in combination) or placebo found all active treatments, including vitamin E alone, slowed progression of AD over two years, as measured by time to occurrence of death, institutionalization, loss of ability to perform basic activities of daily living or severe dementia, but with no effect specifically on cognition (Sano *et al.*, 1997). However, an RCT in which patients at increased risk of developing AD were randomly assigned to receive 2000 IU of vitamin E daily, 10 mg of donepezil daily, or placebo for three years found vitamin E to have no beneficial effect in slowing progression to AD (Petersen *et al.*, 2005; see also Chapter 55, Drug treatments in development for Alzheimer's disease and Chapter 57, Vitamins and complementary therapies used to treat Alzheimer's disease).

58.5　INCREASING NEURONAL RESERVE

58.5.1　Role of cognitive, physical and social activities

A number of cross-sectional and retrospective studies have found an inverse relationship between activities (cognitive, physical or leisure) in midlife and later risk of dementia. The repetition of cognitive skills may improve processing skills such as working memory and perceptual speed by possibly increasing dendritic plasticity. Physical exercise can increase insulin-like growth factor (IGF-1), and somatostatin levels which are decreased in AD. IGF-1 has been shown to reduce tau phosphorylation and have an anti-apoptotic effect. In experiments on rats, environmental enrichment has been shown to inhibit spontaneous apoptosis, increase neurogenesis in dentate gyrus and improve spatial memory (Nilsson *et al.*, 1999; Young *et al.*, 1999). This may suggest a possible link between environment/social stimulation and regenerative brain processes.

58.5.2　Clinical evidence

There are no RCTs, but four large observational studies have shown reduced activities as an independent risk factor for AD. Wilson *et al.* (2002) followed 801 older clergy over four years and 111 developed AD. They recorded seven common activities which involved information processing as a core component (e.g. reading, watching TV, doing crosswords, etc.). The frequency of each activity was rated on a five-point scale (1 = once a year, 5 = everyday) and responses to each item averaged to calculate a composite score (range 1–5). The authors in their previous work had shown this to be a reliable method compared to differential weighing of each item depending on the perceived cognitive demand. After controlling for age, sex and education, a one point increase in cognitive activity was associated with 33 per cent reduction in risk of AD (HR 0.67). The epidemiological evidence for physical activity in prevention of dementia is mixed. Wilson *et al.* (2002) and Verghese *et al.* (2003) suggested that risk reduction was specifically due to cognitively stimulating activities. Friedland *et al.* (2001) found that reduced activity (intellectual, passive or physical) in midlife increased the risk of developing AD by 250 per cent. The mixed results could be partly explained by how each study divided activities into physical, cognitive or social. For example, 'dancing' (Verghese *et al.*, 2003) or 'going to museum' (Wilson *et al.*, 2002) often included as cognitive activities include a strong physical component. Activities, either cognitive or physical, often include social aspects and are done as leisure activities. The social aspect of the activities or rich social network itself may be beneficial in reducing risk of dementia. Wang *et al.* (2002), in their analysis of the Kungsholmen project, found that engagement in stimulating activities (mental, social or productive) reduced the risk of developing dementia over six years by 50 per cent (RR 0.54–0.58). The Cardiovascular Risk Factors, Aging and Incidence of Dementia (CAIDE) study followed 1449 people over 21 years. Of these, 117 developed dementia and 76 AD. Leisure-time physical activity at midlife at least twice a week was associated with a reduced risk of dementia and AD (OR 0.48 (95 per cent CI 0.25–0.91) and 0.38 (0.17–0.85), respectively), even after adjustments for other potential risk factors. The protective effect of midlife activity was more pronounced in those carrying ApoE ε4 carriers (Rovio *et al.*, 2005). Interestingly, the work-related physical activity, including commuting, was not protective (Rovio *et al.*, 2007). However, care has to be taken with interpretation of these studies as activities may be a proxy for some other factors such as education, socioeconomic status and generally healthy lifestyle. Although reduced activities have been shown to exist many years prior to onset of dementia, one cannot completely rule out the possibility of a prolonged prodrome.

There have been two trials targeting patients with cognitive impairment who are at risk of developing dementia. The study from the Netherlands found that a twice-weekly, group-based, moderate-intensity walking programme over one year was associated with small but significant improvements in quality of life measures (van Uffelen *et al.*, 2007). The Australian study randomized 170 participants to receive education and usual care, or a 24-week home-based programme of physical activity (Lautenschlager *et al.*, 2008). At six months the participants in the intervention group were walking about 9000 steps more than those in the usual care group. Participants were followed at six, 12 and 18 months with the Alzheimer's Disease Assessment Scale (ADAS-Cog) as the primary outcome measure. At 18 months, participants in the intervention group's ADAS-Cog changed by −0.73 points (95 per cent CI −1.27 to 0.03) while the usual care group's changed by −0.04 points (95 per cent CI −0.46 to 0.88). The average improvement of 0.69 points on the ADAS-Cog score compared with the usual care group is small but potentially important when one considers the relatively modest amount of physical activity undertaken by participants in the study.

58.6   OTHER FACTORS

There is considerable interest in the role of diet in determining the risk of dementia and AD. A systematic review that included eight cohorts found that adherence to a Mediterranean diet was associated with a number of health-related benefits including reduced mortality and incidence of AD (Sofi et al., 2008). Epidemiological studies suggest that oestrogen may offer some protection against dementia and AD. However, the trials of hormone replacement therapy (HRT) such as the Women's Health Initiative were suspended due to concerns about increased risk of cardiovascular and other morbidities. The subsequent analyses found an increased risk of dementia over two years in the intervention arm but the five-year follow up of the modified trial is ongoing (Sano et al., 2008).

58.7   TARGET POPULATIONS

Many of the risk factors for AD and the beginning of losses in key neuronal receptor systems (Perry et al., 2001) come into play in midlife, 15 to 20 years prior to onset of AD. This would suggest targeting prevention strategies at people with risk factors in their midlife, who may not have any identifiable cognitive impairment. The economics of such trials make them impractical, due to low incident dementia and prolonged follow up over two decades. Identification of surrogate markers of subclinical disease progression is crucial for their viability. Another approach would be to target older people who have developed some cognitive impairment, but which is not severe enough to cause functional impairment and warrant diagnosis of dementia. The somewhat loose and controversial term, MCI, is most widely used to describe this population which has community prevalence of 17–34 per cent with annual 'conversion' to dementia of between 3 and 15 per cent depending upon the population (Burns and Zaudig, 2002; see Chapter 43, Mild cognitive impairment: a historical perspective and Chapter 44, Clinical characteristics of mild cognitive impairment). However, it is essential to operationalize the criteria for MCI to allow comparison between studies (Matthews et al., 2007) and develop surrogate markers to help reduce the size of the study.

58.8   CONCLUSION

The epidemiological evidence suggests that it is possible to delay, if not prevent, the onset of dementia, both AD and VaD. The RCT evidence is building up for antihypertensives but remains sparse for other strategies. There may be a therapeutic time window between midlife and late life during which vascular risk factors increase the risk of dementia. This may explain the dissonance between the epidemiological research that identifies potential risk factor and the RCT that fails to show positive effect of the intervention in older people with MCI. Systolic BP drops around the onset of dementia and lowering BP in patients with MCI, some of whom may have already developed neurodegenerative changes, may not have beneficial effects. In addition, lower the better doctrine applied to BP and cholesterol in cardiovascular and stroke prevention trials may not hold true for cognition in people with MCI. Most RCTs focus on one or two vascular risk factors and assess dementia only as a secondary outcome. There is a need for RCTs, which will target multiple risk factors in at-risk people with MCI or mild vascular cognitive impairment with incident dementia as a primary outcome. The Multidomain Alzheimer prevention Trail (MAPT) is currently recruiting 1200 patients with subjective memory complaint and limitation in one instrumental activity of daily living to investigate the effect of a multidomain (nutrition, physical and cognitive training) intervention with or without omega-3 fatty acid on cognitive decline over three years, with results expected in 2013 (Gillette-Guyonnet et al., 2009).

REFERENCES

Aisen PS, Davis KL, Berg JD et al. (2000) A randomized controlled trial of prednisone in Alzheimer's disease. Alzheimer's Disease Cooperative Study. Neurology 54: 588–93.

Aisen PS, Schafer KA, Grundman M et al. (2003) Alzheimer's Disease Cooperative Study. Effects of rofecoxib or naproxen vs placebo on Alzheimer disease progression: A randomized controlled trial. Journal of American Medical Association 289: 2819–26.

Aisen PS, Schneider LS, Sano M et al. (2008) High-dose B vitamin supplementation and cognitive decline in Alzheimer disease: A randomized controlled trial. Journal of American Medical Association 300: 1774–83.

Applegate WB, Pressel S, Wittes J. (1994) Impact of the treatment of isolated systolic hypertension on behavioral variables. Results from the systolic hypertension in the elderly program. Archives of Internal Medicine 154: 2154–60.

Arvanitakis Z, Schneider JA, Wilson RS et al. (2008) Statins, incident Alzheimer disease, change in cognitive function, and neuropathology. Neurology 70: 1795–802.

Barnes JM, Barnes NM, Costall B et al. (1989) Angiotensin II inhibits the release of [3H]acetylcholine from rat entorhinal cortex in vitro. Brain Research 491: 136–43.

Bosch J, Yusuf S, Pogue J et al. (2002) HOPE Investigators. Heart outcomes prevention evaluation. Use of ramipril in preventing stroke: Double blind randomised trial. British Medical Journal 324: 699–702.

Bottiglieri T, Parnetti L, Arning E et al. (2001) Plasma total homocysteine levels and the C677T mutation in the methylenetetrahydrofolate reductase (MTHFR) gene: A study in an Italian population with dementia. *Mechanism of Ageing and Development* **122**: 2013–23.

Burns A, Zaudig M. (2002) Mild cognitive impairment in older people. *Lancet* **360**: 963–5.

Clarke R, Smith AD, Jobst KA *et al.* (1998) Folate, vitamin B12, and serum total homocysteine levels in confirmed Alzheimer disease. *Archives of Neurology* **55**: 1407–8.

Connelly PJ, Prentice NP, Cousland G, Bonham J. (2008) A randomised double-blind placebo-controlled trial of folic acid supplementation of cholinesterase inhibitors in Alzheimer's disease. *International Journal of Geriatric Psychiatry* **23**: 155–60.

Dufouil C, Alperovitch A, Ducros V *et al.* (2003) Homocysteine, white matter hyperintensities, and cognition in healthy elderly people. *Annals of Neurology* **53**: 214–21.

Dufouil C, Richard F, Fiévet N *et al.* (2005) APOE genotype, cholesterol level, lipid-lowering treatment, and dementia: The Three-City Study. *Neurology* **64**: 1531–8.

Durga J, van Boxtel MP, Schouten EG *et al.* (2007) Effect of 3-year folic acid supplementation on cognitive function in older adults in the FACIT trial: A randomised, double blind, controlled trial. *Lancet* **369**: 208–16.

Etminan M, Gill S, Samii A. (2003) The role of lipid-lowering drugs in cognitive function: A meta-analysis of observational studies. *Pharmacotherapy* **23**: 726–30.

Farris W, Mansourian S, Leissring MA *et al.* (2004) Partial loss-of-function mutations in insulin-degrading enzyme that induce diabetes also impair degradation of amyloid beta-protein. *American Journal of Pathology* **164**: 1425–34.

Fassbender K, Simons M, Bergmann C *et al.* (2001) Simvastatin strongly reduces levels of Alzheimer's disease beta-amyloid peptides Abeta 42 and Abeta 40 *in vitro* and *in vivo*. *Proceedings of the National Academy of Science of the United States of America* **98**: 5856–61.

Flicker L, Martins RN, Thomas J *et al.* (2008) B-vitamins reduce plasma levels of beta amyloid. *Neurobiology of Aging* **29**: 303–5.

Fogari R, Mugellini A, Zoppi A *et al.* (2003) Influence of losartan and atenolol on memory function in very elderly hypertensive patients. *Journal of Human Hypertension* **17**: 781–5.

Forette F, Seux ML, Staessen JA *et al.* (1998) Prevention of dementia in randomised double-blind placebo-controlled systolic hypertension in Europe (Syst-Eur) trial. *Lancet* **352**: 1347–51.

Forette F, Seux ML, Staessen JA *et al.* (2002) The prevention of dementia with antihypertensive treatment: New evidence from the Systolic Hypertension in Europe (Syst-Eur) study. *Archives of Internal Medicine* **162**: 2046–52.

Friedland RP, Fritsch T, Smyth KA *et al.* (2001) Patients with Alzheimer's disease have reduced activities in midlife compared with healthy control-group members. *Proceedings of the National Academy of Science of the United States of America* **98**: 3440–5.

Frosst P, Blom HJ, Milos R *et al.* (1995) A candidate genetic risk factor for vascular disease: A common mutation in methylenetetrahydrofolate reductase. *Nature Genetics* **10**: 111–13.

Gillette-Guyonnet S, Andrieu S, Dantoine T *et al.* (2009) Commentary on 'A roadmap for the prevention of dementia II. Leon Thal Symposium 2008'. The Multidomain Alzheimer Preventive Trial (MAPT): A new approach to the prevention of Alzheimer's disease. *Alzheimer's and Dementia* **5**: 114–21.

Haag MD, Hofman A, Koudstaal PJ *et al.* (2009) Statins are associated with a reduced risk of Alzheimer disease regardless of lipophilicity. The Rotterdam Study. *Journal of Neurology, Neurosurgery, and Psychiatry* **80**: 13–17.

Heart Protection Study Collaborative Group. (2002) MRC/BHF Heart Protection Study of cholesterol lowering with simvastatin in 20 536 high-risk individuals: A randomised placebo-controlled trial. *Lancet* **360**: 7–22.

In't Veld BA, Ruitenberg A, Hofman A *et al.* (2001) Nonsteroidal antiinflammatory drugs and the risk of Alzheimer's disease. *New England Journal of Medicine* **345**: 1515–21.

Johnson KC, Margolis KL, Espeland MA *et al.* (2008) A prospective study of the effect of hypertension and baseline blood pressure on cognitive decline and dementia in postmenopausal women: The Women's Health Initiative Memory Study. *Journal of the American Geriatrics Society* **56**: 1449–58.

Jorm AF, Korten AE, Henderson AS. (1987) The prevalence of dementia: A quantitative integration of the literature. *Acta Psychiatrica Scandinavica* **76**: 465–79.

Kivipelto M, Helkala EL, Laakso MP *et al.* (2002) Apolipoprotein E epsilon4 allele, elevated midlife total cholesterol level, and high midlife systolic blood pressure are independent risk factors for late-life Alzheimer disease. *Annals of Internal Medicine* **137**: 149–55.

Kivipelto M, Ngandu T, Laatikainen T *et al.* (2006) Risk score for the prediction of dementia risk in 20 years among middle aged people: A longitudinal, population-based study. *Lancet Neurology* **5**: 735–41.

Kojro E, Gimpl G, Lammich S *et al.* (2001) Low cholesterol stimulates the nonamyloidogenic pathway by its effect on the alpha-secretase ADAM 10. *Proceedings of the National Academy of Science of the United States of America* **98**: 5815–20.

Lautenschlager NT, Cox KL, Flicker L *et al.* (2008) Effect of physical activity on cognitive function in older adults at risk for Alzheimer disease: A randomized trial. *Journal of the American Medical Association* **300**: 1027–37.

Li G, Rhew IC, Shofer JB *et al.* (2007) Age-varying association between blood pressure and risk of dementia in those aged 65 and older: A community-based prospective cohort study. *Journal of the American Geriatrics Society* **55**: 1161–7.

Lithell H, Hansson L, Skoog I *et al.* (2003) SCOPE Study Group. The Study on Cognition and Prognosis in the Elderly (SCOPE): Principal results of a randomized double-blind intervention trial. *Journal of Hypertension* **21**: 875–86.

McCaddon A, Hudson P, Davies G *et al.* (2001) Homocysteine and cognitive decline in healthy elderly. *Dementia and Geriatric Cognitive Disorders* **12**: 309–13.

McGeer PL, Schulzer M, McGeer EG. (1996) Arthritis and anti-inflammatory agents as possible protective factors for

Alzheimer's disease: A review of 17 epidemiologic studies. *Neurology* **47**: 425–32.

McGuinness B, Craig D, Bullock R, Passmore P. (2009) Statins for the prevention of dementia. *Cochrane Database of Systematic Reviews* (2): CD003160.

Malouf R, Grimley Evans J. (2008) Folic acid with or without vitamin B12 for the prevention and treatment of healthy elderly and demented people. *Cochrane Database Systematic Reviews* (4): CD004514.

Martin BK, Szekely C, Brandt J *et al.* (2008) Cognitive function over time in the Alzheimer's Disease Anti-inflammatory Prevention Trial (ADAPT): Results of a randomized, controlled trial of naproxen and celecoxib. *Archives of Neurology* **65**: 896–905.

Matthews FE, Stephan BC, Bond J *et al.* (2007) Medical Research Council Cognitive Function and Ageing Study. Operationalization of mild cognitive impairment: a graphical approach. *PLoS Medicine* **4**: 1615–19.

Meinert CL, McCaffrey LD, Breitner JC *et al.* (2009) Alzheimer's Disease Anti-inflammatory Prevention Trial: Design, methods, and baseline results. *Alzheimer's and Dementia* **5**: 93–104.

Meyer JS, Judd BW, Tawaklna T *et al.* (1986) Improved cognition after control of risk factors for multi-infarct dementia. *Journal of the American Medical Association* **256**: 2203–9.

Moroney JT, Tang MX, Berglund L *et al.* (1999) Low-density lipoprotein cholesterol and the risk of dementia with stroke. *Journal of the American Medical Association* **282**: 254–60.

Nilsson M, Perfilieva E, Johansson U *et al.* (1999) Enriched environment increases neurogenesis in the adult rat dentate gyrus and improves spatial memory. *Journal of Neurobiology* **39**: 569–78.

Nilsson K, Gustafson L, Hultberg B. (2001) Improvement of cognitive functions after cabolmin/folate supplementation in elderly patients with dementia and elevated plasma homocysteine. *International Journal of Geriatric Psychiatry* **16**: 609–14.

Nordberg A, Hellstrom-Lindahl E, Lee M *et al.* (2002) Chronic nicotine treatment reduces beta-amyloidosis in the brain of a mouse model of Alzheimer's disease (APPsw). *Journal of Neurochemistry* **81**: 655–8.

Peila R, White LR, Petrovich H *et al.* (2001) Joint effect of the APOE gene and midlife systolic blood pressure on late-life cognitive impairment: The Honolulu-Asia aging study. *Stroke* **32**: 2882–9.

Perry EK, Martin-Ruiz CM, Court JA. (2001) Nicotinic receptor subtypes in human brain related to aging and dementia. *Alcohol* **24**: 63–8.

Peters R, Beckett N, Forette F *et al.* (2008a) Incident dementia and blood pressure lowering in the Hypertension in the Very Elderly Trial cognitive function assessment (HYVET-COG): A double-blind, placebo controlled trial. *Lancet Neurology* **7**: 683–9.

Peters R, Peters J, Warner J *et al.* (2008b) Alcohol, dementia and cognitive decline in the elderly: A systematic review. *Age and Ageing* **37**: 505–12.

Petersen RC, Thomas RG, Grundman M *et al.* (2005) Vitamin E and donepezil for the treatment of mild cognitive impairment. *New England Journal of Medicine* **352**: 2379–88.

Petrovitch H, Ross GW, Steinhorn SC *et al.* (2005) AD lesions and infarcts in demented and non-demented Japanese-American men. *Annals of Neurology* **57**: 98–103.

Prince MJ, Bird AS, Blizard RA *et al.* (1996) Is the cognitive function of older patients affected by antihypertensive treatment? Results from 54 months of the Medical Research Council's trial of hypertension in older adults. *British Medical Journal* **312**: 801–5.

Purandare N, Burns A, Daly KJ *et al.* (2006) Cerebral emboli as a potential cause of Alzheimer's disease and vascular dementia: Case-control study. *British Medical Journal* **332**: 1119–24.

Purandare N, Voshaar RC, Morris J *et al.* (2007) Asymptomatic spontaneous cerebral emboli predict cognitive and functional decline in dementia. *Biological Psychiatry* **62**: 339–44.

Qiu C, von Strauss E, Winblad B, Fratiglioni L. (2004) Decline in blood pressure over time and risk of dementia: A longitudinal study from the Kungsholmen project. *Stroke* **35**: 1810–5.

Rockwood K, Kirkland S, Hogan DB *et al.* (2002) Use of lipid-lowering agents, indication bias, and the risk of dementia in community-dwelling elderly people. *Archives of Neurology* **59**: 223–7.

Rovio S, Kåreholt I, Helkala EL *et al.* (2005) Leisure-time physical activity at midlife and the risk of dementia and Alzheimer's disease. *Lancet Neurology* **4**: 705–11.

Rovio S, Kåreholt I, Viitanen M *et al.* (2007) Work-related physical activity and the risk of dementia and Alzheimer's disease. *International Journal of Geriatric Psychiatry* **22**: 874–82.

Sano M, Ernesto C, Thomas RG *et al.* (1997) A controlled trial of selegiline, alpha-tocopherol, or both as treatment for Alzheimer's disease. The Alzheimer's Disease Cooperative Study. *New England Journal of Medicine* **336**: 1216–22.

Sano M, Jacobs D, Andrews H *et al.* (2008) A multi-center, randomized, double blind placebo-controlled trial of estrogens to prevent Alzheimer's disease and loss of memory in women: design and baseline characteristics. *Clinical Trials* **5**: 523–33.

Seshadri S, Beiser A, Selhub J *et al.* (2002) Plasma homocysteine as a risk factor for dementia and Alzheimer's disease. *New England Journal of Medicine* **346**: 466–8.

Seshadri S. (2006) Elevated plasma homocysteine levels: risk factor or risk marker for the development of dementia and Alzheimer's disease? *Journal of Alzheimer's Disease* **9**: 393–8.

Shepherd J, Blauw GJ, Murphy MB *et al.* (2002) Pravastatin in elderly individuals at risk of vascular disease (PROSPER): A randomised controlled trial. *Lancet* **360**: 1623–30.

Simons M, Keller P, De Strooper B *et al.* (1998) Cholesterol depletion inhibits the generation of beta-amyloid in hippocampal neurons. *Proceedings of the National Academy of Sciences of the United States of America* **95**: 6460–4.

Sjogren M, Gustafsson K, Syversen S *et al.* (2003) Treatment with simvastatin in patients with Alzheimer's disease lowers both alpha- and beta-cleaved amyloid precursor protein. *Dementia and Geriatric Cognitive Disorders* **16**: 25–30.

Sofi F, Cesari F, Abbate R *et al.* (2008) Adherence to Mediterranean diet and health status: Meta-analysis. *BMJ* **337**: a1344.

Sun Y, Lu CJ, Chien KL *et al.* (2007) Efficacy of multivitamin supplementation containing vitamins B6 and B12 and folic acid as adjunctive treatment with a cholinesterase inhibitor in

Alzheimer's disease: A 26-week, randomized, double-blind, placebo-controlled study in Taiwanese patients. *Clinical Therapeutics* 29: 2204–14.

Tzourio C, Anderson C, Chapman N *et al.* (2003) PROGRESS Collaborative Group. Effects of blood pressure lowering with perindopril and indapamide therapy on dementia and cognitive decline in patients with cerebrovascular disease. *Archives of Internal Medicine* 163: 1069–75.

Vanhanen M, Koivisto K, Moilanen L *et al.* (2006) Association of metabolic syndrome with Alzheimer disease: A population-based study. *Neurology* 67: 843–7.

van Uffelen JG, Chin A Paw MJ, Hopman-Rock M, van Mechelen W. (2007) The effect of walking and vitamin B supplementation on quality of life in community-dwelling adults with mild cognitive impairment: A randomized, controlled trial. *Quality of Life Research* 16: 1137–46.

Ventura P, Panini R, Verlato C *et al.* (2001) Hyperhomocysteinemia and related factors in 600 hospitalized elderly subjects. *Metabolism* 50: 1466–71.

Verghese J, Lipton RB, Katz MJ *et al.* (2003) Leisure activities and the risk of dementia in the elderly. *New England Journal of Medicine* 348: 2508–16.

Viswanathan A, Raj S, Greenberg SM *et al.* (2009) Plasma Abeta, homocysteine, and cognition: the Vitamin Intervention for Stroke Prevention (VISP) trial. *Neurology* 72: 268–72.

Wang H-X, Karp A, Winblad B *et al.* (2002) Late-life engagement in social and leisure activities is associated with a decreased risk of dementia: A longitudinal study from the Kungsholmen project. *American Journal of Epidemiology* 155: 1081–7.

Weggen S, Eriksen JL, Das P *et al.* (2001) A subset of NSAIDs lower amyloidogenic Abeta42 independently of cyclooxygenase activity. *Nature* 8: 212–16.

Wilson RS, Mendes De Leon CF, Barnes LL *et al.* (2002) Participation in cognitively stimulating activities and risk of incident Alzheimer disease. *Journal of the American Medical Association* 287: 742–8.

Young D, Lawlor PA, Leone P *et al.* (1999) Environmental enrichment inhibits spontaneous apoptosis, prevents seizures and is neuroprotective. *Nature Medicine* 5: 448–53.

Zandi PP, Breitner JC. (2001) Do NSAIDs prevent Alzheimer's disease? And, if so, why? The epidemiological evidence. *Neurobiology of Aging* 22: 811–17.

Zandi PP, Sparks DL, Khachaturian AS *et al.* (2005) Do statins reduce risk of incident dementia and Alzheimer disease? The Cache County Study. *Archives of General Psychiatry* 62: 217–24.

Zhou B, Teramukai S, Fukushima M. (2007) Prevention and treatment of dementia or Alzheimer's disease by statins: A meta-analysis. *Dementia and Geriatric Cognitive Disorders* 23: 194–201.

59

Trial designs

SERGE GAUTHIER

59.1 INTRODUCTION

Any therapy, whether pharmacological or not, requires proof of safety and efficacy. This chapter outlines the various trial designs that have been used for the pharmacological treatment of Alzheimer's disease (AD). The experience gained so far has been predominately in the symptomatic treatment of AD, using parallel group designs over 3–12 months, and rarely a survival design to a disease milestone. A number of randomized clinical studies attempting to modify progression of AD have been completed or are under way, using parallel group designs over 12–18 months.

The natural history of AD is described first (see also Chapter 48, The natural history of Alzheimer's disease), introducing the concepts of disease stages, disease milestones and symptomatic domains that fluctuate in intensity as the disease runs its course. Lessons from symptomatic studies using cholinesterase inhibitors (ChEIs) and memantine are summarized. Current disease modification study designs are then outlined.

59.2 NATURAL HISTORY OF AD

The natural history of AD can be broadly considered as a presymptomatic stage, during which a number of pathological events take place, an early symptomatic or prodromal stage with affective and/or cognitive manifestations, and symptomatic mild, moderate and severe stages (see Chapter 44, Clinical characteristics of mild cognitive impairment; Chapter 46, What is Alzheimer's disease?; Chapter 48, The

natural history of Alzheimer's disease; Chapter 49, The neuropathology of Alzheimer's disease; and Chapter 50, Neurochemistry of Alzheimer's disease). Each of these stages could be targeted for specific treatments, requiring different trial designs and outcomes (**Table 59.1**).

Disease milestones have been defined for AD (**Box 59.1**). Some of these milestones can be targets for treatment, with considerable face validity and impact on care (Galasko *et al.*, 1995). For example, studies in mild cognitive impairment (MCI) of the amnestic type may demonstrate that the diagnosis of dementia (predominately AD) is delayed by six months or longer. Delaying loss of autonomy for self-care and even death in moderate to severe stages of AD using α-tocopherol in only one study of the AD Cooperative Study group (Sano *et al.*, 1997) has influenced clinical practice to use vitamin E in all stages of AD, at least in the USA (see Chapter 57, Vitamins and complementary therapies used to treat Alzheimer's disease). Delaying the loss of autonomy for instrumental activities of daily living (ADL) or the need for nursing home care would reduce the need for supportive care. Delaying emergence of some of the behavioural and psychological symptoms of dementia (BPSD) would reduce caregiver burden and later need for nursing home placement.

Symptomatic domains in dementia include cognition, ADL and behaviour. One can even add a domain of changes in motricity, since patents with AD will manifest some features of parkinsonism late in the disease. In many patients early changes in mood and anxiety precede the formal diagnosis of AD, sometimes with spontaneous improvement as insight into the disease is lost. Cognitive and functional ADL decline are relatively linear over time, whereas BPSD peak midway into the disease course and resolve

Table 59.1   Examples of trial design and outcomes for each stage of Alzheimer's disease.

Stage	Target population	Trial design	Primary outcome
Presymptomatic	Healthy elderly	Survival over 5–7 years	Incident dementia
Prodromal	Mild cognitive impairment; amnestic subtype	Survival over 3 years	Progression to dementia
Mild to moderate	AD in the community	Six months parallel groups	Cognition and global impression of change
Moderate to severe	AD in the community or in assisted living	Six months parallel groups	ADL and global impression of change
Severe	AD in institution	Six months parallel groups	Behaviour

AD, Alzheimer's disease; ADL, activities of daily living.

Box 59.1 Clinical milestones in Alzheimer's disease.

- Emergence of cognitive symptoms
- Progression from amnestic mild cognitive impairment to diagnosable dementia
- Loss of instrumental ADL
- Emergence of behavioural and psychological symptoms of dementia
- Nursing home placement
- Loss of self-care ADL
- Death

---

spontaneously through the severe stage as motricity becomes impaired (Gauthier et al., 2001). These natural fluctuations in the intensity of individual symptomatic domains through the stages of AD have an impact in trial design and outcomes (**Table 59.2**). It should be noted that studies can be of shorter duration and/or of smaller numbers of subjects in moderate compared with mild stages of AD because of the faster rate of decline in the moderate stage, which may be related to the

sensitivity of measurement scales, or to the progression of the AD.

59.3   SYMPTOMATIC CLINICAL TRIALS USING CHEIS AND MEMANTINE

The modern treatment of AD was initiated by the report that tacrine improved some aspects of cognition and daily life. The follow-up confirmatory studies used crossover and parallel group designs. The Food and Drug Administration (FDA) published 'guidelines' (Leber, 1990) which greatly influenced the choice of outcomes for proof of efficacy of drugs improving symptoms in AD: a cognitive performance-based scale such as the Alzheimer's Disease Assessment Scale, cognitive part (ADAS-Cog) and an interview-based impression of change became the primary outcomes in mild to moderate AD, usually defined operationally as scores between 10 and 26 on the Mini-Mental State Examination (MMSE). Unfortunately, as these FDA guidelines cautioned against the 'pseudospecificity' of measurable benefits on neuropsychiatric manifestations in AD, they delayed research in this symptomatic domain. In recent years discussions and publications from the FDA and other regulatory agencies have

---

Table 59.2   Example of impact of symptoms through stages of Alzheimer's disease on trial design and outcomes.

Stage	Prominent features	Types of outcomes	Examples
Mild	Depression may be present; few BPSD; cognitive decline slow but predominant feature; some instrumental ADL losses	Cognition; instrumental ADL	ADAS-Cog, ADCS-ADL, DAD
Moderate	Cognitive decline more rapid; functional decline more rapid; BPSD emerge	Cognition; instrumental and basic ADL; behaviour	ADAS-Cog, DAD, ADCS-ADL, NPI, BEHAVE-AD
Severe	Cognitive losses harder to measure (floor effect); few self-care ADL remaining; BPSD abating; parkinsonism emerging	Cognition; self-care ADL; behaviour; parkinsonism	SIB, ADCS-ADL, NPI, UPDRS

ADAS-Cog, Alzheimer Disease Assessment Scale – cognitive subscale (Rosen et al., 1984); ADCS-ADL, Alzheimer Disease Cooperative Study ADL scale (Galasko et al., 1997); BEHAVE-AD, Behavioural symptoms in Alzheimer's disease (Reisberg et al., 1987); BPSD, behavioural and psychological symptoms of dementia; DAD, Disability Assessment in Dementia (Gélinas et al., 1999); NPI, Neuropsychiatric Inventory (Cummings et al., 1994); SIB, Severe Impairment Battery (Panisset et al., 1994); UPDRS, United Parkinson Disease Rating Scale (Fahn and Elton, 1987).

been more accepting of ADL and behaviour as important outcomes.

The following study designs have been used in the proof of efficacy for ChEIs: parallel groups over 3–12 months and survival to a predefined clinical end point over one year or longer.

Parallel groups offer the possibility of short-term (minimum three months) studies comparing the efficacy of different doses of the drug versus placebo. The primary analysis is done on outcomes at the end of the study using the last observation carried forward (LOCF) or intent to treat (ITT) analyses, which compensate for missing values in case of dropouts. Although LOCF/ITT has been favoured by the FDA, investigators and other regulatory agencies are now suggesting that for studies of 12 months or longer, the primary analysis should be on observed cases (OC), i.e. completers. For practical purposes both types of analysis will usually be performed. Although 'cognitive enhancement' was the main hope for ChEIs as a therapeutic class, the reality has emerged from six-month studies with open-label extensions and the one-year placebo-controlled Nordic study (Winblad et al., 2001) that, although there is a small but statistically significant improvement in cognition peaking at three months with the ChEIs, the most clinically relevant finding has been the stabilization of cognitive decline with 'return to baseline' at 9–12 months for the actively treated groups at the higher therapeutics doses, compared with placebo-treated groups who decline steadily. It should be noted that this natural decline varies greatly between studies in AD, and is even less evident in AD with cerebrovascular disease or in vascular dementia (VaD), where control of vascular risk factors appear to modify progression, at least in studies of six months' duration (Schneider, 2003).

Survival studies have primarily looked at loss of ADL, and have successfully demonstrated a delay in the loss of autonomy for patients on ChEIs compared with placebo. Parallel group six-month studies in patients ranging from mild to moderately severe AD (MMSE 5–26) have also established that ADL are more stable on treatment compared to placebo, but show no reversibility for lost instrumental ADL.

The most difficult domain to study, although very significant clinically, has been behaviour. The availability of general BPSD scales such as the Neuropsychiatric Inventory (NPI) and Behavioural symptoms in Alzheimer's disease (BEHAVE-AD), as well as specific scales such as Cohen-Mansfield Agitation Inventory (Cohen-Mansfield et al., 1989; see Chapter 9, Measurement of behaviour disturbance, non-cognitive symptoms and quality of life, for more information about these three scales), has not yet allowed unequivocal demonstration of benefit in severe stages of AD. New methods of analysis of behaviour have been proposed (Gauthier et al., 2002; Gauthier et al., 2008), and will probably be more successful in defining categories of BPSD symptoms most responsive to ChEIs (anxiety, hallucinations), memantine (agitation) and other drugs.

Memantine has been found to be effective in a range of studies using parallel groups in moderate to severe AD. Scales appropriate for this stage of disease, such as the Severe Impairment Battery (SIB), the Alzheimer Disease Cooperative Study ADL scale (ADCS-ADL) and the NPI have been

used and accepted by the FDA and other regulatory agencies. The trial design of adding memantine or placebo to a stable dose of a ChEI has been used successfully (Tariot et al., 2004), paving the way to a number of studies where novel drugs or placebo are added to 'standard treatment'.

59.4   DISEASE MODIFICATION STRATEGIES

Many studies have been made and others are ongoing with the hope of arresting or significantly slowing disease progression. So far they have used parallel groups designs over 12–18 months in mild to moderate AD, with the new drug or a placebo added to standard treatment with a ChEI and/or memantine. The primary efficacy outcomes are usually the ADAS-Cog and the Clinical Dementia Rating sum of boxes (Hughes et al., 1982), and secondary outcomes include volumetric brain measurement using magnetic resonance imaging at beginning and end of study, looking for a reduced rate of brain (whole brain or hippocampus) atrophy in the actively treated group compared to placebo. Although this design appears promising, there are uncertainties and limitations. For instance, the difference in rate of brain atrophy may be absent or opposite to expectations, with accelerated atrophy in the actively treated group. There may be a discrepancy between a reduced rate of atrophy but no measurable clinical benefit (Gauthier et al., 2009).

One difficult issue in disease modification strategies is the decision of the stage of disease where the proposed drug is most likely to work. On the proof-of-concept phase II/III efficacy and safety study hinges the entire future of the drug. For example, numerous attempts at treating patients with AD in mild to moderate stages using non-steroidal anti-inflammatory drugs have failed, despite the weight of evidence from epidemiological research and the biological plausibility of an inflammatory response to β amyloid deposition. It may be that treatment in the late presymptomatic or in the prodromal stages would be the most appropriate time. On the other hand, studies in these stages of AD would require three to five years, a very long time for a proof-of-concept. Alternative patient groups could be considered for proof-of-concept, such as presenilin or amyloid precursor protein mutation carriers (see Chapter 52, Genetics of Alzheimer's disease), subjects with amnestic MCI that are apolipoprotein E ε4 carriers or subjects with the newly defined 'predementia AD' (Dubois et al., 2007).

59.5   FUTURE STRATEGIES TO DELAY EMERGENCE OF AD

As hypotheses on the pathophysiology of AD emerge from epidemiological research in human populations, post-mortem and biomarker studies in patients, and animal models, we will need to establish whether new therapies can delay the onset of symptoms in asymptomatic people at varying degrees of risk of AD. The prototype of trial designs to establish the safety and efficacy of such therapies are the five to seven year studies comparing Ginkgo biloba to placebo in elderly subjects with or without memory complaints but no measurable impairment, with incident dementia as the primary end point (Vellas *et al.*, 2006; DeKosky *et al.*, 2008). Variations of this design may be possible, by enriching the study population with different levels of risk, such as a positive family history of AD and/or selected gene or biological markers, although enrichment of a study population will limit the applicability of findings to the population as a whole.

Simultaneous multiple interventions may be required to obtain benefit in AD: they are being studied using non-pharmacological interventions such as cognitive training, physical exercise and diet enrichment. The combination of pathological factors in AD (amyloid toxicity, tau pathology, inflammatory responses) may require combinations of drugs in a way similar to cancer chemotherapy. This will need to be carefully thought through with the participation of clinical trialists, regulators and patients' representatives, as was done for a review for scales' measures for AD (Black *et al.*, 2009).

REFERENCES

Black R, Greenberg B, Ryan JM *et al.* (2009) Scales as outcome measures for Alzheimer's disease. *Alzheimer's and Dementia* **5**: 324–39.

Cohen-Mansfield J, Marx MS, Rosenthal AS. (1989) A description of agitation in a nursing home. *Journal of Gerontology* **44**: M77–84.

Cummings JL, Mega M, Gray K *et al.* (1994) Neuropsychiatric Inventory: Comprehensive assessment of psychopathology in dementia. *Neurology* **44**: 2308–14.

DeKosky ST, Williamson JD, Fitzpatrick AL *et al.* (2008) Gingko biloba for prevention of dementia. A randomized controlled trial. *Journal of the American Medical Association* **300**: 2253–62.

Dubois B, Feldman HH, Jacova C *et al.* (2007) Research criteria for the diagnosis of Alzheimer's disease: Revisiting the NINCDS-ADRDA criteria. *Lancet Neurology* **6**: 734–46.

Fahn S, Elton R. (1987) United Parkinson's Disease Rating Scale. In: Fahn S, Marsden C, Golstein M *et al.* (eds). *Recent development in Parkinson's disease.* Florham Park, NJ: Macmillan Health Care, 153–63.

Galasko D, Edland SD, Morris JC *et al.* (1995) The Consortium to establish a Registry for Alzheimer's Disease (CERAD). Part IX. Clinical milestones in patients with Alzheimer's disease followed over 3 years. *Neurology* **45**: 1451–5.

Galasko D, Bennett D, Sano M *et al.* (1997) An inventory to assess activities of daily living for clinical trials in Alzheimer's disease. *Alzheimer Disease and Associated Disorders* **11** (Suppl. 2): S33–9.

Gauthier S, Thal LJ, Rossor MN. (2001) The future diagnosis and management of Alzheimer's disease. In: Gauthier S (ed). *Clinical diagnosis and management of Alzheimer's disease.* London: Martin Dunitz, 369–78.

Gauthier S, Feldman H, Hecker J *et al.* (2002) Efficacy of donepezil on behavioral symptoms in patients with moderate to severe Alzheimer's disease. *International Psychogeriatrics* **14**: 389–404.

Gauthier S, Loft H, Cummings J. (2008) Improvement in behavioral symptoms in patients with moderate to severe Alzheimer's disease by memantine: A pooled data analysis. *International Journal of Geriatric Psychiatry* **23**: 537–45.

Gauthier S, Aisen PS, Ferris SH *et al.* (2009) Effect of tramiprosate in patients with mild-to-moderate Alzheimer's disease: Exploratory analysis of the MRI sub-group of the ALPHASE Study. *Journal of Nutrition, Health and Aging* **13**: 550–7.

Gélinas I, Gauthier L, McIntyre M, Gauthier S. (1999) Development of a functional measure for persons with Alzheimer's disease: The Disability Assessment for Dementia. *American Journal of Occupational Therapy* **53**: 471–81.

Hughes CP, Berg L, Danziger WL *et al.* (1982) A new clinical scale for the staging of dementia. *British Journal of Psychiatry* **140**: 566–72.

Leber P. (1990) *Guidelines for clinical evaluation of antidementia drugs.* Washington DC: US Food and Drug Administration.

Panisset M, Roudier M, Sexton J *et al.* (1994) Severe Impairment Battery: A neuropsychological test for severely demented patients. *Archives of Neurology* **51**: 41–5.

Reisberg B, Borenstein J, Salob SP *et al.* (1987) Behavioral symptoms in Alzheimer's disease. *Journal of Clinical Psychiatry* **48** (Suppl.): 9–15.

Rosen WG, Mohs RC, Davis KL. (1984) A new rating scale for Alzheimer's disease. *American Journal of Psychiatry* **141**: 1356–64.

Sano M, Ernesto C, Thomas RG *et al.* (1997) A controlled trial of selegiline, alpha-tocopherol, or both as treatment for Alzheimer's disease. *New England Journal of Medicine* **336**: 1216–22.

Schneider LS. (2003) Cholinesterase inhibitors for vascular dementia? *Lancet Neurology* **2**: 658–9.

Tariot PN, Farlow MR, Grossberg GT *et al.* (2004) and the Memantine Study Group. Memantine treatment in patients with moderate to severe Alzheimer disease already receiving donepezil: A randomized controlled trial. *Journal of the American Medical Association* **291**: 317–24.

Vellas B, Andrieu S, Ousset PJ *et al.* (2006) The GuidAge study. Methodological issues. A 5-year double-blind randomized trial of the efficacy of EGb 761 for prevention of Alzheimer disease in patients over 70 with a memory complaint. *Neurology* **67** (Suppl. 3): S6–11.

Winblad B, Engedal K, Soininen H *et al.* (2001) Donepezil Nordic Study Group: A 1-year, randomized, placebo-controlled study of donepezil in patients with mild to moderate AD. *Neurology* **57**: 489–95.

PART IV

THE OVERLAP AND INTERACTION BETWEEN ALZHEIMER'S DISEASE AND CEREBROVASCULAR DISEASE

60

Vascular factors and Alzheimer's disease

ROBERT STEWART

60.1 VASCULAR FACTORS IN ALZHEIMER'S DISEASE

The growing recognition of the role of vascular factors in Alzheimer's disease (AD) challenges traditional dementia subclassification. In particular, the assumption that AD and vascular dementia (VaD) are distinguishable clinical disorders in late-onset dementia has become untenable because of the large pathological overlap and poor correlations between diagnosis and pathology. The problems this distinction has caused for research are now well recognized. The system of subclassifying dementia according to presumed AD or vascular aetiology emerged in the 1960s when dementia was occurring earlier in life, when treatment of vascular risk factors was limited and florid cerebrovascular disease was frequently present at post-mortem – i.e. could be assumed to be a single underlying cause. Dementia cases today, particularly in high income nations, are much more frequently arising in later old age (e.g. ninth and tenth decades) where mixed pathology is the norm. Developments in neuroimaging have been a mixed blessing: the ability to detect more minor levels of vascular disturbance is undoubtedly useful in investigating causal pathways; however, detectable 'abnormalities' are now frequently coincidental rather than causal, particularly in older age groups.

'VaD' as a diagnosis implies a single cause and a discrete outcome. However, this has become hard to sustain as a useful entity because of evidence that vascular factors frequently influence dementia occurrence in combination with other pathology (principally AD) – i.e. that most dementia is 'mixed'. The fact that people with 'pure' AD and 'pure' VaD can be identified does not support separate diagnoses if the majority of cases sit somewhere in the middle with combinations of underlying pathologies. Cerebrovascular disease may influence the course and manifestations of dementia but, again, this is better captured by a system which acknowledges its presence as a co morbidity rather than one which assumes it is the only underlying cause. Depressive disorder after bereavement may have different features from depression occurring in other circumstances, but this does not suggest that 'bereavement depression' is helpful as a diagnosis.

A more fundamental challenge to understanding the role of vascular factors in AD is the limited interface between risk factor and outcome research and research into underlying causal pathways. AD can be considered as, in effect, two disorders – one a process of nerve cell death with particular appearances at a cellular level which can only be observed at autopsy, the second a clinical disorder characterized by its symptoms and clinical course. AD, the pathological disorder, is likely to be have been present for a decade or two before AD, the clinical disorder, becomes apparent. However, even these traditions are challenged by the large numbers of people with significant levels of AD pathology who have been found to show no clinical evidence of dementia (Neuropathology Group of the Medical Research Council Cognitive Function and Ageing Study, 2001), and recent evidence suggesting that these changes more poorly predict dementia with advancing old age despite similar associations with cerebral atrophy (Savva et al., 2009).

60.2 VASCULAR FACTORS AND CLINICAL AD

There is now a substantial body of prospective epidemiological research supporting a role for vascular risk factors in the aetiology of AD. Identified risk factors include large vessel atherosclerosis as estimated by carotid ultrasound or the ankle:brachial blood pressure index (Hofman et al., 1997), conventional risk factors for cerebrovascular disease, such as hypertension (Skoog et al., 1996b; Kivipelto et al., 2001), type 2 diabetes (Launer, 2009) and atrial fibrillation (Ott et al., 1997), as well as conventional cardiovascular risk factors, such as raised cholesterol levels (Notkola et al., 1998; Kivipelto et al., 2001), obesity (Gustafson et al., 2003; Hassing et al., 2009) and smoking (Anstey et al., 2007). They also include risk factors such as homocysteine in some studies (Clarke et al., 1998; Seshadri et al., 2002), insulin resistance (Kuusisto et al., 1997) and the metabolic syndrome (Razay et al., 2007), and protective factors such as moderate alcohol intake (Ruitenberg et al., 2002), increased physical activity (Laurin et al., 2001; Scarmeas et al., 2009) and Mediterranean diet (Scarmeas et al., 2009) where other causal pathways may be involved, but whose associations with AD may have a vascular component.

60.3 CHANGES IN VASCULAR RISK FACTORS PRIOR TO DEMENTIA

There is now substantial evidence that associations between vascular factors and dementia change over time, even reversing in some instances. This has been described in most detail for blood pressure. Raised blood pressure in mid-life is associated with later cognitive impairment and dementia (Elias et al., 1993; Launer et al., 1995). However, this has tended to be only apparent in studies with follow-up periods of ten years or more. Studies with shorter follow up often find no association (Posner et al., 2002), and cross-sectional studies frequently show associations between dementia and low rather than high blood pressure (Qiu et al., 2005). This relative hypotension also seems to become more marked at more advanced stages of dementia (Guo et al., 1996). Although a younger age at which blood pressure is measured has been suggested as increasing the likelihood of a positve association with later dementia (Qiu et al., 2005), an analysis of 15-year follow-up data on people aged 70 years at baseline also found that those with AD at the end of the period had raised systolic blood pressure at the start of the study, but lower blood pressure by the time dementia had developed (Skoog et al., 1996b). The interval between measurement of blood pressure and ascertainment of dementia therefore seems to be more important. Two longitudinal studies have now found that blood pressure declines over 3–6 years prior to the clinical onset of dementia (Qiu et al., 2004; Stewart et al., 2009), the second also finding an exaggerated mid- to late-life increase in blood pressure preceding this decline (Stewart et al., 2009).

One possible explanation for this late decline in blood pressure is that early neurodegenerative disease affects regulating centres (Burke et al., 1994) resulting in relative hypotension.

Of relevance, relative weight loss also occurs prior to the onset of dementia over a similar period (Stewart et al., 2005) and different changes in micronutrient levels are observed (Kim et al., 2008), which may reflect similar underlying processes. However, it is also possible that late-life hypotension might be a consequence of earlier sustained hypertension since dementia-associated decline was modified by antihypertensive treatment in one study (Stewart et al., 2009).

Associations between dementia and prior cholesterol levels appear to show a similar pattern to those with blood pressure, i.e. with relatively high mid-life levels, but relatively low or normal contemporaneous levels (Notkola et al., 1998). One study to date has investigated previous changes in cholesterol prior to dementia onset, but found a different pattern to weight and blood pressure changes in that levels appeared to have declined at a much earlier stage, approximately 10–15 years prior to the clinical onset, and then followed a parallel course (Stewart et al., 2007). A possible explanation is that a fall in cholesterol levels accompanied by another event (e.g. an inflammatory or infective event) is associated with very early AD pathology. However, this finding requires replication and further investigation.

60.4 INTERACTIONS WITH APOLIPOPROTEIN E GENOTYPE

The apolipoprotein E (ApoE) ε4 allele was first recognized for its associations with cholesterol metabolism, and in some studies has been associated with stroke (Margaglione et al., 1998; McCarron et al., 1999). However, there has been no evidence that cholesterol levels or other vascular factors explain the association between ε4 and AD (Slooter et al., 1999; Prince et al., 2000). The focus instead has shifted to investigating interactions between vascular factors and ε4 as risk factors, although findings have been conflicting. One community study found that atherosclerosis was more strongly associated with AD in the presence of ApoE ε4 (Hofman et al., 1997). Later examinations in the same study did not support this (Slooter et al., 1999), although other studies have reported similar interactions for cerebrovascular events (Johnston et al., 2000) and atherogenic diet (Laitinen et al., 2006). However, insulin resistance and smoking have been found to be more strongly associated with AD in people without ε4 (Kuusisto et al., 1997; Ott et al., 1998) and, because interactions are frequently not reported as absent, it is difficult to exclude publication bias.

60.5 POTENTIAL UNDERLYING MECHANISMS

60.5.1 The role of stroke and cerebrovascular disease

To what extent are the associations between vascular risk factors and dementia accounted for by stroke or subclinical cerebrovascular disease? Most studies of AD as an outcome have divided these cases into those with and without clinical evidence of co-occurring cerebrovascular disease and most have found that associations remain in the less mixed group. An exception may be atrial fibrillation which appears to be particularly associated with AD co-occurring with stroke (Ott *et al.*, 1997). Furthermore, the following evidence from early studies of clinical stroke and cognitive impairment or dementia suggest at least dual pathology in many cases: (1) most people developing dementia after stroke do so in the absence of further clinical infarction (Tatemichi *et al.*, 1994); (2) post-stroke dementia frequently follows an AD-like clinical course (Kokmen *et al.*, 1996); (3) post-stroke dementia is frequently associated with evidence of pre-stroke cognitive decline (Hénon *et al.*, 2001); (4) cognitive impairment is a risk factor for later first onset of stroke (Ferucci *et al.*, 1996); (5) post-stroke dementia is associated with an increased risk of stroke recurrence (Moroney *et al.*, 1997). These findings suggest that the stroke episode itself, although undoubtedly having an impact on cognitive function, may frequently occur in the context of more insidious and gradual decline. This may reflect co-morbid AD in a substantial number of cases.

There is substantial evidence that vascular factors and AD co-occur in dementia. A community-based neuropathological study found that vascular pathology was frequently present in dementia and that 'pure' AD occurred only in approximately 20 per cent of cases (Fernando and Ince, 2004). In life, white matter hyperintensities (WMH) on magnetic resonance imaging (MRI) are frequently found in association with AD, although are by no means a characteristic feature. Arteriosclerotic changes are often seen in association with white matter alterations, and ischaemia due to small vessel occlusion or hypoperfusion may underlie the dysmyelination and neuronal loss also observed. However, blood–brain barrier disturbance and transient episodes of cerebral oedema may also underlie WMH (Pantoni and Lammie, 2002) as may cortical cell death due to other pathology. Vascular amyloid deposition has been considered as a possible factor accounting for white matter changes in AD, and both cerebral amyloid angiopathy (CAA) and WMH are found in combination in a rare genetic syndrome (Haan *et al.*, 1990); however, in one study, white matter changes were not found to be associated with vascular amyloid in groups with dementia (Erkinjuntti *et al.*, 1996).

Whatever the precise pathology, there is reasonable epidemiological evidence to suggest that WMH represent subclinical cerebrovascular disease in many cases as they have been found to be associated with other risk factors for cerebrovascular disease, such as hypertension (Breteler *et al.*, 1994b; Liao *et al.*, 1997; Dufouil *et al.*, 2001), smoking (Liao *et al.*, 1997), hypercholesterolaemia (Breteler *et al.*, 1994b) and atherosclerosis (Bots *et al.*, 1993). In community samples, they are associated with worse cognitive function (Breteler *et al.*, 1994a; Kuller *et al.*, 1998), in people both with and without dementia (Skoog *et al.*, 1996a). However, although WMH on post-mortem imaging were found to improve the prediction of dementia in life (Fernando and Ince, 2004), they are common findings in older populations and may be present at an apparently severe degree without detectable evidence of cognitive impairment (Fein *et al.*, 1990). WMH, therefore, appear to be insufficient in isolation to give rise to dementia and are likely to require interactions with other pathology.

60.5.2   Vascular pathology in AD

Epidemiological research, as described, supports a role for conventional vascular risk factors in the aetiology of clinical AD. Parallel neurobiological research has suggested that vascular processes may be an important feature of AD at a pathological level. Traditionally, research into the role of amyloid in AD has focused on its deposition in parenchymal neuritic plaques. However, other pathology associated with the disorder has long been recognized. CAA describes the deposition of β-amyloid, among other proteins, in the walls (vascular smooth muscle cell layer) of cortical vessels. CAA increases with age and has been found to be consistently associated with dementia in population-based studies (Keage *et al.*, 2009). It is also recognized to be a risk factor for cerebrovascular disorders, such as small and large vessel haemorrhage, leukoencephalopathy and infarction, and is a feature of some familial early-onset dementia syndromes. CAA is therefore a feature of AD and was associated with cognitive impairment in a community-based autopsy series (Pfeiffer *et al.*, 2002). One possible mechanism underlying its role in AD is that impaired amyloid clearance across the blood–brain barrier (potentially influenced by ApoE genotype) may give rise to CAA; this may in turn compromise vessel wall integrity and give rise to the cerebrovascular disorders listed above which may further exacerbate blood–brain barrier function and AD pathology (Bell and Zlokovic, 2009).

A growing body of evidence suggests that vascular abnormalities in AD are not restricted to arterial and arteriolar amyloid deposition, but are also seen in cerebral microvessels and capillaries. Microangiopathic changes include basement membrane thickening and collagen accumulation (Farkas *et al.*, 2000), as well as smooth muscle cell irregularities, endothelial degeneration and other abnormalities (Kalaria and Skoog, 2002). The underlying causal pathways have yet to be established, although might include toxic effects of accumulating amyloid (Smith and Greenberg, 2009) possibly exacerbated by the microangiopathy itself (de la Torre and Mussivand, 1993; Preston *et al.*, 2003). Another area of uncertainty is whether these 'vascular abnormalities' simply represent a particular feature and byproduct of AD (and a means by which Alzheimer pathology might give rise to cerebrovascular disease) or whether they account for any of the observed associations between vascular risk factors and AD – for example, interacting with and being influenced by the cell damage associated with comorbid cerebrovascular disease (Stewart, 1998). Possible pathways for more direct causal links will be considered in the next sections.

60.5.3   Pathway for vascular 'induction' of AD

The neuropathological findings summarized above suggest that vascular abnormalities are a feature of AD pathology and may be important in its clinical expression. White matter hyperintensities in AD may or may not be a marker of these particular pathological features, but do suggest the involvement of vascular processes because of well-recognized associations with risk factors for cerebrovascular disease. The next question to consider concerns pathways which might explain the association observed in life between vascular risk factors and AD.

Several pathways have been proposed which could potentially explain an association between vascular risk factors and AD and which concern direct causal links at the level of pathological processes. These can be summarized as follows:

- **Ischaemic injury and amyloid deposition**: β-amyloid production appears to be a non-specific response to cerebral trauma, but has been described in particular in the hippocampi of rodents after severe, but transient, ischaemia (Kogure and Kato, 1993), providing a potential link between ischaemia/infarction and AD pathology.
- **Inflammation**: Inflammatory processes are important in mediating cerebral damage following stroke (Emsley and Tyrrell, 2002). Inflammation is also an important feature of AD pathology (Halliday *et al.*, 2000), and might underlie links between the two processes.
- **The blood–brain barrier**: Increased permeability of the blood–brain barrier has been found in association with transient ischaemia (Pluta *et al.*, 1996), and this has been suggested to underlie both perivascular amyloid deposition and white matter changes (Tomimoto *et al.*, 1996).
- **Abnormal protein glycation**: Advance glycation end-products, metabolic oxidation products associated with diabetes and hyperglycaemia (Vlassara *et al.*, 1992) have also been found in association with neurofibrillary tangles and neuritic plaques in AD (Dickson, 1997). These may underlie, at least in part, the association between diabetes and AD which does not appear to be entirely mediated through cerebrovascular disease (Stewart and Liolitsa, 1999).

60.5.4   Exacerbation of cognitive impairment and accelerated age of onset

The mechanisms above concern direct influences of vascular factors on the pathological processes which are believed to underlie AD. However, clinical AD might still be 'caused' without any direct interaction at a pathological level, but instead by interaction in clinical manifestations. Alzheimer pathology develops slowly, possibly over 10–20 years. The chance of someone developing dementia depends a great deal on the extent to which a given level of pathology affects cognition and on the extent to which a person can compensate for this. Alzheimer pathology begins in the hippocampus and manifests in its early stages as declining memory function. Mild levels of cerebrovascular disease on the other hand would be expected to exert most damage on deep white matter and on frontosubcortical connections. The consequent disruption of executive functions, such as selective attention and mental flexibility, may be enough to 'unmask' early AD, which would not otherwise have become apparent for several years. Vascular factors may therefore accelerate the age of onset of clinical AD and precipitate a dementia syndrome at relatively early pathological stages.

60.5.5   Effects on 'functional reserve'

The 'onset' of dementia is defined, at least in research settings, as the point where declining cognitive function starts to interfere with daily functioning. This is an unreliable definition of 'incidence' since it involves considerable subjective judgement on the part of the participant, their family and the research worker. It also assumes a process which can be isolated from all the other factors influencing daily functioning in older people. A given level of cognitive impairment may be more likely to be classified as problematic if daily function is already impaired – for example, because of motor system impairment due to cerebrovascular disease. From the opposite perspective, a person in good physical health may be able to sustain a greater degree of cognitive decline before this can be said to be problematic. Clearly, cerebrovascular disease may have an influence on this component of 'reserve'.

60.6   EVIDENCE FOR CAUSAL LINKS

The hypothetical causal pathways summarized above suggest that vascular factors might act directly to increase the progression of AD pathology, or alternatively they might lower the threshold (cognitive or functional) at which clinical dementia manifests for a given degree of neurodegeneration. These two processes can be tested empirically since they predict different associations between vascular factors and neuropathological findings. Cerebrovascular and Alzheimer pathology overlap substantially in community-derived samples (Fernando and Ince, 2004) and may not in themselves be sufficient to cause dementia since either pathology can be severe with no evidence of dementia in life (Neuropathology Group of the Medical Research Council Cognitive Function and Ageing Study, 2001). The Nun Study and OPTIMA study found that cognitive impairment with mild Alzheimer pathology was much worse if cerebrovascular pathology was also present (Snowdon *et al.*, 1997; Esiri *et al.*, 1999). These findings suggest that mutually deleterious effects on cognitive reserve may be a reason for associations between vascular risk factors and clinical AD risk. However, findings from other studies suggest that there may also be effects on AD pathology itself. In particular, two post-mortem studies have found associations between coronary artery atherosclerosis and Alzheimer pathology (Sparks *et al.*, 1990; Beeri *et al.*, 2006) and one has found higher neurofibrillary tangle counts in association with previous hypertension (Sparks *et al.*, 1995). Neuropathological follow-up studies in a cohort of Japanese–American men have found higher levels of AD pathology associated with increased mid-life blood pressure (Petrovitch *et al.*, 2000) and diabetes (Peila *et al.*, 2002). On the other hand, another neuropathological study of diabetes found no associations with brain pathology in people without dementia, but different dementia-associated pathology between people with and without diabetes (higher β-amyloid load in those without diabetes, higher microvascular infarction and cortical cytokine levels in those with diabetes (Sonnen *et al.*, 2009)).

60.7 COMMON UNDERLYING FACTORS

Associations between vascular factors and AD need not imply direct causal links between the two but might, at least in part, arise from common underlying processes. ApoE genotype has been considered in this respect, although, as discussed earlier, has not been found to explain substantially the co-occurrence of cerebrovascular disease and AD. Both AD and cerebrovascular disease are 'disorders of ageing' – that is, they become more common with increased age. However, 'ageing' as a process is not synonymous with increased chronological age and there is substantial individual variation in the physiological changes which occur in the transition from mid- to late-life. 'Ageing' is likely to be influenced by a variety of factors, both genetic and acquired. Many of these are unknown – for example, genetic factors common to diseases of ageing. Others may be unquantifiable – for example, lifetime exposure to oxidative stress. Dementia is conventionally emphasized as a disorder which is distinct from 'normal ageing'. However, it is likely that there are factors which mediate general vulnerability to ageing processes whether these are experienced in the brain parenchyma or in the vasculature. Finally, both processes can also be said to have common origins in social adversity – increased risk of AD being associated with lower education and reduced 'cognitive reserve', and cardiovascular risk factors known to track with social disadvantage across the life course.

A more specific factor which might link both vascular factors and AD is insulin resistance. This is recognized to be important in underlying the clustering of vascular risk factors, such as hypertension, type 2 diabetes mellitus and hypercholesterolaemia (Reaven, 1988), all of which have been found to be associated with AD, as summarized above. However, insulin levels themselves in theory could have direct effects on cognitive function. Insulin receptors are dense in the hippocampus (Marks et al., 1991). Their role in hippocampal function is not understood, but increased levels of insulin have been found to inhibit hippocampal synaptic activity in vitro (Palovcik et al., 1984). Insulin has also been found to reduce choline acetyl transferase activity (Brass et al., 1992), a key factor in the cognitive impairment associated with AD, and there are links which can be made between insulin growth factor-1 and enzyme pathways which regulate tau protein phosphorylation – and hence neurofibrillary tangle formation (Stewart and Liolitsa, 1999). Several epidemiological studies have investigated markers of insulin resistance in association with dementia/AD risk and findings include associations with hyperinsulinaemia (Kuusisto et al., 1997; Luchsinger et al., 2004; Muller et al., 2007), metabolic syndrome (Razay et al., 2007), and impaired mid-life insulin secretion (Rönnemaa et al., 2008). However, mediating pathways have yet to be established.

60.8 DIRECTION OF CAUSE AND EFFECT

Since vascular risk factors emerge in mid-life and a considerable period before AD incidence begins to increase, it is generally assumed that any causal processes are directed from the vascular risk factor to AD. However, this does not exclude additional adverse effects of AD on the vasculature at a later stage. Links between vascular and Alzheimer pathology have been described above and may be complex and bidirectional. Vascular factors might, therefore, be both a cause and a consequence of AD. At a clinical level, it is likely that worsening cognitive function due to early AD may have adverse effects on risk for vascular disease, particularly through difficulties with adherence to treatment regimes because of declining memory function (Rost et al., 1990). Surprisingly, this has received scant attention despite the frequent co-occurrence of AD and common vascular risk factors, such as hypertension and type 2 diabetes.

60.9 IMPLICATIONS FOR PREVENTING DEMENTIA

This chapter has focused on evidence for the involvement of vascular factors in AD, and on processes which might underlie these associations. Clearly, there are potentially important implications for both prevention and treatment of dementia. A reduction in vascular risk across a population would in theory reduce the risk of later dementia, whether vascular risk factors were acting on AD pathology or reducing cognitive/functional reserve. However, it is doubtful whether the effectiveness of this approach could be demonstrated in a standard randomized controlled trial design given the very long period over which the risk factors may exert their effect. This is likely to be particularly the case for hypertension and to account for the fact that, of the six largest trials of antihypertensive agents with cognitive outcomes (Prince et al., 1996; Starr et al., 1996; Forette et al., 1998; Di Bari et al., 2001; Lithell et al., 2003; Tzourio et al., 2003), only one found significant protective effects in primary analyses (Forette et al., 1998), although these did persist in open label follow up (Forette et al., 2002). Prevention of cognitive decline in diabetes is likely to be a more readily assessible objective, although it is surprising how little research to date has investigated risk factors for cognitive outcomes within people with diabetes. Of studies that have assessed this, one found cognitive impairment to be associated with earlier age of onset, increased duration, insulin treatment and presence of complications (Roberts et al., 2008), while another found occurrence of severe hypoglycaemic episodes to be a risk factor for dementia incidence (Whitmer et al., 2009). For vascular risk factors as a whole, of preventative interventions to date, increased physical activity remains the most supported by randomized controlled trial evidence for cognitive outcomes (Kramer et al., 1999; Lautenschlager et al., 2008).

60.10 IMPLICATIONS FOR TREATING DEMENTIA

Implications for treating AD (i.e. reducing cognitive/functional decline after diagnosis) through modifying vascular risk depend on whether there are direct effects on neurodegenerative processes (i.e. whether vascular risk factors continue to influence cognitive decline rather than simply advance the age of 'dementia' onset). Observational evidence to date has not demonstrated consistent associations between co-occurring cerebrovascular disease and progression of dementia, although there has been little research in this area (Lee *et al.*, 2000; Mungas *et al.*, 2001; Musicco *et al.*, 2009). One observational study found treatment of vascular risk factors to be associated with slower progression (Deschaintre *et al.*, 2009), although a recent randomized controlled trial found no effect of a multi-component vascular care package on cognitive decline in people with both AD and cerebrovascular disease (Richard *et al.*, 2009).

A commonly neglected implication concerns the care of people with dementia. In terms of clinical care, people with AD will commonly have disorders, such as hypertension or diabetes, which require pharmacotherapy and medical review. Neurodegenerative processes themselves may have effects on factors, such as blood pressure and body composition, altering susceptibility to drug effects and side effects, and requiring close attention. In terms of formal and informal social care, people with AD will often also have clinically apparent cerebrovascular disease which may already be affecting non-cognitive areas of functioning, increasing the level of support required. Vascular factors may have an important impact on quality of life for people with AD and their caregivers regardless of whether relationships with AD reflect cause, effect or coincidence. However, this aspect of the interface continues to receive scant attention.

REFERENCES

Anstey KJ, von Sanden C, Salim A, O'Kearney R. (2007) Smoking as a risk factor for dementia and cognitive decline: a meta-analysis of prospective studies. *American Journal of Epidemiology* **166**: 367–78.

Beeri MS, Rapp M, Silverman JM *et al.* (2006) Coronary artery disease is associated with Alzheimer disease neuropathology in APOE4 carriers. *Neurology* **66**: 1399–404.

Bell RD, Zlokovic BV. (2009) Neurovascular mechanisms and blood–brain barrier disorder in Alzheimer's disease. *Acta Neuropathologica* **118**: 103–13.

Bots ML, van Swieten JC, Breteler MMB *et al.* (1993) Cerebral white matter lesions and atherosclerosis in the Rotterdam Study. *Lancet* **341**: 1232–7.

Brass BJ, Nonner D, Barrett JN. (1992) Differential effects of insulin on choline acetyltransferase and glutamic acid decarboxylase activities in neuron-rich striatal cultures. *Journal of Neurochemistry* **59**: 415–24.

Breteler MMB, van Amerongen NM, van Swieten JC *et al.* (1994a) Cognitive correlates of ventricular enlargement and cerebral white matter lesions on magnetic resonance imaging. *Stroke* **25**: 1109–15.

Breteler MMB, van Swieten JC, Bots ML *et al.* (1994b) Cerebral white matter lesions, vascular risk factors, and cognitive function in a population-based study: The Rotterdam Study. *Neurology* **44**: 1246–52.

Burke WJ, Coronado PG, Schmitt CA *et al.* (1994) Blood pressure regulation in Alzheimer's disease. *Journal of the Autonomic Nervous System* **48**: 65–71.

Clarke R, Smith D, Jobst K *et al.* (1998) Folate, vitamin B12, and serum total homocysteine levels in confirmed Alzheimer disease. *Archives of Neurology* **55**: 1449–55.

de la Torre JC, Mussivand T. (1993) Can disturbed brain microcirculation cause Alzheimer's disease? *Neurological Research* **15**: 146–53.

Deschaintre Y, Richard F, Pasquier F. (2009) Treatment of vascular risk factors is associated with slower decline in Alzheimer disease. *Neurology* **73**: 674–80.

Di Bari M, Pahor M, Franse LV *et al.* (2001) Dementia and disability outcomes in large hypertension trials: lessons learned from the systolic hypertension in the elderly program (SHEP) trial. *American Journal of Epidemiology* **153**: 72–8.

Dickson DW. (1997) The pathogenesis of senile plaques. *Journal of Neuropathology and Experimental Neurology* **56**: 321–39.

Dufouil C, de Kersaint-Gilly A, Besançon V *et al.* (2001) Longitudinal study of blood pressure and white matter hyperintensities. *Neurology* **56**: 921–6.

Elias MF, Wolf PA, D'Agostino RB *et al.* (1993) Untreated blood pressure level is inversely related to cognitive functioning: The Framingham study. *American Journal of Epidemiology* **138**: 353–64.

Emsley HCA, Tyrrell PJ. (2002) Inflammation and infection in clinical stroke. *Journal of Cerebral Blood Flow and Metabolism* **22**: 1399–419.

Erkinjuntti T, Benavente O, Eliasziw M *et al.* (1996) Diffuse vacuolization (spongiosis) and arteriosclerosis in the frontal white matter occurs in vascular dementia. *Archives of Neurology* **53**: 325–32.

Esiri MM, Nagy Z, Smith MZ *et al.* (1999) Cerebrovascular disease and threshold for dementia in the early stages of Alzheimer's disease. *Lancet* **354**: 919–20.

Farkas E, De Jong GI, De Vos RA *et al.* (2000) Pathological features of cerebral cortical capillaries are doubled in Alzheimer's disease and Parkinson's disease. *Acta Neuropathologica* **100**: 395–402.

Fein G, Van Dyke C, Davenport L *et al.* (1990) Preservation of normal cognitive functioning in elderly subjects with extensive white-matter lesions of long duration. *Archives of General Psychiatry* **47**: 220–3.

Fernando MS, Ince PG. (2004) MRC Cognitive Function and Ageing Neuropathology Study Group. Vascular pathologies and cognition in a population-based cohort of elderly people. *Journal of the Neurological Sciences* **226**: 13–17.

Ferucci L, Guralnik JM, Salive ME *et al.* (1996) Cognitive impairment and risk of stroke in the older population. *Journal of the American Geriatrics Society* **44**: 237–41.

Forette F, Seux M-L, Staessen JA *et al.* (1998) Prevention of dementia in randomised double-blind placebo-controlled Systolic Hypertension in Europe (Syst-Eur) trial. *Lancet* **352**: 1347–51.

Forette F, Seux M-L, Staessen JA *et al.* (2002) The prevention of dementia with antihypertensive treatment. New evidence from the Systolic Hypertension in Europe (Syst-Eur) study. *Archives of Internal Medicine* **162**: 2046–52.

Guo Z, Viitanen M, Fratiglioni L, Winblad B. (1996) Low blood pressure and dementia in elderly people: the Kungsholmen project. *British Medical Journal* **312**: 805–8.

Gustafson D, Rothenberg E, Blennow K *et al.* (2003) An 18-year follow-up of overweight and risk of Alzheimer disease. *Archives of Internal Medicine* **163**: 1524–8.

Haan J, Roos RA, Algra PR *et al.* (1990) Hereditary cerebral haemorrhage with amyloidosis–Dutch type. Magnetic resonance imaging findings in 7 cases. *Brain* **113**: 1251–67.

Halliday G, Robinson SR, Shepherd C, Kril J. (2000) Alzheimer's disease and inflammation: a review of cellular and therapeutic mechanisms. *Clinical and Experimental Pharmacology and Physiology* **27**: 1–8.

Hassing LB, Dahl AK, Thorvaldsson V *et al.* (2009) Overweight in midlife and risk of dementia: a 40-year follow-up study. *International Journal of Obesity* **33**: 893–8.

Hénon H, Durieu I, Guerouaou D *et al.* (2001) Poststroke dementia: incidence and relationship to prestroke cognitive decline. *Neurology* **57**: 1216–22.

Hofman A, Ott A, Breteler MMB *et al.* (1997) Atherosclerosis, apolipoprotein E, and prevalence of dementia and Alzheimer's disease in the Rotterdam Study. *Lancet* **349**: 151–4.

Johnston JM, Nazar-Stewart V, Kelsey SF *et al.* (2000) Relationships between cerebrovascular events, APOE polymorphism and Alzheimer's disease in a community sample. *Neuroepidemiology* **19**: 320–6.

Kalaria RN, Skoog I. (2002) Pathophysiology: overlap with Alzheimer's disease. In: Erkinjuntti T, Gauthier S (eds). *Vascular cognitive impairment.* London: Martin Dunitz, 145–66.

Keage HAD, Carare RO, Friedland RP *et al.* (2009) Population studies of sporadic cerebral amyloid angiopathy and dementia: a systematic review. *BMC Neurology* **9**: 3.

Kim J-M, Stewart R, Kim S-W *et al.* (2008) Changes in folate, vitamin B$_{12}$, and homocysteine associated with incident dementia. *Journal of Neurology, Neurosurgery and Psychiatry* **79**: 1079–81.

Kivipelto M, Helkala E-L, Laakso MP *et al.* (2001) Midlife vascular risk factors and Alzheimer's disease in later life: longitudinal, population based study. *British Medical Journal* **322**: 1447–51.

Kogure K, Kato H. (1993) Altered gene expression in cerebral ischemia. *Stroke* **24**: 2121–7.

Kokmen E, Whistman JP, O'Fallon WM *et al.* (1996) Dementia after ischemic stroke: a population-based study in Rochester, Minnesota (1960–1984). *Neurology* **19**: 154–9.

Kramer AF, Hahn S, Cohen NJ *et al.* (1999) Ageing, fitness and neurocognitive function. *Nature* **400**: 418–9.

Kuller LH, Shemanski L, Manolio T *et al.* (1998) Relationship between ApoE, MRI findings, and cognitive function in the Cardiovascular Health Study. *Stroke* **29**: 388–98.

Kuusisto J, Koivisto K, Mykkänen L *et al.* (1997) Association between features of the insulin resistance syndrome and Alzheimer's disease independently of apolipoprotein E4 phenotype: cross sectional population based study. *British Medical Journal* **315**: 1045–9.

Laitinen MH, Ngandu T, Rovio S *et al.* (2006) Fat intake at midlife and risk of dementia and Alzheimer's disease: a population-based study. *Dementia Geriatric Cognitive Disorders* **22**: 99–107.

Launer LJ. (2009) Diabetes. Vascular or neurodegenerative: and epidemiologic perspective. *Stroke* **40**: S53–5.

Launer LJ, Masaki K, Petrovitch H *et al.* (1995) The association between midlife blood pressure levels and late-life cognitive function. *Journal of the American Medical Association* **274**: 1846–51.

Laurin D, Verreault R, Lindsay J *et al.* (2001) Physical activity and risk of cognitive impairment and dementia in elderly persons. *Archives of Neurology* **58**: 498–504.

Lautenschlager NT, Cox KL, Flicker L *et al.* (2008) Effect of physical activity on cognitive function in older adults at risk for Alzheimer disease. *Journal of the American Medical Association* **300**: 1027–37.

Lee J-H, Olichney JM, Hansen LA *et al.* (2000) Small concomitant vascular lesions do not influence rates of cognitive decline in patients with Alzheimer disease. *Archives of Neurology* **57**: 1474–9.

Liao D, Cooper L, Cai J *et al.* (1997) The prevalence and severity of white matter lesions, their relationship with age, ethnicity, gender, and cardiovascular disease risk factors: the ARIC study. *Neuroepidemiology* **16**: 149–62.

Lithell H, Hansson L, Skoog I *et al.* (2003) The Study on Cognition and Prognosis in the Elderly (SCOPE): principal results of a randomized double-blind intervention trial. *Journal of Hypertension* **21**: 875–86.

Luchsinger JA, Tang M-X, Shea S, Mayeux R. (2004) Hyperinsulinemia and risk of Alzheimer disease. *Neurology* **63**: 1187–92.

McCarron MO, Delong D, Alberts MJ. (1999) APOE genotype as a risk factor for ischemic cerebrovascular disease. *Neurology* **53**: 1308–11.

Margaglione M, Seripa D, Gravina C *et al.* (1998) Prevalence of apolipoprotein E alleles in healthy subjects and survivors of ischemic stroke. *Stroke* **29**: 399–403.

Marks JL, King MG, Baskin DG. (1991) Localisation of insulin and type 1 IGF receptors in rat brain by *in vitro* autoradiography and in situ hybridisation. *Advances in Experimental Medical Biology* **293**: 459–70.

Moroney JT, Bagiella E, Tatemichi TK *et al.* (1997) Dementia after stroke increases the risk of long-term stroke recurrence. *Neurology* **48**: 1317–25.

Muller M, Tang MX, Schupf N *et al.* (2007) Metabolic syndrome and dementia risk in a multiethnic elderly cohort. *Dementia Geriatric Cognitive Disorders* **24**: 185–92.

Mungas D, Reed BR, Ellis WG, Jaqust WJ. (2001) The effects of age on rate of progression of Alzheimer disease and dementia with associated cerebrovascular disease. *Archives of Neurology* **58**: 1243–7.

Musicco M, Palmer K, Salamone G *et al.* (2009) Predictors of progression of cognitive decline in Alzheimer's disease: the role of vascular and sociodemographic factors. *Journal of Neurology* **256**: 1288–95.

Neuropathology Group of the Medical Research Council Cognitive Function and Ageing Study. (2001) Pathological correlates of late-onset dementia in a multicentre, community-based population in England and Wales. *Lancet* **357**: 169–75.

Notkola I-L, Sulkava R, Pekkanen J *et al.* (1998) Serum total cholesterol, apolipoprotein E4 allele, and Alzheimer's disease. *Neuroepidemiology* **17**: 14–20.

Ott A, Breteler MMB, de Bruyne MC *et al.* (1997) Atrial fibrillation and dementia in a population-based study. *Stroke* **28**: 316–21.

Ott A, Slooter AJC, Hofman A *et al.* (1998) Smoking and the risk of dementia and Alzheimer's disease in a population-based cohort study: The Rotterdam Study. *Lancet* **351**: 1840–3.

Palovcik RA, Philips MI, Kappy MS, Raizada MK. (1984) Insulin inhibits pyramidal neurons in hippocampal slices. *Brain Research* **309**: 187–91.

Pantoni L, Lammie A. (2002) Cerebral small vessel disease: pathological and pathophysiological aspects in relation to vascular cognitive impairment. In: Erkinjuntti T, Gauthier S (eds). *Vascular cognitive impairment.* London: Martin Dunitz, 115–33.

Peila R, Rodriguez BL, Launer LJ. (2002) Type 2 diabetes, APOE gene, and the risk for dementia and related pathologies: The Honolulu-Asia Aging Study. *Diabetes* **51**: 1256–62.

Petrovitch H, White LR, Izmirilian G *et al.* (2000) Midlife blood pressure and neuritic plaques, neurofibrillary tangles, and brain weight at death: the Honolulu Asia Aging Study. *Neurobiology of Aging* **21**: 57–62.

Pfeiffer LA, White LR, Ross GW *et al.* (2002) Cerebral amyloid angiopathy and cognitive function: the HAAS Autopsy Study. *Neurology* **58**: 1587–8.

Pluta R, Barcikowski M, Janusezewski S *et al.* (1996) Evidence of blood–brain barrier permeability/leakage for circulating human Alzheimer's-amyloid-(1-42)-peptide. *Neuroreport* **7**: 1261–5.

Posner HB, Tang M-X, Luchsinger J *et al.* (2002) The relationship of hypertension in the elderly to AD, vascular dementia, and cognitive function. *Neurology* **58**: 1175–81.

Preston SD, Steart PV, Wilkinson A *et al.* (2003) Capillary and arterial cerebral amyloid angiopathy in Alzheimer's disease: defining the perivascular route for the elimination of amyloid beta from the human brain. *Neuropathology and Applied Neurobiology* **29**: 106–17.

Prince MJ, Bird AS, Blizard RA, Mann AH. (1996) Is the cognitive function of older patients affected by antihypertensive treatment? Results from 54 months of the Medical Research Council's treatment trial of hypertension in older adults. *British Medical Journal* **312**: 801–4.

Prince M, Lovestone S, Cervilla J *et al.* (2000) The association between APOE and dementia is mediated neither by vascular disease nor its risk factors in an aged cohort of survivors with hypertension. *Neurology* **54**: 397–402.

Qiu C, von Strauss E, Winblad B, Fratiglioni L. (2004) Decline in blood pressure over time and risk of dementia: a longitudinal study from the Kungsholmen Project. *Stroke* **35**: 1810–15.

Qiu C, Winblad B, Fratiglioni L. (2005) The age-dependent relation of blood pressure to cognitive function and dementia. *Lancet Neurology* **4**: 487–99.

Razay G, Vreugdenhill A, Wilcock G. (2007) The metabolic syndrome and Alzheimer disease. *Archives of Neurology* **64**: 93–6.

Reaven GM. (1988) Role of insulin resistance in human disease. *Diabetes* **37**: 1595–607.

Richard E, Kuiper R, Dijkgraaf MG, Van Gool WA. (2009) Evaluation of vascular care in Alzheimer's disease. Vascular care in patients with Alzheimer's disease with cerebrovascular lesions-a randomized clinical trial. *Journal of the American Geriatrics Society* **57**: 795–805.

Roberts RO, Geda YE, Knopman DS *et al.* (2008) Association of duration and severity of diabetes mellitus with mild cognitive impairment. *Archives of Neurology* **65**: 1066–73.

Rönnemaa E, Zethelius B, Sundelöf J *et al.* (2008) Impaired insulin secretion increases the risk of Alzheimer disease. *Neurology* **71**: 1065–71.

Rost K, Roter D, Quill T, Bertakis K. (1990) Capacity to remember prescription drug changes: deficits associated with diabetes. *Diabetes Research and Clinical Practice* **10**: 183–7.

Ruitenberg A, van Swieten JC, Witteman JCM *et al.* (2002) Alcohol consumption and risk of dementia: the Rotterdam Study. *Lancet* **359**: 281–6.

Savva GM, Wharton SB, Ince PG *et al.* (2009) Medical Research Council Cognitive Function and Ageing Study. Age, neuropathology, and dementia. *New England Journal of Medicine* **360**: 2302–9.

Scarmeas N, Luchsinger JA, Schupf N *et al.* (2009) Physical activity, diet, and risk of Alzheimer disease. *Journal of the American Medical Association* **302**: 627–37.

Seshadri S, Beiser A, Selhub J *et al.* (2002) Plasma homocysteine as a risk factor for dementia and Alzheimer's disease. *New England Journal of Medicine* **346**: 476–83.

Skoog I, Berg S, Johansson B *et al.* (1996a) The influence of white matter lesions on neuropsychological functioning in demented and non-demented 85-year-olds. *Acta Neurologica Scandanavica* **93**: 142–8.

Skoog I, Lernfelt B, Landahl S *et al.* (1996b) 15-year longitudinal study of blood pressure and dementia. *Lancet* **347**: 1141–5.

Slooter AJC, Cruts M, Ott A *et al.* (1999) The effect of APOE on dementia is not through atherosclerosis: The Rotterdam Study. *Neurology* **53**: 1593–5.

Smith EE, Greenberg SM. (2009) β-Amyloid, blood vessels, and brain function. *Stroke* **40**: 2601–6.

Snowdon DA, Greiner LH, Mortimer JA *et al.* (1997) Brain infarction and the clinical expression of Alzheimer disease. *Journal of the American Medical Association* **277**: 813–17.

Sonnen JA, Larson EB, Brickell K *et al.* (2009) Different patterns of cerebral injury in dementia with or without diabetes. *Archives of Neurology* **66**: 315–22.

Sparks DL, Hunsaker JC, Scheff SW *et al.* (1990) Cortical senile plaques in coronary artery disease, aging and Alzheimer's disease. *Neurobiology of Aging* **11**: 601–7.

Sparks DL, Scheff SW, Liu H *et al.* (1995) Increased incidence of neurofibrillary tangles (NFT) in non-demented individuals with hypertension. *Journal of the Neurological Sciences* **131**: 162–9.

Starr JM, Whalley LJ, Deary IJ. (1996) The effects of antihypertensive treatment on cognitive function: results from the HOPE study. *Journal of the American Geriatrics Society* **44**: 411–15.

Stewart R. (1998) Cardiovascular factors in Alzheimer's disease. *Journal of Neurology, Neurosurgery and Psychiatry* **65**: 143–7.

Stewart R, Liolitsa D. (1999) Type 2 diabetes mellitus, cognitive impairment and dementia. *Diabetic Medicine* **16**: 93–112.

Stewart R, Masaki K, Xue Q-L *et al.* (2005) A 32-year prospective study of change in body weight and incident dementia: the Honolulu-Asia Aging Study. *Archives of Neurology* **62**: 55–60.

Stewart R, Xue Q-L, White LR, Launer LJ. (2007) 26-year change in total cholesterol levels and incident dementia. The Honolulu-Asia Aging Study. *Archives of Neurology* **62**: 55–60.

Stewart R, Xue Q-L, Masaki K *et al.* (2009) Change in blood pressure and incident dementia: a 32-year prospective study. *Hypertension* **54**: 233–40.

Tatemichi TK, Paik M, Bagiella E *et al.* (1994) Risk of dementia after stroke in a hospitalised cohort: results of a longitudinal study. *Neurology* **44**: 1885–91.

Tomimoto H, Akiguchi I, Suenaga T *et al.* (1996) Alterations of the blood–brain barrier and glial cells in white-matter lesions in cerebrovascular and Alzheimer's disease patients. *Stroke* **27**: 2069–74.

Tzourio C, Anderson C, Chapman N *et al.* (2003) Effects of blood pressure lowering with perindopril and indapamide therapy on dementia and cognitive decline in patients with cerebrovascular disease. *Archives of Internal Medicine* **163**: 1069–75.

Vlassara H, Fuh H, Makita Z *et al.* (1992) Exogenous advanced glycosylation end products induce complex vascular dysfunction in normal animals: a model for diabetic and aging complications. *Proceedings of the National Academy of Science of the United States of America* **89**: 12043–7.

Whitmer RA, Karter AJ, Yaffe K *et al.* (2009) Hypoglycemic episodes and risk of dementia in older patients with type 2 diabetes mellitus. *Journal of the American Medical Association* **301**: 1565–72.

PART V

CEREBROVASCULAR DISEASE AND COGNITIVE IMPAIRMENT

61

What is vascular cognitive impairment?

TIMO ERKINJUNTTI AND SERGE GAUTHIER

61.1 VASCULAR BURDEN OF THE BRAIN – BACKGROUND

As early as 1896, 'arteriosclerotic dementia' (referring to vascular dementia (VaD)) was separated from 'senile dementia' (referring to Alzheimer's disease (AD)). Alois Alzheimer together with Otto Binswanger recognized the heterogeneity of VaD by describing four clinical pathological subtypes of VaD (Román, 2001), as well as vascular lesions in AD. Nevertheless, until the 1970s, cerebral atherosclerosis causing chronic strangulation of blood supply to the brain, was thought to be the most common cause of dementia, and AD was regarded as a rare cause affecting only younger patients. Tomlinson et al. (Tomlinson et al., 1970) reinvented AD as the more frequent cause of dementia. In 1979, Hachinski and colleagues used the term 'multi-infarct (multistroke) dementia' (MID) to describe the mechanism by which they considered VaD was produced (Hachinski et al., 1974). As the pendulum swung in the direction of AD, vascular forms of dementia became relegated to a position of relative obscurity (Brust, 1988).

During the 1980s and the early 1990s, almost all cerebrovascular disease (CVD) injury leading to dementia was ascribed to large cortical and subcortical infarcts (strokes); so-called MID (Erkinjuntti and Hachinski, 1993). The concept of VaD was introduced to further refine the description of dementias caused by infarcts of varying sizes, including the smaller lacunar and micro-infarcts, as well as white matter lesions (WMLs) (Román et al., 1993). VaD appropriately defined a group of heterogeneous dementia syndromes of CVD origin of which the cortical and subcortical vascular disease was considered as important subtypes (Erkinjuntti and Hachinski, 1993; Román et al., 1993; Román et al., 2002). Although this was an important step forward, it was not adequate to describe fully the vascular causes of early cognitive impairments.

The recognition of AD as the most common cause of dementia led to the development of operational criteria for the diagnosis of dementia in general. The criteria included early and prominent memory loss, progressive cognitive impairment, evidence of irreversibility and presence of cognitive impairment sufficient to affect normal activities of daily living (ADLs) (McKhann et al., 1984; Erkinjuntti et al., 1997). The characteristic episodic memory impairment apparent in AD is attributed to atrophy of the medial temporal lobe. In contrast, CVD lesions do not necessarily have the same regional predilection. The emphasis of the current Alzheimer-type dementia criteria limited to the episodic memory impairment underestimates the vascular burden on cognition. The conventional dementia syndrome concept recognize the vascular burden of the brain too late, when often opportunities to prevent and treat are lost. Accordingly, it was suggested that the 'Alzheimerized' dementia concept should be abandoned in the setting of CVD, and indeed this was one of the motives behind development of the broader category of vascular cognitive impairment (VCI) (Hachinski, 1990; Bowler and Hachinski, 1995; Pasquier and Leys, 1997; O'Brien et al., 2003; Román et al., 2004; Moorhouse and Rockwood, 2008), also referred as vascular cognitive disorder (Román et al., 2004).

61.2   THE MODERN CONCEPT OF VASCULAR COGNITIVE IMPAIRMENT

Until the 1990s, the concept of VaD was of a dementia caused by small or large brain infarcts (strokes), that of MID (Hachinski *et al.*, 1974; Erkinjuntti and Hachinski, 1993). Now, VaD has come full circle with the resurgence of interest in the whole spectrum of vascular causes of cognitive impairment and dementia (Hachinski, 1990; O'Brien *et al.*, 2003). The new term is 'VCI', which reflects an awareness of the importance of the vascular burden of brain and cognition (Bowler and Hachinski, 1995; O'Brien *et al.*, 2003; Moorhouse and Rockwood, 2008). Evidence of complex interactions between vascular aetiologies, changes in the brain, host factors and cognition prompted formulation of the new concepts (Chui, 1989; Tatemichi, 1990; Erkinjuntti and Hachinski, 1993; Desmond, 1996; Pasquier and Leys, 1997), as well as reinvention of the heterogeneity of VaDs and recognition of the small vessel ischaemic subcortical vascular disease and dementia (SIVD) as the cardinal subtype (Román, 1985; Erkinjuntti, 1987; Erkinjuntti and Pantoni, 2000; Erkinjuntti *et al.*, 2000b; Román *et al.*, 2002). The fact that vascular factors relate to and coexist with AD (Kalaria and Ballard, 1999; Skoog *et al.*, 1999; Kivpelto *et al.*, 2006) were important too.

Accordingly, the modern concept of VCI aims to cover the spectrum of cognitive impairments, as well as the spectrum of the aetiologies of vascular burden of the brain (O'Brien *et al.*, 2003; Bowler, 2007; Hachinski, 2008; Moorhouse and Rockwood, 2008). The modern concept of VCI relates to important shifts in thinking (Hachinski, 2008):

- shift from arbitrary thresholds, such as the AD dementia threshold, to a continuum of cognitive impairment;
- shift from the late stages to the early stages of disease;
- shift from the effects to the causes.

The evolution of the new VCI concept is similar to the more recent evolution in degenerative causes of memory diseases, i.e. the new research criteria for the amnestic prodrome of AD (Dubois *et al.*, 2007).

The cognitive syndrome of VCI encompasses all levels of cognitive decline, from the earliest deficits to a severe and broad dementia-like cognitive syndrome (Bowler *et al.*, 1999; O'Brien *et al.*, 2003). VCI cases that do not meet the criteria for dementia can also be labelled as VCI with no dementia or vascular cognitive impairment no dementia (CIND) (Rockwood *et al.*, 2000). These patients have also been labelled as vascular mild cognitive impairment (vMCI) in a similar way to that of amnestic mild cognitive impairment (aMCI) for AD (Petersen *et al.*, 2002).

VCI refers to all aetiologies of CVD, including vascular risks which can result in brain damage leading to cognitive impairment. VCI may include cases with cognitive impairment related to hypertension, diabetes or atherosclerosis, transient ischaemic attacks, cortico-subcortical infarcts, silent infarcts, strategic infarcts, small vessel disease with white matter lesions and lacunae, as well as AD pathology with co-existing CVD. VCI can also encompass those patients who survive intracerebral and other intracranial haemorrhages, but are left with residual cognitive impairment.

61.3   VCI PATHOPHYSIOLOGY

VCI as a general entity includes many syndromes, which themselves reflect a variety of vascular mechanisms and changes in the brain, with different causes and clinical manifestations. The pathophysiology incorporates interactions between vascular aetiologies (CVDs and vascular risk factors), changes in the brain (infarcts, WMLs, atrophy, AD pathology) and host factors (age, education) (Chui, 1989; Tatemichi, 1990; Erkinjuntti and Hachinski, 1993; Desmond, 1996; Pasquier and Leys, 1997; O'Brien *et al.*, 2003) (**Figure 61.1**). Aetiologies of VCI include both CVD and risk factors (**Table 61.1**).

61.3.1   Cerebrovascular diseases

Cerebrovascular diseases (CVDs) include large artery disease, cardiac embolic events, small vessel disease and haemodynamic mechanisms (Erkinjuntti, 1987; Erkinjuntti and Hachinski, 1993; Brun, 1994; Wallin and Blennow, 1994; Pantoni and Garcia, 1995; Amar and Wilcock, 1996).

61.3.2   Risk factors

Risk factors associated with VCI include risks for stroke and ischaemic WMLs. Clinically symptomatic infarcts, clinically silent infarcts and white matter lesions relate to higher dementia risk (Vermeer *et al.*, 2003; Prins *et al.*, 2004; Inzitari *et al.*, 2007; Inzitari *et al.*, 2009). Similarly to AD, the risks for VCI may be considered under demographic, vascular, genetic and ischaemic lesion-related variables (Skoog, 1994; Gorelick, 1997; Skoog, 1998; Kivpelto *et al.*, 2006). Hypoxic ischaemic events giving rise to global cerebrovascular insufficiency are important risk factors for incident dementia in patients with stroke (Sulkava and Erkinjuntti, 1987; Moroney *et al.*, 1996; Moroney *et al.*, 1997a). Furthermore, the traditional vascular risk factors and stroke are also independent factors for the clinical presentation of MCI and AD (Snowdon *et al.*, 1997; Skoog *et al.*, 1999). The important independent mid-life risk-factors of clinical AD include arterial hypertension, high cholesterol, diabetes, obesity and reduced physical activity among others (Skoog *et al.*, 1999; Kivpelto *et al.*, 2006).

61.3.3   Brain changes

Brain changes related to VCI include both ischaemic and non-ischaemic factors (Chui, 1989; Tatemichi, 1990; Erkinjuntti and Hachinski, 1993; Brun, 1994; Erkinjuntti *et al.*, 2000a) (**Table 61.2**). Static ischaemic lesions include arterial territorial infarct, distal field (watershed) infarct, lacunar infarct, ischaemic WMLs and incomplete ischaemic injury. Incomplete ischaemic injury includes focal gliosis and incomplete white matter infarctions in areas of selective vulnerability (Englund *et al.*, 1988; Pantoni and Garcia, 1997). Functional ischaemic changes include both focal (around the ischaemic lesion) and remote (disconnection, diaschisis) effects (Shim *et al.*, 2006). Ischaemia relates also to atrophy without AD pathology (Vinters *et al.*, 2000).

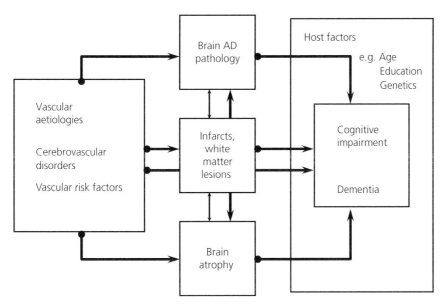

Figure 61.1   Interactions between vascular causes, brain changes and host factors in vascular cognitive impairment.

Table 61.1   Aetiologies of vascular dementia.

Cerebrovascular disorders	Large artery disease	Artery-to-artery embolism
		Occlusion of an extra- or intracranial artery
	Cardiac embolic events	
	Small vessel disease	Lacunar infarcts
		Ischaemic white matter lesions
	Haemodynamic mechanisms	
	Specific arteriopathies	
	Haemorrhages	Intracranial haemorrhage
		Subarachnoidal haemorrhage
	Haematological factors	
	Venous diseases	
	Hereditary entities	
Risk factors	Vascular	Arterial hypertension
		Atrial fibrillation
		Myocardial infarction
		Coronary heart disease
		Diabetes
		Generalized atherosclerosis
		Lipid abnormalities
		Smoking
Demographic factors	High age	
	Low education	
Genetic factors	Family history	
	Specific genetic factors	
Stroke-related factors	Type of cerebrovascular diseases	
	Site and size of infarcts	

61.3.4   Brain mechanisms

Brain mechanisms proposed to be related to VCI include volume of brain infarcts, number of infarcts (additive, synergistic), site of infarcts, WMLs, other ischaemic factors (incomplete ischaemic injury, delayed neuronal death, functional changes), atrophy and additive effects of other pathologies (e.g. AD, etc.) (Erkinjuntti *et al.*, 1988; Chui, 1989; Tatemichi, 1990; Desmond, 1996; Erkinjunti, 1999a; O'Brien *et al.*, 2003; Kalaria *et al.*, 2004). The relationship between vascular factors and cognition is challenging: do the identified vascular factors cause, compound or only coexist

Table 61.2   Brain changes in vascular dementia.

Static lesions	Arterial territorial infarct
	Distal field (watershed) infarct
	Lacunar infarct
	Ischaemic white matter lesions
	Incomplete ischaemic injury
	Atrophy
Functional ischaemic changes	Focal (around the ischaemic lesion)
	Remote (disconnection, diaschisis)

with the VCI syndrome? Small vessel disease with subsequent brain atrophy may well be the cardinal origin of the main subtypes of VCI (Erkinjuntti, 1987; Román, 1987; Pantoni and Garcia, 1995; Román et al., 2002) (see Chapter 60, Vascular factors and Alzheimer's disease and Chapter 62, The neuropathology of vascular dementia). Another important question is whether they contribute to the risk and clinical picture of AD (Snowdon et al., 1997).

61.3.5   Anatomical brain imaging

Computed tomography (CT) and magnetic resonance imaging (MRI) studies on VaD indicate that bilateral ischaemic lesions are of importance (Erkinjuntti and Hachinski, 1993; DeCarli and Scheltens, 2002). A summary of the interaction between lesion and cognition in VaD includes (Román et al., 1993; Erkinjuntti, 1999b; Erkinjuntti et al., 1999; DeCarli and Scheltens, 2002; Román et al., 2002; O'Brien et al., 2003):

- No single feature, but a combination of infarct features, extent and type of WMLs, degree and site of atrophy, and host factors characteristics are correlates of VCI/VaD.
- Infarct features favouring VaD include: bilaterality, multiplicity (>2), location in the dominant hemisphere and location in the frontosubcortical and limbic structures.
- WML features favouring VaD are extensive WMLs (extending periventricular WMLs and confluent to extending WMLs in the deep white matter).
- It is doubtful that only a single small lesion could support a diagnosis of VaD. However, rare cases with strategic infarcts may be exceptions.
- Absence of CVD lesions on CT or MRI are against a diagnosis of VaD.

Examples of MRI findings in the main subtypes of VADs are shown in **Figure 61.2**.

61.4   VCI – THE SIZE OF THE PROBLEM

The size of the VCI problem can be studied by reviewing data on (1) VCI and cognitive impairment no dementia, (2) post-stroke cognitive impairment, (3) post-stroke dementia, (4) VaD, as well as (5) AD with CVD.

61.4.1   VCI

Estimates of the population distribution of VCI and its outcomes are influenced by the variety of definitions used (Erkinjuntti et al., 1997; Pohjasvaara et al., 1997; Lobo et al., 2000; Pohjasvaara et al., 2000b). For example, if AD with CVD or the previously defined VaD with AD pathology is included, then VCI would most certainly be the most common cause of chronic progressive cognitive impairment in elderly people (Rockwood et al., 2000). In a Canadian study, the prevalence of VCI (including CIND) was estimated at 5 per cent in people over age 65 years (Rockwood et al., 2000). The prevalence of vascular CIND was 2.4 per cent, that of AD with CVD was 0.9 per cent and of VaD alone was 1.5 per cent. By comparison, the prevalence of AD without a vascular component, at all ages up to age 85 years, was 5.1 per cent and was less common than VCI (Rockwood et al., 2000).

61.4.2   Post-stroke cognitive impairment

Post-stroke cognitive impairment (PSCI) is a frequent, though neglected, consequence of stroke. An example of a detailed clinical study is the Helsinki Stroke Ageing study (Pohjasvaara et al., 1997). Cognitive impairment three months after ischaemic stroke was present in one domain in 62 per cent and in two domains in 35 per cent of patients aged 55–85 years. The cognitive domains affected included short-term memory (31 per cent), long-term memory (23 per cent), constructive and visuospatial functions (37 per cent), executive functions (25 per cent) and aphasia (14 per cent) (Pohjasvaara et al., 1997).

61.4.3   Post-stroke dementia

The frequency of post-stroke dementia (PSD) vary from 12 to 32 per cent within three months to one year after stroke (Leys et al., 2005). In the Helsinki study, the frequency was 25 per cent three months after incident stroke, and the frequency increased with increasing age: 19 per cent among those aged 55–64 years, and 32 per cent in those aged 75–85 years (Pohjasvaara et al., 1997). The incidence of post-stroke dementia increases with a longer follow-up time from 10 per cent at one year to 32 per cent after five years (Leys et al., 2005). A history of stroke increases the risk of subsequent dementia by a factor of 5 (Linden et al., 2004; Leys et al., 2005).

Determinants of PSD include high age, low education, pre-stroke dependency and cognitive impairment, including pre-stroke dementia (Leys et al., 2005). Risk factors of incident PSD include epileptic seizures, sepsis, cardiac arrhythmias and congestive heart failure (Moroney et al., 1996; Leys et al., 2005). In one large cohort study, the independent clinical correlates of PSD included dysphasia, major dominant stroke syndrome, history of prior CVD and low education (Pohjasvaara et al., 1998). Brain lesion correlates of PSD include a combination of infarcts features (volume, site), presence of WMLs (extent, location), as well as brain

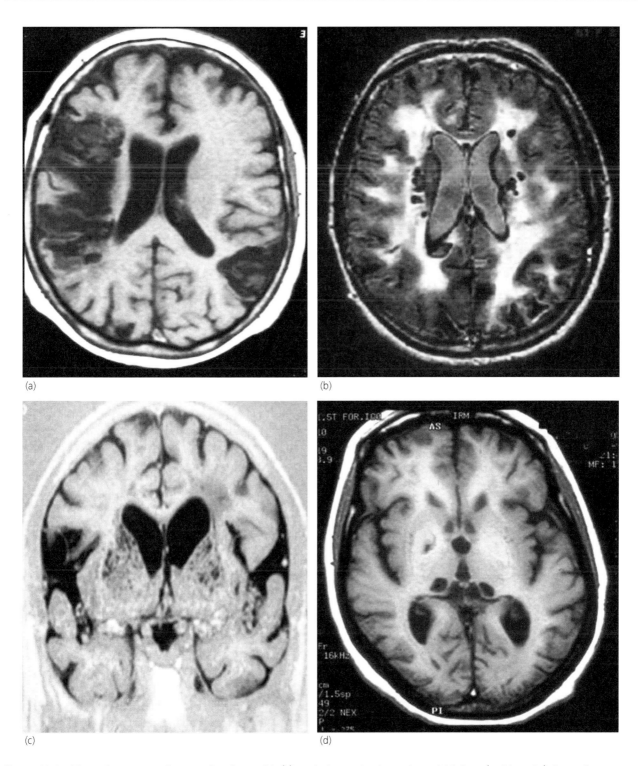

Figure 61.2   Magnetic resonance images of patients with (a) cortical vascular dementia, multi-infarct (multi-stroke) dementia (bilateral infarcts), (b) small vessel ischaemic subcortical vascular disease and dementia (SIVD) with confluent white matter lesions, (c) SIVD with multiple lacunes, and (d) bilateral strategic thalamic infarcts.

atrophy (Pohjasvaara *et al.*, 2000a; Leys *et al.*, 2005). Important critical locations include dominant hemisphere and lesions affecting the prefrontal-subcortical circuit. Lesions mediating executive dysfunction are critical (Vataja *et al.*, 2003).

61.4.4   VaD

VaD, defined as the subset of VCI patients who fulfil traditional AD-type dementia criteria, is considered the second most common cause of dementia accounting for 10–50 per cent cases, but this depends on the geographic location, patient population and the clinical methods used (Lobo *et al.*, 2000). The prevalence of VaD had been reported to range from 1.2 to 4.2 per cent in people aged 65 years and older (Hebert and Brayne, 1995). Using population-based identification of people aged 65 years and older, the European collaborative study reported that the age-standardized prevalence of dementia was 6.4 per cent (all causes), 4.4 per cent for AD and 1.6 per cent for VaD (Lobo *et al.*, 2000). In this study, 15.8 per cent of all cases had VaD and 53.7 per cent AD. However, these studies did not estimate the size of the AD with CVD population in more detail. The incidence of VaD increases with age, without any substantial difference between men and women (Fratiglioni *et al.*, 2000). The reported incidence estimates of VaD vary from 6 to 12 cases per year in 1000 persons aged 70 years and older (Hebert and Brayne, 1995).

61.4.5   AD with CVD

For too long the focus has been the two 'pure' ends of the dementia spectrum: probable AD (McKhann *et al.*, 1984) and probable VaD (Román *et al.*, 1993). One factor has been the need for homogenous patient populations and high antemortem diagnostic specificity for randomized clinical trials. At the same time, combined cases, those with AD and CVD, were neglected. Yet Alois Alzheimer recognized the issue of AD with CVD, which was reinvented by Tomlinson and colleagues (Tomlinson *et al.*, 1970). In the seminal Newcastle series, 8–18 per cent of the patients had AD with CVD (Tomlinson *et al.*, 1970). Accordingly, Roth concluded 'there is evidence that the two types of pathological change augment one another to a statistically significant degree in the production of dementia' (Roth, 1971). Today, based on unselected neuropathological series of patients, we acknowledge that AD with CVD may be the most frequent single cause leading to cognitive impairment: in the brains of cognitively impaired elderly at least 50 per cent show combined AD and CVD changes (Roth, 1971; Snowdon *et al.*, 1997; Neuropathology Group of the Medical Research Council Cognitive Function and Aging Study, 2001). In addition, vascular brain changes relate to a much earlier clinical presentation of the AD syndrome (Snowdon *et al.*, 1997), and vascular risk factors are independent factors related to clinical expression of the AD syndrome (Kivpelto *et al.*, 2006). Importantly, AD and CVD can be seen as secret partners in cognitive and brain health risks; one in every two females aged over 65 years will have in their coming years of life either CVD, AD or AD with CVD (Seshadri and Wolf, 2007).

61.5   WML BURDEN

WMLs, frequently detected on neuroimaging, are associated with cognitive, mood, motor and urinary disorders, all contributing towards disability (Inzitari *et al.*, 2007; Inzitari *et al.*, 2009). In particular, confluent and extensive WMLs relate to cognitive decline, faster progression of disability and death (Inzitari *et al.*, 2009). In addition, confluent WMLs

relate to other important adverse outcomes, including depression, impaired gait and stability and urinary problems. Furthermore, extensive WMLs relate to the dysexecutive syndrome (Jokinen *et al.*, 2005). WMLs are seen as the surrogate of small vessel disease and they relate to the SIVD syndrome, the main subtype of progressive VCI (Erkinjuntti *et al.*, 2000b; Román *et al.*, 2002; Jokinen *et al.*, 2009a). Importantly, the executive small vessel brain network is the largest human endothelial organ (Román, 2008).

61.6   MAIN SUBTYPES OF VCI

VCI encompasses many clinical features, which themselves reflect a variety of vascular mechanisms and changes in the brain, with different causes and neurological outcomes (**Figure 61.3**). The pathophysiology is attributed to interactions between vascular aetiologies (CVD and vascular risk factors), changes in the brain (infarcts, WMLs, atrophy) and host factors (age, education).

The main subtypes of VaD included in current classifications are cortical VaD or MID (also referred as post-stroke VaD), SIVD, small vessel dementia and strategic infarct dementia (Chui *et al.*, 1992; Román *et al.*, 1993; World Health Organization, 1993; American Psychiatric Association, 1994; Erkinjuntti *et al.*, 1997; Chui *et al.*, 2000) (**Table 61.3**). Hypoperfusion dementia resulting from global cerebrovascular insufficiency is also included. Furthermore, subtypes include haemorrhagic dementia, hereditary vascular dementia (e.g. CADASIL) and AD with CVD. The most widely used clinical diagnostic criteria for VaD are the NINDS-AIREN criteria (Román *et al.*, 1993). In addition, research criteria for SIVD have also been proposed (Erkinjuntti *et al.*, 2000b).

61.6.1   Cortical VaD

Cortical VaD (large vessel disease, MID, post-stroke VaD) relates predominantly to large vessel disease and cardiac embolic events. It is a syndrome related to strokes, not a disease entity, and rarely fulfils current criteria modelled on AD-type dementia. It is characterized by predominantly cortical and cortico-subcortical arterial territorial and distal field (watershed) infarcts. It is traditionally characterized by a relative abrupt onset (days to weeks), a step-wise deterioration (some recovery after worsening), and a fluctuating course of cognitive functions (Erkinjuntti, 1987; Erkinjuntti *et al.*, 1988; Chui *et al.*, 1992; Erkinjuntti and Hachinski, 1993; Román *et al.*, 1993). The early cognitive syndrome of cortical VaD includes some memory impairment, which may be mild, and some heteromodal cortical symptom(s), such as aphasia, apraxia, agnosia and visuospatial or constructional difficulty. In addition, most patients have some degree of dysexecutive syndrome (Mahler and Cummings, 1991). Due to the multiple cortico-subcortical infarcts, patients with cortical VaD, often have additional neurological impairments (visual field deficits, lower facial weakness, lateralized sensorimotor changes and/or gait impairment) (Erkinjuntti, 1987).

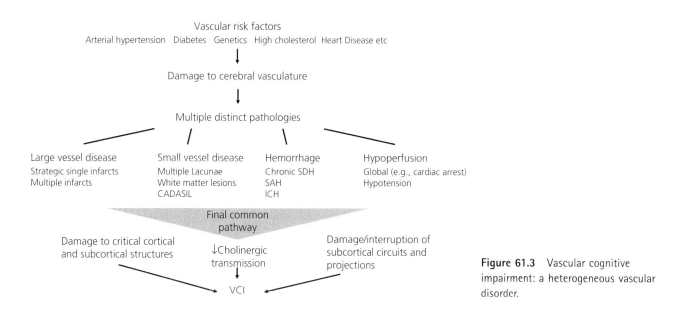

Figure 61.3   Vascular cognitive impairment: a heterogeneous vascular disorder.

Table 61.3   Vascular mechanisms, changes in the brain and clinical heterogeneity in subtypes of traditional vascular dementia (vascular cognitive impairment).

	Cortical VaD/VCI Large vessel disease, MID	Strategic infarct VaD/VCI	Subcortical ischaemic VaD/VCI Small vessel disease (SIVD)
Vascular mechanisms			
Large-vessel disease	+	+	−
Cardiac embolic events	+	+	−
Hypoperfusion	+	+	+
Small-vessel disease	−	+	+
Changes in the brain			
Arterial territorial infarct	+	+	−
Distal field (watershed) infarct	+	+	−
Lacunar infarct	−	+	+
Focal, diffuse WMLs	−	+	+
Incomplete ischaemic injury	−	−	+
Clinical heterogeneity	+ +	+ + +	+

MID, multi-infarct (multi-stroke) dementia; VaD, vascular dementia; WML, white matter lesions.

61.6.2   Subcortical VaD

Subcortical VaD (small vessel disease, SIVD) incorporates two entities: 'the lacunar state' and 'Binswanger's disease' (Erkinjuntti et al, 2000b; Chui, 2001; Román et al., 2002) (**Figure 61.4**). SIVD is attributed to small vessel disease and is characterized by lacunar infarcts, focal and diffuse ischaemic WMLs, and incomplete ischaemic injury (Erkinjuntti, 1987; Erkinjuntti et al., 2000b; Román et al., 2002). SIVD reveals multiple lacunes and extensive WMLs on MRI, supporting the importance of imaging in the diagnostic process (Erkinjuntti et al., 2000b). The onset is variable: as reported by Babikian and Ropper (1987), 60 per cent of the patients had a slow onset, and only 30 per cent an acute onset of cognitive symptoms; the course was gradual without (40 per cent) and with (40 per cent) acute deficits, and fluctuating in only 20 per cent. There is often clinical history of 'prolonged transient ischaemic attcks (TIAs)' or 'multiple TIAs' which mostly are small strokes without residual symptoms, with only mild focal findings. Clinically, SIVD is characterized by a subcortical cognitive syndrome plus pure motor hemiparesis, bulbar signs and dysarthria, gait disorder, variable depressive illness, emotional lability and deficits in executive functioning (Pohjasvaara et al., 2003; Jokinen et al., 2006). The early cognitive syndrome of SIVD is characterized by a dysexecutive syndrome with slowed information processing: usually mild memory deficit and behavioural symptoms. The dysexecutive syndrome in SIVD includes impairment in goal formulation, initiation, planning, organizing, sequencing, executing, set-shifting and set-maintenance, as well as in abstraction (Cummings, 1993; Cummings, 1994; Jokinen et al., 2006; Jokinen et al., 2009a; Jokinen et al., 2009b). The

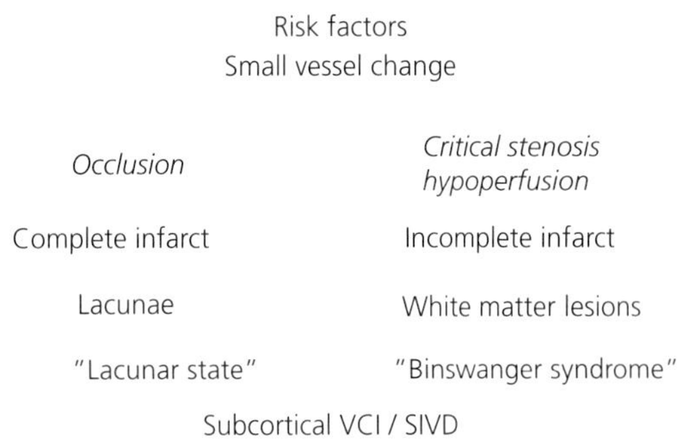

Risk factors
Small vessel change

Occlusion   *Critical stenosis*
                                hypoperfusion

Complete infarct   Incomplete infarct

Lacunae   White matter lesions

"Lacunar state"   "Binswanger syndrome"

Subcortical VCI / SIVD

Figure 61.4 Two main pathways associated with small vessel ischaemic subcortical vascular disease and dementia.

memory deficit in SIVD is usually milder than in AD, and is characterized by impaired recall, relative intact recognition, less severe forgetting and better benefit from cues. Behavioural and psychological symptoms in SIVD include depression, personality change, emotional lability and incontinence, as well as inertia, emotional bluntness and psychomotor retardation. Neurological symptoms and signs in the early phases of SIVD may include subtle episodes of mild upper motor neurone signs (drift, reflex asymmetry, incordination), gait disorder (apractic-atactic or small-stepped), imbalance and falls, urinary frequency and incontinence, dysarthria, dysphagia, as well as extrapyramidal signs, such as hypokinesia and rigidity (Cummings, 1994; Pohjasvaara *et al.*, 2003).

61.6.3   Strategic infarct dementia

Depending on the precise location, the time course and clinical features of strategic infarct dementia are highly variable. Strategic infarct dementia is characterized by focal, often small, ischaemic lesions involving specific sites critical for higher cortical functions. The cortical sites include the hippocampal formation, angular gyrus and cingulate gyrus. The subcortical sites leading to impairment are the thalamus, fornix, basal forebrain, caudate, globus pallidus and the genu or anterior limb of the internal capsule (Tatemichi, 1990; Erkinjuntti and Hachinski, 1993).

61.6.4   AD with CVD

Accumulating evidence shows that different vascular factors, including hypertension and stroke, increase the risk of AD, and frequently CVD coexists with AD (Kalaria and Ballard, 1999; Skoog *et al.*, 1999; DeCarli, 2004; de la Torre, 2004). This overlap is increasingly important in the oldest old (>85 years age). Clinical recognition of patients with AD and CVD is problematic, as evident from recent neuropathological series (Snowdon *et al.*, 1997; Neuropathology Group of the Medical Research Council Cognitive Function and Aging Study, 2001; Schneider *et al.*, 2007). These patients exhibit a history of vascular risk and signs of CVD providing a clinical picture that is close to VaD. However, fluctuating course (odds ratio, OR 0.2) and history of strokes (OR, 0.1) were the

only items differentiating AD from AD with CVD (Moroney *et al.*, 1997b). AD with CVD patients may present clinically either as AD with evidence of CVD lesions on brain imaging, or with features of both AD and VCI (Rockwood *et al.*, 1999). It remains a major clinical undertaking to distinguish dementia due to AD from that arising from CVD in view of the considerable overlap (Langa *et al.*, 2004). Both result in cognitive, functional and behavioural impairments. There are also shared pathophysiological mechanisms (e.g. WMLs, delayed neuronal death and apoptosis) (Pantoni and Garcia, 1995; Snowdon *et al.*, 1997; Skoog *et al.*, 1999), associated risk factors (e.g. age, education, arterial hypertension) (Skoog *et al.*, 1999; DeCarli, 2004) and neurochemical deficits including cholinergic neuronal dysfunction (Wallin *et al.*, 2002; Román and Kalaria, 2006). Based on the findings from the Nun Study, it has been further suggested that CVD may play an important role in determining the presence and severity of clinical symptoms of AD (Snowdon *et al.*, 1997). A better solution to recognizing patients with AD plus CVD would be to discover reliable biological markers of clinical AD. Potential markers include early prominent episodic memory impairment, early and significant medial temporal lobe atrophy on MRI, bilateral parietal hypoperfusion on single photon emission computed tomography or positron emission tomograhy, findings in brain amyloid imaging or low concentrations of cerebrospinal fluid (CSF) Aβ42 peptide with increased phospho tau and tau proteins (Dubois *et al.*, 2007).

61.7   CLINICAL CRITERIA FOR VAD

Since the 1970s, several general clinical criteria for VaD have been used (Wetterling *et al.*, 1996; Pohjasvaara *et al.*, 2000b). Widely used criteria for VaD include the DSM-IV (World Health Organization, 1993; American Psychiatric Association, 1994), ICD-10 (World Health Organization, 1993), ADDTC criteria (Chui *et al.*, 1992), and the NINDS-AIREN criteria (Román *et al.*, 1993).

The two cardinal elements implemented in the clinical criteria for VaD are the definition of the cognitive syndrome of dementia (Erkinjuntti *et al.*, 1997), and the definition of the vascular cause of the dementia (Wetterling *et al.*, 1996; Pohjasvaara *et al.*, 2000b). Variation in defining these two critical elements has caused different definitions in use to give different point prevalence estimates, identify different groups of subjects, and consequently also identify different types and distribution of brain lesions. Furthermore, this heterogeneity may have been a factor in negative results in prior clinical trials on VaD (Inzitari *et al.*, 2000). All the clinical criteria used are consensus criteria, which are neither derived from prospective community-based studies on vascular factors affecting the cognition, nor based on detailed natural histories. All the cited criteria are mainly based on the ischaemic infarct concept and designed to have high specificity, although they have been poorly implemented and validated.

The general NINDS-AIREN criteria: (1) emphasize heterogeneity of VaD syndromes and pathologic subtypes, including not only ischaemic stroke, but also other causes of CVD, including cerebral hypoxic-ischaemic events, WMLs and haemorrhagic strokes; (2) recognize the variability in clinical course, which may be static, remitting, or progressive; (3) highlight the question of the location of ischaemic lesions and the need to establish a causal relationship between vascular brain lesions and cognition; (4) recognize the need to establish a temporal relationship between stroke and dementia onset; (5) include specific findings early in the course that support a vascular rather than a degenerative cause; (6) emphasize the importance of brain imaging to support clinical findings; and (7) give value of neuropsychological testing to document impairments in multiple cognitive domains. The NINDS-AIREN criteria handle VaD as a syndrome with different aetiologies and different clinical manifestations and not as a single entity and list possible subtypes to be used in research studies. The focus is on consequences of CVD, but also the criteria take into account different aetiologies. These criteria incorporate different levels of certainty of the clinical diagnosis (probable, possible, definite). However, in randomized clinical trials using the NINDS-AIREN criteria, all potential subtypes have been lumped together as 'general VaD'. The SIVD criteria of Erkinjuntti *et al.* represent an attempt to define a more homogenous subtype (Erkinjuntti *et al.*, 2000b).

In a neuropathological series, the sensitivity of the NINDS-AIREN criteria for probable and possible VaD was 58 per cent and specificity was 80 per cent (Gold *et al.*, 1997). The criteria succesfully excluded AD in 91 per cent of cases, and the proportion of combined cases misclassified as probable VaD was 29 per cent. Compared to the other modern criteria (the ADDTC criteria), the NINDS-AIREN criteria were more specific and better at excluding combined cases (54 versus 29 per cent). In another series, the sensitivity of the NINDS-AIREN criteria for probable VaD was 20 per cent and specificity 93 per cent; the corresponding figures for probable ADDTC were 25 per cent and 91 per cent (Gold *et al.*, 2002). The inter-rater reliability of the NINDS-AIREN criteria is moderate to substantial (kappa 0.46 to 0.72) (Lopez *et al.*, 1994).

The research criteria of the dysexecutive phenotype of VCI, the SIVD represent a more recent development (Erkinjuntti *et al.*, 2000b; Chui, 2007). In SIVD, the biological markers of small vessel disease are confluent WMLs along with lacunes. Furthermore, changes in the normal appearing white matter, frontal cortical atrophy, as well as microinfacts may be important surrogates (Mungas *et al.*, 2001; Chui, 2007). A similar approach to the small vessel dysexecutive phenotype criteria of SIVD is the more recent criteria for the amnestic phenotype of AD (Dubois *et al.*, 2007).

61.8   CLINICAL CRITERIA FOR VCI

The concept and definition of VCI or vascular CIND are still evolving, but it seems clear that the diagnosis should not be confined to a single aetiology comparable to the traditional 'pure AD' concept. The three main factors to be defined in VCI are the severity of cognitive impairment, the pattern of affected cognitive domains, and the assumed aetiologies and brain changes. It is important to avoid arbitrary new threshold criteria, recognize a continuum of cognitive impairment, focus on causes instead of consequences, and acknowledge complex interactions of coexisting different aetiologies and brain changes. General VCI criteria are probably not needed. It is better to avoid arbitrary clinical threshold criteria such as the old AD-type dementia criteria. General common VCI criteria may hamper discovery of interactive processes related to the continuum of individual cognitive changes. Separate criteria, designed according to the target group, the assumed biological surrogate and the assumed clinical outcomes would be better.

The target groups may be:

- CVD patients at risk of cognitive impairment;
- VCI patients at risk of further cognitive and functional decline;
- SIVD patients at risk of cognitive and functional decline;
- non-demented, non-disabled patients with extensive WMLs at risk of functional decline;
- AD patients with WMLs at risk of cognitive and functional decline;
- elderly with gait instability; or
- depressed elderly with dysexecutive syndrome.

Potential surrogates include white matter burden, lacunar infarct burden, as well as frontal cortical atrophy. The clinical outcomes may relate to cognitive functions, behavioural symptoms, ADLs or gait and stability.

The recent vascular cognitive impairment harmonization standards (Hachinski *et al.*, 2006) are an important step to guide and harmonize VCI studies wordwide. They include a recommendation on minimum, common, clinical and research standards for the description and study of VCI.

61.9   CONCLUSIONS

VCI is the modern term related to vascular burden of the brain, reflecting the all-encompassing effects of CVD on cognition. VCI include all levels of cognitive decline from mild deficits in one or more cognitive domain to a broad dementia-like syndrome. VCI incorporates the complex interactions between vascular risk factors, CVD aetiologies and cellular changes within the brain and cognition. Vascular risk factors towards VCI include arterial hypertension, high cholesterol, and diabetes. VCI includes the common PSD and VaD. The main subtypes of VaD include cortical VaD or MID, also referred as post-stroke VaD and SIVD or small vessel dementia. Traditional vascular risk factors and stroke are also independent factors for the clinical presentation of AD. In addition to these vascular factors, CVD/strokes, infarcts and WMLs may trigger and modify the progression of AD. While CVD is preventable and treatable, it clearly is a major factor in the prevalence of cognitive impairment worldwide. The new VCI harmonization standards are an important step towards international cooperation and innovative studies.

REFERENCES

Amar K, Wilcock G. (1996) Vascular dementia. *British Medical Journal* **312**: 227–31.

American Psychiatric Association. (1994) *Diagnostic and statistical manual of mental disorders*, 4th edn. Washington DC: American Psychiatric Association.

Babikian V, Ropper AH. (1987) Binswanger's disease: a review. *Stroke* **18**: 2–12.

Bowler JV, Hachinski V. (1995) Vascular cognitive impairment: a new approach to vascular dementia. *Baillière's Clinical Neurology* **4**: 357–76.

Bowler JV, Steenhuis R, Hachinski V. (1999) Conceptual background of vascular cognitive impairment. *Alzheimer Disease and Associated Disorders* **13**: S30–7.

Bowler JV. (2007) Modern concept of vascular cognitive impairment. *British Medical Bulletin* **83**: 291–305.

Brun A. (1994) Pathology and pathophysiology of cerebrovascular dementia: pure subgroups of obstructive and hypoperfusive etiology. *Dementia* **5**: 145–7.

Brust JC. (1988) Vascular dementia is overdiagnosed. *Archives of Neurology* **45**: 799–801.

Chui HC. (1989) Dementia: a review emphasizing clinicopathologic correlation and brain–behavior relationships. *Archives in Neurology* **46**: 806–14.

Chui HC. (2001) Vascular dementia, a new beginning. Shifting focus from clinical phenotype to ischemic brain injury. *Neurologic Clinics* **18**: 951–77.

Chui HC. (2007) Subcortical ischemic vascular dementia (SIVD). *Neurologic Clinics* **25**: 717–40.

Chui HC, Victoroff JI, Margolin D *et al.* (1992) Criteria for the diagnosis of ischemic vascular dementia proposed by the State of California Alzheimer's Disease Diagnostic and Treatment Centers. *Neurology* **42**: 473–80.

Chui HC, Mack W, Jackson JE *et al.* (2000) Clinical criteria for the diagnosis of vascular dementia. *Archives in Neurology* **57**: 191–6.

Cummings JL. (1993) Fronto-subcortical circuits and human behavior. *Archives in Neurology* **50**: 873–80.

Cummings JL. (1994) Vascular subcortical dementias: clinical aspects. *Dementia* **5**: 177–80.

de la Torre JC. (2004) Alzheimer's disease is a vasocognopathy: a new term to describe its nature. *Neurological Research* **26**: 517–24.

DeCarli C, Scheltens P. (2002) Structural brain imaging. In: Erkinjunti T, Gauthier S (eds). *Vascular cognitive impairment*, 1st edn. London: Martin Duniz, 433–57.

DeCarli C. (2004) Vascular factors in dementia: an overview. *Journal of the Neurological Sciences* **226**: 19–23.

Desmond DW. (1996) Vascular dementia: a construct in evolution. *Cerebrovascular Brain Metabolism Reviews* **8**: 296–325.

Dubois B, Feldman H, Jacova C *et al.* (2007) Research criteria for the diagnosis of Alzheimer's disease: revising the NINCDS-ADRDA criteria. *Lancet Neurology* **6**: 734–46.

Englund E, Brun A, Alling C. (1988) White matter changes in dementia of Alzheimer's type. Biochemical and neuropathological correlates. *Brain* **111**: 1425–39.

Erkinjuntti T. (1987) Types of multi-infarct dementia. *Acta Neurologica Scandinavica* **75**: 391–9.

Erkinjuntti T, Hachinski VC. (1993) Rethinking vascular dementia. *Cerebrovascular Disorders* **3**: 3–23.

Erkinjunti T. (1999a) Cerebrovascular dementia: A quide to diagnosis and treatment. *CNS Drugs* **12**: 35–48.

Erkinjuntti T. (1999b) Cerebrovascular dementia. Pathophysiology, diagnosis and treatment. *CNS Drugs* **12**: 35–48.

Erkinjuntti T, Pantoni L. (2000) Subcortical vascular dementia. In: Gauthier S, Cummings JL (eds). *Alzheimer's diasease and related disorders annual*. London: Martin Dunitz, 101–33.

Erkinjuntti T, Haltia M, Palo J *et al.* (1988) Accuracy of the clinical diagnosis of vascular dementia: a rospective clinical and post-mortem neuropathological study. *Journal of Neurology, Neurosurgery and Psychiatry* **51**: 1037–44.

Erkinjuntti T, Ostbye T, Steenhuis R, Hachinski V. (1997) The effect of different diagnostic criteria on the prevalence of dementia. *New England Journal of Medicine* **337**: 1667–74.

Erkinjuntti T, Bowler JV, DeCarli C *et al.* (1999) Imaging of static brain lesions in vascular dementia: implications for clinical trials. *Alzheimer Disorders and Associated Disorders* **13** (Suppl. 3): S81–90.

Erkinjuntti T, Inzitari D, Pantoni L *et al.* (2000a) Limitations of clinical critera for the diagnois of vascular dementia in clinical trials: is a focus on subcortical vascular dementia a solution? *Annals of New York Academy of Sciences* **903**: 262–72.

Erkinjuntti T, Inzitari D, Pantoni L *et al.* (2000b) Research criteria for subcortical vascular dementia in clinical trials. *Journal of Neural Transmission* **59** (Suppl. 2): 23–30.

Fratiglioni L, Launer LJ, Andersen K *et al.* (2000) Incidence of dementia and major subtypes in Europe: A collaborative study of population-based cohorts. *Neurology* **54** (Suppl. 5): S10–15.

Gold G, Giannakopoulos P, Montes-Paixao JC *et al.* (1997) Sensitivity and specificity of newly proposed clinical criteria for possible vascular dementia. *Neurology* **49**: 690–4.

Gold G, Bouras C, Canuto A *et al.* (2002) Clinicopathological validation study of four sets of clinical criteria for vascular dementia. *American Journal of Psychiatry* **159**: 82–7.

Gorelick PB. (1997) Status of risk factors for dementia associated with stroke. *Stroke* **28**: 459–63.

Hachinski V. (2008) Shifts in thinking about dementia. *Journal of the American Medical Association* **300**: 2172–3.

Hachinski V, Iadecola C, Petersen CR *et al.* (2006) National Institute of Neurological Disorders and Stoke–Canadian Stroke Network vascular cognitive impairment harmonization standerds. *Stroke* **37**: 2220–41.

Hachinski VC, Lassen NA, Marshall J. (1974) Multi-infarct dementia. A cause of mental deterioration in the elderly. *Lancet* **2**: 207–10.

Hachinski VC. (1990) The decline and resurgence of vascular dementia. *Canadian Medical Association Journal* **142**: 107–11.

Hebert R, Brayne C. (1995) Epidemiology of vascular dementia. *Neuroepidemiology* **14**: 240–57.

Inzitari D, Erkinjuntti T, Wallin A *et al.* (2000) Subcortical vascular dementia as a specific target for clinical trials. *Annals of the New York Academy of Sciences* **903**: 510–21.

Inzitari D, Simoni M, Paracucci G et al. (2007) Risk of rapid global functional decline in elderly patients with severe cerebral age-related white matter changes: the LADIS Study. *Archives of Internal Medicine* **167**: 81–8.

Inzitari D, Pracucci G, Pogessi A et al. (2009) LADIS Study Group. Changes in white matter as determinant of global functional decline in older independent outpatients: three year follow-up of LADIS (leukoaraiosis and disability) study cohort. *British Medical Journal* **339**: b2477.

Jokinen H, Kalska H, Mäntylä R et al. (2005) White matter hyperintesities as a predictor of neuropsychological deficits post-stroke. *Journal of Neurology, Neurosurgery and Psychiatry* **76**: 1229–33.

Jokinen H, Kalska H, Mäntylä R et al. (2006) Cognitive profile of subcortical ischemic vascular disease. *Journal of Neurology, Neurosurgery and Psychiatry* **77**: 28–33.

Jokinen H, Kalska H, Ylikoski R et al. (2009a) LADIS Group. MRI-defined subcortical ischemic vascular disease: baseline clinical and neuropsychological findings. The LADIS study. *Cerebrovascular Diseases* **27**: 336–44.

Jokinen H, Kalska H, Ylikoski R et al. (2009b) LADIS Group. Longitudinal cognitive decline in subcortical ischemic vascular disease. The LADIS study. *Cerebrovascular Diseases* **27**: 384–91.

Kalaria RN, Ballard C. (1999) Overlap between pathology of Alzheimer disease and vascular dementia. *Alzheimer Disease and Associated Disorders* **13** (Suppl. 3): S115–23.

Kalaria RN, Kenny RA, Ballard CG et al. (2004) Towards defining the neuropathological substrates of vascular dementia. *Journal of Neurological Sciences* **226**: 75–80.

Kivpelto M, Ngandu T, Laatikainen T et al. (2006) Risk score for the prediction of dementia risk in 20 years among middle aged people: a longitudinal, population-based study. *Lancet Neurology* **5**: 735–41.

Langa KM, Forster NL, Larson EB. (2004) Mixed dementia: emerging concepts and therapeutic implications. *Journal of the American Medical Association* **292**: 2901–8.

Leys D, Henon H, Mackowiak-Cordoliani M-A, Pasquier F. (2005) Poststroke dementia. *Lancet Neurology* **4**: 752–9.

Linden T, Skoog I, Fagerber B et al. (2004) Cognitive impairment and dementia 20 months after stroke. *Neuroepidemiology* **23**: 45–52.

Lobo A, Launer LJ, Fratiglioni L et al. (2000) Prevalence of dementia and major subtypes in Europe: A collaborative study of population-based cohorts. *Neurology* **54** (Suppl. 5): S4–9.

Lopez OL, Larumbe MR, Becker JT et al. (1994) Reliability of NINDS-AIREN clinical criteria for the diagnosis of vascular dementia. *Neurology* **44**: 1240–5.

McKhann G, Drachman D, Folstein M et al. (1984) Clinical diagnosis of Alzheimer's disease: report of the NINCDS-ADRDA Work Group under the auspices of Department of Health and Human Services Task Force on Alzheimer's Disease. *Neurology* **34**: 939–44.

Mahler ME, Cummings JL. (1991) The behavioural neurology of multi-infarct dementia. *Alzheimer Disease and Associated Disorders* **5**: 122–30.

Moorhouse P, Rockwood K. (2008) Vascular cognitive impairment: current concepts and clinical developments. *Lancet Neurology* **7**: 246–55.

Moroney JT, Bagiella E, Desmond DW et al. (1996) Risk factors for incident dementia after stroke. Role of hypoxic and ischemic disorders. *Stroke* **27**: 1283–9.

Moroney JT, Bagiella E, Desmond DW et al. (1997a) Cerebral hypoxia and ischemia in the pathogenesis of dementia after stroke. *Annals of the New York Academy of Sciences* **826**: 433–6.

Moroney JT, Bagiella E, Hachinski VC et al. (1997b) Misclassification of dementia subtype using the Hachinski Ischemic Score: results of a meta-analysis of patients with pathologically verified dementias. *Annals of the New York Academy of Sciences* **826**: 490–2.

Mungas D, Jagust WJ, Reed BR et al. (2001) MRI predictors of cognition in subcortical ischemic vascular disease and Alzheimer's disease. *Neurology* **57**: 2229–35.

Neuropathology Group. Medical Research Council Cognitive Function and Aging Study. (2001) Pathological correlates of late-onset dementia in a multicentre, community-based population in England and Wales. Neuropathology Group of the Medical Research Council Cognitive Function and Ageing Study (MRC CFAS). *Lancet* **357**: 169–75.

O'Brien JT, Erkinjuntti T, Reisberg B et al. (2003) Vascular cognitive impairment. *Lancet Neurology* **2**: 89–98.

Pantoni L, Garcia JH. (1995) The significance of cerebral white matter abnormalities 100 years after Binswanger's report. A review. *Stroke* **26**: 1293–301.

Pantoni L, Garcia JH. (1997) Pathogenesis of leukoaraiosis: a review. *Stroke* **28**: 652–9.

Pasquier F, Leys D. (1997) Why are stroke patients prone to develop dementia? *Journal of Neurology* **244**: 135–42.

Petersen RC, Doody R, Kurz A et al. (2002) Current concepts in mild cognitive impairment. *Archives of Neurology* **58**: 1985–92.

Pohjasvaara T, Erkinjuntti T, Vataja R, Kaste M. (1997) Dementia three months after stroke. Baseline frequency and effect of different definitions of dementia in the Helsinki Stroke Aging Memory Study (SAM) cohort. *Stroke* **28**: 785–92.

Pohjasvaara T, Erkinjuntti T, Ylikoski R et al. (1998) Clinical determinants of poststroke dementia. *Stroke* **29**: 75–81.

Pohjasvaara T, Mäntylä R, Salonen O et al. (2000a) How complex interactions of ischemic brain infarcts, white matter lesions and atrophy relate to poststroke dementia. *Archives of Neurology* **57**: 1295–300.

Pohjasvaara T, Mäntylä R, Ylikoski R et al. (2000b) Comparison of different clinical criteria for the vascular cause of vascular dementia (ADDTC, DSM-III, DSM-IV, ICD-10, NINDS-AIREN). *Stroke* **31**: 2952–7.

Pohjasvaara T, Mäntylä R, Ylikoski R et al. (2003) Clinical features of MRI-defined subcortical vascular disease. *Alzheimer Disease and Associated Disorders* **17**: 236–42.

Prins ND, van Dijk EJ, den Heijer T et al. (2004) Cerebral white matter lesions and the risk of dementia. *Archives of Neurology* **61**: 1503–4.

Rockwood K, Howard K, MacKnight C, Darvesh S. (1999) Spectrum of disease in vascular cognitive impairment. *Neuroepidemiology* **18**: 248–54.

Rockwood K, Wenzel C, Hachinski V et al. (2000) Prevalence and outcomes of vascular cognitive impairment. *Neurology* **54**: 447–51.

Román GC. (1985) The identity of lacunar dementia and Binswanger disease. *Medical Hypotheses* **16**: 389–91.

Román GC. (1987) Senile dementia of the Binswanger type. A vascular form of dementia in the elderly. *Journal of the American Medical Association* **258**: 1782–8.

Román GC. (2001) Historic evolution of the concept of dementia: a systematic review from 2000 BC to 2000 AD. In: Qizilbash N, Schneider LS, Brodaty H *et al.* (eds). *Evidence-based dementia: a practical guide to diagnosis and management.* Oxford: Blackwell Science.

Román GC, Kalaria RN. (2006) Vascular determinants of cholinergic deficits in Alzheimer disease and vascular dementia. *Neurobiology of Aging* **27**: 1769–85.

Román GC. (2008) Have we forgotten the cerebrovascular circulation. *Alzheimer Disease and Associated Disorders* **22**: 1–3.

Román GC, Tatemichi TK, Erkinjuntti T *et al.* (1993) Vascular dementia: diagnostic criteria for reserach studies. Report of the NINDS-AIREN International Work Group. *Neurology* **43**: 250–60.

Román GC, Erkinjuntti T, Wallin A *et al.* (2002) Subcortical ischaemic vascular dementia. *Lancet. Neurology* **1**: 426–36.

Román GC, Sachdev P, Royall DR *et al.* (2004) Vascular cognitive disorder: a new diagnostic category updating vascular cognitive impairment and vascular dementia. *Journal of Neurological Sciences* **226**: 81–7.

Roth M. (1971) Classification and aetiology in mental disorders of old age: some recent development. In: Kay D, Walk A (eds). *Recent developments in psychogeriatrics.* Ashford: Haedley Brothers, Ashford.

Schneider JA, Arvanitakis Z, Bang W, Bennet DA. (2007) Mixed brain pathologies account for most dementia cases in community-dwelling older persons. *Neurology* **69**: 2197–204.

Seshadri S, Wolf AP. (2007) Lifetime risk of stroke and dementia: current concepts, and estimates from the Framingham Study. *Lancet Neurology* **6**: 1106–14.

Shim YS, Yang DW, Kim BS *et al.* (2006) Comparison of regional cerebral blood flow in two subsets of subcortical ischemic vascular dementia: statistical parametric mapping analysis of SPECT. *Journal of Neurological Sciences* **250**: 85–91.

Skoog I. (1994) Risk factors for vascular dementia: a review. *Dementia* **5**: 137–44.

Skoog I. (1998) Status of risk factors for vascular dementia. *Neuroepidemiology* **17**: 2–9.

Skoog I, Kalaria RN, Breteler MMB. (1999) Vascular factors and Alzheimer's disease. *Alzheimer Disease and Associated Disorders* **13** (Suppl. 3): S106–14.

Snowdon DA, Greiner LH, Mortimer JA *et al.* (1997) Brain infarction and the clinical expression of Alzheimer disease. The Nun Study. *Journal of the American Medical Association* **277**: 813–17.

Sulkava R, Erkinjuntti T. (1987) Vascular dementia due to cardiac arrhythmias and systemic hypotension. *Acta Neurologica Scandinavica* **76**: 123–8.

Tatemichi TK. (1990) How acute brain failure becomes chronic. A view of the echanisms and syndromes of dementia related to stroke. *Neurology* **40**: 1652–9.

Tomlinson BE, Blessed G, Roth M. (1970) Observations on the brains of demented old people. *Journal of Neurological Sciences* **11**: 205–42.

Vataja R, Pohjasvaara T, Mäntylä R *et al.* (2003) MRI correlates of executive dysfunction in patients with ischaemic stroke. *European Journal of Neurology* **10**: 625–31.

Vermeer SE, Prins ND, den Heijer T *et al.* (2003) Silent brain infarcts and the risk of dementia and cognitive decline. *New England Journal of Medicine* **348**: 1215–22.

Vinters HV, Ellis WG, Zarow C *et al.* (2000) Neuropathologic substrates of ischemic vascular dementia. *Journal of Neuropathology and Experimental Neurology* **60**: 658–9.

Wallin A, Blennow K. (1994) The clinical diagnosis of vascular dementia. *Dementia* **5**: 181–4.

Wallin A, Blennow K, Gottfries CG. (2002) Neurochemical abnormalities in vascular dementia. *Dementia* **1**: 120–30.

Wetterling T, Kanitz RD, Borgis KJ. (1996) Comparison of different diagnostic criteria for vascular dementia (ADDTC, DSM-IV, ICD-10, NINDS-AIREN). *Stroke* **27**: 30–6.

World Health Organization. (1993) ICD-10 Classification of Mental and Behavioural Disorders: Diagnostic Criteria for Research, 36–40. Geneva: WHO.

62

The neuropathology of vascular dementia

RAJ N KALARIA

62.1 INTRODUCTION

Cerebrovascular disease (CVD) is responsible for the second most common form of age-related dementia. vascular dementia (VaD), or more concisely vascular cognitive impairment (VCI), is attributed to conditions resulting from a variety of cerebrovascular lesions or impaired brain perfusion (O'Brien *et al.*, 2003). The pathological diagnosis of VaD or VCI requires systematic evaluation of potentially relevant clinical or phenotypic features.

Alois Alzheimer and Emil Kraeplin were among the original neuropsychiatrists who had described gradual strangulation of the blood supply to the brain as the main cause of dementia (Berrios and Freeman, 1991). They surmised that the older age-associated progressive hardening of the arteries lead to arteriosclerotic dementia. Even until the late 1960s (Tomlinson *et al.*, 1970), arteriosclerotic dementia, attributed to cerebral softening with loss of relatively large volume (>50 mL) of tissue was described, but reported to be over-diagnosed clinically in comparison to Alzheimer's disease (AD) (Tomlinson *et al.*, 1970; Román, 2002). However, the first recognition for subclasses of VaD could be credited to Otto Binswanger who described subcortical arteriosclerotic encephalopathy upon pathological verification of cerebral white matter (WM) disorder in a group of eight patients with hypertensive disease (Berrios and Freeman, 1991).

The challenge of defining the neuropathological substrates of VaD is complicated by the heterogeneous localization of lesions and the co-existence of other pathologies, including neurodegenerative changes such as those in AD. Several factors are involved in defining the degree of overall impairment and the VaD phenotype. These include origin and type of vascular occlusion, presence of haemorrhage, distribution of arterial territories and size of vessels as critical factors in defining VaD. Not surprisingly, many brain regions including the territories of the anterior, posterior and middle cerebral arteries, the angular gyrus, caudate and medial thalamus in the dominant hemisphere, the amygdala as well as the hippocampus have been implicated in VaD (Markesbery, 1998). Factors that define subtypes of VaD include multiplicity, size, anatomical location, laterality and age of the lesions besides genetic influences and previous existence of systemic vascular disease (**Box 62.1**). Advances in neuroimaging of CVD and meticulous neuropathological examination have facilitated to define clinical conditions. Multi-infarct dementia is caused by large vessel disease, whereas Binswanger type of VaD involving subcortical regions including the WM results from small vessel changes. It has recently been recognized that subcortical ischaemic VaD is the most significant subtype of VaD (Román, 2002). For the purposes of prevention and treatment, it is imperative to recognize the main subtypes of VaD (Román *et al.*, 1993).

62.2 PREVALENCE OF VAD AT AUTOPSY

The diagnosis of dementia is widely applied upon fulfilment of present DSM-IV criteria after evaluation of information from a range of investigations including clinical history, timing of event, neuropsychometry and neuroimaging, but in the absence of pathological examination. The clinical diagnosis of VaD in impaired patients with evidence of cerebrovascular lesions is considered when other causes of

Box 62.1 Vascular dementia subtypes defined by blood vessel size and pathological process

- Large vessel dementia (multiple infarcts or multi-infarct dementia)
- Small vessel dementia (small vessel disease and microinfarction)
- Strategic infarct dementia (infarcts in strategic locations)
- Hypoperfusive dementia
- Dementia related to angiopathies (hypertension, amyloid)
- Haemorrhagic dementia
- Other causes of vascular dementia (vasculitis)
- Familial VaD (CADASIL, CARASIL, RVCL)

Familial or hereditary forms of cerebral amyloid angiopathy, involving ischaemic strokes and intracerebral haemorrhages may also lead to cognitive impairment and stroke (Natte et al., 2001). CADASIL, cerebral autosomal dominant arteriopathy with subcortical infarcts and leukoencephalopathy (Kalimo and Kalaria, 2005); CARASIL, cerebral autosomal recessive arteriopathy with subcortical infarcts and leukoencephalopahty (Hara et al., 2009); RVCL, autosomal dominant retinal vasculopathy with cerebral leukodystrophy (Kavanagh et al., 2008).

dementia have been discounted (see Chapter 61, What is vascular cognitive impairment?). The current widely used NINDS-AIREN criteria (Román et al., 1993) are additionally biased by the inclusion of deficits in certain cognitive domains, such as memory, that are classed with AD. This concurs with the relatively low sensitivity (0.20), but high specificity (0.93), for probable VaD apparent in clinicopathological validation studies (Gold et al., 2002). As with AD, confirmation of VaD diagnosis is definitive at autopsy derived from appropriate sampling of both cerebral hemispheres and minimal neuropathological examination (Hachinski et al., 2006) to rule out significant pathological changes associated with other dementias. When a range of clinical criteria for VaD, including ADDTC, ICD-10 and DSM-IV (Gold et al., 2002), have been applied in sample sizes of 59 to 1929, autopsy studies show that pathologically diagnosed VaD ranges widely from as low as 0.03 per cent to as high as 58 per cent, with an overall mean rate of 17 per cent (Markesbery, 1998; Jellinger, 2008a) and the range in western countries as 8–15 per cent. In studies where diagnosis was restricted to the currently used NINDS-AIREN (Román et al., 1993) criteria, the frequencies are reported to be lower with a mean of 7 per cent. Taking all these estimates into account, the worldwide frequency of VaD in autopsy-verified cases is calculated to be between 10 and 15 per cent. On the other hand, the incidence of autopsy verified VaD in Japanese studies was 35 per cent (Seno et al., 1999) and 22 per cent (Akatsu et al., 2002). However, to derive more accurate prevalence or incidence estimates of autopsy-verified VaD cases, there must be uniformity of autopsy protocols across centres or departments (Hachinski et al., 2006; Pantoni et al., 2006).

62.3 CRITERIA FOR PATHOLOGICAL DIAGNOSIS OF VAD

Assessing the neuropathological substrates of VaD plainly involves assessment of parenchymal lesions, including infarcts and hemorrhages, and the vascular abnormalities that may have caused them (Kalaria et al., 2004). The vascular lesions that contribute to full-blown dementia syndromes (during life) often show much more severe abnormalities than those contributing to milder conditions (Vinters et al., 2000; Kalaria et al., 2004; Jellinger, 2008b). However, the neuropathological findings could be quantified and related to the progression of cognitive impairment (Mirra, 1997). In addition, systemic factors (e.g. hypotension, hypoglycaemia) may cause brain lesions in the absence of severe vascular disease. Moreover, parenchymal abnormalities of neurodegenerative type may be present that are not obviously associated with either vascular disease or systemic factors; these include Alzheimer or hippocampal lesions. The presence of mixed pathology in terms of concomitant AD and CVD or dementia with Lewy bodies and vascular changes, is particularly challenging in the oldest old (>85 years of age).

Several studies show that high proportions of individuals fulfilling the clinical diagnosis of AD also exhibit cerebrovascular lesions, including lacunes, macroinfarcts, diffuse and periventricular myelin loss, rarefaction, microinfarcts and focal and diffuse gliosis at autopsy (Premkumar et al., 1996; Heyman et al., 1998; Nagy et al., 1998; Kalaria and Ballard, 1999). Conversely, the accuracy of clinically diagnosed VaD is often lacking and invariably autopsy findings reveal subjects with AD-type of pathological changes (Erkinjuntti et al., 1988; Hulette et al., 1997; Kalaria and Ballard, 1999). For example, Nolan et al. (1998) reported that 87 per cent of the patients enrolled in a prospective series to examine VaD in a dementia clinic were found to have AD either alone (58 per cent) or in combination with CVD (42 per cent) at post-mortem. All of the patients with signs of CVD were also found to have some concomitant neurodegenerative disease (**Figure 62.1**). Similarly, another study indicated that large numbers of VaD cases without co-existing neuropathological evidence of AD suggests that 'pure' VaD is very uncommon (Hulette et al., 1997). Thus current clinical diagnostic criteria serve to detect pathology, but not necessarily 'pure' pathology. Unbiased criteria encompassing relevant cognitive domains for VaD still need to be widely tested (Hachinski et al., 2006).

62.4 THE CHALLENGES OF MIXED DEMENTIA AND PATHOLOGIES

The precise population-based prevalence of mixed dementia is unknown, but community studies suggest it may be

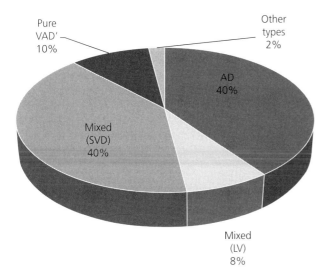

Figure 62.1 Pathological outcomes of clinically diagnosed vascular dementia. Mixed type 1 revealed large infarcts, whereas mixed type 2 predominantly exhibited small vessel disease with microinfarction. Others included Lewy body disease, dementia, mild Parkinson disease and depression. AD, Alzheimer's disease.

frequent (CFAS, 2001). Retrospective and prospective autopsy studies suggest a wide range from 2 to 58 per cent with a reasonable mean range of 6–12 per cent (Jellinger, 2008b). Early validation studies indicated that while mixed dementia could be distinguished from AD, it could not be separated from VaD (Rosen *et al.*, 1980). Recent studies suggest that 30–50 per cent of autopsy-verified mixed AD and VaD cases were misclassified as VaD (Gold *et al.*, 1997; Gold *et al.*, 2002) and the neuroimaging component of the NINDS-AIREN criteria does not distinguish between people with and without dementia in the context of cerebrovascular disease (Ballard *et al.*, 2004). The potential overlap of pathologies is therefore complex, with different types of cerebrovascular lesions, including cortical and subcortical infarction and small vessel disease (SVD) (Esiri *et al.*, 1997; Ballard *et al.*, 2000), and different types and severity of neurodegenerative changes involving tau, amyloid and α-synuclein pathology. While evidence-based pathological criteria for the diagnosis of mixed dementia remains to be perfected, the diagnosis should be made when a primary neurodegenerative disease known to cause dementia exists with one or more of the pathological lesions defining the VaD subtypes (**Box 62.2**). Clinical and pathological evidence indicates that combined neurodegenerative and vascular pathologies act synergistically and worsen outcome of dementia (Snowdon *et al.*, 1997; Esiri *et al.*, 1999; Rossi *et al.*, 2004). However, this is dependent on vascular lesion type and location, as well as severity of concomitant AD-related pathology. In a recent study (Gold *et al.*, 2007) WM lacunes, periventricular and diffuse myelin loss, or cortical gliosis were not associated with cognition, but Braak staging, plaque burden, cortical microinfarcts and thalamic and basal ganglia lacunes predicted the presence of dementia with high sensitivity (0.80) and also distinguished VaD from AD in mixed cases.

Box 62.2 Key variables to define pathology of vascular dementia

- Identify as ischaemic or haemorrhagic infarct(s)
- Presence of lacunes and lacunar infarcts: *état lacunaire* (grey) and *état criblé* (white matter)
- Location of infarcts: cortex, white matter, basal ganglia, brainstem (pontine), cerebellum
- Circulation involved: arterial territories – anterior, middle or posterior
- Laterality: right or left anterior and posterior
- Sizes and number of infarcts = dimension: 0–4 mm, 5–15 mm, 16–30 mm, 31–50 mm and >50 mm; if size <5 mm determine as small or microinfarcts.
- Presence and location of small vessel disease: lipohyalinosis; fibroid necrosis; cerebral amyloid angiopathy
- Presence of white matter disease: rarefaction or incomplete infarction
- Degree of microgliosis and astocytosis: mild, moderate or severe
- Presence of Alzheimer pathology (including NFT and neuritic plaque staging). If degree >stage III, the case is mixed Alzheimer's disease and vascular dementia
- Presence of hippocampal sclerosis

For reporting purposes, each of the above features can be scored numerically to provide a summary (Hachinski *et al.*, 2006). For example, 0 is absent and 1 means present. Less frequent lesions, including watershed infarcts and laminar necrosis. Increasing numerical value may also be assigned to the infarcts. CAA, cerebral amyloid angiopathy; NFT, neurofibrillary tangles.

From the essential information derived at autopsy (**Box 62.2**), we have proposed the neuropathological diagnosis of probable VaD or less popular 'pure VaD' be based on the exclusion of a primary neurodegenerative disease known to cause dementia and the presence of cerebrovascular pathology that defines one or more of the VaD subtypes (**Table 62.1**). These would include dementia among post-stroke survivors who fulfil the NINDS-AIREN (Román *et al.*, 1993) criteria for probable VaD. Those stroke survivors with mild cognitive impairment could be classed as exhibiting VCI, but the criteria for this extension are not widely accepted (O'Brien *et al.*, 2003). The diagnosis of possible VaD may be used when the brain bears significant vascular pathology (Kalaria *et al.*, 2004), which does not fulfil the criteria for one of the subtypes, but where no other explanation for dementia is found. The combination of autopsy-proven AD with multiple vascular or ischaemic lesions with about 30–50 mL of infarcted/damaged brain tissue may be considered mixed. We diagnose mixed pathology when a combination of the nominal three or more infarctions and neurofibrillary pathology above Braak stage III is encountered (Kalaria *et al.*, 2004).

Table 62.1 Dementia associated with different cerebrovascular pathologies.

Vascular dementia subtypes related to:	Subtype
Large infarct or several infarcts (>50 mL loss of tissue); MID	I
Multiple small or microinfarcts (>3 with minimum diameter 5 mm); SVD[a] (involving >3 coronal levels; hyalinization, CAA, lacunar infarcts, perivascular changes)	II
Strategic infarcts (e.g. thalamus, hippocampus)	III
Cerebral hypoperfusion (hippocampal sclerosis, ischaemic–anoxic damage, cortical laminar necrosis, borderzone infarcts involving three different coronal levels)	IV
Cerebral haemorrhages (lobar, ICH or SAH)	V
Cerebrovascular changes with AD pathology (above Braak III); mixed dementia	VI

In all of the above, the age of the vascular lesion(s) should correspond with the time when disease began. The proposed Newcastle categorization includes six subtypes (Kalaria et al., 2004). The post-stroke cases are usually included in subtypes I–III. While these may not be different from other published subtypes (Jellinger, 2008b), they are practical and simple to use. Cases with extensive white matter disease in the absence of significant other features are included under SVD.

AD, Alzheimer's disease; CAA, cerebral amyloid angiopathy; ICH, intracerebral haemorrhage; MID, multi-infarct dementia; SAH, subarachnoid haemorrhage; SVD, small vessel disease.

[a]Subtype I may result from large vessel occlusion (atherothromboembolism), artery to artery embolism or cardioembolism. Subtype II usually involves descriptions of arteriosclerosis, lipohyalinosis, hypertensive, arteriosclerotic, amyloid or collagen angiopathy. Subtypes I–II and V may result from aneurysms, arterial dissections, arteriovenous malformations and various forms of arteritis (vasculitis).

62.5 BRAIN VASCULAR LESIONS AND VAD

Atherothromboembolism is the main cause of infarctions associated with major arterial territories, which may be admixed in cortical and subcortical regions. Thromboembolic events can be responsible for up to 50 per cent of all ischaemic strokes, whereas intracranial SVD causes 25 per cent of the infarcts (Ferrer et al., 2008). Small vessel alterations involve arteriosclerosis and hyalionsis, associated with lacunar infarcts and lacunes predominantly occurring in the subcortical structures. WM disease or subcortical leukoencephalopathy with incomplete infarction and SVD are common pathological changes in cerebrovascular disease. Others features include borderzone (watershed) infarctions, laminar necrosis and amyloid angiopathy (**Box 62.2**). Complicated angiopathies, such as fibromuscular dysplasia, arterial dissections, granulomatous angiitis, collagen vascular disease and giant-cell arteritis, are rarer causes of cerebrovascular disease (Ferrer et al., 2008) and VaD.

Previous studies have recorded ischaemic, oedematous and haemorrhagic lesions affecting the brain circulation or perfusion to be associated with VaD (**Table 62.2**). In ten different studies where VaD was diagnosed, 78 per cent of the cases revealed cortical and subcortical infarcts suggesting other vascular pathologies involving incomplete infarction or borderzone infarcts could be important factors. Among other lesions, a quarter of the cases had cystic infarcts, whereas 50 per cent showed lacunar infarcts or microinfarcts. Lacunar infarcts, however, appear to be a common category of infarcts, and are currently recognized as the most frequent cause of stroke. Severe amyloid angiopathy was present in 10 per cent of the cases. Ischaemic strokes may also lead to hippocampal atrophy which was apparent in 55 per cent of the cases in one study (Vinters et al., 2000). Ischaemic vascular disease appears to also correlate with widespread small ischaemic lesions or microinfarcts distributed throughout the central nervous system (CNS) (Kalaria et al., 2004).

Table 62.2 Types of vascular and hippocampal lesions reported in vascular dementia.

Pathological feature	Cases (%)
Complete infarctions (cortical and subcortical)	78
Lacunar infarcts (mostly WM and BG)	55
Small or microinfarcts	50
Cystic infarcts	26
Cerebral amyloid angiopathy	10
Intracerebral haemorrhages	2
Hippocampal atrophy and sclerosis	55

Data compiled from 214 cases reported in previous studies (Kalaria et al., 2004; Kalaria RN et al., unpublished observations). The percentage of cases are averaged from two or more reported studies. Cystic infarcts (possibly also lacunar) with typically ragged edges were admixed in both cortical and subcortical structures.

BG, basal ganglia; WM, white matter.

62.5.1 Large vessel disease and macroinfarction

Large infarction or macroinfarction is usually defined as that visible upon gross examination of the brain at autopsy. Stenosis arising from atherosclerosis within large vessels is considered to be the main cause of large infarction, which can sometimes extend beyond the arterial territories. The stages of atherosclerosis may vary from accumulation of foam cells causing fatty streaks to complicated atheromas, involving extracellular matrix components and even viral or bacterial infections. Occlusion of the extracranial arteries, such as the internal carotid artery and the main intracranial arteries of the circle of Willis including the middle cerebral artery, leads to multiple infarcts and dementia, which assumes approximately 15 per cent of VaD (Brun, 1994). The differences between the anterior versus posterior portions of the circle of Willis, and left versus right sides may be variable and stenosis of major arteries could be up to 75 per cent in very severe cases. The presence of dolichoectasia and fusiform aneurysms has also been noted in some cases. In severe cases, medium-sized arteries in the leptomeninges and proximal perforating arteries are involved. The damage could be worse depending upon the presence of hypertension. Artery to artery embolism involves breaking of thrombi from the often ulcerated lesions in the extracranial arteries, e.g. at the bifurcation of common carotid artery or the heart. The thrombi may contain in addition to coagulated blood and platelets, cholesterol and calcified deposits from the underlying atheromatous plaque. Various types of cardiogenic emboli may also find their way to the anterior or particularly the posterior cerebral circulation to cause infarcts in the territory of the posterior cerebral artery or superior cerebellar artery.

Arterial territorial infarctions involve four principal areas, particularly those supplied by the major arteries: anterior, middle cerebral artery, posterior artery and the territory between the anterior and middle cerebral artery (Ferrer *et al.*, 2008). The size of these infarctions is determined by assessing the two largest diameters of each lesion (**Box 62.2**). The typical infarct comprises the central core with complete infarction surrounded by a narrow perifocal hypoperfused (or penumbra) zone of incomplete infarction, which may be oedematous, leads into normal appearing tissue. The core may involve both the cortex and underlying WM that is devoid of functional components, such as neurones, axons and oligodendrocytes, and may in time form cavitated lesions or scars, devoid of cells or haemosiderin. Prior to scar formation between 3 and 14 days, infarct cores attract neutrophils, lipid-laden macrophages or microglia and astrocytes in the lesion, which is easily assessed upon routine staining. The intensity of gliosis, both astrocytic and microgliosis, is an important consideration in judging the degree and age of infarction. Degrees of gliosis or glial scars may be noted in brains subjected to global ischaemia, i.e. after transient cardiac arrest where responses may be observed in vulnerable neuronal groups within the hippocampus or neocortical laminae (**Table 62.2**).

62.5.2   Microvascular or small vessel disease

In VaD, arterial disease is considered more significant than venous disease. However, venous adventitial fibrosis has been linked to cognitive abnormalities and neuroradiological lesions (Brown *et al.*, 2002). The smaller vessels of the brain, including intracerebral end arteries and arterioles, undergo progressive age-related changes (Lammie, 2000), which result in lacunar infarcts (cystic lesions generally <1 cm) and microinfarcts. The arteriolar changes range from wall thickening by hyalinosis, reduction or increment of the intima to severe arteriosclerosis and fibroid necrosis (**See p6 of the plate section for Plate 8**). Uncomplicated hyalinosis is characterized by almost complete degeneration of vascular smooth muscle cells (becoming acellular) with concentric accumulation of extracellular matrix components like the collagens and fibroblasts (Lammie, 2000). These changes are most common in the small vasculature of the WM (**See p6 of the plate section for Plate 8**). Small vessel changes likely

promote occlusion or progressive stenosis with consequent acute or chronic ischaemia of the tissue behind it. Alternatively, arteriosclerotic changes located in small vessels in the deep WM and basal ganglia may lose their elasticity to dilate and constrict in response to variations of systemic blood pressure or loss of autoregulation. This, in turn, causes fluctuations in blood flow response and changes in cerebral perfusion. The deep cerebral structures would be rendered most vulnerable because the vessels are end arteries almost devoid of anastomoses. Small vessel pathology could lead also to oedema and damage of the blood–brain barrier (BBB) with chronic leakage of fluid and macromolecules in the WM (Ho and Garcia, 2000). Microvascular disease may also be associated with degrees of inflammation, including the presence of lymphocytes or macrophages centred on blood vessels (and not necessarily a function of brain ischaemia). In the older cases, there may also be evidence of remote haemorrhage in the form of perivascular hemosiderin (Kalaria *et al.*, 2004).

62.5.3   Microinfarction, lacunar infarcts and lacunes

Microinfarcts have been variably described, but widely thought to be small ischaemic lesions visible only upon light microscopy (**See p6 of the plate section for Plate 8**). These lesions of up to 5 mm diameter may or may not involve a small vessel at its centre, but are foci with pallor, neuronal loss, axonal damage (WM) and gliosis. Sometimes, these may include regions of incomplete infarction or rarefied (subacute) change. Microinfarcts have also been described as attenuated lesions of indistinct nature occurring in both cortical or subcortical regions. Such lesions, or combinations of these, should be reported when there are multiple or at least greater than three present in any region (**Table 62.1**). Microinfarcts and lacunar infarcts appear central to the most common cause of VaD and predict poor outcome in the elderly (Ballard *et al.*, 2000; Vinters *et al.*, 2000; White *et al.*, 2002). Interestingly, in the autopsied older Japanese–American men, the importance of microvascular lesions as a likely explanation for dementia was nearly equal to that of Alzheimer lesions (White *et al.*, 2002). Microinfarction in the subcortical structures has been emphasized as substrate of cognitive impairment, and correlated with increased Alzheimer type of pathology, but cortical microinfarcts also appear to contribute significantly to the progression of cognitive deficits in brain ageing (Kovari *et al.*, 2004). Furthermore, microinfarcts even in borderzone (watershed) regions may aggravate the degenerative process as indicated by worsening impairment in AD (Suter *et al.*, 2002). Thus, multiple microinfarction appears strongly correlated with dementia indicated by several studies (Jellinger, 2008a).

Lacunes are complete or cavitating infarcts as defined above, measuring up to 15 mm in diameter seen radiologically and upon gross examination at autopsy (**Box 62.2, See p6 of the plate section for Plate 8**). These lesions are largely confined to the cerebral WM and subcortical structures, including the thalamus, basic ganglia and brainstem. Most lacunes, remnants of small infarcts, are detected in the cystic or chronic stage with no viable central tissue, but could have perifocal regions with incomplete infarction, particularly in the WM. A few lacunes may represent healed or reabsorbed as minute or petechial haemorrhages. Microlacunes have also been described which essentially should be thought of as large cystic microinfarcts. To distinguish perivascular cavities or spaces, it has been suggested that lacunes be classed into three subtypes: lacunar infarcts, lacunar haemorrhages and dilated perivascular spaces (Yamamoto et al., 2009). Lacunar infarcts usually result from progressive SVD manifested as hypertensive angiopathy that may involve stenosis caused by hyalinosis. SVD in a perforating artery for example, may also reveal regions of incomplete infarction, attenuation or rarefaction usually recognized by pallor upon microscopic examination. However, lacunar lesions can also be caused by infections and neoplasms. Lacunes are often associated with small perivascular cavities up to 2 mm in diameter often found in the basal ganglia and the WM. Perivascular spaces or cribriform change (non-infarctive) resulting from distortion or elongation of small arteries, collectively referred to as état lacunaire in the grey matter and état crible in the WM, accompanied by severe myelin loss may be numerous in older subjects.

62.5.4   Cortical microinfarcts

Besides microinfarction in the subcortical structures attributed to SVD, it is becoming increasingly apparent that cortical microinfarcts should be taken into account when defining the neuropathological criteria for VaD or VCI. This is an important substrate in the presence of cerebral amyloid angiopathy (CAA). In a recent study, cortical microinfarcts in watershed regions were frequently detected in AD and associated with CAA, but rarely observed in subcortical VaD linked to SVD (Suter et al., 2002; Okamoto et al., 2009). Microinfarcts in the cerebral cortex associated with severe CAA (**See p6 of the plate section for Plate 8**) may be the primary pathological substrate in a significant proportion of VaD cases (Haglund et al., 2006). Cortical microinfarcts and, to a lesser extent, periventricular demyelination were significantly associated with cognitive decline in individuals at high risk for dementia (Gold et al., 2007). It is proposed that the changes in haemodynamics, e.g. hypotensions, plays a role in the genesis of cortical watershed microinfarcts.

62.5.5   White matter disease

White matter lesions (or subcortical leukoencephalopathy) incorporating myelin loss are considered a consequence of vascular disease (**See p7 of the plate section for Plate 9**). The frequency of WM changes is increased in patients with cerebrovascular disease (Ihara et al., 2010) and those at risk for vascular disease, including arterial hypertension, cardiovascular disease and diabetes mellitus (O'Brien et al., 2003). WM lesions occur in approximately 30 per cent of AD and dementia with Lewy bodies (DLB) cases and may be present irrespective of the focal lesions in VaD (Englund, 1998). It is argued that WM damage in patients with AD might simply

reflect Wallerian changes secondary to cortical loss of neurones. However, this is unlikely since histological changes characteristic of Wallerian degeneration are not evident as WM pallor. Conversely, in AD patients with severe loss of cortical neurones, similar WM lesions are not apparent (Englund, 1998).

Lesions in the deep WM (0.5–1 cm away from ventricle in coronal plane) have been correlated with dementia, including VaD (Kalaria and Ballard, 1999; Pantoni, 2002). Conflicting observations with respect to periventricular lesions may depend on definition of the boundaries between the periventricular and deep WM if the coursing of the fibres are used as markers (Kovari et al., 2007). Lacunar infarcts are produced when the ischaemic damage is focal and of sufficient severity to result in a small area of necrosis, whereas diffuse WM change is considered a form of rarefaction or incomplete infarction where there may be selective damage to some cellular components. Although the U-fibres are often spared (**See p7 of the plate section for Plate 9**), WM disease may comprise several patterns of alterations, including pallor or swelling of myelin, loss of oligodendrocytes, axons and myelin fibres, cavitations with or without presence of macrophages and areas of reactive astrogliosis, where the astrocytic cytoplasm and cell processes may be visible with standard stains. Lesions in the WM also include spongiosis, i.e. vacuolization of the WM structures and widening of the perivascular spaces (Yamamoto et al., 2009). Evidence of periventricular venous collagenosis has also be reported in cases with severe WM changes. Vascular stenosis caused by collagenosis may induce chronic ischaemia or oedema in the deep WM leading to capillary loss and more widespread effects on the brain (Brown et al., 2007; Brown et al., 2009).

62.5.6   Hippocampal atrophy and sclerosis

Hippocampal neurones in the Sommer's sector are highly vulnerable to disturbances in the cerebral circulation or hypoxia caused by systemic or cardiovascular disease. The presence of focal microinfarcts and scars versus diffuse or segmental (CA1, prosubiculum) neurone loss and astrocytic gliosis may vary. Sometimes, the patchy neurone loss and gliosis in a heavily 'Alzheimerized' brain may be difficult or impossible to distinguish from anoxic–ischaemic change. Hippocampal injury resembling hippocampal sclerosis has also been reported in autopsy brain specimens from individuals with frontotemporal dementia, especially the variant associated with motor neurone disease. Severe loss of hippocampal neurones within the CA fields and infarctions along Ammon's horn are evident in a proportion (10–20 per cent) of usually older (>80 years) VaD cases. The loss of cells should be graded when this is evident together with any microinfarctions within the hippocampal formation (Dickson et al., 1994). Hippocampal sclerosis is a likely major contributing factor in the hippocampal atrophy described at gross examination. Hippocampal changes remote to ischaemic injury have also been emphasized in subcortical ischaemic VaD (Vinters et al., 2000). It was also noted that in ischaemic VaD and AD, the loss of CA1 neurones was related to lower hippocampal volume derived by magnetic resonance imaging (MRI) and memory score (Zarow *et al.*, 2005).

62.5.7 Borderzone (watershed) infarcts and incomplete ischaemic injury

The borderzone or watershed infarctions mostly occur from haemodynamic events, usually in patients with severe internal carotid artery stenosis. They could occur bilaterally or unilaterally, and disposed to regions between two main arterial territories, deep and superficial vessel systems. Typical borderzone infarctions may be 5 mm or more wide as wedge-shaped regions of pallor and rarefaction extending into the WM. Larger areas of incomplete infarction may extend into the WM (Hachinski *et al.*, 2006; Ferrer *et al.*, 2008). These are characterized by mild to moderate loss of oligodendrocytes, myelin and axons in areas where there may be hyalinized vessels (Brun, 1994). These features may be accompanied by astrogliosis, some microgliosis and macrophage infiltration. The morphology of incomplete or subinfarctive changes, though suspected to be of clinical importance, is not uniformly described in VaD. It may variably manifest as tissue rarefaction assessed by conventional stains and revealed as injury response, such as microgliosis and astrocytosis, or the presence of other 'reactive' cells or surrogate markers of dendritic, synaptic or axonal damage (Hachinski *et al.*, 2006).

62.5.8 Laminar necrosis

Laminar necrosis is characterized by neuronal ischaemic changes leading to neuronal loss and gliosis in the cortical ribbon. This is particularly apparent in cases where global ischaemia or hypoperfusion has occurred as in cardiac arrest. Typical topographic distribution of spongey form change can be readily apparent with standard stains. They appear more commonly at the arterial border zones (Brun, 1994; Ferrer *et al.*, 2008) that may fall into the subtype IV of VaD pathology (**Table 62.2**).

62.5.9 Cerebral amyloid angiopathy

Cerebral amyloid angiopathy is most common in AD and consistently present in Down syndrome (Premkumar *et al.*, 1996). However, it also occurs in elderly subjects with cerebrovascular disease in the general absence of parenchymal Alzheimer lesions (Cohen *et al.*, 1997). The prevalence of CAA in VaD is not known, but it is an important cause of intracerebral and lobar haemorrhages leading to profound ischaemic damage (Vonsattel *et al.*, 1991). CAA appears also to be causally related to WM changes described by subcortical leukoencephalopathy in patients with CAA, who lacked changes characteristic of AD (Lammie, 2000). Several familial forms of CAA involving ischaemic and haemorrhagic infarcts and cerebral hypoperfusion (Kalaria, 2001) demonstrate the link between CAA and VaD. It is thought that the first stroke-like episode triggers multiple cerebral bleeds which may be preceded by diffuse WM changes that in turn lead to rapid

decline of cognitive functions (Vinters, 1987; Natte *et al.*, 2001; Greenberg, 2002). Amyloid β protein accumulation within or juxtaposed to the vasculature may lead to degeneration of vascular cells in both larger perforating arterial vessels, as well as cerebral capillaries that represent the BBB. These likely lead to vascular dysfunction and cause cortical microinfarctions (Haglund *et al.*, 2006; Okamoto *et al.*, 2009) and perivascular cavities similar to those seen in hyalinized vessels in subcortical structures. Genetic factors, such as the *APOE* ε4 allele associated with severity of CAA may modify or attenuate the perfusion of the WM (Kalaria, 2001).

62.5.10 Alzheimer type of pathology

Alzheimer lesions, including amyloid β plaques and neurofibrillary pathology, occur more often in cases of cerebrovascular disease than normal ageing elderly (Kalaria and Ballard, 1999). Moreover, amyloid deposits and tangles are three times greater in VaD cases with small (<15 mL) compared to larger volume of infarction (Ballard *et al.*, 2000). These findings also corroborate the importance of microvascular disease rather than large vessel disease as the critical substrate in VaD, and in AD (Kalaria, 1996). Recent reports suggest that although conventional histopathology may not reveal the presence of classical Alzheimer type of pathology, tissue accumulation of soluble amyloid β and tau peptides in VaD subjects, revealed by immunochemical methods, may reach up to that in AD by the eighth decade (Lewis *et al.*, 2006). These observations also imply that amyloid β peptides also increase in the brains of patients who succumb to cerebral ischaemia compared to normal elderly free of cerebrovascular disease. The amyloid precursor protein has also been reported to accumulate along WM tracts during cerebral ischaemia in middle-aged subjects (Cochran *et al.*, 1991) and in VaD (Ihara *et al.*, 2010). It is plausible that SVD, along with WM lesions in the brain, causes vascular injury which induces tissue pH changes, oxidative damage, amyloid precursor protein expression and subsequent aggregation of soluble amyloid β. A similar scenario may occur to induce tau-like pathology and related neuronal changes. This is supported by the demonstration that increases in cerebrospinal fluid (CSF) tau are not restricted to AD, but also evident in various forms of VaD (Blennow *et al.*, 1995; Munroe *et al.*, 1995; Skoog *et al.*, 1995). Concentrations of tau in lumbar CSF in patients diagnosed with probable VaD were reported to be comparable to those in AD and were significantly increased compared to those in non-demented elderly controls (Skoog *et al.*, 1995). Similarly, the concentrations of soluble synaptophysin were found to be decreased in VaD, as well as in AD (Zhan *et al.*, 1994). These findings provide evidence for axonal degeneration in VaD as evident in AD, but support the notion that ischaemic or oligaemic events in the elderly are early events leading to increases in known markers of Alzheimer pathology. Other biological markers for AD, such as decreased apolipoprotein E (ApoE) levels in CSF, have also been reported in VaD (Skoog *et al.*, 1997).

Selective transmitter-specific changes have also been described in VaD in some cases different from those found in

AD (Kalaria and Ballard, 1999). Two different groups had previously shown that compared to AD patients, choline acetyltransferase activity was also reduced, albeit to a lesser degree in the temporal cortex and hippocampus in patients diagnosed with multi-infarct dementia or VaD (Perry *et al.*, 1977; Gottfries *et al.*, 1994). However, our recent work showed loss of cholinergic function was only evident in VaD patients with concurrent AD. Conversely, a novel increase in cholinergic activity was identified in patients with infarct dementia (Sharp *et al.*, 2009). Despite these deficits, there do not appear to be pronounced effects in the cholinergic cell bodies of the basal forebrain in VaD (Mann *et al.*, 1986; Keverne *et al.*, 2007). Subsequent studies had reported deficits in monoamines including 5-hydroxytryptamine (5HT) in the basal ganglia and neocortex of VaD subjects (Gottfries *et al.*, 1994). Our new study (Elliott *et al.*, 2009) revealed that 5-HT(1A) and 5-HT(2A) receptors were significantly increased in the temporal cortex of patients with either multi-infarct VaD, but not subcortical VaD compared to controls. These findings reveal an important distinction between the neurochemical pathology of VaD subtypes and suggest pharmacological manipulation of serotonin offers the possibility to develop novel therapies for VaD patients. Thus, there appear similarities and differences in Alzheimer type of changes associated with VaD. The pathological diagnosis of VaD in such cases may be dictated by the degree and location of Alzheimer pathology (**Table 62.2**). If it is restricted to the hippocampus and the density of neuritic plaques or tangles does not exceed stage III of recent criteria (Thal *et al.*, 2002) and Braak (Braak and Braak, 1995), they could be diagnosed as VaD analogous to the probable AD cases exhibiting infarctions or WM changes as defined by CERAD criteria.

62.6 CLINICAL AND PATHOLOGICAL FEATURES OF FAMILIAL SVD AS MODELS OF VAD

Early reports suggest the existence of several familial stroke disorders unrelated to atherosclerotic disease (**Box 62.1**). Most of these disorders may be classed as SVD involving small vessels of the subcortical structures (Kalimo *et al.*, 2002) in view of the striking pathology (**See p6–7 of the plate section for Plates 8 and 9**), including multiple subcortical infarcts, SVD, severe arteriosclerosis, profound WM rarefaction. Cerebral autosomal dominant arteriopathy with subcortical infarcts and leukoencephalopathy (CADASIL) appears the most common form of hereditary SVDs leading to cognitive decline and dementia (Chabriat *et al.*, 1995; Dichgans *et al.*, 1998; Opherk *et al.*, 2004). CADASIL has also been considered a familial form of Binswanger's disease. CADASIL may be manifest well before the first stroke on the basis of characteristic WM hyperintensities upon MRI (Chabriat *et al.*, 1998; Singhal *et al.*, 2004). The key VaD-associated manifestations include transient ischaemic attacks and recurrent subcortical strokes. Motor deficits, an ataxic hemiparesis, hemianopsia and dysarthria may accompany these principal events. Neocortical strokes are rare and they usually do not cover a wide territory (Chabriat *et al.*, 1998).

Large artery infarcts, such as those of the middle or posterior cerebral artery, are uncommon.

Pathological features include severe arteriopathy with the presence of granular osmiophilic material in the arterial walls of both the brain and systemic organs (Lesnik Oberstein *et al.*, 2001). Loss of brain vascular smooth muscle cells leads to wall thickening and fibrosis in small- and medium-sized penetrating arteries. This would reduce both cerebral blood flow and blood volume in affected WM with effects on the haemodynamic reserve by decreasing the vasodilatory response. Affected vessels presumably progress to obliteration or thrombose as evident by the appearance of lacunar infarcts, mainly in the basal ganglia and frontotemporal WM (Lesnik Oberstein *et al.*, 2001). These pathologies initiate cognitive deficits, which progress to dementia of the subcortical vascular type.

Several CADASIL-like disorders not linked to the *NOTCH3* gene have been reported (Sourander and Walinder, 1977). The Maeda syndrome or cerebral autosomal recessive arteriopathy with subcortical infarcts and leukoencephalopathy (CARASIL) is an autosomal recessive disorder similar to CADASIL, described in Japan (Oide *et al.*, 2008). The normotensive affected subjects exhibit not only severe arteriopathy, leukoencephalopathy and lacunar infarcts, but also spinal anomalies and alopecia. Strokes lead to stepwise deterioration with most subjects becoming demented in older age. CARASIL is associated with mutations in the HtrA serine protease 1 (*HTRA1*) gene link between repressed inhibition of signalling by the TGF-beta family (Hara *et al.*, 2009).

SVDs of the brain may also involve progressive visual impairment (Kalimo and Kalaria, 2005). hereditary endotheliopathy with retinopathy, nephropathy and stroke (HERNS), cerebroretinal vasculopathy (CRV) and hereditary vascular retinopathy (HVR) were reported independently, but represent different phenotypes in the same disease spectrum (Jen *et al.*, 1997; Terwindt *et al.*, 1998; Ophoff *et al.*, 2001). They are now described as autosomal dominant retinal vasculopathy with cerebral leukodystrophy (RVCL). RVCL group of SVDs are caused by C-terminal truncations in human *TREX1* gene, encoding DNA-specific 3′–5′ exonuclease DNA III. Renal disease appears to be restricted to HERNS and CRV, whereas HVR is associated with Raynaud phenomenon. The retinopathy involves capillary tortuosity, aneurysms and teleangiectasias that begin in the third and fourth decades with increasing migraine-like episodes. Neurological complications of CRV and HERNS usually lead to death before the age of 55 years, whereas HVR patients live longer.

Cerebral SVD has also been described in association with pseudoxanthoma elasticum, a hereditary connective tissue disorder with abnormalities in the skin and eye and multiple lacunar infarcts in deep WM and pons (Pavlovic *et al.*, 2005). The disease trait cosegregates with mutations in the ATP-binding cassette transporter gene, ABCC6 located on chromosome 16p13.1. Other recently uncovered SVDs include hereditary infantile hemiparesis, retinal arteriolar tortuosity and leukoencephalopathy (Vahedi *et al.*, 2003; Gould *et al.*, 2006) and a novel autosomal dominant SVD of the brain in a large Portuguese–French family. Chabriat and colleagues (Verreault *et al.*, 2006) reported that this SVD was not fully penetrant and distinguished by motor hemiplegia, memory deficits, executive dysfunction and WM changes upon MRI in the general absence of vascular risk.

62.7 CONCLUSIONS

The heterogeneous nature of cerebrovascular disease compels better understanding of the neuropathological substrates of VaD for wide application. The systematic classification of VaD subtypes relies on uniformity in sampling and neuropathological examination. SVD, leading to multiple microinfarcts, small infarcts or lacunes in the subcortical structures, rather than macroinfarction or large vessel disease, appear most robustly related to cognitive impairment in cerebrovascular disease. Diffuse WM changes involving periventricular and deeper regions are frequent in VaD, but need rigorous evaluation to enable correlation with cognitive decline. Concomitant hippocampal pathology including sclerosis and Alzheimer pathology compound disease progression. Further definitions of the neuropathological correlates of VaD and investigation of genetic models would be valuable for exploring the pathogenesis as well as management of VaD through preventative and treatment strategies.

REFERENCES

Akatsu H, Takahashi M, Matsukawa N et al. (2002) Subtype analysis of neuropathologically diagnosed patients in a Japanese geriatric hospital. Journal of Neurological Sciences 196: 63–9.

Ballard C, McKeith I, O'Brien J et al. (2000) Neuropathological substrates of dementia and depression in vascular dementia, with a particular focus on cases with small infarct volumes. Dementia and Geriatric Cognitive Disorders 11: 59–65.

Ballard CG, Burton EJ, Barber R et al. (2004) NINDS AIREN neuroimaging criteria do not distinguish stroke patients with and without dementia. Neurology 63: 983–8.

Berrios GE, Freeman HL. (1991) Alzheimer and the dementias. In: Berrios GE (ed.). Eponymists in medicine series. London: Royal Society of Medicine Services, 69–76.

Blennow K, Wallin A, Agren H et al. (1995) Tau protein in cerebrospinal fluid: a biochemical marker for axonal degeneration in Alzheimer disease? Molecular and Chemical Neuropathology 26: 231–45.

Braak H, Braak E. (1995) Staging of Alzheimer's disease-related neurofibrillary changes. Neurobiology of Aging 16: 271–8; discussion 278–84.

Brown WR, Moody DM, Challa VR et al. (2002) Venous collagenosis and arteriolar tortuosity in leukoaraiosis. Journal of Neurological Sciences 203: 159–63.

Brown WR, Moody DM, Thore CR et al. (2009) Microvascular changes in the white mater in dementia. Journal of the Neurological Sciences 283: 28–31.

Brown WR, Moody DM, Thore CR et al. (2007) Vascular dementia in leukoaraiosis may be a consequence of capillary loss not only in the lesions, but in normal-appearing white matter and cortex as well. Journal of the Neurological Sciences 257: 62–6.

Brun A. (1994) Pathology and pathophysiology of cerebrovascular dementia: pure subgroups of obstructive and hypoperfusive etiology. Dementia 5: 145–7.

CFAS. (2001) Pathological correlates of late-onset dementia in a multicentre, community-based population in England and Wales. Neuropathology Group of the Medical Research Council Cognitive Function and Ageing Study (MRC CFAS). Lancet 357: 169–75.

Chabriat H, Levy C, Taillia H et al. (1998) Patterns of MRI lesions in CADASIL. Neurology 51: 452–7.

Chabriat H, Vahedi K, Iba-Zizen MT et al. (1995) Clinical spectrum of CADASIL: a study of 7 families. Cerebral autosomal dominant arteriopathy with subcortical infarcts and leukoencephalopathy. Lancet 346: 934–9.

Cochran E, Bacci B, Chen Y et al. (1991) Amyloid precursor protein and ubiquitin immunoreactivity in dystrophic axons is not unique to Alzheimer's disease. American Journal of Pathology 139: 485–9.

Cohen DL, Hedera P, Premkumar DR et al. (1997) Amyloid-beta protein angiopathies masquerading as Alzheimer's disease? Annals of the New York Academy of Sciences 826: 390–5.

Dichgans M, Mayer M, Uttner I et al. (1998) The phenotypic spectrum of CADASIL: clinical findings in 102 cases. Annals of Neurology 44: 731–9.

Dickson DW, Davies P, Bevona C et al. (1994) Hippocampal sclerosis: a common pathological feature of dementia in very old (> or =80 years of age) humans. Acta Neuropathologica 88: 212–21.

Elliott MS, Ballard CG, Kalaria RN et al. (2009) Increased binding to 5-HT1A and 5-HT2A receptors is associated with large vessel infarction and relative preservation of cognition. Brain 132: 1858–65.

Englund E. (1998) Neuropathology of white matter changes in Alzheimer's disease and vascular dementia. Dementia and Geriatric Cognitive Disorders 9 (Suppl. 1): 6–12.

Erkinjuntti T, Haltia M, Palo J et al. (1988) Accuracy of the clinical diagnosis of vascular dementia: a prospective clinical and post-mortem neuropathological study. Journal of Neurology, Neurosurgery and Psychiatry 51: 1037–44.

Esiri MM, Nagy Z, Smith MZ et al. (1999) Cerebrovascular disease and threshold for dementia in the early stages of Alzheimer's disease. Lancet 354: 919–20.

Esiri MM, Wilcock GK, Morris JH. (1997) Neuropathological assessment of the lesions of significance in vascular dementia. Journal of Neurology, Neurosurgery and Psychiatry 63: 749–53.

Ferrer I, Kaste M, Kalimo H. (2008) Vascular diseases. In: Love S, Louis D, Ellison D (eds). Greenfield's neuropathology, 8th edn. Oxford: Oxford University Press, 121–240.

Gold G, Bouras C, Canuto A et al. (2002) Clinicopathological validation study of four sets of clinical criteria for vascular dementia. American Journal of Psychiatry 159: 82–7.

Gold G, Giannakopoulos P, Herrmann FR et al. (2007) Identification of Alzheimer and vascular lesion thresholds for mixed dementia. Brain 130: 2830–6.

Gold G, Giannakopoulos P, Montes-Paixao Junior C et al. (1997) Sensitivity and specificity of newly proposed clinical criteria for possible vascular dementia. Neurology 49: 690–4.

Gottfries CG, Blennow K, Karlsson I, Wallin A. (1994) The neurochemistry of vascular dementia. Dementia 5: 163–7.

Gould DB, Phalan FC, van Mil SE et al. (2006) Role of COL4A1 in small-vessel disease and hemorrhagic stroke. New England Journal of Medicine 354: 1489–96.

Greenberg SM. (2002) Cerebral amyloid angiopathy and vessel dysfunction. Cerebrovascular Diseases 13 (Suppl. 2): 42–7.

Hachinski V, Iadecola C, Petersen RC et al. (2006) National Institute of Neurological Disorders and Stroke–Canadian Stroke Network. Vascular cognitive impairment harmonization standards. Stroke 37: 2220–41.

Haglund M, Passant U, Sjobeck M et al. (2006) Cerebral amyloid angiopathy and cortical microinfarcts as putative substrates of vascular dementia. International Journal of Geriatric Psychiatry 21: 681–7.

Hara K, Shiga A, Fukutake T et al. (2009) Association of HTRA1 mutations and familial ischemic cerebral small-vessel disease. New England Journal of Medicine 360: 1729–39.

Heyman A, Fillenbaum GG, Welsh-Bohmer KA et al. (1998) Cerebral infarcts in patients with autopsy-proven Alzheimer's disease: CERAD, part XVIII. Consortium to Establish a Registry for Alzheimer's Disease. Neurology 51: 159–62.

Ho KL, Garcia JH. (2000) Neuropathology of the small blood vessels in selected disease of the cerebral white matter. In: Pantoni L, Inzitari D, Wallin A (eds). The matter of white matter. Current Issues in Neurodegenerative diseases. Utrecht: Academic Pharmaceutical Productions, 247–73.

Hulette C, Nochlin D, McKeel D et al. (1997) Clinical-neuropathologic findings in multi-infarct dementia: a report of six autopsied cases. Neurology 48: 668–72.

Ihara M, Polvikoski TM, Hall R et al. (2010) Quantification of myelin loss in frontal lobe white matter in vascular dementia, Alzheimer's disease, and dementia with Lewy bodies. Acta Neuropathologica 119: 579–89.

Jellinger KA. (2008a) Morphologic diagnosis of 'vascular dementia' – a critical update. Journal of the Neurological Sciences 270: 1–12.

Jellinger KA. (2008b) The pathology of 'vascular dementia': a critical update. Journal of Alzheimer's Disease 14: 107–23.

Jen J, Cohen AH, Yue Q et al. (1997) Hereditary endotheliopathy with retinopathy, nephropathy, and stroke (HERNS). Neurology 49: 1322–30.

Kalaria RN. (1996) Cerebral vessels in ageing and Alzheimer's disease. Pharmacology and Therapeutics 72: 193–214.

Kalaria RN. (2001) Advances in molecular genetics and pathology of cerebrovascular disorders. Trends in Neurosciences 24: 392–400.

Kalaria RN, Ballard C. (1999) Overlap between pathology of Alzheimer disease and vascular dementia. Alzheimer Disease and Associated Disorders 13 (Suppl. 3): S115–123.

Kalaria RN, Kenny RA, Ballard CG et al. (2004) Towards defining the neuropathological substrates of vascular dementia. Journal of the Neurological Sciences 226: 75–80.

Kalimo H, Kalaria RN. (2005) Hereditary forms of vascular dementia. In: Kalimo H (ed.). Cerebrovascular diseases, pathology and genetics. Basel: Neuropath Press, 324–84.

Kalimo H, Ruchoux MM, Viitanen M, Kalaria RN. (2002) CADASIL: a common form of hereditary arteriopathy causing brain infarcts and dementia. Brain Pathology 12: 371–84.

Kavanagh D, Spitzer D, Kothari PH et al. (2008) New roles for the major human 3′–5′ exonuclease TREX1 in human disease. Cell Cycle 7: 1718–25.

Keverne JS, Low WC, Ziabreva I et al. (2007) Cholinergic neuronal deficits in CADASIL. Stroke 38: 188–91.

Kovari E, Gold G, Herrmann FR et al. (2007) Cortical microinfarcts and demyelination affect cognition in cases at high risk for dementia. Neurology 68: 927–31.

Kovari E, Gold G, Herrmann FR et al. (2004) Cortical microinfarcts and demyelination significantly affect cognition in brain aging. Stroke 35: 410–14.

Lammie GA. (2000) Pathology of small vessel stroke. British Medical Bulletin 56: 296–306.

Lesnik Oberstein SA, van den Boom R, van Buchem MA et al. (2001) Cerebral microbleeds in CADASIL. Neurology 57: 1066–70.

Lewis H, Beher D, Cookson N et al. (2006) Quantification of Alzheimer pathology in ageing and dementia: age-related accumulation of amyloid-beta(42) peptide in vascular dementia. Neuropathology and Applied Neurobiology 32: 103–18.

Mann DM, Yates PO, Marcyniuk B. (1986) The nucleus basalis of Meynert in multi-infarct (vascular) dementia. Acta Neuropathologica 71: 332–7.

Markesbery W. (1998) Vascular dementia. In: Markesbery WR (ed.). Neuropathology of dementing disorders. London: Arnold, 293–311.

Mirra SS. (1997) The CERAD neuropathology protocol and consensus recommendations for the postmortem diagnosis of Alzheimer's disease: a commentary. Neurobiology of Aging 18: S91–4.

Munroe WA, Southwick PC, Chang L et al. (1995) Tau protein in cerebrospinal fluid as an aid in the diagnosis of Alzheimer's disease. Annals of Clinical and Laboratory Science 25: 207–17.

Nagy Z, Esiri MM, Joachim C et al. (1998) Comparison of pathological diagnostic criteria for Alzheimer disease. Alzheimer Disease and Associated Disorders 12: 182–9.

Natte R, Maat-Schieman ML, Haan J et al. (2001) Dementia in hereditary cerebral hemorrhage with amyloidosis-Dutch type is associated with cerebral amyloid angiopathy but is independent of plaques and neurofibrillary tangles. Annals of Neurology 50: 765–72.

Nolan KA, Lino MM, Seligmann AW, Blass JP. (1998) Absence of vascular dementia in an autopsy series from a dementia clinic. Journal of the American Geriatrics Society 46: 597–604.

O'Brien JT, Erkinjuntti T, Reisberg B et al. (2003) Vascular cognitive impairment. Lancet Neurology 2: 89–98.

Oide T, Nakayama H, Yanagawa S et al. (2008) Extensive loss of arterial medial smooth muscle cells and mural extracellular matrix in cerebral autosomal recessive arteriopathy with subcortical infarcts and leukoencephalopathy (CARASIL). Neuropathology 28: 132–42.

Okamoto Y, Ihara M, Fujita Y *et al.* (2009) Cortical microinfarcts in Alzheimer's disease and subcortical vascular dementia. *Neuroreport* **20**: 990–6.

Opherk C, Peters N, Herzog J *et al.* (2004) Long-term prognosis and causes of death in CADASIL: a retrospective study in 411 patients. *Brain* **127**: 2533–9.

Ophoff RA, DeYoung J, Service SK *et al.* (2001) Hereditary vascular retinopathy, cerebroretinal vasculopathy, and hereditary endotheliopathy with retinopathy, nephropathy, and stroke map to a single locus on chromosome 3p21.1-p21.3. *American Journal of Human Genetics* **69**: 447–53.

Pantoni L. (2002) Pathophysiology of age-related cerebral white matter changes. *Cerebrovascular Diseases* **13** (Suppl. 2): 7–10.

Pantoni L, Sarti C, Alafuzoff I *et al.* (2006) Postmortem examination of vascular lesions in cognitive impairment: a survey among neuropathological services. *Stroke* **37**: 1005–9.

Pavlovic AM, Zidverc-Trajkovic I, Milovic MM *et al.* (2005) Cerebral small vessel disease in pseudoxanthoma elasticum: three cases. *Canadian Journal of the Neurological Sciences* **32**: 115–18.

Perry EK, Gibson PH, Blessed G *et al.* (1977) Neurotransmitter enzyme abnormalities in senile dementia. Choline acetyltransferase and glutamic acid decarboxylase activities in necropsy brain tissue. *Journal of the Neurological Sciences* **34**: 247–65.

Premkumar DR, Cohen DL, Hedera P *et al.* (1996) Apolipoprotein E-epsilon4 alleles in cerebral amyloid angiopathy and cerebrovascular pathology associated with Alzheimer's disease. *American Journal of Pathology* **148**: 2083–95.

Román GC. (2002) Vascular dementia revisited: diagnosis, pathogenesis, treatment, and prevention. *Medical Clinics of North America* **86**: 477–99.

Román GC, Tatemichi TK, Erkinjuntti T *et al.* (1993) Vascular dementia: diagnostic criteria for research studies. Report of the NINDS-AIREN International Workshop. *Neurology* **43**: 250–60.

Rosen WG, Terry RD, Fuld PA *et al.* (1980) Pathological verification of ischemic score in differentiation of dementias. *Annals of Neurology* **7**: 486–8.

Rossi R, Joachim C, Geroldi C *et al.* (2004) Association between subcortical vascular disease on CT and neuropathological findings. *International Journal of Geriatric Psychiatry* **19**: 690–5.

Seno H, Ishino H, Inagaki T *et al.* (1999) A neuropathological study of dementia in nursing homes over a 17-year period, in Shimane Prefecture, Japan. *Gerontology* **45**: 44–8.

Sharp SI, Francis PT, Elliott MS *et al.* (2009) Choline acetyltransferase activity in vascular dementia and stroke. *Dementia and Geriatric Cognitive Disorders* **28**: 233–8.

Singhal S, Bevan S, Barrick T *et al.* (2004) The influence of genetic and cardiovascular risk factors on the CADASIL phenotype. *Brain* **127**: 2031–8.

Skoog I, Hesse C, Fredman P *et al.* (1997) Apolipoprotein E in cerebrospinal fluid in 85-year-old subjects. Relation to dementia, apolipoprotein E polymorphism, cerebral atrophy, and white matter lesions. *Archives of Neurology* **54**: 267–72.

Skoog I, Vanmechelen E, Andreasson LA *et al.* (1995) A population-based study of tau protein and ubiquitin in cerebrospinal fluid in 85-year-olds: relation to severity of dementia and cerebral atrophy, but not to the apolipoprotein E4 allele. *Neurodegeneration* **4**: 433–42.

Snowdon DA, Greiner LH, Mortimer JA *et al.* (1997) Brain infarction and the clinical expression of Alzheimer disease. The Nun Study. *Journal of the American Medical Association* **277**: 813–17.

Sourander P, Walinder J. (1977) Hereditary multi-infarct dementia. Morphological and clinical studies of a new disease. *Acta Neuropathologica* **39**: 247–54.

Suter OC, Sunthorn T, Kraftsik R *et al.* (2002) Cerebral hypoperfusion generates cortical watershed microinfarcts in Alzheimer disease. *Stroke* **33**: 1986–92.

Terwindt GM, Haan J, Ophoff RA *et al.* (1998) Clinical and genetic analysis of a large Dutch family with autosomal dominant vascular retinopathy, migraine and Raynaud's phenomenon. *Brain* **121**: 303–16.

Thal DR, Rub U, Orantes M, Braak H. (2002) Phases of A beta-deposition in the human brain and its relevance for the development of AD. *Neurology* **58**: 1791–800.

Tomlinson BE, Blessed G, Roth M. (1970) Observations on the brains of demented old people. *Journal of the Neurological Sciences* **11**: 205–42.

Vahedi K, Massin P, Guichard JP *et al.* (2003) Hereditary infantile hemiparesis, retinal arteriolar tortuosity, and leukoencephalopathy. *Neurology* **60**: 57–63.

Verreault S, Joutel A, Riant F *et al.* (2006) A novel hereditary small vessel disease of the brain. *Annals of Neurology* **59**: 353–7.

Vinters HV. (1987) Cerebral amyloid angiopathy. A critical review. *Stroke* **18**: 311–24.

Vinters HV, Ellis WG, Zarow C *et al.* (2000) Neuropathologic substrates of ischemic vascular dementia. *Journal of Neuropathol and Experimental Neurology* **59**: 931–45.

Vonsattel JP, Myers RH, Hedley-Whyte ET *et al.* (1991) Cerebral amyloid angiopathy without and with cerebral hemorrhages: a comparative histological study. *Annals of Neurology* **30**: 637–49.

White L, Petrovitch H, Hardman J *et al.* (2002) Cerebrovascular pathology and dementia in autopsied Honolulu-Asia Aging Study participants. *Annals of the New York Academy of Sciences* **977**: 9–23.

Yamamoto Y, Ihara M, Tham C *et al.* (2009) Neuropathological correlates of temporal pole white matter hyperintensities in CADASIL. *Stroke* **40**: 2004–11.

Zarow C, Vinters HV, Ellis WG *et al.* (2005) Correlates of hippocampal neuron number in Alzheimer's disease and ischemic vascular dementia. *Annals of Neurology* **57**: 896–903.

Zhan SS, Beyreuther K, Schmitt HP. (1994) Synaptophysin immunoreactivity of the cortical neuropil in vascular dementia of Binswanger type compared with the dementia of Alzheimer type and nondemented controls. *Dementia* **5**: 79–87.

63

Therapeutic strategies for vascular dementia and vascular cognitive disorders

GUSTAVO C ROMÁN

63.1 INTRODUCTION

From many viewpoints, the most important advance in the field of dementia in the last decade has been the discovery of the critical contribution of vascular factors affecting the brain to the pathogenesis of Alzheimer's disease (AD) and other forms of dementia (see Chapter 60, Vascular factors and Alzheimer's disease). Population-based autopsy studies show that pure AD and pure cases of vascular dementia (VaD) appear to be uncommon in older demented subjects. In this age group, the neuropathology rule is the presence at autopsy of mixed dementia with a predominant vascular component (Zekry et al., 2002a). According to Matthews et al. (2009), the main attributable-risks at death for dementia are age (18 per cent), small brain (12 per cent), neocortical neuritic plaques (8 per cent) and neurofibrillary tangles (11 per cent), small vessel disease (12 per cent), multiple vascular pathologies (9 per cent), hippocampal atrophy (10 per cent), cerebral amyloid angiopathy (7 per cent) and Lewy bodies (3 per cent). This discovery explains some of the difficulties with criteria for VaD and offers hope for the treatment and prevention of late-life dementia, given the large armamentarium available for the treatment of vascular disease.

The therapeutic management of VaD is particularly challenging because of the multiple types of cerebrovascular injuries and circulatory events that may lead to vascular cognitive decline and eventual dementia. This multiplicity of pathogenetic mechanisms results in a variety of clinical presentations that have hampered the formulation of diagnostic

criteria and the ascertainment of cases for controlled clinical trials. By using strict clinical criteria combined with adequate brain imaging, it is feasible to diagnose and identify patients with clinically unmixed VaD. Subjects recruited for VaD trials disclose clinical features and progression patterns that are clearly different from those observed in populations selected for AD clinical trials.

Although formal modification of existing diagnostic criteria and a clear-cut definition of the role of imaging in VaD trials are still lacking, progress in brain imaging has contributed significantly to the selection of patients for clinical trials in VaD. The latest trial of donepezil in VaD (Román et al., 2010) found that enrolled patients who fulfilled NINDS-AIREN criteria for VaD, but presented evidence of hippocampal atrophy on brain magnetic resonance imaging (MRI), had different clinical progression and treatment response compared to those without atrophy. Also, brain imaging has clarified the pattern of atrophy resulting from normal and pathological ageing (Jagust et al., 2008; Raji et al., 2009), markers of brain amyloid load (Morris et al., 2009), and arterial spin-labelling (ASL) MRI to accurately measure regional cerebral blood flow (rCBF) (Dai et al., 2009), should increase diagnostic accuracy and provide objective end points for future clinical trials.

Moreover, VaD is often complicated by neuropsychiatric symptoms, in particular depression, apathy, aggressiveness and other behavioural changes that require careful management, but very few trials have addressed these issues. Other than symptomatic therapeutic trials, a limited number of studies have shown promise for the prevention of VaD (and AD), giving support to the concept that vigorous treatment of vascular risk factors in patients with early cognitive decline could spare the progression to dementia.

63.2 DEFINITIONS

63.2.1 Vascular cognitive disorder

Sachdev (1999) was the first to indicate the need for a categorical entity – a disorder – to include the large numbers of patients with dementia and cognitive decline of vascular aetiology and proposed the name 'vascular cognitive disorder' (VCD). The diagnostic category of VCD is the preferred umbrella term used here to include all forms of cognitive decline resulting from cerebrovascular disease (CVD) ranging from mild cognitive deficits to VaD (Sachdev, 1999; Román et al., 2004). VCD excludes isolated cognitive dysfunctions resulting from stroke, such as alterations of language (aphasia), intentional gesture (apraxia) or categorical recognition (agnosia), among others. VCD includes specific disease entities, such as syndromes and diseases characterized by cognitive impairment resulting from a cerebrovascular aetiology including post-stroke VaD, CADASIL, Binswanger disease, and AD plus CVD (AD+CVD). Regarding specific aetiologies of VCD, Mendez and Cummings (2003) collected more than 100 potential vascular causes of cognitive impairment and dementia. This conceptual clarification should facilitate epidemiological and pharmacological research in this domain.

63.2.2 Vascular cognitive impairment

A competing umbrella name for VCD is vascular cognitive impairment (VCI) (Bowler and Hachinski, 1995; Erkinjuntti and Gauthier, 2002; O'Brien et al., 2003; Hachinski et al., 2006). However, this term is plagued by inconsistencies (Román et al., 2004). The main problem with the name VCI is the misuse of the term 'impairment'. In medicine, this term, as well as 'disability' and 'handicap', must be used according to the recommendations of the system adopted by the World Health Organization (WHO). Therefore, 'impairment' cannot define a disease or a group of diseases (Román et al., 2004). Moreover, according to Korczyn (2010), VCI cannot be considered a disease, but neither is it a syndrome; and there is disagreement on the definition and limits of VCI ranging from 'the earliest deficit', or a VaD prodrome, to the 'brain at risk stage'.

Bowler and Hachinski (2002) affirmed that in VCI, 'vascular, refers to all causes of CVD, while cognitive impairment encompasses all levels of cognitive decline, from the earliest steps'. Sachdev (1999) pointed out that there is a major problem implicit in this definition of the diagnosis of VCI when the symptoms are subtle: when do cognitive deficits constitute 'impairment'? Is this a statistical concept based on normative data, or a demonstration of decline from an established or putative level in an individual, or indeed a demonstration of functional disability? The distinction between deficits, impairment and disability is quite important because each one has profound and different implications for the patient and the clinician. Sachdev (1999) concluded that although the emphasis on early or minimal dysfunction is laudable, the difficulties in establishing subtle deficits in these patients, who often have comorbid depression, anxiety and other emotional disturbances, should not be under-emphasized. He wrote, 'Clinical interest in subtle CVD runs the danger of becoming so inclusive in the elderly that it could become almost meaningless' (Sachdev, 1999). In addition, the assessment of post-stroke disability is heavily biased by physical and instrumental impairments, quite independently from cognitive dysfunction.

One option proposed by Román et al. (2004) for VCI, is that by analogy to mild cognitive impairment (MCI), considered the earliest manifestation of AD (Petersen et al., 1999) (see Chapter 44, Clinical characteristics of mild cognitive impairment), the definition of VCI could be restricted to vascular forms of cognitive impairment without dementia, also known as VCI-no dementia (VCI-ND). There are no accepted diagnostic criteria for VCI (Leblanc et al., 2006; Hachinski et al., 2006), but the Canadian Study on Health and Aging (2000) successfully implemented a restricted definition of VCI, excluding cases of dementia (i.e. VCI-ND). The Canadian definition and diagnostic criteria (see below under 63.3 Diagnostic criteria and methodology of clinical trials in VaD) could be utilized for future studies of VCI (Canadian Study on Health and Aging, 2000; Tuokko et al., 2001).

Although the use of the word 'dementia' remains highly controversial, nonetheless labelled the VCI-ND syndrome as 'type 2 dementia' to explicitly distinguish it from the neocortical (type 1) clinical syndrome of AD and related disorders. In the setting of ischaemic CVD, type 2 dementia is used to characterize a subset of cases with VCI-ND. Type 2 dementia is sometimes equated with dysexecutive MCI (Winblad et al., 2004). All these various nomenclatures emphasize the clinical absence of Alzheimer's-type dementia.

63.2.3 Vascular dementia

Román (Román, 2002a; Román, 2003a) defined VaD as an aetiological category of dementia characterized by acquired intellectual impairment, severe enough to interfere with social and personal independence, resulting from ischaemic or haemorrhagic stroke, as well as from ischaemic hypoperfusive brain injuries, affecting brain regions important for memory, cognition and behaviour. The most common neuropathological lesions capable of producing VaD are hypoperfusive and ischaemic (occlusive) vascular brain injuries (Brun, 1994; Vinters et al., 2000). These include:

- Hypoxic-hypoperfusion dementia: global anoxia, selective vulnerability, border-zone infarcts and periventricular incomplete white matter ischaemia;
- Ischaemic lesions involving large vessels: strategic single strokes, multi-infarct dementia (MID); small-vessel disease (cortical, subcortical and cortico-subcortical ischaemia), as well as venous occlusions.

63.3 DIAGNOSTIC CRITERIA AND METHODOLOGY OF CLINICAL TRIALS IN VAD

63.3.1 Vascular cognitive impairment

The Canadian Study on Health and Aging (2000) used the following criteria (Rockwood *et al.*, 2000; Ingles *et al.*, 2002) to classify subjects with VCI-ND:

*   The subject's cognitive impairment did not meet the DSM-IIIR criteria for dementia; these criteria require impairment of memory and other cognitive domain causing functional deficits.
*   Cognitive impairment was judged to have a vascular cause as based on the presence of signs of ischaemia/ infarction, e.g. sudden onset, stepwise progression, patchy cortical deficits on cognitive testing, other evidence of atherosclerosis, and a high Hachinski Ischaemic Score (HIS) (Hachinski *et al.*, 1975). Presence of vascular risk factors alone was insufficient for a VCI-ND diagnosis. Global functional impairment was defined as having difficulty in any two of the following domains: performing household chores, managing money, feeding self, dressing, and incontinence.

Using the above criteria in the Canadian cohort of 10 263 randomly selected people aged $\geq$ 65 years, 149 were diagnosed with VCI-ND (Ingles *et al.*, 2002). Follow-up cognitive diagnoses were available for 102 individuals and after five years, 45 patients (44 per cent) developed dementia; institutionalization and mortality rates were equivalent to those of AD (Wentzel *et al.*, 2001; Wentzel *et al.*, 2002). In this study, the progression to dementia was similar to that seen in MCI suggesting that, in all likelihood, the population identified by these criteria was actually a mixture of AD with CVD. Moreover, a number of patients' cognitive scores improved (Wentzel *et al.*, 2002), indicating that VCI-ND, in contrast with VCI, does not follow a unidirectional progression towards dementia.

63.3.2 Vascular dementia

The existence of multiple diagnostic criteria for VaD – and their lack of agreement on patient selection – has been the main argument brandished to deny the existence of VaD as an independent form of dementia, clinically and pathologically separate from AD. The criteria differ since they were designed for different purposes (hospital discharges, research studies, epidemiological surveys, etc.); in addition, they lack sensitivity (particularly when strict imaging criteria are mandatory) since it is difficult to include all forms of VaD within a single set of criteria. Finally, given the importance of CVD in the clinical expression of dementia in patients with AD lesions, the inclusion of mixed dementia (AD+CVD) is a common occurrence with most criteria.

Existing criteria include the HIS (Hachinski *et al.*, 1975); the DSM-IV (American Psychiatric Association, 1994) and DSM-IV-TR (American Psychiatric Association, 2000); the International Classification of Diseases (ICD-10) (World Health Organization, 1992); the California Criteria for ischaemic VaD or ADDTC (Chui *et al.*, 1992), and the Román *et al.* (1993) or NINDS-AIREN consensus criteria. Although all of them are useful in selecting VaD patients with varying degrees of sensitivity and specificity, they are not interchangeable. A critical review by Wiederkehr (Wiederkehr *et al.*, 2008a; Wiederkehr *et al.*, 2008b) studied the comparability of eight sets of diagnostic criteria including the HIS, the Ischaemic Scale of Rosen (Rosen *et al.*, 1980), DSM-III, DSM-IIIR, DSM-IV, ICD-10, ADDTC and NINDS-AIREN. It confirmed that each set of criteria includes different clinical features.

The NINDS-AIREN criteria were developed specifically for research studies in VaD and include a number of vascular aetiologies and clinical manifestations. These criteria have the highest specificity (0.84–0.94) (Gold *et al.*, 2002) and have been used in most modern controlled clinical trials in VaD as they would prevent researchers from including false-positive VaD cases (López-Pousa *et al.*, 1997; Kittner, 1999; Erkinjuntti *et al.*, 2002a; Orgogozo *et al.*, 2002; Wilcock *et al.*, 2002; Black *et al.*, 2003; Wilkinson *et al.*, 2003; Black, 2007). These criteria recognize patients with multiple forms of stroke and CVD (i.e. ischaemic, haemorrhagic, hypoperfusive), but establish strict requirements to classify patients appropriately. Two cardinal elements of the clinical syndrome of VaD must be identified: the cognitive syndrome of dementia and the definition of the vascular cause of the dementia. CVD is defined by the presence of focal neurological signs and detailed brain imaging showing evidence of stroke or ischaemic changes in the brain. A defining element of the criteria is the need for a temporal relationship between dementia and the cerebrovascular disorder, whereby dementia onset should occur within three months following a recognized stroke. The temporal relationship proved to be difficult to fulfil, particularly in patients with silent strokes and in the subcortical form of VaD. These elements are summarized in **Table 63.1**.

63.3.3 Mixed dementia (AD+CVD)

Specific brain pathological lesions define the two most common forms of senile dementia, AD and VaD. Stroke and cerebrovascular disease are the hallmarks of VaD, while senile plaques and neurofibrillary tangles typify AD. When these two pathologies are combined, the neuropathological diagnosis of AD+CVD or 'mixed dementia' is invoked (Zekry *et al.*, 2002a). Coexistent lesions occur in up to one-third of unselected elderly demented patients (Kalaria and Ballard, 1999; Zekry *et al.*, 2002b; Zekry *et al.*, 2002c), or in 10–15 per cent of cases of post-stroke dementia (PSD) (Hénon *et al.*, 1997; Hénon *et al.*, 2001; Barba *et al.*, 2001), but mixed lesions also occur in patients without dementia (Román and Royall, 2004).

Separating AD from VaD is a frequent problem in patients with pre-existing, progressive memory loss worsened by an acute vascular episode. The NINDS-AIREN criteria accurately separate VaD from AD or from AD associated to cerebrovascular lesions (AD+CVD) as demonstrated in validation neuropathological studies comparing various sets

Table 63.1   NINDS–AIREN diagnostic criteria for vascular dementia.[a]

The criteria for the diagnosis of probable VaD include all of the following:

1. **Dementia**: Impairment of memory and two or more cognitive domains (including executive function), interfering with ADLs and not due to physical effects of stroke alone. Exclusion criteria: Alterations of consciousness, delirium, psychoses, severe aphasia or deficits precluding testing, systemic disorders, Alzheimer's disease or other forms of dementia

2. **Cerebrovascular disease**: Focal signs on neurological examination (hemiparesis, lower facial weakness, Babinski sign, sensory deficit, hemianopsia, dysarthria) consistent with stroke (with or without history of stroke, and evidence of relevant CVD by brain CT or MRI including multiple large-vessel infarcts or a single strategically placed infarct (angular gyrus, thalamus, basal forebrain, or PCA or ACA territories), as well as multiple basal ganglia and white matter lacunes or extensive periventricular white matter lesions, or combinations thereof. Exclusion criteria: Absence of cerebrovascular lesions on CT or MRI

I. **A relationship between the above two disorders**: Manifested or inferred by the presence of one or more of the following:

(a) onset of dementia within 3 months following a recognized stroke

(b) abrupt deterioration in cognitive functions; or fluctuating, stepwise progression of cognitive deficits

II. Clinical features consistent with the diagnosis of probable VaD include the following:

(a) Early presence of gait disturbances (small step gait or *marche à petits pas*, or magnetic, apraxic-ataxic or parkinsonian gait)

(b) History of unsteadiness and frequent, unprovoked falls

(c) Early urinary frequency, urgency and other urinary symptoms not explained by urologic disease

(d) Pseudobulbar palsy

(e) Personality and mood changes, abulia, depression, emotional incontinence or other deficits, including psychomotor retardation and abnormal executive function

III. Features that make the diagnosis of VaD uncertain or unlikely include:

(a) Early onset of memory deficit and progressive worsening of memory and other cognitive functions, such as language (transcortical sensory aphasia), motor skills (apraxia) and perception (agnosia), in the absence of corresponding focal lesions on brain imaging

(b) Absence of focal neurological signs, other than cognitive disturbances

(c) Absence of CVD on CT or MRI

ACA, anterior cerebral artery; ADLs, activities of daily living; CT, computered tomography; CVD, cerebrovascular disease; MRI, magnetic resonance imaging; PCA, posterior cerebral artery; VaD, vascular dementia.

[a]From Román *et al.* (1993).

---

of diagnostic criteria. The NINDS-AIREN criteria consistently obtained the highest specificity values, ranging from 0.80 (Gold *et al.*, 1997), 0.86 (Zekry *et al.*, 2002b), 0.93 (Gold *et al.*, 2002), to 0.95 (Holmes *et al.*, 1999). Specificity defines the capacity to identify true negative cases. Therefore, using neuropathology as the gold standard several studies confirmed that the NINDS-AIREN criteria successfully exclude AD cases, and have the lowest proportion of mixed cases misclassified. The NINDS-AIREN criteria for VaD have slightly better specificity than the NINCDS-ADRDA criteria for AD (McKhann *et al.*, 1984; Holmes *et al.*, 1999).

The accuracy of the NINDS-AIREN criteria increases by excluding subjects with pre-existing diagnosis of AD, those with isolated MCI, as well as those with history of obvious progressive cognitive decline prior to a stroke (Hénon *et al.*, 1997; Hénon *et al.*, 2001). VaD typically occurs in patients with stroke and multiple vascular risk factors. The HIS quantifies this profile with high interrater reliability ($\kappa = 0.61$). A score > 4 in the HIS usually excludes AD.

Using the NINDS-AIREN criteria, three international trials of donepezil in VaD (Black *et al.*, 2003; Wilkinson *et al.*, 2003; Román *et al.*, 2010) recruited 2193 patients with relatively pure or unmixed VaD enrolled at 111 investigational sites in the United States, Europe, Canada and Australia (Román *et al.*, 2005). The VaD population selected was older and had a male preponderance, in agreement with population-based epidemiological data on VaD and in contrast with the female preponderance in AD trials (Chan *et al.*, 2008). Furthermore, the six-month progression of the placebo groups selected in the donepezil VaD studies was different

from placebo groups in AD (Román and Rogers, 2004; Chan *et al.*, 2008), as well as in mixed AD plus CVD trials (Erkinjuntti *et al.*, 2002a), further indicating the separate identity of the VaD cases selected (Pratt, 2002). The latest donepezil trial in VaD, recruited 974 patients (mean age, 73.0 years) with probable or possible VaD who were randomized 2:1 to receive donepezil 5 mg/day or placebo (Román *et al.*, 2010). Thus, almost 2200 patients with unmixed VaD identified with the NINDS-AIREN criteria have been studied in clinical trials using one cholinesterase inhibitor (ChEI).

In summary, VaD is a well-defined form of dementia that can be clinically diagnosed with reasonable accuracy. Of all available criteria, the NINDS-AIREN criteria have the highest specificity in neuropathology-confirmed cases, effectively ruling out cases of mixed dementia. The population thus selected is different from that of AD and mixed dementia trials. Several controlled clinical trials on VaD have successfully used the NINDS-AIREN criteria effectively making these criteria the most suitable current choice for VaD studies. Careful interview of relatives and caregivers allows a successful diagnosis of pre-stroke dementia. In most instances, probable AD is a likely aetiology for the progressive memory loss or MCI occurring prior to the ictus (Jagust, 2001).

63.3.4   Methodological aspects of clinical trials in VaD

The methodological requirements for controlled clinical trials in patients with dementia have been reviewed by the

International Working Group on Harmonization of Dementia Drug Guidelines at the Sixth International Congress on AD and Related Disorders in Amsterdam (Whitehouse et al., 1998), and at the 1998 Osaka Conference on VaD (Erkinjuntti and Sawada, 1999; Erkinjuntti et al., 1999); for more recent reviews see Mills and Chow (2003); Mani (2004) and Erkinjuntti et al., (2004). Updated information can also be found in the proceedings of the workshop entitled 'Vascular Cognitive Impairment: Harmonization Criteria' held by the National Institutes of Neurological Disorders and Stroke (NINDS) in Washington DC, in 2005, with USA–Canada co-sponsorship. The proceedings were published as the 'NINDS-Canadian Stroke Network vascular cognitive impairment harmonization standards' (Hachinski et al., 2006).

The first requirement for a valid trial in dementia, and VaD in particular, is the use of appropriate inclusion and exclusion criteria. This is crucial for the selection of a homogeneous population that would allow the generalized application of the trial results. Given the clinical variety of VaD, some authors have suggested limiting trials to patients with subcortical VaD using various sets of criteria (Pantoni et al., 1996; Erkinjuntti et al., 2000; Pantoni et al., 2000a), or to cases of mixed dementia, including AD+CVD (Erkinjuntti et al., 2002a; Erkinjuntti et al., 2002b) or AD plus arterial hypertension (HT) (Kumar et al., 2000). However, as discussed above, the criteria proposed by Román et al. (1993) are appropriate for VaD trials. Several instruments such as the Mini-Mental State Examination (MMSE), the Cambridge Cognitive Examination (CAMCOG), the Alzheimer's Disease Assessment Scale (ADAS-Cog), the Clinical Dementia Rating (CDR) and the Montreal Cognitive Assessment (MoCA) (Nasreddine et al., 2005) are used to ensure that dementia severity is comparable across the trial.

The next requirement is an appropriate sample size. The sample size is a function not only of the effectiveness of the drug, but also of the degree of responsiveness – or lack thereof – of the measuring instruments, as well as of the accuracy of the end points selected for the trial. Instruments that are relatively insensitive to change require larger sample sizes in order to demonstrate a statistically significant difference from the placebo or untreated group. Other requirements include randomization with appropriate group allocation concealment, placebo-controlled, double-blinded design with parallel group, and specific outcome measures, adequate instruments, and well-defined end points. Potential targets for the symptomatic treatment of VaD include: (1) symptomatic improvement of the core symptoms (cognition, function and behaviour); (2) slowing of progression; and (3) treatment of neuropsychiatric symptoms.

All current VaD trials have used the same primary outcome measures used in AD trials, as recommended by the United States Food and Drug Administration (FDA). These instruments include the ADAS-Cog, the Clinician's Interview-Based Impression of change plus caregiver input (CIBIC-plus) (Schneider et al., 1997), or the Clinical Global Impression of Change (CGIC) (Berg, 1988). The European Medicines Agency (EMEA) Committee for Medicinal Products for Human Use (CHMP) also requires positive impact on activities of daily living (ADLs), using scales such as the AD Functional Assessment and Change Scale (ADFACS), that

provides a measure of instrumental and basic ADLs (Mohs et al., 2001), or the Disability Assessment for Dementia (DAD) scale (Gélinas et al., 1999). The CHMP also requires a responder analysis. To the extent that ADAS-Cog and CIBIC-plus assess the multiple cognitive domains affected in all forms of dementia, it is not unreasonable to use the same measures in both AD and VaD patient populations. However, Quinn and colleagues (2000) showed difficulties with CIBIC-plus ratings in instances of clinical improvement; often, the physicians failed to recognize successful disease treatment beyond reversal of progression.

More importantly, current tests are relatively insensitive to frontal/subcortical executive dysfunction, a key cognitive domain in VaD (Román and Royall, 1999). To address this issue, at least two VaD clinical trials, one of donepezil in CADASIL – a genetic, predominantly subcortical form of VaD (Dichgans et al., 2008), and the latest trial of donepezil in VaD (Román et al., 2010), have incorporated tests such as the vascular equivalent of the ADAS-cog, the V-ADAS-Cog (Ferris and Gauthier, 2002), as well as other tests that include formal measurement of executive function. These include among others, CLOX, an executive clock drawing task (Royall et al., 1998) and the EXIT25, an executive interview (Royall et al., 1992). Of interest, ADLs are considered a proxy evaluation of executive function. Pohjasvaara et al. (2002) confirmed that executive dysfunction was the main determinant of abnormalities in both basic and instrumental ADLs in patients with post-stroke VaD.

63.4 RISK FACTORS FOR VASCULAR DEMENTIA

Several case–control studies of PSD provide a quantification of risk factors for VaD (Leys et al., 2005). In the Framingham study, the occurrence of stroke doubled the risk of dementia (Ivan et al., 2004); the prevalence of PSD in stroke survivors is about 30 per cent and the incidence of new onset dementia after stroke increases from 7 per cent after one year to 48 per cent after 25 years (Leys et al., 2005). Other risk factors include diabetes mellitus (Pasquier et al., 2006; Umegaki, 2010), atrial fibrillation (AF) (Lefebvre et al., 2006), as well as conditions resulting in cerebral hypoperfusion (Román, 2004). Johnston and colleagues (2004) observed progressive decline in cognitive function among cardiovascular health study participants with stenosis of the left internal carotid artery (ICA), but not in those with stenosis of the right ICA, in the absence of stroke. Possible explanations include the fact that the left hemisphere has larger cholinergic innervation than the right one; and tests such as the MMSE and the CAMCOG rely heavily on language functions.

PSD risk factors also include current smoking, lower blood pressure, orthostatic hypotension, and larger periventricular white matter ischaemic lesions on brain imaging (Liu et al., 1991; Gorelick et al., 1992). Orthostatic hypotension is an important factor in VaD (Román, 2004) and a strong predictor of periventricular white matter ischaemic lesions (Longstreth et al., 1996). Hypoxic and ischaemic complications of acute stroke are strong and independent risk factors for PSD (Moroney *et al.*, 1996); these complications increase more than four-fold the risk of developing PSD (odds ratio, (OR) 4.3; 95 per cent CI 1.9–9.6, after adjustment for demographic factors, recurrent stroke, and baseline cognitive function). Seizures following stroke (Cordonnier *et al.*, 2007) are independent predictors of new-onset dementia within three years after stroke (hazard ratio (HR) 3.81; 95 per cent CI 1.13–12.82). Pendlebury and Rothwell (2009) reviewed 21 hospital-based and eight population-based cohorts (7511 patients) described in 73 articles and concluded that PSD is associated with multiple strokes rather than with underlying vascular risk factors. However, as noted by Hennerici (2009), most studies were from the 1970s and 1980s, emphasizing the concept of MID and stroke recurrences rather the distinct mechanisms of PSD causation.

PSD is a strong predictor of poor outcome (Desmond *et al.*, 1998; Linden *et al.*, 2004; Leys *et al.*, 2005). In Rochester, MI, 10 per cent of 482 incident cases of dementia had onset or worsening of the dementia within three months of a stroke (Knopman *et al.*, 2003). Overall, patients with VaD had worse mortality than matched subjects (relative risk (RR), 2.7), particularly among cases of PSD (RR, 4.5).

The main correctable population-attributable risk (PAR) factors (Nyenhuis and Gorelick, 2007) include hypertension (PAR = 65 per cent), hypercholesterolaemia (36.5 per cent), smoking (16.7 per cent), diabetes mellitus (7.7 per cent), excessive alcohol drinking (5.4 per cent) and AF (2 per cent).

63.4.1 Hypertension and prehypertension

A large number of prospective studies show that HT increases the risk of dementia. Disruption of diurnal blood pressure (BP) variation is closely associated with cognitive impairment (Sakakura *et al.*, 2007; Nagai *et al.*, 2008). Therefore, there is interest in the diagnosis and treatment of the large population with preHT, defined as BP in the range of >120–139 mmHg systolic or >80–89 mmHg diastolic (Schunkert, 2006). In TROPHY (Trial of Preventing HT), Julius and colleagues (2006) studied the use of the angiotensin-receptor blocker candesartan or placebo for two years in people with preHT (first phase). Then, all participants received placebo for another two years (second phase). TROPHY showed that after two years of active treatment, candesartan may interfere with development of HT and prevent target-organ damage. The end point of the trial was the development of stage 1 HT (BP ≥ 159/99 mmHg). An absolute difference of 9.8 per cent between the two groups and a relative risk reduction of 15.6 per cent for the development of HT was found at the end of four years (Julius *et al.*, 2006). Schunkert (2006) noted that most people with preHT have additional risk factors including obesity, and most of the complications associated with preHT result from these cofactors including diabetes mellitus and chronic kidney disease. Current guidelines (JNC7) recommend antihypertensive treatment of such patients if a trial of lifestyle modification fails to reduce BP below 130/80 mmHg (Chobanian *et al.*, 2003).

Shah *et al.* (2009) reviewed the role of antihypertensive drugs on the incidence and progression of dementia. They analysed 536 publications from 1999 to 2008 that included calcium channel blockers, diuretics and angiotensin-converting enzyme inhibitors (ACE-I). All three drug types appeared to be beneficial in dementia, but only ACE-I plus diuretics showed a significant reduction of dementia risk and progression. A meta-analysis of the SHEP, Syst-Eur and SCOPE trials (McGuinness *et al.*, 2009) showed that antihypertensive therapy resulted in non-statistically significant reduction of the risk of dementia by 11 per cent (OR 0.89; 95 per cent CI 0.69–1.16). Statistically significant reduction of the risk of dementia (HR 0.87; 95 per cent CI: 0.76–1.00) with BP control was found in a meta-analysis of the SHEP, Syst-Eur, PROGRESS and HYVET trials (Peters *et al.*, 2008).

63.4.2 Diuretics

Although diuretics remain the mainstay of HT treatment (Prince, 1997; Chobanian *et al.*, 2003), there were no differences in cognition in those treated with diuretics alone versus controls in the Medical Research Council's (MRC) study (Prince *et al.*, 1996), in the Systolic HT in the Elderly Program (SHEP) cohort (Applegate *et al.*, 1994), nor in HT in the Very Elderly Trial Cognitive Function Assessment (HYVET-cog) trial (Peters *et al.*, 2008). However, at population level, in the Cache County Study (Khachaturian *et al.*, 2006), potassium-sparing diuretics reduced (HR 0.26; 95 per cent CI 0.08–0.64) AD incidence.

63.4.3 Calcium channel blockers

In the Systolic HT in Europe (Syst-Eur) trial (Forette *et al.*, 1998), treatment with the calcium channel blockers (CCB) nitrendipine decreased by 42 per cent the primary endpoint of fatal and nonfatal stroke. Of 2418 participants in the dementia substudy, 60 per cent of the treatment group received nitrendipine alone; the rest also had enalapril and/or a diuretic (hydrochlorothiazide, HCTZ). Compared with the controls, antihypertensive therapy reduced significantly the risk of dementia by 55 per cent (Forette *et al.*, 2002).

63.4.4 Angiotensin–converting enzyme inhibitors

In PROGRESS (Perindopril Protection Against Recurrent Stroke Study) (Tzourio *et al.*, 1999; Tzourio *et al.*, 2003), perindopril plus a diuretic (indapamide) – but not ACE-I alone – caused a relative risk reduction of dementia of 23 per cent (95 per cent CI, 0–41 per cent). In the Heart Outcomes Prevention Evaluation (HOPE) study, ramipril compared with placebo, significantly reduced (RR 0.59; 95 per cent CI, 0.37–0.94) the rate of cognitive decline (Bosch *et al.*, 2002).

63.4.5 Angiotensin II receptor blockers

In the candesartan versus placebo, Study on Cognition and Prognosis in the Elderly (SCOPE) trial (Lithell *et al.*, 2003), and in Prevention Regimen for Effectively Avoiding Second Strokes (PRoFESS) trial of telmisartan versus placebo with over 20 332 subjects (Diener *et al.*, 2008), there were no significant differences in the rate of cognitive decline or dementia with either one of the two angiotensin II receptor blockers (ARBs) compared with placebo. Hanon *et al.* (2008) reported in the Observational Study on Cognitive function And systolic blood pressure (SBP) Reduction (OSCAR), that lowering of SBP by the ARB eprosartan slowed cognitive decline (OR 0.77; 95 per cent CI 0.73–0.82). According to Fogari *et al.* (2006), antihypertensive therapy with an ARB (telmisartan) plus HCTZ, showed significant improvement in cognitive function compared with ACE-I plus diuretic (lisinopril and HCTZ). ARBs have reduce stroke risk, in part independently of their BP-lowering effect (Diener, 2009).

63.4.6 Vascular care and stroke prevention in patients with dementia

Richard *et al.* (2010) in the Evaluation of Vascular Care in AD (EVA) study demonstrated that improved vascular care in patients with AD+CVD slows the progression of white matter lesions (WMLs) on MRI. There was no difference in the number of new lacunes or change in global cortical atrophy or medial temporal lobe atrophy between the standard care and the improved vascular care group.

Savva and Stephan (2010) emphasize the need for stroke prevention, given that a history of stroke doubles the risk of incident dementia in older populations. This increase is not explained by demographic or cardiovascular risk factors or by pre-stroke cognitive decline. The excess risk of incident dementia diminishes with time after stroke and may be higher in those without an ApoE ε4 allele. There is no excess risk of incident dementia in those aged ≥ 85 years with a history of stroke. The effect of stroke on dementia incidence in the population is not explained by common risk factors.

Staekenborg *et al.* (2009) showed that MCI patients who converted to VaD were older and had lower MMSE at baseline than non-converters, and on baseline MRI showed more severe white matter hyperintensities (WMHIs), higher prevalence of lacunes in the basal ganglia and microbleeds. Deep WMLs (HR = 5.7; 95 per cent CI, 1.2–26.7), periventricular hyperintensities (HR = 6.5; 95 per cent CI, 1.4–29.8) and microbleeds (HR = 2.6; 95 per cent CI, 0.9–7.5) increased risk of progression to VaD. Medial temporal lobe atrophy and markers of CVD predict the development of different types of dementia in MCI. It is important to control all vascular risk factors in patients with vascular MCI, particularly when magnetic resonance brain imaging shows WMHIs, lacunes in the basal ganglia and microbleeds.

63.5 PHARMACOLOGICAL THERAPY OF VAD

A review of the history of VaD (Román, 2002b; Román, 2002c) suggests that the prevailing concepts of pathogenesis at a given time influence not only the elaboration of clinical criteria but also the approach to therapy. Until the 1970s,

VaD was believed to be caused by progressive strangulation of blood flow to the brain resulting in chronic cerebral hypoperfusion. Therefore, beginning with nicotinic acid, a number of vasodilating agents were recommended for the treatment of non-specific senile symptoms, cognitive decline and dementia. Following the same logic, Walsh (Walsh, 1968; Walsh *et al.*, 1978) claimed significant improvement of symptoms of presenile and senile dementia with a combination of warfarin anticoagulation and psychotherapy. A vascular pathogenesis mediated by recurrent multiple strokes (MID) also underlay the use of antithrombotic agents, ergot alkaloids, nootropics, TRH-analogue, *Ginkgo biloba* extract, plasma viscosity drugs, hyperbaric oxygen, antioxidants, serotonin and histamine receptor antagonists, vasoactive agents, xanthine derivates, and calcium antagonists (Román, 2000). With increasing recognition of AD and new knowledge of neurotransmitters, neuronal metabolism and biochemical tissue reactions to ischaemia-hypoxia and oxidative stress, more specific medications were developed leading to neuroprotection (Mondadori, 1993). The most recent advance in the treatment of VaD has been the development of medications to enhance specific neurotransmitters, such as acetylcholine. Furthermore, these products have been studied by strict controlled clinical trials. The ChEIs will be discussed first, followed by the NMDA-receptor antagonist, memantine, calcium channel blockers, nootropic agents, xanthines, ergot derivatives, vasodilators, and other treatments for VaD.

With the recent demonstration of reduced regional cerebral blood flow (CBF) in the dementias of the elderly (Román, 2008), the pendulum has returned to the concept of brain hypoperfusion as a critical element in dementia pathogenesis. This has led to a novel form of treatment of VaD using sphenopalatine ganglion (SPG) stimulation to augment CBF (Henninger and Fisher, 2007; Khurana *et al.*, 2009). Clinical trials of this method of treatment are ongoing.

63.5.1 Cholinergic dysfunction in VaD

Cholinergic dysfunction is well documented in VaD, independently of any concomitant AD pathology; these deficits consist of decreased levels of acetylcholine (ACh) in the cerebrospinal fluid (CSF), and reduced cholinergic markers in the brain (Wallin and Gottfries, 1990; Gottfries *et al.*, 1994). Hippocampal choline acetyl transferase (ChAT) deficits of up to 60 per cent were reported in the brains of both AD and VaD patients (Perry *et al.*, 1977; Kalaria *et al.*, 2001). The cholinergic basal forebrain nuclei are irrigated by penetrating arterioles and are susceptible to the effects of HT (Román and Kalaria, 2006). Moreover, ischaemic lesions in the white matter and the basal ganglia can interrupt cholinergic projections (Swartz *et al.*, 2003; Behl *et al.*, 2007). Selden and colleagues (1998) described in the human brain two highly organized and discrete bundles of cholinergic fibres extending from the nucleus basalis of Meynert (nbM) to the cerebral cortex and amygdala. Mesulam *et al.* (2003) demonstrated cholinergic denervation from ischaemic pathway lesions in CADASIL, entirely unmixed with AD lesions.

Cholinergic mechanisms play a role in the modulation of regional CBF (Sato *et al.*, 2001). Stimulation of the nbM results in increased blood flow in the cerebral cortex (Biesold et al., 1989). This cholinergic vasodilatory system relies on activation of both muscarinic and nicotinic cholinergic receptors and the response declines with age (Lacombe et al., 1997; Uchida et al., 2000). Therefore, there is loss of cholinergic function in patients with VaD, and this is associated with reductions in CBF (Court et al., 2002).

These observations provide reasonable arguments to justify the use of ChEIs in VaD, both unmixed with AD, as well as in patients with AD+CVD. Three of the ChEIs approved for use in AD have been studied in VaD.

63.5.2 Donepezil

Donepezil hydrochloride (see Chapter 54, Established treatments for Alzheimer's disease: cholinesterase inhibitors and memantine) is an acetylcholinesterase inhibitor (AChEI) approved for treatment of mild, moderate and advanced AD. The safety and efficacy of donepezil have been studied in three of the largest clinical trials of pure VaD ($n = 2193$) (Goldsmith and Scott, 2003; Román et al., 2005; Román et al., 2010). A total of 1219 subjects were recruited for a 24-week, randomized, placebo-controlled, multicentre, multinational study divided into two identical trials: study 307 (Black et al., 2003) and study 308 (Wilkinson et al., 2003). Patients were randomized to placebo, donepezil at a dosage of 5 mg/day or donepezil at a dosage of 10 mg/day. Most patients (73 per cent) fulfilled diagnosis of probable VaD according to the NINDS-AIREN criteria. All had brain imaging prior to enrolment with demonstration of cerebrovascular lesions. Patients with pre-existing AD and those with 'mixed dementia' (AD plus CVD) were excluded. These two VaD studies enrolled more men than women (58 versus 38 per cent) and their mean age was older than in AD (74.5 ± 0.2 versus 72 ± 0.2 years). The more severe vascular pathology of VaD was reflected in the high HIS score (6.6 ± 0.2 versus <4 in AD); most subjects had HT, hypercholesterolaemia, cardiovascular disease, diabetes, smoking, previous stroke and transient ischaemic attacks (TIAs). The third study (319 trial) recruited 974 subjects (mean age 73.0 years) with probable or possible VaD who were randomized 2:1 to receive donepezil 5 mg/day or placebo. Coprimary outcome measures were the Vascular-Alzheimer's Disease Assessment Scale-cognitive subscale (V-ADAS-Cog) (Ferris and Gauthier, 2002) and the CIBIC-Plus.

There were three main end points: (1) cognition, measured with the ADAS-Cog and the MMSE; (2) global function, evaluated with the CIBIC-plus and with the Sum of Boxes of the Clinical Dementia Rating (CDR-SB); and (3) ADLs, measured with the ADFACS.

In study 307 (Black et al., 2003), both donepezil treatment groups showed statistically significant cognitive improvement measured with the MMSE and the ADAS-Cog; the mean changes from baseline ADAS-Cog scores were: donepezil 5 mg/day, -1.90 ($p = 0.001$); donepezil 10 mg/day, -2.33 ($p < 0.001$). The donepezil 5 mg/day group also showed significant improvement in global function on the CIBIC-plus, but this did not reach significance in the 10 mg/day group ($p = 0.27$). The CDR-SB showed non-significant

benefit in the 5 mg/day group, and statistical significance in the 10 mg/day group ($p = 0.022$). Compared with placebo, there was significant benefit to ADLs ($p < 0.05$) in both donepezil groups on the ADFACS.

Similar results were observed in study 308 (Wilkinson et al., 2003): donepezil treatment resulted in significant improvement in both MMSE and ADAS-Cog scores. For the latter, the mean changes from baseline were: donepezil 5 mg/day, -1.65 ($p = 0.003$); donepezil 10 mg/day, -2.09 ($p = 0.0002$). Global function on the CIBIC-plus was significantly better in the 5 mg/day group ($p = 0.004$), and was barely below significance in the 10 mg/day group ($p = 0.047$). The CDR-SB showed benefits with 5 mg/day (non-significant), and it reached significance with 10 mg/day ($p = 0.03$). ADLs were improved in patients treated with donepezil when compared with placebo using the ADFACS, but did not reach significance at the end of the study. Comparison of cortical versus subcortical forms of VaD showed no differences in the overall results of the trial (Salloway et al., 2003).

In trial 319 (Román et al., 2010), donepezil-treated patients showed significant improvement from baseline to endpoint on the V-ADAS-Cog (least squares mean difference, -1.156; 95 per cent CI, -1.98 to -0.33; $p < 0.01$), but not on the CIBIC-Plus. Donepezil-treated patients with hippocampal atrophy demonstrated stable cognition versus decline in the placebo-treated group; in those without atrophy, cognition improved with donepezil versus relative stability with placebo. Results on secondary efficacy measures were inconsistent. The incidence of adverse events (AEs) was similar across groups. Eleven deaths occurred in the donepezil group (1.7 per cent) – similar to rates previously reported for donepezil trials in VaD – whereas no deaths occurred in the placebo group. Donepezil 5 mg/day showed significant improvement in cognitive, but not global, function, with differential treatment response of VaD patients by hippocampal size. Donepezil was relatively well tolerated; AEs were consistent with current labeling. Mortality in the placebo group was unexpectedly low (Román et al., 2010).

In comparison with AD patients, cognitive decline in untreated patients with VaD during 24 weeks of study in these trials was less severe. These differences were also noted for global effects, measured by the CIBIC-plus. Substantial decline of instrumental ADLs was noted in untreated VaD patients. A combined analysis of the total population confirmed the effects on cognition and global function. Donepezil-treated patients demonstrated statistically significant improvements in instrumental ADLs compared with decline in the placebo group (LS mean change from baseline at end point: placebo, 0.60; 5 mg/day -0.09, $p < 0.05$; 10 mg/day -0.18, $p < 0.01$). These results suggest that donepezil treatment may improve or maintain patients' abilities to perform ADLs. Executive dysfunction is a major component of disability in patients with VaD and the beneficial effect of donepezil on instrumental activities of daily living (IADLs) may be related to improvement or stabilization of executive function.

Donepezil was generally well tolerated, although more adverse effects were reported in the 10 mg/day group than in the 5 mg/day or placebo groups. The adverse effects were assessed as mild to moderate and transient, and were typically diarrhoea, nausea, arthralgia, leg cramps, anorexia and headache. The incidence of bradycardia and syncope was not significantly different from the placebo group. Discontinuation rates were 15 per cent for placebo, 18 per cent for 5 mg, and 28 per cent for the 10 mg group. There was no significant interaction with cardiovascular medications or anti-thrombotic agents. These three trials offer evidence that donepezil is effective and well tolerated in VaD patients.

Dichgans et al. (2008) published the results of a trial of donepezil in patients with CADASIL that randomized 168 patients (mean age 54.8 years) to 10 mg donepezil per day ($n = 86$) or placebo ($n = 82$). Inclusion criteria included a MMSE score of 10–27 or a trail-making test (TMT) B time score at least 1.5 SD below the mean, after adjustment for age and education. The primary end point was the V-ADAS-Cog at 18 weeks. Secondary end points included ADAS-Cog, MMSE, TMT A and B times, Stroop test, EXIT25, CLOX, DAD and CDRS sum-of-boxes. Donepezil (5–10 mg/day) had no effect on V-ADAS-Cog, but had significant effect on two measures of executive function: EXIT25 and TMT-B. These subjects were younger than most VaD patients and most (75 per cent) had no clinically significant memory dysfunction. The positive effect of donepezil on executive function, however, indicates some cholinergic deficit in executive dysfunction.

63.5.3   Galantamine

Galantamine (see Chapter 54, Established treatments for Alzheimer's disease: cholinesterase inhibitors and memantine) is approved for the treatment of mild to moderate AD. Craig and Birks (2006) conducted a Cochrane review of galantamine in VCI. Galantamine has been studied in VaD in the GAL-INT-6 study, a large phase III, randomized, multicentre, double-blind, placebo-controlled clinical trial in patients with probable VaD, or with AD combined with CVD (Erkinjuntti et al., 2002a). Patients received galantamine 24 mg/day ($n = 396$) or placebo ($n = 196$) for six months; patients' ages ranged from 40 to 90 years. Eligible subjects met either the clinical criteria of probable VaD by NINDS-AIREN criteria, or of possible AD according to the NINCDS-ADRDA criteria (McKhann et al., 1984). Radiological evidence of CVD on brain imaging was required (i.e. AD plus CVD), including multiple large-vessel infarcts or a single, strategically placed infarct, or at least two basal ganglia and white-matter lacunes, or white-matter changes involving at least 25 per cent of the total white matter. Mild to moderate dementia was defined by a score of ≥ 12 in the ADAS-Cog/11 and 10–25 on the MMSE. Primary end points were cognition, measured using the ADAS-Cog/11 and global functioning measured with the CIBIC-plus. Secondary end points included assessments of activities of daily living, using the Disability Assessment in Dementia (DAD) (Gélinas et al., 1999), and behavioural symptoms, using the Neuropsychiatric Inventory (NPI) (Cummings et al., 1994).

Galantamine demonstrated greater efficacy than placebo on all outcome measures in analyses of both groups of patients as a whole: ADAS-Cog (2.7 points, $p \leq 0.001$), on the CIBIC-plus (74 versus 59 per cent of patients remained stable or improved, $p \leq 0.001$). ADLs and behavioural symptoms in the NPI were also significantly improved compared with placebo (both $p < 0.05$). Galantamine was safe and well tolerated, but nausea was reported six times as often by VaD patients on galantamine than those on placebo. In comparison, nausea was twice as common in patients with AD treated with galantamine compared with placebo-treated patients (Erkinjuntti et al., 2002a).

In an open-label extension (Erkinjuntti et al., 2003a), the original galantamine group of patients with probable VaD or AD+CVD showed similar sustained benefits in terms of maintenance of or improvement in cognition (ADAS-Cog), functional ability (DAD), and behaviour (NPI) after 12 months. Although not designed to detect differences between subgroups, the subgroup of patients with AD+CVD on galantamine ($n = 188$, 48 per cent) showed greater efficacy than placebo ($n = 97$, 50 per cent) at six months on the ADAS-Cog ($p \leq 0.001$) and the CIBIC-plus ($p = 0.019$) (Erkinjuntti et al., 2002a). In the open-label extension, patients with AD+CVD on galantamine maintained cognition at baseline for 12 months (Erkinjuntti et al., 2003a). The subgroup of patients with probable VaD, compared those on placebo ($n = 81$, 41 per cent) with 171 subjects (43 per cent) on galantamine.

In the subgroup of patients with VaD treated with galantamine for six months the ADAS-Cog scores improved significantly (mean change from baseline, 2.4 points, $p < 0.0001$), compared with no response in placebo group (mean change from baseline, 0.4; treatment difference versus galantamine 1.9, $p = 0.06$). More patients treated with galantamine than with placebo maintained or improved global function (CIBIC-plus, 31 versus 23 per cent, not statistically significant). In these patients, the cognitive benefits of galantamine were maintained at least up to 12 months, demonstrating a mean change of –2.1 in the ADAS-cog score compared to baseline, and the active group was still close to baseline at 24 months. During the 12-month trial, the most frequently reported adverse events were depression (13 per cent), agitation (12 per cent) and insomnia (11 per cent).

Erkinjuntti et al. (2008) performed responder analyses for cognitive, behavioural and functional outcome measures in GAL-INT-6. Galantamine treatment resulted in significant cognitive and functional improvements compared with placebo at six months. Significantly higher percentages of treatment responders were found for the ADAS-Cog/11 (60.5 per cent for galantamine versus 46.0 per cent for placebo, $p = 0.013$); the CIBIC-plus (75 versus 53.6 per cent with placebo, $p = 0.0006$); behaviour (64.9 versus 56.6 per cent, $p = 0.024$), and numerically favourable responder rates were seen with galantamine for ADLs, indicating a broad range of cognitive, functional and behavioural benefits with galantamine across the spectrum of AD and AD+CVD.

In a more recent trial of galantamine in VaD, the GAL-INT-26 study (Auchus et al., 2007), 788 patients with probable VaD and strict centrally-read MRI criteria were randomized to galantamine or placebo. Efficacy was evaluated using measures of cognition, daily function and behaviour using the NPI; EXIT-25 was used to assess executive functioning. Safety and tolerability were monitored. Galantamine showed improvement in ADAS-Cog/11 after 26 weeks compared with placebo (−1.8 versus −0.3; $p < 0.001$), but there was no difference on the ADCS-ADL score (0.7 versus 1.3; $p = 0.783$). Improvement on the CIBIC-plus approached significance ($p = 0.069$). In patients with VaD, galantamine significantly improved cognition, including executive function, but ADLs were similar to the placebo group.

Thavichachart et al. (2006) reported the results of a six-month trial of galantamine in AD in Thai patients with or without CVD and VaD. Galantamine showed favourable effects on ADLs; behavioural symptoms and sleep quality were also significantly improved ($p < 0.05$). Galantamine was well tolerated.

The Cochrane review of galantamine for VaD (Craig and Birks, 2006) concluded that despite some positive evidence of efficacy over placebo in the areas of cognition and executive functioning, more studies are needed before firm conclusions can be drawn; galantamine produced higher rates of gastrointestinal side effects.

63.5.4   Rivastigmine

Rivastigmine (see Chapter 54, Established treatments for Alzheimer's disease: cholinesterase inhibitors and memantine) is approved for use in mild to moderate AD (Farlow, 2003). Rivastigmine was used in small open-label studies of patients with subcortical VaD followed for 12 months (Moretti et al., 2001) and 22 months (Moretti et al., 2002); rivastigmine resulted in stabilization of cognition and ADLs, with slight improvement of executive function and planning, less caregiver stress and improved behaviour. More recently, Moretti et al. (2008) observed significant improvement in behavioural symptoms in two forms of VaD, MID and subcortical VaD, except delusions, suggesting that rivastigmine can reduce concomitant use of neuroleptics and benzodiazepines.

However, rivastigmine effects in VaD remained to be determined in phase III, randomized, double-blind, placebo-controlled clinical trials (Moretti et al., 2004). The first such trial was Vascular Dementia trial studying Exelon (VantagE), a 24-week, multicentre, double-blind study that randomized 710 VaD patients aged 50–85 years to rivastigmine (3–12 mg/day) or placebo (Ballard et al., 2008). Efficacy assessments included global and cognitive performances, ADLs and neuropsychiatric symptoms. Rivastigmine was superior to placebo on three measures of cognitive performance, but not on other outcomes. Cognitive improvement occurred in older patients, likely to have concomitant AD as evidenced by medial temporal atrophy.

Regarding the use of rivastigmine in patients with AD+CVD, Kumar and colleagues (2000) compared the outcomes of AD patients with or without concurrent vascular risk factors; cognitive effects were seen in both groups, but patients with AD and vascular risk had greater clinical benefit. These findings were confirmed by Erkinjuntti and colleagues (2002b) in an open-label extension study of 104 weeks. Compared with non-hypertensive patients with AD, significant treatment differences were observed in the hypertensive subgroup on both the Progressive Deterioration Scale (PDS) and the Global Deterioration Scale (GDS).

Furthermore, Erkinjuntti et al. (2003b) stratified 725 patients with AD treated with rivastigmine, according to the presence or absence of HT at baseline. Rivastigmine 6–12 mg/day provided better outcomes than placebo on the PDS in the hypertensive ($p = 0.031$) and non-hypertensive ($p = 0.035$) subgroups. All patients receiving rivastigmine 6–12 mg/day had superior CIBIC-plus scores than those receiving placebo. The additional apparent benefits on disease progression detected in patients with AD and HT may be linked to drug effects on cerebrovascular risk factors, or to a larger underlying cholinergic deficit in patients with AD and HT.

The problems associated with gastrointestinal side effects requiring slow oral titration of rivastigmine were solved to a large extent with the use of a dermal patch (Winblad and Machado, 2008), but the rivastigmine patch has not been evaluated in VaD.

63.5.5   Memantine

Memantine is a moderate-affinity, voltage-dependent, uncompetitive, potent antagonist of the N-methyl-D-aspartate (NMDA) receptor (Farlow, 2004) (see Chapter 54, Established treatments for Alzheimer's disease: cholinesterase inhibitors and memantine). Memantine has been approved by the FDA for the treatment of moderate to severe AD (Möbius, 2003). Furthermore, Tariot and colleagues (2004) showed that in patients with moderate to severe AD receiving stable doses of donepezil, memantine resulted in significantly better outcomes than placebo in cognition, ADLs, global outcome and behaviour. These findings suggest that this dual therapy could be useful.

Memantine has been used also in patients with VaD based on its experimental efficacy in animal models of ischaemia. The pivotal memantine 9M-Best study by Winblad and Poritis (1999) in severe dementia included both AD and VaD patients. A statistically significant effect was detected in both dementias. Orgogozo and colleagues (2002) and Wilcock and coworkers (2002), completed two randomized, placebo-controlled six-month trials of memantine (20 mg/day) in mild to moderate probable VaD, diagnosed according to the NINDS-AIREN criteria.

In study MMM 300, Orgogozo et al. (2002) randomized 147 patients to memantine and 141 to placebo. After 28 weeks, the mean ADAS-Cog scores were significantly improved relative to placebo: the memantine group gained an average of 0.4 points, versus a decline of 1.6 in the placebo group, a difference of 2.0 points ($p = 0.0016$). The CIBIC-plus that improved or remained stable reached 60 per cent with memantine compared with 52 per cent with placebo ($p = 0.227$). The Gottfries–Bråne–Steen scale (GBS) (Gottfries et al., 1982) and the Nurses' Observation Scale for Geriatric Patients (NOSGER) (Spiegel et al., 1991) total scores at week 28 did not differ significantly between the two groups. However, the GBS scale intellectual function subscore and the NOSGER disturbing behaviour dimension also showed a difference favouring memantine ($p = 0.04$ and $p = 0.07$, respectively).

Wilcock et al. (2002) in study MMM 500 randomized 277 patients to memantine and 271 to placebo. At 28 weeks, the active group had gained 0.53 points and the placebo declined by 2.28 points in ADAS-cog, a significant difference of 1.75 ADAS-Cog points between the groups ($p < 0.05$). There were no differences in CGIC, MMSE, GBS or NOSGER between groups. Memantine was well tolerated in both studies. Möbius and Stoffler (2002) performed a *post hoc* pooled analysis of the above two placebo-controlled trials of memantine in VaD. Baseline severity assessed by MMSE showed larger cognitive benefit in patients with more advanced disease. The cognitive treatment effect for memantine was more pronounced in the small-vessel type group without cortical infarctions by computed tomography (CT) or MRI. The placebo subgroup of patients with large-vessel disease showed less cognitive decline than the other subgroup.

Möbius and Stoffler (Möbius and Stoffler, 2002; Möbius and Stoffler, 2003) reviewed the results of studies of memantine in VaD in a *post hoc* analysis. The small-vessel disease subgroup of VaD accounted for most of the outcome (responders) while the large-vessel disease subgroup (non-responders) was not statistically significant when compared with placebo. Solving this issue would probably require a separate trial of memantine in small-vessel VaD.

In a review, Thomas and Grossberg (2009) concluded that memantine shows promise for the treatment of patients with VaD because of its safety and efficacy. However, Kavirajan and Schneider (2007) performed a meta-analysis of randomized controlled trials (RCTs) of six-month duration in VaD (three donepezil, two galantamine, one rivastigmine and two memantine trials), comprising 3093 patients on the study drugs and 2090 patients on placebo. All drugs produced small but significant cognitive effects of uncertain clinical significance in patients with mild to moderate VaD. Compared with placebo, more dropouts and adverse events (anorexia, nausea, vomiting, diarrhoea and insomnia) occurred with all three ChEIs, but not with memantine. The authors concluded that the data were insufficient to support widespread use of these drugs in VaD. Wong *et al.* (2009) analysed the cost-effectiveness of using ChEIs and memantine in VaD and concluded that treatment with ChEIs or memantine was more effective, but also more costly than standard care for mild to moderate VaD.

63.5.6 Calcium channel blockers

The main calcium channels blockers (CCB) used for the treatment of VaD include nimodipine, nicardipine, lacidipine and fasudil.

63.5.6.1 NIMODIPINE

Nimodipine is a dihydropyridine-type CCB used as an antihypertensive agent. It readily crosses the blood–brain barrier (BBB), affects autoregulation of CBF and produces vasodilatation of small cerebral blood vessels (Jansen *et al.*, 1991). Nimodipine reduces the severity of neurological outcome in patients after subarachnoid haemorrhage (SAH) secondary to ruptured aneurysms, probably by decreasing cerebral vasospasm (Ohman *et al.*, 1991). In addition to its vascular effects, nimodipine appears to have nootropic properties. There is a high density of nimodipine-binding sites in hippocampus, caudate nucleus and cerebral cortex (Traber and Gibsen, 1989). Nimodipine binds to slow L-type calcium receptors, preventing influx of calcium into vascular smooth muscle cells and into ischaemic neurones (Greenberg *et al.*, 1990); experimentally, it provides protection against age-associated microvascular abnormalities in the rat brain (De Jong *et al.*, 1990). Although a neuroprotective effect has been postulated in stroke patients, nimodipine showed only a trend for better outcome when used within the first 12 hours of stroke onset (Gelmers and Hennerici, 1990).

A re-analysis of the Scandinavian Trial of Nimodipine in MID (Pantoni *et al.*, 2000b) showed a beneficial effect in tests of attention and psychomotor performance in the subgroup of patients with subcortical small-vessel VaD, but not in patients with PSD of the MID type. A pilot open-label trial of nimodipine in patients with small-vessel VaD was positive (Pantoni *et al.*, 1996). In this study, subcortical VaD was defined according to ICD-10 criteria (World Health Organization, 1992) and inclusion criteria required the patients to have mild-to-moderate dementia (MMSE, 12–24; GDS, 3–5), as well as CT evidence of extensive leukoaraiosis and at least one lacunar infarct. The primary measure of efficacy was the Sandoz Clinical Assessment–Geriatric (SCAG) scale (Shader *et al.*, 1974).

Using similar criteria and outcome measures, a large multicentre, randomized, double-blind, placebo-controlled trial of nimodipine in subcortical VaD was conducted in Italy and Spain (Pantoni *et al.*, 2005). Of 242 patients randomized to oral nimodipine 90 mg/day or placebo, 230 patients (nimodipine $n = 121$, placebo $n = 109$) were included in the intention-to-treat analysis. At 52 weeks, there was no difference in the primary outcome measure (SCAG scale) between the two groups. However, patients on nimodipine performed better than placebo in lexical production ($p < 0.01$), MMSE ($p < 0.01$) and GDS ($p < 0.05$). More dropouts and adverse events occurred among the placebo group (cardiovascular and cerebrovascular events, and behavioural disturbances requiring intervention). Pantoni *et al.* (2005) concluded that nimodipine offers benefit in subcortical VaD and might protect against cardiovascular and CVD comorbidities in this high-risk group.

A Cochrane review on nimodipine by Lopez-Arrieta and Birks (2002) concluded that there was no convincing evidence for the efficacy of nimodipine in AD, VaD or mixed forms of dementia; and, given the short-term benefits demonstrated in the trials reviewed, use of nimodipine as a long-term antidementia drug could not be justified.

63.5.6.2 NICARDIPINE

Nicardipine is a dihydropyridine-type CCB with high vascular selectivity, strong antihypertensive activity and cerebrovascular effects (Amenta *et al.*, 2008). Nicardipine protects from atherogenesis in experimental vascular injury (Weinstein and Heider, 1989), has anti-oxidant effects, preventing endothelial cell damage from free radical injury (Mak *et al.*, 1992), and inhibits platelet aggregation (Yamada *et al.*,

1990). Nicardipine, like all CCBs, lowers arterial pressure by reducing peripheral vascular resistance; decreasing both systolic and diastolic BP and improving myocardial oxygen supply by vasodilating the coronary arteries (Amenta *et al.*, 2008). Therefore, nicardipine is an anti-angina and cardioprotective agent (Pepine and Lambert, 1990). CCBs are more effective in BP lowering in patients older than 55 years or those of black ethnic origin at any age (Messerli *et al.*, 2007). Amenta *et al.* (2008) recommend nicardipine for the treatment of HT after acute ischaemic stroke or intracerebral haemorrhage, for control of vasospasm in SAH, as well as for stroke prevention (Martí-Massó and Lozano, 1990).

Amenta *et al.* (2008) reviewed the effects of nicardipine on cognition in 24 studies performed on about 6000 patients suffering from 'chronic cerebrovascular insufficiency' due to several forms of CVD, including PSD, and ranging in severity from vascular MCI to VaD. Positive effects of treatment with nicardipine were observed in over 60 per cent of patients; more favourable results were observed in patients with HT, resulting in decreased systolic and diastolic BP, improvement of neurological symptoms and signs, as well as amelioration of cognition assessed with the SCAG scale, MMSE and other batteries.

The Spanish Group of Nicardipine Study in VaD (Grupo Español, 1999) conducted a double-blind, placebo-controlled RCT to investigate the effect of nicardipine on cognitive function in patients with VaD. The effect of daily treatment with nicardipine (20 mg three times a day) for a period of one year was investigated in 156 patients with cognitive impairment of vascular origin, randomized to nicardipine ($n = 81$) or placebo ($n = 75$). A total of 142 subjects completed the study (nicardipine, $n = 73$; placebo, $n = 60$) on intention-to-treat analysis. The primary efficacy variable was the loss of >10 per cent of the MMSE basal score; other end points were the Short Portable Mental Status Questionnaire (SPMSQ) score (Pfeiffer, 1975), functional disability and drug safety. At one year, 21.1 per cent of patients treated with nicardipine had lowered the MMSE score versus 34.6 per cent with placebo. Favourable effects of nicardipine were found on females (40.9 versus 10.5 per cent, $p = 0.01876$), previously untreated subjects (46.2 versus 13.3 per cent, $p = 0.00748$) and patients with concomitant antiplatelet treatment (35.0 versus 15.9; $p = 0.03836$). Survival analysis showed that patients on nicardipine took longer to lose cognitive capacities ($p = 0.031$; RR = 1.15–3.99). Nicardipine significantly delayed cognitive decline, producing better evolution in females. The drug was remarkably safe and was well tolerated for one year; side effects secondary to vasodilatation were short-lived and of low intensity.

The largest ($n ~ 6375$ patients) nicardipine trial on vascular MCI and VaD was an open, prospective, multicentre, six-month study to test the efficacy and tolerability of a single 40 mg/day oral dose of nicardipine retard (slow release) in patients with cognitive deterioration of vascular origin (González-González and Lozano, 2000). BP, ADLs and cognition with the SPMSQ score were obtained. Nicardipine improved functional capacity in 65.5 per cent of the patients; systolic/diastolic BP decreased 11.3/7.4 mmHg in hypertensive patients treated with other antihypertensive drugs and 5.9/4.3 mmHg in those not taking antihypertensives.

Nicardipine was well tolerated and no major side effects were seen.

Amenta *et al.* (2008) concluded that the antihypertensive effect of nicardipine, its safety and effectiveness in improving cognition and functional domains make this a recommended drug in the treatment of cognitive impairment of vascular origin.

63.5.6.3   LACIDIPINE AND LERCANIDIPINE

Lacidipine and lercanidipine are third-generation dihydropyridine calcium antagonists that cause systemic vasodilatation by blocking calcium entry through calcium channels in cell membranes; these agents also improve carotid atherosclerosis (Zanchetti *et al.*, 2004), small-vessel disease (Frishman, 2002) and CBF (Semplicini *et al.*, 2000) in hypertensive patients; their use results in less peripheral oedema than with older dihydropyridine CCBs, and offer some promise for the treatment of VaD.

63.5.6.4   FASUDIL

Fasudil hydrochloride is a novel intracellular calcium antagonist, with Rho-kinase inhibitory activity on arterial walls affecting vessel remodelling (Pearce *et al.*, 2004). Fasudil has been used to prevent and treat vasospasm associated with SAH (Suzuki *et al.*, 2008). Kamei and colleagues (1996) reported the use of fasudil in the treatment of two patients with Binswanger disease (BD) using ^{31}P-magnetic resonance spectroscopy and xenon-computed tomography. Treatment with fasudil at 30 or 60 mg/day orally for 8 weeks controlled the fluctuating symptoms of BD in both patients. Mental tests and imaging also improved during the treatment.

63.5.7   Nootropic agents

The name nootropic (Greek *nous*, mind; *trophikos*, nourishing) describes a category of agents with neuroprotective capacity against anoxic or oxidative injuries.

63.5.7.1   PIRACETAM

Piracetam, the first of the nootropic agents, is a cyclic derivative of γ-aminobutyric acid (GABA) which can cross the BBB (Hitzenberger *et al.*, 1998) to concentrate selectively in the brain cortex (Vernon and Sorkin, 1991). At low doses, piracetam increases both oxygen and glucose utilization via ATP pathways and the release of some neurotransmitters – in particular dopamine metabolites – while at higher dosages, it is associated with platelet anti-aggregation and rheological effects with antithrombotic properties (Moriau *et al.*, 1993). It enhances the microcirculation by promoting erythrocyte deformability and by reducing adherence to endothelial cells. However, studies of piracetam in acute stroke have been inconclusive, although improvement of aphasia in patients treated within 7 hours of stroke onset was seen (Hitzenberger *et al.*, 1998). Several animal studies showed effects of piracetam on memory and facilitation of retention over 24 hours. A Cochrane review (Flicker and Grimley Evans, 2001) concluded that the usefulness of piracetam in patients with AD and VaD in small clinical trials has been unclear, based mainly on subjective Global Impression of Change. These findings are supported by a larger trial in Russia (Batysheva et al., 2009) on 70 patients (37 women and 33 men, mean age 62 years), including 29 (41.5 per cent) with PSD and 41 (58.5 per cent) with chronic cerebral ischaemia. Improvements in cognition (MMSE) and behaviour were better at a dose of 2400 mg/day. Piracetam was well tolerated. A review of 19 trials in patients with several forms of dementia (Waegemans et al., 2002) and a protective effect in patients undergoing coronary artery bypass surgery (Uebelhack et al., 2003) provides some support for a moderate effect of piracetam on cognitive impairment.

63.5.7.2 OXIRACETAM

Oxiracetam is a structural analogue of piracetam. This compound has enhancing effects on vigilance and memory. In comparison with piracetam, oxiracetam exhibits greater improvement in memory (Itil et al., 1986) and has been used extensively for the treatment of dementia, including AD, VaD, MID (Baumel et al., 1989; Dysken et al., 1989) and mixed forms. Green and colleagues (1992) failed to demonstrate a difference with placebo in AD patients. In contrast, Maina et al. (1989) studied 289 patients with MID in a double-blind placebo-controlled trial and after 12 weeks of treatment found that oxiracetam reduced behavioural symptoms.

63.5.7.3 CITICOLINE

Citicoline, also known as CDP-choline or cytidine-5'-diphosphatecholine, is a naturally occurring endogenous nucleoside that functions as an intermediate in three major metabolic pathways (Conant and Schauss, 2004): (1) Synthesis of phosphatidylcholine (lecithin) one of the major cell membrane phospholipids with an important role in the formation of lipoproteins. Citicoline formation is the rate-limiting step in the synthesis of phosphatidylcholine. (2) Synthesis of acetylcholine:citicoline by providing choline for this neurotransmitter could limit choline availability for membrane synthesis (Ulus et al., 1989). (3) Oxidation to betaine, a methyl donor. The main components of citicoline, choline and cytidine, are readily absorbed in the gut and cross the BBB (Secades and Lorenzo, 2006). As a dietary supplement, choline is grouped with the B vitamins. A related product, choline alphoscerate, has been used less frequently (Parnetti et al., 2007).

In animal studies, citicoline is biologically active, enhancing repair of ischaemic neuronal injury and increasing levels of acetylcholine and dopamine (Secades and Frontera, 1995; Secades and Lorenzo, 2006). In aged animals, citicoline increased dopamine release, improving learning and memory tasks (Cacabelos et al., 1993). Lee et al. (2009) showed that citicoline protects against cognitive impairment in a rat model of chronic cerebral hypoperfusion. Silvery et al. (2008) demonstrated by phosphorus magnetic resonance spectroscopy that citicoline treatment for 6 weeks in patients produced significant increases in phosphocreatine (+7 per cent), beta-nucleoside triphosphates – largely ATP in the brain (+14 per cent), and in the ratio of phosphocreatine to inorganic phosphate (+32 per cent), as well as significant changes in membrane phospholipids, observed in the anterior cingulate cortex.

Citicoline can produce regrowth of dendritic spines in an experimental stroke model (Hurtado et al., 2007). In a pooled analysis of clinical trials on acute ischaemic stroke, citicoline was shown to enhance the possibility of recovery (Dávalos et al., 2002; Saver, 2008). Citicoline has been used in a number of trials in patients with AD showing consistent moderate improvement of memory and behaviour (Cacabelos et al., 1993; Alvarez et al., 1999). A recent placebo-controlled trial on 30 patients with VaD showed no evidence of cognitive improvement (Cohen et al., 2003). However, a Cochrane review (Fioravanti and Yanagi, 2005) included 14 studies on aged individuals with symptoms ranging from memory disorders to vascular MCI, VaD or senile dementia. Duration of studies ranged between 20 and 30 days, one study was of 6 weeks' duration, four studies lasted two and three months, and one study lasted 12 months. Multiple doses, inclusion criteria and outcome measures were used. Overall results (884 patients) showed evidence of benefit of CDP-choline on memory and behaviour, but not on attention. There was significant improvement on the Global Impression of Change, in comparison with the placebo group. The effect size was very large (OR = 8.89, 95 per cent CI 5.19–15.22; $p < 0.001$), indicating a strong drug effect (Fioravanti and Yanagi, 2005; Fioravanti and Buckley, 2006) for improvement under active treatment. These authors concluded that the cognitive effects of citicoline are clearly evident at the behavioural level and can be easily appreciated with a clinical observation of patients irrespective of the functional paradigm used to measure them. Citicoline is remarkably well tolerated and more side effects were seen with the placebo than with the active treatment groups (Fioravanti and Yanagi, 2005; Fioravanti and Buckley, 2006).

63.5.8 Xanthine derivatives

The main xanthine derivatives used in the treatment of VaD are pentoxifylline or oxpentifylline, denbufylline (a phosphodiesterase 4 (PDE4) inhibitor) and propentofylline (PPF). Pentoxifylline, derived from theobromine, has haemorheological effects both on the microcirculation and on peripheral vascular disease (in particular for the treatment of intermittent claudication). Pentoxifylline has immunomodulatory properties, increasing the rate of neutrophil migration, suppressing monocyte production of tumour necrosis factor (TNF-α), and inhibiting leukocyte stimulation by TNF-α and interleukin-1 (IL-1). These properties are strong contributors to its haemorheological effects (Samlaska and Winfield, 1994). PPF exhibits adenosine-mediated nootropic properties against post-anoxic neuronal cell damage, and glial-modulation effects with inhibition of microglial activation. Bruno *et al.* (2009) recently showed improvement of neurological and neurochemical deficits in rats subjected to transient brain ischaemia and treated with pentoxifylline.

63.5.8.1 PENTOXIFYLLINE

Haemorheological alterations are found in patients with AD and in some forms of VaD, such as BD, in comparison with age-matched controls (Solerte *et al.*, 2000). Abnormalities included hyperviscosity, increased sedimentation rate, hyperfibrinogenemia and increased acute-phase reactants; these changes correlate with increased levels of TNF-α and IFN-γ. Pentoxifylline treatment lowers fibrinogen and TNF-α levels. Black and colleagues (1992) demonstrated beneficial effects of pentoxifylline in patients with MID. These preliminary findings were confirmed in the larger, multicentre European Pentoxifylline Multi-Infarct Dementia Study (1996) that demonstrated significant cognitive improvement in the MID form of VaD in comparison with placebo. Sha and Callahan (2003) reviewed 20 articles on the use of pentoxifylline in VaD, but only four studies met criteria for a systematic review. A trend towards improved cognitive function was found in patients treated with pentoxifylline. A subgroup analysis of three studies of VaD noted statistically significant improvement in cognitive function with pentoxifylline compared with placebo and suggested a potential therapeutic role for pentoxifylline in VaD.

63.5.8.2 PROPENTOFYLLINE

Beneficial effects on learning and memory were observed in several European and Canadian double-blind, placebo-controlled, parallel group RCTs of PPF in AD and VaD (Kittner *et al.*, 1997; Mielke *et al.*, 1998; Pischel, 1998; Kittner, 1999). Most studies included patients with mild-to-moderate VaD according to NINDS-AIREN criteria. Significant symptomatic improvement and long-term efficacy in ADAS-Cog and CIBIC-plus were noted up to 48 weeks of treatment compared to placebo. Sustained treatment effects for at least 12 weeks after withdrawal suggested an effect on disease progression (Pischel, 1998; Rother *et al.*, 1998). Despite these positive results, the clinical development of PPF was halted in 2000.

63.5.8.3 DENBUFYLLINE

Denbufylline, a xanthine derivative and PDE4 inhibitor, has effects such as vasodilatation of cerebral vessels (Willette *et al.*, 1997) and potent activation of the hypothalamo–pituitary–adrenal axis. PDE4 is one of the cyclic AMP (cAMP) specific phosphodiesterases whose tissue distribution is important in pathologies related to the central nervous and immune systems. In the experimental animal, denbufylline increases ACTH, circulating corticosterone, luteinizing hormone, corticotrophin-releasing hormone, and cAMP content of the hypothalamic tissue, but is without effect on arginine vasopressin (Kumari *et al.*, 1997). Treves and Korczyn (1999) studied a group of patients with AD, mixed dementia and

VaD treated with denbufylline. No significant differences were found in comparison with placebo for the treatment of AD or VaD, although patients who received denbufylline tended to improve their cognitive scores.

63.5.9 Vasodilators

Yesavage and colleagues (1979) reviewed 102 studies from the literature on the use of vasodilating agents in senile dementias; the postulated effect of these agents was to counteract 'hardening of the arteries'. Recommendations for most of these agents were based on trials invalidated by the small number of participants, short open treatment periods, and variations in diagnostic criteria and clinical end points. In 1979, Cochrane himself strongly criticized the poor quality of the evidence thus obtained.

The principal pharmacological agents with primary effect on smooth muscle resulting in vasodilatation include cyclandelate, papaverine, isoxsuprine, cinnarizine and nafronyl. No significant effects have been demonstrated with the use of vasodilating agents in VaD (Cook and James, 1981).

Nicotinic acid (niacin), used for many years for its vasodilating properties, has received renewed attention due to its effects in the treatment of primary hypercholesterolaemia and mixed dyslipidaemia. Nicotinic acid is the only drug that primarily lowers concentrations of non-sterified fatty acids and thereby lowers very low density lipoprotein (VLDL) triglycerides. Nicotinic acid also seems to improve insulin resistance and to stimulate cholesterol mobilization from macrophages, offering an avenue for regression of the vascular lesions of atherosclerosis (Karpe and Frayn, 2004).

63.5.10 Ergot derivatives

The main ergot derivatives used for the treatment of VaD are nicergoline and codergocrine or ergoloid mesylates – a mixture (in a 3:3:2:1 ratio) of four dehydrogenated mesylated ergot peptide derivatives, dihydroergocornine, dihydroergocristine, dihydro-α-ergocryptine, and dihydro-β-ergocryptine (Wadworth and Chrisp, 1992).

63.5.10.1 ERGOLOID MESYLATES

The metabolic effects of ergoloid mesylates are incompletely understood; however, enhancement of noradrenergic, dopaminergic and serotoninergic neurotransmission (Weil, 1988) and reduction of free radical formation (Favit *et al.*, 1995) have been proposed. Schneider and Olin (1994) reviewed 151 reports on the use of ergoloid mesylates (Hydergine) in senile dementia, but only 47 of these trials (31 per cent) met strict criteria for meta-analysis. The review by Schneider and Olin (1994) and a subsequent Cochrane report (Olin *et al.*, 2001) confirmed that patients with VaD appeared to benefit more from Hydergine than patients with AD in terms of cognition, clinical global ratings and combined measures. However, compared with placebo, efficacy was very modest, and there are at present no grounds to recommend its use.

63.5.10.2   NICERGOLINE

Nicergoline is an ergot derivative used for the treatment of cognitive, affective and behavioural disorders of the elderly. Although initially considered a vasoactive drug indicated for CVD, nicergoline appears to have protective effects against degeneration of cholinergic neurones (Giardino et al., 2002). Nicergoline has a broad spectrum of action (Winblad et al., 2008): (1) as α1-adrenoceptor antagonist, it induces vasodilatation and increases arterial blood flow; (2) enhances cholinergic and catecholaminergic neurotransmission; (3) inhibits platelet aggregation; (4) promotes metabolic activity, resulting in increased utilization of oxygen and glucose; and (5) has neurotrophic and anti-oxidant properties.

Nicergoline has been used for the treatment of various forms of dementia, including AD and VaD (Fioravanti and Flicker, 2001). The therapeutic effects of nicergoline were evident by two months of treatment and were maintained for 6–12 months. Cognitive assessment (MMSE) was performed in 261 patients. The difference between treatment and control groups on the MMSE favoured nicergoline; at 12 months, the effect size was 2.86. Herrmann and colleagues (1997) conducted a double-blind placebo-controlled RCT involving 136 MID patients. After six months of treatment, the nicergoline group was significantly better than the placebo group. Another placebo-controlled pilot study by Bes and colleagues (1999), recruited 72 elderly hypertensive patients with VCI and evidence of leukoaraiosis, randomly assigned to either nicergoline ($n = 36$) or placebo ($n = 36$) for 24 months. Nicergoline (30 mg twice a day for 24 months) was well tolerated and attenuated the cognitive decline of elderly hypertensive patients. A recent review of clinical trials by Winblad et al. (2008) showed that up to 89 per cent of patients treated with nicergoline 30 mg twice daily showed improvements in cognition and behaviour; patients remained stable after 12 months of treatment. Nicergoline has a favourable safety and tolerability profile.

63.5.10.3   POSATIRELIN

Posatirelin is a thyrotropin-releasing hormone (TRH) analogue. In an experimental model of brain cholinergic deficit in the rat by lesion of the nucleus basalis magnocellularis (nbM), posatirelin treatment was shown to rescue cholinergic neurons of the nbM and their cholinergic projections to the cerebral cortex (Sabbatini et al., 1998). Posatirelin has been used in patients with AD and VaD (Parnetti et al., 1995; Parnetti et al., 1996). VaD patients treated with posatirelin showed significant improvements in intellectual performance, orientation, motivation and memory, as compared to controls. The drug was well tolerated.

63.5.11   Antithrombotic agents

Antiplatelet drugs effectively prevent TIAs and ischaemic stroke (Easton, 2003). Aspirin provides a relative reduction of 19 per cent in the rate of major vascular events in patients with arterial disease in general, and 13 per cent in patients with ischaemic CVD (van Gijn and Algra, 2003). Other antiplatelet agents, such as sulfinpyrazone, ticlopidine, clopidogrel, dipyridamole, and orally administered IIb/IIIa inhibitors, have similar effects, although the combination of aspirin and dipyridamole may be more efficacious than aspirin alone. The Antithrombotic Trialists' Collaboration (Easton, 2003) assessed the effect of antiplatelet therapy in 135 000 patients. Antiplatelet therapy reduces the combined odds of stroke, myocardial infarction or vascular death by 22 per cent, and antiplatelet agents reduce the odds of a nonfatal stroke by 25 per cent in patients with or without a history of stroke. Likewise, among patients with nonvalvular AF, anticoagulation (INR $\geq$ 2.0) reduces not only the frequency and severity, but also the mortality of ischaemic stroke (Hart, 2003; Hylek et al., 2003).

63.5.11.1   ASPIRIN

A population-based study by Sturmer and colleagues (1996) showed that aspirin (ASA) users have a slight protection against cognitive decline (OR = 0.97 to 0.87). A single randomized trial used ASA (325 mg daily) in patients with mild MID-type of VaD (Meyer et al., 1989). Cognitive tests and CBF were performed at onset and one year later. Stabilization or mild improvement was seen in the active group compared with untreated controls. However, a Cochrane review (Williams et al., 2000) concluded that there is no evidence that aspirin is effective in treating patients with VaD.

63.5.11.2   TRIFLUSAL

Triflusal is an antiplatelet agent structurally related to the salicylates, but it is not derived from ASA. Triflusal and its active metabolite (3-hydroxy-4-trifluoro-methylbenzoic acid or HTB) produce specific inhibition of platelet arachidonic acid metabolism (McNeely and Goa, 1998). A single open-label 12-month trial of triflusal in 73 patients with VaD (López-Pousa et al., 1997) showed fewer declines in MMSE scores in the active group compared with the untreated subjects. More recently, triflusal was used in patients with amnesic MCI, 257 patients were randomized to receive 900 mg of triflusal or placebo for 18 months. Triflusal therapy was associated with a significantly lower rate of conversion to dementia (Gómez-Isla et al., 2008).

63.5.11.3   GINKGO

Ginkgo, extract EGb 761 from the *Ginkgo biloba* tree, has been widely used in several European countries and in North America for the treatment of 'chronic cerebral circulatory insufficiency' (Kleijnen and Knipschild, 1992; Gertz and Kiefer, 2004). Ginkgo biloba extracts are considered to have vasodilating and anti-oxidant properties, as well as haemorheological and nootropic effects, and to decrease platelet aggregability and blood viscosity, but the mechanism of action remains poorly understood (Zimmermann et al., 2002; Gertz and Kiefer, 2004). Several trials have used ginkgo in patients with MID or with AD plus CVD, with modest positive results (Le Bars et al., 1997; Kanowski and Hoerr, 2003; van Dongen et al., 2003). Using Cochrane data, Kurz and Van Baelen (2004) showed significant benefit versus placebo with ginkgo treatment only when all doses were pooled, although the effects appeared to be minimal. Ginkgo treatment in the elderly has been associated with subarachnoid haemorrhage and other haemorrhagic complications, such as subdural haematoma, intracranial and intraocular bleeding (Vale, 1998; Fong and Kinnear, 2003; Meisel et al., 2003). Snitz et al. (2009) conducted the Ginkgo Evaluation of Memory (GEM) trial and concluded that compared with placebo, the use of G. biloba, 120 mg twice daily, did not prevent cognitive decline in older adults with normal cognition or with MCI. A recent review by Brown et al. (2010) emphasized that the mild therapeutic results obtained with ginkgo should be tempered by the potential side effects.

63.5.11.4 CHOTO–SAN

Choto-san (Gouteng-san) is a Japanese (Kampo) herbal medicine with apparent neuroprotective effect against glutamate-induced neuronal death (Itoh et al., 1999; Watanabe et al., 2003). Choto-san was administered for 12 weeks to ten patients with post-stroke VCI; P3 event-related brain potentials, MMSE, and verbal fluency tests significantly improved with treatment (Yamaguchi et al., 2004). In a larger trial, Choto-san improved ADLs, global rating and subjective and psychiatric symptoms (Itoh et al., 1999).

63.5.11.5 JIANNAO YIZHI

Zhang and colleagues (2002) evaluated the safety and efficiency of Jiannao yizhi, a Chinese herbal medicine, in the treatment of VaD. A multicentre, double-blind, placebo-controlled RCT studied 242 patients with mild to moderate VaD; 89 cases were randomized to the active group (Jiannao yizhi granules), 106 cases to the western medicine group and 47 to the placebo group. MMSE and Blessed dementia scale were used to evaluate the therapeutic effect after 60 days of therapy. Treatment with Jiannao yizhi was superior to western medicine and to placebo.

63.5.11.6 VINPOCETINE

Vinpocetine is a synthetic ethyl ester of apovincamine, a vinca alkaloid. For many years, vinpocetine has been used for the treatment of cognitive impairment, but the mechanism of action remains unclear (Szatmari and Whitehouse, 2003). A Cochrane review of three short-term studies involving 583 patients with dementia (AD, VaD, mixed) treated with vinpocetine or placebo, concluded that patients treated with vinpocetine (30–60 mg/day) showed modest benefit compared to placebo (Szatmari and Whitehouse, 2003).

63.5.11.7 DEHYDROEPIANDROSTERONE

Dehydroepiandrosterone (DHEA) is a weakly androgenic adrenal steroid and an intermediary in the biosynthesis of androgens and oestrogens. Small quantities of DHEA are produced in the brain (Knopman and Henderson, 2003). DHEA or its sulphate ester metabolite dehydroepiandrosterone sulphate (DHEAS) is the most abundant circulating steroid and declines in serum and CSF with age. Bicikova and colleagues (2004) suggest that variations in levels of these neurohormones could discriminate between AD and VaD. However, Kim et al. (2003) observed that DHEAS levels in the CSF were significantly decreased in both AD and VaD.

DHEA is classified as a dietary supplement; its effect on dementia could result from a direct action, or through testosterone, oestradiol and other metabolites. However, there is no association between DHEAS levels and duration or severity of symptoms in AD. Wolkowitz and coworkers (2003) conducted a six-month, double-blind RCT of DHEA for AD. A modest improvement was seen with DHEA, but increasing confusion, agitation and paranoid reactions were seen among DHEA-treated participants. A high dropout may have compromised the study. DHEA alone seems unlikely to be superior to currently available ChEIs for AD. A single open-label trial of DHEA in the MID type of VaD (Azuma et al., 1999) used intravenous DHEAS (200 mg/day) for 4 weeks; the treatment markedly increased serum and CSF levels of DHEAS in seven MID patients, but improvement of ADL and emotional disturbances was seen in only three patients.

63.5.12 Cerebrolysin

Cerebrolysin is a peptidergic drug produced from purified porcine brain proteins, with postulated neurotrophic activity (Windisch, 2000; Windisch et al., 1998) and probable neuroprotective effects (Rockenstein et al., 2003). A small open-label trial in patients with AD and VaD (Rainer et al., 1997) showed minimal improvement in cognitive tests and clinical global impression. The main side effects are nausea and vertigo. A recent review by Plosker and Gauthier (2009) emphasized the need for further clinical trials in AD and VaD.

63.5.13 Sulodexide

Sulodexide is a glycosaminoglycan with effects on plasma viscosity by lowering plasma fibrinogen concentrations (Lunetta and Salanitri, 1992). Sulodexide differs from other glycosaminoglycans, like heparin, by having a longer half-life, reduced effect on systemic clotting and bleeding, and increased lipolytic activity. Oral administration of sulodexide results in the release of tissue plasminogen activator and an increase in fibrinolytic activities. Sulodexide is effective and well tolerated in peripheral occlusive arterial disease with claudication (Shustov, 1997) and diabetic nephropathy (Vilayur and Harris, 2009). Parnetti and colleagues (1997) conducted a trial of sulodexide in patients that fulfilled NINDS-AIREN criteria for probable VaD; 46 patients were included in the active treatment group, compared with 40 in the pentoxifylline group. Larger reductions of plasma fibrinogen levels were seen with sulodexide, and both groups showed a slight reduction in activated factor VII levels. Dementia scores improved more in the sulodexide group.

63.5.14 Thrombin inhibitors

Hypercoagulable states could result in increased risk of dementia (Mari *et al.*, 1996). Bots and colleagues (1998) from the Dutch Vascular Factors in Dementia Study in Rotterdam found that dementia, particularly post-stroke VaD, was associated with increased thrombin generation. In this population, increased levels of thrombin–antithrombin complex (TAT), cross-linked D-dimer and tissue-type plasminogen activator (tPA) activity were associated with increased risk of dementia. In addition, coagulation abnormalities have been described in patients with BD. Schneider and colleagues (1987) found increased fibrinogen levels and hyperviscosity in patients with BD. Iwamoto *et al.* (1995) demonstrated increased platelet activation in BD that was manifested by increased plasma β-thromboglobulin levels. Tomimoto *et al.* (Tomimoto *et al.*, 1999; Tomimoto *et al.*, 2001) found coagulation activation leading to hypercoagulable state in Japanese patients with BD; levels of fibrinogen, TAT complex, prothrombin fragment 1+2, and D-dimer were found to be significantly increased, particularly in patients with recent aggravation of their deficits.

There are no controlled clinical trials in BD, but the above results point toward several potential therapeutic options (Román, 1999a). Iwamoto *et al.* (1995) reported that the use of ticlopidine hydrochloride in eight patients with BD resulted in lower levels of platelet activation, without major clinical change. There is a need for controlled trials of ticlopidine and other antiplatelet agents, such as aspirin, dipyridamole and clopidogrel, alone or in combination, in BD.

Hyperfibrinogenaemia has deleterious effects on haemorheological conditions in the cerebral microcirculation that result in hyperviscosity and slowing of blood flow in deep border-zone territories in BD. Therefore, the use of medications, such as pentoxifylline ancrod (Sherman, 2002) or bezafibrate (Tanne *et al.*, 2001) to lower fibrinogen levels could be indicated.

63.5.14.1 ANCROD

Ancrod, a defibrinating enzyme (Sherman, 2002), was used by Ringelstein *et al.* (1988) in ten patients with BD. Treatment with subcutaneous ancrod decreased plasma levels of fibrinogen from 3.26 g/L (SD 1.3) prior to treatment (normal 2.5–4.0 g/L), to 1.52 g/L (SD 0.53) after one month of therapy. Treatment improved retinal arteriovenous circulation time (abnormally slow prior to treatment) and increased CO_2-induced cerebral vasomotor response by transcranial Doppler. However, clinical condition and neuropsychological tests were unchanged, and there was no decrease in stroke recurrences over six months.

63.5.14.2 ARGATROBAN

In 1968, Walsh (Walsh, 1968; Walsh *et al.*, 1978) observed improved dementia symptoms with a treatment based on warfarin anticoagulation. Direct thrombin inhibitors are equally effective; they inhibit fibrin-bound thrombin, produce a predictable anticoagulant response that is unaffected by platelet factor 4, and require no long-term monitoring and no dose adjustment (Weitz and Crowther, 2002; Donnan *et al.*, 2004). There are three parenteral direct thrombin inhibitors, hirudin, bivalirudin and argatroban, and one oral agent, ximelagatran (Francis *et al.*, 2003; Schulman *et al.*, 2003).

Argatroban was successfully used by Akiguchi and colleagues (1999) for the treatment of a Japanese patient with BD with antiphospholipid antibody syndrome, and a hypercoagulable state with abnormally high levels of TAT and fibrinogen. A long-term therapeutic regimen with argatroban (20 mg i.v. daily for 28 days), improved gait disturbances and mental dysfunction. Argatroban reduced TAT and improved levels of fibrinogen and other coagulation markers to normal limits. Kario *et al.* (1999) also reported similar positive effects with the use of argatroban in reducing silent ischaemic strokes in a patient with VaD.

63.6.14.3 HEPARIN–MEDIATED EXTRACORPOREAL LDL/FIBRINOGEN PRECIPITATION

Since 1993, Walzl (Walzl, 1993; Walzl, 2000) has developed a haemorheological treatment called HELP (heparin-mediated extracorporeal LDL/fibrinogen precipitation) to reduce elevated fibrinogen levels and increased lipid fractions, to control hyperviscosity of plasma and whole blood, and to reduce aggregability or sludging of red blood cells. HELP was used in 141 patients with the MID type of VaD. Laboratory and clinical evaluations were performed before and after treatment. Each HELP treatment reduced whole blood and plasma viscosity and red cell transit time. Total cholesterol, low-density lipoproteins and triglycerides were reduced significantly. Neurological improvement was documented by improved scores in MMSE, Mathew scale and ADL.

63.5.15 Hyperbaric oxygen treatment

Vila *et al.* (1999) reported on the use of hyperbaric oxygen treatment (HOT) in four patients with BD. Patients received daily sessions of HOT at 2.5 atmospheres absolute (ATA) for 45 minutes, for a total of ten days. Controls received room air at 1.1 ATA. The procedure was well tolerated. After active treatment, noticeable improvements in gait, urinary symptoms and cognitive tests were observed in all subjects, with increase in independence. This improvement persisted for up to five months, after which the previous deficits reappeared, but responded again to repeated HOT treatment. Despite the promise of the method, there has been no independent confirmation of the benefits of HOT in BD (Román, 1999b).

63.5.16 Sphenopalatine ganglion stimulation

The sphenopalatine ganglion (SPG) is the source of parasympathetic innervation to the anterior cerebral circulation. Animal studies have demonstrated that electrical stimulation of SPG neurones leads to profound ipsilateral increase in CBF, augmenting tissue perfusion (Henninger and Fisher, 2007; Khurana *et al.*, 2009). This method was successfully used in the treatment of acute stroke in ImPACT-I, a prospective, multinational, open-label, pilot study, that evaluated the safety and effectiveness of SPG-stimulation using the Ischemic Stroke System (ISS) and culminated with promising results leading to an ongoing pivotal trial, ImPACT-24.

Based on those results, an ongoing pilot study investigated the safety, tolerability and effectiveness of the ISS in the treatment of small vessel ischaemic subcortical vascular disease and dementia (SIVD). The ISS includes a 1-inch long implant, the implantable neurostimulator (INS). The INS is implanted to all patients through the greater palatine canal, in a minimally invasive, oral procedure under local anaesthesia. Study patients are unilaterally implanted with the INS and treated daily for up to 90 days. Treatment is expected to augment CBF, improve cerebral perfusion, and halt cognitive deterioration and progression of WML. The study end points include safety, CBF and WML progression by positron emission tomography (PET) and MRI; cognitive functions are assessed by a tests including MMSE, V-ADAS-cog and the Luria Hand Test with assessments at baseline, 45 and 90 days. Preliminary results in the first ten patients (Alladi *et al.*, 2009) confirmed significant increase in CBF ipsilateral to the stimulated side and in the contralateral cerebellum by fluorodeoxy-glucose (FDG) PET scan, along with significant improvement in attention, orientation, memory, ability to execute verbal commands and executive function (Alladi *et al.*, 2009). Results of a large, double-blind trial are awaited.

63.6 GENERAL MEDICAL MANAGEMENT OF THE PATIENT WITH VAD

Epidemiological studies have confirmed the increased risk of dementia associated with vascular risk factors, in particular HT. Other important risk factors, include diabetes mellitus, raised homocysteine and smoking (see Chapter 60, Vascular factors and Alzheimer's disease; Chapter 61, What is vascular cognitive impairment? and Chapter 62, The neuropathology of vascular dementia). These vascular risk factors increase the risk of both VaD and AD. Other than the ApoE gene, other genetic and racial factors are probably important. In Alabama, Zamrini and colleagues (2004a) showed that blacks had higher rates of HT than whites, whereas whites had a higher incidence of AF, coronary artery disease and higher cholesterol. Therefore, primary and secondary prevention of stroke and CVD appears to be mandatory for the prevention of dementia (Lechner, 1998; Erkinjuntti and Gauthier, 2002; O'Brien *et al.*, 2003). There are clear guidelines for the use of anticoagulants (Hart, 2003) and antiplatelet medication in the prevention of stroke (Elkind, 2004). The reader is referred to the Guidelines for Primary Stroke Prevention of the American Heart Association and the American Stroke Association Stroke Council (Goldstein *et al.*, 2006).

63.6.1 Treatment of hypertension

Treatment of HT protects against cognitive decline even in the absence of stroke (Forette *et al.*, 1998; Clarke, 1999;

Forette *et al.*, 2002). No deleterious effects on cognition, mood and quality of life have been demonstrated with the treatment of HT in the elderly (Applegate *et al.*, 1994; Prince *et al.*, 1996; Starr *et al.*, 1996; Prince, 1997). On the contrary, Forette and collaborators (2002) confirmed that treatment of systolic hypertension with nitrendipine, a calcium channel blocker, protects against dementia in older patients. Compared with placebo, long-term antihypertensive therapy reduced the risk of dementia by 55 per cent, from 7.4 to 3.3 cases per 1000 patient-years. After adjustment for sex, age, education and entry BP, the relative hazard rate associated with the use of nitrendipine was 0.38 (95 per cent CI, 0.23–0.64; $p < 0.001$). Treatment of 1000 patients for five years can prevent 20 cases of dementia (95 per cent CI, 7–33) (Forette *et al.*, 1998; Forette *et al.*, 2002). The most appropriate levels of BP control remain undecided. The results of the ongoing SPS3 study should help solve this issue (Benavente, 2003).

The SCOPE confirmed that treatment of mild to moderate HT in the elderly prevents stroke and dementia (Lithell *et al.*, 2003). SCOPE enrolled 4964 patients aged 70–89 years, with systolic BP of 160–179 mmHg and/or diastolic blood pressure of 90–99 mmHg, and an MMSE score ≥ 24; patients were treated with candesartan, an angiotensin-receptor blocker, or with placebo, plus open-label active antihypertensive therapy added as needed. Blood pressure reduction was slightly better with candesartan therapy, compared with control therapy; this was associated with a modest, statistically non-significant, reduction in major cardiovascular events and with a marked reduction in non-fatal stroke. Cognitive function was well maintained in both treatment groups in the presence of substantial BP reductions. Current guidelines (JNC7) should be consulted for the recommend antihypertensive treatments (Chobanian *et al.*, 2003).

Finally, control of HT in patients with stroke (secondary prevention) is also helpful in preventing dementia. The PROGRESS trial (2001), a RCT of perindopril, an angiotensin-converting enzyme (ACE) inhibitor, and a diuretic (indapamide) used in 6105 individuals with previous stroke or TIA, showed that after a 3.9-year follow up, BP was reduced, lowering the risks of stroke and other major vascular events. Dementia was decreased too, with a relative risk reduction of 12 per cent (Tzourio *et al.*, 2003). Cognitive decline occurred in 9.1 per cent of the actively treated group and 11.0 per cent of the placebo group (risk reduction, 19 per cent).

63.6.2 Treatment of hyperlipidaemia with statins

The most recent recommendations for the management of hyperlipidaemia suggest a reduction of low-density lipoprotein (LDL) cholesterols to below 100 mg/dL, and drug therapy for high-risk patients whose LDL ranges from 100 to 129 mg/dL (Grundy *et al.*, 2004). High-risk patients have coronary heart disease or peripheral vascular disease in the extremities or the vessels to the brain, or diabetes, or multiple (two or more) risk factors that give them a greater than 20 per cent chance of having a heart attack within ten years. Very high-risk patients are those who have cardiovascular disease together with either multiple risk factors (especially diabetes), or severe and poorly controlled risk factors, or metabolic syndrome (a constellation of risk factors associated with obesity including high triglycerides and low high-density lipoprotein (HDL)). Patients hospitalized for acute coronary syndromes or strokes are at very high risk (Grundy *et al.*, 2004).

There are indications that the use of statins can reduce the risk of dementia (Jick *et al.*, 2000; Rockwood *et al.*, 2002; Zamrini *et al.*, 2004b). In Boston, Jick and colleagues (2000) studied 284 patients with dementia and 1080 controls older than 50 years of age; the adjusted relative risk for those prescribed statins was 0.29 (95 per cent CI, 0.13–0.63; $p = 0.002$) indicating a substantially lowered risk of developing dementia, independent of the presence or absence of untreated hyperlipidaemia. Furthermore, between 1997 and 2001, Zamrini and coworkers (2004b) conducted a study of veterans in Birmingham, AL, USA; patients with a new diagnosis of AD ($n = 309$) were compared with age-matched non-AD controls ($n = 3088$). In this group, statin users had a 39 per cent lower risk of AD relative to non-statin users (odds ratio 0.61, 95 per cent CI 0.42–0.87). These results indicate a possible antidementia effect of statins, perhaps related to anti-inflammatory effects. However, the use of statins in non-demented, non-hyperlipidaemic patients cannot be recommended yet (Miller and Chacko, 2004).

63.6.3   Control of diabetes

Abnormalities in carbohydrate, lipid and protein metabolism resulting from diabetes mellitus produce injury of blood vessels, nerves and other tissues. Diabetes increases up to four-fold the relative risk for cardiovascular and CVD due to vascular complications. Diabetes produces cognitive decline with doubling of the overall risk of dementia (see Chapter 60, Vascular factors and Alzheimer's disease; Chapter 61, What is vascular cognitive impairment? and Chapter 62, The neuropathology of vascular dementia).

Diabetes increases blood viscosity via hyperglycaemia, endothelial oxidative damage, loss of NO-mediated endothelial functions, and alterations of the BBB (Moordian *et al.*, 1997). The result is the impairment of perfusion through the cerebral and retinal microcirculation. In addition, stress-activated pathways such as the Jun-kinases play a major role in diabetic microangiopathy (Evans *et al.*, 2002). The most current guidelines for treatment are the 2004 American Diabetes Association Clinical Practice Recommendations and those of the U.S.A. Veterans Hospitals (Pogach *et al.*, 2004).

63.6.4   Cessation of smoking

Smokers double the risk of coronary artery disease, congestive heart failure, and peripheral vascular disease, and increase 1.5 times the risk of stroke and dementia (see Chapter 60, Vascular factors and Alzheimer's disease; Chapter 61, What is vascular cognitive impairment? and Chapter 62, The neuropathology of vascular dementia). Smoke, in addition to nicotine and carbon monoxide, contains a complex mixture of free radicals including quinone/hydroquinone, NO and NO_2 that cause morphological irregularities of the endothelium, formation of blebs, leakage of macromolecules and increased endothelial cell death (Pittilo, 2000). Smoke reduces prostacyclin release, enhances endothelium-derived vasodilatation and decreases nitric oxide concentrations and cGMP production, increasing aggregation of platelets and leukocytes. Smoking worsens atheromatous plaque formation, increases HT, blood coagulability, serum viscosity and fibrinogen. Smokers have worse cognitive performances than non-smokers, including reduced psychomotor speed and reduced cognitive flexibility. This effect is observed in subjects as young as 45 years (Kalmijn *et al.*, 2002).

63.6.5   Diet

Dietary change with reduced sodium intake is a crucial component of the treatment of HT. The Dietary Approaches to Stop HT (DASH) diet, rich in magnesium, potassium, calcium, protein and fibre and low in saturated fat, cholesterol and total fat (Sacks *et al.*, 2001), is recommended by the US Department of Health and Human Services. A recent clinical trial (McGuire *et al.*, 2004) randomized hypertensive patients to advice-only group; to a group treated with weight loss, increased physical activity and reduced sodium and alcohol intake; and, a third group that included the latter plus the DASH diet. At six months, compared with the advice-only group, the second group had a decline of mean systolic BP of 3.7 mmHg ($p < 0.001$) and 4.3 mmHg for the DASH diet group ($p < 0.001$). The study confirmed that HT control requires multiple lifestyle changes, including an appropriate eating plan.

Epidemiological data suggest an association between dietary factors, in particular anti-oxidants and cognition (Deschamps *et al.*, 2001). Similarities in the diets of patients with AD and VaD have been reported in Japan (Otsuka *et al.*, 2002), with higher energy intake from fats, in particular polyunsaturated fatty acids and decrease in anti-oxidant vitamins B, C and carotene. However, in the Honolulu–Asia Aging Study, mid-life intakes of anti-oxidants, such as beta-carotene, flavonoids, and vitamins E and C, did not modify the risk for late-life dementia, including AD and VaD (Laurin *et al.*, 2004); nor was any effect of fat intake in the development of dementia found in the Rotterdam study (Engelhart *et al.*, 2002).

Wald and colleagues (2002) concluded, based on evidence from genetic and prospective studies, that the association between increased homocysteine and cardiovascular disease is causal. On this basis, lowering homocysteine concentrations by 3 µmol/L from current levels (achievable by increasing folic acid intake) would reduce the risk of ischaemic heart disease (IHD) by 16 per cent (11–20 per cent), deep vein thrombosis by 25 per cent (8–38 per cent), and stroke by 24 per cent (15–33 per cent). However, meta-analysis of observational studies suggests that elevated homocysteine is at most a modest independent predictor of IHD and stroke risk in healthy populations (Homocysteine Studies Collaboration, 2002).

Moreover, folic acid/vitamin B_{12} is not an effective treatment of dementia; a Cochrane review (Malouf *et al.*, 2003) concluded that in older patients with mild to moderate cognitive decline, supplementation with 750 μg/day of folic acid, with or without B_{12}, had no beneficial effects on measures of cognition or mood, although folic acid plus vitamin B_{12} reduced serum homocysteine concentrations. A trial on the use of vitamins to prevent recurrent stroke also gave negative results (Toole *et al.*, 2004).

Nonetheless, a diet rich in anti-oxidant phytophenols appears effectively to inhibit endothelial adhesion molecule expression, explaining in part the protection from atherosclerosis afforded by Mediterranean diets (Carluccio *et al.*, 2003; Scarmeas *et al.*, 2009a; Scarmeas *et al.*, 2009b).

63.6.6   Chronic inflammation

Markers of inflammation such as C-reactive protein (CRP) are important predictors of atherosclerotic disease, particularly in patients with diabetes (Rader, 2000). Chronic infections, including periodontal disease and persistent intracellular infection with *Chlamydia pneumoniae* are associated with increased risk of vascular events (Kalayoglu *et al.*, 2002).

63.7   PUBLIC HEALTH ASPECTS OF VAD

Population ageing will lead to increasing incidence of stroke and heart disease in the near future. It is predicted that VaD will become the most common cause of senile dementia, both by itself and as a contributor to other degenerative dementias (Román, 2002d).

There is evidence that preventive measures to decrease the vascular burden on the brain may decrease VaD. VaD and AD share with stroke a number of vascular risk factors demonstrated in large epidemiological studies. The most important of the modifiable factors is HT, a treatable risk factor that explains at least half of the attributable risk of stroke. Three large controlled trials (Forette *et al.*, 1998; Forette *et al.*, 2002; Lithell *et al.*, 2003; Tzourio *et al.*, 2003) demonstrate that BP lowering significantly decreases the risk of dementia. Thus, interventions aiming at reducing the level of vascular risk factors might prevent dementia. The expected benefit of these interventions could be estimated from data provided by epidemiological studies; but there is a dearth of large population-based controlled studies to demonstrate the efficacy of preventive interventions (Román, 2003b; Alperovitch *et al.*, 2004; Williams, 2004). Prevention appears to be the most promising avenue for decreasing the incidence of the two most common forms of senile dementia, AD and VaD.

REFERENCES

Akiguchi I, Tomimoto H, Kinoshita M *et al.* (1999) Effects of antithrombin on Binswanger's disease with antiphospholipid antibody syndrome. *Neurology* 52: 398–401.

Alladi S, Panigrahi M, Tripathi M *et al.* (2009) for the Ischemic Stroke System (ISS) trial. A pilot study evaluating the safety, tolerability and effectiveness of the ischemic stroke system (ISS) for treatment of subcortical ischemic vascular disease. Barcelona: International Congress on Vascular Dementia, Abstr.

Alperovitch A, Schwarzinger M, Dufouil C *et al.* (2004) Towards a prevention of dementia. *Revue Neurologique* 160: 256–60.

Amenta F, Tomassoni D, Traini E *et al.* (2008) Nicardipine: a hypotensive dihydropyridine-type calcium antagonist with a peculiar cerebrovascular profile. *Clinical and Experimental Hypertension* 30: 808–26.

American Psychiatric Association. (1994) *Diagnostic and statistical manual of mental disorders*, 4th edn. DSM-IV. Washington DC: American Psychiatric Association.

American Psychiatric Association. (2000) *Diagnostic and statistical manual of mental disorders*, 4th edn. text revision, (DSM-IV-TR).Washington DC: American Psychiatric Association.

Applegate WB, Pressel S, Wittes J *et al.* (1994) Impact of the treatment of isolated systolic hypertension on behavioral variables. Results from the systolic hypertension in the elderly program. *Archives of Internal Medicine* 154: 2154–60.

Auchus AP, Brashear HR, Salloway S *et al.* (2007) Galantamine treatment of vascular dementia: a randomized trial. GAL-INT-26 Study Group. *Neurology* 69: 448–58.

Azuma T, Nagai Y, Saito T *et al.* (1999) The effect of dehydroepiandrosterone sulfate administration to patients with multi-infarct dementia. *Journal of the Neurological Sciences* 162: 69–73.

Ballard C, Sauter M, Scheltens P *et al.* (2008) Efficacy, safety and tolerability of rivastigmine capsules in patients with probable vascular dementia: the VantagE study. *Current Medical Research Opinion* 24: 2561–74.

Barba R, Castro MD, del Mar Morin M *et al.* (2001) Prestroke dementia. *Cerebrovascular Diseases* 11: 216–24.

Batysheva TT, Bagir LV, Kostenko EV *et al.* (2009) Experience of the out-patient use of memotropil in the treatment of cognitive disorders in patients with chronic progressive cerebrovascular disorders. *Neuroscience and Behavioral Physiology* 39: 193–7.

Baumel B, Eisner L, Karukin M *et al.* (1989) Oxiracetam in the treatment of multi-infarct dementia. *Progress in Neuropsychopharmacology and Biological Psychiatry* 13: 673–82.

Behl P, Bocti C, Swartz RH *et al.* (2007) Strategic subcortical hyperintensities in cholinergic pathways and executive function decline in treated Alzheimer patients. *Archives of Neurology* 64: 266–72.

Benavente O. (2003) Antithrombotic therapy in small subcortical strokes (lacunar infarcts). *Advances in Neurology* 92: 275–80.

Bes A, Orgogozo JM, Poncet M *et al.* (1999) A 24-month, double-blind, placebo-controlled multicentre pilot study of the efficacy and safety of nicergoline 60 mg per day in elderly hypertensive patients with leukoaraiosis. *European Journal of Neurology* 6: 313–22.

Bicikova M, Ripova D, Hill M *et al.* (2004) Plasma levels of 7-hydroxylated dehydroepiandrosterone (DHEA) metabolites and selected amino-thiols as discriminatory tools of Alzheimer's disease and vascular dementia. *Clinical Chemistry Laboratory Medicine* 42: 518–24.

Biesold D, Inanami O, Sato A, Sato Y. (1989) Stimulation of the nucleus basalis of Meynert increases cerebral cortical blood flow in rats. *Neuroscience Letters* 98: 39–44.

Black SE. (2007) Therapeutic issues in vascular dementia: Studies, designs and approaches. *Canadian Journal of Neurological Sciences* 34 (Suppl. 1): S125–30.

Black RS, Barclay LL, Nolan KA et al. (1992) Pentoxifylline in cerebrovascular dementia. *Journal of the American Geriatrics Society* 40: 237–44.

Black S, Román GC, Geldmacher DS et al. (2003) for the Donepezil 307 Vascular Dementia Study Group. Efficacy and tolerability of donepezil in vascular dementia. Positive results of a 24-week, multicenter, international, randomized, placebo-controlled clinical trial. *Stroke* 34: 2323–32.

Bosch J, Yusuf S, Pogue J et al. (2002) for the HOPE Investigators. Heart outcomes prevention evaluation. Use of ramipril in preventing stroke: double blind randomised trial. *British Medical Journal* 324: 699–702.

Bots ML, Breteler MM, van Kooten F et al. (1998) Coagulation and fibrinolysis markers and risk of dementia. The Dutch Vascular Factors in Dementia Study. *Haemostasis* 28: 216–22.

Bowler JV, Hachinski V. (1995) Vascular cognitive impairment: a new approach to vascular dementia. *Baillière's Clinical Neurology* 4: 357–76.

Brown LA, Riby LM, Reay JL. (2010) Supplementing cognitive aging: a selective review of the effects of ginkgo biloba and a number of everyday nutritional substances. *Experimental Aging Research* 36: 105–22.

Brun A. (1994) Pathology and pathophysiology of cerebrovascular dementia: pure subgroups of obstructive and hypoperfusive etiology. *Dementia* 5: 145–7.

Bruno R de B, Marques TF, Batista TM et al. (2009) Pentoxifylline treatment improves neurological and neurochemical deficits in rats subjected to transient brain ischemia. *Brain Research* 1260: 55–64.

Cacabelos R, Alvarez XA, Franco-Maside A et al. (1993) Effect of CDP-choline on cognition and immune function in Alzheimer's disease and multi-infarct dementia. *Annals of the New York Academy of Sciences* 695: 321–3.

Canadian Study of Health and Aging Working Group. (2000) The incidence of dementia in Canada. *Neurology* 55: 66–73.

Carluccio MA, Siculella L, Ancora MA et al. (2003) Olive oil and red wine antioxidant polyphenols inhibit endothelial activation: antiatherogenic properties of Mediterranean diet phytochemicals. *Arteriosclerosis, Thrombosis, and Vascular Biology* 23: 622–9.

Chan M, Lim WS, Sahadevan S. (2008) Stage-independent and stage-specific phenotypic differences between vascular dementia and Alzheimer's Disease. *Dementia and Geriatric Cognitive Disorders* 26: 513–21.

Chobanian AV, Bakris GL, Black HR et al. (2003) The Seventh Report of the Joint National Committee on Prevention, Detection, Evaluation, and Treatment of High Blood Pressure: The JNC 7 report. *Journal of the American Medical Association* 289: 2560–72.

Chui HC, Victoroff JI, Margolin D et al. (1992) Criteria for the diagnosis of ischemic vascular dementia proposed by the State of California Alzheimer's Disease Diagnostic and Treatment Centers. *Neurology* 42: 473–80.

Clarke CE. (1999) Does the treatment of isolated hypertension prevent dementia? *Journal of Human Hypertension* 13: 357–8.

Cochrane AL. (1979) Concluding remarks. In: Tognoni G, Garattini S (eds). *Treatment and prevention in cerebrovascular disorders.* Amsterdam: Elsevier, 453–5.

Cohen RA, Browndyke JN, Moser DJ et al. (2003) Long-term citicoline (cytidine diphosphate choline) use in patients with vascular dementia: neuroimaging and neuropsychological outcomes. *Cerebrovascular Diseases* 16: 199–204.

Conant R, Schauss AG. (2004) Therapeutic applications of citicoline for stroke and cognitive dysfunction in the elderly: a review of the literature. *Alternative Medicine Review* 9: 17–31.

Cook P, James I. (1981) Drug therapy: cerebral vasodilators. *New England Journal of Medicine* 305: 1508–13; 1560–4.

Cordonnier C, Hénon H, Derambure P et al. (2007) Early epileptic seizures after stroke are associated with increased risk of new-onset dementia. *Journal of Neurology Neurosurgery and Psychiatry* 78: 514–6.

Court JA, Perry EK, Kalaria RN. (2002) Neurotransmitter control of the cerebral vasculature and abnormalities in vascular dementia. In: Erkinjuntti T, Gauthier S (eds). *Vascular cognitive impairment.* London: Martin Dunitz, 167–85.

Craig D, Birks J. (2006) Galantamine for vascular cognitive impairment. *Cochrane Database of Systematic Reviews* (1): CD004746.

Cummings JL, Mega M, Gray K et al. (1994) The Neuropsychiatric Inventory. Comprehensive assessment of psychopathology in dementia. *Neurology* 44: 2308–14.

Dai W, Lopez OL, Carmichael OT et al. (2009) Mild cognitive impairment and Alzheimer disease: Patterns of altered cerebral blood flow at MR imaging. *Radiology* 250: 856–66.

Dávalos A, Castillo J, Alvarez-Sabin J et al. (2002) Oral citicoline in acute ischemic stroke: an individual patient data pooling analysis of clinical trials. *Stroke* 33: 2850–7.

De Jong GI, de Weerd H, Schuurman T et al. (1990) Microvascular changes in aged rat forebrain. Effects of chronic nimodipine treatment. *Neurobiology of Aging* 11: 381–9.

Desmond DW, Moroney JT, Bagiella E et al. (1998) Dementia as a predictor of adverse outcomes following stroke. An evaluation of diagnostic methods. *Stroke* 29: 69–74.

Dichgans M, Markus HS, Salloway S et al. (2008) Donepezil in patients with subcortical vascular cognitive impairment: a randomised double-blind trial in CADASIL. *Lancet Neurology* 7: 310–8.

Diener HC. (2009) Preventing stroke: the PRoFESS, ONTARGET, and TRANSCEND trial programs. *Journal of Hypertension* 27 (Suppl. 5) S31–6.

Diener HC, Sacco RL, Yusuf S et al. (2008) for the Prevention Regimen for Effectively Avoiding Second Strokes (PRoFESS) study group. (2008) Effects of aspirin plus extended release dipyridamole versus clopidogrel and telmisartan on disability and cognitive function after recurrent stroke in patients with ischaemic stroke in the Prevention Regimen for Effectively

Avoiding Second Strokes (PRoFESS) trial: A double-blind, active and placebo-controlled study. *Lancet Neurology* 7: 875–84.

Donnan GA, Dewey HM, Chambers BR. (2004) Warfarin for atrial fibrillation: the end of an era? *Lancet Neurology* 3: 305–8.

Dysken MW, Katz R, Stallone F, Kuskowski M. (1989) Oxiracetam in the treatment of multi-infarct dementia and primary degenerative dementia. *Journal of Neuropsychiatry and Clinical Neurosciences* 1: 249–52.

Easton D. (2003) Evidence with antiplatelet therapy and ADP-receptor antagonists. *Cerebrovascular Diseases* 16 (Suppl. 1): 20–6.

Elkind MS. (2004) Secondary stroke prevention: review of clinical trials. *Clinical Cardiology* 27 (Suppl. 2): II25–35.

Engelhart MJ, Geerlings MI, Ruitenberg A *et al.* (2002) Diet and risk of dementia: Does fat matter?: The Rotterdam Study. *Neurology* 59: 1915–21.

Erkinjuntti T, Gauthier S. (eds) (2002) *Vascular cognitive impairment.* London: Martin Dunitz.

Erkinjuntti T, Sawada T. (eds) (1999) Summary of the First International Conference on Development of Drug Treatment for Vascular Dementia, by the International Working Group on Harmonization of Dementia Drug Guidelines. October 7–9, 1998, Osaka, Japan. *Alzheimer Disease and Associated Disorders* 13 (Suppl. 3): S1–212.

Erkinjuntti T, Sawada T, Whitehouse PJ. (1999) Osaka Conference on Vascular Dementia 1998. *Alzheimer Disease and Associated Disorders* 13 (Suppl.): S1–3.

Erkinjuntti T, Inzitari D, Pantoni L *et al.* (2000) Research criteria for subcortical vascular dementia in clinical trials. *Journal of Neural Transmission* 59 (Suppl. 1): 23–30.

Erkinjuntti T, Kurz A, Gauthier S *et al.* (2002a) Efficacy of galantamine in probable vascular dementia and Alzheimer's disease combined with cerebrovascular disease: a randomized trial. *Lancet* 359: 1283–90.

Erkinjuntti T, Skoog I, Lane R, Andrews C. (2002b) Rivastigmine in patients with Alzheimer's disease and concurrent hypertension. *International Journal of Clinical Practice* 56: 791–6.

Erkinjuntti T, Kurz A, Small GW *et al.* (2003a) An open-label extension trial of galantamine in patients with probable vascular dementia and mixed dementia. *Clinical Therapeutics* 25: 1765–82.

Erkinjuntti T, Skoog I, Lane R, Andrews C. (2003b) Potential long-term effects of rivastigmine on disease progression may be linked to drug effects on vascular changes in Alzheimer brains. *International Journal of Clinical Practice* 57: 756–60.

Erkinjuntti T, Román G, Gauthier S *et al.* (2004) Emerging therapies for vascular dementia and vascular cognitive impairment. *Stroke* 35: 1010–7.

Erkinjuntti T, Gauthier S, Bullock R *et al.* (2008) Galantamine treatment in Alzheimer's disease with cerebrovascular disease: Responder analyses from a randomized, controlled trial (GAL-INT-6). *Journal of Psychopharmacology* 22: 761–8.

European Pentoxifylline Multi-Infarct Dementia Study. (1996) *European Neurology* 36: 315–21.

Evans JLK, Goldfine ID, Maddux BA, Grodsky GM. (2002) Oxidative stress and stress-activated signaling pathways: a unifying hypothesis of type 2 diabetes. *Endocrine Reviews* 23: 599–622.

Farlow MR. (2003) Update on rivastigmine. *The Neurologist* 9: 230–4.

Farlow MR. (2004) NMDA receptor antagonists. A new therapeutic approach for Alzheimer's disease. *Geriatrics* 59: 22–7.

Fogari R, Mugellini A, Zoppi A *et al.* (2006) Effect of telmisartan/hydrochlorothiazide vs. lisinopril/hydrochlorothiazide combination on ambulatory blood pressure and cognitive function in elderly hypertensive patients. *Journal of Human Hypertension* 20: 177–85.

Favit A, Sortino MA, Aleppo G *et al.* (1995) The inhibition of peroxide formation as a possible substrate for the neuroprotective action of dehydroergocryptine. *Journal of Neural Transmission* 45 (Suppl.): 297–305.

Ferris S, Gauthier S. (2002) Cognitive outcome measures in vascular dementia. In: Erkinjuntii T, Gauthier S (eds). *Vascular cognitive impairment.* London: Martin Dunitz, 395–400.

Fioravanti M, Flicker L. (2001) Efficacy of nicergoline in dementia and other age associated forms of cognitive impairment. *Cochrane Database of Systematic Reviews* (4): CD003159.

Fioravanti M, Yanagi M. (2000) Cytidinediphosphocholine (CDP choline) for cognitive and behavioural disturbances associated with chronic cerebral disorders in the elderly. *Cochrane Database of Systematic Reviews* (4): CD000269.

Flicker L, Grimley Evans G. (2001) Piracetam for dementia or cognitive impairment. *Cochrane Database of Systematic Reviews* (2): CD001011.

Fogari R, Mugellini A, Zoppi A *et al.* (2006) Effect of telmisartan/hydrochlorothiazide vs. lisinopril/hydrochlorothiazide combination on ambulatory blood pressure and cognitive function in elderly hypertensive patients. *Journal of Human Hypertension* 20: 177–85.

Folstein MF, Folstein SE, McHugh PH. (1975) Mini-mental state. A practical method for grading the cognitive state of patients for the clinician. *Journal of Psychiatric Research* 12: 189–98.

Fong KC, Kinnear PE. (2003) Retrobulbar haemorrhage associated with chronic Gingko biloba ingestion. *Postgraduate Medical Journal* 79: 531–2.

Forette F, Seux ML, Staessen JA *et al.* (1998) for the Syst-Eur investigators. Prevention of dementia in randomised double-blind placebo-controlled Systolic Hypertension in Europe (Syst-Eur) trial. *Lancet* 352: 1347–51.

Forette F, Seux ML, Staessen JA *et al.* (2002) for the Syst-Eur investigators. The prevention of dementia with antihypertensive treatment: new evidence from the Systolic Hypertension in Europe (Syst-Eur) study. *Archives of Internal Medicine* 162: 2046–52.

Francis CW, Berkowitz SD, Comp PC *et al.* (2003) for the EXULT A Study Group. Comparison of ximelagatran with warfarin for the prevention of venous thromboembolism after total knee replacement. *New England Journal of Medicine* 349: 1703–12.

Frishman WH. (2002) Are antihypertensive agents protective against dementia? A review of clinical and preclinical data. *Heart Diseases* 4: 380–6.

Gélinas I, Gauthier L, McIntyre M, Gauthier S. (1999) Development of a functional measure for persons with Alzheimer's disease: the Disability Assessment for Dementia. *American Journal of Occupational Therapy* 53: 471–81.

Gelmers HJ, Hennerici M. (1990) Effect of nimodipine on acute ischemic stroke. Pooled results from five randomized trials. *Stroke* 21 (Suppl. 12): IV81–4.

Gertz HJ, Kiefer M. (2004) Review about ginkgo biloba special extract EGb 761 (Ginkgo). *Current Pharmaceutical Design* 10: 261–4.

Giardino L, Giuliani A, Battaglia A et al. (2002) Neuro-protection and aging of the cholinergic system: a role for the ergoline derivative nicergoline (Sermion). *Neuroscience* 109: 487–97.

Gold G, Giannakopoulos P, Montes-Paixao Junior C et al. (1997) Sensitivity and specificity of newly proposed clinical criteria for possible vascular dementia. *Neurology* 49: 690–4.

Gold G, Bouras C, Canuto A et al. (2002) Clinicopathological validation study of four sets of clinical criteria for vascular dementia. *American Journal of Psychiatry* 159: 82–7.

Goldsmith DR, Scott LJ. (2003) Donepezil in vascular dementia. *Drugs and Aging* 20: 1127–36.

Goldstein LB, Adams R, Alberts MJ et al. (2006) for the American Heart Association; American Stroke Association Stroke Council. Primary prevention of ischemic stroke: A guideline from the American Heart Association/American Stroke Association Stroke Council: cosponsored by the Atherosclerotic Peripheral Vascular Disease Interdisciplinary Working Group; Cardiovascular Nursing Council; Clinical Cardiology Council; Nutrition, Physical Activity, and Metabolism Council; and the Quality of Care and Outcomes Research Interdisciplinary Working Group. *Circulation* 113: 873–923.

Gómez-Isla T, Blesa R, Boada M et al. (2008) for the TRIMCI Study Group. A randomized, double-blind, placebo controlled-trial of triflusal in mild cognitive impairment: the TRIMCI study. *Alzheimer Disease and Associated Disorders* 22: 21–9.

González-González JA, Lozano RA. (2000) Estudio sobre la tolerabilidad y efectividad del nimodipino retard en el deterioro cognitivo de origen vascular [Study of the tolerability and effectiveness of nicardipine retard in cognitive deterioration of vascular origin]. *Revista de Neurología* 30: 719–28.

Gorelick PB, Chatterjee A, Patel D et al. (1992) Cranial computed tomographic observations in multi-infarct dementia: a controlled study. *Stroke* 23: 804–11.

Gottfries CG, Bråne G, Steen G. (1982) A new rating scale for dementia syndromes. *Gerontology* 28 (Suppl. 2): 20–31.

Gottfries CG, Blennow K, Karlsson I, Wallin A. (1994) The neurochemistry of vascular dementia. *Dementia* 5: 163–7.

Green RC, Goldstein FC, Auchus AP et al. (1992) Treatment trial of oxiracetam in Alzheimer's disease. *Archives of Neurology* 49: 1135–6.

Greenberg JH, Uematsu D, Araki N et al. (1990) Cytosolic free calcium during focal cerebral ischemia and the effects of nimodipine on calcium and histological damage. *Stroke* 21 (Suppl. 2): IV72–7.

Grundy SM, Cleeman JI, Bairey Merz CN et al. (2004) for the Coordinating Committee of the National Cholesterol Education Program. Implications of recent clinical trials for the National Cholesterol Education Program Adult Treatment Panel III guidelines. *Circulation* 110: 227–39.

Grupo Español de Estudio de Nicardipino en Demencia Vascular. (1999) Ensayo clínico experimental, doblemente ciego, aleatorizado, controlado con placebo, del efecto de nicardipino en la función cognitiva en pacientes afectos de demencia vascular [Spanish group of nicardipine study in vascular dementia. An experimental, randomized, double-blind, placebo-controlled clinical trial to investigate the effect of nicardipine on cognitive function in patients with vascular dementia.] *Revista de Neurología* 28: 835–45.

Hachinski VC, Iliff LD, Zilhka E et al. (1975) Cerebral blood flow in dementia. *Archives of Neurology* 32: 632–7.

Hachinski V, Iadecola C, Petersen RC et al. (2006) National Institute of Neurological Disorders and Stroke–Canadian Stroke Network vascular cognitive impairment harmonization standards. *Stroke* 37: 2220–41.

Hanon O, Berrou JP, Negre-Pages L et al. (2008) Effects of hypertension therapy based on eprosartan on systolic arterial blood pressure and cognitive function: primary results of the Observational Study on Cognitive Function and Systolic Blood Pressure Reduction open-label study. *Journal of Hypertension* 26: 1642–50.

Hennerici MG. (2009) What are the mechanisms of post-stroke dementia? *Lancet Neurology* 8: 973–5.

Henninger N, Fisher M. (2007) Stimulating circle of Willis nerve fibers preserves the diffusion–perfusion mismatch in experimental stroke. *Stroke* 38: 2779–86.

Hénon H, Pasquier F, Durieu I et al. (1997) Preexisting dementia in stroke patients. Baseline frequency, associated factors, and outcome. *Stroke* 28: 2429–36.

Hénon H, Durieu I, Guerouaou D et al. (2001) Poststroke dementia: incidence and relationship to prestroke cognitive decline. *Neurology* 57: 1216–22.

Herrmann WM, Stephan K, Gaede K, Apeceche M. (1997) A multicenter randomized double-blind study on the efficacy and safety of nicergoline in patients with multi-infarct dementia. *Dementia and Geriatric Cognitive Disorders* 8: 9–17.

Hitzenberger G, Rameis H, Manigley C. (1998) Pharmacological properties of piracetam. *Central Nervous System Drugs* 9 (Suppl. 1): 19–27.

Holmes C, Cairns N, Lantos P, Mann A. (1999) Validity of current clinical criteria for Alzheimer's disease, vascular dementia and dementia with Lewy bodies. *British Journal of Psychiatry* 174: 45–50.

Homocysteine Studies Collaboration. (2002) Homocysteine and risk of ischemic heart disease and stroke: a meta-analysis. *Journal of the American Medical Association* 288: 2015–22.

Hurtado O, Cárdenas A, Pradillo JM et al. (2007) A chronic treatment with CDP-choline improves functional recovery and increases neuronal plasticity after experimental stroke. *Neurobiology of Disease* 26: 105–11.

Hylek EM, Go AS, Chang Y et al. (2003) Effect of intensity of oral anticoagulation on stroke severity and mortality in atrial fibrillation. *New England Journal of Medicine* 349: 1019–26.

Ingles JL, Wentzel C, Fisk JD, Rockwood K. (2002) Neuropsychological predictors of incident dementia in patients with vascular cognitive impairment, without dementia. *Stroke* 33: 1999–2002.

Itil TM, Menon GN, Songar A, Itil KZ. (1986) CNS pharmacology and clinical therapeutic effects of oxiracetam. *Clinical Neuropharmacology* 9 (Suppl. 3): S70–2.

Itoh T, Shimada Y, Terasawa K. (1999) Efficacy of Choto-san on vascular dementia and the protective effect of the hooks and stems of *Uncaria sinensis* on glutamate-induced neuronal death. *Mechanisms of Ageing and Development* 111: 155–73.

Ivan CS, Seshadri S, Beiser A *et al.* (2004) Dementia after stroke: the Framingham Study. *Stroke* 35: 1264–8.

Iwamoto T, Kubo H, Takasaki M. (1995) Platelet activation in the cerebral circulation in different subtypes of ischemic stroke and Binswanger's disease. *Stroke* 26: 52–6.

Jagust W. (2001) Untangling vascular dementia. *Lancet* 358: 2097–8.

Jagust WJ, Zheng L, Harvey DJ *et al.* (2008) Neuropathological basis of magnetic resonance images in aging and dementia. *Annals of Neurology* 63: 72–80.

Jansen I, Tfelt-Hansen P, Edvinsson L. (1991) Comparison of the calcium entry blockers nimodipine and flunarizine on human cerebral and temporal arteries: role in cerebral disorders. *European Journal of Clinical Pharmacology* 40: 7–15.

Jick H, Zornberg GL, Jick SS *et al.* (2000) Statins and the risk of dementia. *Lancet* 356: 1627–31.

Johnston SC, O'Meara ES, Manolio TA *et al.* (2004) Cognitive impairment and decline are associated with carotid artery disease in patients without clinically evident cerebrovascular disease. *Annals of Internal Medicine* 140: 237–47.

Julius S, Nesbitt SD, Egan BM *et al.* (2006) Feasibility of treating prehypertension with an angiotensin-receptor blocker. *New England Journal of Medicine* 354: 1685–97.

Khachaturian AS, Zandi PP, Lyketsos CG *et al.* (2006) Antihypertensive medication use and incident Alzheimer disease: the Cache County Study. *Archives of Neurology* 63: 686–92.

Kalaria RN, Ballard C. (1999) Overlap between pathology of Alzheimer disease and vascular dementia. *Alzheimer Disease and Associated Disorders* 13 (Suppl. 3): S115–23.

Kalaria RN, Ballard CG, Ince PG *et al.* (2001) Multiple substrates of late-onset dementia: implications for brain protection. *Novartis Foundation Symposium* 235: 49–60.

Kalayoglu MV, Libby P, Byrne GI. (2002) *Chlamydia pneumoniae* as an emerging risk factor in cardiovascular disease. *Journal of the American Medical Association* 288: 2724–31.

Kalmijn S, van Boxtel MP, Verschuren MW *et al.* (2002) Cigarette smoking and alcohol consumption in relation to cognitive performance in middle age. *American Journal of Epidemiology* 156: 936–44.

Kamei S, Oishi M, Takasu T. (1996) Evaluation of fasudil hydrochloride treatment for wandering symptoms in cerebrovascular dementia with ^{31}P-magnetic resonance spectroscopy and Xe-computed tomography. *Clinical Neuropharmacology* 19: 428–38.

Kanowski S, Hoerr R. (2003) Ginkgo biloba extract EGb 761 in dementia: intent-to-treat analyses of a 24-week, multi-center, double-blind, placebo-controlled, randomized trial. *Pharmacopsychiatry* 36: 297–303.

Kario K, Matsuo T, Hoshide S *et al.* (1999) Effect of thrombin inhibition in vascular dementia and silent cerebrovascular disease. An MR spectroscopy study. *Stroke* 30: 1033–7.

Karpe F, Frayn KN. (2004) The nicotinic acid receptor – a new mechanism for an old drug. *Lancet* 363: 1892–4.

Kavirajan H, Schneider LS. (2007) Efficacy and adverse effects of cholinesterase inhibitors and memantine in vascular dementia: A meta-analysis of randomized controlled trials. *Lancet Neurology* 6: 782–92.

Khurana D, Kaul S, Bornstein NM. (2009) for the ImpACT-1 Study Group. Implant for augmentation of cerebral blood flow trial. 1: A pilot study evaluating the safety and effectiveness of the Ischaemic Stroke System for treatment of acute ischaemic stroke. *International Journal of Stroke* 4: 480–5.

Kilander L, Nyman H, Boberg M *et al.* (1998) Hypertension is related to cognitive impairment: a 20-year follow-up of 999 men. *Hypertension* 31: 780–6.

Kim SB, Hill M, Kwak YT *et al.* (2003) Neurosteroids: Cerebrospinal fluid levels for Alzheimer's disease and vascular dementia diagnostics. *Journal of Clinical Endocrinology and Metabolism* 88: 5199–206.

Kittner B. (1999) Clinical trials of propentofylline in vascular dementia. The European/Canadian Propentofylline Study Group. *Alzheimer Disease and Associated Disorders* 13 (Suppl. 3): S166–71.

Kittner B, Rossner M, Rother M. (1997) Clinical trials in dementia with propentofylline. *Annals of the New York Academy of Sciences* 826: 307–16.

Kleijnen J, Knipschild P. (1992) Ginkgo biloba. *Lancet* 340: 1136–9.

Knopman D, Henderson VW. (2003) DHEA for Alzheimer's disease: a modest showing by a superhormone. *Neurology* 60: 1060–1.

Knopman DS, Rocca WA, Cha RH *et al.* (2003) Survival study of vascular dementia in Rochester, Minnesota. *Archives of Neurology* 60: 85–90.

Korczyn AD. (2010) Book review: Vascular cognitive impairment in clinical practice. *Journal of Neurology, Neurosurgery and Psychiatry* 81: 126.

Kumar V, Anand R, Messina J *et al.* (2000) An efficacy and safety analysis of Exelon in Alzheimer's disease patients with concurrent vascular risk factors. *European Journal of Neurology* 7: 159–69.

Kumari M, Cover PO, Poyser RH, Buckingham JC. (1997) Stimulation of the hypothalamo–pituitary–adrenal axis in the rat by three selective type-4 phosphodiesterase inhibitors: *in vitro* and *in vivo* studies. *British Journal of Pharmacology* 121: 459–68.

Kurz A, Van Baelen B. (2004) Ginkgo biloba compared with cholinesterase inhibitors in the treatment of dementia: A review based on meta-analyses by the Cochrane Collaboration. *Dementia and Geriatric Cognitive Disorders* 18: 217–26.

Lacombe P, Sercombe R, Vaucher E, Seylaz J. (1997) Reduced cortical vasodilatory response to stimulation of the nucleus basalis of Meynert in the aged rat and evidence for a control of the cerebral circulation. *Annals of the New York Academy of Sciences* 826: 410–5.

Laurin D, Masaki KH, Foley DJ *et al.* (2004) Midlife dietary intake of antioxidants and risk of late-life incident dementia: the Honolulu-Asia Aging Study. *American Journal of Epidemiology* **159**: 959–67.

Le Bars PL, Katz MM, Berman N *et al.* (1997) for the North American EGb Study Group. A placebo-controlled, double-blind, randomized trial of an extract of Ginkgo biloba for dementia. *Journal of the American Medical Association* **278**: 1327–32.

Leblanc GG, Meschia JF, Stuss DT, Hachinski V. (2006) Genetics of vascular cognitive impairment: the opportunity and the challenges. *Stroke* **37**: 248–55.

Lechner H. (1998) Status of treatment of vascular dementia. *Neuroepidemiology* **17**: 10–13.

Lee HJ, Kang JS, Kim YI. (2009) Citicoline protects against cognitive impairment in a rat model of chronic cerebral hypoperfusion. *Journal of Clinical Neurology* **5**: 33–8.

Lefebvre C, Deplanque D, Hénon H *et al.* (2006) for the SAFE II investigators. Influence of dementia on antithrombotic therapy prescribed before stroke in patients with atrial fibrillation. *Cerebrovascular Disease* **21**: 401–7.

Li L, Sengupta A, Haque N *et al.* (2004) Memantine inhibits and reverses the Alzheimer type abnormal hyperphosphorylation of tau and associated neurodegeneration. *FEBS Letters* **566**: 261–9.

Linden T, Skoog I, Fagerberg B *et al.* (2004) Cognitive impairment and dementia 20 months after stroke. *Neuroepidemiology* **23**: 45–52.

Lithell H, Hansson L, Skoog I *et al.* (2003) for the SCOPE Study Group. The Study on Cognition and Prognosis in the Elderly (SCOPE): principal results of a randomized double-blind intervention trial. *Journal of Hypertension* **21**: 875–86.

Liu CK, Miller BL, Cummings JL *et al.* (1991) A quantitative MRI study of vascular dementia. *Neurology* **42**: 138–43.

Longstreth Jr WT, Manolio TA, Arnold A *et al.* (1996) for the Cardiovascular Health Study. (1996) Clinical correlates of white matter findings on cranial magnetic resonance imaging of 3301 elderly people. *Stroke* **27**: 1274–82.

Lopez-Arrieta JM, Birks J. (2002) Nimodipine for primary degenerative, mixed and vascular dementia. *Cochrane Database of Systematic Reviews* (3): CD000147.

López-Pousa S, Mercadal-Dalmau J, Marti-Cuadros AM *et al.* (1997) Triflusal in the prevention of vascular dementia. *Revista de Neurología* **25**: 1525–8.

Lunetta M, Salanitri T. (1992) Lowering of plasma viscosity by the oral administration of the glycosaminoglycan sulodexide in patients with peripheral vascular disease. *Journal of International Medical Research* **20**: 45–53.

McGuinness B, Todd S, Passmore P, Bullock R. (2009) Blood pressure lowering in patients without prior cerebrovascular disease for prevention of cognitive impairment and dementia. *Cochrane Database of Systematic Reviews* (2): CD004034.

McGuire HL, Svetkey LP, Harsha DW *et al.* (2004) Comprehensive lifestyle modification and blood pressure control: a review of the PREMIER trial. *Journal of Clinical Hypertension* **6**: 383–90.

McKhann G, Drachman D, Folstein M *et al.* (1984) Clinical diagnosis of AD: report of the NINCDS-ADRDA Work Group under the auspices of Department of Health and Human Services Task Force on AD. *Neurology* **34**: 939–44.

McNeely W, Goa KL. (1998) Triflusal. *Drugs* **55**: 823–33.

Mak IT, Boehme P, Weglicki WB. (1992) Antioxidant effects of calcium channel blockers against free radical injury in endothelial cells. Correlation with preservation of glutathione levels. *Circulation Research* **70**: 1099–103.

Maina G, Fiori L, Torta R *et al.* (1989) Oxiracetam in the treatment of primary degenerative and multi-infarct dementia: a double-blind, placebo-controlled study. *Neuropsychobiology* **21**: 141–5.

Malouf R, Birks J. (2004) Donepezil for vascular cognitive impairment. *Cochrane Database of Systematic Reviews* (1): CD004395.

Malouf M, Grimley EJ, Areosa SA. (2003) Folic acid with or without vitamin B_{12} for cognition and dementia. *Cochrane Database of Systematic Reviews* ; (4): CD004514.

Mani RB. (2004) The evaluation of disease modifying therapies in Alzheimer's disease: a regulatory viewpoint. *Statistics in Medicine* **23**: 305–14.

Mari D, Parnetti L, Coppola R *et al.* (1996) Hemostasis abnormalities in patients with vascular dementia and Alzheimer's disease. *Thrombosis and Haemostasis* **75**: 216–8.

Martí-Massó JF, Lozano R. (1990) Nicardipine in the prevention of cerebral infarction. *Clinical Therapeutics* **12**: 344–51.

Matthews FE, Brayne C, Lowe J *et al.* (2009) Epidemiological pathology of dementia: Attributable-risks at death in the Medical Research Council Cognitive Function and Ageing Study. *PLoS Medicine* **6**: e1000180.

Messerli FH, Williams B, Ritz E. (2007) Essential hypertension. *Lancet* **370**: 591–603.

Meisel C, Johne A, Roots I. (2003) Fatal intracerebral mass bleeding associated with Ginkgo biloba and ibuprofen. *Atherosclerosis* **167**: 367.

Mendez MF, Cummings JL. (2003) *Dementia. A clinical approach.* Philadelphia: Butterworth-Heinemann, 142–6.

Mesulam M, Siddique T, Cohen B. (2003) Cholinergic denervation in a pure multi-infarct state: observations on CADASIL. *Neurology* **60**: 1183–5.

Meyer JS, Rogers RL, McClintic K *et al.* (1989) Randomized clinical trial of daily aspirin therapy in multi-infarct dementia. A pilot study. *Journal of the American Geriatrics Society* **37**: 549–55.

Mielke R, Möller H-J, Erkinjunti T *et al.* (1998) Propentofylline in the treatment of vascular dementia and Alzheimer-type dementia: overview of phase I and phase II clinical trials. *Alzheimer Disease and Associated Disorders* **12** (Suppl. 2): 29–35.

Miller LJ, Chacko R. (2004) The role of cholesterol and statins in Alzheimer's disease. *Annals of Pharmacotherapy* **38**: 91–8.

Mills EJ, Chow TW. (2003) Randomized controlled trials in long-term care residents with dementia: a systematic review. *Journal of the American Medical Directors Association* **4**: 302–7.

Möbius HJ. (2003) Memantine: update on the current evidence. *International Journal of Geriatric Psychiatry* **18** (Suppl. 1): S47–54.

Möbius HJ, Stoffler A. (2002) New approaches to clinical trials in vascular dementia: memantine in small vessel disease. *Cerebrovascular Diseases* **13** (Suppl. 2): 61–6.

Möbius HJ, Stoffler A. (2003) Memantine in vascular dementia. *International Psychogeriatrics* 15 (Suppl. 1): 207–13.

Mohs RC, Doody RS, Morris JC *et al.* (2001) A 1-year placebo-controlled preservation of function survival study of donepezil in AD patients. *Neurology* 57: 481–8.

Mondadori C. (1993) The pharmacology of the nootropics: new insights and new questions. *Behavioural Brain Research* 59: 1–9.

Mooradian AD. (1997) Central nervous system complications of diabetes mellitus-a perspective from the blood–brain barrier. *Brain Research and Brain Research Reviews* 23: 210–8.

Moretti R, Torre P, Antonello RM, Cazzato G. (2001) Rivastigmine in subcortical vascular dementia: a comparison trial on efficacy and tolerability for 12 months follow-up. *European Journal of Neurology* 8: 361–2.

Moretti R, Torre P, Antonello RM *et al.* (2002) Rivastigmine in subcortical vascular dementia: an open 22-month study. *Journal of the Neurological Sciences* 203: 141–6.

Moretti R, Torre P, Antonello RM *et al.* (2004) Rivastigmine in vascular dementia. *Expert Opinion in Pharmacotherapy* 5: 1399–410.

Moretti R, Torre P, Antonello RM *et al.* (2008) Different responses to rivastigmine in subcortical vascular dementia and multi-infarct dementia. *American Journal of Alzheimer's Disease and Other Dementias* 23: 167–76.

Moriau M, Crasborn L, Lavenne-Pardonge E *et al.* (1993) Platelet antiaggregant and rheological properties of piracetam. A pharmacodynamic study in normal subjects. *Arzneimittel-Forschung/Drug Research* 43: 110–8.

Moroney JT, Bagiella E, Desmond DW *et al.* (1996) Risk factors for incident dementia after stroke. Role of hypoxic ischemic disorders. *Stroke* 27: 1283–9.

Morris JC, Roe CM, Grant EA *et al.* (2009) Pittsburgh Compound B imaging and prediction of progression from cognitive normality to symptomatic Alzheimer disease. *Archives of Neurology* 66: 1469–75.

Nagai M, Hoshide S, Ishikawa J *et al.* (2008) Ambulatory blood pressure as an independent determinant of brain atrophy and cognitive function in elderly hypertension. *Journal of Hypertension* 26: 1636–41.

Nasreddine ZS, Phillips NA, Bedirian V *et al.* (2005) The Montreal cognitive assessment (MoCA): A brief screening tool for mild cognitive impairment. *Journal of the American Geriatric Society* 53: 695–9.

Nyenhuis DL, Gorelick PB. (2007) Diagnosis and management of vascular cognitive impairment. *Current Atherosclerosis Reports* 9: 326–32.

O'Brien JT, Erkinjuntti T, Reisberg B *et al.* (2003) Vascular cognitive impairment. *Lancet Neurology* 2: 89–98.

Ohman J, Servo A, Heiskanen O. (1991) Long-term effects of nimodipine on cerebral infarcts and outcome after aneurysmal subarachnoid hemorrhage and surgery. *Journal of Neurosurgery* 74: 8–13.

Olin J, Schneider I, Novit A, Luczak S. (2001) Hydergine for dementia. *Cochrane Database of Systematic Reviews* (2): CD000359.

Orgogozo J-M, Rigaud AS, Stoffler A *et al.* (2002) Efficacy and safety of memantine in patients with mild to moderate vascular dementia: a randomized, placebo-controlled trial (MMM 300). *Stroke* 33: 1834–9.

Otsuka M, Yamaguchi K, Ueki A. (2002) Similarities and differences between Alzheimer's disease and vascular dementia from the viewpoint of nutrition. *Annals of the New York Academy of Sciences* 977: 155–61.

Pantoni L, Carosi M, Amigoni S *et al.* (1996) A preliminary open trial with nimodipine in patients with cognitive impairment and leukoaraiosis. *Clinical Neuropharmacology* 19: 497–506.

Pantoni L, Bianchi C, Beneke M *et al.* (2000a) The Scandinavian Multi-Infarct Dementia Trial: a double-blind, placebo-controlled trial on nimodipine in multi-infarct dementia. *Journal of the Neurological Sciences* 175: 116–23.

Pantoni L, Rossi R, Inzitari D *et al.* (2000b) Efficacy and safety of nimodipine in subcortical vascular dementia: a subgroup analysis of the Scandinavian Multi-Infarct Dementia Trial. *Journal of the Neurological Sciences* 175: 124–34.

Pantoni L, del Ser T, Soglian AG *et al.* (2005) Efficacy and safety of nimodipine in subcortical vascular dementia: a randomized placebo-controlled trial. *Stroke* 36: 619–24.

Parnetti L, Ambrosoli L, Abate G *et al.* (1995) Posatirelin for the treatment of late-onset Alzheimer's disease: a double-blind multicentre study vs citicoline and ascorbic acid. *Acta Neurologica Scandinavica* 92: 135–40.

Parnetti L, Ambrosoli L, Agliati G *et al.* (1996) Posatirelin in the treatment of vascular dementia: a double-blind multicentre study vs placebo. *Acta Neurologica Scandinavica* 93: 456–63.

Parnetti L, Mari D, Abate G *et al.* (1997) Vascular dementia Italian sulodexide study (VaDISS). Clinical and biological results. *Thrombosis Research* 87: 225–33.

Parnetti L, Mignini F, Tomassoni D *et al.* (2007) Cholinergic precursors in the treatment of cognitive impairment of vascular origin: Ineffective approaches or need for re-evaluation? *Journal of the Neurological Sciences* 257: 264–9.

Pasquier F, Boulogne A, Leys D, Fontaine P. (2006) Diabetes mellitus and dementia. *Diabetes and Metabolism* 32: 403–14.

Pearce JD, Li J, Edwards MS *et al.* (2004) Differential effects of Rho-kinase inhibition on artery wall mass and remodeling. *Journal of Vascular Surgery* 39: 223–8.

Pendlebury ST, Rothwell PM. (2009) Prevalence, incidence, and factors associated with pre-stroke and post-stroke dementia: a systematic review and meta-analysis. *Lancet Neurology* 8: 1006–18.

Pepine CJ, Lambert CR. (1990) Cardiovascular effects of nicardipine. *Angiology* 41: 978–86.

Perry EK, Gibson PH, Blessed G *et al.* (1977) Neurotransmitter enzyme abnormalities in senile dementia. Choline acetyltransferase and glutamic acid decarboxylase activities in necropsy brain tissue. *Journal of the Neurological Sciences* 34: 247–65.

Peters R, Beckett N, Forette F *et al.* (2008) for the HYVET investigators. Incident dementia and blood pressure lowering in the Hypertension in the Very Elderly Trial cognitive function assessment (HYVETCOG): A double-blind, placebo controlled trial. *Lancet Neurology* 7: 683–9.

Petersen RC, Smith GE, Waring SC *et al.* (1999) Mild cognitive impairment: clinical characterization and outcome. *Archives of Neurology* **56**: 303–8.

Pfeiffer E. (1975) A short portable mental status questionnaire for the assessment of organic brain deficit in elderly patients. *Journal of the American Geriatrics Society* **23**: 433–41.

Pischel T. (1998) Long-term-efficacy and safety of propentofylline in patients with vascular dementia. Results of a 12 months placebo-controlled trial. *Neurobiology of Aging* **19** (Suppl. 4): S182.

Pittilo RM. (2000) Cigarette smoking, endothelial injury and cardiovascular disease. *International Journal of Experimental Pathology* **81**: 219–30.

Plosker GL, Gauthier S. (2009) Cerebrolysin: A review of its use in dementia. *Drugs in Aging* **26**: 893–915.

Pogach LM, Brietzke SA, Cowan Jr CL *et al.* (2004) for the VA/DoD Diabetes Guideline Development Group. Development of evidence-based clinical practice guidelines for diabetes: the Department of Veterans Affairs/Department of Defense guidelines initiative. *Diabetes Care* **27** (Suppl. 2): B82–9.

Pohjasvaara T, Leskela M, Vataja R *et al.* (2002) Post-stroke depression, executive dysfunction and functional outcome. *European Journal of Neurology* **9**: 269–75.

Pratt RD. (2002) Patient populations in clinical trials of the efficacy and tolerability of donepezil in patients with vascular dementia. *Journal of the Neurological Sciences* **203**: 57–65.

Prince MJ. (1997) The treatment of hypertension in older people and its effect on cognitive function. *Biomedicine and Pharmacotherapy* **51**: 208–12.

Prince MJ, Bird AS, Blizard RA, Mann AH. (1996) Is the cognitive function of older patients affected by antihypertensive treatment? Results from 54 months of the Medical Research Council's trial of hypertension in older adults. *British Medical Journal* **312**: 801–5.

PROGRESS Collaborative Group. (2001) Randomised trial of a perindopril-based blood-pressure-lowering regimen among 6,105 individuals with previous stroke or transient ischaemic attack. *Lancet* **358**: 1033–41.

Quinn J, Moore M, Benson DF *et al.* (2000) A videotaped CIBIC for dementia patients: Validity and reliability in a simulated clinical trial. *Neurology* **58**: 433–7.

Rader DJ. (2000) Inflammatory markers of coronary risk. *New England Journal of Medicine* **343**: 1179–82.

Rainer M, Brunnbauer M, Dunky A *et al.* (1997) Therapeutic results with Cerebrolysin in the treatment of dementia. *Wiener Medizinische Wochenschrift* **147**: 426–31.

Raji CA, Lopez OL, Kuller LH *et al.* (2009) Age, Alzheimer disease and brain structure. *Neurology* **73**: 1899–905.

Richard E, Gouw AA, Scheltens P, van Gool WA. (2010) Vascular care in patients with Alzheimer disease with cerebrovascular lesions slows progression of white matter lesions on MRI. The Evaluation of Vascular Care in Alzheimer's disease (EVA) Study. *Stroke* **41**: 544–6.

Ringelstein EB, Mauckner A, Schneider R *et al.* (1988) Effects of enzymatic blood defibrination in subcortical arteriosclerotic encephalopathy. *Journal of Neurology, Neurosurgery and Psychiatry* **51**: 1051–7.

Rockenstein E, Adame A, Mante M *et al.* (2003) The neuroprotective effects of Cerebrolysin in a transgenic model of Alzheimer's disease are associated with improved behavioral performance. *Journal of Neural Transmission* **110**: 1313–27.

Rockwood K, Wentzel C, Hachinski V *et al.* (2000) Prevalence and outcomes of vascular cognitive impairment. Vascular Cognitive Impairment Investigators of the Canadian Study on Health and Aging. *Neurology* **54**: 447–51.

Rockwood K, Kirkland S, Hogan DB. (2002) Use of lipid-lowering agents, indication bias, and the risk of dementia in community-dwelling elderly people. *Archives of Neurology* **59**: 223–7.

Román GC. (1999a) Editorial: New insight into Binswanger disease. *Archives of Neurology* **56**: 1061–2.

Román GC. (1999b) [Hyperbaric oxygenation: a promising treatment for Binswanger's disease]. *Revista de Neurología* **28**: 707.

Román GC. (2000) Perspectives in the treatment of vascular dementia. *Drugs of Today* **36**: 641–53.

Román GC. (2002a) Defining dementia: Clinical criteria for the diagnosis of vascular dementia. *Acta Neurologica Scandinavica* **178** (Suppl.): 6–9.

Román GC. (2002b) On the history of lacunes, état criblé, and the white matter lesions of vascular dementia. *Cerebrovascular Diseases* **13** (Suppl. 2): 1–6.

Román GC. (2002c) Historical evolution of the concept of dementia: a systematic review from 2000 BC to AD 2000. In: Qizilbash N, Schneider LS, Chui H *et al.* (eds). *Evidence-based dementia practice.* Oxford: Blackwell Science, 199–227.

Román GC. (2002d) Vascular dementia may be the most common form of dementia in the elderly. *Journal of the Neurological Sciences* **203**: 7–10.

Román GC. (2003a) Vascular dementia: Distinguishing characteristics, treatment, and prevention. *Journal of the American Geriatrics Society* **51** (Suppl. 5): S296–304.

Román GC. (2003b) Stroke, cognitive decline and vascular dementia: the silent epidemic of the 21st century. *Neuroepidemiology* **22**: 161–4.

Román GC. (2004) Brain hypoperfusion: a critical factor in vascular dementia. *Neurological Research* **26**: 454–8.

Román GC. (2008) Alzheimer disease research: have we forgotten the cerebrovascular circulation? *Alzheimer Disease and Associated Disorders* **22**: 1–3.

Román GC, Kalaria RN. (2006) Vascular determinants of cholinergic deficits in Alzheimer disease and vascular dementia. *Neurobiology of Aging* **27**: 1769–85.

Román GC, Royall DR. (1999) Executive control function: a rational basis for the diagnosis of vascular dementia. *Alzheimer Disease and Associated Disorders* **13** (Suppl. 3): S69–80.

Román GC, Royall DR. (2004) A diagnostic dilemma: is 'Alzheimer's dementia' Alzheimer's disease, vascular dementia, or both? *Lancet Neurology* **3**: 141.

Román GC, Tatemichi TK, Erkinjuntti T *et al.* (1993) Vascular dementia: diagnostic criteria for research studies. Report of the NINDS-AIREN International Workshop. *Neurology* **43**: 250–60.

Román GC, Sachdev P, Royall DR *et al.* (2004) Vascular cognitive disorder: a new diagnostic category updating vascular cognitive impairment and vascular dementia. *Journal of the Neurological Sciences* 226: 81–7.

Román GC, Wilkinson DG, Doody RS *et al.* (2005) Donepezil in vascular dementia: combined analysis of two large-scale clinical trials. *Dementia and Geriatric Cognitive Disorders* 20: 338–44.

Román GC, Salloway S, Black SE, *et al.* (2010) A randomized, placebo-controlled clinical trial of donepezil in vascular dementia: Differential effects by hippocampal size. *Stroke* (accepted for publication).

Rosen WG, Terry RD, Fuld PA *et al.* (1980) Pathological verification of ischemic score in differentiation of dementias. *Annals of Neurology* 7: 486–8.

Rother M, Erkinjuntti T, Roessner M *et al.* (1998) Propentofylline in the treatment of Alzheimer's disease and vascular dementia: a review of phase III trials. *Dementia and Geriatric Cognitive Disorders* 9 (Suppl. 1): 36–43.

Royall DR, Mahurin RK, Gray KF. (1992) Bedside assessment of executive cognitive impairment: the executive interview. *Journal of the American Geriatric Society* 40: 1221–6.

Sabbatini M, Coppi G, Maggioni A *et al.* (1998) Effect of lesions of the nucleus basalis magnocellularis and of treatment with posatirelin on cholinergic neurotransmission enzymes in the rat cerebral cortex. *Mechanisms of Ageing and Development* 104: 183–94.

Sachdev P. (1999) Vascular cognitive disorder. *International Journal of Geriatric Psychiatry* 14: 402–3.

Sacks FM, Svetkey LP, Vollmer WM *et al.* (2001) for the DASH-Sodium Collaborative Research Group. Effects on blood pressure of reduced dietary sodium and the Dietary Approaches to Stop Hypertension (DASH) diet. *New England Journal of Medicine* 344: 3–10.

Sakurada T, Alufuzoff I, Winblad B, Nordberg A. (1990) Substance P-like immunoreactivity, choline acetyltransferase activity and cholinergic muscarinic receptors in Alzheimer's disease and multi-infarct dementia. *Brain Research* 521: 329–32.

Salloway S, Pratt RD, Perdomo CA. (2003) for the Donepezil 307 and 308 Study Groups. A comparison of the cognitive benefits of donepezil in patients with cortical versus subcortical vascular dementia: a subanalysis of two 24-week, randomized, double-blind, placebo-controlled trials. *Neurology* 60 (Suppl. 1): A141–2.

Sakakura K, Ishikawa J, Okuno M *et al.* (2007) Exaggerated ambulatory blood pressure variability is associated with cognitive dysfunction in the very elderly and quality of life in the younger elderly. *American Journal of Hypertension* 20: 720–7.

Samlaska CP, Winfield EA. (1994) Clinical review: Pentoxifylline. *Journal of the American Academy of Dermatology* 30: 603–21.

Saver JL. (2008) Citicoline. Update on a promising and widely available agent for neuroprotection and neurorepair. *Reviews in Neurological Diseases* 5: 167–77.

Savva GM, Stephan BCM. (2010) for the Alzheimer's Society Vascular Dementia Systematic Review Group. Epidemiological studies of the effect of stroke on incident dementia: A systematic review. *Stroke* 41: e41–6.

Scarmeas N, Stern Y, Mayeux R *et al.* (2009a) Mediterranean diet and mild cognitive impairment. *Archives of Neurology* 66: 216–25.

Scarmeas N, Luchsinger JA, Schupf N *et al.* (2009b) Physical activity, diet, and risk of Alzheimer disease. *Journal of the American Medical Association* 302: 627–37.

Schneider LS, Olin JT. (1994) Overview of clinical trials of Hydergine in dementia. *Archives of Neurology* 51: 787–98.

Schneider LS, Olin JT, Doody RS *et al.* (1997) Validity and reliability of the Alzheimer's Disease Cooperative Study – Clinical global impression of change. *Alzheimer Disease and Associated Disorders* 11: S22–32.

Schneider R, Ringelstein EB, Kiesewetter H, Jung F. (1987) The role of plasma hyperviscosity in subcortical arteriosclerotic encephalopathy (Binswanger's disease). *Journal of Neurology* 234: 67–73.

Schunkert H. (2006) Pharmacotherapy for prehypertension – Mission accomplished? *New England Journal of Medicine* 354: 1742–4.

Schulman S, Wahlander K, Lundstrom T *et al.* (2003) for the THRIVE III Investigators. Secondary prevention of venous thromboembolism with the oral direct thrombin inhibitor ximelagatran. *New England Journal of Medicine* 349: 1713–21.

Secades JJ, Frontera G. (1995) CDP-choline: pharmacological and clinical review. *Methods and Findings in Experimental and Clinical Pharmacology* 17 (Suppl. B): 1–54.

Secades JJ, Lorenzo JL. (2006) Citicoline: pharmacological and clinical review, 2006 update. *Methods and Findings in Experimental and Clinical Pharmacology* 28 (Suppl. B): 1–56.

Selden NR, Gitelman DR, Salamon-Murayama N *et al.* (1998) Trajectories of cholinergic pathways within the cerebral hemispheres of the human brain. *Brain* 121: 2249–57.

Semplicini A, Maresca A, Simonella C *et al.* (2000) Cerebral perfusion in hypertensives with carotid artery stenosis: a comparative study of lacidipine and hydrochlorothiazide. *Blood Pressure* 9: 34–9.

Shader RI, Harmatz JS, Salzman C. (1974) A new scale for clinical assessment in geriatric populations: Sandoz Clinical Assessment – Geriatric (SCAG). *Journal of the American Geriatric Society* 22: 107–13.

Sha MC, Callahan CM. (2003) The efficacy of pentoxifylline in the treatment of vascular dementia: a systematic review. *Alzheimer Disease and Associated Disorders* 17: 46–54.

Shah K, Qureshi SU, Johnson M *et al.* (2009) Does use of antihypertensive drugs affect the incidence or progression of dementia? A systematic review. *American Journal of Geriatric Pharmacotherapy* 7: 250–61.

Sherman DG. (2002) Ancrod. *Current Medical Research and Opinion* 18 (Suppl. 2): S48–52.

Shustov SB. (1997) Controlled clinical trial on the efficacy and safety of oral sulodexide in patients with peripheral occlusive arterial disease. *Current Medical Research and Opinion* 13: 573–82.

Silveri MM, Dikan J, Ross AJ *et al.* (2008) Citicoline enhances frontal lobe bioenergetics as measured by phosphorus magnetic resonance spectroscopy. *NMR in Biomedicine* 21: 1066–75.

Snitz BE, O'Meara ES, Carlson MC *et al.* (2009) for the Ginkgo Evaluation of Memory (GEM) Study Investigators. Ginkgo biloba for preventing cognitive decline in older adults: a randomized trial. *Journal of the American Medical Association* 302: 2663–70.

Solerte SB, Ceresini G, Ferrari E, Fioravanti M. (2000) Hemorreological changes and overproduction of cytokines from immune cells in mild to moderate dementia of the Alzheimer's type: adverse effects on cerebromicrovascular system. *Neurobiology of Aging* 21: 271–81.

Spiegel R, Brunner C, Ermini-Funfschilling D et al. (1991) A new behavioral assessment scale for geriatric out- and in-patients: the NOSGER (Nurses' Observation Scale for Geriatric Patients). *Journal of the American Geriatrics Society* 39: 339–47.

Staekenborg SS, Koedam EL, Henneman WJP et al. (2009) Progression of mild cognitive impairment to dementia: Contribution of cerebrovascular disease compared with medial temporal lobe atrophy. *Stroke* 40: 1269–74.

Starr JM, Whalley LJ, Deary IJ. (1996) The effects of antihypertensive treatment on cognitive function: results from the HOPE study. *Journal of the American Geriatrics Society* 44: 411–5.

Sturmer T, Glynn RJ, Field TS et al. (1996) Aspirin use and cognitive function in the elderly. *American Journal of Epidemiology* 143: 683–91.

Suzuki Y, Shibuya M, Satoh S et al. (2008) Safety and efficacy of fasudil monotherapy and fasudil-ozagrel combination therapy in patients with subarachnoid hemorrhage: Sub-analysis of the post-marketing surveillance study. *Neurologia Medico-Chirurgica* 48: 241–7.

Swartz RH, Sahlas DJ, Black SE et al. (2003) Strategic involvement of cholinergic pathways and executive dysfunction: does location of white matter signal hyperintensity matter? *Journal of Stroke and Cerebrovascular Diseases* 12: 29–36.

Szatmari SZ, Whitehouse PJ. (2003) Vinpocetine for cognitive impairment and dementia. *Cochrane Database of Systematic Reviews* (1): CD003119.

Tanne D, Benderly M, Goldbourt U et al. (2001) for the Bezafibrate Infarction Prevention Study Group. A prospective study of plasma fibrinogen levels and the risk of stroke among participants in the bezafibrate infarction prevention study. *American Journal of Medicine* 111: 457–63.

Tariot PN, Farlow MR, Grossberg GT et al. (2004) for the Memantine Study Group. Memantine treatment in patients with moderate to severe Alzheimer disease already receiving donepezil: a randomized controlled trial. *Journal of the American Medical Association* 291: 317–24.

Thavichachart N, Phanthumchinda K, Chankrachang S et al. (2006) Efficacy study of galantamine in possible Alzheimer's disease with or without cerebrovascular disease and vascular dementia in Thai patients: a slow-titration regimen. *International Journal of Clinical Practice* 60: 533–40.

Thomas SJ, Grossberg GT. (2009) Memantine: a review of studies into its safety and efficacy in treating Alzheimer's disease and other dementias. *Clinical Interventions on Aging* 4: 367–77.

Tomimoto H, Akiguchi I, Wakita H et al. (1999) Coagulation activation in patients with Binswanger disease. *Archives of Neurology* 56: 1104–8.

Tomimoto H, Akiguchi I, Ohtani R et al. (2001) The coagulation-fibrinolysis system in patients with leukoaraiosis and Binswanger disease. *Archives of Neurology* 58: 1620–5.

Toole JF, Malinow MR, Chambless LE et al. (2004) Lowering homocysteine in patients with ischemic stroke to prevent recurrent stroke, myocardial infarction, and death: the Vitamin Intervention for Stroke Prevention (VISP) randomized controlled trial. *Journal of the American Medical Association* 291: 565–75.

Traber WH, Gibsen J. (1989) *Nimodipine and central nervous system function: new vistas.* Stuttgart: Schattauaer-Verlag.

Treves TA, Korczyn AD. (1999) Denbufylline in dementia: a double-blind controlled study. *Dementia and Geriatric Cognitive Disorders* 10: 505–10.

Tuokko HA, Frerichs RJ, Kristjansson B. (2001) Cognitive impairment, no dementia: concepts and issues. *International Psychogeriatrics* 13: 183–202.

Tzourio C, Anderson C, Chapman N et al. (2003) for the PROGRESS Collaborative Group. Effects of blood pressure lowering with perindopril and indapamide therapy on dementia and cognitive decline in patients with cerebrovascular disease. *Archives of Internal Medicine* 163: 1069–75.

Uchida S, Suzuki A, Kagitani F, Hotta H. (2000) Effects of age on cholinergic vasodilation of cortical cerebral blood vessels in rats. *Neuroscience Letters* 294: 109–12.

Uebelhack R, Vohs K, Zytowski M et al. (2003) Effect of piracetam on cognitive performance in patients undergoing bypass surgery. *Pharmacopsychiatry* 36: 89–93.

Ulus IH, Wurtman RJ, Mauron C, Blusztajn JK. (1989) Choline increases acetylcholine release and protects against the stimulation-induced decrease in phosphatide levels within membranes of rat corpus striatum. *Brain Research* 484: 217–27.

Umegaki H. (2010) Pathophysiology of cognitive dysfunction in older people with type 2 diabetes: Vascular changes or neurodegeneration? *Age and Ageing* 39: 8–10.

Vale S. (1998) Subarachnoid haemorrhage associated with ginkgo biloba. *Lancet* 352: 36.

van Dongen M, van Rossum E, Kessels A et al. (2003) Ginkgo for elderly people with dementia and age-associated memory impairment: a randomized clinical trial. *Journal of Clinical Epidemiology* 56: 367–76.

van Gijn J, Algra A. (2003) Aspirin and stroke prevention. *Thrombosis Research* 110: 349–53.

Vernon MW, Sorkin EM. (1991) Piracetam: An overview of its pharmacological properties and a review of its therapeutic use in senile cognitive disorders. *Drugs and Aging* 1: 17–35.

Vila JF, Balcarce PE, Abiusi GR et al. (1999) [Hyperbaric oxygenation in subcortical frontal syndrome due to small artery disorders with leukoaraiosis]. *Revista de Neurología* 28: 655–60.

Vilayur E, Harris DC. (2009) Emerging therapies for chronic kidney disease: What is their role? *Nature Reviews, Nephrology* 5: 375–83.

Vinters HV, Ellis WG, Zarow C et al. (2000) Neuropathological substrate of ischemic vascular dementia. *Journal of Neuropathology and Experimental Neurology* 59: 931–45.

Wadworth AN, Chrisp P. (1992) Co-dergocrine mesylate. A review of its pharmacodynamic and pharmacokinetic properties and therapeutic use in age-related cognitive decline. *Drugs and Aging* **2**: 153–73.

Waegemans T, Wilsher CR, Danniau A *et al.* (2002) Clinical efficacy of piracetam in cognitive impairment: a meta-analysis. *Dementia and Geriatric Cognitive Disorders* **13**: 217–24.

Wald DS, Law M, Morris JK. (2002) Homocysteine and cardiovascular disease: evidence on causality from a meta-analysis. *British Medical Journal* **325**: 1202.

Wallin A, Gottfries CG. (1990) Biochemical substrates in normal aging and Alzheimer's disease. *Pharmacopsychiatry* **23**: 37–43.

Walsh AC. (1968) Anticoagulant therapy as potentially effective method for the prevention of presenile dementia: two case reports. *Journal of the American Geriatrics Society* **16**: 472–81.

Walsh AC, Walsh BH, Melaney C. (1978) Senile-presenile dementia: follow-up data on an effective psychotherapy-anticoagulant regimen. *Journal of the American Geriatrics Society* **26**: 467–70.

Walzl M. (1993) Effect of heparin-induced extracorporeal low-density lipoprotein precipitation and bezafibrate on hemorheology and clinical symptoms in cerebral multi-infarct disease. *Haemostasis* **23**: 192–202.

Walzl M. (2000) A promising approach to the treatment of multi-infarct dementia. *Neurobiology of Aging* **21**: 283–7.

Watanabe H, Zhao Q, Matsumoto K *et al.* (2003) Pharmacological evidence for antidementia effect of Choto-san (Gouteng-san), a traditional Kampo medicine. *Pharmacology Biochemistry and Behavior* **75**: 635–43.

Weil C. (1988) *Hydergine: Pharmacologic and clinical facts.* Berlin: Springer-Verlag.

Weinstein DB, Heider JG. (1989) Protective action of calcium channel antagonists in atherogenesis and experimental vascular injury. *American Journal of Hypertension* **2**: 205–12.

Weitz JI, Crowther M. (2002) Direct thrombin inhibitors. *Thrombosis Research* **106**: V275–84.

Wentzel C, Rockwood K, MacKnight C *et al.* (2001) Progression of impairment in patients with vascular cognitive impairment without dementia. *Neurology* **57**: 714–6.

Wentzel C, Fisk JD, Rockwood K. (2002) Neuropsychological predictors of incident dementia in patients with vascular cognitive impairment, without dementia. *Stroke* **33**: 1999–2002.

Whitehouse PJ, Kittner B, Roessner M *et al.* (1998) Clinical trial designs for demonstrating disease-course-altering effects in dementia. *Alzheimer Disease and Associated Disorders* **12**: 281–94.

Wiederkehr S, Simard M, Fortin C, van Reekum R. (2008a) Comparability of the clinical diagnostic criteria for vascular dementia: a critical review. Part I. *Journal of Neuropsychiatry and Clinical Neurosciences* **20**: 150–61.

Wiederkehr S, Simard M, Fortin C, van Reekum R. (2008b) Validity of the clinical diagnostic criteria for vascular dementia: a critical review. Part II. *Journal of Neuropsychiatry and Clinical Neurosciences* **20**: 162–77.

Wilcock G, Möbius HJ, Stoffler A. and the MMM 500 group. (2002) A double-blind, placebo-controlled multicentre study of memantine in mild to moderate vascular dementia (MMM 500). *International Clinical Psychopharmacology* **17**: 297–305.

Wilkinson D, Doody R, Helme R *et al.* (2003) Donepezil in vascular dementia. A randomized, placebo-controlled study. *Neurology* **61**: 479–86.

Willette RN, Shiloh AO, Sauermelch CF *et al.* (1997) Identification, characterization, and functional role of phosphodiesterase type IV in cerebral vessels: effects of selective phosphodiesterase inhibitors. *Journal of Cerebral Blood Flow and Metabolism* **17**: 210–9.

Williams B. (2004) Protection against stroke and dementia: an update on the latest clinical trial evidence. *Current Hypertension Reports* **6**: 307–13.

Williams PS, Rands G, Orrel M, Spector A. (2000) Aspirin for vascular dementia. *Cochrane Database of Systematic Reviews* ; (4): CD001296.

Winblad B, Machado JC. (2008) Use of rivastigmine transdermal patch in the treatment of Alzheimer's disease. *Expert Opinion on Drug Delivery* **5**: 1377–86.

Winblad B, Poritis N. (1999) Memantine in severe dementia: results of the 9M-Best Study (Benefit and efficacy in severely demented patients during treatment with memantine). *International Journal of Geriatric Psychiatry* **14**: 135–46.

Winblad B, Palmer K, Kivipelto M *et al.* (2004) Mild cognitive impairment: Beyond controversies, towards a consensus. Report of the International Working Group on Mild Cognitive Impairment. *Journal of International Medicine* **256**: 240–6.

Winblad B, Fioravanti M, Dolezal T *et al.* (2008) Therapeutic use of nicergoline. *Clinical Drug Investigation* **28**: 533–52.

Windisch M. (2000) Approach towards an integrative drug treatment of Alzheimer's disease. *Journal of Neural Transmission* **59**: 301–13.

Windisch M, Gschanes A, Hutter-Paier B. (1998) Neurotrophic activities and therapeutic experience with a brain derived peptide preparation. *Journal of Neural Transmission* **53** (Suppl.): 289–98.

Wolkowitz OM, Kramer JH, Reus VI *et al.* (2003) for the DHEA-Alzheimer's Disease Collaborative Research. DHEA treatment of Alzheimer's disease: a randomized, double-blind, placebo-controlled study. *Neurology* **60**: 1071–6.

Wong CL, Bansback N, Lee PE, Anis AH. (2009) Cost-effectiveness: cholinesterase inhibitors and memantine in vascular dementia. *Canadian Journal of Neurological Sciences* **36**: 735–9.

World Health Organization. (2008) ICD-10, International Statistical Classification of Diseases and Related Health Problems, 10th rev. Geneva: WHO.

Yamada Y, Furui H, Furumichi T *et al.* (1990) Inhibitory effects of endothelial cells and calcium channel blockers on platelet aggregation. *Japanese Heart Journal* **31**: 201–5.

Yamaguchi S, Matsubara M, Kobayashi S. (2004) Event-related brain potential changes after Choto-san administration in stroke patients with mild cognitive impairments. *Psychopharmacology* **171**: 241–9.

Yesavage JA, Tinkleberg JR, Hollister LE, Berger PA. (1979) Vasodilators in senile dementia: a review of the literature. *Archives of General Psychiatry* **36**: 220–3.

Zamrini E, Parrish JA, Parsons D, Harrell LE. (2004a) Medical comorbidity in black and white patients with Alzheimer's disease. *Southern Medical Journal* **97**: 2–6.

Zamrini E, McGwin G, Roseman JM. (2004b) Association between statin use and Alzheimer's disease. *Neuroepidemiology* 23: 94–8.

Zanchetti A, Bond MG, Hennig M *et al.* (2004) for the ELSA Investigators. (2004) Absolute and relative changes in carotid intima-media thickness and atherosclerotic plaques during long-term antihypertensive treatment: further results of the European Lacidipine Study on Atherosclerosis (ELSA). *Journal of Hypertension* 22: 1201–12.

Zekry D, Hauw J-J, Gold G. (2002a) Mixed dementia: epidemiology, diagnosis, and treatment. *Journal of the American Geriatrics Society* 50: 1431–8.

Zekry D, Duyckaerts C, Belmin J *et al.* (2002b) Alzheimer's disease and brain infarcts in the elderly. Agreement with neuropathology. *Journal of Neurology* 249: 1529–34.

Zekry D, Duyckaerts C, Moulias R *et al.* (2002c) Degenerative and vascular lesions of the brain have synergistic effects in dementia of the elderly. *Acta Neuropathologica* 103: 481–7.

Zhang BL, Wang YY, Chen RX. (2002) Clinical randomized double-blinded study on treatment of vascular dementia by jiannao yizhi granule. *Zhongguo Zhong Xi Yi Jie He Za Zhi* 22: 577–80.

Zimmermann M, Colciaghi F, Cattabeni F, Di Luca M. (2002) Ginkgo biloba extract: from molecular mechanisms to the treatment of Alzheimer's disease. *Cellular and Molecular Biology* 48: 613–23.

PART VI

DEMENTIA WITH LEWY BODIES AND PARKINSON'S DISEASE

Dementia with Lewy bodies: a clinical and historical overview

IAN G MCKEITH

64.1 INTRODUCTION

64.1.1 Dementia with Lewy bodies: what's in a name?

dementia with Lewy bodies (DLB) is now the preferred term (McKeith *et al.*, 1996) for a variety of clinical diagnoses including diffuse LB disease (DLBD) (Kosaka *et al.*, 1984; Dickson *et al.*, 1987; Lennox *et al.*, 1989), LB dementia (LBD) (Gibb *et al.*, 1987), dementia associated with cortical Lewy bodies (DCLB) (Byrne *et al.*, 1991), the LB variant of Alzheimer's disease (LBVAD) (Hansen *et al.*, 1990; Förstl *et al.*, 1993), and senile dementia of LB type (SDLT) (Perry *et al.*, 1990). **Figure 64.1** provides a simple schematic of the relationship between the various Lewy body terminologies recommended currently and consistency of use is essential to a full understanding of the disorder. This chapter considers the evolution of diagnostic concepts and methods; the pathology and management of DLB are considered in subsequent chapters.

DLB is important in clinical practice because:

- It usually has a clinical presentation and course which differs from Alzheimer's disease (AD) and other non-AD dementias.
- Functional disability and impairment in quality of life are greater in DLB than AD and generate significantly higher costs of care.
- The management of psychosis and behavioural disturbances, which are common in DLB, is complicated by sensitivity to neuroleptic medication.
- It may be particularly amenable to cholinesterase inhibitor treatment.

64.1.2 Scale of the problem

Several studies in a range of settings have suggested that DLB accounts for just under 20 per cent of all cases of dementia referred for neuropathological autopsy (McKeith *et al.*, 2005). Community-based estimates are much more variable ranging from 0 to 30.5 per cent (Zaccai *et al.*, 2005). A community study of over 85 year olds found 5.0 per cent to meet

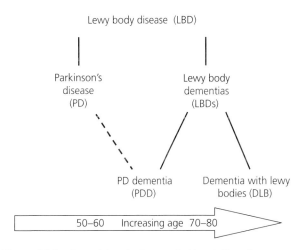

Figure 64.1 Correct terminology and abbreviations for describing dementia with Lewy bodies.

diagnostic criteria for DLB representing 22 per cent of all demented cases (Rahkonen *et al.*, 2003), similar to other clinical estimates (Stevens *et al.*, 2002; Aarsland *et al.*, 2008). In clinical practice, however, it is likely that only 2–5 per cent of dementia cases referred for specialist assessment are given a DLB diagnosis suggesting significant under-detection. Survival in DLB was initially reported as being significantly reduced compared with AD, but more recent series have not confirmed a general tendency to reduced survival or more rapid cognitive decline. Risk factors for DLB are unclear as prevalence studies have been too small.

64.2 DEVELOPMENT OF CLINICAL DIAGNOSTIC CRITERIA FOR DLB

64.2.1 Early case reports

When Friedrich Lewy first described the eosinophilic, neuronal inclusions which we now call Lewy bodies (LBs), in the brainstem of patients with paralysis agitans, he did not associate the inclusions with cognitive impairment and psychiatric disorder (Forster and Lewy, 1912). This was despite half of his sample being clinically demented and a quarter having mood disorders, hallucinations and paranoid delusions (Förstl and Levy, 1991). The first case reports specifically describing patients with dementia and LBs did not appear until 1961 when Okazaki published two cases, both elderly men presenting with cognitive decline and subsequently developing severe dementia (Okazaki *et al.*, 1961). Over the next 20 years, 34 similar cases were reported. Kosaka *et al.* (1984) noted a 3:1 male predominance, with memory disturbance as the presenting feature in 67 per cent, psychotic states (*sic*) in 17 per cent and dizziness due to orthostatic hypotension in 17 per cent. Progressive dementia with muscular rigidity occurred eventually in 80 per cent, although only 25 per cent of cases were diagnosed with parkinsonism. The first substantial listing of these Japanese cases in the western literature was in 1987 by Gibb *et al.* who added four new UK cases.

64.2.2 Early diagnostic criteria

The following year, Burkhardt *et al.* (1988) listed 34 US cases and carried out a simple meta-analysis. The most common presentation was a 'neurobehavioural syndrome'; memory impairment and other cognitive deficits were typical, all but one eventually becoming demented. Psychotic features, such as depression, hallucinations and paranoia, were seen in ten (29 per cent), two patients being psychotic for many years before developing other symptoms. Parkinsonian features, the most common of which was rigidity, were usually overshadowed by dementia; in only five cases (15 per cent) were no extrapyramidal features present. Duration of illness was very variable (1–20 years) with an end state of severe dementia, rigidity, akinetic mutism, quadriparesis in flexion and emaciation. The most common reported cause of death was aspiration pneumonia. Based upon these observations, Burkhardt *et al.* (1988) were the first to attempt a general

description of the clinical syndrome associated with diffuse Lewy body disease, distinguishing it as separate from PD with dementia. They concluded that 'DLBD should be suspected in any elderly patient who presents with a rapidly progressive dementia, followed in short order by rigidity and other parkinsonian features. Myoclonus may be present.'

Crystal *et al.* (1990), in a paper entitled 'Antemortem diagnosis of diffuse Lewy body disease', criticized this approach on the grounds that 'extrapyramidal features occur in many patients with severe AD and since dementia occurs in many subjects with PD, the clinical criteria for the diagnosis of DLBD remain unclear'. The authors proposed alternative criteria of 'progressive dementia with gait disorder, psychiatric symptoms and a burst pattern on electroencephalogram (EEG) at the time of moderate dementia'. No particular characteristics of the pattern of cognitive impairment were noted.

Although these early clinical definitions were important in drawing attention to the existence of DLB and describing some of its salient characteristics, neither could be regarded as satisfactory for clinical diagnostic purposes, since they lacked detail and were not operationalized in a way which would allow acceptable inter-rater reliability (Hansen and Galasko, 1992).

64.2.3 The Nottingham Group for the Study of Neurodegenerative Disorders

The Nottingham group reported the clinical characteristics of 15 new UK cases in considerable detail, the largest individual series published at that time (Byrne *et al.*, 1989) leading to the first formal proposal of operational criteria for dementia associated with cortical Lewy bodies (Byrne *et al.*, 1991). Seven were men, the mean age at onset was 72 years and the mean duration of illness, 5.5 years. Forty per cent presented with symptoms and signs of idiopathic PD, with cognitive impairment occurring one to four years later. A further 20 per cent had parkinsonism and mild cognitive impairment at presentation and the remaining 40 per cent showed motor features later in their illnesses, gait disturbance and postural abnormalities being most common. These latter cases presented with neuropsychiatric features only, in various combinations of cognitive impairment, paranoid delusions and visual or auditory hallucinations. Fourteen of the 15 were demented before death, the exception presenting with classical PD and later becoming depressed, irritable and mildly forgetful with frequent falls. Fluctuating cognition with episodic confusion for which no adequate underlying cause could be found, was observed in 80 per cent of the Nottingham cases. Byrne also drew attention to the frequent occurrence of depression (20 per cent) and psychosis (33 per cent).

64.2.4 The Newcastle studies

At around the same time, the Newcastle upon Tyne group identified 14 UK cases with the neuropathological features of 'senile dementia of Lewy body type' (Perry *et al.*, 1990) accounting for 15 per cent of a series of dementia autopsies.

These SDLT cases had been regarded during lifetime as clinically atypical 'causing much diagnostic perplexity'. Acute onset, fluctuating course, more rapid deterioration, early and prominent hallucinatory and behavioural disturbances, and associated mild parkinsonian features were present. Two further Newcastle series were reported soon after (McKeith et al., 1992a; McKeith et al., 1992b) and depressive symptoms, unexplained falls, observed disturbances of consciousness and excessive sensitivity to side effects of neuroleptic medication were added to the list of clinical characteristics with potential to distinguish DLB pathology cases from AD.

Based upon these observations, new clinical diagnostic criteria were proposed with an emphasis upon cognitive dysfunction and neuropsychiatric features which could occur in the absence of extrapyramidal motor signs and an attempt was made to describe the typical course of illness.

The first stage is often recognized only in retrospect and may extend back one to three years pre-presentation with occasional minor episodes of forgetfulness, sometimes described as lapses of concentration or 'switching off'. A brief period of delirium is sometimes noted for the first time, often associated with genuine physical illness and/or surgical procedures. Disturbed sleep, nightmares and daytime drowsiness often persist after recovery.

Progression to the second stage frequently prompts psychiatric or medical referral. A more sustained cognitive impairment is established, albeit with marked fluctuations in severity. Recurrent confusional episodes are accompanied by vivid hallucinatory experiences, visual misidentification syndromes and topographical disorientation. Extensive medical screening is usually negative. Attentional deficits are apparent as apathy, and daytime somnolence and sleep behaviour disorder may be severe. Gait disorder and bradykinesia are often overlooked, particularly in elderly subjects. Frequent falls occur due either to postural instability or syncope.

The third and final stage often begins with a sudden increase in behavioural disturbance leading to requests for sedation or hospital admission by perplexed and exhausted carers. The natural course from this point is variable and obscured by the high incidence of adverse reactions to neuroleptic medication. For patients not receiving or tolerating neuroleptics, a progressive decline into severe dementia with dysphasia and dyspraxia occurs over months or years, with death usually due to cardiac or pulmonary disease. During this terminal phase, patients show continuing behavioural disturbance, including vocal and motor responses to hallucinatory phenomena. Lucid intervals with some retention of recent memory function and insight may still be apparent. Neurological disability is often profound with fixed flexion deformities of the neck and trunk and severe gait impairment (McKeith et al., 1992a).

64.2.5   International consensus criteria

64.2.5.1   FIRST REPORT OF THE DLB CONSORTIUM

By the early 1990s, it was becoming apparent that DLB was a relatively common cause of dementia in old age and that the

several research groups investigating it were adopting different terminologies. The Consortium on DLB met in October 1995 to agree common clinical and pathological methods and nomenclature. The Consensus Criteria (McKeith et al., 1996) described the particular characteristics of the cognitive impairments of DLB in some detail as differing from the dementia syndrome of AD, in which memory deficits predominate. In DLB, attentional deficits and prominent visuospatial dysfunction are the main features (Salmon and Galasko, 1996). Probable DLB could be diagnosed if any two of the three key symptoms were present, namely fluctuation, visual hallucinations or spontaneous motor features of parkinsonism, and possible DLB if only one was present.

Several retrospective and two prospective studies have examined the predictive accuracy of these original consensus clinical criteria for probable DLB (McKeith et al., 2000; Litvan et al., 2003). They suggest that sensitivity of case detection is generally low at around 40 per cent, whereas specificity is much higher, typically around 90 per cent suggesting that the criteria are most useful for confirmation of diagnosis (low false-positive rate), but less helpful for case finding.

64.2.5.2   SECOND REPORT OF THE DLB CONSORTIUM

The Second International DLB Workshop met in July 1998 (McKeith et al., 1999). The objectives were to review developments since publication of the consensus guidelines and to determine whether these yet require to be modified. It was recommended that the clinical consensus criteria should continue to be used in their current format with the addition of two new supportive features, namely rapid eye movement (REM) sleep behaviour disorder (RBD) (3.1.3.3) and depression (3.1.3.4).

64.2.5.3   THIRD REPORT OF THE DLB CONSORTIUM

In order to address the perceived shortcomings of the original diagnostic criteria, the DLB Consortium met again in 2003 to resolve improved methods of identifying cases antemortem (McKeith et al., 2005). No major amendments to the three core features of DLB were proposed, but better methods for their clinical assessment were recommended. A new category of features 'suggestive' of DLB was described comprising REM sleep behaviour disorder (RBD), severe neuroleptic sensitivity and abnormal dopamine transporter neuroimaging imaging. If one or more of these suggestive features is present, in addition to one or more core features, a diagnosis of probable DLB can be made (see **Box 64.1**). Possible DLB can be diagnosed if one or more suggestive features are present in a patient with dementia even in the absence of any core features. The revised criteria are also more explicit about the importance to be attached to clinical and radiological evidence of cerebrovascular disease.

These improved criteria have been suggested to detect 25 per cent more DLB cases than the previous version (Aarsland et al., 2008), although a retrospective application of the new criteria to an autopsy-verified sample reported that cases with Braak stage 5 and 6 AD pathology were still unlikely to be detected ante-mortem. Such cases tend to lack core or

Box 64.1 Criteria for the clinical diagnosis of dementia with Lewy bodies

1. **Central feature** (essential for a diagnosis of possible or probable DLB):
Dementia defined as progressive cognitive decline of sufficient magnitude to interfere with normal social or occupational function. Prominent or persistent memory impairment may not necessarily occur in the early stages, but is usually evident with progression. Deficits on tests of attention, executive function and visuospatial ability may be especially prominent.

2. **Core features** (two core features are sufficient for a diagnosis of probable DLB, one for possible DLB):
   - fluctuating cognition with pronounced variations in attention and alertness;
   - recurrent visual hallucinations that are typically well formed and detailed;
   - spontaneous features of parkinsonism.

3. **Suggestive features** (if one or more of these is present in the presence of one or more core features, a diagnosis of probable DLB can be made. In the absence of any core features, one or more suggestive features is sufficient for possible DLB. Probable DLB should not be diagnosed on the basis of suggestive features alone):
   a. REM sleep behaviour disorder;
   b. severe neuroleptic sensitivity;
   c. low dopamine transporter uptake in basal ganglia demonstrated by SPECT or PET imaging.

4. **Supportive features** (commonly present, but not proven to have diagnostic specificity):
   a. repeated falls and syncope;
   b. transient, unexplained loss of consciousness;
   c. severe autonomic dysfunction, e.g. orthostatic hypotension, urinary incontinence;
   d. hallucinations in other modalities;
   e. systematized delusions;
   f. depression;
   g. relative preservation of medial temporal lobe structures on CT/MRI scan;
   h. generalized low uptake on SPECT/PET perfusion scan with reduced occipital activity;
   i. abnormal (low uptake) MIBG myocardial scintigraphy;
   j. prominent slow wave activity on EEG with temporal lobe transient sharp waves.

5. A diagnosis of DLB is less likely:
   - in the presence of cerebrovascular disease, evident as focal neurological signs or on brain imaging;
   - in the presence of any other physical illness or brain disorder sufficient to account in part or in total for the clinical picture;
   - if parkinsonism only appears for the first time at a stage of severe dementia.

6. Temporal sequence of symptoms:

DLB should be diagnosed when dementia occurs before or concurrently with parkinsonism (if it is present). The term Parkinson's disease dementia (PDD) should be used to describe dementia that occurs in the context of well-established Parkinson's disease. In a practice setting, the term that is most appropriate to the clinical situation should be used and generic terms, such as LB disease, are often helpful. In research studies in which distinction needs to be made between DLB and PDD, the existing one-year rule between the onset of dementia and parkinsonism DLB continues to be recommended. Adoption of other time periods will simply confound data pooling or comparison between studies. In other research settings that may include clinicopathologic studies and clinical trials, both clinical phenotypes may be considered collectively under categories such as LB disease or alpha-synucleinopathy.

suggestive DLB features and clinically resemble AD (Weisman *et al.*, 2007). This is consistent with the proposal made by the third consortium group that the likelihood of a patient having the typical DLB clinical syndrome is 'directly related to the severity of Lewy-related pathology and inversely related to the severity of concurrent AD-type pathology'. Given that AD-type pathology is frequently present in DLB, there will therefore be a significant number of patients who will always prove very difficult to identify solely on clinical grounds. This group, who are best described pathologically as AD+LB or as LB variant of Alzheimer's disease (LBVAD) (Hansen *et al.*, 1990), can probably only be reliably identified

by additional investigations and biomarkers (see below under 64.4. Clinical investigation).

64.3 DIFFERENTIAL DIAGNOSIS OF DLB IN CLINICAL PRACTICE

64.3.1 Clinical presentations of DLB

DLB patients may present to psychiatric services (cognitive impairment, psychosis or behavioural disturbance), internal medicine (acute confusional state or syncope) or neurology (movement disorder or disturbed consciousness). The details of clinical assessment and differential diagnoses will be shaped to a large extent by these symptom and specialty biases (McKeith *et al.*, 1995). In all cases, a detailed history from patient and reliable informants should document the time of onset of relevant key symptoms, the nature of their progression, and their effects on social, occupational and personal function. Functional disability in DLB is generally greater than in AD patients with similar severity of cognitive impairment. Most of the extra burden is due to motor impairments that cause difficulty with mobility, feeding and toileting (McKeith *et al.*, 2006). Given the additional disabilities associated with DLB, it is not suprising that care costs have been estimated at twice those for patients with AD (Boström *et al.*, 2007a) and that carers rate DLB patients' quality of life as significantly worse than in AD (Boström *et al.*, 2007b).

64.3.2   Cognitive impairment

Although brief bedside tests of mental status (e.g. Mini-Mental State Examination (MMSE)) may confirm the presence of cognitive impairment in DLB, total scores are usually equivalent to AD and unhelpful in differential diagnosis. More detailed psychometric examination is usually required to reveal a profile of deficits that helps to identify DLB from AD or other dementias (Ferman *et al.*, 2006). Prominent deficits on tests of executive function and problem-solving, such as the Trail Making Test and verbal fluency for categories and letters, may be useful clinical discriminators (Salmon and Galasko, 1996), as may disproportionate impairment on tests of visuospatial performance, present in up to three-quarters of DLB patients at first evaluation (Tiraboschi *et al.*, 2006). Although total CAMCOG scores were identical in DLB and AD, significant differences were found in mean scores for the delayed recall subtest (DLB performing better) and the visuospatial praxis subtest (DLB performing worse) (Walker *et al.*, 1996). With the progression of dementia, this selective pattern of cognitive deficits may be lost, making differential diagnosis based on neuropsychological examination difficult during the later stages.

DLB is particularly characterized by increased variability in performance on cognitive tasks, within and between patients and when compared to age-matched controls and patients with AD. This variability is most evident in executive and attentional tasks. Wide test–retest variation in performance of timed computer-based tasks (Walker *et al.*, 2000a) has been proposed as a reliable and widely applicable quantified measure which is well correlated with clinical expert estimates of fluctuating performance.

64.3.3   Core features

A review of nine studies which report clinical details on 190 autopsy confirmed DLB cases and compares them with 261 AD cases, provides a useful source of frequency rates of the core features of DLB (Byrne *et al.*, 1989; McKeith *et al.*, 1992a; McKeith *et al.*, 1992b; Förstl *et al.*, 1993; Galasko *et al.*, 1996; Hely *et al.*, 1996; Klatka *et al.*, 1996; Weiner *et al.*, 1996; Ala *et al.*, 1997). The wide ranges reported most likely reflect sampling biases and different methods of symptom ascertainment.

64.3.3.1   FLUCTUATION

Fluctuations in cognitive function, which may vary over minutes, hours or days, occur in 58 per cent of DLB cases at the time of presentation (range 8–85 per cent) and are observed at some point during the course of the illness in 75 per cent (45–90 per cent). Substantial changes in mental state and behaviour may be seen within the duration of a single interview or between consecutive examinations. Fluctuation includes, and indeed may be based on, pronounced variations in attention and alertness. Excessive daytime drowsiness with transient confusion on waking commonly occurs. Episodes may last from a few seconds to several hours and can be ascertained by caregiver report, observer rating (Walker *et al.*, 2000b) or using computer-based measures of variation in attentional performance (Walker *et al.*, 2000a). Questions such as 'are there episodes when his/her thinking seems quite clear and then becomes muddled?' may be useful opening probes, although up to 75 per cent of carers will respond in the affirmative regardless of AD/DLB diagnosis (Bradshaw *et al.*, 2004; Ferman *et al.*, 2004). Objective questions about daytime drowsiness and lethargy, daytime sleep of 2 or more hours, staring into space for long periods and episodes of disorganized speech are more informative. The presence of three or four features of this composite occurred in 63 per cent of DLB patients compared with 12 per cent of AD patients and 0.5 per cent of normal elderly persons (Ferman *et al.*, 2004).

64.3.3.2   VISUAL HALLUCINATIONS

Visual hallucinations are present in 33 per cent of DLB cases at the time of presentation (range 11–64 per cent) and occur at some point during the course of the illness in 46 per cent (13–80 per cent). Most patients experience complex hallucinations daily, normally lasting for at least several minutes. They commonly see people or animals and the experiences are usually perceived as unpleasant. Simple hallucinations are rare. Neuropsychiatric symptoms commonly coexisting with hallucinations are apathy, sleep disturbance and anxiety (Mosimann *et al.*, 2006). Carers are more likely than mild or moderately demented patients to give 'don't know' answers about visual hallucinations and the use of a semi-structured interview can increase both the quantity and quality of information about a symptom which is present early and strongly predictive of a DLB diagnosis (Tiraboschi *et al.*, 2006; Mosimann *et al.*, 2008). It is the persistence of visual hallucinations in DLB (McShane *et al.*, 1995) that helps distinguish them from the episodic perceptual disturbances that occur transiently in dementias of other aetiology or during a delirium provoked by an external cause. It has been suggested that they arise from a combination of faulty perceptual processing of environmental stimuli, and less detailed recollection of experience, combined with intact image generation (Collerton *et al.*, 2005). Visual hallucinations in DLB are associated with greater deficits in cortical acetylcholine (Perry *et al.*, 1991) and predict better response to cholinesterase inhibitors (McKeith *et al.*, 2004b).

64.3.3.3 MOTOR PARKINSONISM

extrapyramidal signs (EPS) are reported in 25–50 per cent of DLB cases at diagnosis and the majority develop some EPS during the natural course. Up to 25 per cent of autopsy-confirmed cases may, however, have no record of EPS indicating that parkinsonism is not necessary for a clinical diagnosis of DLB. Initial suggestions that parkinsonism in DLB is mild has not been supported by studies finding equal severity with non-demented PD patients (Louis *et al.*, 1997; Aarsland *et al.*, 2001) with similar annual progression rates in motor Unified Parkinson's Disease Rating Scale (UPDRS) scores (Ballard *et al.*, 2000). The pattern of EPS in DLB shows an axial bias with greater postural instability and facial impassivity and a tendency towards less tremor consistent with greater 'non-dopaminergic' motor involvement (Burn *et al.*, 2003). The degree of cognitive impairment appears to have no influence on the occurrence of EPS, although more demented patients may have difficulty in following instructions on formal motor tests. A modified version of the Unified Parkinson's Disease Rating Scale which allows for this has been developed (Ballard *et al.*, 1997).

64.3.4 Suggestive features

64.3.4.1 REM SLEEP BEHAVIOUR DISORDER

REM sleep behaviour disorder is a parasomnia characterized by loss of normal skeletal muscle atonia during REM sleep with resultant motor activity and 'acting out of dreams'. Patients demonstrate a variety of movements ranging from verbal outbursts to pugilistic movements and even more dramatic motor activity. Injuries to patients and bed partners are common. Estimates from prospective studies in specialist centres place the frequency of RBD at 50–80 per cent in DLB (Boeve *et al.*, 2004) and it is uncommon in patients with AD. The diagnosis is made on clinical grounds and careful questioning of bed partners is therefore vital. Use of a validated instrument, such as the Mayo Sleep Questionnaire, is recommended since techniques such as polysomnography (PSG), utilizing audiovisual footage to confirm the physical features of RBD in addition to electromyography, electro-oculography, EEG and oxygen saturation recordings during sleep are generally unavailable for most patients. The history of RBD may precede the diagnosis of dementia by several years and may either persist or diminish following the onset of cognitive decline. REM sleep–wakefulness dissociations characteristic of narcolepsy may explain several features of DLB including daytime hypersomnolence, visual hallucinations and cataplexy. Sleep disorders may contribute to fluctuations typical of DLB and their treatment may improve fluctuations and quality of life.

64.3.4.2 SEVERE NEUROLEPTIC SENSITIVITY

The hypothesis of an abnormal sensitivity to adverse effects of neuroleptic medication was based upon the observation that 57 per cent of a series of DLB patients deteriorated rapidly after either receiving neuroleptics for the first time, or following a dose increase (McKeith *et al.*, 1992a; McKeith *et al.*, 1992b). Mortality risk, estimated by survival analysis, was increased by a factor of 2.7. A severe adverse reaction to neuroleptic medication may be an important diagnostic indicator of underlying LB disorder, but tolerance of neuroleptics does not rule out DLB. Neuroleptic challenge is never justified as a diagnostic test and neuroleptic prescribing is routinely and desirably avoided in patients suspected of having DLB. Newer atypical antipsychotics used at low dose may be safer in this regard, but sensitivity reactions have been documented with most and they should be used with great caution (McKeith *et al.*, 2004a; Aarsland *et al.*, 2005).

64.3.4.3 LOW DOPAMINE TRANSPORTER UPTAKE IN BASAL GANGLIA

Functional imaging of the dopamine transporter (DAT) defines integrity of the nigrostriatal dopaminergic system and was originally developed to assist diagnosis of patients with tremor of uncertain aetiology (Marshall and Grosset, 2003). positron emission tomography (PET) and single photon emission computed tomography (SPECT) ligands are available for this purpose and both have subsequently been shown also to be useful in the discrimination of DLB from AD. ^{123}I-radiolabelled FP-CIT (2 beta-carbomethoxy-3 beta-(4-iodophenyl)-N-(3-fluoropropyl) nortropane) has been the most investigated and a sensitivity of 78 per cent for detecting probable DLB with a specificity of 85 per cent for AD and 94 per cent for controls has been reported (O'Brien *et al.*, 2004) (**see p8 of the plate section for Plates 10a and 10b**). A multicentre clinical trial subsequently demonstrated similar results across a wide variety of settings (McKeith *et al.*, 2007) and regulatory approval for distinguishing probable DLB from AD with FP-CIT imaging now exists in Europe. The most useful clinical application of the test, however, is probably in cases of possible DLB or where diagnostic uncertainty is high. A longitudinal study found that of 12/19 people (63 per cent) who had a diagnosis of possible DLB accompanied by an abnormal DAT scan were rediagnosed with probable DLB at a one year clinical follow up. By contrast, 100 per cent of cases initially diagnosed as possible DLB, but reclassified as AD a year later had normal DAT scans at first evaluation (O'Brien *et al.*, 2009).

64.3.5 Supportive features

A detailed discussion of every feature identified as supportive of a diagnosis of DLB is beyond the scope of this chapter. Clinical symptoms are summarized briefly below and investigations, including neuroimaging, are discussed below under 64.4 Clinical investigation.

64.3.5.1   REPEATED FALLS, SYNCOPE AND TRANSIENT LOSSES OF CONSCIOUSNESS

Dementia of any aetiology is probably a risk factor for all three of these clinical features and it can be difficult to clearly distinguish between them. Repeated falls may be due to posture, gait and balance difficulties in DLB and are a significant cause of hospitalization contributing to reduced survival (Hanyu *et al.*, 2009). Syncopal attacks in DLB with complete loss of consciousness and muscle tone and transient episodes of unresponsiveness without loss of muscle tone are probably related phenomena representing one extreme of fluctuating attention and cognition. Episodes of each type occur in about 20 per cent of DLB cases at presentation and up to a half during the whole course of illness (McKeith *et al.*, 1992a; McKeith *et al.*, 1992b). Such episodes frequently lead to a misdiagnosis of vascular dementia because of the suspicion of transient ischaemic attack.

64.3.5.2   AUTONOMIC DYSFUNCTION

Autonomic dysfunction which affects both sympathetic and parasympathetic systems is a significant, common and often early feature of DLB presenting as orthostatic hypotension, carotid sinus hypersensitivity, reduced secretions (lacrimal, mouth, sweat), urinary retention, erectile dysfunction and bowel problems, both constipation and diarrhoea (Del-Ser *et al.*, 1996). Orthostatic hypotension and carotid sinus sensitivity appear to occur more commonly in DLB than AD or age-matched controls (Kenny *et al.*, 2004; Allan *et al.*, 2007) and probably contribute to the high rates of syncope and falls that occur in this population.

64.3.5.3   SYSTEMATIZED DELUSIONS AND HALLUCINATIONS IN OTHER MODALITIES

Delusions are common in DLB, occurring in about half of patients. They are usually based on recollections of hallucinations and perceptual disturbances and consequently often have a fixed, complex and bizarre content that contrasts with the mundane and often poorly formed persecutory ideas encountered in AD which are based on forgetfulness and confabulation. Auditory, olfactory and tactile hallucinations occur much less often, but can be striking presenting features in some DLB cases leading to initial diagnoses of late onset psychosis (Birkett *et al.*, 1992) and temporal lobe epilepsy (McKeith *et al.*, 1992a). In such circumstances, severe neuroleptic sensitivity reactions may indicate the true underlying cause.

64.3.5.6   DEPRESSION

Depressive symptoms are frequent in most neuropsychiatric syndromes and often of little differential diagnostic value. However, depression was diagnosed at first consultation in 38 per cent of DLB patients compared with 16 per cent with AD ($p < 0.05$), and was the primary reason for referral in 60 per cent of the patients in whom it was present (McKeith *et al.*, 1992a). Klatka *et al.* (1996) found depression in 14/28 (50 per cent) DLB, 8/58 (14 per cent) AD and 15/26 (58 per cent) PD cases with autopsy confirmation. No particular characteristics of depression have been described in DLB, but apathy and psychomotor retardation are to be expected in this population and may confound the assessment of affective state.

64.3.6   Differential diagnosis

There are four main categories of disorder that should be considered in the differential diagnosis of DLB. These are:

1. other dementia syndromes;
2. other causes of delirium;
3. other neurological syndromes, including Parkinson's disease;
4. other psychiatric disorders.

64.3.6.1   OTHER DEMENTIA SYNDROMES

Sixty-five per cent of autopsy confirmed DLB cases meet the NINCDS-ADRDA clinical criteria for probable or possible AD (McKeith *et al.*, 1994) and this is the most frequent clinical misdiagnosis of DLB. Conversely, 12–36 per cent of cases meeting NINCDS criteria for a clinical diagnosis of AD are unexpectedly found to have LB pathology at autopsy (Burns *et al.*, 1990; Hansen *et al.*, 1990). There is a large 'overlap' group of patients who have both LB and AD pathologies and who cannot easily be classified by clinical criteria alone (see above under 64.2.5.3 Third report of the DLB Consortium). Up to a third of DLB cases can be misclassified as having vascular dementia by virtue of items such as fluctuating nature and course of illness. Pyramidal and focal neurological signs are, however, usually absent.

64.3.6.2   OTHER CAUSES OF DELIRIUM

In patients with intermittent delirium, appropriate examination and laboratory tests should be performed during the acute phase to maximize the chances of detecting infective, metabolic, inflammatory or other aetiological factors. Pharmacological causes are particularly common in elderly patients. Although the presence of any of these features makes a diagnosis of DLB less likely, comorbidity is not unusual in elderly patients and the diagnosis should not be excluded simply on this basis.

64.3.6.3   PATIENTS WITH A PREVIOUS DIAGNOSIS OF PARKINSON'S DISEASE

Dementia in PD (see Chapter 67, Cognitive impairment and dementia in Parkinson's disease) is often similar to DLB with respect to fluctuating neuropsychological function and neuropsychiatric features. Such patients who only develop the typical features of DLB after many years of motor disability present some problems of classification. Anti-parkinsonian medications are usually held responsible for hallucinations and confusion in PD, but research findings do not fully support this clinical impression. There has been considerable debate as to whether PD, PDD and DLB are simply different clinical presentations of the same underlying biological process, i.e. Lewy body disease, and indeed whether Lewy body disease might be a better clinical term to use for the whole spectrum of phenotypes (O'Brien, 2009). The current recommendation is to apply an arbitrary one-year rule that proposes that the onset of dementia within 12 months of the onset of parkinsonism qualifies as DLB, and more than 12 months of parkinsonism before the onset of dementia qualifies as PDD (McKeith et al., 2005). Using diagnostic labels, such as PDD and DLB that describe the order of onset of symptoms, is generally helpful in the diagnosis and management of most clinical cases and the majority of patients and carers (and clinicans) are able to understand that the diagnosis given, e.g. DLB, is 'caused by' Lewy body disease. In some patients, particularly those with an admixture of neurological and psychiatric symptoms occurring in relatively short order, a single label of LB disease may serve as the best primary diagnosis, qualified by a secondary descriptive epithet, for example, LB disease with parkinsonism, or LB disease with dementia, or LB disease with parkinsonism and dementia. Clinicians need to decide which term is the most appropriate for each individual patient, and carefully explain the terminology to the patient and his or her caregivers.

64.3.6.4 OTHER NEUROLOGICAL SYNDROMES

Other atypical parkinsonian syndromes, associated with poor levodopa response, cognitive impairment and postural instability, include progressive supranuclear palsy (Fearnley et al. 1991), multisystem atrophy and corticobasal degeneration. The development of myoclonus in patients with a rapidly progressive form of DLB may lead the clinician to suspect Creutzfeldt–Jacob disease. Syncopal episodes in DLB are often incorrectly attributed to transient ischaemic attacks, despite an absence of focal neurological signs. Recurrent disturbances in consciousness accompanied by complex visual hallucinations may suggest complex partial seizures (temporal lobe epilepsy) and vivid dreaming with violent movements during sleep may meet criteria for REM sleep behaviour disorder.

64.3.6.5 OTHER PSYCHIATRIC DISORDERS

If a patient spontaneously develops parkinsonian features or cognitive decline, or shows excessive sensitivity to neuroleptic medication, in the course of late onset delusional disorder, depressive psychosis or hypomania (Birkett et al., 1992; Mullan et al., 1996), DLB should be considered.

64.4 CLINICAL INVESTIGATION

Detailed psychometric testing and expert neurological examination are likely to be informative as outlined in the previous sections and should be carried out whenever DLB is suspected. Although it is premature to conclude that specific biomarkers for DLB have yet been identified, significant progress has been made in developing neuroimaging investigations that can be helpful in supporting the clinical diagnosis and there are promising developments in other modalities.

64.4.1 Neuroimaging – structural and functional

Prominent atrophy of the medial temporal lobes on computed tomography (CT) or magnetic resonance imaging (MRI) is indicative of AD pathology, rather than DLB (Burton et al., 2009). Periventricular lesions and white matter hyperintensities are often present in DLB cases (Barber et al., 2000), but like measures of generalized atrophy and rates of progression of whole brain tissue loss (O'Brien et al., 2001) are similar to those also seen in AD. Functional imaging of dopamine transporter loss in the caudate and putamen by PET or SPECT has been reported as more accurate in predicting neuropathological diagnosis of DLB than the application of clinical consensus criteria (Walker et al., 2007) and low dopamine transporter uptake in basal ganglia is listed as a suggestive feature for the clinical diagnosis of DLB (discussed in more detail above under 64.3.4.3 Low dopamine transporter uptake in basal ganglia). Another potentially useful imaging modality is that of cardiac scintigraphy with [123]iodine metaiodobenzyl guanidine (^{123}I-MIBG), which is markedly reduced in DLB compared to AD (Suzuki et al., 2006), particularly if SPECT perfusion imaging is equivocal (Hanyu et al., 2006).

64.4.2 Electroencephalogram

The electroencephalogram is diffusely abnormal in over 90 per cent of DLB patients and abnormalities often appear early in the disease course. Since it is not yet possible to reliably differentiate DLB and AD subjects on the basis of the EEG, the presence of prominent slow wave activity with temporal lobe sharp waves is listed only as a supportive feature of DLB.

64.4.3 Genotyping

No specific genetic markers for DLB have been identified and genetic testing cannot presently be recommended as part of the diagnostic process. DLB patients have an elevated Apolipoprotein ε4 allele frequency (Benjamin et al., 1994; Pickering-Brown et al., 1994) similar to that reported in AD so a positive ε4 test does not provide additional information in the differential diagnosis of AD and DLB. Reports are emerging of abnormalities in the genes encoding for glucocerebrosidase and alpha-synuclein. A gene–dose effect has been suggested for alpha-synuclein with triplication of the gene giving rise to familial variants of DLB and PDD, whereas duplication is associated only with motor PD. Genetic testing cannot yet be recommended for use in clinical practice.

64.4.4 Cerebrospinal fluid and plasma markers

Cerebrospinal fluid (CSF) levels of alpha-synuclein species have been proposed as potential markers of DLB (Mollenhauer and Trenkwalder, 2009), but these are not yet sufficiently developed for clinical application. Since amyloid deposition in the brain is similar in DLB and AD, it is unlikely that measuring CSF amyloid will distinguish the two disorders and there is also some overlap in measures of p-tau. Recently, serum proteomic array methods which identify multiple potential diagnostic protein markers have been used to diagnostically separate DLB from AD (Wada-Isoe et al., 2007) and efforts continue to find less invasive biomarkers.

REFERENCES

Aarsland D, Ballard C, McKeith I et al. (2001) Comparison of extrapyramidal signs in dementia with Lewy bodies and Parkinson's disease. Journal of Neuropsychiatry and Clinical Neurosciences 13: 374–9.

Aarsland D, Ballard C, Larsen JP et al. (2005) Marked neuroleptic sensitivity in dementia with Lewy bodies and Parkinson's disease. Journal of Clinical Psychiatry 66: 633–7.

Aarsland D, Rongve A, Nore SP et al. (2008) Frequency and case identification of dementia with Lewy bodies using the revised consensus criteria. Dementia and Geriatric Cognitive Disorders 26: 445–52.

Ala TA, Yang K-H, Sung JH, Frey WHI. (1997) Hallucinations and signs of Parkinsonism help distinguish patients with dementia and cortical Lewy bodies from patients with Alzheimer's disease. Journal of Neurology, Neurosurgery and Psychiatry 62: 16–21.

Allan LM, Ballard CG, Allen J et al. (2007) Autonomic dysfunction in dementia. Journal of Neurology, Neurosurgery and Psychiatry 78: 671–7.

Ballard CG, McKeith I, Burn D et al. (1997) The UPDRS scale as a means of identifying extrapyramidal signs in patients suffering from dementia with Lewy bodies. Acta Neurologica Scandinavica 96: 366–71.

Ballard C, O'Brien J, Swann A et al. (2000) One year follow-up of parkinsonism in dementia with Lewy bodies. Dementia and Geriatric Cognitive Disorders 11: 219–22.

Barber R, Ballard C, McKeith IG et al. (2000) MRI volumetric study of dementia with Lewy bodies. A comparison with AD and vascular dementia. Neurology 54: 1304–9.

Benjamin R, Leake A, Edwardson JA et al. (1994) Apolipoprotein E genes in Lewy body and Parkinson's disease. Lancet 343: 1565.

Birkett DP, Desouky A, Han L, Kaufman M. (1992) Lewy bodies in psychiatric patients. International Journal of Geriatric Psychiatry 7: 235–40.

Boeve BF, Silber MH, Ferman TJ. (2004) REM sleep behavior disorder in Parkinson's disease and dementia with Lewy bodies. Journal of Geriatric Psychiatry and Neurology 17: 146–57.

Boström F, Jonsson L, Minthon L, Londos E. (2007a) Patients with Lewy body dementia use more resources than those with Alzheimer's disease. International Journal of Geriatric Psychiatry 22: 713–19.

Boström F, Jonsson L, Minthon L, Londos E. (2007b) Patients with dementia with Lewy bodies have more impaired quality of life than patients with Alzheimer disease. Alzheimer Disease and Associated Disorders 21: 150–4.

Bradshaw J, Saling M, Hopwood M et al. (2004) Fluctuating cognition in dementia with Lewy bodies and Alzheimer's disease is qualitatively distinct. Journal of Neurology, Neurosurgery and Psychiatry 75: 382–7.

Burkhardt CR, Filley CM, Kleinschmidt-DeMasters BK et al. (1988) Diffuse Lewy body disease and progressive dementia. Neurology 38: 1520–8.

Burn DJ, Rowan EN, Minett T et al. (2003) Extrapyramidal features in Parkinson's disease with and without dementia and dementia with Lewy bodies: A cross-sectional comparative study. Movement Disorders 18: 884–9.

Burns A, Luthert P, Levy R et al. (1990) Accuracy of clinical diagnosis of Alzheimer's disease. British Medical Journal 301: 1026.

Burton EJ, Barber R, Mukaetova-Ladinska EB et al. (2009) Medial temporal lobe atrophy on MRI differentiates Alzheimers disease from dementia with Lewy bodies and vascular cognitive impairment: a prospective study with pathological verification of diagnosis. Brain 132: 195–203.

Byrne EJ, Lennox G, Lowe J, Godwin-Austen RB. (1989) Diffuse Lewy body disease: clinical features in 15 cases. Journal of Neurology, Neurosurgery and Psychiatry 52: 709–17.

Byrne EJ, Lennox G, Godwin-Austen RB et al. (1991) Dementia associated with cortical Lewy bodies. Proposed diagnostic criteria. Dementia 2: 283–4.

Collerton D, Perry E, McKeith I. (2005) Why people see things that are not there: a novel Perception and Attention Deficit model for recurrent complex visual hallucinations. Behavioral and Brain Sciences 28: 737–57.

Crystal HA, Dickson DW, Lizardi JE et al. (1990) Antemortem diagnosis of diffuse Lewy body disease. Neurology 40: 1523–8.

Del-Ser T, Munoz DG, Hachinski V. (1996) Temporal pattern of cognitive decline and incontinence is different in Alzheimer's disease and diffuse Lewy body disease. Neurology 46: 682–6.

Dickson DW, Davies P, Mayeux R et al. (1987) Diffuse Lewy body disease. Neuropathological and biochemical studies of six patients. Acta Neuropathologica 75: 8–15.

Fearnley JM, Revesz T, Brooks DJ et al. (1991) Diffuse Lewy body disease presenting with a supranuclear gaze palsy. Journal of Neurology, Neurosurgery and Psychiatry 54: 159–61.

Ferman T, Smith GE, Boeve BF et al. (2004) DLB fluctuations: specific features that reliably differentiate from AD and normal aging. Neurology 62: 181–7.

Ferman TJ, Smith GE, Boeve BF et al. (2006) Neuropsychological differentiation of dementia with Lewy bodies from normal aging and Alzheimer's disease. Clinical Neuropsychologist 20: 623–36.

Forster E, Lewy FH. (1912) Paralysis agitans. I. Pathologische Anatomie. In: Lewandowsky M (ed.). Handbuch der neurologie. Berlin: Springer, 920–33.

Förstl H, Levy R. (1991) FH Lewy on Lewy bodies, Parkinsonism and dementia. *International Journal of Geriatric Psychiatry* 6: 757–66.

Förstl H, Burns A, Luthert P *et al.* (1993) The Lewy-body variant of Alzheimer's disease. Clinical and pathological findings. *British Journal of Psychiatry* 162: 385–92.

Galasko D, Katzman R, Salmon DP *et al.* (1996) Clinical and neuropathological findings in Lewy body dementias. *Brain and Cognition* 31: 166–75.

Gibb WRG, Esiri MM, Lees AJ. (1987) Clinical and pathological features of diffuse cortical Lewy body disease (Lewy body dementia). *Brain* 110: 1131–53.

Hansen L, Salmon D, Galasko D *et al.* (1990) The Lewy body variant of Alzheimer's disease: A clinical and pathologic entity. *Neurology* 40: 1–8.

Hansen LA, Galasko D. (1992) Lewy body disease. *Current Opinion in Neurology and Neurosurgery* 5: 889–94.

Hanyu H, Shimizu S, Hirao K *et al.* (2006) Comparative value of brain perfusion SPECT and [123I]MIBG myocardial scintigraphy in distinguishing between dementia with Lewy bodies and Alzheimer's disease. *European Journal of Nuclear Medicine and Molecular Imaging* 33: 248–53.

Hanyu H, Sato T, Hirao K *et al.* (2009) Differences in clinical course between dementia with Lewy bodies and Alzheimer's disease. *European Journal of Neurology* 16: 212–17.

Hely MA, Reid WGJ, Halliday GM *et al.* (1996) Diffuse Lewy body disease: clinical features in nine cases without coexistent Alzheimer's disease. *Journal of Neurology, Neurosurgery and Psychiatry* 60: 531–8.

Kenny RA, Shaw FE, O'Brien JT *et al.* (2004) Carotid sinus syndrome is common in dementia with Lewy bodies and correlates with deep white matter lesions. *Journal of Neurology, Neurosurgery and Psychiatry* 75: 966–71.

Klatka LA, Louis ED, Schiffer RB. (1996) Psychiatric features in diffuse Lewy body disease: Findings in 28 pathologically diagnosed cases. *Neurology* 47: 1148–52.

Kosaka K, Yoshimura M, Ikeda K, Budka H. (1984) Diffuse type of Lewy body disease: progressive dementia with abundant cortical Lewy bodies and senile changes of varying degree-A new disease? *Clinical Neuropathology* 3: 185–92.

Lennox G, Lowe J, Byrne EJ *et al.* (1989) Diffuse Lewy body disease. *Lancet* 1: 323–4.

Litvan I, Bhatia KP, Burn DJ *et al.* (2003) SIC Task Force Appraisal of clinical diagnostic criteria for parkinsonian disorders. *Movement Disorders* 18: 467–86.

Louis E, Klatka L, Lui Y *et al.* (1997) Comparison of extrapyramidal features in 31 pathologically confirmed cases of diffuse Lewy body disease and 34 pathologically confirmed cases of Parkinson's disease. *Neurology* 48: 376–80.

McKeith IG, Perry RH, Fairbairn AF *et al.* (1992a) Operational criteria for senile dementia of Lewy body type (SDLT). *Psychological Medicine* 22: 911–22.

McKeith I, Fairbairn A, Perry R *et al.* (1992b) Neuroleptic sensitivity in patients with senile dementia of Lewy body type. *British Medical Journal* 305: 673–8.

McKeith IG, Fairbairn AF, Perry RH, Thompson P. (1994) The clinical diagnosis and misdiagnosis of senile dementia of Lewy body type (SDLT). *British Journal of Psychiatry* 165: 324–32.

McKeith IG, Galasko D, Wilcock GK, Byrne EJ. (1995) Lewy body dementia – diagnosis and treatment. *British Journal of Psychiatry* 167: 709–17.

McKeith IG, Galasko D, Kosaka K *et al.* (1996) Consensus guidelines for the clinical and pathologic diagnosis of dementia with Lewy bodies (DLB): Report of the consortium on DLB international workshop. *Neurology* 47: 1113–24.

McKeith IG, Perry EK, Perry RH. (1999) Report of the second dementia with Lewy body international workshop. *Diagnosis and treatment. Neurology* 53: 902–5.

McKeith IG, Ballard CG, Perry RH *et al.* (2000) Prospective validation of Consensus criteria for the diagnosis of dementia with Lewy bodies. *Neurology* 54: 1050–8.

McKeith I, Mintzer J, Aarsland D *et al.* (2004a) Dementia with Lewy bodies. *Lancet Neurology* 3: 19–28.

McKeith IG, Wesnes KA, Perry E, Ferrara R. (2004b) Hallucinations predict attentional improvements with rivastigmine in dementia with Lewy bodies. *Dementia and Geriatric Cognitive Disorders* 18: 94–100.

McKeith IG, Dickson DW, Lowe J *et al.* (2005) Diagnosis and management of dementia with Lewy bodies. Third report of the DLB consortium. *Neurology* 65: 1863–72.

McKeith IG, Rowan E, Askew K *et al.* (2006) More severe functional impairment in dementia with Lewy bodies than Alzheimer disease is related to extrapyramidal motor dysfunction. *American Journal of Geriatric Psychiatry* 14: 582–8.

McKeith I, O'Brien J, Walker Z *et al.* (2007) Sensitivity and specificity of dopamine transporter imaging with (123)I-FP-CIT SPECT in dementia with Lewy bodies: a phase III, multicentre study. *Lancet Neurology* 6: 305–13.

McShane R, Gedling K, Reading M *et al.* (1995) Prospective study of relations between cortical Lewy bodies, poor eyesight, and hallucinations in Alzheimer's disease. *Journal of Neurology, Neurosurgery and Psychiatry* 59: 185–8.

Marshall V, Grosset D. (2003) Role of dopamine transporter imaging in routine clinical practice. *Movement Disorders* 18: 1415–23.

Mollenhauer B, Trenkwalder C. (2009) Neurochemical biomarkers in the differential diagnosis of movement disorders. *Movement Disorders* 24: 1411–26.

Mosimann UP, Rowan EN, Partington CE *et al.* (2006) Characteristics of visual hallucinations in Parkinson disease dementia and dementia with Lewy bodies. *American Journal of Geriatric Psychiatry* 14: 153–60.

Mosimann UP, Collerton D, Dudley R *et al.* (2008) A semi-structured interview to assess visual hallucinations in older people. *International Journal of Geriatric Psychiatry* 23: 712–18.

Mullan E, Cooney C, Jones E. (1996) Mania and cortical Lewy body dementia. *International Journal of Geriatric Psychiatry* 11: 837–9.

O'Brien JT. (2009) DLB and PDD: the same or different? Is there a debate? *International Psychogeriatrics* 21: 220–4.

O'Brien JT, Paling S, Barber R *et al.* (2001) Progressive brain atrophy on serial MRI in dementia with Lewy bodies, AD, and vascular dementia. *Neurology* 56: 1386–8.

O'Brien JT, Colloby SJ, Fenwick J *et al.* (2004) Dopamine transporter loss visualised with FP-CIT SPECT in Dementia with Lewy bodies. *Archives of Neurology* **61**: 919–25.

O'Brien JT, McKeith IG, Walker Z *et al.* (2009) Diagnostic accuracy of 123I-FP-CIT SPECT in possible dementia with Lewy bodies. *British Journal of Psychiatry* **194**: 34–9.

Okazaki H, Lipton LS, Aronson SM. (1961) Diffuse intracytoplasmic ganglionic inclusions (Lewy type) associated with progressive dementia and quadrapesis in flexion. *Journal of Neurology, Neurosurgery and Psychiatry* **20**: 237–44.

Perry RH, Irving D, Blessed G *et al.* (1990) Senile dementia of Lewy body type. A clinically and neuropathologically distinct form of Lewy body dementia in the elderly. *Journal of Neurological Sciences* **95**: 119–39.

Perry EK, McKeith I, Thompson P *et al.* (1991) Topography, extent, and clinical relevance of neurochemical deficits in dementia of Lewy body type, Parkinson's disease and Alzheimer's disease. *Annals of the New York Academy of Sciences* **640**: 197–202.

Pickering-Brown SM, Mann DMA, Bourke JP *et al.* (1994) Apolipoprotein E4 and Alzheimer's disease pathology in Lewy body disease and in other beta-amyloid-forming diseases. *Lancet* **343**: 1155.

Rahkonen T, Eloniemi-Sulkava U, Rissanen S *et al.* (2003) Dementia with Lewy bodies according to the consensus criteria in a general population aged 75 years or older. *Journal of Neurology, Neurosurgery and Psychiatry* **74**: 720–4.

Salmon D, Galasko D. (1996) Neuropsychological aspects of Lewy body dementia. In: Perry R, McKeith I, Perry E (eds). *Dementia with Lewy bodies*. New York: Cambridge University Press, 99–114.

Stevens T, Livingston G, Kitchen G *et al.* (2002) Islington study of dementia subtypes in the community. *British Journal of Psychiatry* **180**: 270–6.

Suzuki M, Kurita A, Hashimoto M *et al.* (2006) Impaired myocardial ^{123}I-metaiodobenzylguanidine uptake in Lewy body disease: Comparison between dementia with Lewy bodies and Parkinson's disease. *Journal of the Neurological Sciences* **240**: 15–19.

Tiraboschi P, Salmon DP, Hansen LA *et al.* (2006) What best differentiates Lewy body from Alzheimer's disease in early-stage dementia? *Brain* **129**: 729–35.

Wada-Isoe K, Michio K, Imamura K *et al.* (2007) Serum proteomic profiling of dementia with Lewy bodies: diagnostic potential of SELDI-TOF MS analysis. *Journal of Neural Transmission* **114**: 1579–83.

Walker MP, Ayre GA, Cummings JL *et al.* (2000a) Quantifying fluctuation in dementia with Lewy bodies, Alzheimer's disease, and vascular dementia. *Neurology* **54**: 1616–24.

Walker MP, Ayre GA, Cummings JL *et al.* (2000b) The Clinician Assessment of Fluctuation and the One Day Fluctuation Assessment Scale. Two methods to assess fluctuating confusion in dementia. *British Journal of Psychiatry* **177**: 252–6.

Walker Z, Allen RL, Shergill S, Katona C. (1996) Neuropsychological performance in Lewy body dementia and Alzheimer's disease. *British Journal of Psychiatry* **170**: 156–8.

Walker Z, Jaros E, Walker RWH *et al.* (2007) Dementia with Lewy bodies: a comparison of clinical diagnosis, FP-CIT single photon emission computed tomography imaging and autopsy. *Journal of Neurology Neurosurgery and Psychiatry* **78**: 1176–81.

Weiner MF, Risser RC, Cullum CM *et al.* (1996) Alzheimer's disease and its Lewy body variant: A clinical analysis of postmortem verified cases. *American Journal of Psychiatry* **153**: 1269–73.

Weisman D, Cho M, Taylor C *et al.* (2007) In dementia with Lewy bodies, Braak stage determines phenotype, not Lewy body distribution. *Neurology* **69**: 356–9.

Zaccai J, McCracken C, Brayne C. (2005) A systematic review of prevalence and incidence studies of dementia with Lewy bodies. *Age and Ageing* **34**: 561–6.

65

Pathology of dementia with Lewy bodies

PAUL INCE AND GLENDA HALLIDAY

65.1 INTRODUCTION

The pathology of dementia with Lewy bodies (DLB) is of a primary degenerative dementia sharing features of both Alzheimer's disease (AD) and Parkinson's disease (PD). The diagnosis of DLB is challenging and requires clinicopathological correlation. There is a variable burden of Alzheimer-type pathology (ATP), together with Lewy bodies (LB) in both cortical and subcortical regions. Neocortical Alzheimer senile plaque formation is equivalent to that found in AD, but neocortical neurofibrillary tangles are variable and often infrequent (Dickson et al., 1989; Kosaka et al., 1988; Perry et al., 1990d). DLB patients with only minimal plaque and paired helical filament (PHF)-tau pathology are referred to as 'pure DLB' as opposed to the 'common form' in which AD pathology is more prominent.

The relationship of DLB to AD and PD is unresolved. Pathology data in the literature reflect the variable provenance of cases from clinical practice based in neurology and old age psychiatry. Problems remain in defining the relationship between DLB and PD with dementia (PDD), although the pathological definition of PD has been reviewed recently (Dickson et al., 2009).

LB are a coincidental pathology in many conditions (**Table 65.1**), but characteristically are associated with idiopathic PD (Gibb, 1986) and other conditions now grouped as α-synucleinopathies. The concept of α-synucleinopathy comes from the discovery of causal mutations in the gene encoding α-synuclein (αS) in familial PD (Polymeropoulos et al., 1997), and of αS as the major filamentous protein within LB (Spillantini et al., 1997). The range of clinical syndromes in which α-synucleinopathy predominates ranges from cognitive impairment, through extrapyramidal movement disorders, to autonomic dysfunction (**Table 65.2**). A spectrum of α-synucleinopathies, among which PD is the best known disorder (Ince et al., 1998), reflects this phenotypic diversity. Determinants of the clinical manifestation of α-synucleinopathy are not understood, but must involve the severity and anatomical distribution of pathology in the nervous system interacting with comorbidity, environmental factors and genetic determinants of individual susceptibility.

Table 65.1 Disorders in which 'incidental' Lewy bodies have been described.

Ataxia telangiectasia
Corticobasal degeneration
Down syndrome
Familial early-onset Alzheimer's disease
Frontotemporal lobar degeneration
Hallervorden–Spatz disease
Lysosomal storage disorders
Motor neurone disease
Multiple system atrophy
Neuroaxonal dystrophy
Neuroferritinopathy
Progressive supranuclear palsy
Subacute sclerosing panencephalitis
Neurofibrillary tangles with calcification

Table 65.2   Spectrum of α-synucleinopathy.

Syndrome	Neocortex	Limbic cortex	Substantia nigra	Dorsal vagus nucleus	Lateral grey horn/ sympathetic ganglia	Myenteric ganglia
Dementia with Lewy bodies	++/+++	+++	+/++	+/+++	+	+
Parkinson's disease	+/++	++/+++	+++	+/+++	+/++	+/++
Pure autonomic failure	0	0	0/+	+/++	++/+++	+
LB dysphagia	0	0	0/+	0/+	0/+	++/+++

0, no LB; +, mild LB formation/neuronal loss; ++, moderate LB and neuronal loss; +++, severe LB and neuronal loss. LB, Lewy body.

The pathogenesis of different syndromes within this spectrum is not understood. Inclusion body formation in α-synucleinopathy involves the ubiquitin/proteasome system and aberrant phosphorylation of αS. αS immunocytochemistry (ICC) shows extensive neuritic accumulation of fibrillar αS, the 'neuritic dystrophy hypothesis' (Duda, 2004). More recently, a key role for oligomeric species of αS, associated with synaptic loss, has been proposed (Kramer and Schulz-Schaeffer, 2007). Pathology highlights the co-occurrence of α-synucleinopathy and ATP in the same patient. DLB continues to pose major questions:

- What are the clinical, pathological and aetiological relationships among α-synucleinopathies? Should we regard them as diseases, disorders or syndromes?
- How does DLB relate to AD?

Consensus guidelines have been formulated to compare diagnosis and research between centres (McKeith et al., 1996; McKeith et al., 2005). The pathological guidelines were originally designed to generate uniform semi-quantitative data about the distribution and severity of LB pathology and allocate cases to three categories: (1) neocortical, (2) limbic (transitional) and (3) brainstem predominant. There was no assumption or requirement that any specific category should be classified as DLB. Subsequent revisions of the DLB consensus guidelines have moved towards pathological 'criteria for diagnosis' rather than simply a framework for the evaluation of lesions. Pathology in α-synucleinopathy may evolve as an anatomical hierarchy, beginning in medulla oblongata (Braak et al., 2003). However, data from large cohorts of older brain donors, including population-based studies, undermine the validity of this concept (Parkkinen et al. 2003; Zaccai et al. 2008), and suggest an alternate pathway through olfactory and limbic brain regions (Beach et al. 2009).

Neurochemical pathology research has attempted to identify key brain structures where pathology underpins the major and minor clinical features of DLB. Parkinsonism is securely attributable to degeneration of the nigrostriatal dopaminergic pathway, and the tendency to falls is probably related to peripheral autonomic involvement. Neurochemical and anatomical substrates for visual hallucination, fluctuating consciousness and rapid eye movement (REM) behavioural sleep

disorder remain poorly characterized. Finally, the diagnosis of DLB does not preclude other diagnoses. ATP especially should be assessed, according to established diagnostic criteria for AD to judge whether there is sufficient pathology to also warrant that diagnosis. Vascular pathology is also frequent given the age range in which DLB predominantly occurs.

65.2   DEVELOPMENT AND VALIDATION OF CLINICAL DIAGNOSTIC CRITERIA FOR DLB

The DLB Consortium pathological guidelines for DLB have evolved over more than a decade of research and clinical practice (McKeith et al., 2005), while the recent new staging scheme suggested for Lewy body disorders (Beach et al., 2009) is yet to be validated. The validated consensus method proposed is shown in **Table 65.3a** and **Table 65.3b** and includes a protocol for anatomical sampling. It evokes the hierarchic concept of the spread of α-synucleinopathy of Braak et al. (2003). Additional workers suggested simplified methods (Harding and Halliday, 1998), most recently specifically for dementia patients (Leverenz et al., 2008). The sensitivity (83 per cent) and specificity (92 per cent) of the consensus diagnostic criteria compared with 78 and 87 per cent for a diagnosis of 'probable AD' in the same study (McKeith et al., 2000). These guidelines involve the identification of pathology, and semiquantitative evaluation within anatomical areas, but a semiquantitative approach is problematic in terms of interobserver reproducibility. The European Brain Net Europe Consortium (www.brainnet-europe.org) has developed and validated a purely anatomical approach, but this has not yet been tested in terms of clinicopathological diagnostic performance (Alafuzoff et al., 2009).

65.3   PREVALENCE OF DLB AND OF α-SYNUCLEINOPATHY IN AGEING POPULATIONS

The population-prevalence of α-synucleinopathy can only be established from pathology studies because the associated clinical phenotypes (e.g. PD and DLB) do not predict the

Table 65.3a   Methods for the pathological diagnosis of dementia with Lewy bodies (DLB). Assignment of Lewy body type based upon pattern of Lewy-related pathology in brainstem, limbic and neocortical regions.

	Brainstem regions			Basal forebrain/limbic regions				Neocortical regions		
	IX–X	LC	SN	nbM	Amygdala	Transentorhinal	Cing–ulate	Temporal	Frontal	Parietal
Lewy body type										
Brainstem predominant	1–3	1–3	1–3	0–2	0–2	0–1	0–1	0	0	0
Limbic (transitional)	1–3	1–3	1–3	2–3	2–3	1–3	1–3	0–2	0–1	0
Diffuse neocortical	1–3	1–3	1–3	2–3	3–4	2–4	2–4	2–3	1–3	0–2

LC, locus ceruleus; nbM, nucleus basalis of Meynert; SN, substantia nigra; IX, 9th cranial nerve nucleus; X, 10th cranial nerve nucleus.
Brain regions are as defined anatomically in the original Consensus report.

Table 65.3b   Methods for the pathological diagnosis of dementia with Lewy bodies (DLB). Assessment of the likelihood that the pathologic findings are associated with a DLB clinical syndrome

	Alzheimer type pathology		
	NIA-Reagan Low (Braak stage 0–II)	NIA-Reagan Intermediate (Braak stage III–IV)	NIA-Reagan High (Braak stage V–VI)
Lewy body-type pathology			
Brainstem-predominant	Low	Low	Low
Limbic (transitional)	High	Intermediate	Low
Diffuse neocortical	High	High	Intermediate

underlying pathologic substrate better than four of five cases, and α-synucleinopathy can be asymptomatic (Parkkinen et al., 2005). The concept of DLB as a disease, and its associated pathology, arises from clinical practice-based cohorts selected by disease phenotypes. Synucleinopathy looks very different from a population-based perspective. The main category of α-synucleinopathy that lies outside the Braak scheme is the so-called 'amygdala-predominant' form when nigrostriatal, brainstem and neocortical involvement is limited or absent (Uchikado et al., 2006). A UK population-based study showed some degree of synucleinopathy in 37 per cent of 207 elderly people (Zaccai et al., 2008). A Japanese population-based study reported prevalence of α-synucleinopathy in 22.5 per cent at autopsy, comprising 41 per cent of demented people (Wakisaka et al., 2003), similar to findings from Finland (Parkkinen et al., 2003).

65.4   PATHOLOGICAL PHENOTYPES

65.4.1   Spectrum of α-synucleinopathy

DLB is part of a spectrum that can be interpreted in part on the basis of the anatomical distribution and severity of α-synucleinopathy (**Table 65.2**). The concept of DLB originates from cases of atypical dementia with parkinsonism and cortical LB first described by Okazaki et al. (1961). Peripheral and central nervous system involvement by LB is well recognized in PD, including the hypothalamic nuclei, nucleus basalis of Meynert, dorsal raphé, locus ceruleus, substantia

nigra, dorsal vagus nucleus and intermediolateral nucleus (Den Hartog Jager and Bethlem, 1960). The concept of a spectrum of LB diseases categorized into three types (brainstem, transitional and diffuse) forms the basis for the DLB Consortium categories (McKeith et al., 1996; McKeith et al., 2005). A 'cerebral' subtype of LB disease with progressive dementia and no detectable parkinsonism (Kosaka et al., 1996) shows widespread cortical, and minimal subcortical, involvement, with no significant ATP. Classification of α-synucleinopathy is problematic unless the concept of 'amygdala-predominant' disease is included (Uchikado et al., 2006; Zaccai et al., 2008; Beach et al., 2009). Gut motility is impaired in PD related to α-synucleinopathy of the myenteric nerve plexus and there are reports of pure gut motility disorders (LB dysphagia) (Jackson et al., 1995). Synucleinopathy may also cause primary autonomic failure.

Given this spectrum, the role of pathology is to address two questions:

1. Is the disorder associated with α-synucleinopathy?
2. What is the anatomical distribution and regional severity of α-synucleinopathy?

65.4.2   Alzheimer, vascular and other pathologies

Both ATP and cerebrovascular pathology are found in DLB at autopsy. DLB cases can usually be assigned to one of two broad groups: (1) the numerically more numerous show sufficient ATP to satisfy pathological criteria for AD (Mirra *et al.*, 1991) or (2) enough such that ATP has likely contributed to the neuropsychiatric phenotype. This 'common form' of DLB has been called 'LB variant of Alzheimer's disease' (Hansen *et al.*, 1990). The second group of cases show mild to negligible ATP, a 'pure form' of DLB called 'diffuse LB disease' (Hansen and Samuel, 1997). Patients with more severe ATP are likely to resemble AD clinically (Ballard *et al.*, 2004), may have more intense cortical LB formation than 'pure' DLB, and may show more severe dementia (Serby *et al.*, 2003).

In common with AD cases, microvascular pathology is a frequent finding in DLB at autopsy (Ince *et al.*, 1995; Londos *et al.*, 2002). Exclusion of cases with vascular features may be of value for research studies, but not in a routine clinical diagnostic setting.

TDP43 proteinopathy is the basis for many cases of frontotemporal dementia (FTD) (Neumann *et al.*, 2006). TDP43 deposition is commonly present as a minor component of the pathology of AD, especially in hippocampus and amygdala (Amador-Ortiz *et al.*, 2007). TDP43 FTD cases can present with clinical features mimicking DLB (Claassen *et al.*, 2008) and up to 60 per cent of DLB show pathological deposition of TDP43 as a minor pathological feature (Nakashima-Yasuda *et al.*, 2007).

65.5 PATHOLOGY OF DLB

The pathological lesions encountered in DLB are listed in **Table 65.4**. None of these is exclusive to this disorder.

65.5.1 Alpha-synucleinopathy

LB develop in many grey matter regions. In the pigmented brainstem nuclei, LB show an eosinophilic core and peripheral halo. In the cortex, they are diffusely granular, eosinophilic spheroids with no halo. Antibodies to αS are the optimum marker of LB throughout the central and peripheral nervous systems (Spillantini *et al.*, 1997).

LB frequency in the substantia nigra may be low in DLB and the loss of neurones not as severe compared to PD (Perry *et al.*, 1990d; Ince *et al.*, 1995). Some DLB cases show substantia nigra neurone loss in the PD range. The cholinergic

pedunculopontine tegmental nucleus is regularly affected in DLB (Schmeichel *et al.*, 2008) and patients vary in the involvement of serotonergic raphé nucleus subdivisions. The locus ceruleus is severely affected by neuronal loss (Zweig *et al.*, 1993).

PD cases show cortical LB involvement in 75–95 per cent of cases whether or not the patient has dementia (Mattila *et al.*, 1998). The difference between cortical LB pathology in PD and DLB is quantitative. In both clinical phenotypes, cortical LB are most frequent in limbic areas (Perry *et al.*, 1990d). The amygdala complex, insular, hippocampal, entorhinal and transentorhinal cortices are sites of predilection for LB formation. Neocortical involvement is usually most severe in the temporal lobe and follows the gradient: temporal > parietal = frontal > occipital (Kosaka *et al.*, 1984; Perry *et al.*, 1990d).

LB are found predominantly in deeper cortical layers (4, 5 and 6) within small and medium-sized neurones (Kosaka *et al.*, 1984). Cortical LB frequency may correlate with the intensity of dementia (Samuel *et al.*, 1996). There is extensive pathological change in addition to classical LB, including a neuritic component and diffuse cytoplasmic granular staining, but these are not always present (Duda *et al.*, 2002). 'Lewy neurites' were first described in the CA2 sector of the hippocampus in DLB (Dickson *et al.*, 1994) possibly related to disease in the medial septum and diagonal band projections (Fujishiro *et al.*, 2006). Neuritic α-synucleinopathy is now considered the most consistent feature of LB diseases and in PD concentrates in the amygdala (Braak *et al.* 1994), basal forebrain, substantia nigra, pedunculopontine nucleus, raphé nuclei, dorsal efferent vagal nucleus and neocortex (Gai *et al.*, 1995; Pellise *et al.*, 1996), but does not predict dementia (de Vos *et al.*, 1995). Neurites do not colocalize with tyrosine hydroxylase, suggesting that they do not arise in distal projections of the substantia nigra.

65.5.2 Alzheimer-type pathology

Many cases of DLB have ATP, but there are pathological observations that support the distinction of DLB from AD:

- There are cases with no significant ATP.
- Quantitative and qualitative analysis of the ATP shows differences between DLB and AD.

Table 65.4 Pathological features associated with dementia with Lewy bodies (DLB).

	Feature
Essential for the diagnosis of DLB	Lewy bodies
Associated with DLB but not essential	Lewy neurites
	Alzheimer-type pathology
	Senile plaques
	Neurofibrillary tangles
	Regional neuronal loss, especially affecting substantia nigra, locus ceruleus, and nucleus basalis of Meynert
	Microvacuolation
	Synapse loss
	Neurochemical abnormalities/neurotransmitter deficits

- The similarity is predominantly related β-amyloid deposition, not neuronal inclusion pathology.

Most cases of DLB have αS accumulation without extensive PHF-tau accumulation (**Table 65.3**). The picture is reversed in AD, where αS is often in the amygdala only (Hamilton, 2000; Leverenz et al., 2008). If tauopathy and α-synucleinopathy are both present, the likelihood of clinical expression of DLB is greater at lower Braak NFT stages (Ballard et al., 2004; Fujishiro et al., 2008), although Braak stage does not predict dementia status in PD and DLB (Jellinger, 2009). The burden of senile plaques in most DLB cases and age-matched AD patients is similar (Gentleman et al., 1992; McKenzie et al., 1996). DLB cases with little ATP are clinically indistinguishable from other DLB cases.

DLB cases have excess hippocampal ATP when compared with age-matched controls and demented and non-demented PD patients (Harding et al., 2002b; Ince et al., 1991). Morphological markers of the integrity of the perforant pathway also show changes in DLB of lesser severity than in AD (Lippa et al., 1997; Wakabayashi et al., 1997). These changes may contribute to neuropsychological features, such as defective short-term memory, but do not account for much of the clinical picture of DLB.

Problems in defining the relationship between AD and DLB include the pathological criteria used to define AD. Criteria have evolved through the CERAD criteria (Mirra et al., 1991), which rely on neuritic plaques, to the National Institute on Aging (NIA)-Reagan Institute guidelines, which combine CERAD and Braak stage (National Institute on Aging, 1997). Whether DLB cases are a variant of AD is dependent on which diagnostic criteria are used. A plaque-based method assigns most DLB patients as meeting AD criteria. Most DLB patients will fall short of AD if there is a requirement for significant neocortical tangles.

65.5.3   Regional neuronal loss

The major clinical features of DLB include the presence of mild Parkinsonism. In contrast to the cognitive features of DLB, the pathological and neurochemical substrate for this is well characterized. DLB patients have substantia nigra degeneration intermediate between that seen in PD and normal control individuals of the same age (Perry et al., 1990d). Depigmentation of the substantia nigra is often only moderate neurone loss, and incontinence of pigment is usually less than in PD, and the cellular pathology includes classical LB, pale bodies and a variable background of neuritic changes. Pale bodies contain ubiquitin and αS and are regarded as a precursor of LB (Dale et al., 1992). Atypical AD patients may attract an erroneous clinical diagnosis of DLB due to the prominence of parkinsonism (McKeith et al., 2000). Erroneous clinical diagnosis of DLB occurs in other tau-related neurodegenerative disorders, including progressive supranuclear palsy and corticobasal degeneration (Chin and Goldman, 1996; Feany et al., 1996). The locus ceruleus is routinely affected and is often totally depigmented to the naked eye. LB are usually frequent in the surviving neurones.

Other brainstem and midbrain nuclei contain LB including the raphé (serotonergic) and pedunculopontine (cholinergic) nuclei (Schmeichel et al., 2008). Neuronal loss in the cholinergic nucleus basalis of Meynert has been reported in PD, DLB and AD (Jellinger and Bancher, 1996) and, in DLB cases with significant AD pathology, this neuronal population may contain both LB and neurofibrillary tangles.

65.5.3.1   MICROVACUOLATION

Early reports of DLB emphasized the presence of cortical spongiform changes in the temporal cortex (Hansen et al., 1989). This pathology was said to resemble prion disease, but this has been excluded on the basis of failed animal transmission experiments and lack of ICC for prion protein. There is no clear relationship between spongiosis and the distribution or severity of cortical LB pathology in individual cases.

65.5.3.2   SYNAPTIC LOSS

Synaptic loss has been proposed to be a major process in the pathogenesis of DLB linked to the role of oligomeric αS acting as a synaptotoxin (Kramer and Schulz-Schaeffer, 2007). Cortical synaptic loss of 50 per cent is reported in AD (Masliah et al., 1991) as a major substrate for reduced cognitive function. Significant synaptic loss was reported in the 'common form' of DLB, compared to a non-significant decrease in 'pure' DLB (Samuel et al. 1997). Hippocampal synaptic loss in DLB is also related to ATP not α-synucleinopathy (Revuelta et al., 2008).

65.5.4   Neurotransmitters and neurochemistry in DLB

Neuronal loss occurs in specific subcortical nuclei in DLB as it does in AD and PD. The cholinergic and dopaminergic systems have received most neurochemical research attention in DLB.

65.5.4.1   CHOLINERGIC SYSTEMS

Cortical cholinergic abnormalities and degeneration of basal forebrain nuclei are considered to contribute to cognitive impairment in AD. In PD, cortical cholinergic activity and nucleus basalis neurone counts are lower in demented compared with non-demented individuals. In DLB, neocortical choline acetyltransferase (ChAT) is lower than in AD and similar to that in demented PD (Perry et al. 1994). Cholinergic activity is lower in hallucinating compared with non-hallucinating DLB cases, whereas 5HT activity is relatively preserved (Perry et al., 1990b).

Loss of striatal ChAT in DLB (Langlais et al., 1993) may account for the reduced severity of extrapyramidal clinical symptoms in some DLB patients who have equivalent loss of dopaminergic substantia nigra neurones as PD patients. Selective dendritic degeneration of striatal medium spiny neurons in DLB has been linked to executive dysfunction (Zaja-Milatovic et al., 2006).

In DLB and PD, the muscarinic M1 subtype is elevated in the cortex, in contrast to AD (Perry et al., 1990c), reflecting upregulation of postsynaptic receptors in response to cholinergic denervation. Normal receptor coupling via G proteins suggests that cholinoceptive neurones are intact in DLB. In contrast, striatal M1 receptor density is lower in DLB, and parallels low D2 receptor density, which may relate to the relatively mild movement disorder (Piggott et al., 2003).

Cortical nicotinic receptors are reduced equally in DLB compared with AD and PD (Perry et al., 1990c). In the substantia nigra, receptor binding is equally depleted in DLB and PD, despite the greater loss of neurones in PD (Perry et al., 1995) suggesting that loss or downregulation of the receptor may precede neurodegeneration. Unchanged expression of various receptor subunits ($\alpha2$, $\alpha7$, $\beta2$, $\beta3$) in DLB suggests a problem at the level of receptor assembly (Martin-Ruiz et al., 2000). Therapeutic implications of the cholinergic neurochemical pathology in DLB include:

- Since cortical cholinergic abnormalities exist in most cases in the absence of tangle pathology, and muscarinic receptors are functionally intact, cholinergic replacement therapy (anticholinesterases, muscarinic or nicotinic agonists) is likely to be more effective than in AD.
- Since the cortical cholinergic deficits in DLB relate more to psychiatric than cognitive symptoms, therapy may be more effective in alleviating the former.

65.5.4.2 DOPAMINERGIC SYSTEMS

Loss of pigmented substantia nigra neurones and clinical evidence of parkinsonism in DLB indicate disruption of the dopaminergic input to the striatum. Striatal presynaptic dopamine transporter (DT) is lowered in both PD and DLB and is the basis for the use of single photon emission computed tomography (SPECT) imaging as a diagnostic test to distinguish AD from DLB (Walker et al., 2007). There is much lower dopaminergic neurotransmission in the cortex compared to striatum and no changes have been observed (Perry et al., 1993). Although L-dopa may induce hallucinations in PD, there are no dopaminergic parameters that distinguish between patients with and without hallucinations.

Striatal dopaminergic D2 receptors are upregulated in PD but not DLB, suggesting that basal ganglia pathology may be distinct between the two diseases. Clinical evidence supports this possibility (Louis et al., 1997) and that DLB patients are unusually sensitive to typical neuroleptic D2 antagonists (McKeith et al., 1992). A profound loss of D2 receptors in DLB cerebral cortex, compared to AD, may underlie this sensitivity to neuroleptic D2 antagonist drugs (Piggott et al. 2007b).

65.6 MOLECULAR AND ANATOMICAL PATHOLOGY CORRELATES OF CLINICAL FEATURES IN DLB

65.6.1 Cognitive decline in DLB

Attributing specific molecular pathological changes as the substrate of cognitive decline in DLB is complicated by the frequent coexistence of significant ATP (Jellinger and Attems, 2008b). ATP and α-synucleinopathy may interact synergistically. How the anatomical distribution and the burden of α-synucleinopathy influence cognitive decline is not fully resolved (Jellinger, 2006). The consensus guidelines for evaluating LB pathology (McKeith et al., 1996; McKeith et al., 2005) are often interpreted as diagnostic guidelines implying that dementia is associated with at least the 'limbic' stage. Evidence suggests that increased neocortical LB pathology is associated with cognitive decline in DLB and Parkinson's disease (Kovari et al., 2003).

65.6.2 Visual hallucinations

The obvious candidate regions expected to correlate with visual hallucinations in DLB are the components of the visual pathways. Cortical cholinergic activity is lower in patients with hallucinations, while serotonergic neurotransmission is relatively preserved (Perry et al., 1990a). The occipital neocortex is relatively spared from α-synucleinopathy in terms of LB formation (Perry et al., 1990d), but occipital hypometabolism has been consistently demonstrated in DLB compared to AD (Shimada et al., 2009). An increased burden of α-synucleinopathy in the medial temporal lobe (parahippocampus, amygdala) (Harding et al., 2002a), claustrum (Yamamoto et al., 2007; Kalaitzakis et al., 2009), and secondary visual pathway (pulvinar, BA18/19 and inferior temporal cortex) (Yamamoto et al., 2006) are potential correlates of visual hallucination and it has been proposed that an intrinsic α-synucleinopathy of the retina may contribute (Maurage et al., 2003).

65.6.3 Parkinsonism

The pathological and neurochemical basis of mild parkinsonism in DLB are the most satisfactorily characterized aspect of DLB pathology. The presence of nigral dopamine neurone loss with reduced presynaptic dopamine transporter activity in the striatum now form the basis for a clinical diagnostic strategy (Walker et al., 2007) to distinguish DLB from other dementia syndromes. Rather less well resolved is the relationship between DLB and Parkinson's disease with dementia (McKeith, 2009). Findings which show few differences between DLB and PDD include the extent of α-synucleinopathy, amyloid plaques (Jellinger and Attems, 2008b), cerebral amyloid angiopathy (Jellinger and Attems, 2008a), and the extent and progression of white matter hyperintensities (Burton et al., 2006). Differences between PDD and DLB are reported in relation to striatal tauopathy (Jellinger and Attems, 2006), increased cortical atrophy in DLB (Beyer et al. 2007), and the contrast between thalamic D2 receptor upregulation in PDD compared to DLB cases (Piggott et al., 2007a), although DLB cases with parkinsonism were not distinguishable from PDD so the phenomenon seems to relate primarily to the movement disorder component.

Harding AJ, Halliday GM. (1998) Simplified neuropathological diagnosis of dementia with Lewy bodies. *Neuropathology and Applied Neurobiology* 24: 195–201.

Hashimoto M, Hsu LJ, Sisk A *et al.* (1998) Human recombinant NACP/α-synuclein is aggregated and fibrillated *in vitro*: Relevance for Lewy body disease. *Brain Research* 799: 301–6.

Henderson JM, Carpenter K, Cartwright H, Halliday GM. (2000) Degeneration of the centré median-parafascicular complex in Parkinson's disease. *Annals of Neurology* 47: 345–52.

Ince P, Irving D, MacArthur F, Perry RH. (1991) Quantitative neuropathology in the hippocampus: comparison of senile dementia of Alzheimer type, senile dementia of Lewy body type, Parkinson's disease and non-demented elderly control patients. *Journal of the Neurological Sciences* 106: 142–52.

Ince P, Morris C, Perry E. (1998) Dementia with Lewy bodies: a distinct non-Alzheimer dementia? *Brain Pathology* 8: 299–324.

Ince PG, McArthur FK, Bjertness E *et al.* (1995) Neuropathological diagnoses in elderly patients in Oslo: Alzheimer's disease, Lewy body disease and vascular lesions. *Dementia* 6: 162–8.

Jackson M, Lennox G, Balsitis M *et al.* (1995) Lewy body dysphagia. *Neuropathology and Applied Neurobiology* 21: 18–26.

Jellinger KA. (2006) Pathological substrate of dementia in Parkinson's disease – its relation to DLB and DLBD. *Parkinson's Disease and Related Disorders* 12: 119–20.

Jellinger KA. (2009) A critical evaluation of current staging of alpha-synuclein pathology in Lewy body disorders. *Biochimica Biophysica Acta* 1792: 730–40.

Jellinger KA, Attems J. (2006) Does striatal pathology distinguish Parkinson disease with dementia and dementia with Lewy bodies? *Acta Neuropathologica* 112: 253–60.

Jellinger KA, Attems J. (2008a) Cerebral amyloid angiopathy in Lewy body disease. *Journal of Neural Transmission* 115: 473–82.

Jellinger KA, Attems J. (2008b) Prevalence and impact of vascular and Alzheimer pathologies in Lewy body disease. *Acta Neuropathologica* 115: 427–36.

Jellinger KA, Bancher C. (1996) Dementia with Lewy bodies: relationships to Parkinson's and Alzheimer's diseases. In: Perry RH, McKeith IG, Perry EK (eds). *Dementia with Lewy bodies*. Cambridge: Cambridge University Press, 268–86.

Jensen PH, Nielsen MS, Jakes R *et al.* (1998) Binding of α-synuclein to brain vesicles is abolished by familial Parkinson's disease mutation. *Journal of Biological Chemistry* 273: 26292–4.

Kalaitzakis ME, Pearce RK, Gentleman SM. (2009) Clinical correlates of pathology in the claustrum in Parkinson's disease and dementia with Lewy bodies. *Neuroscience Letters* 461: 12–15.

Kosaka K, Yoshimura M, Ikeda K, Budka H. (1984) Diffuse type of Lewy body disease: progressive dementia with abundant cortical Lewy bodies and senile changes of varying degree – A new disease? *Clinical Neuropathology* 3: 185–92.

Kosaka K, Tsuchiya K, Yoshimura M. (1988) Lewy body disease with and without dementia: a clinicopathological study of 35 cases. *Clinical Neuropathology* 7: 299–305.

Kosaka K, Iseki E, Odawara T *et al.* (1996) Cerebral type of Lewy body disease. *Neuropathology* 16: 32–5.

Kovari E, Gold G, Herrmann FR *et al.* (2003) Lewy body densities in the entorhinal and anterior cingulate cortex predict cognitive deficits in Parkinson's disease. *Acta Neuropathologica* 106: 83–8.

Kramer ML, Schulz-Schaeffer WJ. (2007) Presynaptic alpha-synuclein aggregates, not Lewy bodies, cause neurodegeneration in dementia with Lewy bodies. *Journal of Neuroscience* 27: 1405–10.

Langlais PJ, Thal L, Hansen L *et al.* (1993) Neurotransmitters in basal ganglia and cortex of Alzheimer's disease with and without Lewy bodies. *Neurology* 43: 1927–34.

Leverenz JB, Hamilton R, Tsuang DW *et al.* (2008) Empirical refinement of the pathological assessment of Lewy-related pathology in the dementia patient. *Brain Pathology* 18: 220–4.

Lippa CF, Pulaski-Salo D, Dickson DW, Smith TW. (1997) Alzheimer's disease, Lewy body disease and aging: a comparative study of the perforant pathway. *Journal of the Neurological Sciences* 147: 161–6.

Londos E, Passant U, Risberg J *et al.* (2002) Contributions of other brain pathologies in dementia with Lewy bodies. *Dementia and Geriatric Cognitive Disorders* 13: 130–48.

Louis ED, Klatka LA, Lui Y, Fahn S. (1997) Comparison of extrapyramidal features in 31 pathologically confirmed cases of diffuse Lewy body disease and 34 pathologically confirmed cases of Parkinson's disease. *Neurology* 48: 376–80.

McKeith I. (2009) Commentary: DLB and PDD: the same or different? Is there a debate? *International Psychogeriatrics* 21: 220–4.

McKeith I, Del-Ser T, Anand R *et al.* (2004) International Psychogeriatric Association Expert Meeting on Dementia with Lewy bodies. *Lancet Neurology* 3: 19–28.

McKeith IG, Fairbairn A, Perry R *et al.* (1992) Neuroleptic sensitivity in patients with senile dementia of Lewy body type. *British Medical Journal* 305: 673–8.

McKeith IG, Galasko D, Kosaka K *et al.* (1996) Consensus guidelines for the clinical and pathological diagnosis of dementia with Lewy bodies (DLB): report of the consortium on DLB International Workshop. *Neurology* 47: 1113–24.

McKeith IG, Ballard CG, Perry RH *et al.* (2000) Prospective validation of consensus criteria for the diagnosis of dementia with Lewy bodies. *Neurology* 54: 1050–8.

McKeith IG, Dickson DW, Lowe J *et al.* (2005) Diagnosis and management of dementia with Lewy bodies: Third report of the DLB consortium. *Neurology* 65: 1863–72.

McKenzie JE, Edwards R, Gentleman SM *et al.* (1996) A quantitative comparison of plaque types in Alzheimer's disease and senile dementia of the Lewy body type. *Acta Neuropathologica* 91: 526–9.

Martin-Ruiz C, Court J, Lee M *et al.* (2000) Nicotinic receptors in dementia of Alzheimer. Lewy body and vascular types. *Acta Neurologica Scandanaciva* 176 (Suppl.): 34–41.

Masliah E, Terry RD, Alford M *et al.* (1991) Cortical and subcortical patterns of synaptophysin-like immunoreactivity in Alzheimer's disease. *American Journal of Pathology* 138: 235–46.

Mattila PM, Roytta M, Torikka H *et al.* (1998) Cortical Lewy bodies and Alzheimer-type changes in patients with Parkinson's disease. *Acta Neuropathologica* 95: 576–82.

Maurage C, Ruchoux MM, de Vos R *et al.* (2003) Retinal involvement in dementia with Lewy bodies: a clue to hallucinations? *Annals of Neurology* 54: 542–7.

Miller VM, Kenny RA, Oakley AE *et al.* (2009) Dorsal motor nucleus of vagus protein aggregates in Lewy body disease with autonomic dysfunction. *Brain Research* 1286: 165–73.

Minguez-Castellanos A, Chamorro CE, Escamilla-Sevilla F *et al.* (2007) Do alpha-synuclein aggregates in autonomic plexuses predate Lewy body disorders?: a cohort study. *Neurology* 68: 2012–18.

Mirra SS, Heyman A, McKeel DW *et al.* (1991) The consortium to establish a registry of Alzheimer's disease (CERAD) Part II. Standardization of the neuropathologic assessment of Alzheimer's disease. *Neurology* 41: 479–86.

Nakashima-Yasuda H, Uryu K, Robinson J *et al.* (2007) Co-morbidity of TDP-43 proteinopathy in Lewy body related diseases. *Acta Neuropathologica* 114: 221–9.

National Institute on Aging and Reagan Institute Working Group on Diagnostic Criteria for the Neuropathological Assessment of Alzheimer's Disease. (1997) Consensus recommendations for the postmortem diagnosis of Alzheimer's disease. *Neurobiology of Aging* 18: S1–S2.

Neumann M, Sampathu DM, Kwong LK *et al.* (2006) Ubiquitinated TDP-43 in Frontotemporal Lobar Degeneration and Amyotrophic Lateral Sclerosis. *Science* 314: 130–3.

Okazaki H, Lipkin LS, Aronson SM. (1961) Diffuse intracytoplasmic ganglionic inclusions (Lewy type) associated with progressive dementia and quadriparesis in flexion. *Journal of Neuropathlogy and Experimental Neurology* 20: 237–44.

Orimo S, Amino T, Itoh Y *et al.* (2005) Cardiac sympathetic denervation precedes neuronal loss in the sympathetic ganglia in Lewy body disease. *Acta Neuropathologica* 109: 583–8.

Parkkinen L, Soininen H, Alfuzoff I. (2003) Regional distribution of alpha-synuclein pathology in unimpaired aging and Alzheimer's disease. *Journal Neuropathology and Experimental Neurology* 62: 363–7.

Parkkinen L, Pirttila T, Tervahauta M, Alafuzoff I. (2005) Widespread and abundant alpha-synuclein pathology in a neurologically unimpaired subject. *Neuropathology* 25: 304–14.

Pellise A, Roig C, Barraquer-Bordas Ll, Ferrer I. (1996) Abnormal ubiquitinated cortical neurites in patients with diffuse Lewy body disease. *Neuroscience Letters* 206: 85–8.

Perry EK, Marshall E, Kerwin J *et al.* (1990a) Evidence of a monoaminergic:cholinergic imbalance related to visual hallucinations in Lewy body dementia. *Journal of Neurochemistry* 55: 1454–6.

Perry EK, Curtis M, Dick DJ *et al.* (1990b) Cholinergic and dopaminergic activities in senile dementia of Lewy body type. *Alzheimer Disease and Related Disorders* 4: 87–95.

Perry EK, Smith CJ, Court JA, Perry RH. (1990c) Cholinergic nicotinic and muscarinic receptors in dementia of Alzheimer, Parkinson and Lewy body types. *Journal of Neural Transmission* 2: 149–58.

Perry RH, Irving D, Blessed G *et al.* (1990d) Senile dementia of Lewy body type: a clinically and neuropatholgically distinct form of Lewy body dementia in the elderly. *Journal of the Neurological Sciences* 95: 119–39.

Perry EK, Irving D, Kerwin JM *et al.* (1993) Cholinergic transmitter and neurotrophic activities Lewy body dementia: similarity to Parkinson's disease and distinction form Alzheimer's disease. *Alzheimer Disease and Related Disorders* 7: 69–79.

Perry EK, Haroutunian V, Davis KL *et al.* (1994) Neocortical cholinergic activities differentiate Lewy body dementia from classical Alzheimer's disease. *Neuroreport* 5: 747–9.

Perry EK, Morris CM, Court JA *et al.* (1995) Alteration in nicotine binding sites in Parkinson's disease, Lewy body dementia and Alzheimer's disease: possible index of early neuropathology. *Neuroscience* 64: 385–95.

Piggott M, Owens J, O'Brien J *et al.* (2003) Muscarinic receptors in basal ganglia in dementia with Lewy bodies, Parkinson's disease and Alzheimer's disease. *Journal of Chemical Neuroanatomy* 25: 161–73.

Piggott MA, Ballard CG, Kickinson HO *et al.* (2007a) Thalamic D2 receptors in dementia with Lewy bodies, Parkinson's disease, and Parkinson's disease dementia. *International Journal of Neuropsychopharmacology* 10: 231–44.

Piggott MA, Ballard CG, Rowan E *et al.* (2007b) Selective loss of dopamine D2 receptors in temporal cortex in dementia with Lewy bodies, association with cognitive decline. *Synapse* 61: 903–11.

Polymeropoulos MH, Lavedan C, Leroy E *et al.* (1997) Mutation in the α-synuclein gene identified in families with Parkinson's disease. *Science* 276: 2045–7.

Revuelta GJ, Rosso A, Lippa CF. (2008) Neuritic pathology as a correlate of synaptic loss in dementia with lewy bodies. *American Journal of Alzheimer's Disease* 23: 97–102.

Samuel W, Galasko D, Masliah E, Hansen LA. (1996) Neocortical Lewy body counts correlate with dementia in the Lewy body variant of Alzheimer's disease. *Journal of Neuropathology and Experimental Neurology* 55: 44–52.

Samuel W, Alford M, Hofstetter CR, Hansen L. (1997) Dementia with Lewy bodies versus pure Alzheimer's disease: differences in cognition, neuropathology, cholinergic dysfunction, and synaptic density. *Journal of Neuropathology and Experimental Neurology* 56: 499–508.

Schmeichel AM, Buchhalter LC, Low PA *et al.* (2008) Mesopontine cholinergic neuron involvement in Lewy body dementia and multiple system atrophy. *Neurology* 70: 368–73.

Serby M, Brickman AM, Haroutunian V *et al.* (2003) Cognitive burden and excess Lewy-body pathology in the Lewy-body variant of Alzheimer's disease. *American Journal of Geriatric Psychiatry* 11: 371–4.

Shimada H, Hirano S, Shinotoh H *et al.* (2009) Mapping of brain acetylcholinesterase alterations in Lewy body disease by PET. *Neurology* 73: 273–8.

Spillantini MG, Schmidt ML, Lee VM *et al.* (1997) Alpha-synuclein in Lewy bodies. *Nature* 388: 839–40.

Uchikado H, Lin WL, DeLucia MW, Dickson DW. (2006) Alzheimer disease with amygdala Lewy bodies: a distinct form of alpha-synucleinopathy. *Journal of Neuropathology and Experimental Neurology* 65: 685–97.

Wakabayashi K, Hansen L A, Vincent I *et al.* (1997) Neurofibrillary tangles in the dentate granule cells of patients with Alzheimer's disease, Lewy body disease and progressive supranuclear palsy. *Acta Neuropathologica* **93**: 7–12.

Wakisaka Y, Furuta A, Tanizaki Y *et al.* (2003) Age-associated prevalence and risk factors of Lewy body pathology in a general population: the Hisayama study. *Acta Neuropathologica* **106**: 374–82.

Walker Z, Jaros E, Walker RW *et al.* (2007) Dementia with Lewy bodies: a comparison of clinical diagnosis, FP-CIT single photon emission computed tomography imaging and autopsy. *Journal of Neurology, Neurosurgery and Psychiatry* **78**: 1176–81.

Yamamoto R, Iseki E, Murayama N *et al.* (2006) Investigation of Lewy pathology in the visual pathway of brains of dementia with Lewy bodies. *Journal of the Neurological Sciences* **246**: 95–101.

Yamamoto R, Iseki E, Murayama N *et al.* (2007) Correlation in Lewy pathology between the claustrum and visual areas in brains of dementia with Lewy bodies. *Neuroscience Letters* **415**: 219–24.

Zaccai J, Brayne C, McKeith I *et al.* (2008) Patterns and stages of alpha-synucleinopathy: Relevance in a population-based cohort. *Neurology* **70**: 1042–8.

Zaja-Milatovic S, Keene CD, Montine KS *et al.* (2006) Selective dendritic degeneration of medium spiny neurons in dementia with Lewy bodies. *Neurology* **66**: 1591–3.

Zweig RM, Cardillo JE, Cohen M *et al.* (1993) The locus ceruleus and dementia in Parkinson's disease. *Neurology* **43**: 986–91.

66

The treatment of dementia with Lewy bodies

E JANE BYRNE AND JOHN O'BRIEN

66.1 INTRODUCTION

The treatment of dementia with Lewy bodies (DLB) presents the clinician with several challenges. Some of the most persistent and troublesome symptoms can be made worse by 'conventional' therapies. A complex balance often has to be struck, as treatments to improve motor symptoms can make neuropsychiatric symptoms worse, and vice versa. Although many treatments are given empirically, there are now some well-conducted clinical trials emerging which can aid treatment decisions in the area.

66.2 PRIMARY PREVENTION

In a condition whose nosological status is uncertain, it may seem premature to discuss therapies or strategies that may prevent or delay its onset. The pathological features of DLB are, however, increasingly well described. The controversy lies in the interpretation of the histological features, for example whether they indicate a variant of Alzheimer's disease (AD), Parkinson's disease (PD), the coexistence of the two, a distinct entity, or as part of a group of 'synucleinopathies'. Clinically, about 20 per cent of those diagnosed with DLB present with a syndrome indistinguishable from idiopathic PD, 40 per cent with parkinsonism and dementia and 20 per cent with dementia alone (Lennox, 1992). Pure DLB cases without significant Alzheimer histological change are more likely to be young (under 70 years) and male with prominent early parkinsonian features (Kosaka, 1990; Hely et al., 1996). Putative strategies to prevent PD might therefore be expected to be effective in these cases.

Exposure to pesticides has been postulated as a risk factor for the development of PD (Liou et al., 1997; Herishanu et al., 1998). Hubble et al. (1998) have reported a possible gene–toxin interaction as a putative risk factor for PD with dementia (PDD). They found that subjects who had exposure to pesticides and at least one copy of the CYP2D629B+ allele had an 83 per cent predicted probability of the development of dementia in association with PD.

Apoptotic-like changes have been described in nigral cells in PD and DLB (Tompkins et al., 1997). One mechanism whereby this may occur is through the actions of nitric oxide (NO) (Snyder, 1996). NO is formed from arginine by NO synthase (NOS) which has three forms each with different genetic derivation and glutamate neurones form synapses with neuronal NOS (nNOS) neurons. Glutamate in excess causes a release of NO which leads to cell death (Dawson et al., 1996). NOS inhibitors prevent this NO-mediated cell death in MPTP-treated baboons (Hantraye et al., 1996). As NO has also been implicated as a cause of cell damage in AD and in DLB (Molina et al., 2002), the use of NOS inhibitors in DLB has some theoretical justification, which is also supported by the suggestion that polymorphisms in the NOS2A gene may predispose individuals to the development of DLB (Xu et al., 2000). This rationale might also suggest the potential of excitatory amino acid antagonists as putative treatments in DLB. However, these remain theoretical possibilities at present.

Strategies to prevent the accumulation of alpha-synuclein have been suggested (Beyer and Ariza, 2008). Cholesterol metabolites may accelerate alpha-synuclein fibrillization and cholesterol-lowering agents, such as statins, may thus reduce alpha-synuclein accumulation (Koob et al., 2010). In transgenic mice which overexpress neuronal alpha-synuclein,

Koob and colleagues (2010) found that lovostatin reduced the levels of neuronal alpha-synuclein aggregates when compared to saline-treated controls. Wei and colleagues (2009) suggest a protective role for endogenous gangliosides against lysosomal abnormalities in a cellular model of synucleinopathy. As DLB has pathological features of both PD and AD, it is highly likely that preventative strategies developed for both disorders may have relevance.

66.3 SYMPTOMATIC TREATMENTS

There is accumulating evidence that DLB and dementia which occurs in established PD (PDD, defined by convention as dementia occurring one year or more after the onset of motor features of parkinsonism) are closely related and overlapping, though not identical, clinical entities (Byrne, 1995). Given these findings, it is not unreasonable to suggest that treatments that are effective in the treatment of PDD may be useful in the treatment of DLB and vice versa. Thus, some studies on the treatment of PDD are included in this chapter.

66.3.1 Cholinesterase inhibitors

In DLB, there is a severe choline acetyl transferase deficiency (ChAT), even greater than that seen in AD (Dickson et al., 1987; Perry et al., 1990). The Newcastle group were the first to suggest the use of cholinesterase inhibitors (ChEIs) for the treatment of DLB. Evidence from the early placebo-controlled trials of tacrine supported this suggestion when the first three responders in the London trial were found to have cortical Lewy bodies (CLB) (Levy et al., 1994). Others found that response to tacrine was not limited to those AD cases with CLB (Wilcock and Scott, 1994). Lebert et al. (1998) have studied the effects of tacrine (120 mg/day) in clinically diagnosed AD and DLB cases. They found that while the ratio of AD and DLB cases did not differ between responders and

non-responders, the pattern of response was different between the two groups. In the DLB group, cognitive performance improved on tests of attention (digit span and verbal initiation), while the AD group improved on tests of conceptualization. In this study, tacrine was apparently not associated with adverse effects on the mental state of DLB patients, although case reports suggest there may be possible adverse effects of tacrine in clinically diagnosed DLB (Witjeratne et al., 1995).

Early case reports of the use of 'second-generation' ChEIs suggested that this class of drugs might improve some of the core features of DLB (Lanctôt and Herrmann, 2000). However, few clinical trials have been performed in DLB subjects and while some have focused on the outcome of the treatment on single symptoms, an emerging literature suggests that it might be more useful to examine the effect of a treatment on 'clusters' of symptoms instead, which may be stable across dementia diagnosis (Robert et al., 2005; Robert et al., 2007; Aalten et al., 2007; Aalten et al., 2008). While such 'clusters' are derived by statistical analysis, they may have a resonance in clinical practice and there is some evidence to suggest that ChEIs treat 'clusters' of neuropsychiatric symptoms like psychosis (McKeith et al., 2000; Herrmann et al., 2005; Gauthier et al., 2005). In addition to their supposedly symptomatic clinical effects, ChEIs may play a role in disease modification, for example by reducing cortical β-amyloid (Ballard et al., 2007), although this has not yet been clearly demonstrated in controlled studies and remains speculative.

Table 66.1 summarizes some studies of ChEIs in the treatment of DLB. Only one randomized controlled trial (RCT) of a ChEI (rivastigmine) in the treatment of DLB has been reported (McKeith et al., 2000). The difficulties of conducting such trials are shown by the low completion rate (44 per cent) in this study, although this did not differ between placebo and active treatment groups. In all three studies (**Table 66.1**), the most significant effects of the ChEI were on neuropsychiatric symptoms. **Table 66.2** summarizes some studies which compare the efficacy of ChEIs in DLB

Table 66.1 Studies of cholinesterase inhibitors in dementia with Lewy bodies.

Study	No. (completed study)	Drug (duration)	Design	Outcome measures	Results
McKeith et al. (2000)	120 (55)	Rivastigmine (20 weeks)	RCT	NPI CGIC	Significant improvement in sub-scale of NPI (NPI-4) versus controls
Edwards et al. (2007)	50 (42)	Galantamine (24 weeks)	Open label	NPI, CGIC, CDRCAT	Significant improvement in NPI-12 scores and CGIC ratings versus baseline
Mori et al. (2006)	12	Donepezil (12 weeks)	Open label	NPI, ADAS-J Cog, UPDRS	Significant improvement in NPI-11 scores versus baseline (12 weeks) Significant improvement in ADAS-J Cog scores at 4 weeks versus baseline

ADAS-J Cog, Japanese version of Alzheimer's Disease Assessment Scale; CDRCAT, Cognitive Drug Research Computerised Attentional Tasks; CGIC, Clinicians Global Impression of Change; NPI, Neuropsychiatric Inventory; RCT, randomized (placebo) controlled trial; UPDRS, Unified Parkinson's Disease Rating Scale.

Table 66.2   Studies comparing the efficacy of cholinesterase inhibitors in dementia with Dewy bodies versus Alzheimer's disease or Parkinson's disease with dementia.

Study	No. (total)	Drug(s) (duration)	Comparison groups	Design	Outcome measures	Results
Samuel et al. (2000)	16	Rivastigmine (6 months)	AD (n = 12), DLB (n = 4)	Open label, blinded ratings	MMSE, Behave-AD	DLB significant increase in mean MMSE score, no difference in Behave-AD
Thomas et al., 2005	70	Donepezil (20 weeks)	PDD (n = 40), DLB (n = 30)	Open label	MMSE, NPI, UPDRS 111 (motor)	Both groups improved on MMSE and NPI versus baseline
Touchon et al., 2006	994	Rivastigmine or donepezil (2 years)	AD (n = 945), AD + DLB (n = 49)	Retrospective analysis of clinical population	SIB, MMSE, GDS, NPI, ADCS-ADL	AD/DLB on rivastigmine significantly greater improvement in SIB, MMSE and ADCS-ADL versus donepezil
Rowan et al., 2007	45	Donepezil (20 weeks)	PDD (n = 23), DLB (n = 22), controls (n = 183)	Open label	CDRCAT (measure of attention)	Power of attention and continuity of attention improved in both PDD and DLB versus controls

AD, Alzheimer's disease, DLB, dementia with Lewy bodies; PDD, Parkinson's disease dementia.
ADCDS-ADL, Alzheimer's Disease Cooperative Study Activities of Daily Living Scale; Behave-AD, Behavioural Symptoms in Alzhemer's Disease Scale; CDRCAT, Cognitive Drug Research Computerised Attentional Tasks; GDS, Global Deterioration Scale; MMSE, Mini Mental State Examination; NPI, Neuropsychiatric Inventory; SIB, Severe Impairment Battery; UPDRS 111, Unified Parkinson's Disease Rating Scale (motor subscale).

versus either PDD or AD. While all these studies were open label and had differing designs, there is a trend towards a significant benefit of ChEIs for the treatment of neuropsychiatric symptoms in DLB or PDD over and above their effect on cognition. The neuropsychiatric symptoms responsive to ChEIs include psychotic symptoms (hallucinations and delusions), depression and apathy.

Bhasin and colleagues (2007) have undertaken a secondary analysis comparing the efficacy of rivastigmine, galantamine and donepezil in the treatment of DLB (using the studies in **Table 66.1**). They found, on the basis of these limited data, that donepezil reduced neuropsychiatric symptoms to a greater extent than either rivastigmine or galantamine. Caution is needed as there are no controlled prospective comparative studies, and the only RCT has been undertaken with rivastigmine. However, given that there is good evidence from neurochemical studies that psychotic symptoms in DLB have a cholinergic basis, it is reasonable to conclude that ChEIs as a class are appropriate treatments for non-cognitive symptoms in DLB. As with AD, there is also little evidence to guide the clinician on the potential benefits of switching between one ChEI or another, or on when to cease treatment.

Other putative therapeutic agents aimed at enhancing cholinergic function in DLB are muscarinic agonists (Harrison and McKeith, 1995) and nicotinic agonists (Perry and Perry, 1996). Xanomeline, an M1 muscarinic receptor agonist, has been subject to a controlled trial in AD. While significant improvement in both cognitive function and behavioural abnormalities were found, in oral form the drug was poorly tolerated (Bodick et al., 1997) and this has been a

problem with several other agonists. Loss of nicotinic receptors has been described in both AD and PD (Newhouse et al., 1997). Sahakian et al. (1989) reported improvement of attention in AD patients treated with nicotine, although two later trials of short duration (up to 4 weeks) using transdermal administration of nicotine in AD found no improvement in cognitive function (Wilson et al., 1995; Snaedal et al., 1996).

66.3.2   Memantine

Memantine is an N-methyl-D-aspartate (NMDA) receptor antagonist which has clinical efficacy in moderate to severe AD (Reisberg et al., 2003; Winblad et al., 2007) and may be useful in the treatment of agitation in such cases (Wilcock et al., 2008). In DLB and PDD, it has been used as an adjunctive therapy (Sabbagh et al., 2005) and also as a primary treatment with studies shown in **Table 66.3**. Aarsland et al. (2009) included patients with either PDD or DLB who were randomized to treatment or to placebo. In the other study (Leroi et al., 2009), only patients with PDD were included. This was a small study, and while results were negative, no major adverse events were reported. Aarsland et al. (2009) found a significant benefit for memantine over placebo in global outcome, the primary outcome measure, although there was no effect on neuropsychiatric symptoms or activities of daily living (ADLs). An attentional speed measure also showed an improvement on memantine, while parkinsonian symptoms did not worsen. Further studies are needed, but from the evidence available memantine may have

Table 66.3   Trials of memantine in PDD and DLB.

Study	No.	Dose in treatment group	Design	Outcome measures	Response	Adverse effects
Aarsland et al. (2009)	72	20 mg/day	Parallel group, randomized controlled trial, in patients with PDD or DLB	GCIC (primary)	Treatment group significantly ($p = 0.03$) improved on primary outcome measure versus controls	Included. No significant difference in adverse events between groups. 78% ($n = 56$) completed study
Leroi et al. (2009)	25	20 mg/day	Parallel group, randomized controlled trial in patients with PDD	DRS-cognition (primary)	No significant difference on primary outcome measure between groups	No major adverse events. 96% ($n = 24$) completed study

DLB, dementia with Lewy bodies; DRS, Mattis Dementia Rating Scale; GCIC, clinical global impression of change; PDD, Parkinson's disease dementia.

some mild global benefits in DLB. Some caution may be needed, however, as increased agitation has been reported as a side effect of memantine in some DLB subjects (Ridha et al., 2005), although this was not observed in the studies of Aarsland and Leroi.

66.3.3   Dopaminergic therapy

Although dopamine levels are reduced in post-mortem studies DLB (Perry et al., 1990) and cerebrospinal fluid (CSF) homovanillic acid levels are reduced in autopsy-confirmed cases of DLB (Weiner et al., 1996), there has been little systematic enquiry into the effects of levadopa therapy in DLB. Some early studies found little or no levadopa response in those who were treated (Hansen et al., 1990; Perry et al., 1990; Mark et al., 1992), while others found response to be variable (Byrne et al., 1989; Gibb et al., 1989; Kosaka, 1990).

In eight autopsy-diagnosed cases of DLB reported by Louis et al. (1995), four were treated with levadopa in life and all showed a response to treatment. In clinically diagnosed cases of DLB reported by Gnanalingham et al. (1997), 12/15 received levadopa and all responded to it.

One of the earliest open trials of levadopa in DLB was that of Williams et al. (1993). Five cases which fulfilled clinical criteria for DLB (Byrne et al., 1991) were longitudinally assessed in terms of motor function, cognitive function and ADLs, during an open trial of levadopa and selegiline. The dose of levadopa (with carbidopa) was commenced at a low level and slowly titrated upwards to reach best-response (defined as a 2-week plateau in motor response). Three cases showed considerable improvement in motor function and two cases modest improvement. In no case was there an adverse effect on mental state. The results of two recent open trials of dopaminergic drugs are shown in **Table 66.4**. Around a third of subjects responded to levadopa in both studies. It is

Table 66.4   Treatment of motor features with levodopa in DLB.

Study	No.	Design	Outcome measures	Response (>10% increase in UPDRS 111)	Adverse effects
Molloy et al. (2005)	14	Open label; acute challenge L-dopa in 'off' state after 6 months treatment	UPDRS III, NPI	30%	Cognition worse, GI symptoms
Goldman et al. (2008)	19	Open label, measures before and after an increase in dopaminergic drugs	UPDRS III	36%	Psychotic symptoms worse, (only L-dopa increased)

NPI, Neuropsychiatric Inventory; UPDRS 111, Unified Parkinson's Disease Rating Scale (motor subscale).

likely motor symptoms in DLB are undertreated, although acute confusional states (delirium) and other adverse effects are not uncommon with levadopa therapy. This may (together with the perception that parkinsonian symptoms are atypical or mild) lead to a lack of enthusiasm for using these drugs in DLB. However, a significant group of DLB cases may benefit from levadopa therapy, especially those in whom parkinsonian symptoms are especially troublesome and in whom neuropsychiatric symptoms are less prominent. It should be noted that there are, as yet, no predictors of a favourable response to dopaminergic agents. A pragmatic strategy is to start with low doses and titrate upwards having made a careful record of the mental state (non-cognitive and cognitive features) and the range of fluctuation in symptoms both before and during treatment. Only then can one assess whether the treatment is beneficial or harmful (McKeith et al., 2005).

66.4   OTHER TREATMENTS FOR SPECIFIC SYMPTOMS

66.4.1   Psychotic symptoms

Psychotic symptoms, especially recurrent visual hallucinations, are common and troublesome in DLB. The Newcastle group were the first to draw attention to the phenomenon of neuroleptic sensitivity (NS) in DLB (McKeith et al., 1992). They noted a high rate of adverse responses (over 50 per cent severe) in 16/20 DLB cases diagnosed at post-mortem. Only one of 21 AD cases showed severe adverse reaction. The nature of the adverse response was comprised of worsening motor function, aggravation or precipitation of cognitive dysfunction or non-cognitive features and drowsiness, together with some features of neuroleptic malignant syndrome (NMS) with fever, generalized rigidity and raised serum creatinine kinase. In some cases, the NS response was life threatening. Survival analysis of the seven cases with severe reactions showed increased mortality compared to those with no or mild neuroleptic sensitivity.

A more detailed report from the same group (Ballard et al., 1998) is of 80 longitudinally assessed cases, 40 of AD and 40 of DLB (matched for age and sex) with post-mortem diagnoses. Severe neuroleptic sensitivity only occurred in the DLB cases (29 per cent) and in all such cases occurred within 2 weeks of a new neuroleptic prescription or a dose change. In this series, 47 per cent of the neuroleptics were the newer, atypical compounds compared to 16 per cent in the 1992 series (McKeith et al., 1992). This neuroleptic sensitivity is additional to other known deleterious effects of antipsychotics which have been described in dementia, including cognitive decline, sedation, increased mortality and increased risk of cerebrovascular events (McShane et al., 1997; Schneider et al., 2005).

However, neuroleptic sensitivity is not an inevitable consequence of neuroleptic medication in DLB, but it is certainly common and severe in DLB (Aarsland et al., 2005). There is also evidence that antipsychotics can be effective in treating psychotic symptoms in DLB. Risperidone has been used in DLB with benefit (remission of psychotic features) by Allen et al. (1995), Lee et al. (1994) and Shiwach and Woods (1998). Some have advocated quetiapine for the treatment of psychosis in DLB (Baskys, 2004; Poewe, 2005); however, the evidence on which this is based is limited. One small trial of quetiapine in the treatment of DLB ($n = 11$) in comparison to patients with PD and psychosis ($n = 87$) found at least partial (and in some cases total) resolution of psychosis in 90 per cent DLB and 80 per cent PD subjects (Fernandez et al., 2002). Olanzapine in the treatment of psychosis in DLB has been examined with conflicting results. For example, Cummings and colleagues (2002) found that the psychosis in 19 patients with DLB treated with olanzapine (in doses from 5 to 15 mg/day) improved in all patients (to some degree) when compared to a placebo group of DLB patients ($n = 10$), whereas Walker and colleagues (1999) found that olanzapine (at doses from 2.5 to 7.5 mg/day) was poorly tolerated in three of eight patients, tolerated but not beneficial in three of eight patients and beneficial in only two of eight patients. In some cases, clozapine may be beneficial in treating psychotic symptoms in DLB (Abelskov and Torpdahl, 1993; Chacko et al., 1993), but others report worsening of cognition and behaviour with clozapine treatment in DLB (Burke et al., 1998).

The mechanism by which antipsychotics induce NS is not completely understood, Piggott et al. (1994) suggest it is due to a failure to upregulate D_2 receptors in DLB. Unfortunately, no features have been identified which distinguish those cases of DLB likely to develop neuroleptic sensitivity. Ballard et al. (1998) found that age nor sex nor severity nor clinical profile did so. Furthermore, of the six cases with severe reactions, four were on novel or atypical neuroleptics and all were on low doses. Two of these six cases died within 2 weeks of the prescription. Neuroleptic sensitivity in DLB has been reported in patients treated with risperidone (Sechi et al., 2000) and quetiapine (Kobayashi et al., 2006).

The treatment of troublesome psychotic symptoms in DLB with neuroleptics thus presents a challenge to the clinician. The pragmatic approach would suggest that neuroleptics should not be first-line treatments in such cases, should only be used in patients with severe psychotic symptoms who have not responded to alternative therapies and should only be prescribed by specialists after a careful risk/benefit analysis and under very close supervision. An atypical antipsychotic with low D_2 potency would be preferred over typical agents in DLB, both should be used with extreme caution and only under specialist advice, at low dose for short periods with frequent review.

Other empirical treatments for psychotic symptoms in DLB include chlormethiazole and carbamazepine, although the evidence base is weak. The use of chlomethiazole was suggested because of its effectiveness in delirium tremens and because some patients with DLB have delirious-like episodes. In addition, there is some evidence that chlomethiazole has neuroprotective effects (Cross et al., 1991; Baldwin et al., 1993). In clinical practice, it may reduce or obviate visual hallucinations and may be helpful in sleep disorders in DLB. Carbamazepine, an anti-epileptic drug with antidepressant actions has also been used empirically to treat psychotic features in DLB. Lebert *et al.* (1996) found great benefit in two cases of DLB treated with 100–400 mg/day. Both chlormethiazole and carbamazepine are GABAergic agents. GABA has been suggested as an important transmitter in delirium (Ross *et al.*, 1991), and GABA has an important function in motor control.

66.4.2   Sleep disorders

Disturbance of sleep is common in dementia, but has only relatively recently been associated with DLB. Some early case reports (Schenck *et al.*, 1997; Turner *et al.*, 1997) linked DLB with (rapid eye movement, REM) REM sleep behaviour disorder (RBD). RBD is 'a parasomnia defined by intermittent loss of electromyographic atonia during REM sleep with emergence of complex and vigorous behaviours' (Schenck *et al.*, 1997). Behaviours include kicking, punching and leaping from bed. Such behaviours are very commonly associated with harm (in up to 96 per cent of cases) to the patient or to their sleep partner (Schenck *et al.*, 1987; Boeve *et al.*, 1998; Boeve *et al.*, 2001; Gugger and Wagner, 2007). Boeve and colleagues (1998) found 37 patients with dementia and RBD confirmed by polysomnography, of whom 92 per cent (32 cases) met criteria (McKeith *et al.*, 1996) for DLB. Three patients underwent necropsy; all had limbic Lewy bodies with or without cortical Lewy bodies.

The strong association of RBD with neurodegenerative disorders, especially the synucleinopathies (including DLB), has been confirmed by more recent studies (Grace *et al.*, 2000; Boeve *et al.*, 2001; Boeve *et al.*, 2003a). The risk of a person with RBD developing a neurodegenerative disorder has recently been assessed. In two studies in which patients with RBD were followed up, 45 per cent of patients developed a neurodegenerative disorder, most commonly PD or DLB (Iranzo *et al.*, 2006; Hickey *et al.*, 2007). In both these studies the time of onset of RBD preceded the onset of the neurodegenerative disorder by an identical mean duration of time 11.5 years. A lower (30 per cent), but nevertheless substantial, risk of patients with RBD developing a neurodegenerative disorder was found by Postuma and colleagues (2009). This group estimated the risk of a person with RBD (time of onset of RBD to time of onset of a neurodegenerative disorder) developing a neurodegenerative disorder by time at five years as 17.7 per cent, at ten years as 40.6 per cent and at 12 years as 52.4 per cent.

RBD can be successfully treated with clonazepam (Schenck *et al.*, 1987; Gugger and Wagner, 2007), although in a minority of patients there is no response. Potential problems with clonazepam (even at low dosage) are daytime sedation (in up to 58 per cent of patients (Anderson and Shneerson, 2009) and loss of efficacy over time. In those unresponsive or unable to tolerate clonazepam alternative treatments include desimipramine and zopiclone (Schenck *et al.*, 1987; Anderson and Shneerson, 2009). Melatonin has been used to treat RBD both as a primary and as an adjunctive therapy (Boeve *et al.*, 2003b; Gugger and Wagner, 2007).

Other sleep disorders, including excessive daytime sleepiness (EDS), are frequent in DLB (Grace *et al.*, 2000). EDS or hypersomnolence may be responsive to ChEIs (Catt and Kaufer, 1998; Grace *et al.*, 2000; Maclean *et al.*, 2001).

66.4.3   Depression

Although depression is very common in DLB, there are no well-conducted clinical trials of antidepressants. Reviews of the treatment of DLB (Fernandez *et al.*, 2003; McKeith *et al.*, 2005) suggest the use of selective serotonin re-uptake inhibitors (SSRIs), which have an evidence base in both AD and PD. Electroconvulsive therapy has been used with efficacy and safety in a few DLB patients with severe depression (Rasmussen *et al.*, 2003; Takahashi *et al.*, 2009).

66.4.4   Autonomic symptoms

The involvement of the autonomic nervous system in the pathology of DLB was suggested by reports of orthostatic hypotension in some early case series of DLB (Kosaka, 1990) and by Jackson and colleagues (1995) who reported a case of DLB presenting with dysphagia. Orthostatic hypotension is common in DLB (up to 70 per cent) and in other causes of dementia (Allan *et al.*, 2007; Andersson *et al.*, 2008) and is an important cause of falls in some DLB patients (Allan *et al.*, 2009). Management strategies for the treatment of orthostatic hypotension have been suggested by the European Federation of Neurological Societies (EFNS) (Lahrmann *et al.*, 2006) and by Allan and colleagues (2009). Such strategies include ensuring adequate hydration, the use of support stockings and drug therapy, such as fludrocortisone or midodrine. Cardiac sympathetic innervation is compromised in PD and DLB (Kenny *et al.*, 2004; Oka *et al.*, 2007) leading to syncope in some patients which, in some cases, may require a cardiac pacemaker. This is especially pertinent given the cardiac problems, including bradycardia and heart block, associated with ChEI use.

66.5   OTHER PUTATIVE TREATMENTS

A number of other putative treatments for DLB have been suggested. Ondansetron, a selective $5HT_3$ antagonist, has been suggested as a treatment for DLB because of the relative serotonergic overactivity in the condition (Perry *et al.*, 1993; Sagar *et al.*, 1996). In PD, ondansetron at a dose of 12–24 mg daily reduced psychotic symptoms in the majority of 16 patients with severe disease in an open trial (Zoldan *et al.*, 1993). Benzodiazepines have been reported as being of use in the management of anxiety and restlessness in DLB (Lennox, 1992; McKeith *et al.*, 1996). Neurotrophins, because of their neuroprotective effect, have been postulated as a therapy for AD and other neurodegenerative disorders, although little is known about the neurotrophic factors in DLB (Wilcock, 1996). The use of non-pharmacological therapies or interventions in the management of DLB has rarely been investigated. Bright light therapy may improve agitation in some patients with DLB (Burns *et al.*, 2009).

66.6 CARERS

The carers of patients with DLB experience high levels of stress (Ricci *et al.*, 2009) and depression (Lowery *et al.*, 2000). There is, therefore, a particular need to consider carer stress when DLB is the diagnosis, and to consider interventions at an early stage. Interventions to reduce these symptoms in carers may also benefit patients. There is a need for well-conducted trials in this area, as none to date have focused on carers of DLB subjects.

66.7 CONCLUSION

The evidence base for the treatment of DLB is beginning to emerge, but many more studies are needed. ChEI remain the mainstay of treatment, but a host of other symptoms ranging from depression and motor symptoms to dysautonomia and carer stress can successfully be managed with appropriate interventions. Greater understanding of the neuropathological mechanisms underlying DLB will lead to treatments targeted at basic processes. Until that time, the treatment of DLB presents great challenges to the physician in which art as much as science still plays a part and the needs of the patient and their carers have to be central to what are often difficult and challenging management decisions.

REFERENCES

Aalten P, Verhey FRJ, Boziki M *et al.* (2007) Neuropsychiatric syndromes in dementia. Results from the European Alzheimer's Disease Consortium (EADC): Part I. *Dementia and Geriatric Cognitive Disorders* 24: 457–63.

Aalten P, Verhey FRJ, Boziki M *et al.* (2008) Consistency of neuropsychiatric syndromes across dementias: results from the European Alzheimer Disease Consortium. Part II. *Dementia and Geriatric Cognitive Disorders* 25: 1–8.

Aarsland D, Perry R, Larsen JP *et al.* (2005) Neuroleptic sensitivity in Parkinson's disease and parkinsonian dementias. *Journal of Clinical Psychiatry* 66: 633–7.

Aarsland D, Ballard C, Walker Z *et al.* (2009) Memantine in patients with Parkinson's disease dementia or dementia with Lewy bodies: a double-blind, placebo-controlled, multicentre trial. *Lancet Neurology* 8: 613–18.

Abelskov KE, Torpdahl P. (1993) Lewy body demens – en ny sygdomsenied. [Lewy-body dementia – a new disease entity]. *Ugeskr Laeger* 155: 457–9.

Allan LM, Ballard CG, Allen J *et al.* (2007) Autonomic dysfunction in dementia. *Journal of Neurology, Neurosurgery and Psychiatry* 78: 671–7.

Allan LM, Ballard CG, Rowan EN, Kenny RA. (2009) Incidence and prediction of falls in dementia: a prospective study in older people. *PLoS One* 4: e5521.

Allen RL, Walter Z, D'Ath PJ, Katona CLE. (1995) Risperidone for psychotic and behavioural symptoms in Lewy body dementia. *Lancet* 346: 185.

Anderson KN, Shneerson JM. (2009) Drug treatment of REM sleep behavior disorder: the use of drug therapies other than clonazepam. *Journal of Clinical Sleep Medicine* 5: 235–9.

Andersson M, Hansson O, Minthon L *et al.* (2008) The period of hypotension following orthostatic challenge is prolonged in dementia with Lewy bodies. *International Journal of Geriatric Psychiatry* 23: 192–8.

Baldwin HA, Jones JA, Cross AJ *et al.* (1993) Histological, biochemical and behavioural evidence for the neuroprotective action of chlormethiazole following prolonged carotid artery occlusion. *Neurodegeneration* 2: 139–46.

Ballard C, Grace J, McKeith IG, Holmes C. (1998) Neuroleptic sensitivity in dementia with Lewy bodies and Alzheimer's disease. *Lancet* 351: 1032–3.

Ballard CG, Chalmers KA, Todd C *et al.* (2007) Cholinesterase inhibitors reduce cortical Abeta in dementia with Lewy bodies. *Neurology* 68: 1726–9.

Baskys A. (2004) Lewy body dementia: the litmus test for neuroleptic sensitivity and extrapyramidal symptoms. *Journal of Clinical Psychiatry* 65 (Suppl. 11): 16–22.

Beyer K, Ariza A. (2008) The therapeutical potential of alpha-synuclein antiaggregatory agents for dementia with Lewy bodies. *Current Medicinal Chemistry* 15: 2748–59.

Bhasin M, Rowan E, Edwards K, McKeith I. (2007) Cholinesterase inhibitors in dementia with Lewy bodies: a comparative analysis. *International Journal of Geriatric Psychiatry* 22: 890–5.

Bodick NC, Offen WW, Shannon AE *et al.* (1997) The selective muscarinic agonist xanomeline improves bath the cognitive deficits and behavioural symptoms of Alzheimer's disease. *Alzheimer's Disease Association and Disorders* 11 (Suppl. 4): S16–22.

Boeve BF, Silber MH, Ferman TJ *et al.* (1998) REM sleep behaviour disorder and degenerative dementia: an association likely reflecting Lewy body disease. *Neurology* 51: 363–70.

Boeve BF, Silber MH, Ferman TJ *et al.* (2001) Association of REM sleep behavior disorder and neurodegenerative disease may reflect an underlying synucleinopathy. *Movement Disorders* 16: 622–30.

Boeve BF, Silber MH, Parisi JE *et al.* (2003a) Synucleinopathy pathology and REM sleep behavior disorder plus dementia or parkinsonism. *Neurology* 61: 40–5.

Boeve BF, Silber MH, Ferman TJ. (2003b) Melatonin for treatment of REM sleep behavior disorder in neurologic disorders: results in 14 patients. *Sleep Medicine* 4: 281–4.

Burke WJ, Pfeipfer RF, McComb RD. (1998) Neuroleptic sensitivity to clozapine in dementia with Lewy bodies. *Journal of Neuropsychiatry and Clinical Neurosciences* 10: 227–9.

Burns A, Allen H, Tomenson B *et al.* (2009) Bright light therapy for agitation in dementia: a randomized controlled trial. *International Psychogeriatrics* 21: 711–21.

Byrne EJ. (1995) Cortical Lewy body disease: An alternative view. In: Howard R, Levy R (eds). *Developments in dementia and functional disorders in the elderly*. Stroud: Wrightson, 21–7.

Byrne EJ, Lennox G, Lowe J, Godwin-Austen RB. (1989) Diffuse Lewy body disease: clinical features in 15 cases. *Journal of Neurology, Neurosurgery and Psychiatry* 52: 709–17.

Byrne EJ, Lennox G, Godwin-Austen RB et al. (1991) Dementia associated with cortical Lewy bodies: proposed clinical diagnostic criteria. *Dementia* 2: 283–4.

Catt K, Kaufer D. (1998) Dementia with Lewy bodies: response of psychosis and hypersomnolence to Donepezil. *Journal of the American Geriatric Society* 46 (Suppl.): 581.

Chacko RC, Hyrley RA, Jonkovic J. (1993) Clozapine use in diffuse Lewy body disease. *Journal of Neuropsychiatry and Clinical Neurosciences* 5: 206–8.

Cross AJ, Jones JA, Baldwin HA et al. (1991) Neuroprotective activity of chlormethiazole following transient forebrain ischaemic in the gerbil. *British Journal of Pharmacology* 104: 406–11.

Cummings JL, Street J, Masterman D, Clark WS. (2002) Efficacy of olanzapine in the treatment of psychosis in dementia with lewy bodies. *Dementia and Geriatric Cognitive Disorders* 13: 67–73.

Dawson VL, Kizushi VM, Huang PL et al. (1996) Resistance to neurotoxicity in cortical cultures from neuronal nitric oxide synthase-deficient mice. *Journal of Neurosciences* 16: 2479–87.

Dickson DW, Davies P, Mayeux R et al. (1987) Diffuse Lewy body disease: neuropathological and biochemical studies in 6 patients. *Acta Neuropathologica* 75: 8–15.

Edwards K, Royall D, Hershey L et al. (2007) Efficacy and safety of galantamine in patients with dementia with Lewy bodies: a 24-week open-label study. *Dementia and Geriatric Cognitive Disorders* 23: 401–5.

Fernandez HH, Trieschmann ME, Burke MA, Friedman JH. (2002) Quetiapine for psychosis in Parkinson's disease versus dementia with Lewy bodies. *Journal of Clinical Psychiatry* 63: 513–15.

Fernandez HH, Wu CK, Ott BR. (2003) Pharmacotherapy of dementia with Lewy bodies (review). *Expert Opinion on Pharmacotherapy* 4: 2027–37.

Gauthier S, Wirth Y, Mobius HJ. (2005) Effects of memantine on behavioural symptoms in Alzheimer's disease patients: an analysis of the Neuropsychiatric Inventory (NPI) data of two randomised, controlled studies. *International Journal of Geriatric Psychiatry* 20: 459–64.

Gibb WRG, Luthert PJ, Janota I, Lantos PL. (1989) Cortical Lewy body dementia: clinical features and classification. *Journal of Neurology, Neurosurgery and Psychiatry* 52: 185–92.

Gnanalingham KK, Byrne EJ, Thornton A et al. (1997) Motor and cognitive function in Lewy body dementia: comparison with Alzheimer's and Parkinson's disease. *Journal of Neurology, Neurosurgery and Psychiatry* 62: 243–52.

Goldman JG, Goetz CG, Brandabur M et al. (2008) Effects of dopaminergic medications on psychosis and motor function in dementia with Lewy bodies. *Movement Disorders* 23: 2248–50.

Grace JB, Walker MP, McKeith IG. (2000) A comparison of sleep profiles in patients with dementia with lewy bodies and Alzheimer's disease. *International Journal of Geriatric Psychiatry* 15: 1028–33.

Gugger JJ, Wagner ML. (2007) Rapid eye movement sleep behavior disorder. *Annals of Pharmacotherapy* 41: 1833–41.

Hansen I, Salmon D, Galasko D et al. (1990) The Lewy body variant of Alzheimer's disease: a clinical and pathologic entity. *Neurology* 40: 1–8.

Hantraye P, Brouillet E, Ferrante E et al. (1996) Inhibition of neuronal nitric oxide synthase prevents MPTP-induced parkinsonism in baboons. *Nature Medicine* 2: 1017–21.

Harrison RWS, McKeith IG. (1995) Senile dementia of Lewy body type – A review of clinical and pathological features: Implications for treatment. *International Journal of Geriatric Psychiatry* 10: 919–26.

Hely MA, Reid WG, Halliday GM et al. (1996) Diffuse Lewy body disease: Clinical features in nine cases without co-existent Alzheimer's disease. *Journal of Neurology, Neurosurgery and Psychiatry* 60: 531–8.

Herishanu YO, Kordysh E, Goldmith JR. (1998) A case-referent study of extrapyramidal signs. (pre-parkinsonism) in rural communities of Israel. *Canadian Journal of Neurological Sciences* 25: 127–33.

Herrmann N, Rabheru K, Wang J, Binder C. (2005) Galantamine treatment of problematic behavior in Alzheimer disease: post-hoc analysis of pooled data from three large trials. *American Journal of Geriatric Psychiatry* 13: 527–34.

Hickey MG, Demaerschalk BM, Caselli RJ et al. (2007) 'Idiopathic' rapid-eye-movement (REM) sleep behavior disorder is associated with future development of neurodegenerative diseases. *Neurologist* 13: 98–101.

Hubble JP, Kurth JH, Glatt SL et al. (1998) Gene–toxin interaction as a putative risk factor for Parkinson's disease with dementia. *Neuro-epidemiology* 17: 96–104.

Iranzo A, Molinuevo JL, Santamaría J et al. (2006) Rapid-eye-movement sleep behaviour disorder as an early marker for a neurodegenerative disorder: a descriptive study. *Lancet Neurology* 5: 572–7.

Jackson M, Lennox G, Balsitis M, Lowe J. (1995) Lewy body dysphagia. *Journal of Neurology, Neurosurgery and Psychiatry* 58: 756–8.

Kenny RA, Shaw FE, O'Brien JT et al. (2004) Carotid sinus syndrome is common in dementia with Lewy bodies and correlates with deep white matter lesions. *Journal of Neurology, Neurosurgery and Psychiatry* 75: 966–71.

Kobayashi A, Kawanishi C, Matsumura T et al. (2006) Quetiapine-induced neuroleptic malignant syndrome in dementia with Lewy bodies: a case report. *Progress in Neuropsychopharmacology and Biological Psychiatry* 30: 1170–2.

Koob AO, Ubhi K, Paulsson JF et al. (2010) Lovastatin ameliorates alpha-synuclein accumulation and oxidation in transgenic mouse models of alpha-synucleinopathies. *Experimental Neurology* 221: 267–74.

Kosaka D. (1990) Diffuse Lewy body disease in Japan. *Journal of Neurology* 237: 197–204.

Lahrmann H, Cortelli P, Hilz M et al. (2006) EFNS guidelines on the diagnosis and management of orthostatic hypotension. *European Journal of Neurology* 13: 930–6.

Lanctôt KL, Herrmann N. (2000) Donepezil for behavioural disorders associated with Lewy bodies: a case series. *International Journal of Geriatric Psychiatry* 15: 338–45.

Lebert F, Souliez L, Pasquier F. (1996) Tacrine and symptomatic treatment. In: Perry R, McKeith I, Perry E (eds). *Dementia with Lewy bodies.* Cambridge: Cambridge University Press, 439–48.

Lebert F, Pasquier F, Souliez L, Petit H. (1998) Tacrine efficacy in Lewy body dementia. *International Journal of Geriatric Psychiatry* 13: 516–19.

Lee H, Cooney JM, Lawlor BA. (1994) Case report: The use of Risperidone, an atypical neuroleptic in Lewy body disease. *International Journal of Geriatric Psychiatry* 9: 415–17.

Lennox G. (1992) Lewy body dementia. *Bailliere's Clinical Neurology* 1: 653–76.

Leroi I, Overshott R, Byrne EJ et al. (2009) Randomized controlled trial of memantine in dementia associated with Parkinson's disease. *Movement Disorders* 24: 1217–21.

Levy R, Eagger S, Griffiths M et al. (1994) Lewy bodies and response to tacrine in Alzheimer's disease. *Lancet* 343: 176.

Liou HH, Tsai MC, Chen CJ et al. (1997) Environmental risk factors and Parkinson's disease: A case–control study in Taiwan. *Neurology* 48: 1583–8.

Louis ED, Goldman JE, Powers JM, Fahns S. (1995) Parkinsonian features of eight pathologically diagnosed cases of diffuse Lewy body disease. *Movement Disorders* 10: 188–94.

Lowery K, Mynt P, Aisbett J et al. (2000) Depression in the carers of dementia sufferers: a comparison of the carers of patients suffering from dementia with Lewy bodies and the carers of patients with Alzheimer's disease. *Journal of Affective Disorders* 59: 61–5.

McKeith IG, Fairbairn A, Perry RH et al. (1992) Neuroleptic sensitivity in patients with senile dementia of Lewy body type. *British Medical Journal* 305: 673–8.

McKeith IG, Galasko D, Kosaka K et al. (1996) Consensus guidelines for the clinical and pathologic diagnosis of dementia with Lewy bodies (DLB): report of the consortium on DLB international workshop. *Neurology* 47: 1113–24.

McKeith I, Del Ser T, Spano P et al. (2000) Efficacy of rivastigmine in dementia with Lewy bodies: a randomised, double-blind, placebo-controlled international study. *Lancet* 356: 2031–6.

McKeith IG, Dickson DW, Lowe J et al. (2005) Diagnosis and management of dementia with Lewy bodies: third report of the DLB Consortium. *Neurology* 65: 1863–72.

Maclean LE, Collins CC, Byrne EJ. (2001) Dementia with Lewy bodies treated with Rivastigmine: effects on cognitive neuropsychiatric symptoms and sleep. *International Journal of Psychogeriatrics* 13: 277–88.

McShane R, Keene J, Gedling K et al. (1997) Do neuroleptic drugs hasten cognitive decline in dementia? Prospective study with necropsy follow up. *British Medical Journal* 314: 266–70.

Mark MH, Sage JI, Dickson DW et al. (1992) Levodopa-non responsive Lewy body parkinsonism: clinicopathologic study of two cases. *Neurology* 42: 1323–7.

Molina JA, Leza JC, Ortiz S et al. (2002) Cerebrospinal fluid and plasma concentrations of nitric oxide metabolites are increased in dementia with Lewy bodies. *Neuroscience Letters* 333: 151–3.

Molloy S, McKeith IG, O'Brien JT, Burn DJ. (2005) The role of levodopa in the management of dementia with Lewy bodies. *Journal of Neurology, Neurosurgery and Psychiatry* 76: 1200–3.

Mori S, Mori E, Iseki E, Kosaka K. (2006) Efficacy and safety of donepezil in patients with dementia with Lewy bodies: preliminary findings from an open-label study. *Psychiatry and Clinical Neurosciences* 60: 190–5.

Newhouse PA, Potter A, Levin ED. (1997) Nicotinic system involvement in Alzheimer's and Parkinson's diseases. Implications for therapeutics. *Drugs and Ageing* 11: 206–28.

Oka H, Morita M, Onouchi K et al. (2007) Cardiovascular autonomic dysfunction in dementia with Lewy bodies and Parkinson's disease. *Journal of the Neurological Sciences* 254: 72–7.

Perry EK, Perry RH. (1996) Altered consciousness and transmitter signalling in Lewy body dementia. In: Perry R, McKeith I, Perry E (eds). *Dementia with Lewy bodies*. Cambridge: Cambridge University Press, 397–413.

Perry RH, Irvin D, Blessed G et al. (1990) Senile dementia of the Lewy body type: a clinically and neuropathologically distinct form of Lewy body dementia in the elderly. *Journal of the Neurological Sciences* 95: 119–39.

Perry EK, Irvin D, Kerwin JM et al. (1993) Cholinergic neurotransmitter and neurotrophic activities in Lewy body dementia. Similarity to Parkinson's and distinctions from Alzheimer's disease. *Alzheimer's Disease Association and Disorders* 7: 62–79.

Piggott MA, Perry EK, McKeith IG et al. (1994) Dopamine D2 receptors in demented patients with severe neuroleptic sensitivity. *Lancet* 343: 1044–5.

Poewe W. (2005) Treatment of dementia with Lewy bodies and Parkinson's disease dementia. *Movement Disorders* 20 (Suppl. 12): S77–82.

Postuma RB, Gagnon JF, Vendette M et al. (2009) Quantifying the risk of neurodegenerative disease in idiopathic REM sleep behavior disorder. *Neurology* 72: 1296–300.

Rasmussen Jr KG, Russell JC, Kung S et al. (2003) Electroconvulsive therapy for patients with major depression and probable Lewy body dementia. *Journal of ECT* 19: 103–9.

Reisberg B, Doody R, Stöffler A et al. (2003) Memantine Study Group. Memantine in moderate-to-severe Alzheimer's disease. *New England Journal of Medicine* 348: 1333–41.

Ricci M, Guidoni SV, Sepe-Monti M et al. (2009) Clinical findings, functional abilities and caregiver distress in the early stage of dementia with Lewy bodies (DLB) and Alzheimer's disease (AD). *Archives of Gerontology and Geriatrics* 49: e101–4.

Ridha BH, Josephs KA, Rossor MN. (2005) Delusions and hallucinations in dementia with Lewy bodies: worsening with memantine. *Neurology* 65: 481–2.

Robert PH, Verhey FR, Byrne EJ et al. (2005) Grouping for behavioral and psychological symptoms in dementia: clinical and biological aspects. Consensus paper of the European Alzheimer disease consortium. *European Psychiatry* 20: 490–6.

Robert P, Verhey FR, Aalten P et al. (2007) Neuropsychiatric outcome for clinical trials. *The Journal of Nutrition Health and Aging* 11: 345–7.

Ross CA, Peyser CE, Shapiro I et al. (1991) Delirium: Phenomenologic and etiologic subtypes. *International Journal of Psychogeriatrics* 3: 135–47.

Rowan E, McKeith IG, Saxby BK et al. (2007) Effects of donepezil on central processing speed and attentional measures in Parkinson's disease with dementia and dementia with Lewy bodies. *Dementia and Geriatric Cognitive Disorders* 23: 161–7.

Sabbagh MN, Hake AM, Ahmed S, Farlow MR. (2005) The use of memantine in dementia with Lewy bodies. *Journal of Alzheimer's Disease* 7: 285–9.

Sagar HJ, Jonsen ENH, Perry EK. (1996) Resumé of treatment workshop sessions. In: Perry R, McKeith I, Perry E (eds). *Dementia with Lewy bodies.* Cambridge: Cambridge University Press, 487–90.

Sahakian B, Jones G, Levy R et al. (1989) The effects of nicotine on attention, information processing and short-term memory in patients with dementia of the Alzheimer type. *British Journal of Psychiatry* **154**: 797–800.

Samuel W, Caligiuri M, Galasko D et al. (2000) Better cognitive and psychopathologic response to donepezil in patients prospectively diagnosed as dementia with Lewy bodies: a preliminary study. *International Journal of Geriatric Psychiatry* **15**: 794–802.

Schenck CH, Bundle SR, Patterson AL, Mahowald NW. (1987) Rapid eye movement sleep behaviour disorder. A treatable parasomnia affecting older adults. *Journal of the American Association* **257**: 1786–9.

Schenck CH, Mahowald MW, Anderson ML et al. (1997) Lewy body variant of Alzheimer's disease (AD) identified by post-mortem ubiquitin staining in a previously reported case of AD associated with REM sleep behaviour disorder. *Biological Psychiatry* **42**: 527–8.

Schneider LS, Dagerman KS, Insel P. (2005) Risk of death with atypical antipsychotic drug treatment for dementia: meta-analysis of randomized placebo-controlled trials. *Journal of the American Medical Association* **294**: 1934–43.

Sechi G, Agnetti V, Masuri R et al. (2000) Risperidone, neuroleptic malignant syndrome and probable dementia with Lewy bodies. *Progress in Neuropsychopharmacology and Biological Psychiatry* **24**: 1043–51.

Shiwach RS, Woods S. (1998) Risperidone and withdrawal bruxism in Lewy body dementia. *International Journal of Geriatric Psychiatry* **13**: 64–7.

Snaedal J, Johannesson T, Jansson JE, Gottfries G. (1996) Nicotine in dermal plasters did not improve cognition in Alzheimer's disease. *Dementia* **7**: 47–52.

Snyder SH. (1996) No NO prevents parkinsonism. *Nature Medicine* **2**: 965–6.

Takahashi S, Mizukami K, Yasuno F, Asada T. (2009) Depression associated with dementia with Lewy bodies (DLB) and the effect of somatotherapy. *Psychogeriatrics* **9**: 56–61.

Thomas AJ, Burn DJ, Rowan EN et al. (2005) A comparison of the efficacy of donepezil in Parkinson's disease with dementia and dementia with Lewy bodies. *International Journal of Geriatric Psychiatry* **20**: 938–44.

Tompkins MM, Basgall EJ, Zamrini E, Hill WD. (1997) Apoptotic-like changes in Lewy-body-associated disorders and normal ageing

in substantia nigral neurons. *American Journal of Pathology* **150**: 119–31.

Touchon J, Bergman H, Bullock R et al. (2006) Response to rivastigmine or donepezil in Alzheimer's patients with symptoms suggestive of concomitant Lewy body pathology. *Current Medical Research and Opinion* **22**: 49–59.

Turner RS, Chervin RD, Frey KA et al. (1997) Probable diffuse Lewy body disease presenting as REM sleep behaviour disorder. *Neurology* **49**: 523–7.

Walker Z, Grace J, Overshot R et al. (1999) Olanzapine in dementia with Lewy bodies: a clinical study. *International Journal of Geriatric Psychiatry* **14**: 459–66.

Wei J, Fujita M, Nakai M et al. (2009) Protective role of endogenous gangliosides for lysosomal pathology in a cellular model of synucleinopathies. *American Journal of Pathology* **174**: 1891–909.

Weiner MF, Risser RC, Cullum M et al. (1996) Alzheimer's disease and its Lewy body variant: A clinical analysis of post-mortem verified cases. *American Journal of Psychiatry* **153**: 1269–73.

Wilcock GK. (1996) Neurotrophins and the cholinergic system in dementia. In: Perry R, McKeith I, Perry E (eds). *Dementia with Lewy bodies.* Cambridge: Cambridge University Press, 468–76.

Wilcock GK, Scott I. (1994) Tacrine for senile dementia of Alzheimer's or Lewy body type. *Lancet* **344**: 544.

Wilcock GK, Ballard CG, Cooper JA, Loft H. (2008) Memantine for agitation/aggression and psychosis in moderately severe to severe Alzheimer's disease: a pooled analysis of 3 studies. *Journal of Clinical Psychiatry* **69**: 341–8.

Williams SW, Byrne EJ, Stokes P. (1993) The treatment of diffuse Lewy body disease: a pilot study. *International Journal of Geriatric Psychiatry* **8**: 731–9.

Wilson AL, Longley LK, Monley J et al. (1995) Nicotine patches in Alzheimer's disease: Pilot study on learning, memory and safety. *Pharmacology, Biochemistry and Behavior* **51**: 509–14.

Winblad B, Jones RW, Wirth Y et al. (2007) Memantine in moderate to severe Alzheimer's disease: a meta-analysis of randomised clinical trials. *Dementia and Geriatric Cognitive Disorders* **24**: 20–7.

Witjeratne C, Bandyopadhyay D, Howard R. (1995) Failure of tacrine treatment in a case of cortical Lewy body dementia. *International Journal of Geriatric Psychiatry* **10**: 808.

Xu W, Liu L, Emson P et al. (2000) The CCTTT polymorphism in the NOS2A gene is associated with dementia with Lewy bodies. *Neuroreport* **11**: 297–9.

Zoldan J, Freidberg G, Goldberg-Stern H, Melamed E. (1993) Ondansetron for hallucinosis in advanced Parkinson's disease. *Lancet* **341**: 562–3.

67

Cognitive impairment and dementia in Parkinson's disease

DAG AARSLAND, CARMEN JANVIN AND KOLBJØRN BRØNNICK

67.1 INTRODUCTION

Parkinson's disease (PD) is a common neurodegenerative disorder affecting about 1.5 per cent of people aged 65 years or older (de Rijk et al., 1997). PD is defined pathologically as cell loss in the pigmented dopaminergic cells of substantia nigra, pars compacta and synuclein pathology (Lewy neurites and Lewy bodies) in the surviving cells. In addition, cholinergic forebrain nuclei and other brain stem nuclei, including the serotonergic raphe nuclei and the noradrenergic locus coeruleus, are usually affected. The topographical progression subsequently involves the anteromedial temporal mesocortex, including the transentorhinal region, and reaches into adjoining high-order sensory association areas and important limbic structures, such as amygdalae and hippocampus (Braak et al., 2003; Jellinger, 2003a). In addition, amyloid plaques and even neurofibrillary tangles are found in most cases at autopsy (Jellinger et al., 2002). The cardinal clinical features of PD are resting tremor, bradykinesia, rigidity and postural abnormalities. However, owing to the wide distribution of neurodegeneration, it is not surprising that a wide range of non-motor symptoms occur as well, including neuropsychiatric symptoms and autonomic dysfunction.

The treatment of PD involves dopamine replacement therapy with L-dopa and several dopamine agonists, including the selective dopamine D3 receptor agonists, ropinirole and pramipexole. In addition, the monoamine oxidase inhibitors selegiline and rasagiline with a potential neuroprotective effect may slow disease progression. Deep cerebral stimulation with implantation of electrodes can be very helpful for selected patients. A wide range of behavioural side effects can occur during drug and surgical treatments.

It is now increasingly recognized that PD is a neuropsychiatric disorder and not merely a movement disorder. Independent of the motor symptoms of PD, dementia and other neuropsychiatric symptoms affect quality of life, contribute to caregiver distress and increased risk of nursing home placement, and is associated with more psychiatric symptoms, such as depression and hallucinations, higher mortality and functional disability, and higher risk for drug toxicity. This chapter discusses the epidemiology, pathophysiologic mechanism, clinical presentation and management of cognitive impairment and dementia in patients with PD.

67.2 MILD COGNITIVE IMPAIRMENT IN PARKINSON'S DISEASE

Impairment on a range of neuropsychological tests was found in 16 per cent of recently diagnosed PD patients (Reid et al., 1996). Three more recent studies of recently diagnosed patients supported these early findings. In the CamPaign study, 36 per cent were considered to have cognitive impairment (Foltynie et al., 2004), although normal control subjects were not included. In another study, including a wide range of neuropsychological tests, 24 per cent of PD patients fulfilled criteria for impairment compared to only 4 per cent of the control group (Muslimovic et al., 2005). In one study based on an incidence cohort of unmedicated people with recently diagnosed PD, 19 per cent of the PD patients without dementia were cognitively impaired compared to 9 per cent of the controls (Aarsland *et al.*, 2009a).

The cognitive profile in non-demented PD varies, but executive control impairment is paramount, including deficits in working memory (Possin *et al.*, 2008), set-shifting, planning, error monitoring (Willemssen *et al.*, 2009), response inhibition (Wylie *et al.*, 2005) and dual tasking (Brown and Marsden, 1991). While there is also memory impairment (Whittington *et al.*, 2006), it is probable that executive/attentional deficits to a large degree explain such deficits (Higginson *et al.*, 2003). Visuospatial dysfunction is a hallmark of dementia in PD, but such deficits are not very pronounced in early, non-demented PD (Aarsland *et al.*, 2009a).

67.2.1 Mechanisms underlying mild cognitive impairment in PD

The heterogeneous cognitive deficits in PD probably reflect differing forms and location of neuropathological involvement. Executive impairment is most likely related to the dopaminergic deficits, caused by either disruption of nigrostriatal circuitry with altered outflow of the caudate nuclei to frontal cortex via thalamus (Rinne *et al.*, 2000) or diminished dopamine activity in the frontal projections consequent to degeneration of mesocortical projections (Mattay *et al.*, 2002). There is also evidence linking the cortical noradrenergic system to extradimensional shift performance, whereas visual memory may be dependent on acetylcholine rather than dopamine (Robbins *et al.*, 2003).

A positron emission tomography (PET) study revealed that non-demented PD patients had widespread cortical glucose hypometabolism, involving mainly frontal, but also left temporal and parietal regions, compared with a more marked and global reduction, including severe bilateral temporoparietal defects, in PD patients with dementia (Peppard *et al.*, 1992). In a more recent PET study, even mild cognitive impairment (MCI) in PD was found to be associated with discrete regional changes and abnormal metabolic network activity (Huang *et al.*, 2008). In addition to functional changes, there is also evidence of cortical atrophy in PD with MCI (Beyer *et al.*, 2007).

67.2.2 The course of MCI in PD

The annual decline on the Mini-Mental State Examination (MMSE) score in PD is 1 point, but with wide interindividual variations (Aarsland *et al.*, 2004). Mild executive and memory impairments are predictors of subsequent dementia in PD, independent of age and stage of PD (Levy *et al.*, 2002a). Recent studies have demonstrated that PD patients with mild cognitive impairment have a shorter time to dementia than those with normal cognition (Janvin *et al.*, 2006). In a larger study based on incident PD, an interesting dissociation between cognitive domains and dementia risk was reported. Tests with a putative more posterior cortical basis predicted more rapid cognitive decline, but not tests suggesting frontostriatal dysfunction (Williams-Gray *et al.*, 2007). This

cognitive dissociation was paralleled by a genetic dissociation: polymorphism of the microtubule-associated protein tau gene, but not catechol O-methyltransferase (COMT) gene, was associated with dementia (Goris *et al.*, 2007), whereas a polymorphism of the COMT gene was associated with attentional dysfunction and underlying frontal activiation, but not dementia risk (Williams-Gray *et al.*, 2008).

67.3 DEMENTIA

67.3.1 Epidemiology

In addition to the MCI discussed above, dementia develops in a considerable proportion of patients with PD. In a systematic review including 13 studies with 1767 patients, a prevalence of 31.3 per cent (95 per cent confidence interval, 29.2–33.6), was found, and between 3 and 4 per cent of patients with dementia in the general population were due to PD, with an estimated prevalence of PD dementia in the general population aged 65 years and over of 0.3–0.5 per cent (Aarsland *et al.*, 2005).

In two community-based studies, the annual incidence was 95.3 (Aarsland *et al.*, 2001) and 112.5 per thousand (Marder *et al.*, 1995), indicating that about 10 per cent of PD patients develop dementia per year, although during the first years the incidence may be lower (Williams-Gray *et al.*, 2007). The risk for developing dementia in PD is nearly six times higher than in non-PD subjects (Aarsland *et al.*, 2001). In the Sydney study, *de novo* PD patients were followed for up to 20 years, with 75 per cent being diagnosed with dementia (Hely *et al.*, 2008). Since differential mortality among demented and non-demented were not adjusted for, the cumulative prevalence is likely to be even higher. In the Stavanger study, based on a prevalence sample, the eight-year cumulative prevalence of dementia was calculated to be 78 per cent after controlling for attrition due to death (Aarsland *et al.*, 2003), and a high likelihood of dementia and mortality for the higher age-groups has been shown (Buter *et al.*, 2008).

67.3.1.1 RISK FACTORS FOR DEMENTIA

The median time to dementia in PD is ten years, but there are wide variations, and age, advanced parkinsonism and mild cognitive impairment are predictors of dementia in PD (Levy *et al.*, 2002b; Aarsland *et al.*, 2003). Rigidity and symptoms mediated mainly by non-dopaminergic systems, such as speech, gait and postural disorders, are particularly related to subsequent development of dementia, whereas patients with a tremor-dominant pattern have a lower risk (Alves *et al.*, 2005). The relationship with age and severity of parkinsonism seems to be related to their combined effect rather than separate effects (Levy *et al.*, 2002b).

67.3.1.2 GENETICS AND DEMENTIA IN PD

Some, but not all, studies have found an association between dementia and Apolipoprotein (ApoE) ε4 in PD (Williams-Gray *et al.*, 2009). In addition to the association with Alzheimer-type and vascular pathologies, an association of the ε4 allele with the severity of Lewy body pathology has been reported. Finally, a positive association of dementia with the H1 haplotype of the tau-gene has been noted (Goris *et al.*, 2007).

67.3.2   Diagnosis of dementia in PD

The motor symptoms and apathy can make the diagnosis of cognitive impairment and dementia difficult in PD, and both over- and under-diagnosis may occur (Litvan *et al.*, 1998). Cognitive rating scales should be used, taking into account the disabilities from motor symptoms. Screening tests, such as the MMSE, may be employed, although instruments including executive dysfunction, such as the Dementia Rating Scale and the Montreal Cognitive Assessment (MoCA) seem to be more sensitive to the cognitive disorders in PD. Particular care should be taken to distinguish between dementia and confusional states from drug toxicity. Criteria to diagnose dementia in PD have been proposed (Emre *et al.*, 2007), although have not yet been validated. A practical guide to assist in the diagnostic process has been published (Dubois *et al.*, 2007).

There is considerable clinical and pathological overlap between dementia with Lewy bodies (DLB) and PD dementia. A diagnosis of Parkinson's disease dementia (PDD) should be made in patients who are diagnosed as PD and develop dementia after at least one year with motor symptoms. If dementia develops before or within one year after the diagnosis of PD, a diagnosis of DLB should be made (McKeith *et al.*, 2005), although this time-window is rather arbitrary. There is debate whether they represent distinct diseases or rather two syndromes on a spectrum of Lewy body diseases, and there are no major clinical consequences related to this differentiation.

67.3.2.1   IMAGING

Reduced hippocampal volumes have been shown in PD patients with dementia (Laakso *et al.*, 1996). Volume loss in the temporal and frontal cortices has also been reported (Beyer *et al.*, 2007; Burton *et al.*, 2004). Rate of atrophy is also higher in PDD compared to PD and controls (Burton *et al.*, 2005). Some, but not all, studies have reported more marked white-matter hyperintensities in demented compared to non-demented PD patients. A few studies using proton magnetic resonance spectroscopy have reported changes in PDD in cingulated or occipital cortex (Summerfield *et al.*, 2002).

Several recent studies have explored amyloid pathology in PD *in vivo* using ^{11}C-PIB PET. In a subgroup of patients with dementia in PD, increased amyloid load has been found, and seems to be associated with Alzheimer-like characteristics both for clinical phenotype and CSF (Maetzler *et al.*, 2009). Although both structural and functional imaging techniques may assist in the diagnostic work up of patients with parkinsonism and cognitive impairment, the final diagnosis must be based on the history and clinical examination, including routine supplementary tests.

67.3.3   Mechanisms

The heterogeneous cognitive profile of dementia in PD, with features of both subcortical and cortical dementia, is consistent with the various neuropathological and neurochemical involvements in PD. Cortical Lewy bodies are associated with dementia in PD (Aarsland *et al.*, 2005b), although may occur in the cortex also of non-demented PD patients (Colosimo *et al.*, 2003). There is also evidence that Alzheimer-like changes contribute to dementia in PD (Jellinger *et al.*, 2002), and in elderly patients, vascular changes may contribute as well (Jellinger, 2003b; Jellinger and Adams, 2008). Consistent with the heterogeneous clinical pattern, the underlying pathology is heterogeneous, with some patients exhibiting early and widespread cortical neurodegeneration and an aggressive clinical course, whereas others have less cortical involvement and a slower decline (Ballard *et al.*, 2006; Halliday *et al.*, 2008).

Neurochemical changes involving dopamine, noradrenaline and acetylcholine, may influence cognition in PD. In particular, much interest has focused on the relationship between cholinergic deficits and dementia in PDD. Selective loss of cells in the cholinergic nucleus basalis of Meynert and cortical cholinergic losses of similar degrees as in AD have been reported, and these changes are more pronounced in PD patients with dementia compared with non-demented patients (Perry *et al.*, 1993; Tiraboschi *et al.*, 2000).

67.4   TREATMENT

The cholinergic loss in dementia in PD, an increase of muscarinic receptor binding (Perry *et al.*, 1993) and less neurodegenerative changes in neocortex compared with AD, indicate that cholinergic drugs may be useful. Two early small placebo-controlled trials suggested that the cholinesterase inhibitor donepezil may be useful (Aarsland *et al.*, 2002; Leroi *et al.*, 2004). A large-scale placebo-controlled trial over 24 weeks showed that rivastigmine can improve cognition, activities of daily living and neuropsychiatric symptoms in patients with PDD (Emre *et al.*, 2004). The response is particularly marked in those with visual hallucinations (Burn *et al.*, 2006), and an open-label extension study suggest sustained benefits for up to 48 weeks (Poewe *et al.*, 2006). In addition to the typical side effects, including gastrointestinal problems, worsening of tremor does occur in some patients, but is usually mild and transient. Changes in the glutamatergic system have been reported in PD. Case reports of memantine, a partial NMDA antagonist, suggested benefit in PDD, and a significant effect was found in a small placebo-controlled study (Aarsland *et al.*, 2009b). Memantine was well tolerated, but larger studies are needed to confirm these early promising findings.

Neuropsychiatric symptoms such as psychosis, apathy and depression, are common in PD in PD dementia. The only evidence-based treatment for neuropsychiatric symptoms in PD is the use of clozapine for hallucinations, although patients with dementia were not included. Non-specific measures, such as reviewing and removing drugs that may cause worsening of cognition, i.e. anticholinergic agents, and treating comorbid conditions, are thus of importance. Informing the patient and family about the risk of progressive worsening of cognitive functioning and emergence of psychiatric symptoms is also important.

67.5 CONCLUSIONS

Cognitive impairment and dementia are very common in PD patients, with important clinical consequences for them and their carers. Clinicians need to focus on these and other neuropsychiatric symptoms in addition to the motor symptoms in order to provide optimal care for patients. The underlying aetiology and the clinical presentation of cognitive impairment in PD are highly variable, and the nosological classification of dementia in PD and its relationship to other dementias, in particular DLB, is not yet clarified. The complex clinical presentation in these frail and elderly individuals poses considerable challenges for the clinical management. Rivastigmine is approved for treatment of dementia in PD, and emerging evidence indicates that memantine is useful as well.

REFERENCES

Aarsland D, Andersen K, Larsen JP *et al.* (2001) Risk of dementia in Parkinson's disease: a community-based, prospective study. *Neurology* **56**: 730–6.

Aarsland D, Laake K, Larsen JP, Janvin C. (2002) Donepezil for cognitive impairment in Parkinson's disease: a randomised controlled study. *Journal of Neurology, Neurosurgery, and Psychiatry* **72**: 708–12.

Aarsland D, Andersen K, Larsen JP *et al.* (2003) Prevalence and characteristics of dementia in Parkinson disease: an 8-year prospective study. *Archives of Neurology* **60**: 387–92.

Aarsland D, Andersen K, Larsen JP *et al.* (2004) The rate of cognitive decline in Parkinson's disease. *Archives of Neurology* **61**: 1906–11.

Aarsland D, Zaccai J, Brayne C. (2005a) A systematic review of prevalence studies of dementia in Parkinson's disease. *Movement Disorders* **20**: 1255–63.

Aarsland D, Perry R, Brown A *et al.* (2005b) Neuropathology of dementia in Parkinson's disease: a prospective, community-based study. *Annals of Neurology* **58**: 773–6.

Aarsland D, Bronnick K, Larsen JP *et al.* (2009a) Cognitive impairment in incident, untreated Parkinson disease: the Norwegian ParkWest study. *Neurology* **72**: 1121–6.

Aarsland D, Ballard C, Walker Z *et al.* (2009b) Memantine in patients with Parkinson's disease dementia or dementia with Lewy bodies: a double-blind, placebo-controlled, multicentre trial. *Lancet Neurology* **8**: 613–8.

Alves G, Wentzel-Larsen T, Aarsland D, Larsen JP. (2005) Progression of motor impairment and disability in Parkinson disease: a population-based study. *Neurology* **65**: 1436–41.

Ballard C, Ziabreva I, Perry R *et al.* (2006) Differences in neuropathologic characteristics across the Lewy body dementia spectrum. *Neurology* **67**: 1931–4.

Beyer MK, Janvin CC, Larsen JP, Aarsland D. (2007) A magnetic resonance imaging study of patients with Parkinson's disease with mild cognitive impairment and dementia using voxel-based morphometry. *Journal of Neurology, Neurosurgery and Psychiatry* **78**: 254–9.

Braak H, Del Tredici K, Rub U *et al.* (2003) Staging of brain pathology related to sporadic Parkinson's disease. *Neurobiological Aging* **24**: 197–211.

Brown RG, Marsden CD. (1991) Dual task performance and processing resources in normal subjects and patients with Parkinson's disease. *Brain* **114**: 215–31.

Burn D, Emre M, McKeith I *et al.* (2006) Effects of rivastigmine in patients with and without visual hallucinations in dementia associated with Parkinson's disease. *Movement Disorders* **21**: 1899–907.

Burton EJ, McKeith IG, Burn DJ *et al.* (2004) Cerebral atrophy in Parkinson's disease with and without dementia: a comparison with Alzheimer's disease, dementia with Lewy bodies and controls. *Brain* **127**: 791–800.

Burton EJ, McKeith IG, Burn DJ, O'Brien JT. (2005) Brain atrophy rates in Parkinson's disease with and without dementia using serial magnetic resonance imaging. *Movement Disorders* **20**: 1571–6.

Buter TC, van den Hout A, Matthews FE *et al.* (2008) Dementia and survival in Parkinson disease: a 12-year population study. *Neurology* **70**: 1017–22.

Colosimo C, Hughes AJ, Kilford L, Lees AJ. (2003) Lewy body cortical involvement may not always predict dementia in Parkinson's disease. *Journal of Neurology, Neurosurgery, and Psychiatry* **74**: 852–6.

de Rijk MC, Tzourio C, Breteler MM *et al.* (1997) Prevalence of parkinsonism and Parkinson's disease in Europe: the EUROPARKINSON Collaborative Study. European Community Concerted Action on the Epidemiology of Parkinson's disease. *Journal of Neurology, Neurosurgery, and Psychiatry* **62**: 10–15.

Dubois B, Burn D, Goetz C *et al.* (2007) Diagnostic procedures for Parkinson's disease dementia: recommendations from the movement disorder society task force. *Movement Disorders* **22**: 2314–24.

Emre M, Aarsland D, Albanese A *et al.* (2004) Rivastigmine for dementia associated with Parkinson's disease. *New England Journal of Medicine* **351**: 2509–18.

Emre M, Aarsland D, Brown R *et al.* (2007) Clinical diagnostic criteria for dementia associated with Parkinson's disease. *Movement Disorders* **22**: 1689–707; quiz 1837.

Foltynie T, Brayne CE, Robbins TW, Barker RA. (2004) The cognitive ability of an incident cohort of Parkinson's patients in the UK. The CamPaIGN study. *Brain* **127**: 550–60.

Goris A, Williams-Gray CH, Clark GR *et al.* (2007) Tau and alpha-synuclein in susceptibility to, and dementia in, Parkinson's disease. *Ann Neurology* **62**: 145–53.

Halliday G, Hely M, Reid W, Morris J. (2008) The progression of pathology in longitudinally followed patients with Parkinson's disease. *Acta Neuropathologica* **115**: 409–15.

Hely MA, Reid WG, Adena MA *et al.* (2008) The Sydney multicenter study of Parkinson's disease: the inevitability of dementia at 20 years. *Movement Disorders* 23: 837–44.

Higginson CI, King DS, Levine D *et al.* (2003) The relationship between executive function and verbal memory in Parkinson's disease. *Brain Cognition* 52: 343–52.

Huang C, Mattis P, Perrine K *et al.* (2008) Metabolic abnormalities associated with mild cognitive impairment in Parkinson disease. *Neurology* 70: 1470–7.

Janvin CC, Larsen JP, Aarsland D, Hugdahl K. (2006) Subtypes of mild cognitive impairment in Parkinson's disease: progression to dementia. *Movement Disorders* 21: 1343–9.

Jellinger KA. (2003a) Alpha-synuclein pathology in Parkinson's and Alzheimer's disease brain: incidence and topographic distribution – a pilot study. *Acta Neuropathologica (Berlin)* 106: 191–201.

Jellinger KA. (2003b) Prevalence of cerebrovascular lesions in Parkinson's disease. A postmortem study. *Acta Neuropathologica (Berlin)* 105: 415–9.

Jellinger KA, Attems J. (2008) Prevalence and impact of vascular and Alzheimer pathologies in Lewy body disease. *Acta Neuropathologica* 115: 427–36.

Jellinger KA, Seppi K, Wenning GK, Poewe W. (2002) Impact of coexistent Alzheimer pathology on the natural history of Parkinson's disease. *Journal of Neural Transmission* 109: 329–39.

Laakso MP, Partanen K, Riekkinen P *et al.* (1996) Hippocampal volumes in Alzheimer's disease, Parkinson's disease with and without dementia, and in vascular dementia: an MRI study. *Neurology* 46: 678–81.

Leroi I, Brandt J, Reich SG *et al.* (2004) Randomized placebo-controlled trial of donepezil in cognitive impairment in Parkinson's disease. *International Journal of Geriatric Psychiatry* 19: 1–8.

Levy G, Jacobs DM, Tang MX *et al.* (2002a) Memory and executive function impairment predict dementia in Parkinson's disease. *Movement Disorders* 17: 1221–6.

Levy G, Schupf N, Tang MX *et al.* (2002b) Combined effect of age and severity on the risk of dementia in Parkinson's disease. *Annals of Neurology* 51: 722–9.

Litvan I, MacIntyre A, Goetz CG *et al.* (1998) Accuracy of the clinical diagnoses of Lewy body disease, Parkinson disease, and dementia with Lewy bodies: a clinicopathologic study. *Archives of Neurology* 55: 969–78.

McKeith IG, Dickson DW, Lowe J *et al.* (2005) Diagnosis and management of dementia with Lewy bodies: third report of the DLB Consortium. Consortium on DLB. *Neurology* 65: 1863–72.

Marder K, Tang MX, Cote L *et al.* (1995) The frequency and associated risk factors for dementia in patients with Parkinson's disease. *Archives of Neurology* 52: 695–701.

Mattay VS, Tessitore A, Callicott JH *et al.* (2002) Dopaminergic modulation of cortical function in patients with Parkinson's disease. *Annals of Neurology* 51: 156–64.

Maetzler W, Liepelt I, Reimold M *et al.* (2009) Cortical PIB binding in Lewy body disease is associated with Alzheimer-like characteristics. *Neurobiology of Disease* 34: 107–12.

Muslimovic D, Post B, Speelman JD, Schmand B. (2005) Cognitive profile of patients with newly diagnosed Parkinson disease. *Neurology* 65: 1239–45.

Peppard RF, Martin WR, Carr GD *et al.* (1992) Cerebral glucose metabolism in Parkinson's disease with and without dementia. *Archives of Neurology* 49: 1262–8.

Perry EK, Irving D, Kerwin JM *et al.* (1993) Cholinergic transmitter and neurotrophic activities in Lewy body dementia: similarity to Parkinson's and distinction from Alzheimer disease. *Alzheimer Disease and Associated Disorders* 7: 69–79.

Poewe W, Wolters E, Emre M *et al.* (2006) EXPRESS Investigators. Long-term benefits of rivastigmine in dementia associated with Parkinson's disease: an active treatment extension study. *Movement Disorders* 21: 456–61.

Possin KL, Filoteo JV, Song DD, Salmon DP. (2008) Spatial and object working memory deficits in Parkinson's disease are due to impairment in different underlying processes. *Neuropsychology* 22: 585–95.

Reid WG, Hely MA, Morris JG *et al.* (1996) A longitudinal study of Parkinson's disease: clinical and neuropsychological correlates of dementia. *Journal of Clinical Neuroscience* 3: 327–33.

Rinne JO, Portin R, Ruottinen H *et al.* (2000) Cognitive impairment and the brain dopaminergic system in Parkinson disease: [18F]fluorodopa positron emission tomographic study. *Archives of Neurology* 57: 470–5.

Robbins TW, Crofts HS, Cools R, Roberts AC. (2003) Evidence for DA-dependent neural dissociations in cognitive performance in PD. In: Bedard MA (eds). *Mental and behavioral dysfunction in movement disorders.* Totowa, NJ: Humana Press, 194–7.

Summerfield C, Gómez-Ansón B, Tolosa E *et al.* (2002) Dementia in Parkinson disease: a proton magnetic resonance spectroscopy study. *Archives of Neurology* 59: 1415–20.

Tiraboschi R, Hansen LA, Alford M *et al.* (2000) Cholinergic dysfunction in diseases with Lewy bodies. *Neurology* 54: 407–11.

Whittington CJ, Podd J, Stewart-Williams S. (2006) Memory deficits in Parkinson's disease. *Journal of Clinical and Experimental Neuropsychology* 28: 738–54.

Willemssen R, Muller T, Schwarz M *et al.* (2009) Response monitoring in *de novo* patients with Parkinson's disease. *PLoS One* 4: e4898.

Williams-Gray CH, Foltynie T, Brayne CE *et al.* (2007) Evolution of cognitive dysfunction in an incident Parkinson's disease cohort. *Brain* 130: 1787–98.

Williams-Gray CH, Hampshire A, Barker RA, Owen AM. (2008) Attentional control in Parkinson's disease is dependent on COMT val 158 met genotype. *Brain* 131: 397–408.

Williams-Gray CH, Goris A, Saiki M *et al.* (2009) Apolipoprotein E genotype as a risk factor for susceptibility to and dementia in Parkinson's disease. *Journal of Neurology* 256: 493–8.

Wylie SA, Stout JC, Bashore TR. (2005) Activation of conflicting responses in Parkinson's disease: evidence for degrading and facilitating effects on response time. *Neuropsychologia* 43: 1033–43.

Zaccai J, McCracken C, Brayne C. (2005) A systematic review of prevalence and incidence studies of dementia with Lewy bodies. *Age and Ageing* 34: 561–6.

PART VII

FOCAL DEMENTIAS AND RELATED ISSUES

68

Frontotemporal dementia

DAVID NEARY

68.1 INTRODUCTION

Frontotemporal dementia (FTD) is the most common of a group of clinical syndromes, associated with degeneration of the frontal and temporal lobes and non-Alzheimer pathology, and collectively referred to as frontotemporal lobar degeneration (FTLD). Behavioural change dominates the clinical picture of FTD at onset and throughout the disease course. However, cognitive impairments, particularly in executive functions, and qualitative changes in language also occur. The paucity of neurological signs and findings of focal abnormalities in the frontotemporal lobes on neuroimaging contribute to the diagnosis. Recent years have seen improved clinical recognition of the disorder and dramatic advances in understanding of its neurobiology.

68.2 TERMINOLOGY AND DIAGNOSTIC CRITERIA

The term 'frontotemporal dementia' was introduced by workers in Lund, Sweden and Manchester, United Kingdom (Lund and Manchester groups, 1994) to refer specifically to the behavioural disorder described in this chapter. The term superseded labels such as 'frontal-lobe dementia', reflecting the fact that the behavioural disorder almost invariably affects anterior temporal, as well as frontal lobes. The behavioural disorder of FTD was subsequently distinguished from the two

other prototypical forms of FTLD, progressive non-fluent aphasia and semantic dementia and clinical diagnostic criteria for each syndrome were formulated (Neary et al., 1998). Consensus criteria for FTD are shown in **Table 68.1**. Pathological links between the distinct syndromes of FTLD have led some workers to use the label FTD in a generic sense to encompass all FTLD syndromes (McKhann et al., 2001). This chapter uses the term FTD in its original sense. The syndromes of progressive aphasia and semantic dementia are described in detail in Chapter 71, Semantic dementia and Chapter 72, Primary progressive aphasia and posterior cortical atrophy.

Studies of the usefulness of the clinical criteria shown in **Table 68.1**, based respectively on a large pathological series (Knopman et al., 2005) and a memory clinic population (Pijnenburg et al., 2008) have reported high specificity (99 and 90 per cent), suggesting that the criteria effectively distinguish FTD from other forms of dementia. Sensitivity levels are rather lower (85 and 79 per cent, respectively), suggesting that all core diagnostic features may not invariably be present. One study (Piguet et al., 2009) reported a sensitivity of only 56 per cent at initial presentation (based on the presence of all core features) rising to 73 per cent with progression, although interpretation is complicated by the fact that fewer than half the presumed FTD cases had pathological confirmation of diagnosis. Proposed revisions to these criteria include indicating levels of probability of diagnosis based on number of features present and elevating the status of atrophy on magnetic resonance imaging (MRI) from supportive to core feature.

Table 68.1 Clinical diagnostic features of frontotemporal dementia.

I. Core diagnostic features	Insidious onset and gradual progression		
	Early decline in social interpersonal conduct		
	Early impairment in regulation of personal conduct		
	Early emotional blunting		
	Early loss of insight		
II. Supportive diagnostic features	A. Behavioural disorder	Decline in personal hygiene and grooming	
		Mental rigidity and inflexibility	
		Distractibility and impersistence	
		Hyperorality and dietary changes	
		Perseverative and stereotyped behaviour	
		Utilization behaviour	
	B. Speech and language	Altered speech output	Aspontaneity and economy of speech
			Press of speech
		Stereotypy of speech	
		Echolalia	
		Perseveration	
		Mutism	
	C. Physical signs	Primitive reflexes	
		Incontinence	
		Akinesia, rigidity and tremor	
		Low and labile blood pressure	
	D. Investigations	Neuropsychology: significant impairment on frontal lobe tests in the absence of severe amnesia, aphasia or perceptuospatial disorder	
		Electroencephalography: normal on conventional EEC despite clinically evident dementia	
		Brain imaging (structural and/or functional): predominant frontal and/or anterior temporal abnormality	

68.3 EPIDEMIOLOGY AND DEMOGRAPHICS

Prevalence data are limited. One study, based on 17 patients with clinical FTD in the area of Cambridge, UK (Ratnavalli *et al.*, 2002) reported a prevalence of 15 per 100 000 in people aged 45–64 years. A larger study of 245 FTD patients in the Netherlands (Rosso *et al.*, 2003) yielded lower estimates: 3.6 per 100 000 at age 50–59, increasing to 9.4 per 100 000 at age 60–69 and reducing to 3.8 per 100 000 at 70–79 years. The high prevalence in the Cambridge study led the authors to conclude that FTD may be as common as Alzheimer's disease (AD) before the age of 60 years. However, clinical referral rates to centres in Manchester, UK and Matsuyama, Japan suggest that AD is more common even before 60 years. In a pathological series of 524 dementia patients, covering the full age spectrum, examined in Lund, Sweden over a 30-year period (Brunnström *et al.*, 2009), 4 per cent had FTD and 42 per cent AD.

A positive family history is present in up to 40 per cent of cases, although reports vary. The familial incidence is likely to be influenced by geography: FTD families with +16 exon 10 splice-site mutations have been traced to a common founder in North Wales (Pickering-Brown *et al.*, 2004).

There is an equal incidence for men and women (Rosso *et al.*, 2003). Onset of symptoms is most commonly 45–65 years (**Table 68.2**). However, there is a wide range, the youngest recorded onset being 21 years (Snowden *et al.*, 2004). Age at onset in familial and sporadic cases does not differ (Piguet *et al.*, 2004). The length of illness varies from 2 to 20 years, median 6–8 years (Snowden *et al.*, 1996; Hodges *et al.*, 2003), very short durations being associated with the presence of motor neurone disease (MND).

68.4 BEHAVIOUR AND AFFECT

68.4.1 Personal and social

The overriding presenting feature is breakdown in social conduct (Neary *et al.*, 1988; Neary *et al.*, 2005). Patients

Table 68.2 Demographic features in frontotemporal dementia.

Usual onset 45–65 years
Earliest recorded onset 21 years
Equal sex incidence
Mean illness duration eight years, range 2–20 years
Family history in up to 50%
No known geographical or environmental influences

neglect personal responsibilities, mismanage domestic and financial affairs and underperform occupationally, leading to demotion or dismissal from work. Patients show a decline in manners, social graces and decorum. Some patients are overactive, distractible and socially disinhibited. They talk to strangers, laugh or sing inappropriately. They make social faux-pas, such as drinking from the wine bottle in a restaurant. They may pace restlessly and wander. Other patients are apathetic and avolitional. There is a lack of insight into mental change.

Patients lose interest in their appearance, neglect personal hygiene and need prompting to wash and change their clothes. Behaviour becomes inflexible and patients may adopt a fixed daily routine. They are unable to see another's point of view.

68.4.2   Eating and oral behaviours

Changes in eating and drinking patterns are common and may be early symptoms (Miller *et al.*, 1995; Bathgate *et al.*, 2001). Patients are gluttonous, eat indiscriminately, cram food and steal food from others' plates. Relatives have to ration food to prevent obesity. Patients show a preference for sweet foods, which they seek out and hoard. Hyperorality (Kluver–Bucy syndrome), involving ingestion of inedible objects, is observed in some patients, usually in late stage disease. In some patients, excessive eating or drinking is attributable to gluttony, whereas in others it reflects stimulus-boundedness and environmental dependency.

68.4.3   Sleeping and sexual behaviour

Increased somnolence occurs, particularly in apathetic patients. Altered sexual behaviour most often takes the form of a loss of libido, particularly in apathetic, inert patients. Sexual disinhibition is usually secondary to patients' general behavioural disinhibition and lack of social awareness. However, a minority of patients do become hypersexual and exhibit interest in sexual perversions.

68.4.4   Repetitive behaviours, compulsions and rituals

Repetitive, stereotyped behaviours are common. They may comprise simple motor mannerisms, such as hand rubbing, foot tapping or grunting or complex behavioural routines. Patients may pace and wander a fixed route, repeat

incessantly a favoured word, phrase or anecdote, repeat the same puns, ditties or dance steps, or clap a favoured rhythm. Hygiene and dress and toileting may themselves be the source of stereotypies.

A striking form of repetitive behaviour, present in a small minority of patients, is that of forced utilization. Objects elicit the motor actions appropriate to those objects, even though the action may be contextually inappropriate: an empty cup elicits a repeated drinking action.

68.4.5   Affect

The onset of FTD is insidious and may sometimes be heralded by affective changes that include depression, anxiety and excessive sentimentality, as well as hypochondriasis and somatic preoccupation (Lund and Manchester groups, 1994). In some cases, discrete episodes of treatable mood disturbances may occur several months or even years before the emergence of gross behavioural change. Commonly, however, subtle mood disturbances are the precursor to the progressive alterations in personality, social conduct and affect that characterize the disease.

In established FTD, affect is typically bland, shallow and indifferent. Patients lack empathy, sympathy and compassion and seem selfish and self-centred. Relatives may be perturbed by the patient's absence of grief on the death of a loved one or callous response to a tragedy. Patients no longer exhibit shame or embarrassment, and may lack personal modesty. Disinhibited patients may display a fatuous jocularity.

Patients may fail to respond to painful stimuli, with indifference to scalds and burns. However, sometimes patients respond in an exaggerated, melodramatic way to non-threatening tactile stimuli, such as casual touching. Paradoxically, the two may co-occur: the patient tolerates the pain of a needle without comment, yet recoils in apparent agony as a person brushes past. FTD patients may avoid social contact, both physical and eye contact.

68.5   PHYSICAL FINDINGS

68.5.1   General physical examination

Patients are typically physically well. However, low and labile blood pressure may be noted. Incontinence, without embarrassment, is a relatively early feature.

68.5.2   Typical neurological signs

Patients typically remain neurologically intact, even in the presence of gross behavioural and cognitive change. Signs are generally limited to primitive reflexes, such as grasping, pouting, sucking and extensor plantar responses. Extrapyramidal signs of akinesia, rigidity and tremor, become evident, in most cases, only after many years and reflect breakdowns in nigrostriatal dopaminergic function (Rinne *et al.*, 2002). Myoclonus does not occur.

68.5.3 FTD with motor neurone disease

About 10 per cent of FTD patients develop symptoms and signs of motor neurone disease (MND) of the amyotrophic type (Neary et al., 1990; Strong et al., 2009). Patients exhibit bulbar palsy, weakness and wasting of the limbs, widespread muscular fasciculations in the tongue, limbs and trunk and primitive reflexes. With disease progression, muscular wasting increases and dysarthria and ineffective coughing lead to death, commonly within three years. The physical signs of MND may precede, coincide with or follow the development of behavioural change.

68.6 INVESTIGATIONS

68.6.1 Electrophysiology

Routine electroencephalogram (EEG) typically remains normal even in the context of severe dementia, a feature that helps to distinguish FTD from AD, in which there is slowing of wave forms. In patients with symptoms and signs of MND electrophysiological studies of neuromuscular function reveal normal nerve conduction studies, multifocal muscular fasciculations, reduced muscular firing rates and giant motor units, compatible with widespread muscular denervation due to anterior horn cell death.

68.6.2 Structural and functional brain imaging

Computed tomography (CT) reveals non-specific cerebral atrophy or widening of the interhemispheric and sylvian fissures suggesting a frontotemporal distribution of atrophy. Emphasis of atrophy in the frontal and anterior temporal lobes is more reliably demonstrated on MRI (Varma et al., 2002; Whitwell et al., 2004).

Frontotemporal hypoperfusion/metabolism is demonstrated using single photon emission tomography (SPECT) (Varma et al., 2002) and positron emission tomography (PET) (Diehl et al., 2004), ventromedial frontal cortex being identified as the critical affected area (Salmon et al., 2003). The pattern of anterior hemisphere dysfunction contrasts with the prototypical pattern of posterior hemisphere dysfunction seen in AD (Talbot et al., 1998; Varrone et al., 2002; Foster et al., 2007). Functional MRI has shown loss of frontal activation in early FTD cases in whom structural MRI is normal (Rombouts et al., 2003).

68.7 NEUROPSYCHOLOGY OF FTD

68.7.1 Historical reports

Personality and behavioural changes are prominent and outweigh cognitive symptoms. Relatives may comment on alterations in the patient's language: sparse conversation, stereotyped iteration of words, phrases or anecdotes, echoing

of others' speech (echolalia). They may describe variable, self-centred memory disturbances (the patient may seem selectively to remembers what he wants to remember), absent-mindedness and faulty attention. Symptoms of visuospatial disorientation are notably absent. Relatives are surprised when the patient wanders miles from the home, yet finds his way back.

68.7.2 Quality of neuropsychological test performance

Some patients are markedly distractible and restless and may attempt to leave the room during a testing session, and compliance may be lost. Economy of mental effort and cursory, superficial responses characterize test performance in apathetic, inert patients. The lack of concerted application is an important feature, because it effectively impairs performance across a wide range of tests that are purportedly designed to evaluate a spectrum of psychological functions (Thompson et al., 2005). Test scores taken at face value may lead to spurious interpretations of the nature of the patient's psychological deficit.

Performance may be compromised too by verbal and motor perseveration, which may occur at either an elementary (repetition of a single movement) or higher-order (repetition of a complete programme of actions) level. Concreteness of thought can compromise interpretation of verbal instructions, pictures and stories. Patients may fail to abstract an underlying narrative or draw inferences that go beyond the elements physically present.

68.7.3 Language

Speech output is characteristically reduced. Patients do not initiate conversation, and responses to questions are brief and unelaborated, with minimal application of mental effort. Verbal stereotypies may be present, constituting favoured words or phrases, or sometimes an entire well-rehearsed repertoire. Echolalia, verbal perseverations and concrete responses are common. Despite speech economy, utterances are fluent and effortless, without pronunciation difficulties. However, hypophonia and loss of prosody may become evident. Mutism ensues in late-stage disease. The reduction in generative language or 'adynamia' bears resemblance to the 'dynamic aphasia' described by Luria and Tsvetkova (1968).

The attenuation of conversational discourse contrasts with the relative preservation of overlearnt, 'automatic' aspects of language. Patients may repeat phrases, recite series such as the months of the year, complete nursery rhymes and join in songs at a time when spontaneous utterances are virtually absent.

Comprehension is typically relatively well preserved at a single word level, but impaired for complex syntax and sequential commands. Performance on tests of comprehension is governed by the mental demands of the task. Naming to confrontation can be relatively well preserved. Open-ended verbal fluency tasks, involving generation of words from a semantic category or beginning with a specified letter are typically disproportionately impaired compared to object naming.

Reading aloud is relatively preserved and patients may develop a habit of reading aloud road signs and advertising hoardings, even when their spontaneous conversation is minimal. In a test setting, virtually mute patients may read aloud test material accurately, much to the surprise of their relatives. Errors in reading typically arise secondary to patients' poor attention, rather than to primary linguistic deficits. Reading for comprehension characteristically mirrors comprehension of spoken language. In reading a complete narrative, such as a fable-like short story, patients typically show poor abstractive and synthetic powers.

Written output is typically reduced and patients tend to write single words or brief phrases, rather than complete sentences. Spelling may be erratic, reflecting lack of checking. Markedly perseverative responses characterize the writing of a proportion of patients.

The ability to communicate non-verbally by symbolic gesture, conveying actions such as waving, saluting and beckoning, may be preserved, at least initially. However, just as speech output decreases, so too do the patient's body movements, and in late-stage disease it may be impossible to elicit any gestures, either to command or by demonstration. Buccofacial movements typically fail to convey a range of facial expression: a bland or fatuous expression predominates.

68.7.4   Visual perception and spatial skills

Patients typically have no difficulty in the perceptual recognition of objects, do not make perceptual errors on naming tests involving pictorial material, and for the most part use objects appropriately. There is no convincing evidence moreover of 'parietal'-type deficits, even with advanced disease. Clinical observation suggests that patients have no difficulty localizing objects, can manipulate and orientate clothing correctly, and negotiate their environment, without becoming lost. Even when patients become formally untestable and are mute, they may fixate and reach for objects without difficulty, and may show behaviours as part of a stereotypic repertoire that demonstrate preserved spatial localization skills, such as repeated folding of a handkerchief or aligning of papers. Impairments on formal neuropsychological tests of perceptuospatial function arise secondary to patients' poor attention, organizational and strategic skills and lack of concern for accuracy. The notable preservation of spatial skills in FTD patients contrasts with the severe impairment common in AD.

68.7.5   Memory

Patients often perform poorly on formal tests of memory. However, recall is enhanced by the use of specific, directed rather than broad open-ended questions, performance benefits from provision of multiple-choice alternatives and there is no abnormal loss of information over a delay. These features suggest a 'frontal'-type of memory impairment, arising secondary to impairments in attention, strategic functioning and active information generation, rather than a classical amnesia. Patients are typically oriented and can provide appropriate information about autobiographical events.

68.7.6   Motor skills

Patients have normal manual dexterity and can manipulate objects, use feeding implements and carry out complex actions, such as lighting a cigarette, until relatively late in the disease. Occasionally, patients exhibit 'utilization behaviour', in which objects placed within reach of the patient elicits the motor actions appropriate to those objects even though those behaviours are contextually inappropriate. Performance on motor tasks may be compromised by perseveration and impersistence.

With progression of disease, it may become increasingly difficult in inert, apathetic patients to elicit motor responses. However, actions may be more easily evoked by imitation than through verbal command, and a minority of patients exhibit frank echopraxia, copying actions of the examiner without being requested to do so.

68.7.7   Frontal executive functions

Patients show impairments in a range of executive skills, including abstraction, planning, organizational and strategic functioning, sustained, selective and switching of attention. 'Frontal lobe' tests that are sensitive to such changes include the Wisconsin card sorting test, Weigls test, Stroop test, Trail making test, verbal fluency, design fluency, Haylings and Brixton test, and Test of Everyday Attention. Details of test administration can be found in Lezak (2002).

68.7.8   Social cognition

FTD patients shown impairments on tests of social cognition and emotion recognition (Lough et al., 2001; Snowden et al., 2003; Torralva et al., 2009). Such socially based skills may be impaired even in patients who perform relatively well on standard executive tasks (Lough et al., 2001; Torralva et al., 2009), a factor likely to contribute to patients' severe breakdown in social, interpersonal conduct.

68.7.9   Performance on standard tests of intelligence

Some patients who present with disinhibition and over-activity may initially perform normally on standard test batteries, such as the Wechsler Adult Intelligence Scale, highlighting a dissociation between the profound alteration in personality and behaviour and breakdown in social competence, and relative preservation of cognitive skills. Often, however, performance is impaired, and becomes so in all individuals with progression of disease. A pattern of test scores may be evident which points to a predominant frontal lobe dysfunction: disproportionate impairment for the comprehension, similarities and picture arrangement subtests. A verbal-performance discrepancy, occurring in a

Table 68.3   Cognitive characteristics of frontotemporal dementia.

Characteristics	
Language	Economy of mental effort and output
	Perseveration, echolalia, stereotypy
	Concreteness
	Late mutism
Perceptuospatial function	Preserved. Errors on constructional tasks arise secondary to organizational deficits
Memory	Variable, idiosyncratic day to day memory
	Preserved orientation in time and place
	Poor information retrieval
	Recall enhanced by cues and directed probes
Motor skills	Poor temporal sequencing
	Perseveration
Abstraction and planning	Concrete responses
	Poor set shifting
	Organizational and sequencing failure
	Perseveration

Table 68.4   Clinical subtypes of frontotemporal dementia.

Subtype	
Disinhibited	Restless, overactive, disinhibited
	Fatuous, jocular, unconcerned
	Profound social breakdown
	Behavioural disorder more prominent than cognitive disorder
Apathetic	Inert, aspontaneous, avolitional
	Bland, apathetic, unconcerned
	Mentally rigid and perseverative
	Severely impaired on frontal-lobe cognitive tests
Stereotypic	Stereotypic, ritualistic, compulsive
	Bland, unconcerned
	Mentally rigid
	Behavioural disorder salient feature

minority of patients, will tend to favour performance items. However, commonly, performance is impoverished across all subtests, with no clear pattern of deficits emerging across tasks. This profile, which appears to arise as a consequence of patients' lack of effortful application to tasks and cursory mode of responding, may misleadingly give rise to the interpretation of a 'generalized' dementia.

The principle cognitive characteristics are summarized in **Table 68.3**.

68.8   PHENOTYPIC VARIATION IN FTD

68.8.1   Behavioural subtypes

FTD patients all share the core features of change in personality and altered social conduct. Nevertheless, the precise behavioural characteristics of the disorder may vary (Snowden *et al.*, 2001) (**Table 68.4**).

68.8.1.1   DISINHIBITED TYPE

Some patients present with features reminiscent of hypomania. They are overactive, restless, inattentive and distractible, rushing unproductively from one activity to another, with marked lack of application and persistence. Their demeanour is fatuous, inappropriately jocular, disinhibited and socially inappropriate. Such patients may perform relatively well on cognitive tasks, at least in the early stages of disease. In such patients, functional imaging typically reveals relatively circumscribed tracer deficits involving the orbitofrontal and anterior temporal lobes.

68.8.1.2   APATHETIC TYPE

Some patients present with an apathetic, amotivational, pseudo-depressed state. Their behaviour is characterized by

loss of volition and inertia, so that if left to their own devices they would spend their day in bed or sitting unoccupied. All behaviours are economical, with minimal expenditure of mental effort. With disease progression, the patient becomes increasingly unresponsive, so that virtually no verbal or motor behaviour can be elicited. It is in these patients that perseverative behaviour, both verbal and motor, is the most pronounced, and in whom executive deficits are most severe. Imaging shows widespread frontal lobe involvement, including dorsolateral convexity regions. Disinhibited patients typically show increased apathy with disease progression. Nevertheless, behavioural distinctions at initial presentation suggest that the disinhibition–apathy spectrum is not merely a product of disease severity.

68.8.1.3   STEREOTYPIC TYPE

Occasionally, the striking presenting characteristic is of repetitive, ritualistic and idiosyncratic behaviours (e.g. repeated sequential tapping of the walls of a room). Such patients typically exhibit parkinsonian signs at a relatively early stage of the illness and imaging shows severe striatal involvement.

68.8.2   Mixed FTD phenotypes

Some patients do not present a 'pure' picture of FTD, but rather an overlapping clinical phenotype in which the behavioural disorder and frontal executive impairments of FTD are combined with language impairments of progressive aphasia or the conceptual impairments of semantic dementia (see Chapter 71, Semantic dementia and Chapter 72, Primary progressive aphasia and posterior cortical atrophy).

68.9   THE NEUROPATHOLOGY OF FTD

The principle atrophy in FTD involves the frontal and anterior temporal neocortices, the amygdala and basal ganglia (Brun, 1987; Brun, 1993; Mann and South, 1993;

Mann *et al.*, 1993). Within the neocortex, the histological changes principally involve layers II and III, the origin of cortico-cortical associational neurones, sparing layer V, the major source of cortico-subcortical neurones.

The underlying histopathology is not uniform (Cairns *et al.*, 2007; Mackenzie *et al.*, 2009) (see Chapter 70, The genetics and molecular pathology of frontotemporal lobar degeneration, for a full account). Cases can be classified broadly as tau-positive (FTLD-tau) or tau-negative, ubiquitin-positive (FTLD-U). In tau-positive cases, there are insoluble tau proteins in the brain in the form of intraneuronal neurofibrillary tangles or Pick bodies. In tau-negative cases, the ubiquitinated target protein is, in the majority of cases, the transactive response DNA-binding protein, TDP-43 (FTLD-TDP). Ubiquitin histology has been further divided into three major subtypes on the basis of the relative preponderance of neuronal cytoplasmic inclusions, dystrophic neurites and neuronal intranuclear inclusions.

Whereas language-related clinical syndromes of FTLD, namely semantic dementia and progressive non-fluent aphasia, are preferentially associated with certain histopathological subtypes (Snowden *et al.*, 2007; Josephs *et al.*, 2009), the behavioural disorder of FTD appears to occur with comparable frequencies in association with tau and non-tau pathology and with each subtype of tau-negative, ubiquitin-positive pathology. Notably, however, FTD-MND is invariably associated with tau-negative, ubiquitin/TDP positive pathology and the ubiquitin subtype characterized by numerous neuronal cytoplasmic inclusions in both superficial and deep cortical laminae (type 3 according to Mackenzie *et al.* (2006); type 2 according to Sampathu *et al.* (2006)).

68.10 MOLECULAR GENETICS

In familial forms of FTD, the mode of inheritance appears to be autosomal dominant. Missense and splice-site mutations have been identified in the *tau* gene on chromosome 17 in some familial FTD cases (Hutton *et al.*, 1998; Poorkaj *et al.*, 1998; Janssen *et al.*, 2002; Pickering-Brown *et al.*, 2002). Such cases are associated with tau pathology. In other familial cases, as well as in a small number of patients without obvious family

history, mutations have been identified in the *progranulin* gene on chromosome 17 (Baker *et al.*, 2006). Such cases are associated with tau-negative, TDP-43 pathology, and more specifically with the subtype characterized by neuronal cytoplasmic inclusions, dystrophic neurites and neuronal intranuclear inclusions (Mackenzie type 1; Sampathu type 3). Linkage to chromosome 3 has been reported in an extended Danish family (Brown *et al.*, 1995; Gydesen *et al.*, 2002) and to chromosome 9 in patients with FTD/MND (Hosler *et al.*, 2000; Le Ber *et al.*, 2009). See Chapter 70, The genetics and molecular pathology of frontotemporal lobar degeneration for a detailed description of the genetics and molecular pathology of FTD.

68.11 TREATMENT AND MANAGEMENT

The severe behavioural disorder of FTD places an enormous emotional and practical burden on families. Pharmacological treatments are, however, limited and symptomatic (Huey *et al.*, 2006; Boxer and Boeve, 2007). There is evidence of abnormalities in serotonergic function (Procter *et al.*, 1999; Franceschi *et al.*, 2005). Selective serotonin reuptake inhibitors (SSRIs) are sometimes used to manage behavioural symptoms, although their reported effectiveness is variable. Serotonergic abnormalities affect the postsynaptic rather than presynaptic system and it has been suggested (Bowen *et al.*, 2008) that treatment with a $5-HT_{1A}$ receptor antagonist might be warranted. In FTD, there is no cholinergic deficit, so there is no rational basis for use of conventional AD therapies.

Management of patients concentrates largely on construction of a support network through social, psychiatric and voluntary services to provide day, respite and ultimately residential care. Services are often best provided by old age psychiatry services, although access to those services by younger, behaviourally disturbed people may be problematic. Specialist facilities for younger dementia sufferers are urgently required. Within the setting of a hospital environment, repetitive behaviours can sometimes be turned to the advantage of the group by harnessing the stereotypic activity to socially useful ends.

Table 68.5 Comparison of clinical features in frontotemporal dementia and Alzheimer's disease.

	Frontotemporal dementia	Alzheimer's disease
Demographics	Typically early onset	Typically late onset
History	Early personality change	Memory loss
	Social breakdown	Spatial disorientation
	Altered eating habits	Aphasia
Affect	Blunted, fatuous	Concerned, anxious
Neurology	Early primitive reflexes	Akinesia and rigidity, myoclonus
Language	Adynamic speech, mutism	Aphasia
Visuospatial skills	Preserved	Impaired
Memory	'Frontal-type' amnesia	'Limbic-type' amnesia
EEG	Normal	Abnormal, slow
SPECT	Anterior cerebral abnormality	Posterior cerebral abnormality

EEC, electroencephalogram; SPECT, single photon emission tomography.

68.12 DIFFERENTIAL DIAGNOSIS

Features that distinguish FTD from AD are summarized in **Table 68.5**. However, in the very early stages patients with both FTD and AD may show few neurological symptoms or signs. Moreover, disinhibited FTD patients may perform relatively well on standard neuropsychological tests, including 'frontal lobe' tests, so that neuropsychological assessment is not invariably informative. Neuroimaging techniques are not available in all centres. Differential diagnosis is, therefore, crucially dependent on the evaluation of the patient's behaviour and affect, hence the emphasis on behavioural features in diagnostic criteria. Informant-based behavioural interviews can elicit information that is highly discriminating (Bozeat *et al.*, 2000; Bathgate *et al.*, 2001; Ikeda *et al.*, 2002). In a comparative study of FTD and AD (Bozeat *et al.*, 2000), behavioural stereotypies, altered eating habits and loss of social awareness best discriminated the two groups. Similarly, in a comparative study of FTD, AD and vascular dementia (Bathgate *et al.*, 2001), the best discriminators included changes in eating habits, especially overeating and the presence of repetitive, stereotyped behaviours. Particularly discriminating also was the reduced capacity of FTD patients to demonstrate both primary and social emotions (e.g. sadness, fear, sympathy, embarrassment), and the loss of emotional insight (i.e. a lack of distress or concern when confronted by deficits). Informant-based interviews have been found to have discriminatory value even when carried out retrospectively several years after the patient's death (Barber *et al.*, 1995).

68.13 CONCLUSION

Frontotemporal dementia is a relatively common form of early-onset dementia. It is characterized by profound alteration in personality and social conduct, and by cognitive defects in attention, abstraction planning, judgement, organization and strategic functioning. In contrast, instrumental tools of cognition, particularly spatial navigational skills, are relatively preserved. The neuropsychological disorder, indicative of anterior hemisphere dysfunction, is the converse of that seen in AD, in which profound breakdown in the tools of cognition: memory, language and perceptuospatial abilities, occur in the context of remarkably well-preserved social skills. The paucity of neurological signs in FTD and in particular the absence of myoclonus, the normal electroencephalogram and the selective anterior hemisphere abnormalities seen on brain imaging also help to separate FTD from the relatively more common dementia of AD. FTD is neither clinically nor pathologically uniform. Molecular genetic advances have distinguished mutations responsible for FTD in some familial cases and other mutations are likely to be identified. Such advances are beginning to clarify nosological issues relating the status of the different histopathologies associated with FTLD and the relationship between FTD and language/conceptual syndromes of progressive aphasia and semantic dementia. Genetic advancement also holds the prospect of future treatment for this devastating form of dementia.

REFERENCES

Baker M, Mackenzie IRA, Pickering-Brown SM *et al.* (2006) Mutations in Progranulin cause tau-negative frontotemporal dementia linked to chromosome 17. *Nature* 442: 916–19.

Barber RA, Snowden JS, Craufurd D. (1995) Retrospective differentiation of frontotemporal dementia and Alzheimer's disease using information from informants. *Journal of Neurology, Neurosurgery and Psychiatry* 59: 61–70.

Bathgate D, Snowden JS, Varma A *et al.* (2001) Behaviour in frontotemporal dementia, Alzheimer's disease and vascular dementia. *Acta Neurologica Scandinavica* 103: 367–78.

Bowen DM, Procter AW, Mann DM *et al.* (2008) Imbalance of a serotonergic system in frontotemporal dementia: implications for pharmacotherapy. *Psychopharmacology (Berl)* 196: 603–10.

Boxer AL, Boeve BF. (2007) Frontotemporal dementia treatment: current symptomatic therapies and implications of recent genetic, biochemical and neuroimaging studies. *Alzheimer's disease and Associated Disorders* 21: S79–87.

Bozeat S, Gregory CA, Lambon Ralph MA, Hodges JR. (2000) Which neuropsychiatric and behavioural features best distinguish frontal and temporal variants of frontotemporal dementia from Alzheimer's disease. *Journal of Neurology, Neurosurgery and Psychiatry* 69: 178–86.

Brown J, Ashworth A, Gydesen S. (1995) Familial nonspecific dementia maps to chromosome 3. *Human Molecular Genetics* 4: 1625–8.

Brun A. (1987) Frontal lobe degeneration of non-Alzheimer type. I. Neuropathology. *Archives of Gerontolology and Geriatrics* 6: 193–208.

Brun A. (1993) Frontal lobe degeneration of non-Alzheimer type revisited. *Dementia* 4: 126–31.

Brunnström H, Gustafson L, Passant U, Englund E. (2009) Prevalence of dementia subtypes: a 30 year retrospective survey. *Archives of Gerontology and Geriatrics* 49: 146–9.

Cairns NJ, Biggio EH, Mackenzie IRA *et al.* (2007) Neuropathological diagnostic criteria and nosology of the frontotemporal lobar degenerations: consensus criteria of the Consortium for Frontotemporal Lobar Degenerations. *Acta Neuropathologica* 114: 5–22.

Diehl J, Grimmer T, Drzezga A *et al.* (2004) Cerebral metabolic patterns at early states of frontotemporal dementia and semantic dementia: a PET study. *Neurobiology of Aging* 25: 1051–6.

Foster NL, Heidebrink JL, Clark CM *et al.* (2007) FDG-PET improves accuracy of distinguishing frontotemporal and Alzheimer's disease. *Brain* 130: 2616–35.

Franceschi M, Anchisi D, Pelati O *et al.* (2005) Glucose metabolisms and serotonin receptors in the frontotemporal lobar degeneration. *Annals of Neurology* 57: 216–25.

Gydesen S, Brown JM, Brun A *et al.* (2002) Chromosome 3 linked frontotemporal dementia (FTD-3). *Neurology* 59: 1585–94.

Hodges JR, Davies R, Xuereb J *et al.* (2003) Survival in frontotemporal dementia. *Neurology* 61: 349–54.

Hosler BA, Siddique T, Sapp PC *et al.* (2000) Linkage of familial amyotrophic lateral sclerosis with frontotemporal dementia to chromosome 9q21-q22. *Journal of the American Neurological Association* 284: 1664–9.

Huey ED, Putman KT, Grafman J. (2006) A systematic review of neurotransmitter deficits and treatments in frontotemporal dementia. *Neurology* 66: 17–22.

Hutton M, Lendon CL, Rizzu P *et al.* (1998) Association of missense and 5′-splice-site mutations in tau with the inherited dementia FTDP-17. *Nature* 393: 702–5.

Ikeda M, Brown J, Holland AJ *et al.* (2002) Changes in appetite, food preference and eating habits in frontotemporal dementia and Alzheimer's disease. *Journal of Neurology, Neurosurgery and Psychiatry* 73: 371–6.

Janssen JC, Warrington EK, Morris HR *et al.* (2002) Clinical features of frontotemporal dementia due to the intronic tau 10^{+16} mutation. *Neurology* 58: 1161–8.

Josephs KA, Stroh A, Dugger B, Dickson DW. (2009) Evaluation of subcortical pathology and clinical correlations in FTLD-U subtypes. *Acta Neuropathologica* 118: 349–58.

Knopman DS, Boeve BF, Parisi JE *et al.* (2005) Antemortem diagnosis of frontotemporal lobar degeneration. *Annals of Neurology* 57: 480–8.

Le Ber I, Camazat A, Berger E *et al.* (2009) Chromosome 9p-linked families with frontotemporal dementia associated with motor neuron disease. *Neurology* 72: 1669–76.

Lezak MD. (2002) *Neuropsychological assessment*, 4th edn. Oxford: Oxford University Press.

Lough S, Gregory C, Hodges JR. (2001) Dissociation of social cognition and executive function in frontal variant frontotemporal dementia. *Neurocase* 7: 123–30.

Lund and Manchester groups. (1994) Consensus statement. Clinical and neuropathological criteria for frontotemporal dementia. *Journal of Neurology, Neurosurgery and Psychiatry* 4: 416–18.

Luria AR, Tsvetkova LS. (1968) The mechanism of 'dynamic aphasia'. *Foundations of Language* 4: 296–307.

Mackenzie IRA, Barborie A, Pickering-Brown S *et al.* (2006) Heterogeneity of ubiquitin pathology in frontotemporal lobar degeneration: classification and relation to clinical phenotype. *Acta Neuropathologica* 112: 539–49.

Mackenzie IRA, Neumann M, Bigio EH *et al.* (2009) Nomenclature for neuropathologic subtypes of frontotemporal lobar degeneration: consensus recommendations. *Acta Neuropathologica* 117: 15–18.

Mann DMA, South PW. (1993) The topographic distribution of brain atrophy in frontal lobe dementia. *Acta Neuropathologica* 85: 334–40.

Mann DMA, South PW, Snowden JS, Neary D. (1993) Dementia of frontal lobe type; neuropathology and immunohistochemistry. *Journal of Neurology, Neurosurgery and Psychiatry* 56: 605–14.

McKhann GM, Albert MS, Grossman M *et al.* (2001) Clinical and pathological diagnosis of frontotemporal dementia: report of the Working Group on Fronotemporal Dementia and Pick's disease. *Archives of Neurology* 58: 1803–9.

Miller BL, Darby AL, Swartz JR *et al.* (1995) Dietary changes, compulsions and sexual behaviour in frontotemporal degeneration. *Dementia* 6: 195–9.

Neary D, Snowden JS, Northen B, Goulding PJ. (1988) Dementia of frontal lobe type. *Journal of Neurology, Neurosurgery and Psychiatry* 51: 353–61.

Neary D, Snowden JS, Mann DMA *et al.* (1990) Frontal lobe dementia and motor neuron disease. *Journal of Neurology, Neurosurgery and Psychiatry* 53: 23–32.

Neary D, Snowden JS, Gustafson L *et al.* (1998) Frontotemporal lobar degeneration. A consensus on clinical diagnostic criteria. *Neurology* 51: 1546–54.

Neary D, Snowden J, Mann D. (2005) Frontotemporal dementia. *Lancet Neurology* 4: 771–80.

Pickering-Brown SM, Richardson AMT, Snowden JS *et al.* (2002) Inherited frontotemporal dementia in nine British families associated with intronic mutations in the tau gene. *Brain* 125: 732–51.

Pickering-Brown S, Baker M, Bird T *et al.* (2004) Evidence for a founder effect in families with frontotemporal dementia that harbour the tau +16 splice mutation. *Americal Journal of Medical Genetics B Neuropsychiatric Genetics* 125B: 79–82.

Piguet OW, Brooks S, Halliday GM *et al.* (2004) Similar early clinical presentations in familial and non-familial frontotemporal dementia. *Journal of Neurology, Neurosurgery and Psychiatry* 75: 1743–5.

Piguet O, Hornberger M, Shelley BP *et al.* (2009) Sensitivity of current criteria for the diagnosis of behavioural variant frontotemporal dementia. *Neurology* 72: 732–7.

Pijnenburg YA, Mulder JL, van Swieten JC *et al.* (2008) Diagnostic accuracy of consensus diagnostic criteria for frontotemporal dementia in a memory clinic population. *Dementia and Geriatric Cognitive Disorders* 25: 157–64.

Poorkaj P, Bird TD, Wijsman E *et al.* (1998) Tau is a candidate gene for chromosome 17 frontotemporal dementia. *Annals of Neurology* 43: 815–25.

Procter AW, Qume M, Francis PT. (1999) Neurochemical features of frontotemporal dementia. *Dementia and Geriatric Cognitive Disorders* 10 Suppl. 1: 80–4.

Ratnavalli E, Brayne C, Dawson K, Hodges JR. (2002) The prevalence of frontotemporal dementia. *Neurology* 58: 1615–21.

Rinne JO, Laine M, Kaasinen V *et al.* (2002) Striatal dopamine transporter and extrapyramidal symptoms in frontotemporal dementia. *Neurology* 58: 1489–93.

Rombouts SA, Van Swieten JC, Pijnenburg YA *et al.* (2003) Loss of frontal fMRI activation in early frontotemporal dementia compared to early AD. *Neurology* 60: 1904–8.

Rosso SM, Donker Kaat L, Baks T *et al.* (2003) Frontotemporal dementia in the Netherlands: patient characteristics and prevalence estimates from a population-based study. *Brain* 126: 2016–22.

Salmon E, Garraux G, Delbeuck X *et al.* (2003) Predominant ventromedial frontopolar metabolic impairment in frontotemporal dementia. *Neuroimage* 20: 435–40.

Sampathu DM, Neumann M, Kwong LK *et al.* (2006) Pathological heterogeneity of frontotemporal lobar degeneration with ubiquitin-positive inclusions delineated by ubiquitin immunohistochemistry and novel monoclonal antibodies. *American Journal of Pathology* 169: 1343–52.

Snowden JS, Neary D, Mann DMA. (1996) *Frontotemporal lobar degeneration: frontotemporal dementia, progressive aphasia, semantic dementia.* London: Churchill Livingstone.

Snowden JS, Bathgate D, Varma A *et al.* (2001) Distinct behavioural profiles in frontotemporal dementia and semantic dementia. *Journal of Neurology, Neurosurgery and Psychiatry* 70: 323–32.

Snowden JS, Gibbons ZC, Blackshaw A *et al.* (2003) Social cognition in frontotemporal dementia and Huntington's disease. *Neuropsychologia* 41: 688–701.

Snowden JS, Neary D, Mann DMA. (2004) Autopsy proven, sporadic frontotemporal dementia, due to microvacuolar histology, with onset at 21 years of age. *Journal of Neurology, Neurosurgery and Psychiatry* 75: 1337–9.

Snowden JS, Neary D, Mann D. (2007) Frontotemporal lobar degeneration: clinical and pathological relationships. *Acta Neuropathogica* 114: 31–8.

Strong MJ, Grace GM, Freedman M *et al.* (2009) Consensus criteria for the diagnosis of frontotemporal cognitive and behavioural symptoms in amyotrophic lateral sclerosis. *Amyotrophic Lateral Sclerosis* 10: 131–46.

Talbot PR, Lloyd JJ, Snowden JS *et al.* (1998) A clinical role for 99mTc-HMPAO SPECT in the investigation of dementia? *Journal of Neurology, Neurosurgery and Psychiatry* 64: 306–13.

Thompson JC, Stopford CL, Snowden JS, Neary D. (2005) Qualitative neuropsychological performance characteristics in frontotemporal dementia and Alzheimer's disease. *Journal of Neurology, Neurosurgery and Psychiatry* 76: 920–7.

Torralva T, Roca M, Geichgerrcht E *et al.* (2009) A neuropsychological battery to detect specific executive and social cognitive impairments in early frontotemporal dementia. *Brain* 132: 1299–309.

Varma AR, Adams W, Lloyd JJ *et al.* (2002) Diagnostic patterns of regional atrophy on MRI and regional cerebral blood flow change on SPECT in young onset patients with Alzheimer's disease, frontotemporal dementia and vascular dementia. *Acta Neurologica Scandinavica* 105: 261–9.

Varrone A, Pappata S, Caraco C *et al.* (2002) Voxel-based comparison of rCBF SPET images in frontotemporal dementia and Alzheimer's disease highlights involvement of different cortical networks. *European Journal of Nuclear Medicine and Molecular Imaging* 29: 1447–54.

Whitwell JL, Anderson VM, Scahill RI *et al.* (2004) Longitudinal patterns of regional change on volumetric MRI in frontotemporal lobar degeneration. *Dementia and Geriatric Cognitive Disorders* 17: 307–10.

Pick's disease: its relationship to progressive aphasia, semantic dementia and frontotemporal dementia

JOHN HODGES

69.1 INTRODUCTION

Considerable advances continue to be made in our understanding of the group of neurodegenerative diseases that present with focal cognitive deficits arising from circumscribed pathology of the frontal and/or temporal lobes, most commonly referred to collectively as Pick's disease (PiD) or frontotemporal dementia (FTD). However, the literature on these conditions is filled with a confusing plethora of terms, which can make these developments difficult to follow for the non-expert. Central to the problem is a lack of clarity as to the intended level of description (clinical syndrome versus clinicopathological entity versus specific histological diagnosis) and a lack of concordance between these levels. For example, while some labels denote a clinical syndrome without specific histological implications (e.g. progressive aphasia, semantic dementia or dementia of frontal type), others denote specific neuropathological entities (e.g. PiD or familial tauopathy), hybrid clinicopathological entities (e.g. FTD), or even specific genetic disorders (e.g. FTD with parkinsonism linked to chromosome 17). Recent differences in opinion over terminology are well illustrated by the titles of the following books, all published in the last decade: *Pick's disease and Pick complex* (Kertesz and Munoz, 1998), *Frontotemporal dementia*

(Pasquier *et al.*, 1996), *Frontotemporal lobar degeneration: frontotemporal dementia, progressive aphasia, semantic dementia* (Snowden *et al.*, 1996) and *Frontotemporal dementia syndromes* (Hodges, 2007). This lack of clarity is acknowledged, and efforts to rationalize terminology and achieve clinicopathological and nosological consensus have been made (Brun *et al.*, 1994; Neary *et al.*, 1998; McKhann *et al.*, 2001). Even at a recent meeting of experts, agreement over terms was far from universal (Kertesz *et al.*, 2003b).

The aims of this chapter are to review the evolution of the terms used to describe this spectrum of disorders, to highlight recent advances and examine areas of continuing controversy. While the author's bias is to prefer the term 'Pick's disease' for this group of disorders – which is more readily understood by carers and parallels use of the label Alzheimer's disease (AD) – the current tide of opinion is to use 'frontotemporal dementia' as an umbrella term for the overall clinical syndrome.

69.2 WHAT DID PICK ACTUALLY DESCRIBE?

In 1892, Arnold Pick, working in Prague, reported a 71-year-old man with progressive mental deterioration and unusually severe aphasia who at post-mortem had marked atrophy of the cortical gyri of the left temporal lobe (Pick, 1892; Girling and Berrios, 1994). Pick wanted to draw attention to the fact that local accentuation of progressive brain atrophy may lead to symptoms of local disturbance (in this instance, aphasia). He also made specific and, as we will see below, highly perceptive predictions regarding the role of the mid-temporal region of the left hemisphere in the representation of word meaning. In subsequent papers, he described four further patients with left temporal atrophy (Pick, 1904; Girling and Berrios, 1997) or frontotemporal atrophy (Pick, 1901; Girling and Markova, 1995), again stressing their progressive language disturbance. It was only in his 1906 publication that Pick turned his attention to bilateral frontal atrophy with resultant behavioural disturbance (Pick, 1906). Spatt (2003) has reviewed Pick's approach to cognitive disorders and his concept of dementia.

Several points should be emphasized:

- Pick's primary interest in these patients was their language disorder, particularly the clinicoanatomical correlates of aphasia.
- He did not claim to have discovered a new disease, merely novel phenomena arising from asymmetric degeneration.
- He did not describe distinct neuropathological changes in his patients with focal atrophy.
- Both the major syndromes now included under the rubric of FTD (dementia of frontal type and semantic dementia) were clearly reported by Pick.

In view of these monumental contributions, it is sad that Pick has been relegated to a minor place in the modern terminology of FTD.

The histological abnormalities associated with PiD were, in fact, described a few years later by Alzheimer (1911) who recognized changes distinct from those found in the form of cerebral degeneration later associated with his name. Alzheimer recognized both argyrophilic intracytoplasmic inclusions (Pick bodies) and diffusely staining ballooned neurones (Pick cells) in association with focal lobar atrophy. It is interesting to note that a comprehensive review of 20 patients from the literature with aphasia owing to focal lobar atrophy written soon after Alzheimer's description (Mingazzini, 1914) did not use the label 'Pick's disease', which was introduced by Gans some eight years later (Gans, 1922). The term was then taken up by Onari and Spatz (1926), but Carl Schneider (Schneider, 1927; Schneider, 1929) is probably most responsible for its popularization. Unfortunately, however, Schneider concentrated on the frontal lobe component of the syndrome and thus began the neglect of the temporal lobe syndromes. He distinguished three clinical phases, the first characterized by impaired judgement and behaviour, the second by local symptoms, and the third by generalized dementia. Many papers describing PiD then appeared in the 1930s and 1940s (Ferrano and Jervis, 1936; Lowenberg and Arbor, 1936; Nichols and Weigner, 1938; Lowenberg et al., 1939; Neumann, 1949), which again mainly focused on the frontal lobe aspects of the disorder.

After the Second World War, interest in PiD faded, together with a general waning of interest in the cognitive aspects of neurology in the English-speaking world. The focus of interest in English-language publications became the neuropathology, and latterly the genetics, of PiD. This resulted in a gradual change in the criteria for PiD, which evolved to include the necessity for specific pathological changes (i.e. focal atrophy with Pick cells and or Pick bodies). Indeed, many authors went as far as to claim that AD and PiD were clinically indistinguishable in life (Katzman, 1986; Kamo et al., 1987). In continental Europe, however, there remained a strong interest in the clinical phenomena of the dementias; PiD remained an *in vivo* diagnosis based on a combination of clinical features suggestive of frontal and/or temporal lobe dysfunction and focal lobar atrophy (Mansvelt, 1954; Tissot et al., 1975). This controversy continues and has contributed to the adoption of the many labels to describe patients with the clinical syndrome of progressive frontal or temporal lobe degeneration (Baldwin and Förstl, 1993).

69.3 REDISCOVERING PICK'S DISEASE: FROM DEMENTIA OF THE FRONTAL TYPE AND PROGRESSIVE APHASIA TO FRONTOTEMPORAL DEMENTIA

69.3.1 Dementia of frontal type

A renaissance of interest in the focal dementias occurred in the 1980s. Workers from Lund (Gustafson, 1987; Brun, 1987) reported on a large series of patients with dementia and found that of 158 patients studied prospectively, who came to post-mortem, 26 had evidence of frontal lobe degeneration. Since only a small proportion had Pick cells and Pick bodies – the remainder had very similar findings, but without specific inclusions (i.e. focal lobar atrophy with severe neuronal loss and spongiosis) – the Lund group preferred to adopt the term 'frontal degeneration of non-Alzheimer type'. At approximately the same time, Neary and coworkers (1986) in Manchester began a series of important clinicopathological studies of patients with presenile dementia. They, likewise, found a high proportion of cases with a progressive frontal lobe syndrome that had neither specific changes of AD (plaques and tangles) nor specific Pick pathology. They introduced the term 'dementia of frontal type'. Over the next few years, other groups described very similar cases under the labels 'frontal lobe degeneration' (Miller et al., 1991) and 'dementia lacking distinct histological features' (Knopman et al., 1990). The author's own preferred term for this group of patients is 'behavioural variant FTD' (bvFTD) (Davies et al., 2006; Kipps et al., 2007; Rascovsky et al., 2007; Hornberger et al., 2008; Kipps et al., 2009).

In the advanced stages of the disease, patients with this disorder present no diagnostic difficulty. They have the triad of:

- a profound change in personality and behaviour;
- neuropsychological impairments indicative of selective or disproportionate frontal pathology; and
- appropriate changes on structural and/or functional brain imaging.

Diagnosing early cases is by no means easy and one of the challenges is to develop better methods of early, accurate detection (Gregory et al., 1999). Since patients are typically unaware of the insidious changes noted by others, we rely upon carer-based assessments. One undoubted advance in the area has, therefore, been the development of standardized carer interviews such as the Neuropsychiatric Inventory (Cummings et al., 1994), which appears to differentiate patients with FTD and AD (Levy et al., 1996). In an attempt to develop a local instrument capable of early diagnosis, we identified key symptoms that occurred very commonly in patients with bvFTD (Gregory and Hodges, 1993; Gregory and Hodges, 1996) which became the foundation for the Cambridge Behavioural Inventory (Wedderburn et al., 2008). Kertesz and his group have developed a tool specifically aimed at frontal behaviours, the Frontal Behaviour Inventory, which appears to discriminate patients with FTD from those with AD or depression (Kertesz et al., 1997; Kertesz et al., 2000; Kertesz et al., 2003a). Recent work has focused on specific behaviours that can discriminate patients with bvFTD and semantic dementia from patients with AD, such as changes in appetite, food preferences and eating habits (Ikeda et al., 2002), or the presence of stereotypies (Nyatsanza et al., 2003).

Many patients with bvFTD present to psychiatrists and acquire a label of functional psychiatric disorder (including simple schizophrenia, depression and obsessive–compulsive disorder) because despite gross behavioural changes other aspects of cognition are typically preserved (Ames et al., 1994; Tonkonogy et al., 1994; Gregory and Hodges, 1996; Miller et al., 1997). This is understandable in terms of the site of pathology in bvFTD, the orbital and mesial frontal lobes, which are critically involved in social judgement, motivation, risk assessment and the pathophysiology of obsessive–compulsive behaviour (Cummings, 1999). By contrast, dorsolateral frontal regions, which have been the focus of classic neuropsychological studies, are spared in the early stages of the disease. The development of quantifiable tasks sensitive to orbital and mesial frontal function has begun with paradigms involving probability and gambling (Rogers et al., 1998; Rahman et al., 1999), emotion processing (Keane et al., 2002), and 'theory of mind' (ToM) tasks, such as detection of social faux pas (Gregory et al., 2002; Torralva et al., 2007) and the discrimination of sincere from sarcastic statements (Kipps et al., 2009; Rankin et al., 2009). An important recent development has been the identification of a subgroup of patients with clinical features of bvFTD, but who show little or no progression often over many years of follow up (Davies et al., 2006; Kipps et al., 2007; Kipps et al., 2008). Such patients are almost universally men and can be distinguished on the basis of a number of factors: normal performance on executive and social cognition tasks (Hornberger et al., 2008; Kipps et al., 2009), preservation of activities of daily living (Mioshi and Hodges, 2007; Mioshi et al., 2007), absence of brain atrophy on magnetic resonance imaging (MRI) (Davies et al., 2006; Kipps et al., 2009) and normal FDG-PET (Kipps et al., 2009). The aetiology of the so-called bvFTD phenotype syndrome remains unclear, a proportion of such patients have a decompensated personality disorders and others a functional psychiatric disorder, but much work remains to be done in this area.

69.3.2 Progressive aphasia and semantic dementia

The other strand of the story concerns the rediscovery of the syndrome of progressive aphasia in association with focal left perisylvian or temporal lobe atrophy. In 1982, Mesulam reported six patients with a long history of insidiously worsening aphasia in the absence of signs of more generalized cognitive failure. One of these patients underwent a brain biopsy, which revealed non-specific histology without specific markers of either AD or PiD (Mesulam, 1982). Following Mesulam's seminal paper, approximately 100 patients with progressive aphasia were reported over the next 15 years (for reviews, see Mesulam and Weintraub, 1992; Hodges and Patterson, 1996; Snowden et al., 1996; Garrard and Hodges, 1999). From this literature it became clear that, although the language impairment in patients with progressive aphasia is heterogeneous, there are two identifiable and distinct aphasia syndromes: progressive non-fluent aphasia and progressive fluent aphasia. In the latter syndrome, speech remains fluent and well articulated, but becomes progressively devoid of content words. The language and other non-verbal cognitive deficits observed in these patients reflect a breakdown in semantic memory that has led many authors to apply the label of 'semantic dementia' (Snowden et al., 1989; Hodges et al., 1992; Hodges et al., 1994; Saffran and Schwartz, 1994; Hodges and Patterson, 1996) (see also Chapter 71, Semantic dementia).

Although the term 'semantic dementia' is recent, the syndrome has, as discussed above, been recognized under different labels for many years. Pick (Pick, 1892; Pick, 1904) and a number of other early authors (Rosenfeld, 1909; Mingazzini, 1914; Stertz, 1926; Schneider, 1927) recognized that the chief clinical manifestations of temporal lobe atrophy were 'amnesic aphasia' or 'transcortical sensory aphasia', together attributed to atrophy of the middle and inferior temporal gyri leaving Wernicke's area intact. These language impairments were typically associated with a type of dementia variously described as a reduction in categorical or abstract thinking, sensory or 'associative agnosia' (Malamud and Boyd, 1940; Robertson et al., 1958). These features – amnesic aphasia and associative agnosia – can now be united by the concept of 'semantic memory loss'.

Warrington (1975) was the first to clearly delineate the syndrome of semantic memory impairment in three patients. Drawing on the work of Tulving (Tulving, 1972; Tulving, 1983), Warrington recognized that the progressive anomia in her patients was not simply a linguistic deficit, but reflected a fundamental loss of semantic memory (or knowledge) about the items, which thereby affected naming, word comprehension and object recognition. 'Semantic memory' is the term applied to the component of long-term memory that contains the permanent representation of our knowledge about things in the world and their interrelationship, facts and concepts, as well as words and their meaning (Hodges et al., 1992; Garrard et al., 1997; Hodges and Patterson, 1997; Hodges et al., 1998). Cases of semantic dementia have also been recognized for many years in Japan as cases of 'gogi (word meaning) aphasia' (Imura et al., 1971; Sasanuma and Mondi, 1975; Morita et al., 1987; Tanabe, 1992; Tanabe et al., 1992).

Our original paper reported five cases with progressive loss of semantic memory and focal temporal atrophy (Hodges *et al.*, 1992). All five presented with a fluent aphasia and all the characteristics of semantic memory loss: empty speech with word-finding difficulty and occasional semantic paraphasias (mother for father), a severe reduction in the generation of exemplars on category fluency tests (in which subjects are asked to produce as many examples as possible from defined semantic categories, such as animals or musical instruments, within 1 minute), impaired single word comprehension on picture-pointing tests, a loss of fine-grained attribution knowledge about a range of items with preservation of broad superordinate information on verbal and pictorial tests of knowledge. By contrast, other aspects of language competency (phonology and syntax) were strikingly preserved. In contrast to AD, the patients also had good day-to-day (episodic) memory, although we have more recently shown that this sparing of autobiographical memory applies to fairly recent memories only (Graham and Hodges, 1997; Hodges and Graham, 1998). They also showed no impairment on tests of immediate (working) memory, visually based problem solving or visuoperceptual abilities. Four of the five patients showed severe and circumscribed temporal lobe atrophy on computed tomography (CT) scanning or MRI. Since 1992, we have studied many further such patients and have confirmed the association with focal atrophy of the temporal lobe – involving the temporal pole and inferolateral neocortex (particularly the peri-rhinal cortex and fusiform gyrus), with relative sparing of the hippocampal formation. In many cases, the atrophy is strikingly asymmetric, but always involves the left side (Hodges *et al.*, 1998; Mummery *et al.*, 1999; Garrard and Hodges, 1999; Galton *et al.*, 2001; Hodges and Patterson, 2007).

This lateralization raises the issue of what are the cognitive and/or behavioural signatures of isolated right temporal atrophy. In 1994, we reported a patient (VH) with progressive prosopagnosia followed by a specific loss of knowledge about people (Evans *et al.*, 1995). VH was unable to identify from face or name even very famous people, yet had intact general semantic and autobiographical memory (Kitchener and Hodges, 1999). In a more recent study, Thompson *et al.* (2004) reported a dissociation of person-specific from general semantic knowledge in two patients with contrasting patterns of temporal atrophy. Subject MA, with predominantly left temporal atrophy, showed impairment of general semantics with relative preservation of knowledge about people, while subject JP, with predominantly right temporal atrophy, showed the opposite pattern of impairments with severely impaired person-specific knowledge in the context of relatively preserved knowledge about objects and animals. The group, led by Miller, have also drawn attention to the bizarre behaviours (including irritability, impulsiveness, alterations in dress, limited and fixed ideas, and decreased facial expression) exhibited by patients with predominantly right temporal lobe atrophy (Edwards Lee *et al.*, 1997; Miller *et al.*, 1997). A recent review of 47 patients with semantic dementia identified distinct behavioural and cognitive profiles associated with the left and right temporal variants of the disease (Thompson *et al.*, 2003). Social awkwardness, job loss, lack of

insight and difficulty with person identification were all more likely to be associated with major right temporal atrophy; while word-finding difficulties and reduced comprehension were all more likely to be associated with predominantly left-sided atrophy.

There are a number of compelling reasons to consider semantic dementia as part of the same disease spectrum as bvFTD. The first is pathological: in early clinicopathological studies of cases fulfilling criteria for semantic dementia, all had either classic PiD (i.e. Pick bodies and/or Pick cells) or non-specific spongiform change of the type found in the majority of cases with the frontal form of lobar atrophy (Wechsler, 1977; Wechsler *et al.*, 1982; Holland *et al.*, 1985; Poeck and Luzzatti, 1988; Graff-Radford *et al.*, 1990; Snowden *et al.*, 1992; Scholten *et al.*, 1995; Harasty *et al.*, 1996; Hodges *et al.*, 1998; Schwarz *et al.*, 1998). More recently, a broader spectrum of pathology has been described, particularly FTD with tau-negative ubiquitin-positive inclusions discussed more fully below (Rossor *et al.*, 2000; Hodges *et al.*, 2004; Davies *et al.*, 2005). Second is the evolution of the pattern of cognitive and behavioural changes over time: although semantic dementia patients present with progressive anomia and other linguistic deficits, on follow up the features that characterize the frontal form of FTD emerge (Hodges and Patterson, 1996; Edwards Lee *et al.*, 1997). Indeed, semantic dementia and bvFTD may share many behavioural features even on presentation (Bozeat *et al.*, 2000). Third is the fact that modern neuroimaging techniques demonstrate subtle involvement of the orbitofrontal cortex in the majority of cases presenting with prominent temporal atrophy and semantic dementia (Mummery *et al.*, 2000; Rosen *et al.*, 2002a; Williams *et al.*, 2005).

The status of patients with the non-fluent form of progressive aphasia within the spectrum of FTD is more complex. Clinically, such cases are clearly separable from cases of semantic dementia. Speech is faltering and distorted with frequent phonological substitutions and grammatical errors. Other non-language-based aspects of cognition remain well preserved, as do activities of daily living. Changes in behaviour and personality of the type that typify dementia of frontal type, and are seen in the later stages of semantic dementia, are rare, but after a number of years, global cognitive decline occurs (Green *et al.*, 1990; Hodges and Patterson, 1996). Some patients with progressive non-fluent aphasia have Alzheimer pathology at post-mortem, albeit with an atypical distribution; that is to say, marked involvement of perisylvian language areas, but sparing of medial temporal structures (Greene *et al.*, 1996; Croot *et al.*, 1997; Galton *et al.*, 2000; Knibb *et al.*, 2006), while others have tau-positive inclusion pathology with classic Pick bodies or more diffuse neuronal and glial tau inclusions (Weintraub *et al.*, 1990; Mesulam and Weintraub, 1992; Knibb *et al.*, 2006). Recent functional neuroimaging studies have implicated the anterior insula as the key abnormal region (Nestor *et al.*, 2003).

A potentially important recent development has been the separation of non-fluent aphasic patients into two subgroups. The first characterized by apraxia of speech and or agrammatism who have severe anomia, dysfluency because of word-finding pauses, occasional phonological errors and markedly impaired sentence repetition have been termed 'logopenic progressive aphasia' with emerging evidence of largely AD pathology at post-mortem (Gorno-Tempini *et al.*, 2008; Mesulam, 2008).

69.3.3   Frontotemporal dementia and frontotemporal lobar degeneration

The final terms to be considered are those of FTD and frontotemporal lobar degeneration (FTLD). In 1994, the Lund and Manchester groups introduced the term FTD and suggested tentative criteria for the diagnosis (Brun *et al.*, 1994). The term 'FTD' was subsequently replaced by 'FTLD', and consensus clinical diagnostic criteria were published (Neary *et al.*, 1998). The adoption of the terms FTD or FTLD has the advantage of avoiding specific pathological implications; it also brings to attention the fact that patients with the same disease may present with different clinical syndromes and that with time both types of deficit are likely to emerge. Three main clinical syndromes are recognized: FTD, progressive non-fluent aphasia and semantic dementia (Neary *et al.*, 1998) (see **Figure 69.1**). However, disadvantages of the term FTLD are the blurring of levels of description and the amalgamation of distinct clinical syndromes. In particular, confusion may occur between FTD (now referring only to the behavioural variant of the disorder) and FTLD (the new term for the overall spectrum of presentations). **Figure 69.2** presents the preferred Cambridge nomenclature.

It remains to be established which of the long list of phenomena listed as 'criteria' actually separate FTD and AD, although a study by Miller *et al.* (1997), using SPECT as the gold standard, suggested that loss of personal awareness (self-care), disordered eating, perseverative behaviour and reduction in speech most clearly differentiate FTD from AD. We have also looked at a wide range of neurobehavioural symptoms in a large group of patients with FTD (frontal variant of FTD (FvFTD) and semantic dementia) and AD and identified four distinct clusters of symptoms by factor analysis: stereotypic and eating behaviours, executive function and self-care, mood changes and loss of social awareness (Bozeat *et al.*, 2000).

In this study, stereotypic and eating behaviours together with loss of social awareness reliably differentiated FTD from AD. At the level of individual symptoms, patients with semantic dementia showed increased rates of mental rigidity and depression compared with patients with bvFTD, while conversely, the latter group showed more disinhibition.

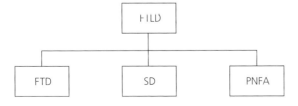

Figure 69.1   Clinical classification of frontotemporal dementia according to the Lund–Manchester criteria. FTD, frontotemporal dementia; FTLD, frontotemporal lobar degeneration; PNFA, progressive non-fluent aphasia; SD, semantic dementia.

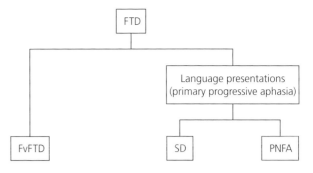

Figure 69.2   Clinical classification of frontotemporal dementia according to the Cambridge group. FTD, frontotemporal dementia; fvFTD, frontal or behavioural variant of FTD; PNFA, progressive non-fluent aphasia; SD, semantic dementia.

69.4   FAMILIAL CHROMOSOME 17-LINKED FRONTOTEMPORAL DEMENTIA

The term FTD increased in usage with the discovery of a specific gene mutation in familial cases. Linkage had been established in a number of families in which FTD was inherited as an autosomal dominant trait to chromosome 17q21-22, a region which contains the gene for the microtubule-associated protein tau (Wilhelmsen, 1997).

The story of the chromosome 17 linkage is extraordinary in a number of ways. Families around the world with what has become known as FTD with parkinsonism linked to chromosome 17 (Spillantini *et al.*, 1998a) had originally been reported under a range of headings including: disinhibition–dementia–parkinsonism–amyotrophy complex (DDPAC) (Wilhelmsen *et al.*, 1994); rapidly progressive autosomal dominant parkinsonism and dementia with pallidopontonigral degeneration (Wszolek *et al.*, 1992); familial progressive subclinical gliosis (Petersen *et al.*, 1995); hereditary dysphasic dementia (Morris *et al.*, 1984); hereditary FTD (Heutink *et al.*, 1997); multiple system tauopathy with presenile dementia (Spillantini *et al.*, 1997); familial presenile dementia with psychosis (Sumi *et al.*, 1992) and Pick's disease (Schenk, 1951). In 1996, a meeting of representatives from all of the groups identifying linkage to chromosome 17 was held in Ann Arbor, MI (Foster *et al.*, 1997). Comparison of clinical and pathological data revealed a great deal of similarity between the families who all shared the characteristics of predominately frontotemporal distribution of pathology with marked behavioural changes. Extrapyramidal dysfunction was present in most. In some families, psychotic symptoms were a major feature and a number had amyotrophy. It was recognized at that time that some of the families shared the common pathology with microtubule-associated protein tau-positive inclusions. Progress in the field was then rapid. It was soon discovered that most, if not all, families had tau inclusions with a distinctive morphological pattern leading to the coining of the term 'familial tauopathy' and the suggestion that the disease might reflect a mutation in the tau gene known to be located in the 17q21-22 region (Spillantini *et al.*, 1998a). Within two years of the Ann Arbor meeting, the first mutations were identified (Dumanchin *et al.*, 1998; Hutton *et al.*, 1998; Poorkaj *et al.*, 1998; Spillantini *et al.*, 1998b).

Subsequent progress has been rapid: more than 50 different tau mutations have been reported in association with familial FTD, differing according to their positions in the tau gene, their effects on tau mRNA and protein, and the type of tau pathology they cause (Ingram and Spillantini, 2002).

Not all cases of familial FTD are caused by tau mutations. In one large Danish family with autosomal dominant FTD, linkage has been established to chromosome 3 (Brown et al., 1995; Brown, 1998) and, in some families with FTD-motor neurone disease, linkage has been established to chromosome 9. In a series of 22 cases of familial FTD only, 11 (50 per cent) had tau mutations (Morris et al., 2001).

In 2006, another major breakthrough established mutations of the progranulin gene also on chromosome 17 which results in dominantly inherited FTD with ubiquitin-positive tau-negative pathology (Baker et al., 2006). Mutations of the progranulin gene account for a substantial proportion of familial cases not caused by tau gene mutations (Gass et al., 2006). Even more recently, mutations of progranulin have been linked to abnormalities of the TAR-DNA binding protein 43 (TDP43) identified as the pathological protein in both FTLD-U and in motor neuron disease (Neumann et al., 2006).

69.5 CORTICOBASAL DEGENERATION, PROGRESSIVE SUPRANUCLEAR PALSY AND FRONTOTEMPORAL DEMENTIA

In 1967, Rebeiz and colleagues described three patients with a neurodegenerative illness affecting both cortex and basal ganglia (Rebeiz et al., 1968). Each patient presented with a progressive asymmetrical akinetic-rigid syndrome and apraxia; on the basis of neuropathology findings Rebeiz et al. called the disorder 'corticodentatonigral degeneration with neuronal achromasia', later renamed 'corticobasal degeneration' (CBD). Initially, CBD was conceptualized as a distinct clinicopathological entity, but in the early 1990s it was recognized that considerable clinical and pathological heterogeneity existed within the disorder. Clinically, cases of pathologically proven CBD were described presenting with the clinical syndromes of frontotemporal dementia (Mathuranath et al., 2000) or progressive aphasia (Lippa et al., 1991). Conversely, it was recognized that other pathologies might underlie the clinical syndrome of CBD; in a review of 32 consecutive cases of clinically diagnosed CBD (Boeve et al., 1999), the underlying pathological diagnosis was CBD in 18, AD in three, PiD in two, progressive supranuclear palsy in six, and dementia lacking specific histology in two. A distinction has been drawn by some authors between the corticobasal syndrome (the constellation of clinical features characteristically associated with CBD) and corticobasal degeneration (the histopathological disorder itself). There is growing awareness of the overlap between the clinical syndrome of CBD and progressive non-fluent aphasia (PNFA): many patients with PNFA develop apraxia and parkinsonian features and conversely many CBD patients have subtle language production deficits that worsen as the disease progresses (Graham et al., 2003).

The related disorder progressive supranuclear palsy (PSP), originally described by Steele et al. in 1964, is classically characterized by progressive axial rigidity, bradykinesia, vertical gaze palsy and dysarthria. Pathologically, tau-positive neurofibrillary tangles and threads are found in the substantia nigra, the subthalamic nucleus and the dentate nucleus. It is increasingly recognized that pathological PSP may present with the clinical features of CBD, or even progressive aphasia or a frontal lobe syndrome. Conversely, the PSP phenotype may result from tau gene mutations (Morris et al., 2003; Soliveri et al., 2003). Both CBD and PSP share an identified genetic risk factor, the H1 haplotype of the tau gene, and the tau deposits in both these diseases consist of the four-repeat isoforms of tau.

In their original case report, Rebeiz et al. (1968) recognized the similarity of the neuropathology in CBD to that seen in PiD. The Work Group on Frontotemporal Dementia and Pick's Disease (McKhann et al., 2001) now includes both CBD and PSP among the pathological causes of the FTD syndromes.

69.6 FRONTOTEMPORAL DEMENTIA WITH MOTOR NEURONE DISEASE

Although motor neurone disease (MND) has traditionally been regarded as a disorder which spares higher cognitive abilities, it has become clear since early reports from Japan (Mitsuyama and Takamiya, 1979) that the rate of dementia in MND is significantly greater than expected. Indeed, up to 10 per cent of patients with MND might show features of dementia and/or aphasia if such features are systematically elicited (Rakowicz and Hodges, 1998; Lillo and Hodges, 2009). Neuroimaging in MND with cognitive impairment demonstrates widespread frontal and temporal atrophy. Conversely, a significant minority of patients with FTD develop features of MND (Neary et al., 1990; Caselli et al., 1993; Rakowicz and Hodges, 1998; Bak and Hodges, 1999; Strong et al., 2003). Such patients present with cognitive symptoms, either FvFTD or progressive aphasia, which then progresses rapidly, followed by the emergence of bulbar features and mild limb amyotrophy. Such cases have a characteristic pattern of histological change with ubiquitin (and TDP43)-positive, tau-negative, inclusions in cortical regions and the dentate gyrus. One interesting observation is that such patients almost invariably have disproportionately greater impairment of verb rather than noun processing, which affects both production and comprehension (Bak et al., 2001).

From a practical perspective, this variant of FTD should be suspected in any cases with rapidly progressive disease or the emergence of bulbar symptoms. The overlap in clinical presentation between FTD and related disorders is illustrated schematically in **Figure 69.3**.

69.7 CORRELATION BETWEEN CLINICAL SYNDROMES AND NEUROPATHOLOGY

The definitive diagnosis of FTD depends upon neuropathological examination. Unlike other dementia syndromes, notably AD, FTD encompasses considerable pathological

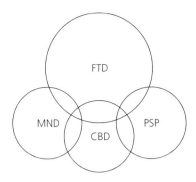

Figure 69.3 Overlap in clinical presentation of frontotemporal dementia and related disorders. CBD, corticobasal degeneration; FTD, frontotemporal dementia; MND, motor neurone disease; PSP, progressive supranuclear palsy.

heterogeneity. There have been considerable developments in the past few years. Three broad subdivisions have been recognized depending on the profile of immunohistochemical staining and the pattern of intracellular inclusions (Jackson and Lowe, 1996; Dickson, 1998; McKhann *et al.*, 2001; Hodges *et al.*, 2003). First, patients with tau-positive pathology, which in turn comprise a number of subvariants including those with classic argyrophilic, tau-positive, intraneuronal Pick bodies; those with MAP tau gene mutations (FTDP-17) and diffuse tau-positive neuronal and astrocytic immunoreactivity; those characterized by tau-positive astrocytic plaques and ballooned achromatic neurones (CBD); and those with tau-positive argyrophilic grain disease (AGD). Second, cases ubiquitin-positive and TDP43-positive inclusions in the dentate gyrus and brain stem motor nuclei which include cases with associated motor neurone disease and those with progranulin gene mutations. Third, dementia lacking distinctive histology (DLDH) which now constitutes a very small proportion of cases (**Figure 69.4**).

The question as to whether distinct pathological subtypes map on to distinct clinical syndromes is of great interest (see **Figure 69.4**). Relatively few clinicopathological series have been reported to date (Rascovsky *et al.*, 2002; Rosen *et al.*, 2002b; Hodges *et al.*, 2003; Josephs *et al.*, 2006; Mesulam *et al.*, 2008). In summary, it appears that the majority of patients with semantic dementia have tau-negative, TDP43-positive

pathology with relatively few cases having tau positive inclusions. The converse is true of PNFA which is typically associated with tau-positive forms of FTD or alternatively with AD pathology. Pathology in the common bvFTD is least predictable with approximately half having tau-positive FTD and the other half having TDP43-positive FTD.

69.8 HOW COMMON IS FRONTOTEMPORAL DEMENTIA?

Historically, it has long been recognized that FTD is less common than AD. Until recently, however, most estimates of the prevalence of FTD were based on reports from specialist units where FTD tended to be over-represented as a diagnosis. This has changed with the publication of a number of community-based studies that give a clearer picture of the true prevalence of FTD.

Ratnavalli *et al.* (2002) conducted a prevalence survey aiming to ascertain all cases of early-onset dementia (age of onset less than 65 years) in a UK region with a total population of 326 000. The overall prevalence for early-onset dementia was 81 per 100 000 for patients aged 45–64 years, with equivalent prevalences of AD and FTD at 15 per 100 000. Of 185 cases seen by the study group, 23 (12 per cent) fulfilled the Lund–Manchester criteria for FTD, suggesting that, although FTD is by no means rare, it still represents only a minority of cases of dementia in those under 65 years. (For comparison, AD was diagnosed in 34 per cent, vascular dementia in 18 per cent, alcohol-related dementia in 10 per cent and dementia with Lewy bodies in 7 per cent.)

Similar figures were obtained by Harvey *et al.* (2003), who surveyed three London boroughs with a total population of 567 500 people and calculated an overall prevalence for early onset-dementia of 98 per 100 000 for patients aged 45–64 years.

The prevalence of FTD in those over 65 years is largely unknown. Recent prospective investigation of 451 85-year-olds in Sweden found that 86 (19 per cent) fulfilled the criteria for a frontal lobe syndrome and 14 (3 per cent) fulfilled the Lund–Manchester criteria for FvFTD (Gislason *et al.*, 2003).

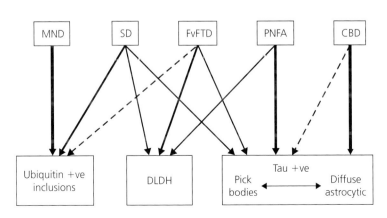

Figure 69.4 Relationship between clinical syndrome and underlying pathology for frontotemporal dementia and related disorders. CBD, corticobasal degeneration; DLDH, dementia lacking distinctive histology; fvFTD, frontal or behavioural variant of FTD; MND, motor neurone disease; PNFA, progressive non-fluent aphasia; SD, semantic dementia. Thickness of arrow lines denotes the relative strengths of relationships between clinical syndromes and pathology.

REFERENCES

Alzheimer A. (1911) Über eigenartige Krankheitsfälle des späteren Alters (About peculiar cases of disease in old age). *Zeitschrift für die gesamte Neurologie und Psychiatrie* 4: 356–85.

Ames D, Cummings JL, Wirshing WC *et al.* (1994) Repetitive and compulsive behavior in frontal lobe degenerations. *Journal of Neuropsychiatry and Clinical Neurosciences* 6: 100–13.

Bak T, Hodges JR. (1999) Cognition, language and behaviour in motor neurone disease: evidence of frontotemporal dementia. *Dementia and Geriatric Cognitive Disorders* 10: 29–32.

Bak TH, O'Donovan DG, Xuereb JH *et al.* (2001) Selective impairment of verb processing associated with pathological changes in the Brodman areas 44 and 45 in the motor neurone disease/dementia/aphasia syndrome. *Brain* 124: 103–24.

Baker M, Mackenzie IR, Pickering-Brown SM *et al.* (2006) Mutations in progranulin cause tau-negative frontotemporal dementia linked to chromosome 17. *Nature* 442: 916–9.

Baldwin B, Förstl H. (1993) Pick's disease – 101 years. Still there but in need of reform. *British Journal of Psychiatry* 163: 100–5.

Boeve BF, Maraganore DM, Parisi JE *et al.* (1999) Pathologic heterogeneity in clinically diagnosed corticobasal degeneration. *Neurology* 53: 795–800.

Bozeat S, Gregory CA, Lambon Ralph MA *et al.* (2000) Which neuropsychiatric and behavioural features distinguish frontal and temporal variants of frontotemporal dementia from Alzheimer's disease? *Journal of Neurology, Neurosurgery, and Psychiatry* 69: 178–86.

Brown J. (1998) Chromosome 3-linked frontotemporal dementia. *Cellular and Molecular Life Sciences* 54: 925–7.

Brown J, Ashworth A, Gydesen S *et al.* (1995) Familial nonspecific dementia maps to chromosome 3. *Human Molecular Genetics* 4: 1625–8.

Brun A. (1987) Frontal lobe degeneration of non-Alzheimer's type. I. Neuropathology. *Archives of Gerontology and Geriatrics* 6: 209–33.

Brun A, Englund B, Gustafson L *et al.* (1994) Clinical and neuropathological criteria for frontotemporal dementia. *Journal of Neurology, Neurosurgery, and Psychiatry* 57: 416–8.

Caselli RJ, Windebank AJ, Petersen RC *et al.* (1993) Rapidly progressive aphasic dementia and motor neuron disease. *Annals of Neurology* 33: 200–7.

Croot K, Patterson K, Hodges JR. (1997) Phonological disruption in atypical dementia of the Alzheimer's type. *Brain and Cognition* 32: 186–90.

Cummings JL. (1999) Principles of neuropsychiatry: towards a neuropsychiatric epistemology. *Neurocase* 5: 181–8.

Cummings JL, Mega M, Gray K *et al.* (1994) The neuropsychiatric inventory: comprehensive assessment of psychopathology in dementia. *Neurology* 44: 2308–14.

Davies RR, Hodges JR, Kril J *et al.* (2005) The pathological basis of semantic dementia. *Brain* 128: 1984–95.

Davies RR, Kipps CM, Mitchell J *et al.* (2006) Progression in frontotemporal dementia: identifying a benign behavioral variant by magnetic resonance imaging. *Archives of Neurology* 63: 1627–31.

Dickson DW. (1998) Pick's disease: a modern approach. *Brain Pathology* 8: 339–54.

Dumanchin C, Camuzat A, Campion D *et al.* (1998) Segregation of a missense mutation in the microtubule-associated protein tau gene with familial frontotemporal dementia and parkinsonism. *Human Molecular Genetics* 7: 1825–9.

Edwards Lee T, Miller B, Benson F *et al.* (1997) The temporal variant of frontotemporal dementia. *Brain* 120: 1027–40.

Evans JJ, Heggs AJ, Antoun N *et al.* (1995) Progressive prosopagnosia associated with selective right temporal lobe atrophy: a new syndrome? *Brain* 118: 1–13.

Ferrano A, Jervis GA. (1936) Pick's disease. *Archives of Neurology and Psychiatry* 36: 739–67.

Foster NL, Wilhelmsen K, Sima AAF *et al.* (1997) Frontotemporal dementia and parkinsonism linked to chromosome 17: a consensus conference. *Annals of Neurology* 41: 706–15.

Galton CJ, Patterson K, Xuereb JH *et al.* (2000) Atypical and typical presentations of Alzheimer's disease: a clinical, neuropsychological, neuroimaging and pathological study of 13 cases. *Brain* 123: 484–98.

Galton CJ, Patterson K, Graham KS *et al.* (2001) Differing patterns of temporal atrophy in Alzheimer's disease and semantic dementia. *Neurology* 57: 216–25.

Gans A. (1922) Betrachtungen über Art und Ausbreitung des krankhaften Prozesses in einem fall von Picksher Atrophie des Stirhirns. *Zeitschrift für die gesamte Neurologie und Psychiatrie* 80: 10–28.

Garrard P, Hodges JR. (1999) Semantic dementia: implications for the neural basis of language and meaning. *Aphasiology* 13: 609–23.

Garrard P, Perry R, Hodges JR. (1997) Disorders of semantic memory. *Journal of Neurology, Neurosurgery, and Psychiatry* 62: 431–5.

Gass J, Cannon A, Boeve B *et al.* (2006) Mutations in progranulin are a major cause of ubiquitin-positive frontotemporal lobar degeneration. *Human Molecular Genetics* 15: 2988–3001.

Girling DM, Berrios GE. (1994) On the relationship between senile cerebral atrophy and aphasia (translation of Pick A. (1802) Über die Beziehungen der senilen Atrophie zur Aphasie. *Prager Medizinische Wochenschrift* 17: 165–7). *History of Psychiatry* 8: 542–7.

Girling DM, Berrios GE. (1997) On the symptomatology of left-sided temporal lobe atrophy (translation of Pick A. Zur (1904) Symptomatologie der linksseitigen Schäfenlappenatrophie. *Monatschrift für Psychiatrie und Neurologie* 16: 378–88). *History of Psychiatry* 8: 149–59.

Girling DM, Markova IS. (1995) Senile atrophy as the basis for focal symptoms (translation of Pick A. (1901) Senile Hirnatrophie als Grundlage für Herderescheinungen. *Wiener Klinische Wochenschrift* 14: 403–4). *History of Psychiatry* 6: 533–7.

Gislason TB, Sjogren M, Larsson L *et al.* (2003) The prevalence of frontal variant frontotemporal dementia and the frontal lobe syndrome in a population based sample of 85 year olds. *Journal of Neurology, Neurosurgery, and Psychiatry* 74: 867–71.

Gorno-Tempini ML, Brambati SM, Ginex V *et al.* (2008) The logopenic/phonological variant of primary progressive aphasia. *Neurology* 71: 1227–34.

Graff-Radford NR, Damasio AR, Hyman BT *et al.* (1990) Progressive aphasia in a patient with Pick's disease: a neuropsychological, radiologic, and anatomic study. *Neurology* 40: 620–6.

Graham KS, Hodges JR. (1997) Differentiating the roles of the hippocampal complex and the neocortex in long-term memory storage: evidence from the study of semantic dementia and Alzheimer's disease. *Neuropsychology* 11: 77–89.

Graham NL, Bak TH, Hodges JR. (2003) Corticobasal degeneration as a cognitive disorder. *Movement Disorders* 18: 1224–32.

Green J, Morris JC, Sandson J *et al.* (1990) Progressive aphasia: a precursor of global dementia? *Neurology* 40: 423–9.

Greene JDW, Patterson K, Xuereb J *et al.* (1996) Alzheimer disease and nonfluent progressive aphasia. *Archives of Neurology* 53: 1072–8.

Gregory C, Lough S, Stone V *et al.* (2002) Theory of mind in patients with frontal variant frontotemporal dementia and Alzheimer's disease: theoretical and practical implications. *Brain* 125: 752–64.

Gregory CA, Hodges JR. (1993) Dementia of frontal type and the focal lobar atrophies. *International Review of Psychiatry* 5: 397–406.

Gregory CA, Hodges JR. (1996) Frontotemporal dementia use of consensus criteria and prevalence of psychiatric features. *Neuropsychiatry, Neuropsychology and Behavioural Neurology* 9: 145–53.

Gregory CA, Serra-Mestres J, Hodges JR. (1999) Early diagnosis of the frontal variant of frontotemporal dementia: how sensitive are standard neuroimaging and neuropsychologic tests? *Neuropsychiatry, Neuropsychology and Behavioral Neurology* 12: 128–35.

Gustafson L. (1987) Frontal lobe degeneration of non-Alzheimer's type II: clinical picture and differential diagnosis. *Archives of Gerontology and Geriatrics* 6: 209–23.

Harasty JA, Halliday GM, Code C *et al.* (1996) Quantification of cortical atrophy in a case of progressive fluent aphasia. *Brain* 119: 181–90.

Harvey RJ, Skelton-Robinson M, Rossor MN. (2003) The prevalence and causes of dementia in people under the age of 65 years. *Journal of Neurology, Neurosurgery, and Psychiatry* 74: 1206–9.

Heutink P, Stevens M, Rizzu P *et al.* (1997) Hereditary frontotemporal dementia is linked to chromosome 17q21-q22: a genetic and clinicopathological study of three Dutch families. *Annals of Neurology* 41: 150–9.

Hodges JR. (2007) *Frontotemporal dementia syndromes.* Cambridge: Cambridge University Press.

Hodges JR, Graham KS. (1998) A reversal of the temporal gradient for famous person knowledge in semantic dementia. Implications for the neural organization of long-term memory. *Neuropsychologia* 36: 803–25.

Hodges JR, Patterson K. (1996) Non-fluent progressive aphasia and semantic dementia a comparative neuropsychological study. *Journal of the International Neuropsychological Society* 2: 511–24.

Hodges JR, Patterson KE. (1997) Semantic memory disorders. *Trends in Cognitive Science* 1: 67–72.

Hodges JR, Patterson K. (2007) Semantic dementia: a unique clinicopathological syndrome. *Lancet Neurology* 6: 1004–14.

Hodges JR, Patterson K, Oxbury S *et al.* (1992) Semantic dementia progressive fluent aphasia with temporal lobe atrophy. *Brain* 115: 1783–806.

Hodges JR, Patterson K, Tyler LK. (1994) Loss of semantic memory: implications for the modularity of mind. *Cognitive Neuropsychology* 11: 505–42.

Hodges JR, Garrard P, Patterson K. (1998) Semantic dementia. In: A Kertesz A, Munoz DG (eds). *Pick's disease and Pick complex.* New York: Wiley-Liss, 83–104.

Hodges JR, Davies R, Xuereb J *et al.* (2003) Survival in frontotemporal dementia. *Neurology* 61: 349–54.

Hodges JR, Davies R, Xuereb J *et al.* (2004) Clinicopathological correlates in frontotemporal dementia. *Annals of Neurology* 56: 399–406.

Holland AL, McBurney DH, Moossy J *et al.* (1985) The dissolution of language in Pick's disease with neurofibrillary tangles: a case study. *Brain and Language* 24: 36–58.

Hornberger M, Piguet O, Kipps C, Hodges JR. (2008) Executive function in progressive and nonprogressive behavioral variant frontotemporal dementia. *Neurology* 71: 1481–8.

Hutton M, Lendon CL, Rizzu P *et al.* (1998) Association of missense and 5′-splice-site mutations in tau with the inherited dementia FTDP-17. *Nature* 18: 702–5.

Ikeda M, Brown J, Holland AJ *et al.* (2002) Changes in appetite, food preference, and eating habits in frontotemporal dementia and Alzheimer's disease. *Journal of Neurology, Neurosurgery, and Psychiatry* 73: 371–6.

Imura T, Nogami Y, Asakawa K. (1971) Aphasia in Japanese Language. *Nihon University Journal of Medicine* 13: 69–90.

Ingram EM, Spillantini MG. (2002) Tau gene mutations: dissecting the pathogenesis of FTDP-17. *Trends in Molecular Medicine* 8: 555–62.

Jackson M, Lowe J. (1996) The new neuropathology of degenerative frontotemporal dementias. *Acta Neuropathologica* 91: 127–34.

Josephs KA, Duffy JR, Strand EA *et al.* (2006) Clinicopathological and imaging correlates of progressive aphasia and apraxia of speech. *Brain* 129: 1385–98.

Kamo H, McGeer PL, Harrop R *et al.* (1987) Positron emission tomography and histopathology in Pick's disease. *Neurology* 37: 439–45.

Katzman R. (1986) Differential diagnosis of dementing illnesses. *Neurologic Clinics* 4: 329–40.

Keane J, Calder AJ, Hodges JR *et al.* (2002) Face and emotion processing in frontal variant frontotemporal dementia. *Neuropsychologia* 40: 655–65.

Kertesz A, Munoz DG. (1998) *Pick's disease and Pick complex.* New York: Wiley-Liss

Kertesz A, Davidson W, Fox H. (1997) Frontal behavioral inventory: diagnostic criteria for frontal lobe dementia. *Canadian Journal of Neurological Sciences* 24: 29–36.

Kertesz A, Nadkarni N, Davidson W *et al.* (2000) The frontal behavioral inventory in the differential diagnosis of frontotemporal dementia. *Journal of the International Neuropsychological Society* 6: 460–8.

Kertesz A, Davidson W, McCabe P *et al.* (2003a) Behavioral quantitation is more sensitive than cognitive testing in frontotemporal dementia. *Alzheimer Disease and Associated Disorders* 17: 223–9.

Kertesz A, Munoz DG, Hillis A. (2003b) Preferred terminology. *Annals of Neurology* 54 (Suppl.): S3–S6.

Kipps CM, Nestor PJ, Fryer TD, Hodges JR. (2007) Behavioural variant frontotemporal dementia: not all it seems? *Neurocase* 13: 237–47.

Kipps CM, Nestor PJ, Dawson CE et al. (2008) Measuring progression in frontotemporal dementia: Implications for therapeutic interventions. *Neurology* 70: 2046–52.

Kipps CM, Nestor PJ, Acosta-Cabronero J et al. (2009) Understanding social dysfunction in the behavioural variant of frontotemporal dementia: the role of emotion and sarcasm processing. *Brain* 132: 592–603.

Kitchener E, Hodges JR. (1999) Impaired knowledge of famous people and events and intact autobiographical knowledge in a case of progressive right temporal lobe degeneration: implications for the organization of remote memory. *Cognitive Neuropsychology* 16: 589–607.

Knibb JA, Xuereb JH, Patterson K, Hodges JR. (2006) Clinical and pathological characterization of progressive aphasia. *Annals of Neurology* 59: 156–65.

Knopman DS, Mastri AR, Frey WH et al. (1990) Dementia lacking distinctive histological features: a common non-Alzheimer degenerative disease. *Neurology* 40: 251–6.

Levy ML, Miller BL, Cummings JL et al. (1996) Alzheimer disease and frontotemporal dementias: behavioral distinctions. *Archives of Neurology* 53: 687–90.

Lillo P, Hodges J. (2009) Frontotemporal dementia and motor neurone disease: Overlapping clinic-pathological disorders. *Journal of Clinical Neuroscience* 16: 1131–5.

Lippa CF, Cohen R, Smith TW et al. (1991) Primary progressive aphasia with focal neuronal achromasia. *Neurology* 41: 882–6.

Lowenberg K, Arbor A. (1936) Pick's disease: a clinicopathologic contribution. *Archives of Neurology and Psychiatry* 36: 768–89.

Lowenberg K, Boyd DA, Salon DD et al. (1939) Occurence of Pick's disease in early adult years. *Archives of Neurology and Psychiatry* 41: 1004–20.

McKhann GM, Albert MS, Grossman M et al. (2001) Clinical and pathological diagnosis of frontotemporal dementia report of the Work Group on Frontotemporal Dementia and Pick's Disease. *Archives of Neurology* 58: 1803–9.

Malamud N, Boyd DA. (1940) Pick's disease with atrophy of the temporal lobes: a clinicopathologic study. *Archives of Neurology and Psychiatry* 43: 210–21.

Mansvelt JV. (1954) 'Pick's disease: a syndrome of lobar cerebral atrophy, its clinico-anatomical and histopathological types'. Thesis, Utrecht University.

Mathuranath PS, Xuereb JH, Bak T et al. (2000) Corticobasal ganglionic degeneration and/or frontotemporal dementia? A report of two overlap cases and review of literature. *Journal of Neurology, Neurosurgery, and Psychiatry* 68: 304–12.

Mesulam M. (2008) Representation, interference, and transcendent encoding in neurocognitive networks of the human brain. *Annals of Neurology* 64: 367–78.

Mesulam M, Wicklund A, Johnson N et al. (2008) Alzheimer and frontotemporal pathology in subjects of primary progressive aphasia. *Annals of Neurology* 63: 709–19.

Mesulam MM. (1982) Slowly progressive aphasia without generalised dementia. *Annals of Neurology* 11: 592–8.

Mesulam MM, Weintraub S. (1992) Primary progressive aphasia. In: Boller F (ed.) *Heterogeneity of Alzheimer's disease.* Berlin: Springer-Verlag, 43–66.

Miller BL, Cummings JL, Villanueva-Meyer J et al. (1991) Frontal lobe degeneration: clinical, neuropsychological, and SPECT characteristics. *Neurology* 41: 1374–82.

Miller BL, Darby A, Benson DF et al. (1997) Aggressive, socially disruptive and antisocial behaviour associated with frontotemporal dementia. *British Journal of Psychiatry* 170: 150–5.

Mingazzini G. (1914) On aphasia due to atrophy of the cerebral convolutions. *Brain* 36: 493–524.

Mioshi E, Hodges JR. (2007) Activities of daily living in frontotemporal dementia and Alzheimer disease – Reply. *Neurology* 69: 2110.

Mioshi E, Kipps CM, Dawson K et al. (2007) Activities of daily living in frontotemporal dementia and Alzheimer disease. *Neurology* 68: 2077–84.

Mitsuyama Y, Takamiya S. (1979) Presenile dementia with motor neuron in Japan. *Archives of Neurology* 36: 592–3.

Morita K, Kaiya H, Ikeda T et al. (1987) Presenile dementia combined with amyotrophy: a review of 34 Japanese cases. *Archives of Gerontology and Geriatrics* 6: 263–77.

Morris HR, Khan MN, Janssen JC et al. (2001) The genetic and pathological classification of familial frontotemporal dementia. *Archives of Neurology* 58: 1813–6.

Morris HR, Osaki Y, Holton J et al. (2003) Tau exon 10+16 mutation FTDP-17 presenting clinically as sporadic young onset PSP. *Neurology* 61: 102–4.

Morris JC, Cole M, Banker BQ et al. (1984) Hereditary dysphasic dementia and the Pick–Alzheimer spectrum. *Annals of Neurology* 16: 455–66.

Mummery CJ, Patterson K, Wise RJS et al. (1999) Disrupted temporal lobe connections in semantic dementia. *Brain* 122: 61–73.

Mummery CJ, Patterson K, Price CJ et al. (2000) A voxel based morphometry study of semantic dementia. The relationship between temporal lobe atrophy and semantic dementia. *Annals of Neurology* 47: 36–45.

Neary D, Snowden JS, Bowen DM et al. (1986) Neuropsychological syndromes in presenile dementia due to cerebral atrophy. *Journal of Neurology, Neurosurgery, and Psychiatry* 49: 163–74.

Neary D, Snowdon JS, Mann DMA et al. (1990) Frontal lobe dementia and motor neuron disease. *Journal of Neurology, Neurosurgery, and Psychiatry* 53: 23–32.

Neary D, Snowden JS, Gustafson L et al. (1998) Frontotemporal lobar degeneration: a consensus on clinical diagnostic criteria. *Neurology* 51: 1546–54.

Nestor PJ, Graham NL, Fryer TD et al. (2003) Progressive non-fluent aphasia is associated with hypometabolism centred on the left anterior insula. *Brain* 126: 2406–18.

Neumann M, Sampathu DM, Kwong LK *et al.* (2006) Ubiquitinated TDP-43 in frontotemporal lobar degeneration and amyotrophic lateral sclerosis. *Science* **314**: 130–3.

Neumann MA. (1949) Pick's disease. *Journal of Neuropathology and Experimental Neurology* **8**: 255–82.

Nichols IC, Weigner WC. (1938) Pick's disease – a specific type of dementia. *Brain* **3**: 237–49.

Nyatsanza S, Shetty T, Gregory C *et al.* (2003) A study of stereotypic behaviours in Alzheimer's disease and frontal and temporal variant frontotemporal dementia. *Journal of Neurology, Neurosurgery, and Psychiatry* **74**: 1398–402.

Onari K, Spatz H. (1926) Anatomische Beitrage zur Lehre von der Pickschen umschriebenen Grosshirnrindenatrophie (Piscksche Krankheit). *Zeitschrift für die gesamte Neurologie und Psychiatrie* **101**: 470–511.

Pasquier F, Lebert F, Scheltens P. (1996) *Frontotemporal dementia.* The Netherlands: ICG Publications.

Petersen RB, Tabaton M, Chen SG *et al.* (1995) Familial progressive subcortical gliosis: presence of prions and linkage to chromosome 17. *Neurology* **45**: 1062–7.

Pick A. (1892) Über die Beziehungen der senilen Atrophie zur Aphasie. *Prager Medizinische Wochenschrift* **17**: 165–7.

Pick A. (1901) Senile Hirnatrophie als Grundlage für Hernderscheinungen. *Wiener Klinische Wochenschrift* **14**: 403–4.

Pick A. (1904) Zur symptomatologie der linksseitigen Schläfenlappenatrophie. *Monatschrift für Psychiatrie und Neurologie* **16**: 378–88.

Pick A. (1906) Über einen weiteren symptomenkomplex im Rahmen der Dementia senilis, bedingt durch umschriebene starkere Hirnatrophie. *Monatschrift für Psychiatrie und Neurologie* **19**: 97–108.

Poeck K, Luzzatti C. (1988) Slowly progressive aphasia in three patients: the problem of accompanying neuropsychological deficit. *Brain* **111**: 151–68.

Poorkaj P, Bird TD, Wijsman E *et al.* (1998) Tau is a candidate gene for chromosome 17 frontotemporal dementia. *Annals of Neurology* **43**: 815–25.

Rahman S, Sahakian BJ, Hodges JR *et al.* (1999) Specific cognitive deficits in mild frontal variant frontotemporal dementia. *Brain* **122**: 1469–93.

Rakowicz Z, Hodges JR. (1998) Dementia and aphasia in motor neurone disease: an under recognised association. *Journal of Neurology, Neurosurgery, and Psychiatry* **65**: 881–9.

Rankin KP, Salazar A, Gorno-Tempini ML *et al.* (2009) Detecting sarcasm from paralinguistic cues: anatomic and cognitive correlates in neurodegenerative disease. *Neuroimage* **47**: 2005–15.

Rascovsky K, Salmon DP, Ho GJ *et al.* (2002) Cognitive profiles differ in autopsy-confirmed frontotemporal dementia and AD. *Neurology* **58**: 1801–8.

Rascovsky K, Hodges JR, Kipps CM *et al.* (2007) Diagnostic criteria for the behavioral variant of frontotemporal dementia (bvFTD): current limitations and future directions. *Alzheimer Disease and Associated Disorders* **21**: S14–8.

Ratnavalli E, Brayne C, Dawson K *et al.* (2002) The prevalence of frontotemporal dementia. *Neurology* **58**: 1615–21.

Rebeiz JJ, Kolodny EH, Richardson EP. (1968) Corticodentatonigral degeneration with neuronal achromasia. *Archives of Neurology* **18**: 20–33.

Robertson EE, Le Roux A, Brown JH. (1958) The clinical differentiation of Pick's disease. *Journal of Mental Science* **104**: 1000–24.

Rogers RD, Sahakian BJ, Hodges JR *et al.* (1998) Dissociating executive mechanisms of task control following frontal lobe damage and Parkinson's disease. *Brain* **121**: 815–42.

Rosen HJ, Gorno-Tempini ML, Goldman WP *et al.* (2002a) Patterns of brain atrophy in frontotemporal dementia and semantic dementia. *Neurology* **58**: 198–208.

Rosen HJ, Hartikainen KM, Jagust W *et al.* (2002b) Utility of clinical criteria in differentiating frontotemporal lobar degeneration (FTLD) from AD. *Neurology* **58**: 1608–15.

Rosenfeld M. (1909) Die partielle Grosshirnatrophie. *Journal für Psychologie und Neurologie* **14**: 115–30.

Rossor MN, Revesz T, Lantos PL *et al.* (2000) Semantic dementia with ubiquitin-positive tau-negative inclusion bodies. *Brain* **123**: 267–76.

Saffran EM, Schwartz MF. (1994) Of cabbages and things: semantic memory from a neuropsychological perspective – a tutorial review. In: C Umilta C, Moscovitch M (eds). *Attention and performance XV.* Hove: Lawrence Erlbaum, 507–36.

Sasanuma S, Mondi H. (1975) The syndrome of Gogi (word meaning) aphasia. *Neurology* **25**: 627–32.

Schenk VWS. (1951) Maladie de Pick: etude anatomo-clinique de 8 cas. *Annales Medico-Psychologiques (Paris)* **109**: 574–87.

Schneider C. (1927) Über Picksche Krankheit. *Monatschrift für Psychologie und Neurologie* **65**: 230–75.

Schneider C. (1929) Weitere Beitrage zur Lehre von der Pickschen Krankheit. *Zeitschrift für die gesamte Neurologie und Psychiatrie* **120**: 340–84.

Scholten IM, Kneebone AC, Denson LA *et al.* (1995) Primary progressive aphasia: serial linguistic, neuropsychological and radiological findings with neuropathological results. *Aphasiology* **9**: 495–516.

Schwarz M, De Bleser R, Poeck K *et al.* (1998) A case of primary progressive aphasia: a 14-year follow-up study with neuropathological findings. *Brain* **121**: 115–26.

Snowden JS, Goulding PJ, Neary D. (1989) Semantic dementia a form of circumscribed cerebral atrophy. *Behavioural Neurology* **2**: 167–82.

Snowden JS, Neary D, Mann DMA *et al.* (1992) Progressive language disorder due to lobar atrophy. *Annals of Neurology* **31**: 174–83.

Snowden JS, Neary D, Mann DMA. (1996) *Fronto-temporal lobar degeneration: Fronto-temporal dementia, progressive aphasia, semantic dementia.* New York: Churchill Livingstone.

Soliveri P, Rossi G, Monza D *et al.* (2003) A case of dementia parkinsonism resembling progressive supranuclear palsy due to mutation in the tau protein gene. *Archives of Neurology* **60**: 1454–6.

Spillantini MG, Bird TD, Ghetti B. (1998a) Frontotemporal dementia and parkinsonism linked to chromosome 17. A new group of tauopathies. *Brain Pathology* **8**: 387–402.

Spatt J. (2003) Arnold Pick's concept of dementia. *Cortex* **39**: 525–31.

Spillantini MG, Goedert M, Crowther RA *et al.* (1997) Familial multiple system tauopathy with presenile dementia a disease with abundant neuronal and glial tau filaments. *Proceedings of the National Academy of Sciences of the United States of America* **94**: 4113–8.

Spillantini MG, Murrell JR, Goedert M *et al.* (1998b) Mutation in the tau gene in familial multiple system tauopathy with presenile dementia. *Proceedings of the National Academy of Sciences of the United States of America* **95**: 7737–41.

Steele JC, Richardson JC, Olszewski J. (1964) Progressive supranuclear palsy. A heterogeneous degeneration involving the brain stem, basal ganglia and cerebellum with vertical gaze and pseudobulbar palsy, nuchal dystonia and dementia. *Archives of Neurology* **10**: 333–59.

Stertz G. (1926) Über die Picksche atrophie. *Zeitschrift für die gesamte Neurologie und Psychiatrie* **101**: 729–47.

Strong MJ, Lomen-Hoerth C, Caselli RJ *et al.* (2003) Cognitive impairment, frontotemporal dementia, and the motor neuron diseases. *Annals of Neurology* **54** (Suppl. 5): S20–3.

Sumi SM, Bird TD, Nochlin D *et al.* (1992) Familial presenile dementia with psychosis associated with cortical neurofibrillary tangles and degeneration of the amygdala. *Neurology* **42**: 120–7.

Tanabe H. (1992) Personality of typical Gogi (word meaning) aphasics. *Japanese Journal of Neuropsychology* **8**: 34–42.

Tanabe H, Ikeda M, Nakagawa Y *et al.* (1992) Gogi (word meaning) aphasia and semantic memory for words. *Higher Brain Function Research* **12**: 153–69.

Thompson SA, Patterson K, Hodges JR. (2003) Left/right asymmetry of atrophy in semantic dementia behavioral-cognitive implications. *Neurology* **61**: 1196–203.

Thompson SA, Graham KS, Williams G *et al.* (2004) Dissociating person-specific from general semantic knowledge: roles of the left and right temporal lobes. *Neuropsychologia* **42**: 359–70.

Tissot R, Constantanidis J, Richard J. (1975) *La maladie de Pick.* Paris: Masson.

Tonkonogy JM, Smith TW, Barreira PJ. (1994) Obsessive-compulsive disorders in Pick's disease. *Journal of Neuropsychiatry and Clinical Neurosciences* **6**: 176–80.

Torralva T, Kipps CM, Hodges JR *et al.* (2007) The relationship between affective decision-making and theory of mind in the frontal variant of fronto-temporal dementia. *Neuropsychologia* **45**: 342–9.

Tulving E. (1972) Episodic and semantic memory. In: Tulving E, Donaldson W (eds). *Organization of memory.* New York: Academic Press, 381–403.

Tulving E. (1983) *Elements of episodic memory.* New York: Oxford University Press.

Warrington EK. (1975) Selective impairment of semantic memory. *Quarterly Journal of Experimental Psychology* **27**: 635–57.

Wechsler A. (1977) Presenile dementia presenting as aphasia. *Journal of Neurology, Neurosurgery, and Psychiatry* **40**: 303–5.

Wechsler AF, Verity MA, Rosenscheim S *et al.* (1982) Pick's disease: a clinical, computed tomographic and histological study with Golgi impregnation observations. *Archives of Neurology* **39**: 3287–90.

Wedderburn C, Wear H, Brown J *et al.* (2008) The utility of the Cambridge Behavioural Inventory in neurodegenerative disease. *Journal of Neurology, Neurosurgery and Psychiatry* **79**: 500–3.

Weintraub S, Rubin NP, Mesulam M-M. (1990) Primary progressive aphasia: longitudinal course, profile, and language features. *Archives of Neurology* **47**: 1329–35.

Wilhelmsen KC. (1997) Frontotemporal dementia is on the MAP. *Annals of Neurology* **41**: 139–40.

Wilhelmsen KC, Lynch T, Pavlou E *et al.* (1994) Localization of disinhibition–dementia–parkinsonism–amyotrophy complex to 17q21-22. *American Journal of Human Genetics* **55**: 1159–65.

Williams GB, Nestor PJ, Hodges R. (2005) The neural correlates of semantic and behavioural deficits in frontotemporal dementia. *Neuroimage* **24**: 1042–51.

Wszolek ZK, Pfeiffer RF, Bhatt MH *et al.* (1992) Rapidly progressive autosomal dominant parkinsonism and dementia with pallido-ponto-nigral degeneration. *Annals of Neurology* **32**: 312–20.

70

The genetics and molecular pathology of frontotemporal lobar degeneration

DAVID MA MANN

70.1 INTRODUCTION

The term frontotemporal lobar degeneration (FTLD) is used here to describe a clinically and pathologically heterogeneous group of non-Alzheimer forms of dementia arising from degeneration of the frontal and temporal lobes. The prototypical, and most common, clinical syndrome is frontotemporal dementia (FTD), manifesting as behavioural and personality changes, involving disinhibition, stereotypy, unsocial acts and language disorder, leading to apathy, mutism and late neurological (frontal release or extrapyramidal) signs (Neary *et al.*, 1998; Neary *et al.*, 2005; Neary *et al.*, 2007). However, the spectrum of illness is wider, involving cases where movement disorder, with relatively mild dementia, is the major disabling feature (Cordes *et al.*, 1992; Wszolek *et al.*, 1992; Lynch *et al.*, 1994) or others with the linguistic disorders of semantic dementia (SD) and progressive non-fluent aphasia (PNFA) (Snowden *et al.*, 1992; Neary *et al.*, 1998; Neary *et al.*, 2005; Neary *et al.*, 2007). FTD can be accompanied by clinical motor neurone disease (MND) in about 10 per cent cases giving the syndrome of frontotemporal dementia with motor neurone disease (FTD+MND) (Neary *et al.*, 1998; Neary *et al.*, 2005; Neary *et al.*, 2007). Onset of illness is usually before 65 years of age, with duration being between six and nine years, though up to 15 years is not uncommon (Neary *et al.*, 1998; Rosso *et al.*, 2003; Neary *et al.*, 2005; Neary *et al.*, 2007).

Outward inspection of the brain in FTLD gives few clues to pathogenesis, but can be a useful index of clinical presentation. Hence, FTD is associated with bilateral atrophy of the frontal and anterior temporal lobes and SD is associated with bitemporal lobe atrophy, often asymmetric, but usually favouring the left side. PNFA is associated with marked asymmetry, most often of the left cerebral hemisphere (Neary *et al.*, 2005; Neary *et al.*, 2007). Routine histology has contributed little to our understanding of the disorder, beyond the early identification of the 'classic' inclusion bodies (Pick bodies) and swollen neurones (Pick cells) (Pick, 1892), and the characteristic, though nonspecific, features of microvacuolation of outer cortical laminae marking the site of the principal molecular changes (Knopman *et al.*, 1990).

The recognition in about 40 per cent of patients of a previous family history of a similar disorder consistent with autosomal dominant inheritance (Stevens *et al.*, 1998; Rosso *et al.*, 2003) paved the way for the breakthroughs in knowledge and understanding of the molecular pathology of the disorder that have come through the wealth of genetic investigations performed over the past decade. By 1997, genetic linkage had identified a locus on the long arm of chromosome 17 (17q21–22) in some families, and because parkinsonism usually accompanied the dementia, these cases came to be snappily described as 'frontotemporal dementia and parkinsonism linked to chromosome 17' (FTDP-17) (Foster *et al.*, 1997). In 1998, mutational events in the tau gene, *MAPT*, were identified (Hutton *et al.*, 1998; Poorkaj *et al.*, 1998; Spillantini *et al.*, 1998). The prevalence of *MAPT* mutations within FTLD varies between 6 and 18 per cent depending on the population studied (Dumanchin *et al.*, 1998; Houlden *et al.*, 1999a; Rizzu *et al.*, 1999; Kowalska *et al.*, 2001; Poorkaj *et al.*, 2001; Binetti *et al.*, 2003; Rosso *et al.*, 2003).

Nonetheless, despite exhaustive genetic analyses, there remained a number of linked families in whom no mutations in *MAPT* could be found. This paradox was resolved in 2006 when mutations within the progranulin gene (*PGRN*), located just 1.8 cM from *MAPT*, were identified (Baker *et al.*, 2006; Cruts *et al.*, 2006). Collectively, *MAPT* and *PGRN* mutations likely account for no more than 20 per cent of all cases of FTLD, less than 50 per cent of all autosomally dominant inherited forms, and further causative mutations or genetic risk factors remain to be defined or confirmed.

Over the past decade, numerous immunohistochemical studies have identified aggregated or accumulated proteins within the brain in neurodegenerative diseases, not only to improve diagnostic power and criteria, but also to understand better the basic pathology and devise experimental approaches to enhance knowledge of pathogenesis. About 45 per cent cases of FTLD display insoluble tau proteins in their brains in the form of intraneuronal neurofibrillary tangles or Pick bodies; about half are associated with *MAPT* mutations (Taniguchi *et al.*, 2004; Shi *et al.*, 2005). However, a tau-negative, but ubiquitin-positive pathology, known as FTLD-U, accounts for the other 55 per cent of cases (Lipton *et al.*, 2004; Taniguchi *et al.*, 2004; Mott *et al.*, 2005; Shi *et al.*, 2005; Forman *et al.*, 2006a); in most, the ubiquitinated target protein is the transactive response (TAR) DNA binding protein, TDP-43.

70.2 THE TAU GENE (*MAPT*) AND TAU PATHOLOGY IN FTLD

70.2.1 The structure of *MAPT* and the function of tau proteins

The tau gene (*MAPT*) has 15 coding regions (exons), and transcripts are alternatively spliced to produce six different isoforms ranging from 352 to 441 amino acids in length.

Tau is normally located in axons and regulates microtubule assembly/disassembly and axonal transport of proteins and organelles. All six isoforms play a role in maintenance of microtubular structure. If one or more fails, or if there is a stoichiometric imbalance in the different variants, microtubule formation will become more difficult or the stability of microtubules formed will become compromised. Any excess of tau (of any isoform composition) can be bundled into indigestible residues (neurofibrillary tangles or Pick bodies) that choke the cell, but may also induce neurotoxicity.

70.2.2 *MAPT* mutations in FTLD

To date, about 44 *MAPT* mutations in around 131 families have been identified (see AD and FTD mutation database: www.molgen.ua.ac.be/FTDmutations). Typically, patients with *MAPT* mutations display FTD with early signs of

disinhibition, loss of initiative, stereotypic behaviours and linguistic changes of a semantic nature (Pickering-Brown *et al.*, 2002), although other patients display a phenotype resembling progressive supranuclear palsy (PSP) or corticobasal degeneration (CBD) (Bugiani *et al.*, 1999; Wszolek *et al.*, 2001).

70.2.3 Pathology and biochemistry

All cases with MAPT mutations are characterized by the deposition of insoluble, aggregated tau proteins within neurones and glial cells in the cerebral cortex and other brain regions. Nevertheless, there are two histological patterns: those mutations in and around the stem loop structure produce an excess of 4R tau, and hence, the insoluble tau aggregates are composed predominantly of 4R tau isoforms (Clark *et al.*, 1998; Hong *et al.*, 1998; Hasegawa *et al.*, 1999; Pickering-Brown *et al.*, 2002; De Silva *et al.*, 2006), appearing as neurofibrillary tangle-like structures within large and smaller pyramidal cells of cortical layers III and V (**See p9–10 of the plate section for Plate 11**), and prominent within glial cells in the deep white matter, globus pallidus and internal capsule (**See p9–10 of the plate section for Plate 11**) (Pickering-Brown *et al.*, 2002). Neurones within subcortical structures, such as corpus striatum, medial thalamus, nucleus basalis of Meynert, dorsal raphe, pontine and dentate nuclei, locus caeruleus and substantia nigra can likewise be affected, but less severely so (Pickering-Brown *et al.*, 2002).

70.3 PROGRANULIN GENE (*PGRN*) AND TDP-43 PATHOLOGY

70.3.1 *PGRN* mutations in FTLD

MAPT mutations account for only 10 per cent of cases of FTLD at most (Houlden *et al.*, 1999a; Rizzu *et al.*, 1999; Poorkaj *et al.*, 2001; Rosso *et al.*, 2003), although the frequency may reach 20 per cent when only cases consistent with autosomal dominance are considered (Rizzu *et al.*, 1999). Indeed, following the identification of *MAPT* mutations, there remained at least five chromosome 17-linked families for which no mutational event in *MAPT* could be determined. Moreover, no insoluble aggregates of tau were seen biochemically or histopathologically (Foster *et al.*, 1997; Rosso *et al.*, 2001; Rademakers *et al.*, 2002; Froelich Fabre *et al.*, 2003), although ubiquitin-positive inclusions were variably present (Rosso *et al.*, 2001; Rademakers *et al.*, 2002; Froelich Fabre *et al.*, 2003). Such cases became known as FTLD-ubiquitinated (FTLD-U). In 2006, causative mutations in these families were identified (Baker *et al.*, 2006; Cruts *et al.*, 2006). Many subsequent studies identified mutations in *PGRN*, with 66 different mutations within 199 families recorded to date (see AD and FTD mutation database: www.molgen.ua.ac.be/FTDmutations).

PGRN mutations in FTLD include missense mutations generating premature stop codons, insertion or deletion mutations resulting in frameshifts, or changes within initiation codons precluding transcription (Baker *et al.*, 2006; Cruts *et al.*, 2006). Some are located within or close to splice donor sites, resulting in splicing out of particular exons (Baker *et al.*, 2006; Cruts *et al.*, 2006; Masellis *et al.*, 2006; Le Ber *et al.*, 2007). Missense mutations in exon 0 lead to nuclear degradation, and mutations that affect the Kosak sequence prevent translation (Cruts *et al.*, 2006; Le Ber *et al.*, 2007). One particular mutation, Ala9Asp, affects the hydrophobic core of the signal peptide sequence disrupting the normal insertion of the protein into the endoplasmic reticulum leading to a trapping of the (transcribed and translated) mutated protein within the Golgi apparatus (Mukherjee *et al.*, 2006). Whole deletions of *PGRN* occur, but only rarely (Gijselinck *et al.*, 2008; Rovelet-Lecrux *et al.*, 2008). Nonetheless, all mutations, irrespective of type, ultimately generate the same functional effect – a null allele – with at least 50 per cent loss of translated protein giving haploinsufficiency. Most transcripts are immediately destroyed through nonsense-mediated decay, and it is unlikely that any, or perhaps only a small proportion, become translated into mutated proteins, thereby explaining the lack of mutated PGRN protein within the ubiquitinated lesions (Baker *et al.*, 2006). The biological effects would therefore seem to be ones of a 'loss of function effect', although the brain accumulation of abnormal ubiquitinated proteins may also confer a neurotoxic 'gain of function', or some combination of the two is possible.

In contrast to *MAPT*, *PGRN* mutations may not be fully penetrant. In one family (DR8), several unaffected carriers have been reported to live well beyond the obligate onset age for the mutation, one as late as 81 years (Cruts *et al.*, 2006). In R493X mutation, there is delayed onset age in patients carrying the rare rs9897528 allele on the wild-type *PGRN* allele (Rademakers *et al.*, 2007), suggesting genetic variability on the wild-type allele might influence the age-related disease penetrance of *PGRN* mutations. Bruni *et al.* (2007) also reported a potential influence of the wild-type allele upon age-associated disease penetrance. Common polymorphisms on the normal allele may impact on disease expression through (further) lowering of PGRN protein. Conversely, *MAPT* haplotype or *APOE* genotype do not influence either age at onset or disease penetrance (Cruts *et al.*, 2006; Gass *et al.*, 2006; Bruni *et al.*, 2007; Rademakers *et al.*, 2007).

70.3.2   The structure and function of progranulin

PGRN contains 13 exons and encodes a full length protein (predicted molecular weight 68 kDa) secreted as a glycosylated 85 kDa precursor which can be cleaved by elastase-like activity into a series of 6 kDa cysteine-rich fragments called granulins (GRNs) (Zhu *et al.*, 2002; He *et al.*, 2003). Both PGRN and the GRNs are biologically active with roles in tissue remodelling processes (Ahmed *et al.*, 2007; van Swieten and Heutink, 2008). In peripheral tissues, PGRN plays a role in development, wound repair and inflammation, by activating signalling cascades that control cell cycle progression and cell motility (He and Bateman, 2003). In the brain, PGRN is expressed in both neurons and microglia. Reduced

levels of this secreted mitogenic factor induce neurodegeneration in *FTLD*, indicating an important role in neuronal survival. As with *VCP* and *CHMP2B* mutations, loss of PGRN may be associated with defects in protein degradation through cytoplasmic organelles (Ahmed *et al.*, 2007). Suppression of *PGRN* expression results in caspase-dependent cleavage of TDP-43, with cellular accumulation of C-terminal fragments (Zhang *et al.*, 2007).

70.3.3   Pathology of *PGRN* mutations

Consistent with observations that *PGRN* mutations do not result in the translation of mutated proteins, pathological changes in FTLD are not reflected by changes in biochemistry or structure of PGRN, but are witnessed as brain accumulations of ubiquitinated protein devoid of PGRN, principally in the cerebral cortex and hippocampus, as neuronal cytoplasmic inclusion (NCI) bodies or dystrophic neurites (DN) (Baker *et al.*, 2006; Cruts *et al.*, 2006). neuronal intranuclear inclusions (NII) of a 'cat's eye' or 'lentiform' appearance have been described (Baker *et al.*, 2006; Cruts *et al.*, 2006; Mackenzie *et al.*, 2006b; Pickering-Brown *et al.*, 2006; Snowden *et al.*, 2006; Snowden *et al.*, 2007; Pickering-Brown *et al.*, 2008), although these occur in FTLD-U cases where no *PGRN* mutation has been determined (Davidson *et al.*, 2007). The ubiquitinated NCI and DN contain TDP-43 (Arai *et al.*, 2006; Neumann *et al.*, 2006). TDP-43 is a 43 kDa nuclear protein, 414 amino acids long, first identified as a binding partner to the TAR DNA element of the human immunodeficiency virus. The TDP-43 gene (*TARDBP*), located on chromosome 1p36.2, contains six exons and is ubiquitously expressed. It has two highly conserved RNA recognition motifs (RRM1 and RRM2) and a C-terminal, glycine-rich tail which mediates protein–protein interactions, including interactions with other heterogeneous ribonuclear protein (hnRNP) family members. Although, under physiological conditions, TDP-43 is mostly present within the nucleus, although low levels occur within the cytoplasm (Ayala *et al.*, 2008; Buratti and Baralle, 2008; Thorpe *et al.*, 2008; Turner *et al.*, 2008; Winton *et al.*, 2008). It is believed that TDP-43 shuttles continuously between nucleus and cytoplasm, a process regulated by nuclear localization, and nuclear export, signal motifs. Ultrastructural studies show TDP-43 to be enriched within euchromatin domains, specifically within perichromatin fibrils (Casafont *et al.*, 2009), which are nuclear sites of transcription and transcriptional splicing. TDP-43 may therefore function as a transcription repressor or an initiator of exon skipping in the alternative splicing of mRNA (Wang *et al.*, 2004; Buratti and Baralle, 2008).

Most cases of FTLD-U, however, are not associated with *PGRN* mutations, although the majority of these still display TDP-43 pathological changes. There are qualitative differences in the relative burdens of TDP-43 immunoreactive NCI, DN and NII across the FTLD-U cases, and four major histological types have been independently described (Mackenzie *et al.*, 2006a; Sampathu *et al.*, 2006), now unified under a single classification (Cairns *et al.*, 2007a; Mackenzie *et al.*, 2009). In this, type 1 histology describes cases with a preponderance of DN within neocortical regions (**See p11 of** the plate section for Plate 12a) with rounded, solid (Pick body-like) NCI within the hippocampus dentate gyrus (DG) granule cells. Type 2 histology describes cases with a preponderance of neuronal NCI and few, if any, DN within the neocortex (See p11 of the plate section for Plate 12b), with more granular NCI within the hippocampus. In type 3 histology, numerous NCI and DN are present within the neocortex (See p11 of the plate section for Plate 12c), and in many cases lentiform NII are seen (See p11 of the plate section for Plate 12d). Granular NCI are again seen within the hippocampus.

These histological variations are not without clinical significance. Type 1 histology is common in SD, whereas type 2 histology describes FTD with MND. Type 3 histology is present in *PGRN* mutation, but not exclusively so, and can describe either a 'straightforward' FTD presentation or often, PNFA (Mackenzie *et al.*, 2006b; Davidson *et al.*, 2007; Josephs *et al.*, 2009). In addition to these diagnostically characteristic changes in cerebral cortex and hippocampus, similar changes are widespread throughout other neocortical regions, including insular and anterior parietal cortex and cingulate gyrus; posterior parietal and occipital cortex are rarely affected. Non-cortical regions regions, such as amygdala and corpus striatum (See p12 of the plate section for Plate 12f) are frequently and severely affected, although thalamus, substantia nigra, and inferior olives (See p12 of the plate section for Plate 12g) are variably and mildly involved (Brandmeir *et al.*, 2008; Geser *et al.*, 2008a; Davidson *et al.*, 2009; Josephs *et al.*, 2009). Because of their regional variations in distribution of TDP-43 pathological changes throughout the neuraxis, these histological subtypes might represent distinct clinicopathological entities with separate pathogenesis (Josephs *et al.*, 2009).

When TDP-43, NCI are present in the cell, TDP-43 immunostaining is absent from the nucleus, possibly having been sequestered into NCI. Perturbation of trafficking of TDP-43 between nucleus and cytoplasm may be a functional consequence of its incorporation into these cytoplasmic aggregates (Winton *et al.*, 2008), although it is still unclear whether disease is due to a toxic gain of function relating to these pathological aggregates, or stems from loss of normal nuclear functions, or some combination of the two.

70.4   OTHER TAU AND TDP-43 NEGATIVE FTLD CASES

70.4.1   Pathology

Although about 95 per cent of FTLD cases can be accounted by tauopathy or TDP-43 proteinopathy (See p13 of the plate section for Plate 13), there still remains a small proportion of cases where alternative target proteins are involved or remain undetermined.

In some of these, ubiquitinated, Pick body-like inclusions are present in neurones of frontal and temporal cortex, and basal ganglia. These are negative for tau, TDP-43 and α-synuclein but (variably) immunoreactive for all class IV intermediate filaments (IF), light, medium and heavy

neurofilament subunits (Bigio *et al.*, 2003; Cairns *et al.*, 2003; Josephs *et al.*, 2003; Cairns *et al.*, 2004a) and α-internexin (Cairns *et al.*, 2004b). Consequently, the disorder became known as neuronal intermediate filament inclusion disease (NIFID) and was classed as FTLD-IF (Mackenzie *et al.*, 2009).

70.4.2   FUSopathies

Very recent work (Munoz *et al.*, 2009; Neumann *et al.*, 2009a; Neumann *et al.*, 2009b) has shown that in the majority of these tau-negative, TDP-43-negative FTLD cases, the ubiquitinated inclusion bodies are immunoreactive to a protein called fused in sarcoma (FUS) (also known as translocation in liposarcoma (TLS)), and may be part of a newly identified 'family' of proteinopathies, termed 'FUSopathies' (Munoz *et al.*, 2009; Neumann *et al.*, 2009a; Neumann *et al.*, 2009b). In the context of FTLD, these should be known as FTLD-FUS (Mackenzie *et al.*, 2009).

70.4.3   Pathogenetic considerations

TDP-43 and FUS are both transcription factors involved in the transport of mRNA to dendritic spines for local translation in relation to synaptic activity. This process requires the involvement of several types of RNA-containing granules – ribonuclearprotein particles (RNP), processing bodies (PB) and stress granules (SG) (Bramham and Wells, 2007). However, while TDP-43 appears to be associated with PB, FUS relates to SG (Bramham and Wells, 2007; Wang *et al.*, 2008). PB are associated with mRNA decay processes, and decapping enzyme1 protein – a marker for PB – is absent from NCI in basophilic inclusion body disease (BIBD) (Fujita *et al.*, 2008), explaining the lack of TDP-43 in such inclusions. In contrast, NCI in BIBD contain mRNA-binding proteins poly(A) binding protein 1 and T cell intracellular antigen 1 indicating their association with SG, rather than RNP or PB (Fujita *et al.*, 2008). Hence, TDP-43 and FUS play different, although complementary, roles in the processing of RNA.

While for purposes of classification it is logical to clump aFTLD-U, NIFID and BIBD into the broad brush category of FTLD-FUS, this might hide mechanistic differences. The disorders clearly differ in neuropathology – the NCI in NIFID and aFTLD-U do not contain RNA, vermiform NII are commonplace in NIFID and aFTLD-U, but rare or absent in BIBD, loss of lower motor neurons, giving MND phenotype, is frequent in BIBD but less common in aFTLD-U (Munoz *et al.*, 2009) – all features pointing to distinctions in pathogenesis. The challenge will be to understand how changes in the metabolism of TDP-43 and FUS dictate patterns of neurodegeneration and clinical expression of disease.

70.5   OTHER TDP-43 PROTEINOPATHIES

TDP-43 pathological changes colocalize within the ubiquitinated NCI in various other neurodegenerative disorders.

Such changes occur in 20–30 per cent patients with Alzheimer's disease (AD) (Amador-Ortiz *et al.*, 2007; Hu *et al.*, 2008; Uryu *et al.*, 2008) or dementia with Lewy bodies (DLB) (Nakashima-Yasuda *et al.*, 2007; Arai *et al.*, 2009), in some cases of CBD (Uryu *et al.*, 2008), PSP and in others with Parkinson's disease (Uryu *et al.*, 2008) and parkinsonism–dementia complex of Guam (Guam PDC) (Hasegawa *et al.*, 2007; Geser *et al.*, 2008b), argyrophilic grain disease, Perry syndrome (Farrer *et al.*, 2009) and familial British dementia (FBI) (Schwab *et al.*, 2009). TDP-43 protein has not been (consistently) found in tangles in AD (Amador-Ortiz *et al.*, 2007; Uryu *et al.*, 2008), in Pick bodies (Davidson *et al.*, 2007; Uryu *et al.*, 2008, but see Arai *et al.*, 2006; Freeman *et al.*, 2008) or in the ubiquitinated inclusions of FTD-3 (Holm *et al.*, 2007). Elsewhere, TDP-43 pathological changes occur in Rosenthal fibres and granular eosinophilic bodies in low-grade tumours and reactive brain tissue (but not in anoxic or ischaemic lesions) (Lee *et al.*, 2008), indicating pathological alterations in the structure or function of TDP-43 may occur across a wide range of neurodegenerative diseases and other disorders, and might result from a variety of mechanistic disturbances.

70.6   OTHER GENETIC CHANGES

70.6.1   Chromosome 9

Linkage to chromosome 9p in several families clinically sharing an FTD and MND phenotype has been claimed (Hosler *et al.*, 2000; Morita *et al.*, 2006; Vance *et al.*, 2006), but not confirmed (Ostojic *et al.*, 2003). A sequence variation in the intraflagellar transport 74 gene (*IFT74*) was reported to segregate with disease in one family, but similar variations were not found in other linked families (Momeni *et al.*, 2006; Xiao *et al.*, 2007). Nonetheless, the pathology in such cases that have been reported is that of FTLD-TDP, type 2 (Cairns *et al.*, 2007b), consistent with expectations given the clinical phenotype.

UBAP1 encodes a protein of 502 residues, predicted to have a molecular weight of 55 kDa, originally cloned from a tumour suppressor locus (Qian *et al.*, 2001). While little is known of the actual function of the protein, the gene is a likely member of the ubiquitin-activated enzymes family which includes proteins with connections to ubiquitin and the ubiquitination pathway, suggesting a link between the UPS and this condition.

70.6.2   Chromosome 3

Linkage to chromosome 3p11-12 has been reported in a Danish family (Brown *et al.*, 1995) showing FTD with fronto-temporal atrophy, neuronal loss and gliosis (Gydesen *et al.*, 1987; Gydesen *et al.*, 2002). The gene responsible for disease in this pedigree (Skibinski *et al.*, 2005), and in three smaller families with FTD+MND (Parkinson *et al.*, 2006), has been identified as *CHMP2B*, which encodes the endosomal sorting complex required for transport III (ESCRTIII-complex sub-unit). CHMP2B is part of the chromatin-modifying protein/

charged multivesicular body protein family and is involved in the degradation of surface receptor proteins and the formation of endocytotic multivesicular bodies, and forms a component of the ubiquitin proteasome system. The neuropathology is that of FTLD-U. The ubiquitinated inclusions contain p62 protein, but not TDP-43 or FUS, occurring mostly as granular NCI within the hippocampal DG granule cells (Holm *et al.*, 2007). Such cases are thus presently classified as FTLD-UPS (Mackenzie *et al.*, 2009). In some family members, a few tau tangles are seen, without senile (amyloid) plaques (Yancopoulou *et al.*, 2003), but less common than is usual for cases of FTLD with *MAPT* mutations. To date, only four families have been identified with this particular mutation (see AD and FTD mutation database: wwww.mol gen.ua.ac.be/FTDmutations) and the significance of this particular genetic change to the broader pathogenesis of FTLD remains unknown.

70.6.3   Other genetic risk factors for FTLD

Although it is well established that *ApoE* ε4 allele is a risk factor for late onset sporadic and familial AD (Corder *et al.*, 1993), whether this plays a role in FTLD is still unclear. There have been many claims that *ApoE* ε4 allele frequency is elevated in FTLD (Czech *et al.*, 1994; Frisoni *et al.*, 1994; Farrer *et al.*, 1995; Schneider *et al.*, 1995; Stevens *et al.*, 1997; Fabre *et al.*, 2001), although other (usually larger) studies generally have not substantiated this in either Caucasian (Minthon *et al.*, 1997; Geschwind *et al.*, 1998; Pickering-Brown *et al.*, 2001; Riemenschneider *et al.*, 2002; Short *et al.*, 2002; Verpillat *et al.*, 2002; Binetti *et al.*, 2003) or non-Caucasian (Kowalska *et al.*, 2001) populations. Indeed, a meta-analysis involving most of these studies (Verpillat *et al.*, 2002) found no overall association between *ApoE* ε4 allele frequency and FTLD (but see Srinivasan *et al.*, 2006). In patients with *MAPT* mutations, *ApoE* ε4 allele frequency is not different from controls (Houlden *et al.*, 1999b; Pickering-Brown *et al.*, 2002). Nonetheless, Srinivasan *et al.* (2006) reported that *ApoE* ε4 allele frequency might be selectively increased in males with FTLD, thereby doubling their chances of developing disease. It is also possible that clinical subgroups under FTLD umbrella might be differentially affected. Short *et al.* (2002) reported *ApoE* ε4 allele frequency to be increased in SD, compared FTD and PA, although Pickering-Brown *et al.* (2001) found this to be normal in FTD and SD, but tended to be increased in PA. However, in both studies the number of patients with PA and SD was relatively small and the present variability in findings could be a reflection of this.

In contrast to AD, possession of *ApoE* ε4 allele does not appear to affect age at onset of disease (or duration of illness) in sporadic FTLD (Pickering-Brown *et al.*, 2001; Short *et al.*, 2002; Srinivasan *et al.*, 2006) or in cases with *MAPT* mutations (Houlden *et al.*, 1999b; Janssen *et al.*, 2002; Pickering-Brown *et al.*, 2002; Riemenschneider *et al.*, 2002). Hence it seems unlikely that *ApoE* ε4 allele acts as a risk factor or disease modifier in FTLD generally, but could play a role in other clinical subtypes, such as SD or PA.

Results from small series of FTLD patients suggest *APOE* ε2 allele could act as a risk factor (Lehmann *et al.*, 2000; Verpillat *et al.*, 2002), but again this remains to be substantiated (Kowalska *et al.*, 2001; Pickering-Brown *et al.*, 2001; Riemenschneider *et al.*, 2002; Binetti *et al.*, 2003). Meta-analysis, nevertheless, suggested increased *APOE* ε2 allele frequency.

70.7   FOUNDER EFFECTS

70.7.1   *MAPT*

P301L is the most common *MAPT* mutation found to date, being present in many families worldwide (Clark *et al.*, 1998; Dumanchin *et al.*, 1998; Hutton *et al.*, 1998; Houlden *et al.*, 1999a; Mirra *et al.*, 1999; Rizzu *et al.*, 1999; Binetti *et al.*, 2003; Rosso *et al.*, 2003). Four of five families with P301L mutation shared the less common H2 haplotype on the disease gene (Houlden *et al.* 1999a). These four families were of Dutch origin (Rizzu *et al.*, 1999) and might therefore stem from a founder within this population (Rosso *et al.*, 2003). Two other families with P301L mutation on the same H2 haplotype background (Sobrido *et al.*, 2003) indicate this same founder probably underlies other North American/French Canadian families with French/Dutch ancestry (Bird *et al.*, 1999). However, P301L mutation has been reported in other North American families with no known Dutch/French or French Canadian ancestry (Mirra *et al.*, 1999) raising the possibility of a separate founder. Japanese families with P301L mutation do not share the same extended H2 haplotype, again implying separate founders. However, despite sharing H1 haplotype, several other *MAPT* polymorphisms, unique to Japanese individuals, differed between two Japanese subjects with P301L mutation suggesting separate founders.

Haplotype analysis (Pickering-Brown *et al.*, 2004) has shown a likely founder effect for British (Janssen *et al.*, 2002; Pickering-Brown *et al.*, 2002), North American (Yamaoka *et al.*, 1996; Hulette *et al.*, 1999) and Australian families (Dark, 1997; Hutton *et al.*, 1998) with +16 splice site mutation. Subsequent analysis (Colombo *et al.*, 2009) dates this particular mutation back to an origin around 1300AD within North Wales, a rural and relatively remote region, some 23 generations ago. It is likely that the founder lived in this part of the United Kingdom with 'spread' of the mutation into more industrialized regions during the Industrial Revolution with further spread to other parts of the world, particularly Commonwealth countries through emigration in the eighteenth to twentieth centuries. The identification of this large extended pedigree may be useful for identifying disease-modifying loci.

All other *MAPT* mutations appear to exist within single families, or single family members, and may represent mutational events that have remained 'private' to that family or to have 'spread' less extensively to other countries.

70.7.2   *PGRN*

R493X is the most commonly reported *PGRN* mutation to date, explaining the disease in 2.2 per cent of FTLD cases, and ascertained in 13 genealogically unrelated FTLD families (Gass *et al.*, 2006; Huey *et al.*, 2006; Pickering-Brown *et al.*, 2006;

Spina *et al.*, 2007). Patients have a wide onset age range (44–69 years) and variable clinical diagnoses including FTD, PNFA, CBD and AD (Rademakers *et al.*, 2007). Haplotype analysis has suggested two separate founding events. A single common founder, most likely originating in the UK approximately 300 years ago, implicated 27 present day families. As with *MAPT* +16 mutation, patients with R493X founder haplotype have been observed in countries of British migration, including the United States and Australia. Significantly, neither the *PGRN* R493X nor the *MAPT* +16 mutations have been identified in FTLD series from continental Europe (including The Netherlands, Belgium, Poland, France, Italy and Spain) consistent with the view that the likely founders were from the UK, the appearance of patients in other countries following patterns of British migration. Founder effects have also been suggested for Gln415X (Pickering-Brown *et al.*, 2008) and Cys31LeufsX35 (Mackenzie *et al.*, 2006b) mutations, both again relating to British stock.

70.8   BIOMARKERS FOR FTLD

Although clinicopathological correlations have suggested that certain clinical FTLD subtypes are strongly associated with one particular kind of histology, or even histological subtype, these associations are not perfect, particularly for FTD which can be associated with all known histological forms of FTLD (including FUS pathology), and for PNFA where tauopathy (Pick histology) can sometimes be present. While the determination of genotype (i.e. identification of *MAPT/PGRN/CHMP2B/VCP* mutations) can unequivocally point towards the relevant histology, such cases are still relatively few and the full range of genetic involvement is unclear. Conversely, although particular clinical phenotypes are frequently associated with particular mutational events (for example, certain *MAPT* mutations usually present with FTD, often with linguistic changes (Pickering-Brown *et al.*, 2008), and *PGRN* mutations with FTD or PNFA phenotype (Snowden *et al.*, 2006; Snowden *et al.*, 2007; Pickering-Brown *et al.*, 2008), the mutation present in familial autosomal dominantly inherited FTLD cannot be precisely inferred without gene analysis. Hence, a straightforward laboratory test, based on easily accessible body fluids or tissues, that would identify patients with FTLD from other neurodegenerative disorders, or perhaps more importantly discriminate cases with underlying FTLD-tau from those with FTLD-TDP without the requirement of complex genetic investigations, would be a major adjunct to diagnostic precision. It could also act as a predictive test, having great practical value in directing therapeutic strategies aimed at preventing or removing tau or TDP-43 pathological changes from the brain in FTLD and other TDP-43 proteinopathies. The recent identification of key molecular changes in the pathogenesis of FTLD (and MND) should open the way to progress in these respects.

70.9   CONCLUSION

The past three years has seen a sea change in appreciation of the genetics and molecular pathology of FTLD. The twin discoveries of the presence of gene mutations in progranulin as a cause of FTLD, and the identification of the ubiquitinated proteins, TDP-43 and FUS in the pathological lesions of non-tauopathy forms of FTLD, has opened new vistas into the causes and effects of those tissue changes that are the pathological markers of disease, even if they may not be the actual damaging agents. However, what we have seen so far, and what meagre clues have been gained, is likely to be only the tip of the iceberg. There is still a whole world of basic neurobiology relating to PGRN, TDP-43 and FUS waiting to be discovered, and with that it will become increasingly clear as to the roles these molecules play not only in FTLD, or even in other neurodegenerative disorders such as AD, but perhaps most importantly in terms of how they might maintain a watchful surveillance over the health and well-being of the nervous system ensuring proper brain function. These data will not be won easily. It has been nearly two decades since the discovery of the amyloid precursor protein (APP), yet a definitive role for this protein in the brain is still elusive. Likewise, the prion protein has long been known, yet its precise brain function remains unclear. PGRN, like APP and prion protein, may subserve a variety of roles concerned with regulating the fundamental health, environment and infrastructure of the brain. Although AD and prion disease are pathologically characterized by accumulations of aggregated proteins, with presumed neurotoxic effects, it may be loss of the parent protein that is vital. The loss of function effect of *PGRN* mutations in FTLD is instructive in this latter context.

REFERENCES

Ahmed Z, Mackenzie IR, Hutton ML, Dickson DW. (2007) Progranulin in frontotemporal lobar degeneration and neuroinflammation. *Journal of Neuroinflammation* 4: 7.

Amador-Ortiz C, Lin W-L, Ahmed Z et al. (2007) TDP-43 immunoreactivity in hippocampal sclerosis and Alzheimer's disease. *Annals of Neurology* 61: 435–45.

Arai T, Hasegawa M, Akiyama H et al. (2006) TDP-43 is a component of ubiquitin-positive tau-negative inclusions in frontotemporal lobar degeneration and amyotrophic lateral sclerosis. *Biochemical Biophysical Research Communications* 351: 602–11.

Arai T, Mackenzie IRA, Hasegawa M et al. (2009) Phosphorylated TDP-43 in Alzheimer's disease and dementia with Lewy bodies. *Acta Neuropathologica* 117: 125–36.

Ayala YM, Misteli T, Baralle FE. (2008) TDP-43 regulates retinoblastoma protein phosphorylation through the repression of cyclindependent kinase 6 expression. *Proceedings of the National Academy of Sciences of the United States of America* 105: 3785–9.

Baker M, Mackenzie IRA, Pickering-Brown SM et al. (2006) Mutations in Progranulin cause tau-negative frontotemporal dementia linked to chromosome 17. *Nature* 442: 916–19.

Bigio EH, Lipton AM, White CL et al. (2003) Frontotemporal and motor neurone degeneration with neurofilament inclusion

bodies: additional evidence for overlap between FTD and ALS. *Neuropathology and Applied Neurobiology* 29: 239–53.

Binetti G, Nicosia F, Benussi L et al. (2003) Prevalence of *TAU* mutations in an Italian clinical series of familial frontotemporal patients. *Neuroscience Letters* 338: 85–7.

Bird TD, Nochlin D, Poorkaj P et al. (1999) A clinical pathological comparison of 3 families with frontotemporal dementia and identical mutations in the tau gene (P301L). *Brain* 122: 741–56.

Bramham CR, Wells DG. (2007) Dendritic mRNA: transport, translation and function. *Nature Reviews in Neuroscience* 8: 776–89.

Brandmeir NJ, Geser F, Kwong LK et al. (2008) Severe subcortical TDP-43 pathology in sporadic frontotemporal lobar degeneration with motor neuron disease. *Acta Neuropathologica* 115: 123–31.

Brown J, Ashworth A, Gydesen S et al. (1995) Familial non-specific dementia maps to chromosome 3. *Human Molecular Genetics* 4: 1625–8.

Bruni AC, Momeni P, Bernardi L et al. (2007) Heterogeneity within a large kindred with frontotemporal dementia: a novel progranulin mutation. *Neurology* 69: 140–7.

Bugiani O, Murrell JR, Giaccone G et al. (1999) Frontotemporal dementia and corticobasal degeneration in a family with a P301S mutation in tau. *Journal of Neuropathology and Experimental Neurology* 58: 667–77.

Buratti E, Baralle FE. (2008) Multiple roles of TDP-43 in gene expression, splicing regulation, and human disease. *Frontiers in Bioscience* 13: 867–78.

Cairns NJ, Perry RH, Jaros E et al. (2003) Patients with a novel neurofilamentopathy: dementia with neurofilament inclusions. *Neuroscience Letters* 341: 177–80.

Cairns NJ, Grossman M, Arnold SE et al. (2004a) Clinical and neuropathologic variation in neuronal intermediate filament inclusion disease. *Neurology* 63: 1376–84.

Cairns NJ, Zhuckareva V, Uryu K et al. (2004b) Alpha-internexin is present in the pathological inclusions of neuronal intermediate filament inclusion disease. *American Journal of Pathology* 164: 2153–61.

Cairns NJ, Bigio EH, Mackenzie IRA et al. (2007a) Neuropathologic diagnostic and nosologic criteria for frontotemporal lobar degeneration: consensus of the Consortium for Frontotemporal Lobar Degeneration. *Acta Neuropathologica* 114: 5–22.

Cairns NJ, Neumann M, Bigio EH et al. (2007b) TDP-43 in familial and sporadic frontotemporal lobar degeneration with ubiquitin inclusions. *American Journal of Pathology* 171: 227–40.

Casafont I, Bengoechea R, Tapia O et al. (2009) TDP-43 localises in mRNA transcription and processing sites in mammalian neurones. *Journal of Structural Biology* 167: 235–41.

Clark LN, Poorkaj P, Wzsolek Z et al. (1998) Pathogenic implications of mutations in the tau genein pallido-ponto-nigral degeneration and related neurodegenerative disorders linked to chromosome 17. *Proceedings of the National Academy of Sciences of the United States of America* 95: 13103–7.

Colombo R, Tavian D, Baker MC et al. (2009) Recent origin and spread of a common Welsh MAPT splice mutation causing frontotemporal lobar degeneration. *Neurogenetics* 10: 313–18.

Corder EH, Saunders AM, Strittmatter WJ et al. (1993) Gene dose of Apolipoprotein E type 4 allele and the risk of Alzheimer's disease in late onset families. *Science* **261**: 921–3.

Cordes M, Wszolek WK, Calne DB et al. (1992) Magnetic resonance imaging studies in rapidly progressive autosomal dominant Parkinsonism and dementia with pallido-ponto-nigral degeneration. *Neurodegeneration* **1**: 217–24.

Cruts M, Gijselinck I, van der Zee J et al. (2006) Null mutations in progranulin cause ubiquitin-positive frontotemporal dementia linked to chromosome 17q21. *Nature* **442**: 920–4.

Czech C, Forstl H, Monning U et al. (1994) ApoEε4 in clinically diagnosed Alzheimer's disease, frontal lobe degeneration and non-demented controls. *Neurobiology of Ageing* **15** (Suppl 1): S132.

Dark F. (1997) A family with autosomal dominant, non-Alzheimer's presenile dementia. *Australian/New Zealand Journal of Psychiatry* **31**: 139–44.

Davidson Y, Kelley T, Mackenzie IR et al. (2007) Ubiquitinated pathological lesions in frontotemporal lobar degeneration contain the TAR DNA-binding protein, TDP-43. *Acta Neuropathologica* **113**: 521–33.

Davidson Y, Amin H, Kelley T et al. (2009) TDP-43 in ubiquitinated inclusions in the inferior olives in frontotemporal lobar degeneration and in other neurodegenerative diseases; a degenerative process distinct from normal ageing. *Acta Neuropathologica* **118**: 359–69.

De Silva R, Lashley T, Strand K et al. (2006) An immunohistochemical study of cases of sporadic and inherited frontotemporal lobar degeneration using 3R- and 4R-specific tau monoclonal antibodies. *Acta Neuropathologica* **111**: 329–40.

Dumanchin C, Camuzat C, Campion D et al. (1998) Segregation of a missense mutation in the microtubule-associated protein tau gene with familial frontotemporal dementia with parkinsonism. *Human Molecular Genetics* **7**: 1825–9.

Fabre SF, Forsell C, Viitanen M et al. (2001) Clinic-based cases with frontotemporal dementia show increased cerebrospinal fluid tau and high Apolipoprotein E ε4 frequency, but no tau gene mutations. *Experimental Neurology* **168**: 413–18.

Farrer LA, Abraham CR, Volicer L et al. (1995) Allele ε4 of Apolipoprotein E shows a dose effect on age at onset of Pick disease. *Experimental Neurology* **136**: 162–70.

Farrer MJ, Hulihan MM, Kachergus JM et al. (2009) *DCTN1* mutations in Perry syndrome. *Nature Genetics* **41**: 163–5.

Forman MS, Farmer J, Johnson JK et al. (2006a) Frontotemporal dementia: clinicopathological correlations. *Annals of Neurology* **59**: 952–62.

Foster NL, Wilhelmsen K, Sima AAF et al. (1997) Frontotemporal dementia and Parkinsonism linked to chromosome 17: A consensus conference. *Annals of Neurology* **41**: 706–15.

Freeman SF, Spires-Jones T, Hyman BT et al. (2008) TAR-DNA binding protein 43 in Pick disease. *Journal of Neuropathology and Experimental Neurology* **67**: 62–7.

Frisoni GB, Calabresi L, Geroldi C et al. (1994) Apolipoprotein E ε4 allele in Alzheimer's disease and vascular dementia. *Dementia* **5**: 240–2.

Froelich Fabre S, Axelman P, Almkvist A et al. (2003) Extended investigation of tau and mutation screening of other candidate genes on chromosome 17q21 in a Swedish FTDP-17 family. *American Journal of Medical Genetics Part B (Neuropsychiatric Genetics)* **121B**: 112–18.

Fujita K, Ito H, Nakano S et al. (2008) Immunohistochemical identification of messenger RNA-related proteins in basophilic inclusions of adult-onset atypical motor neuron disease. *Acta Neuropathologica* **116**: 439–45.

Gass J, Cannon A, Mackenzie IR et al. (2006) Mutations in progranulin are a major cause of ubiquitin-positive frontotemporal lobar degeneration. *Human Molecular Genetics* **55**: 2988–3001.

Geser F, Brandmeir NJ, Kwong LK et al. (2008a) Evidence of multisystem disorder in whole-brain map of pathological TDP-43 in amyotrophic lateral sclerosis. *Archives of Neurology* **65**: 636–41.

Geser F, Winton MJ, Kwong LW et al. (2008b) Pathological TDP-43 in parkinsonism–dementia complex and amyotrophic lateral sclerosis. *Acta Neuropathologica* **115**: 133–46.

Geschwind D, Karrim J, Nelson SF, Miller B. (1998) The Apolipoprotein E epsilon4 allele is not a significant risk factor for frontotemporal dementia. *Annals of Neurology* **44**: 134–8.

Gijselinck I, van der Zee J, Engelborghs S et al. (2008) Progranulin locus deletion in frontotemporal dementia. *Human Mutation* **29**: 53–8.

Gydesen S, Brown JM, Brun A et al. (2002) Chromosome 3 linked frontotemporal dementia (FTD-3). *Neurology* **59**: 1585–94.

Hasegawa M, Smith MJ, Iijima M et al. (1999) FTDP-17 mutations N279K and S305N in tau produce increased splicing of exon 10. *FEBS Letters* **443**: 93–6.

Hasegawa M, Arai T, Akiyama H et al. (2007) TDP-43 is deposited in the Guam parkinsonism–dementia complex brains. *Brain* **130**: 1386–94.

He Z, Bateman A. (2003) Progranulin (granulin-epithelin precursor, PC-cell-derived growth factor, acrogranin) mediates tissue repair and tumorigenesis. *Journal of Molecular Medicine* **81**: 600–12.

He Z, Ong CH, Halper J, Bateman A. (2003) Progranulin is a mediator of the wound response. *Nature Medicine* **9**: 225–9.

Holm IE, Englund E, Mackenzie IRA et al. (2007) A reassessment of the neuropathology of frontotemporal dementia linked to chromosome 3 (FTD-3). *Journal of Neuropathology and Experimental Neurology* **66**: 884–91.

Hong M, Zhukareva V, Vogelsberg-Ragaglia V et al. (1998) Mutation-specific functional impairments in distinct tau isoforms of hereditary FTDP-17. *Science* **282**: 1914–17.

Hosler B, Siddique T, Sapp PC et al. (2000) Linkage of familial amyotrophic lateral sclerosis with frontotemporal dementia to chromosome 9q21-22. *Journal of the American Medical Association* **284**: 1664–9.

Houlden H, Baker M, Adamson J et al. (1999a) Frequency of tau mutations in three series of non-Alzheimer's degenerative dementia. *Annals of Neurology* **46**: 243–8.

Houlden H, Rizzu P, Stevens M et al. (1999b) Apolipoprotein E genotype does not affect age at onset of dementia in families with defined tau mutations. *Neuroscience Letters* **260**: 193–5.

Hu WT, Josephs KA, Knopman DS et al. (2008) Temporal lobar predominance of TDP-43 neuronal cytoplasmic inclusions in Alzheimer's disease. Acta Neuropathologica 116: 215–20.

Huey ED, Grafman J, Wassermann EM et al. (2006) Characteristics of frontotemporal dementia patients with a Progranulin mutation. Annals of Neurology 60: 374–80.

Hulette CM, Pericak-Vance MA, Roses AD et al. (1999) Neuropathological features of frontotemporal dementia with parkinsonism linked to chromosome 17q21-22(FTDP-17). Journal of Neuropathology and Experimental Neurology 58: 859–66.

Hutton M, Lendon CL, Rizzu P et al. (1998) Association of missense and 5′-splice-site mutations in tau with the inherited dementia FTDP-17. Nature 393: 702–5.

Josephs KA, Holton JL, Rossor MN et al. (2003) Neurofilament inclusion body disease: a new proteinopathy? Brain 126: 2291–303.

Josephs KA, Stroh A, Dugger B, Dickson DW. (2009) Evaluation of subcortical pathology and clinical correlations in FTLD-U subtypes. Acta Neuropathologica 118: 349–58.

Knopman DS, Mastri AR, Frey WH et al. (1990) Dementia lacking distinctive histologic features: a common non-Alzheimer degenerative dementia. Neurology 40: 251–6.

Kowalska A, Asada T, Arima K et al. (2001) Genetic analysis in patients with familial and sporadic frontotemporal dementia: two tau mutations in only familial cases and no association with Apolipoprotein ε4. Dementia and Geriatric Cognitive Disorders 12: 387–92.

Le Ber I, van der Zee J, Hannequin D et al. (2007) Progranulin null mutations in both sporadic and familial frontotemporal dementia. Human Mutation 28: 846–55.

Lee EB, Lee VM-Y, Trojanowski JQ, Neumann M. (2008) TDP-43 immunoreactivity in anoxic, ischaemic and neoplastic lesions of the central nervous system. Acta Neuropathologica 115: 305–10.

Lehmann DJ, Smith AD, Combrinck M et al. (2000) Apolipoprotein E ε2 may be a risk factor for sporadic frontotemporal dementia. Journal of Neurology, Neurosurgery and Psychiatry 69: 404–5.

Lipton AM, White CL III, Bigio EH. (2004) Frontotemporal lobar degeneration with motor neuron disease-type inclusions predominates in 76 cases of frontotemporal degeneration. Acta Neuropathologica 108: 379–85.

Lynch T, Sano M, Marder KS et al. (1994) Clinical characteristics of a family with chromosome 17-linked disinhibition–dementia–parkinsonism–amyotrophy complex. Neurology 44: 187–94.

Mackenzie IRA, Baker M, Pickering-Brown S et al. (2006a) The neuropathology of frontotemporal lobar degeneration caused by mutations in the progranulin gene. Brain 129: 3081–90.

Mackenzie IRA, Shi J, Shaw CL et al. (2006b) Dementia lacking distinctive histology (DLDH) revisited. Acta Neuropathologica 112: 551–9.

Mackenzie IRA, Neumann M, Bigio E et al. (2009) Nomenclature for neuropathologic subtypes of frontotemporal lobar degeneration: consensus recommendations. Acta Neuropathologica 117: 15–18.

Masellis M, Momeni P, Meschino W et al. (2006) Novel splicing mutation in the progranulin gene causing familial corticobasal syndrome. Brain 129: 3115–23.

Minthon L, Hesse C, Sjogren M et al. (1997) The Apolipoprotein E ε4 allelefrequency is normal in fronto-temporal dementia, but correlates with age at onset of disease. Neuroscience Letters 226: 65–7.

Mirra SS, Murrell JR, Gearing M et al. (1999) Tau pathology in a family with dementia and a P301L mutation in tau. Journal of Neuropathology and Experimental Neurology 58: 335–45.

Momeni P, Schymick J, Jain S et al. (2006) Analysis of IFT74 as a candidate gene for chromosome 9p-linked ALS-FTD. BMC Neurology 6: 44.

Morita M, Al-Chalabi A, Andersen PM et al. (2006) A locus on chromosome 9p confers susceptibility to ALS and frontotemporal dementia. Neurology 66: 839–44.

Mott RT, Dickson DW, Trojanowski JQ et al. (2005) Neuropathologic, biochemical, and molecular characterization of the frontotemporal dementias. Journal of Neuropathology and Experimental Neurology 64: 420–8.

Mukherjee O, Pastor P, Cairns NJ et al. (2006) HDDD2 is a familial frontotemporal lobar degeneration with ubiquitin-positive, tau-negative inclusions caused by a missense mutation in the signal peptide of progranulin. Annals of Neurology 60: 314–22.

Munoz D, Neumann M, Kusaka H et al. (2009) FUS pathology in basophilic inclusion body disease (BIBD). Acta Neuropathologica 118: 617–27.

Nakashima-Yasuda H, Uryu K, Robinson J et al. (2007) Co-morbidity of TDP-43 proteinopathy in Lewy body related diseases. Acta Neuropathologica 114: 221–9.

Neary D, Snowden JS, Gustafson L et al. (1998) Frontotemporal lobar degeneration: A consensus on clinical diagnostic criteria. Neurology 51: 1546–54.

Neary D, Snowden JS, Mann DMA. (2005) Frontotemporal dementia. Lancet Neurology 4: 771–9.

Neary D, Snowden JS, Mann DMA. (2007) Frontotemporal lobar degeneration: clinical and pathological relationships. Acta Neuropathologica 114: 31–8.

Neumann M, Sampathu DM, Kwong LK et al. (2006) Ubiquitinated TDP-43 in frontotemporal lobar degeneration and amyotrophic lateral sclerosis. Science 314: 130–3.

Neumann M, Rademakers R, Roeber S et al. (2009a) A new subtype of frontotemporal lobar degeneration with FUS pathology. Brain 132: 2922–31.

Neumann M, Roeber S, Kretzschmar H, Mackenzie IRA. (2009b) Abundant FUS pathology in neuronal intermediate filament inclusion disease. Acta Neuropathologica 118: 605–16.

Ostojic J, Axelman K, Lannfelt L, Froelich-Fabre S. (2003) No evidence of linkage to chromosome 9q21-22 in a Swedish family with frontotemporal dementia and amyotrophic lateral sclerosis. Neuroscience Letters 340: 245–7.

Parkinson N, Ince PG, Smith MO et al. (2006) ALS phenotypes with mutations in CHMP2B (charged multivesicular body 2B). Neurology 67: 1074–7.

Pick A. (1892) Uber die Bejiehungen des senilen Hirnatrophie zur Aphasie. Prager Med Wochenschrift 17: 165–7.

Pickering-Brown SM, Owen F, Snowden JS *et al.* (2001) Apolipoprotein E E4 allele has no effect on age at onset or duration of disease in cases of frontotemporal dementia with Pick- or microvacuolar-type histology. *Experimental Neurology* **163**: 452–6.

Pickering-Brown SM, Richardson AMT, Snowden JS *et al.* (2002) Inherited frontotemporal dementia in nine British families associated with intronic mutations in the tau gene. *Brain* **125**: 732–51.

Pickering-Brown S, Baker M, Bird T *et al.* (2004) Evidence of a founder effect in families with frontotemporal dementia that harbour the tau +16 splice mutation. *American Journal of Medical Genetics (Part B Neuropsychiatric Genetics)* **125B**: 79–82.

Pickering-Brown SM, Baker M, Gass J *et al.* (2006) Mutations in progranulin explain atypical phenotypes with variants in MAPT. *Brain* **129**: 3124–6.

Pickering-Brown S, Rollinson S, Du Plessis D *et al.* (2008) Frequency and clinical characteristics of progranulin (PGRN) mutation carriers in the Manchester frontotemporal lobar degeneration cohort: comparison to patients with tau (MAPT) and no known mutation. *Brain* **131**: 721–31.

Poorkaj P, Bird T, Wijsman E *et al.* (1998) Tau is a candidate gene for chromosome 17 frontotemporal dementia. *Annals of Neurology* **43**: 815–25.

Poorkaj P, Grossman M, Steinbart E *et al.* (2001) Frequency of tau gene mutations in familial and sporadic cases of non-Alzheimer dementia. *Archives of Neurology* **58**: 383–7.

Qian J, Yang J, Zhang X *et al.* (2001) Isolation and characterization of a novel cDNA, UBAP1, derived from the tumor suppressor locus in human chromosome 9p21-22. *Journal of Cancer Research and Clinical Oncology* **127**: 613–18.

Rademakers R, Cruts M, Dermaut B *et al.* (2002) Tau-negative frontal lobe dementia at 17q21: significant fine mapping of the candidate region to a 4.8-cm interval. *Molecular Psychiatry* **7**: 1064–74.

Rademakers R, Baker M, Gass J *et al.* (2007) An international initiative to study phenotypic variability associated with progranulin haploinsufficiency in patients with the common c.1477c>t (p.R493X) mutation mutation. *Lancet Neurology* **6**: 857–68.

Riemenschneider M, Diehl J, Muller U *et al.* (2002) Apolipoprotein E polymorphism in German patients with frontotemporal degeneration. *Journal of Neurology, Neurosurgery and Psychiatry* **72**: 639–43.

Rizzu P, Van Swieten JC, Joosse M *et al.* (1999) High prevalence of mutations in the microtubule-associated protein tau in a population study of frontotemporal dementia in the Netherlands. *American Journal of Human Genetics* **64**: 414–21.

Rosso SM, Kamphorst W, de Graaf B *et al.* (2001) Familial frontotemporal dementia with ubiquitin positive inclusions is linked to chromosome 17q21-22. *Brain* **124**: 1948–57.

Rosso SM, Donker Kaat L, Baks T *et al.* (2003) Frontotemporal dementia in the Netherlands: patient characteristics and prevalence estimates from a population based study. *Brain* **126**: 2016–22.

Rovelet-Lecrux A, Deramecourt V, Legallic S *et al.* (2008) Deletion of the progranulin gene in patients with frontotemporal lobar degeneration or Parkinson disease. *Neurobiology of Disease* **31**: 41–5.

Sampathu DM, Neumann M, Kwong LK *et al.* (2006) Pathological heterogeneity of frontotemporal lobar degeneration with ubiquitin-positive inclusions delineated by ubiquitin immunohistochemistry and novel monoclonal antibodies. *American Journal of Pathology* **169**: 1343–52.

Schneider JA, Gearing M, Robbins RS *et al.* (1995) Apolipoprotein E genotype in diverse neurodegenerative disorders. *Annals of Neurology* **38**: 131–5.

Schwab C, Arai T, Hasegawa M *et al.* (2009) TDP-43 pathology in familial British dementia. *Acta Neuropathologica* **118**: 303–11.

Shi J, Shaw CL, Richardson AMT *et al.* (2005) Histopathological changes underlying frontotemporal lobar degeneration with clinicopathological correlation. *Acta Neuropathologica* **110**: 501–12.

Short RA, Graff-Radford NR, Adamson J *et al.* (2002) Differences in tau and Apolipoprotein E polymorphism frequencies in sporadic frontotemporal lobar degeneration syndromes. *Archives of Neurology* **59**: 611–15.

Skibinski G, Parkinson NJ, Brown JM *et al.* (2005) Mutations in the endosomal ESCRTIII-complex subunit CHMP2B in frontotemporal dementia. *Nature Genetics* **37**: 806–8.

Snowden JS, Neary D, Mann DMA *et al.* (1992) Progressive language disorder due to lobar atrophy. *Annals of Neurology* **31**: 174–83.

Snowden JS, Pickering-Brown SM, Mackenzie IR *et al.* (2006) Progranulin gene mutations associated with frontotemporal dementia and progressive aphasia. *Brain* **129**: 3091–102.

Snowden JS, Pickering-Brown SM, Du Plessis D *et al.* (2007) Progressive anomia revisited: Focal degeneration associated with progranulin gene mutation. *Neurocase* **13**: 366–77.

Sobrido M-J, Miller BL, Havlioglu N *et al.* (2003) Novel tau polymorphisms, tau haplotypes and splicing in familial and sporadic frontotemporal dementia. *Archives of Neurology* **60**: 698–702.

Spillantini MG, Murrell JR, Goedert M *et al.* (1998) Mutation in the tau gene in familial multiple system tauopathy with presenile dementia. *Proceedings of the National Academy of Sciences of the United States of America* **95**: 7737–41.

Spina S, Murrell JR, Huey ED *et al.* (2007) Clinicopathologic features of frontotemporal dementia with Progranulin sequence variation. *Neurology* **68**: 820–7.

Srinivasan R, Davidson Y, Gibbons L *et al.* (2006) The Apolipoprotein E ε4 allele selectively increases the risk of frontotemporal lobar degeneration in males. *Journal of Neurology, Neurosurgery and Psychiatry* **77**: 154–8.

Stevens M, van Duijn CM, de Knijff P *et al.* (1997) Apolipoprotein E gene and sporadic frontal lobe dementia. *Neurology* **48**: 1526–9.

Stevens M, van Duijn CM, Kamporst W *et al.* (1998) Familial aggregation in frontotemporal dementia. *Neurology* **50**: 1541–5.

Taniguchi S, McDonagh AM, Pickering-Brown SM *et al.* (2004) The neuropathology of frontotemporal lobar degeneration with respect to the cytological and biochemical characteristics of tau protein. *Neuropathology and Applied Neurobiology* **30**: 1–18.

Thorpe JR, Tang H, Atherton J, Cairns NJ. (2008) Fine structural analysis of the neuronal inclusions in frontotemporal lobar degeneration with TDP-43 proteinopathy. *Journal of Neural Transmission* **115**: 1661–71.

Turner BJ, Baumer D, Parkinson NJ *et al.* (2008) TDP-43 expression in mouse models of amyotrophic lateral sclerosis and spinal muscular atrophy. *BMC Neuroscience* **9**: 104–14.

Uryu K, Nakashima-Yasuda H, Forman MS *et al.* (2008) Concomitant TAR-DNA-binding protein 43 pathology is present in Alzheimer disease and corticobasal degeneration but not in other tauopathies. *Journal of Neuropathology and Experimental Neurology* **67**: 555–64.

Vance C, Al-Chalabi A, Ruddy D *et al.* (2006) Familial amyotrophic lateral sclerosis with frontotemporal dementia is linked to a locus on chromosome 9p13.2-21.3. *Brain* **129**: 868–76.

Van Swieten JC, Heutink P. (2008) Mutations in progranulin (GRN) within the spectrum of clinical and pathological phenotypes of frontotemporal dementia. *Lancet Neurology* **7**: 965–74.

Verpillat P, Camuzat A, Hannequin D *et al.* (2002) Association between the extended tau haplotype and frontotemporal dementia. *Archives of Neurology* **59**: 935–9.

Wang HY, Wang IF, Bose J, Shen CK. (2004) Structural diversity and functional implications of the eukaryotic TDP gene family. *Genomics* **83**: 130–9.

Wang IF, Wu LS, Chang HY, Shen CK. (2008) TDP-43, the signature protein of FTLD-U, is a neuronal activity-responsive factor. *Journal of Neurochemistry* **105**: 797–806.

Winton MJ, Igaz IM, Wong MM *et al.* (2008) Disturbance of nuclear and cytoplasmic TAR DNA-binding protein (TDP-43) induces disease-like redistribution, sequestration, and aggregate formation. *Journal of Biological Chemistry* **283**: 13302–9.

Wszolek ZK, Pfeiffer RF, Bhatt MH *et al.* (1992) Rapidly progressive autosomal dominant Parkinsonism and dementia with pallido-ponto-nigral degeneration. *Annals of Neurology* **32**: 312–20.

Wszolek ZK, Tsuboi Y, Uitti RJ *et al.* (2001) Progressive supranuclear palsy as a disease phenotype caused by S305S tau gene mutation. *Brain* **124**: 1666–70.

Xiao S, Sato C, Kawarai T *et al.* (2007) Genetic studies of GRN and IFT74 in amyotrophic lateral sclerosis. *Neurobiology of Aging* **29**: 1279–82.

Yamaoka LH, Welsh-Bohmer KA, Hulette CM *et al.* (1996) Linkage of frontotemporal dementia to chromosome 17: Clinical and neuropathological characterization of phenotype. *American Journal of Human Genetics* **59**: 1306–12.

Yancopoulou D, Crowther A, Chakrabarti L *et al.* (2003) Tau protein in frontotemporal dementia linked to chromosome 3 (FTD-3). *Journal of Neuropathology and Experimental Neurology* **62**: 878–82.

Zhang YJ, Xu YF, Dickey CA *et al.* (2007) Progranulin mediates caspase-dependent cleavage of TAR DNA binding protein-43. *Journal of Neuroscience* **27**: 10530–4.

Zhu J, Nathan C, Jin W *et al.* (2002) Conversion of proepithelin to epithelins: roles of SLPI and elastase in host defense and wound repair. *Cell* **111**: 867–78.

71

Semantic dementia

JULIE S SNOWDEN

71.1 INTRODUCTION

Semantic dementia is a disorder of conceptual knowledge, resulting from temporal lobe neurodegeneration (Snowden et al. 1989; Hodges et al. 1992). It is one of the distinct clinical syndromes, along with the behavioural disorder of frontotemporal dementia (FTD) and expressive language disorder of progressive non-fluent aphasia (PNFA), encompassed under the umbrella of frontotemporal lobar degeneration (FTLD) (**Table 71.1**) (Neary et al., 1998). Patients with semantic dementia lose the ability to name and understand words, to recognize faces, and to understand the significance of objects, non-verbal sounds, tastes and smells (Snowden et al., 1996; Bozeat et al., 2000). Non-semantic aspects of cognition are largely preserved. It is the dramatic, yet selective nature of the semantic disorder, together with characteristic behavioural alterations, that distinguishes semantic dementia from Alzheimer's disease (AD). Although relatively rare, recognition of the disorder is important because of its distinct implications for management. Moreover, in recent years it has attracted considerable academic interest because of its potential to shed light on the organization and neural basis of semantic memory. From a neurobiological perspective, a central interest is the relationship between semantic dementia and other forms of FTLD.

71.2 BACKGROUND

The term 'semantic dementia' was introduced in 1989 (Snowden et al., 1989) to encapsulate the multi-modal loss of knowledge that typifies the syndrome. Prior to this, there were seminal reports in the literature of patients, with circumscribed impairments of semantic memory associated with neurodegenerative disease, who would now be classified as having semantic dementia (Warrington, 1975; Schwartz et al., 1979). Moreover, in the classical neurological and psychiatric literature, there are patient descriptions (Pick, 1892; Rosenfeld, 1909) that appear prototypical of semantic dementia (Snowden, 2001). It is clear that semantic dementia has long existed.

Semantic dementia is frequently described within the context of primary progressive aphasia (Amici et al., 2006; see also Chapter 72, Primary progressive aphasia and posterior cortical atrophy). Since the earliest descriptions of progressive aphasia (Mesulam, 1982) it has been recognized that the language disorder is not uniform (Basso et al., 1988; Poeck and Luzzatti, 1988; Snowden, et al., 1992; Tyrrell et al., 1990a). Whereas some patients have non-fluent or hesitant speech production, others speak fluently and effortlessly. Patients with the fluent form commonly have a disorder of semantics that, on close examination, is found to extend beyond the verbal domain and is consistent with semantic

Table 71.1 Clinical diagnostic features of semantic dementia (Neary *et al.*, 1998).

I. Core diagnostic features	A. Insidious onset and gradual progression	
	B. Language disorder characterized by:	(i) progressive, fluent, empty spontaneous speech
		(ii) loss of word meaning, manifest by impaired naming and comprehension
		(iii) semantic paraphasias
	and/or	
	C. Perceptual disorder characterized by:	(i) prosopagnosia: impaired recognition of identity of familiar faces and/or
		(ii) associative agnosia: impaired recognition of object identity
	D. Preserved perceptual matching and drawing reproduction	
	E. Preserved single word repetition	
	F. Preserved ability to read aloud and write to dictation orthographically regular words	
II. Supportive diagnostic features	A. Speech and language	(i) press of speech
		(ii) idiosyncratic word usage
		(iii) absence of phonemic paraphasias
		(iv) surface dyslexia and dysgraphia
		(v) preserved calculation
	B. Behaviour	(i) loss of sympathy and empathy
		(ii) narrowed preoccupations
		(iii) parsimony
	C. Physical signs	(i) absent or late primitive reflexes
		(iii) akinesia, rigidity and tremor
	D. Neuropsychological testing	(i) profound semantic loss, manifest in failure of word comprehension and naming and/or face and object recognition
		(ii) preserved phonology and syntax, elementary perceptual processing, spatial skills and day-to-day memorizing
	E. Electrophysiology	normal
	F. Brain imaging (structural and/or functional)	predominant anterior temporal abnormality (symmetric or asymmetric)

dementia (Adlam *et al.*, 2006). Cases of progressive proso-pagnosia (Tyrrell *et al.*, 1990b; Evans *et al.*, 1995) are likely to represent right hemisphere presentations of semantic dementia (Josephs *et al.*, 2008).

71.3 DEMOGRAPHIC FEATURES

Semantic dementia most commonly presents between the ages of 50 and 70, affecting men and women equally. The median illness duration has been estimated at eight years (Snowden *et al.*, 1996), although some authors suggest that it may be longer (Hodges and Patterson, 2007). What is clear is that there is wide variation, with durations as short as three years and as long as 15 years. Most cases are sporadic, a positive family history being less common than in other forms of FTLD (Goldman *et al.*, 2005). There are no known geographical or socioeconomic factors which affect incidence. Accurate incidence and prevalence data are not currently available. In an analysis of patient referrals to a specialist dementia clinic in Manchester, patients with prototypical, 'pure' semantic dementia accounted for approximately 10 per cent of cases of frontotemporal lobe degeneration, which in turn accounted for about 25 per cent

of cases of primary degenerative dementia presenting before the age of 65 years.

71.4 PRESENTING COMPLAINTS

The presenting complaint is typically of a difficulty 'with words' or 'remembering things'. Careful history-taking reveals that the problem in 'remembering' is not one of memory loss in the traditional sense. Patients are able to remember day-to-day events, keep track of time, remember appointments, find their way around without becoming lost, and retain a degree of functional independence that would be incompatible with a classical amnesia. The problem lies in remembering what words mean, who people are and what objects are for. The presenting symptoms are most often in the verbal domain, manifest by patients' difficulty in the understanding and use of words, but occasionally are in the visual realm, manifest by a difficulty recognizing faces. Relatives may also report a failure of object recognition: for example, an inability to recognize fruits and vegetables in the supermarket. Medical referral is sometimes precipitated by accompanying behavioural alterations. Patients are typically physically well, without neurological symptoms.

71.5 COGNITIVE CHARACTERISTICS

71.5.1 Language

Patients speak fluently and effortlessly, with normal articulation and grammar and without phonological (sound-based) errors, giving the superficial impression of normal language. Indeed, patients are often garrulous (**Table 71.2**). Nevertheless, there is typically a reduction in content words, with reliance on broad generic terms and stereotyped usage of words and phrases Semantic errors (e.g. 'sock' for glove) may be present.

The semantic impairment, which may be scarcely apparent at clinical interview, becomes strikingly evident on formal testing of naming and word comprehension. Patients may score close to floor level on standard picture naming tasks and derive no benefit from first-letter cues. Word comprehension is also affected. Expressions of lack of understanding of previously familiar words (e.g. 'Tiger, tiger, what's a tiger? I don't know what that is') are a revealing demonstration of the loss of word meaning. There are known influences on naming performance. Common words are more likely to be named than low frequency terms (Lambon Ralph *et al.*, 1998) and items typical of a category better than atypical items (Woollams *et al.*, 2008). There is a tendency for vocabulary relating to patients' daily life to be better preserved than non-personally relevant vocabulary (Snowden, *et al.*, 1994; Snowden, *et al.*, 1995). Word comprehension and naming tests should therefore not be restricted to the common objects and body parts typically used in bedside testing, but should include names of animals, foods and objects, such as 'sheep', 'plum', 'violin' which are unlikely to relate directly to the patient's daily routine. Loss of knowledge about a word's meaning may not be absolute. The patient may, for example, know that a lemon is a food rather than an animal, but not know how it differs from an apple or banana. Assessment of word understanding should therefore probe knowledge of attributes, as well as broad category knowledge.

Language comprehension problems arise principally at the single word level. Comprehension of syntactic rules of language is typically relatively well preserved. Thus, a patient may respond with ease to the question, 'If the tiger is killed by the lion which animal is dead?', because it depends on syntactic understanding, while failing the apparently simpler question, 'Is a tiger bigger than a mouse?', which depends on understanding of nouns. Patients' ability to read aloud and write to dictation is relatively well preserved for words with regular spellings. However, patients read phonetically rather than for meaning, so produce 'regularization' errors (e.g. 'glove' pronounced to rhyme with 'rove' and 'stove'; 'pint' to rhyme with 'mint'), consistent with surface dyslexia (Patterson *et al.*, 1985). Parallel errors occur in writing (e.g. 'caught' written as 'cort').

With progression of disease, speech content is increasingly empty and stereotyped, but at no time is speech production non-fluent or effortful: conversational repertoire simply becomes progressively reduced until only a few stereotyped words or phrases remain.

71.5.2 Face and object recognition

Problems in recognizing familiar faces occur early in the course of disease. Difficulties are most profound for impersonal faces, such as those of celebrities, and least marked for family and friends with whom the patient maintains daily contact. Perceptual discrimination of faces (i.e. whether two faces are the same or different) is preserved.

Object recognition difficulties may not be apparent initially, but invariably emerge with disease progression. Recognition failure is not all or none. Thus, patients may be able to distinguish edible from non-edible objects, but fail to distinguish foods that are normally cooked (e.g. potatoes) and those normally eaten raw (e.g. lettuce). Patients may recognize a picture of a camel as an animal, but not know how it differs from a dog. Moreover, they may recognize and use entirely appropriately their own belongings while failing to recognize other examples of those same objects or pictures of those objects (Snowden *et al.*, 1994; Bozeat *et al.*, 2002). This latter feature helps to explain the clinical observation that patients function reasonably well within the narrow confines of their familiar environment and repertoire of daily activities at a time when abstract semantic knowledge is profoundly impaired. In time, even highly familiar objects may no longer be recognized.

Non-semantic aspects of object perception are well preserved. Patients can copy drawings normally, sometimes to a strikingly proficient level (Snowden *et al.*, 1996). They also have no difficulty carrying out perceptual matching tasks, which are not dependent upon recognition of object meaning.

Table 71.2 Characteristics of language disorder in semantic dementia.

Spontaneous speech	Fluent, effortless, often garrulous
	Empty content, reduced nominal terms
	Semantic paraphasias
	Substitution of generic terms
	Verbal stereotypies
	Preserved use of syntax
	Preserved phonology
	Normal articulation and prosody
Comprehension	Impaired word understanding
	Good understanding of syntax
Repetition	Relatively preserved
Naming	Profound anomia
	Semantic errors present (e.g. 'dog' for elephant)
	No benefit from phonemic cues
Reading	Fluent reading aloud
	Accurate reading of regular words
	Regularization of irregular words (surface dyslexia)
	Impaired comprehension of written material
Writing	Fluent, effortless execution
	Regularization of irregular words (e.g. 'cort' for caught) (surface dysgraphia)

71.5.3 Numeracy

Understanding of number concepts and the ability to carry out arithmetical procedures often appear remarkably well preserved (Cappelletti et al., 2001; Cappelletti et al., 2002; Crutch and Warrington, 2002), perhaps explaining why semantic dementia patients commonly enjoy number puzzles such as sudoku and television quiz shows involving numbers. Nevertheless, number concepts are not entirely normal (Julien et al., 2008). Eventually, arithmetical skills become compromised and patients cease to understand the meaning of spoken and written numerals.

71.5.4 Spatial skills

Spatial and navigational skills are generally excellent. Patients are able to find their way without becoming lost and may use spatial cues to compensate for object recognition difficulties (for example, by recalling the spatial location of food items on a supermarket shelf). On neuropsychological testing, patients typically perform well on traditional spatial tests, such as line orientation (Benton, et al., 1978), dot counting, position discrimination and cube estimation (Warrington and James, 1991), although in late stage disease performance may be compromised secondarily by their semantic disorder (e.g. failure to recall the names of numbers). Nevertheless, even in advanced disease, patients negotiate their environment skilfully, may recall the location of their chair or bed on a hospital ward, localize and manipulate with ease objects in the environment and spatially align objects perfectly.

71.5.5 Memory

A feature that is striking on clinical grounds and that helps to distinguish semantic dementia from other forms of dementia is the apparent preservation of patients' current autobiographical memory (Warrington, 1975; Snowden et al., 1996). Patients remember appointments and personally relevant events and keep track of time. They negotiate the environment without becoming lost. If they move home, they have no difficulty learning their new surroundings. In contrast, they show gross breakdown in impersonal, factual (semantic) knowledge, including knowledge about public figures and important world events. The preservation of autobiographical memory is not easily captured by standard memory tests, which typically involve lists of words, faces or line drawings that may have little meaning for the patient. Moreover, routine bedside questions, designed to probe orientation, such as 'What town are we in?' demand naming skills and thus may be compromised in semantic dementia. Time orientation scores are typically superior to those for place orientation, reflecting better preservation of number-related vocabulary. Testing of memory needs to include test materials which are meaningful to the patients and questions regarding the patient's own daily life. Episodic memory, assessed in a naturalistic setting, has been shown to be well preserved (Adlam et al., 2009).

71.5.6 Touch, taste, smell and hearing

Primary sensory abilities are well preserved, so patients have no difficulty detecting the presence of tactile, gustatory, olfactory and auditory stimuli and discriminating whether two stimuli are the same or different. However, the disorder of meaning extends to all sensory modalities (Snowden et al., 1996; Bozeat et al., 2000; Luzzi et al., 2007). Patients may have difficulty recognizing the identity of textures, tastes, smells and non-verbal sounds, such as the ringing of a telephone or doorbell, despite perceiving those stimuli normally.

71.6 BEHAVIOURAL CHANGES

Although the semantic deficits are the defining characteristic of the disorder, there are also accompanying behavioural changes (Snowden et al., 1996; Snowden et al., 2001), which are a source of great stress for families (**Table 71.3**). Patients become more self-centred, lacking in empathy, inflexible and intransigent. Their behavioural repertoire becomes narrowed and they frequently become preoccupied with one or two activities (e.g. painting, doing jigsaws, doing sudoku puzzles), which they pursue relentlessly and at which they are adept (Green and Patterson, 2009). Similarly, they may become mentally preoccupied by particular themes (e.g. the withdrawal of their driving licence), which they repeat incessantly to the exasperation of family members. Behaviour acquires a markedly stereotyped, compulsive quality. Patients adopt a fixed routine, will clock-watch, and carry out specific activities at precisely the same time each day. They often have a preference for order and may align objects, straighten out folds in the curtains and plump up the cushions as soon as a person rises from an armchair. Nevertheless, the affective responses of anxiety and release from anxiety associated with obsessional-compulsive disorder are typically absent.

Semantic dementia patients may show hypersensitivity to sensory stimuli and overact to light touch or to ostensibly innocuous environmental sounds. They may be oblivious to danger, probably linked to their loss of conceptual understanding of the world. They commonly show narrowed food preferences and usually favour sweet foods.

71.6.1 Insight

Patients are aware of and may become preoccupied by their difficulties. However, they frequently provide trivial

Table 71.3 Behavioural changes in semantic dementia.

Self-centredness (narrowed world view)
Inflexibility and intransigence
Preoccupation with limited range of activities
Preference for routine, clockwatching
Stereotypies, rituals and compulsions
Hyper-reactivity to sensory stimuli
Loss of awareness of danger
Food fads
Preference for sweet foods

explanations for them, such as being 'out of practice with talking' by virtue of being alone all day, and they demonstrate little real distress or concern. A likely reason is the absence of an internal 'model' of prior conceptual knowledge. Patients have no comparator by which to appreciate the magnitude of what they have lost.

71.7 NEUROLOGICAL SIGNS

Patients are generally physically well and free from neurological signs until late in the disease. Extrapyramidal signs of akinesia and rigidity, and frontal release phenomena may emerge in advanced disease. As in other forms of FTLD, neurological signs of motor neurone disease may occur in a minority of patients. Myoclonus does not occur.

71.8 BRAIN IMAGING

71.8.1 Structural brain imaging

Magnetic resonance imaging (MRI) shows cerebral atrophy, particularly marked in the anterior temporal lobes, and affecting inferior more than superior temporal gyri (Mummery *et al.*, 2000; Chan *et al.*, 2001; Rohrer *et al.*, 2008; Rohrer *et al.*, 2009). Although bilateral, the temporal lobe atrophy is often asymmetric (**Figure 71.1**), the left or right predominance being associated with clinical presentations emphasizing word meaning or face recognition disorder, respectively. With progression, there is atrophy spread within both hemispheres (Brambati *et al.*, 2009), although asymmetries may be manifest even at end-stage disease.

71.8.2 Functional brain imaging

positron emission tomography (PET) (Diehl *et al.*, 2004; Desgranges *et al.*, 2007) and single photon emission tomography (SPECT) show abnormalities in the anterior cerebral hemispheres, particularly the temporal regions. Appearances may be asymmetrical, affecting disproportionately the left or right hemisphere.

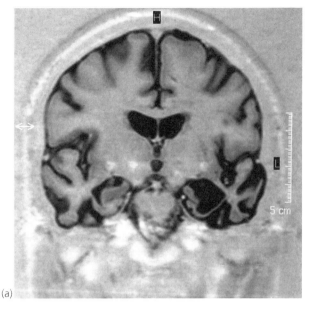

(a)

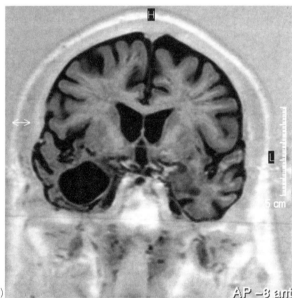

(b)

Figure 71.1 Magnetic resonance images of two patients with semantic dementia showing severe temporal lobe atrophy. In one case (a) atrophy is more marked on the left side and in the other case (b) on the right.

71.9 NEUROPATHOLOGY

The striking feature on macroscopic examination is atrophy of the temporal lobes. Atrophy is bilateral, but often asymmetrical and affects particularly anterior and inferior parts of the temporal lobes (Snowden *et al.*, 1996). Frontal cortex is affected to a lesser degree. There is relative sparing of superior temporal gyrus, parietal and occipital cortex.

The histopathological changes found in FTLD are now known to be heterogeneous (see Chapter 70, The genetics and molecular pathology of frontotemporal lobar degeneration). A primary distinction is between tau-positive and tau-negative, ubiquitin-positive cases, TDP-43 being identified as the

target protein in the majority of ubiquitin positive cases (Cairns *et al.*, 2007; Mackenzie *et al.*, 2009). Ubiquitin histology has been further divided into three major subtypes on the basis of the relative preponderance of neuronal cytoplasmic inclusions, dystrophic neurites and neuronal intranuclear inclusions. Interestingly, in the light of this pathological diversity, the underlying pathology in semantic dementia is remarkably uniform. Pure semantic dementia cases are consistently associated with tau-negative, TDP-43 positive histology (Rossor *et al.*, 2000; Snowden *et al.*, 2007; Josephs *et al.*, 2009) and the ubiquitin subtype characterized by a preponderance of dystrophic neurites within cerebral cortex (Snowden *et al.*, 2007; Josephs *et al.*, 2009).

Tau pathology has been associated with a mixed clinical picture in which the frontal behavioural disorder of FTD is combined with the multimodal semantic impairment of semantic dementia (Pickering-Brown *et al.*, 2002).

In some series, a minority of patients clinically diagnosed with semantic dementia have proven ultimately to have AD pathology (Davies *et al.*, 2005). Such findings exemplify the fact that semantic impairment may be a prominent feature in some AD patients and so can be mistaken for semantic dementia. Such patients are typically differentiable clinically on the basis of the presence of classical amnesia in addition to their semantic impairment.

71.10 MOLECULAR GENETICS

Semantic dementia, in its pure form, has not been linked to mutations in either the *tau* or *progranulin* gene on chromosome 17, as found in a proportion of cases of FTD and PNFA (see Chapter 70, The genetics and molecular pathology of frontotemporal lobar degeneration). However, +16 tau mutations have been associated with a mixed clinical picture, in which a prominent 'frontal' behavioural disorder consistent with FTD is combined with semantic loss (Pickering-Brown *et al.*, 2002).

71.11 RELATIONSHIP BETWEEN SEMANTIC DEMENTIA AND OTHER FORMS OF FTLD

The established association between semantic dementia and the 'frontal' behavioural disorder of FTD and the expressive language disorder of PNFA comes from several sources: (1) the existence of mixed/overlapping clinical phenotypes (e.g. Pickering-Brown *et al.*, 2002), (2) the association of each syndrome with motor neurone disease (Neary, *et al.*, 1990; Caselli, *et al.*, 1993), (3) common underlying pathologies. This latter point requires elaboration. The assumption until recently was that the clinical syndrome of FTLD reflected the anatomical distribution of pathological change within the anterior hemispheres (the temporal lobes in semantic dementia, the frontal lobes and temporal poles in FTD and perisylvian regions of the left hemisphere in PNFA), but

could not predict the underlying pathology (tau or non-tau), which could be associated with each syndrome. Nevertheless, refinement of histopathological characterization has challenged this assumption. There is a closer mapping between clinical phenotype and underlying histopathology than previously thought. Whereas non-tau, TDP-43 pathology is characteristic in semantic dementia (Snowden *et al.*, 2007; Josephs *et al.*, 2009) tau pathology is common in PNFA (Josephs *et al.*, 2006; Knibb *et al.*, 2006). Among TDP-43 cases, semantic dementia cases are almost invariably associated with the ubiquitin subtype in which dystrophic neurites predominate (Snowden *et al.*, 2007; Josephs *et al.*, 2009), whereas neuronal intranuclear inclusions are found in PNFA (Snowden *et al.*, 2007; Josephs *et al.*, 2009). Such findings suggest that clinical phenotype has significant implications for underlying neurobiology.

71.12 DIFFERENTIATION FROM FTD

Semantic dementia is unlikely to be confused with the behavioural syndrome of FTD on cognitive grounds (see Chapter 68, Frontotemporal dementia). The problems in word and object recognition are quite distinct from the frontal executive failures of FTD. Nevertheless, both semantic dementia and FTD involve behavioural change, which may appear superficially similar, leading to confusion in classification of phenotype. Closer examination does, however, reveal differences between the 'temporal' behaviours of semantic dementia and the 'frontal' behaviours of FTD (**Table 71.4**) (Snowden *et al.*, 1996; Snowden *et al.*, 2001).

- In FTD, behaviour tends to be unproductive and lacking in goal direction, whereas in semantic dementia behavioural routines may be remarkably complex.
- In FTD, there is poor mental application and impersistence, whereas patients with semantic dementia frequently show dogged persistence, albeit on a narrowed range of activities.
- FTD patients show generalized blunting of emotions. In semantic dementia, affective changes are more selective, typically affecting particularly the capacity to show fear.

Table 71.4 Behavioural differences between semantic dementia and frontotemporal dementia.

	Semantic dementia	Frontotemporal dementia
Affect	Restricted impairment	Pervasive loss of emotions
	Concern for illness	Unconcern
Social behaviour	Exaggerated sociability	Reduced sociability
Interest and motivation	Narrowed interests	General loss of interest
Response to sensory stimuli	Exaggerated	Diminished
Eating	Food fads	Gluttony, indiscriminate eating
Wandering	No wandering	Wandering common
Pacing fixed route	Absent	May be present
Repetitive behaviours	Complex routines common	Simple motor stereotypies more likely
	Repetitive themes	No repetitive themes
	Clockwatches	Unconcerned by time
	Compulsive quality	No compulsive quality

- Patients with FTD show a lack of concern with personal appearance and hygiene, whereas the latter may become a source of preoccupation in patients with semantic dementia.
- FTD patients may show reduced sensitivity to pain, whereas semantic dementia patients are more likely to show an exaggerated response to sensory stimuli.
- FTD patients commonly exhibit gluttony and indiscriminate eating, whereas semantic dementia patients are more likely to show food fads.
- Repetitive behaviours have a more compulsive quality in semantic dementia than FTD, particulary the apathetic form. Disinhibited FTD patients with more circumscribed atrophy of the orbitofrontal lobes and temporal pole may show some overlap with semantic dementia.

To complicate classification, some patients show, from the outset or with progression of disease, a mixed clinical phenotype, combining the 'frontal' behaviour of FTD with the semantic impairment of semantic dementia.

71.13 DIFFERENTIATION FROM AD

Semantic dementia is most likely to be confused with AD. This is unsurprising because presenting complaints in both are commonly of 'memory' problems and signs of semantic disorder may not be obvious at initial interview (**Table 71.5**). Nevertheless, the typical clinical profiles are very different (**Table 71.6**).

- In semantic dementia, 'memory loss' refers to loss of impersonal, conceptual knowledge about the world, whereas personal, autobiographical memories remain relatively well preserved. In AD, the converse is true.
- In semantic dementia, speech production is fluent and effortless. In AD, it is typically hesitant, suggesting a difficulty in retrieving words, and sentences may be unfinished reflecting loss of train of thought. There may be phonological errors and in later stages a festinant speech quality.
- In semantic dementia, comprehension is most impaired for words and better preserved for syntax, whereas in AD the reverse is the case.
- Numerical skills are well preserved in semantic dementia, whereas calculation problems are affected early in AD.
- Spatial abilities are well preserved in semantic dementia, whereas AD patients commonly show difficulty orientating clothing when dressing and topographical disorientation within a familiar environment.
- Patients with both semantic dementia and AD may have object recognition problems. In semantic dementia, the difficulty lies in assigning meaning to objects that are perceived normally (associative agnosia). They can copy drawings of objects that they cannot recognize. In AD, perceptual breakdown lies at the level of achieving an integrated percept (apperceptive agnosia). Patients may interpret elements of a figure instead of the overall outline (e.g. a pair of scissors identified as a bowl on the basis of the circular handle). They have difficulty copying line drawings, their copies often being fragmented with loss of the spatial relationships between elements of the figure.

Table 71.5 Five factors affecting poor recognition of semantic dementia.

1. Rare disorder
2. Historical reports of 'memory' disorder
3. Semantic disorder may not be evident at clinical interview
4. Semantic impairments may be misinterpreted as classical amnesia
5. Need explicit tests of word comprehension and naming, face and object recognition

Table 71.6 Clinical differences between semantic dementia and Alzheimer's disease.

	Semantic dementia	Alzheimer's disease
Age of onset	Most common in middle age	Most common in elderly
Language	Selective semantic disorder	No selective semantic disorder
	Impaired single word comprehension	Impaired sentence comprehension
Perception	Associative agnosia	Apperceptive agnosia
Calculation	Preserved early in course	Impaired early in course
Spatial orientation	Preserved	Impaired early in course
Constructional skills	Preserved	Impaired early in course
Memory	Autobiographical memory preserved	Autobiographical memory impaired
Neurological signs	Akinesia and rigidity relatively late	Akinesia and rigidity relatively early
	Myoclonus absent	Myoclonus may be present
Electroencephalography	Normal	Slowing of wave forms
Structural brain imaging	Focal temporal lobe atrophy typical	Focal atrophy rare
	Hippocampi relatively preserved	Hippocampi atrophic
	Marked hemispheric asymmetry common	Marked asymmetry rare
Functional brain imaging	Anterior hemisphere abnormalities	Posterior hemisphere abnormalities
	Marked hemispheric asymmetry common	Marked asymmetry rare

Notwithstanding these distinct profiles, there are some patients in whom diagnosis can be difficult. Semantic impairment may occur in AD (Hodges and Patterson, 1995; Rogers and Friedman, 2008) and in some patients it is a prominent feature (Alladi *et al.*, 2007). Diagnostic differentiation in such cases is likely to lie in the degree of accompanying amnesia.

71.14 TREATMENT AND MANAGEMENT

Pharmacological therapies for AD do not have a rational role in semantic dementia, because there is no demonstrated evidence of abnormalities in the cholinergic system (Francis *et al.*, 1993). In patients with problematic behavioural changes, symptomatic treatment may be warranted. Repetitive, stereotypic behaviours may respond to serotonin reuptake inhibitors.

With regard to practical management, it is of relevance that concepts (of words, object meaning, etc.), relevant to the patient's daily life appear to be better retained than those which have no personal relevance (Snowden *et al.*, 1994; Snowden *et al.*, 1995; Westmacott *et al.*, 2003). It has been argued that this feature results from patients' preserved autobiographical memory: concepts, which would otherwise be lost in their abstract sense, have some meaning to the patient if they are framed within the context of the patient's ongoing daily experience. By implication, input from speech therapists is more likely to be beneficial if this takes place in the patient's own surroundings using as referents patients' own belongings, than in the abstract setting of a clinical consulting room using standard pictorial materials.

There is clinical evidence in semantic dementia that some learning is possible. Patients may, for example, effectively learn the names of new acquaintances and the names of medicines prescribed to them. They may also succeed in relearning lost vocabulary (Graham *et al.*, 1999; Snowden and Neary, 2002; Henry *et al.*, 2008). However, such reacquired knowledge is tenuous and vocabulary can be maintained only as long as those words are used regularly and are linked to patients' ongoing daily experience.

71.15 THEORETICAL ISSUES

Semantic dementia has attracted considerable theoretical interest from neuropsychologists. Because of its circumscribed nature, it is a natural experimental model for understanding how the brain represents conceptual knowledge.

Issues that have been addressed include:

- The role of the two hemispheres in meaning representation. The traditional view has been that semantic memory is particularly dependent on the left hemisphere. However, patients with semantic dementia provide evidence that both hemispheres contribute and may have different roles (Thompson *et al.*, 2003; Thompson *et al.*, 2004; Snowden *et al.*, 2004).

- The representation of different categories of information. Patients with semantic dementia may show disproportionate impairment in their knowledge of some categories (e.g. animals and vegetables) compared to others (e.g. household objects) (Basso *et al.*, 1988; Cardebat *et al.*, 1996). Such findings have been interpreted by some in terms of a distributed model in which different properties of objects, such as sensory features and functional attributes are represented separately (Warrington and McCarthy, 1987; Warrington and Shallice, 1984). Others (Caramazza and Shelton, 1998; Martin, 2007) have argued for a categorical organization of conceptual knowledge.

- The relationship between semantic memory and episodic memory. Semantic memory is regarded as abstract knowledge independent of experience. However, findings in semantic dementia patients (Snowden *et al.*, 1994; Snowden *et al.*, 1995; Westmacott *et al.*, 2003) suggest a closer relationship between knowledge and personal experience and interdependence between memory systems than generally recognized.

- Multimodal versus amodal accounts of semantic representation. The existence of a distributed semantic network is generally accepted. More contentious is whether semantic concepts are represented by modality-specific patterns of connectivity alone (Lauro-Grotto *et al.*, 1997) or whether there is an additional supramodal or 'amodal' level of representation, the anterior temporal lobes constituting an amodal 'hub' (Patterson *et al.*, 2007).

71.16 CONCLUSION

Semantic dementia is a striking disorder, clinically distinct from AD and other forms of dementia. Patients exhibit unique patterns of cognitive and behavioural symptomatology, which demand novel approaches to treatment and management. Neuropsychological studies are required to improve understanding of the cognitive characteristics of the disorder. Meanwhile, advances in molecular genetic research ought to shed light on the underlying aetiology of this and other clinical manifestations of frontotemporal lobar degeneration.

REFERENCES

Adlam AL, Patterson K, Rogers YY *et al.* (2006) Semantic dementia and fluent primary progressive aphasia: two sides of the same coin? *Brain* **129**: 3066–80.

Adlam AL, Patterson K, Hodges JR. (2009) 'I remember it as if it were yesterday'. Memory for recent events in patients with semantic dementia. *Neuropsychologia* **47**: 1344–51.

Alladi S, Xuereb J, Bak T *et al.* (2007) Focal cortical presentations of Alzheimer's disease. *Brain* **130**: 2636–45.

Amici S, Gorno-Tempini ML, Ogar JM *et al.* (2006) An overview of primary progressive aphasia and its variants. *Behavioural Neurology* **17**: 77–87.

Basso A, Capitani E, Laiacona M. (1988) Progressive language impairment without dementia: a case with isolated category specific semantic defect. *Journal of Neurology, Neurosurgery and Psychiatry* **51**: 1201–7.

Benton AL, Varney NR, Hamsher KD. (1978) Visuo-spatial judgement: a clinical test. *Archives of Neurology* **35**: 364–7.

Bozeat S, Lambon Ralph MA, Patterson K et al. (2000) Non-verbal semantic impairment in semantic dementia. *Neuropsychologia* **38**: 1207–15.

Bozeat S, Lambon Ralph MA, Patterson K, Hodges J. (2002) The influence of personal familiarity and context on object use in semantic dementia. *Neurocase* **8**: 127–34.

Brambati SM, Rankin KP, Narvid J et al. (2009) Atrophy progression in semantic dementia with asymmetric temporal involvement: a tensor-based morphometry study. *Neurobiology of Aging* **30**: 103–11.

Cairns NJ, Biggio EH, Mackenzie IRA et al. (2007) Neuropathological diagnostic criteria and nosology of the frontotemporal lobar degenerations: consensus criteria of the Consortium for Frontotemporal Lobar Degenerations. *Acta Neuropathologica* **114**: 5–22.

Cappelletti M, Butterworth B, Kopelman M. (2001) Spared numerical abilities in a case of semantic dementia. *Neuropsychologia* **39**: 1224–39.

Cappelletti M, Kopelman M, Butterworth B. (2002) Why semantic dementia drives you to the dogs (but not to the horses): a thoeretical account. *Cognitive Neuropsychology* **19**: 483–503.

Caramazza A, Shelton J. (1998) Domain-specific knowledge in the brain: the animate–inanimate distinction. *Journal of Cognitive Neuroscience* **10**: 1–34.

Cardebat D, Demonet JF, Celsis P, Puel M. (1996) Living/non-living dissociation in a case of semantic dementia: A SPECT activation study. *Neuropsychologia* **34**: 1175–9.

Caselli RJ, Windebank AJ, Petersen RC et al. (1993) Rapidly progressive aphasic dementia with motor neuron disease. *Annals of Neurology* **33**: 200–7.

Chan D, Fox NC, Scahill RI et al. (2001) Patterns of temporal lobe atrophy in semantic dementia and Alzheimer's disease. *Annals of Neurology* **49**: 433–42.

Crutch SJ, Warrington EK. (2002) Preserved calculation skills in a case of semantic dementia. *Cortex* **38**: 389–99.

Davies RR, Hodges JR, Kril J et al. (2005) The pathological basis of semantic dementia. *Brain* **128**: 1984–95.

Desgranges B, Matuszewski V, Piolino P et al. (2007) Anatomical and functional alterations in semantic dementia: a voxel-based MRI and PET study. *Neurobiology of Aging* **28**: 1904–13.

Diehl J, Grimmer T, Drzezga A et al. (2004) Cerebral metabolic patterns at early states of frontotemporal dementia and semantic dementia: a PET study. *Neurobiology of Aging* **25**: 1051–6.

Evans JJ, Heggs AJ, Antoun N, Hodges JR. (1995) Progressive prosopagnosia associated with selective right temporal lobe atrophy: a new syndrome? *Brain* **118**: 1–13.

Francis PT, Holmes C, Webster M-T et al. (1993) Preliminary neurochemical findings in non-Alzheimer dementia due to lobar atrophy. *Dementia* **4**: 172–7.

Goldman JS, Farmer JM, Wood EM et al. (2005) Comparison of family histories in FTLD subtypes and related tauopathies. *Neurology* **65**: 1817–19.

Graham KS, Patterson K, Pratt KH, Hodges JR. (1999) Relearning and subsequent forgetting of semantic category exemplars in a case of semantic dementia. *Neuropsychology* **13**: 359–80.

Green HA, Patterson K. (2009) Jigsaws – A preserved ability in semantic dementia. *Neuropsychologia* **47**: 569–76.

Henry ML, Beeson PM, Rapcsak SZ. (2008) Treatment for anomia in semantic dementia. *Seminars in Speech and Language* **29**: 60–70.

Hodges JR, Patterson K. (1995) Is semantic memory consistently impaired early in the course of Alzheimer's disease? Neuroanatomical and diagnostic implications. *Neuropsychologia* **33**: 441–59.

Hodges JR, Patterson K. (2007) Semantic dementia: a unique clinicopathological syndrome. *Lancet Neurology* **6**: 1004–14.

Hodges JR, Patterson K, Oxbury S, Funnell E. (1992) Semantic dementia. Progressive fluent aphasia with temporal lobe atrophy. *Brain* **115**: 1783–806.

Josephs KA, Duffy JR, Strand EA et al. (2006) Clinicopathological and imaging correlates of progressive aphasia and apraxia of speech. *Brain* **129**: 1385–98.

Josephs KA, Whitwell JL, Vemuri P et al. (2008) The anatomic correlate of prosopagnosia in semantic dementia. *Neurology* **71**: 1628–33.

Josephs KA, Stroh A, Dugger B, Dickson DW. (2009) Evaluation of subcortical pathology and clinical correlations in FTLD-U subtypes. *Acta Neuropathologica* **118**: 349–58.

Julien CL, Thompson JC, Neary D, Snowden JS. (2008) Arithmetic knowledge in semantic dementia: is it invariably preserved? *Neuropsychologia* **46**: 2732–44.

Knibb JA, Xuereb JH, Patterson K, Hodges JR. (2006) Clinical and pathological characterization of progressive aphasia. *Annals of Neurology* **59**: 156–65.

Lambon Ralph MA, Graham KS, Ellis AW, Hodges JR. (1998) Naming in semantic dementia – what matters? *Neuropsychologia* **36**: 775–84.

Lauro-Grotto R, Piccini C, Shallice T. (1997) Modality-specific operations in semantic dementia. *Cortex* **33**: 593–622.

Luzzi S, Snowden JS, Neary D et al. (2007) Distinct patterns of olfactory impairment in Alzheimer's disease, semantic dementia, frontotemporal dementia and corticobasal degeneration. *Neuropsychologia* **45**: 1823–31.

Mackenzie IRA, Neumann M, Bigio EH et al. (2009) Nomenclature for neuropathologic subtypes of frontotemporal lobar degeneration: consensus recommendations. *Acta Neuropathologica* **117**: 15–18.

Martin A. (2007) The representation of object concepts in the brain. *Annual Review of Psychology* **58**: 25–45.

Mesulam M. (1982) Slowly progressive aphasia without generalised dementia. *Annals of Neurology* **11**: 592–8.

Mummery CJ, Patterson K, Price CJ et al. (2000) A voxel-based morphometry study of semantic dementia: relationship between temporal lobe atrophy and semantic memory. *Annals of Neurology* **47**: 36–45.

Neary D, Snowden JS, Mann DMA *et al.* (1990) Frontal lobe dementia and motor neuron disease. *Journal of Neurology, Neurosurgery and Psychiatry* **53**: 23–32.

Neary D, Snowden JS, Gustafson L *et al.* (1998) Frontotemporal lobar degeneration. A consensus on clinical diagnostic criteria. *Neurology* **51**: 1546–54.

Patterson KE, Marshall JC, Coltheart M. (1985) *Surface dyslexia: Neuropsychological and cognitive studies of phonological reading.* Hove: Erlbaum.

Patterson K, Nestor PJ, Rogers TT. (2007) Where do you know what you know? The representation of semantic knowledge in the human brain. *Nature* **8**: 976–87.

Pick A. (1892) Uber die Beziehungen der senilen Hirnatrophie zur Aphasie. *Prager Medizinische Wochenschrift* **17**: 165–7.

Pickering-Brown SM, Richardson AM, Snowden JS *et al.* (2002) Inherited frontotemporal dementia in nine British families associated with intronic mutations in the tau gene. *Brain* **125**: 732–51.

Poeck K, Luzzatti C. (1988) Slowly progressive aphasia in three patients. The problem of accompanying neuropsychological deficit. *Brain* **111**: 151–68.

Rogers SL, Friedman RB. (2008) The underlying mechanisms of semantic memory loss in Alzheimer's disease and semantic dementia. *Neuropsychologia* **46**: 12–21.

Rohrer JD, McNaught E, Foster J *et al.* (2008) Tracking progression in frontotemporal lobar degeneration: serial MRI in semantic dementia. *Neurology* **71**: 1445–51.

Rohrer JD, Warren JD, Modat M *et al.* (2009) Patterns of cortical thinning in the language variants of frontotemporal lobar degeneration. *Neurology* **72**: 1562–9.

Rosenfeld M. (1909) Die partielle Grosshirnatrophie. *Zeitschrift für Psychologie und Neurologie* **14**: 115–30.

Rossor MN, Revesz T, Lantos PL, Warrington EK. (2000) Semantic dementia with ubiquitin-positive tau-negative inclusion bodies. *Brain* **123**: 267–76.

Schwartz MF, Marin OSM, Saffran EM. (1979) Dissociations of language function in dementia: a case study. *Brain and Language* **7**: 277–306.

Snowden JS. (2001) Commentary on Liepmann 1908 and Rosenfeld 1909. *Cortex* **37**: 563–71.

Snowden JS, Neary D. (2002) Relearning of verbal labels in semantic dementia. *Neuropsychologia* **40**: 1715–28.

Snowden JS, Goulding PJ, Neary D. (1989) Semantic dementia: a form of circumscribed atrophy. *Behavioural Neurology* **2**: 167–82.

Snowden JS, Neary D, Mann DMA *et al.* (1992) Progressive language disorder due to lobar atrophy. *Annals of Neurology* **31**: 174–83.

Snowden JS, Griffiths H, Neary D. (1994) Semantic dementia: autobiographical contribution to preservation of meaning. *Cognitive Neuropsychology* **11**: 265–88.

Snowden JS, Griffiths HL, Neary D. (1995) Autobiographical experience and word meaning. *Memory* **3**: 225–46.

Snowden JS, Neary D, Mann DMA. (1996) *Frontotemporal lobar degneration: frontotemporal dementia, progressive aphasia, semantic dementia.* London: Chuchill-Livingstone.

Snowden JS, Bathgate D, Varma A *et al.* (2001) Distinct behavioural profiles in frontotemporal dementia and semantic dementia. *Journal of Neurology, Neurosurgery and Psychiatry* **70**: 323–32.

Snowden JS, Thompson JC, Neary D. (2004) Knowledge of famous faces and names in semantic dementia. *Brain* **127**: 860–72.

Snowden JS, Neary D, Mann D. (2007) Frontotemporal lobar degeneration: clinical and pathological relationships. *Acta Neuropathogica* **114**: 31–8.

Thompson SA, Patterson K, Hodges JR. (2003) Left/right asymmetry of atrophy in semantic dementia: behavioural–cognitive implications. *Neurology* **61**: 1196–203.

Thompson SA, Graham KS, Williams G *et al.* (2004) Dissociating person-specific from general semantic knowledge: roles of the left and right temporal lobes. *Neuropsychologia* **42**: 359–70.

Tyrrell PJ, Warrington EK, Frackowiak RSJ, Rossor MN. (1990a) Heterogeneity in progressive aphasia due to focal cortical atrophy. A clinical and PET study. *Brain* **113**: 1321–36.

Tyrrell PJ, Warrington EK, Frackowiak RSJ, Rossor MN. (1990b) Progressive degeneration of the right temporal lobe studied with positron emission tomography. *Journal of Neurology, Neurosurgery and Psychiatry* **53**: 1046–50.

Warrington EK. (1975) The selective impairment of semantic memory. *Quarterly Journal of Experimental Psychology* **27**: 635–7.

Warrington EK, James M. (1991) *The visual object and space perception battery.* Bury St Edmonds: Thames Valley Test Company.

Warrington EK, McCarthy RA. (1987) Categories of knowledge: further fractionations and an attempted integration. *Brain* **110**: 1273–96.

Warrington EK, Shallice T. (1984) Category specific semantic impairments. *Brain* **107**: 829–54.

Westmacott R, Black SE, Freedman M, Moscovitch M. (2003) The contribution of autobiographical significance to semantic memory: evidence from Alzheimer's disease, semantic dementia and amnesia. *Neuropsychologia* **42**: 25–48.

Woollams AM, Cooper-Pye E, Hodges JR, Patterson K. (2008) Anomia: a doubly typical signature of semantic dementia. *Neuropsychologia* **46**: 2503–14.

Primary progressive aphasia and posterior cortical atrophy

JONATHAN D ROHRER, SEBASTIAN J CRUTCH, JASON D WARREN AND MARTIN N ROSSOR

72.1 INTRODUCTION

This chapter has two sections covering the focal dementia syndromes of primary progressive nonfluent aphasia and posterior cortical atrophy.

72.2 PROGRESSIVE NONFLUENT APHASIA AND THE LOGOPENIC/PHONOLOGICAL VARIANT OF PRIMARY PROGRESSIVE APHASIA

72.2.1 Introduction and nosology

The term 'primary progressive aphasia' (PPA) has been used to encompass all patients with progressive language impairment as the initial feature of a degenerative disorder (Mesulam, 1982; Mesulam, 2001; Mesulam, 2003). There is genetic and pathological overlap with the frontotemporal lobar degeneration (FTLD) spectrum (Neary et al., 1998; Mackenzie and Rademakers, 2007). Although some researchers have classified all language disorders under this one term (Mesulam, 2001; Mesulam et al., 2003), a number of subtypes can be identified (Grossman et al., 2004; Amici et al., 2006; Hodges and Patterson, 2007; Mesulam et al., 2007; Rohrer et al., 2008a). The fluency of speech output forms the basis for a simple clinical descriptive sub-classification of PPA i.e. 'fluent' and 'nonfluent' aphasias. Although fluency is hard to operationalize, nonfluency has generally been used to refer to reduced, effortful or sparse speech. Semantic dementia (SD) is an homogeneous clinicopathological entity with characteristic clinical, neuropsychological and radiological findings (see Chapter 71, Semantic dementia). SD presents usually with a 'fluent' aphasia (Adlam et al., 2006); however two other major PPA syndromes are associated with 'nonfluent' language output: these nonfluent disorders, progressive nonfluent aphasia (PNFA) and logopenic/phonological aphasia (LPA), are discussed below. It is unclear if these are the only subtypes of PPA and how this heterogeneous group of conditions maps on to the underlying genetic and pathological causes. While early PNFA can resemble Broca's aphasia and early LPA may resemble conduction aphasia (Hachisuka et al., 1999; reviewed in Rohrer et al., 2008a), the PPA subtypes do not correspond closely with the acute aphasia syndromes of stroke, due both to differing neuroanatomical patterns of involvement and the progressive nature of the disease. Although there are 'consensus' criteria for PNFA and SD (Neary et al., 1998) and other criteria for PPA as a unitary syndrome (Mesulam, 2001; Mesulam, 2003), these are not universally agreed. Descriptive clinical criteria for PNFA, SD and LPA are under revision.

72.2.2 Synonyms

- Progressive nonfluent aphasia (PNFA), nonfluent progressive aphasia (NFPA), progressive apraxia of speech, agrammatic variant of PPA.
- Logopenic/phonological aphasia (LPA), logopenic aphasia (LPA), progressive logopenic aphasia (PLA), logopenic variant of PPA.
- Semantic dementia (SD), fluent variant of PPA, semantic variant of PPA, 'Gogi aphasia'.

72.2.3   Epidemiology

The PPA variants are uncommon, although there are no large epidemiological studies. There are no clearly associated non-genetic risk factors for PPA, although one study showed an increased frequency of learning disability in PPA patients and their first-degree relatives (Rogalski *et al.*, 2008).

72.2.4   Genetics

PNFA is usually sporadic, but can rarely be familial (Krefft *et al.*, 2003; Goldman *et al.*, 2005). In one study, PNFA was associated with an autosomal dominant family history of PPA or FTLD in 6.9 per cent of cases (Goldman *et al.*, 2005). The heritability of LPA is less clear. Many familial PPA patients have mutations in the progranulin (*GRN*) gene (Snowden *et al.*, 2006; Mesulam *et al.*, 2007; Snowden *et al.*, 2007a; Beck *et al.*, 2008) which is associated with FTLD-TDP type 3 pathology (Sampathu/Cairns classification). However, some familial PPA cases lack *GRN* mutations (Janssen *et al.*, 2005; Beck *et al.*, 2008). In contrast, SD is very rarely familial. There have been inconsistent results from studies investigating apolipoprotein E (ApoE) and prion protein (*PRNP*) codon 129 genotypes, as well as microtubule associated protein tau (*MAPT*) haplotype in PPA, and no clear genetic risk factors have emerged (Mesulam *et al.*, 1997; Sobrido *et al.*, 2003; Gorno-Tempini *et al.*, 2004; Li *et al.*, 2005; Acciarri *et al.*, 2006; Rohrer *et al.*, 2006; Daniele *et al.*, 2009).

72.2.5   Pathology

The main pathological causes of PPA fall into three categories: the two major FTLD pathologies known as FTLD-tau and FTLD-TDP (where TDP is the TAR DNA-binding protein) and Alzheimer's disease (AD) pathology. SD is typically a FTLD-TDP type 1 disorder (Sampathu/Cairns classification), but can rarely be caused by FTLD-tau Pick's disease or AD pathology (Knibb *et al.*, 2006; Snowden *et al.*, 2007b; Pereira *et al.*, 2009). In contrast, PNFA can be caused by all three pathologies, although patients with a prominent motor speech impairment are associated particularly with the FTLD-tau pathologies, corticobasal degeneration, progressive supranuclear palsy and Pick's disease (Josephs *et al.*, 2006), rather than FTLD-TDP. However, a single case of progressive motor speech impairment and AD pathology is reported (Gerstner *et al.*, 2007). LPA is most commonly associated with AD pathology, although some cases have FTLD-TDP inclusions (Mesulam *et al.*, 2008). Prior to the detailed description of LPA, a number of researchers described an atypical language variant of AD, many cases of which might now be characterized as LPA (Greene *et al.*, 1996; Galton *et al.*, 2000; Alladi *et al.*, 2007; Josephs *et al.*, 2008). Those PPA cases associated with *GRN* mutations fall within the FTLD-TDP spectrum pathologically (see **Figure 72.1** for a schematic diagram of the clinicopathological associations of PPA).

72.2.6   Clinical and neuropsychological features

Table 72.1 summarizes the clinical and neuropsychological features of the PPA syndromes; SD is included for comparison.

72.2.7   Progressive nonfluent aphasia

72.2.7.1   SPONTANEOUS SPEECH

The characteristic features of PNFA are the presence of agrammatism and hesitant, effortful speech secondary to a motor speech impairment characterized as an apraxia of speech (AOS) (Weintraub *et al.*, 1990; Tyrrell *et al.*, 1991; Turner *et al.*, 1996; Westbury and Bub, 1997; Neary *et al.*, 1998; Gorno-Tempini *et al.*, 2004; Ogar *et al.*, 2007). Either of these features may dominate at presentation. There is controversy as to which is the core deficit and how they relate to each other. Cases of pure progressive apraxia of speech have been described, but most such cases with longitudinal follow up appear to develop agrammatism/aphasia. Similarly, there are patients who initially have pure agrammatism. Both symptoms are neuroanatomically related to left inferior frontal/insular atrophy and it is unsurprising that they commonly co-occur. Nonetheless, some authorities exclude pure motor speech impairment in the absence of other speech and language deficits from the PPA spectrum (Mesulam *et al.*, 2007). One other difficulty lies in defining apraxia of speech (a problem of planning articulation) so that it is uniformly applied by different centres (Ogar *et al.*, 2005); the key features are difficulty initiating speech and trial and error groping towards the correct word leading to dysprosodic, hesitant and effortful speech output. Errors in patients with apraxia of speech are sound distortions (often additions) and are termed 'apraxic' or 'phonetic' errors. In practice, these can be difficult to distinguish from phonemic errors due to the incorrectly selected sound, although it is likely that both phonetic and phonemic errors occur in PNFA. The importance of defining patients as PNFA with or without motor speech impairment is the association with a particular pathology; AOS is likely to predict tau-positive histopathology (Josephs *et al.*, 2006). In imaging studies, apraxia of speech is associated with premotor and supplementary motor areas (Josephs *et al.*, 2006), as well as the insula and basal ganglia (Ogar *et al.*, 2007). Most patients eventually become mute, although non-speech vocalizations, such as laughter, may be present even when there is no speech (Rohrer *et al.*, 2009b). Early mutism in PNFA has been associated with left pars opercularis and basal ganglia atrophy (Gorno-Tempini *et al.*, 2006).

72.2.7.2   NAMING AND SINGLE WORD COMPREHENSION

Other features include anomia (initially mild). Verb naming may be affected more than nouns (broadly, the reverse pattern to that seen in SD) (Hillis *et al.*, 2002; Hillis *et al.*, 2004). The underlying cognitive deficit causing anomia has not been fully established in PNFA and, although there is some evidence to

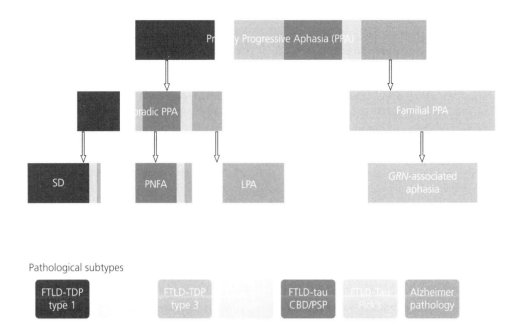

Figure 72.1   Clinicopathological and clinicogenetic associations in primary progressive aphasia. Primary progressive aphasia (PPA) as a syndrome has heterogeneous genetic and pathological associations. However, the importance of subtyping PPA is indicated by the third row of boxes which show in a schematic manner the pathological associations with semantic dementia (SD), progressive nonfluent aphasia (PNFA), logopenic/phonological aphasia (LPA) and with the familial GRN-associated form of PPA, where one pathological subtype tends to dominate. Each of the pathological subtypes are indicated by a separate coloured box: FTLD-TDP types 1 to 3 or type unclear if subtyping has not been performed, FTLD-tau (corticobasal degeneration, (CBD), progressive supranuclear palsy (PSP) and Pick's disease) and Alzheimer's disease (AD) pathology.

implicate a primary word retrieval deficit, this may not be the only or even the primary domain (Rogalski *et al.*, 2008). Imaging studies implicate a network of brain areas in association with anomia in PNFA, particularly inferior frontal, lateral temporal and anterior parietal lobes (Grossman *et al.*, 2004; McMillan *et al.*, 2004; Amici *et al.*, 2007). Single word comprehension is essentially normal early in the disease, but becomes affected some years into the illness (Blair *et al.*, 2007). The cause of single word comprehension impairment in advancing PNFA is unclear. This may partly reflect a more generalized auditory agnosia associated with posterior perisylvian damage (Uttner *et al.*, 2006; Goll *et al.*, 2010).

72.2.7.3   GRAMMAR AND SENTENCE COMPREHENSION

As well as expressive agrammatism, PNFA patients also have receptive agrammatism and a sentence comprehension deficit. This has been studied in detail by Grossman and colleagues (Cooke *et al.*, 2003; Grossman and Moore, 2005; Peelle *et al.*, 2007). Patients perform poorly on complex sentences, but relatively normally with simple sentence structures. One small functional magnetic resonance imaging (fMRI) study showed decreased activation in left ventral inferior frontal lobe areas associated with grammatical processing (Cooke *et al.*, 2003).

72.2.7.4   REPETITION

PNFA patients have early difficulty with repetition of polysyllabic words and sentences. This progresses so that later on

even monosyllabic word repetition becomes difficult. Impaired polysyllabic word repetition with intact single word comprehension has been proposed as a simple bedside measure to distinguish nonfluent aphasias from SD (e.g. asking the patient to repeat 'hippopotamus' and then to identify a picture of a hippopotamus) (Hodges *et al.*, 2008).

72.2.7.5   LITERACY

Patients with PNFA often have phonological dyslexia. Writing may be agrammatic with phonological errors, but tends to be affected later than speech.

72.2.7.6   OTHER COGNITIVE DOMAINS

Other domains including calculation and limb praxis may be affected (Joshi *et al.*, 2003). Episodic memory, visuospatial and visuoperceptual skills generally remain relatively intact in PNFA patients.

72.2.7.7   BEHAVIOURAL FEATURES

Although language impairment is the dominant feature early in the disease patients do develop behavioural features, similar to the behavioural variant of FTLD as the disease progresses. There may be a coexisting depression early (Medina and Weintraub, 2007) with subsequent emergence of apathy, anxiety and, in particular, irritability (Marczinski

Table 72.1   Summary of language, neuropsychological and imaging features in primary progressive aphasia (PPA).

	Semantic dementia	Progressive nonfluent aphasia	Logopenic/phonological aphasia
Speech rate/pauses	Normal	Slow with hesitancy, effortfulness secondary to motor speech disorder and/or agrammatism	Slow with word-finding pauses
Speech errors	Semantic	Phonetic/apraxic errors Phonemic errors	Occasional phonemic errors, rare semantic errors
Apraxia of speech	None	Present	None
Dysarthria	None	Can be present as the disease progresses	None
Naming	Anomia	Initially can be normal, but anomic as disease progresses	Anomia
Single word comprehension	Impaired secondary to verbal semantic impairment	Initially intact, but in late disease becomes affected	Initially relatively intact, but becomes affected as disease progresses
Sentence comprehension	Normal initially, but becomes impaired as single word comprehension deteriorates	Impaired for complex sentences	Impaired for simple and complex sentences
Single word repetition	Normal	Impaired with phonetic/apraxic errors	Impaired with occasional phonemic errors
Sentence repetition	Often normal initially, but can make transposition errors	Can be impaired	Very impaired
Reading	Surface dyslexia	Phonological dyslexia	Phonological dyslexia
Other cognitive domains involved	Non-verbal semantic impairment, can develop object agnosia/ prosopagnosia	Can later develop dominant parietal impairment (dyscalculia, limb apraxia) particularly if associated with CBS	Verbal short-term (phonological) memory and other dominant parietal functions – dyscalculia, limb apraxia
Behaviour	Disinhibition, appetite change	Depression, apathy	Apathy, anxiety
Additional neurological abnormalities	Usually none	Can be associated with CBS, hemiparkinsonism, PSP-syndrome	Usually none
Neuroanatomy	Asymmetrical anteroinferior temporal lobes	Asymmetrical L>R inferior frontal lobe/insula	Asymmetrical L>R posterior temporal-inferior parietal lobes

et al., 2004; Rosen *et al.*, 2006; Banks and Weintraub, 2008).

72.2.7.8   ADDITIONAL NEUROLOGICAL FEATURES

The presence of a motor speech disorder, particularly AOS, predicts the pathological diagnosis of a tauopathy, either corticobasal degeneration or progressive supranuclear palsy (Josephs *et al.*, 2008). Similarly, during life a corticobasal degeneration (CBD) or progressive supranuclear palsy (PSP) syndrome often accompanies PNFA (Kertesz *et al.*, 1999; Mochizuki *et al.*, 2003; Gorno-Tempini *et al.*, 2004b; McMonagle *et al.*, 2006a; Josephs *et al.*, 2008). Dysphagia can occur late in PNFA (Fuh *et al.*, 1994).

Rarely, PNFA can be associated with motor neurone disease (MND) (Caselli *et al.*, 1993; Tsuchiya *et al.*, 2000; Bak *et al.*, 2001; Catani *et al.*, 2004; da Rocha *et al.*, 2007), although there are no systematic studies of MND in PPA. Limited evidence suggests that selective impairment of verb processing may be an aphasic hallmark of PPA/MND (Bak *et al.*, 2001).

72.2.8   Logopenic/phonological aphasia

72.2.8.1   SPONTANEOUS SPEECH

The spontaneous speech of patients with LPA is slow with long word-finding pauses, but without agrammatism or motor speech impairment. When the patient does actually produce speech, output is relatively 'fluent' (non-effortful); an important bedside distinction from PNFA.

72.2.8.2   NAMING AND SINGLE WORD COMPREHENSION

Naming is affected to a greater extent than in PNFA (but less prominently than with SD). Single word comprehension is relatively intact initially, but may become affected later.

72.2.8.3   GRAMMAR AND SENTENCE COMPREHENSION

LPA patients have difficulty with both simple and complex sentence comprehension. This is thought to be secondary to a verbal short-term (phonological) memory deficit rather than a primary grammatical deficit (Gorno-Tempini *et al.*, 2008).

72.2.8.4   REPETITION

Sentence repetition is particularly affected in patients with LPA with single word repetition relatively intact early in the disease (Gorno-Tempini *et al.*, 2008).

72.2.8.5   LITERACY

One study suggested that LPA patients have greater difficulty reading nonsense or pseudo-words which they characterized as phonological dyslexia, associated neuroanatomically with left temporoparietal atrophy (Brambati *et al.*, 2009a; Brambati *et al.*, 2009b).

72.2.8.6   OTHER COGNITIVE DOMAINS

Verbal or phonological short-term memory appears to be a key cognitive domain affected in LPA. This is reflected in the poor forwards digit span exhibited by these patients and may underpin linguistic deficits, such as impaired sentence repetition and sentence comprehension (Gorno-Tempini *et al.*, 2008). Consistent with underlying AD pathology in many cases, episodic memory is frequently affected later in the disease (Gorno-Tempini *et al.*, 2004), although less prominently than in typical AD.

72.2.8.7   BEHAVIOURAL FEATURES

As in PNFA, behavioural features are generally not salient early in LPA, but may emerge later. One study identified depression, anxiety and apathy as behavioural features of LPA (Rosen *et al.*, 2006).

72.2.8.8   ADDITIONAL NEUROLOGICAL FEATURES

There are usually no additional neurological features in LPA, and in particular (in contrast to PNFA) associated parkinsonism or motor neurone disease appear rare.

72.2.9   Progranulin–associated PPA

There have been few detailed studies of the aphasia associated with mutations in the *GRN* gene. Initial reports suggested a nonfluent aphasia (Baker *et al.*, 2006; Cruts *et al.*, 2006), but more detailed studies have reported cases with a prominent early anomia, no motor speech impairment and an early single word comprehension deficit (Snowden *et al.*, 2006; Snowden *et al.*, 2007a; Rohrer *et al.*, 2008b).

72.2.10   Other focal speech and language syndromes

A number of other speech and language syndromes have been described that do not clearly fit into the current scheme of the progressive aphasias. As these lack defined pathological or genetic associations, it is unclear exactly how they are related to SD, PNFA and LPA. Progressive articulatory disorders associated with cortical disease have been described as 'progressive dysarthria' (Soliveri *et al.*, 2003), 'slowly progressive anarthria' (Broussolle *et al.*, 1996; Lucchelli and Papagno, 2005) or 'pure progressive aphemia' (Cohen *et al.*, 1993). While dysarthria commonly occurs as an accompaniment to apraxia of speech and aphasia in PNFA (Gorno-Tempini *et al.*, 2004a; Ogar *et al.*, 2007), it remains unclear whether isolated 'cortical dysarthrias' eventually evolve into the same syndrome, or may remain isolated. Similarly, progressive impairment of prosody has been described as a selective deficit (Ghacibeh and Heilman, 2003; Luzzi *et al.*, 2008), but probably occurs more frequently as part of a PPA syndrome (Tsao *et al.*, 2004). So-called 'dynamic aphasia', a selective disorder of verbal planning, may manifest as a progressive disorder independent of a widespread apathy or abulia (Warren *et al.*, 2003).

72.2.11   Neuroimaging

Numerous imaging studies have investigated the neuroanatomical patterns of atrophy or hypometabolism in PNFA and LPA (Nestor *et al.*, 2003; Gorno-Tempini *et al.*, 2004a; Grossman *et al.*, 2004; Clark *et al.*, 2005; Zahn *et al.*, 2005; Josephs *et al.*, 2006; Nestor *et al.*, 2007; Ogar *et al.*, 2007; Schroeter *et al.*, 2007; Gorno-Tempini *et al.*, 2008; Lindberg *et al.*, 2009; Rohrer *et al.*, 2009a). Findings in PPA have been heterogeneous indicating involvement mainly of the left hemisphere frontotemporoparietal language network (Sonty *et al.*, 2003; Vandenbulcke *et al.*, 2005; Sonty *et al.*, 2007). This is largely attributable to a scarcity of well-defined, uniform clinicopathological cohorts; most studies have been performed in clinically defined cohorts likely to contain patients with heterogeneous tissue pathologies. Nonetheless, in most studies of PNFA, the most significantly affected areas are in the left inferior frontal lobe and anterior insula (Nestor *et al.*, 2003; Gorno-Tempini *et al.*, 2004a; Ogar *et al.*, 2007; Rohrer *et al.*, 2009a), with the left middle and superior frontal and superior temporal lobes also commonly affected as the disease evolves (Gorno-Tempini *et al.*, 2004a; Gorno-Tempini *et al.*, 2004b; Ogar *et al.*, 2007; Rohrer *et al.*, 2009a). Anterior parietal lobe involvement is less common, but may occur particularly with disease progression and when there is an accompanying corticobasal syndrome (Gorno-Tempini *et al.*, 2004b; Rohrer *et al.*, 2009a). Most pathologically confirmed studies of PNFA are based on mixed pathological groups (tau-positive but a mixture of PSP, CBD and/or Pick's disease), but have also shown broadly similar involvement of anterior insula and inferior frontal lobe (Josephs *et al.*, 2006; Rohrer *et al.*, 2009a). Metabolic (positron emission tomography (PET)/single photon emission tomography (SPECT)) brain imaging may help to distiguish nonfluent patients with AD pathology from others with FTLD pathology (Nestor *et al.*, 2007). There are few longitudinal studies of PNFA (Gorno-Tempini *et al.*, 2004b; Knopman *et al.*, 2009); with disease progression, there is spread from the left inferior frontal and insular cortex to involve superior temporal, middle and superior frontal and anterior parietal lobes (Gorno-Tempini *et al.*, 2004b; Rohrer *et al.*, 2009a) and whole brain atrophy rates are similar to other neurodegenerative diseases (1.6 per cent per year) (Knopman *et al.*, 2009).

LPA has been less studied than PNFA (Gorno-Tempini *et al.*, 2004; Gorno-Tempini *et al.*, 2008; Wilson *et al.*, 2009); however, most studies have shown most significant involvement of the left posterior superior temporal and inferior parietal lobes with spread to the posterior cingulate and middle/inferior temporal lobe as the disease unfolds. Consistent with the hypothesis that most patients with LPA have AD pathology, a study using the ^{13}C-PIB-PET amyloid binding ligand showed that all LPA patients (4/4) had a positive PIB scan (compared to only 1/6 PNFA and 1/5 SD patients) (Rabinovici *et al.*, 2008).

There are few neuroimaging studies of *GRN*-associated PPA (Borroni *et al.*, 2008; Cruchaga *et al.*, 2008; Rohrer *et al.*, 2008b). There tends to be asymmetrical left greater than right hemisphere atrophy affecting frontal, temporal and (to a lesser extent) parietal lobes with more prominent posterior atrophy than usually occurs in PNFA and more anterior temporal lobe atrophy than in LPA.

Little information is available for PNFA associated with MND. In single cases, bilateral (often greater on the left) frontal or frontotemporal atrophy/hypometabolism has been reported (Bak *et al.*, 2001; Catani *et al.*, 2004; da Rocha *et al.*, 2007).

72.2.12   Management

There are no symptomatic or curative pharmacological therapies for PPA. Small trials have yielded inconclusive results (bromocriptine: Reed *et al.*, 2004; galantamine: Kertesz *et al.*, 2008) and there are unsubstantiated single case reports of the use of a variety of drugs. Although there is little evidence, many patients find speech and language therapy helpful for communication strategies. Low-technology input, such as communication notebooks, are generally favoured over such devices as hand-held computers (Rogers *et al.*, 2000; Beukelman *et al.*, 2007). Genetic counselling is important in those with a family history and/or a known *GRN* mutation.

72.2.13   Conclusions

The progressive aphasias provide unique neurobiological perspectives on the processes of focal neurodegeneration, yet there is continuing controversy within the field. How many subtypes of nonfluent PPA are there? How can motor speech disorders/apraxia of speech best be operationalized? Is the first symptom of agrammatism compared to a motor speech disorder significant? What are the clinicopathological correlates of the different subtypes? How do patterns of brain atrophy change over time? Only studies with larger cohorts of patients followed over a longer period of time will resolve these issues. None of the PPA syndromes has yet achieved consensus criteria for diagnosis. Although new criteria are in development, it seems likely that only future research with detailed anatomical, pathological and genetic correlation will

yield sufficiently robust criteria. The arrival of disease-modifying therapy and molecular biomarkers is likely to accelerate this process.

72.3   POSTERIOR CORTICAL ATROPHY

72.3.1   Introduction and nosology

The term 'posterior cortical atrophy' (PCA) refers to a progressive neurodegenerative condition involving prominent tissue loss in posterior brain regions. Most individuals with PCA exhibit a progressive, dramatic and relatively selective decline in higher visual processing and other posterior cortical functions. PCA is a descriptive term, introduced in the absence of pathological data identifying the cause of the earliest cases of the syndrome (Cogan, 1985; De Renzi, 1986; Benson *et al.*, 1988). Subsequent histopathological studies have identified amyloid plaques and neurofibrillary tangles as the most common underlying pathology, leading to PCA being considered frequently as a variant of AD. However, the occurrence of PCA associated with alternative aetiologies has led to renewed calls for PCA to be considered as a distinct nosological entity with its own diagnostic criteria (Tang-Wai and Mapstone, 2006). Others suggest that, at least among patients with underlying AD, focal presentations such as PCA should be considered extremes of a continuum of variation in AD (Stopford *et al.*, 2007).

Many questions remain over whether PCA should be considered a unitary clinico-anatomical syndrome or as a collection of related, but distinct syndromic subtypes. Extrapolating from basic neuroscience evidence of distinct cortical streams which process different kinds of visual information (Ungerleider and Mishkin, 1982; Goodale and Milner, 1992), it has been suggested that separate parietal (dorsal), occipitotemporal (ventral) and primary visual (posterior) forms of PCA exist (Galton *et al.*, 2000). Such claims are based on the observation of patterns of impairment in single cases, and the existence of an occipitotemporal variant has not been supported by larger group studies (McMonagle *et al.*, 2006b). These anterior–posterior and superior–inferior distinctions also fail to capture the pronounced asymmetry apparent in the neuropsychological and neuroimaging profiles of many PCA patients (Freedman *et al.*, 1991; Snowden *et al.*, 2007c). It is noteworthy that with a relative preservation of episodic memory, individuals with PCA do not meet all established criteria for dementia.

72.3.2   Synonyms

Synonyms for posterior cortical atrophy are Benson's syndrome, progressive posterior cortical dysfunction, biparietal AD and visual variant of AD.

72.3.3   Epidemiology

The exact prevalence and incidence of PCA are unknown and are likely to be underestimated because of sparse knowledge of the syndrome's existence. However, in a study of 523 patients with AD at a single specialist centre, a visual presentation (also labelled PCA) was reported in 5 per cent of the cohort (Snowden et al., 2007c). Studies comparing PCA and amnestic AD suggest few epidemiological differences apart from age of disease onset, which tends to be earlier in PCA (mid-50s and early 60s) (Mendez et al., 2002; McMonagle et al., 2006b), although some studies report a wide distribution (40–86 years; Tang-Wai et al., 2004). Group studies and reviews indicate either no sex difference in prevalence (Mendez et al., 2002; Renner et al., 2004; McMonagle et al., 2006b) or over-representation among women (Tang-Wai et al., 2004; Snowden et al., 2007c; Lehmann et al., 2009).

72.3.4   Genetics

The proportion of PCA patients with a family history of dementia is not significantly different to individuals with typical AD (Mendez et al., 2002). There have been no reports of an autosomal dominant inheritance pattern in PCA, and of the 11 PCA patients (27.5 per cent) in the Tang-Wai et al. (2004) study who had a family history of dementia, none of those family members had a posterior cortical syndrome. These studies also report no difference in the ApoE status of PCA relative to typical AD. However, a difference between the ApoE status of individuals with posterior cortical presentations of AD and amnestic AD has been suggested (Schott et al., 2006; van der Flier et al., 2006; Snowden et al., 2007b). Schott et al. (2006) reported that fewer patients with biparietal AD than typical AD have one or more ε4 alleles (20 and 86 per cent, respectively). In a larger study examining the relationship between cognitive profile and ApoE status in 302 patients with typical or atypical AD (Snowden et al., 2007b), the percentage of patients with a visual presentation possessing at least one ε4 allele was significantly lower than patients with an amnestic presentation (30 and 82 per cent, respectively; typical AD: 55 per cent) and no different to a population of 756 healthy individuals from the same region (27 per cent; Payton et al., 2003), suggesting that risk factors other than ApoE underpin posterior cortical syndromes in AD.

72.3.5   Pathology

Histopathological studies show that AD is the most common underlying cause of PCA (Hof et al., 1989; Hof et al., 1990; Ross et al., 1996; Galton et al., 2000; Renner et al., 2004; Tang-Wai et al., 2004; Alladi et al., 2007; Snowden et al., 2007b). The distinction between PCA and typical AD lies in the distribution of this pathology. Compared to individuals with typical AD, PCA patients show a much greater density of senile plaques and neurofibrillary tangles in occipital cortex and regions of posterior parietal cortex and temporo-occipital junction, and fewer pathological changes in more anterior areas (Levine et al., 1993; Ross et al., 1996; Hof et al., 1997). However, AD is not the only aetiology responsible for the syndrome, with a small number of cases attributable to corticobasal degeneration (Tang-Wai et al., 2003a;

Renner et al., 2004), dementia with Lewy bodies (DLB) (Tang-Wai et al., 2003b; Renner et al., 2004), prion disease (Victoroff et al., 1994; Renner et al., 2004) and 'subcortical gliosis' (Victoroff et al., 1994).

72.3.6   Clinical and neuropsychological features

72.3.6.1   PROPOSED DIAGNOSTIC FEATURES

Two broadly comparable sets of diagnostic criteria have been proposed (Mendez et al., 2002; Tang-Wai et al., 2004). Suggested core features include (1) insidious onset and gradual progression; (2) presentation with visual complaints in the absence of ocular disease; (3) relatively preserved episodic memory, verbal fluency and personal insight; (4) presence of symptoms including visual agnosia, simultanagnosia, optic ataxia, ocular apraxia, dyspraxia and environmental disorientation; (5) absence of stroke or tumour. Supportive features include alexia, ideomotor apraxia, agraphia, acalculia, onset before the age of 65 years and neuroimaging evidence of posterior cortical atrophy or hypoperfusion.

72.3.6.2   ADDITIONAL NEUROLOGICAL FEATURES

Neurological signs have been inconsistently reported in PCA, and estimates of symptom frequency depend on the study population's composition. However, among 24 PCA patients with probable AD, the frequency of extrapyramidal signs (41 per cent), myoclonus (24 per cent) and grasp reflex (26 per cent) was comparable to individuals with typical AD (Snowden et al., 2007c). Up to 25 per cent of PCA patients may also experience visual hallucinations (Tang-Wai et al., 2004; McMonagle et al., 2006b). In 59 patients with PCA, visual hallucinations were observed in 13 (22 per cent) and were associated with parkinsonism, REM-sleep behaviour disorder, myoclonic jerks and both atrophy of occipitoparietal regions and disruption of thalamocortical circuits (Josephs et al., 2006).

72.3.6.3   NEUROPSYCHOLOGICAL PROFILES

The most frequent neuropsychological deficits in PCA are visuospatial and visuoperceptual, including some or all of the features of Balint's syndrome (simultanagnosia, oculomotor apraxia, optic ataxia, environmental agnosia), Gerstmann's syndrome (acalculia, agraphia, finger agnosia, left/right disorientation), alexia, agraphia, acalculia and apraxia (Mendez et al., 2002; Renner et al., 2004; Tang-Wai et al., 2004; Charles and Hillis, 2005; McMonagle et al., 2006b; Whitwell et al., 2007). The most detailed neuropsychological study of PCA suggests that of these symptoms, alexia, agraphia, simultanagnosia and optic ataxia are the most consistent. Additional features reported in a proportion of patients include agnosia for objects, faces and colours, but overall the pattern of impairments is suggestive of greater impairment of the dorsal than ventral visual processing streams (McMonagle et al., 2006b). However, a clear distinction exists between patients who show predominantly parietal deficits and those with early impairments of early visual processing skills (Crutch and Warrington, 2007) associated with atrophy of the striate and extrastriate cortex (Galton *et al.*, 2000). Overall, the plethora of associated posterior cognitive deficits have predictable consequences for the performance of PCA patients on more general neuropsychological tests, such as performance IQ (often up to 30–40 points lower than verbal IQ scores) and constructional tasks. Longitudinal studies demonstrate that anterograde memory functions, linguistic skills and frontal lobe functions, which are sometimes strikingly preserved in the earlier stages of the condition, gradually deteriorate as individuals develop a more global dementia state (Levine *et al.*, 1993; McMonagle *et al.*, 2006b). The aphasic difficulties are characterized by progressive anomia and phonological impairment and increasingly resemble the LPA syndrome.

72.3.6.4   UNUSUAL SYMPTOMS

Whilst individuals with PCA experience the loss of many visual functions, many also describe unusual new experiences. These phenomena include abnormally prolonged colour afterimages (Chan *et al.*, 2001), reverse size phenomena (Stark *et al.*, 1997), the perception of movement among static stimuli, and even the 180° upside-down reversal of vision (Crutch *et al.*, submitted). Anecdotally, individuals with PCA also report a range of localized sensory and pain phenomena, and disturbances of balance and bodily orientation potentially linked to deranged visuovestibular interactions.

72.3.7   Other focal posterior cortical syndromes

The proposed diagnostic criteria for PCA (Mendez *et al.*, 2002; Tang-Wai *et al.*, 2004) both consider 'presentation with visual complaints' as a core syndrome feature. However, some AD patients present initially with focal deterioration in other cognitive domains, such as praxis or spelling (De Renzi, 1986; Green *et al.*, 1995; Aharon-Peretz *et al.*, 1999; Snowden *et al.*, 2007a) with relative sparing of visual function. Often, these individuals progress to a more general posterior cortical syndrome with memory relatively spared until later in the disease, and could be considered to fall within the spectrum of PCA phenotypes. Given the increasing awareness of non-AD pathologies underpinning PCA and the move toward considering PCA as a distinct nosologic entity in its own right, diagnostic criteria for PCA may require expansion to include posterior cortical presentations which are not primarily visual.

72.3.8   Neuroimaging

As the term PCA suggests, the syndrome is associated with tissue loss primarily of the occipital, parietal and temporo-occipital cortices. This atrophy pattern is often evident from magnetic resonance imaging (MRI) or computed

tomography (CT) images, but less specific radiological findings, such as generalized atrophy or normal volume for age are also common (Della Sala *et al.*, 1996; Galton *et al.*, 2000; Mendez *et al.*, 2002). Only two systematic evaluations of brain structure in PCA using automated methods have been conducted, with voxel-based morphometry revealing greater right parietal and less left medial temporal and hippocampal atrophy in PCA patients compared with those with typical AD (Whitwell *et al.*, 2007; Lehmann *et al.*, 2009). Direct cortical thickness comparisons between PCA and typical AD revealed greater cortical thinning in the right superior parietal lobe and less thinning in the left entorhinal cortex among PCA patients (Lehmann *et al.*, 2009) (**See p14 of the plate section for Plate 14**).

Consistent with structural findings of atrophic changes, functional imaging often reveals hypoperfusion and hypometabolism in dorsal occipitoparietal more than ventral occipitotemporal regions (Pietrini *et al.*, 1996; Aharon-Peretz *et al.*, 1999; Goethals and Santens, 2001). In addition to posterior regions, FDG-PET shows specific areas of hypometabolism in the frontal eye fields bilaterally which may occur secondary to loss of input from occipitoparietal regions and underpin ocular apraxia in PCA (Nestor *et al.*, 2003). Pathophysiological fMRI studies are lacking in PCA, but may be pertinent as the positive perceptual phenomena described by these patients suggest not merely loss of activity but aberrant activity in affected cortical areas.

72.3.9   Management

No studies have examined the effectiveness of cholinesterase inhibitor therapy in PCA. However, anecdotal and limited single case reports suggest that donepezil, rivastigmine and galantamine produce symptomatic benefit in a proportion of the patients (Kim *et al.*, 2005), probably those with underlying AD or DLB.

A lack of widespread understanding of PCA limits access to relevant services, and the care and advice provided are often inappropriate, catering to problems that are not significant (e.g. memory deficits), while failing to cater to functionally critical perceptual deficits (many activities in day centres and nursing homes are visually mediated). Owing to the relative preservation of memory, language and personal insight, particularly in the mild and moderate stages of the condition, individuals with PCA are well disposed to take advantage of peer support meetings and psychological therapies. Peer support meetings provide an important opportunity for reducing social isolation, sharing the experience of what is often a long and difficult route to diagnosis, and for exchanging tips and advice for managing problems associated with the condition. PCA patients often benefit from resources designed for the blind and partially sighted, such as talking watches, mobile phones with simplified displays, voice recognition software, talking books, culinary aids and lamps to increase ambient light levels. Referral to an ophthalmologist may be required for an individual to register as partially sighted under statutory invalidity schemes, which can enable access to benefits and services.

72.3.10   Conclusions

PCA is a debilitating and under-recognized condition, associated with a range of different disease pathologies. Analogies can be drawn between the key focal dementia syndromes of PCA and PPA: like PPA, PCA provides a crucial window on the neurobiology of neurodegeneration and raises substantial nosological difficulties. The PCA syndrome justifies independent nosological status, but with AD as the most common underlying cause, a lack of consistency between studies regarding the classification of PCA is likely to continue until more detailed diagnostic criteria and terminology are available. Better understanding and awareness of the syndrome is necessary to improve support services and information provided to PCA patients and their families. Clinical trials to assess pharmacological and non-pharmacological interventions are required in this patient population.

REFERENCES

Acciarri A, Masullo C, Bizzarro A et al. (2006) Apoe epsilon2–epsilon4 genotype is a possible risk factor for primary progressive aphasia. *Annals of Neurology* **59**: 436–7.

Adlam AL, Patterson K, Rogers TT et al. (2006) Semantic dementia and fluent primary progressive aphasia: two sides of the same coin? *Brain* **129**: 3066–80.

Aharon-Peretz J, Israel O, Goldsher D, Peretz A. (1999) Posterior cortical atrophy variants of Alzheimer's disease. *Dementia and Geriatric Cognitive Disorders* **10**: 483–7.

Alladi S, Xuereb J, Bak T et al. (2007) Focal cortical presentations of Alzheimer's disease. *Brain* **130**: 2636–45.

Amici S, Gorno-Tempini ML, Ogar JM et al. (2006) An overview on primary progressive aphasia and its variants. *Behavioural Neurology* **17**: 77–87.

Amici S, Ogar J, Brambati SM et al. (2007) Performance in specific language tasks correlates with regional volume changes in progressive aphasia. *Cognitive Behavioural Neurology* **20**: 203–11.

Bak TH, O'Donovan DG, Xuereb JH et al. (2001) Selective impairment of verb processing associated with pathological changes in Brodmann areas 44 and 45 in the motor neurone disease-dementia-aphasia syndrome. *Brain* **124**: 103–20.

Baker M, Mackenzie IR, Pickering-Brown SM et al. (2006) Mutations in progranulin cause tau-negative frontotemporal dementia linked to chromosome 17. *Nature* **442**: 916–19.

Banks SJ, Weintraub S. (2008) Neuropsychiatric symptoms in behavioral variant frontotemporal dementia and primary progressive aphasia. *Journal of Geriatric Psychiatry and Neurology* **21**: 133–41.

Beck J, Rohrer JD, Campbell T et al. (2008) A distinct clinical, neuropsychological and radiological phenotype is associated with progranulin gene mutations in a large UK series. *Brain* **131**: 706–20.

Benson F, Davis J, Snyder BD. (1988) Posterior cortical atrophy. *Archives of Neurology* **45**: 789–93.

Beukelman DR, Fager S, Ball L, Dietz A. (2007) AAC for adults with acquired neurological conditions: A review. *Augmentative and Alternative Communication* **23**: 230–42.

Blair M, Marczinski CA, Davis-Faroque N, Kertesz A. (2007) A longitudinal study of language decline in Alzheimer's disease and frontotemporal dementia. *Journal of the International Neuropsychological Society* **13**: 237–45.

Borroni B, Alberici A, Premi E et al. (2008) Brain magnetic resonance imaging structural changes in a pedigree of asymptomatic progranulin mutation carriers. *Rejuvenation Research* **11**: 585–95.

Brambati SM, Ogar J, Neuhaus J et al. (2009a) Reading disorders in primary progressive aphasia: a behavioral and neuroimaging study. *Neuropsychologia* **47**: 1893–900.

Brambati SM, Rankin KP, Narvid J et al. (2009b) Atrophy progression in semantic dementia with asymmetric temporal involvement: a tensor-based morphometry study. *Neurobiology of Aging* **30**: 103–11.

Broussolle E, Bakchine S, Tommasi M et al. (1996) Slowly progressive anarthria with late anterior opercular syndrome: a variant form of frontal cortical atrophy syndromes. *Journal of the Neurological Sciences* **144**: 44–58.

Caselli RJ, Windebank AJ, Petersen RC et al. (1993) Rapidly progressive aphasic dementia and motor neuron disease. *Annals of Neurology* **33**: 200–7.

Catani M, Piccirilli M, Geloso MC et al. (2004) Rapidly progressive aphasic dementia with motor neuron disease: a distinctive clinical entity. *Dementia and Geriatric Cognitive Disorders* **17**: 21–8.

Chan D, Crutch SJ, Warrington EK. (2001) A disorder of colour perception associated with abnormal colour after-images: a defect of the primary visual cortex. *Journal of Neurology, Neurosurgery and Psychiatry* **71**: 515–7.

Charles RF, Hillis AE. (2005) Posterior cortical atrophy: clinical presentation and cognitive deficits compared to Alzheimer's disease. *Behavioural Neurology* **16**: 15–23.

Clark DG, Charuvastra A, Miller BL et al. (2005) Fluent versus nonfluent primary progressive aphasia: a comparison of clinical and functional neuroimaging features. *Brain and Language* **94**: 54–60.

Cogan DG. (1985) Visual disturbances with focal progressive dementing disease. *American Journal of Ophthalmology* **100**: 68–72.

Cohen L, Benoit N, Van Eeckhout P et al. (1993) Pure progressive aphemia. *Journal of Neurology, Neurosurgery and Psychiatry* **56**: 923–4.

Cooke A, DeVita C, Gee J et al. (2003) Neural basis for sentence comprehension deficits in frontotemporal dementia. *Brain and Language* **85**: 211–21.

Cruchaga C, Fernández-Seara MA, Seijo-Martínez M et al. (2008) Cortical atrophy and language network reorganization associated with a novel progranulin mutation. *Cerebral Cortex*. Available from: cercor.oxfordjournals.org/cgi/content/full/bhn202v2.

Crutch SJ, Warrington EK. (2007) Foveal crowding in posterior cortical atrophy: a specific early-visual-processing deficit affecting word reading. *Cognitive Neuropsychology* **24**: 843–66.

Crutch S, Lehmann M, Gorgoraptis N et al. (In press) Abnormal visual phenomena in posterior cortical atrophy. Neurocase.

Cruts M, Gijselinck I, van der Zee J et al. (2006) Null mutations in progranulin cause ubiquitin-positive frontotemporal dementia linked to chromosome 17q21. Nature 442: 920–4.

da Rocha AJ, Valério BC, Buainain RP et al. (2007) Motor neuron disease associated with non-fluent rapidly progressive aphasia: case report and review of the literature. European Journal of Neurology 14: 971–5.

Daniele A, Matera MG, Seripa D et al. (2009) APOE epsilon2/ epsilon4 genotype a risk factor for primary progressive aphasia in women. Archives of Neurology 66: 910–2.

DellaSala S, Spinnler H, Trivelli C. (1996) Slowly progressive impairment of spatial exploration and visual perception. Neurocase 2: 299–323.

De Renzi E. (1986) Slowly progressive visual agnosia or apraxia without dementia. Cortex 22: 171–80.

Freedman L, Selchen DH, Black SE et al. (1991) Posterior cortical dementia with alexia: neurobehavioural, MRI, and PET findings. Journal of Neurology, Neurosurgery and Psychiatry 54: 443–8.

Fuh JL, Liao KK, Wang SJ, Lin KN. (1994) Swallowing difficulty in primary progressive aphasia: a case report. Cortex 30: 701–5.

Galton CJ, Patterson K, Xuereb JH, Hodges JR. (2000) Atypical and typical presentations of Alzheimer's disease: a clinical, neuropsychological, neuroimaging and pathological study of 13 cases. Brain 123: 484–98.

Gerstner E, Lazar RM, Keller C et al. (2007) A case of progressive apraxia of speech in pathologically verified Alzheimer disease. Cognitive Behavioural Neurology 20: 15–20.

Ghacibeh GA, Heilman KM. (2003) Progressive affective aprosodia and prosoplegia. Neurology 60: 1192–4.

Goethals M, Santens P. (2001) Posterior cortical atrophy. Two case reports and a review of the literature. Clinical Neurology and Neurosurgery 103: 115–9.

Goldman JS, Farmer JM, Wood EM et al. (2005) Comparison of family histories in FTLD subtypes and related tauopathies. Neurology 65: 1817–9.

Goll JC, Crutch SJ, Loo J et al. (2010) Non-verbal sound processing in the primary progressive aphasias. Brain 133: 272–85.

Goodale MA, Milner AD. (1992) Separate visual pathways for perception and action. Trends in Neuroscience 15: 20–5.

Gorno-Tempini ML, Dronkers NF, Rankin KP et al. (2004a) Cognition and anatomy in three variants of primary progressive aphasia. Annals of Neurology 55: 335–46.

Gorno-Tempini ML, Murray RC, Rankin KP et al. (2004b) Clinical, cognitive and anatomical evolution from nonfluent progressive aphasia to corticobasal syndrome: a case report. Neurocase 10: 426–36.

Gorno-Tempini ML, Ogar JM, Brambati SM et al. (2006) Anatomical correlates of early mutism in progressive nonfluent aphasia. Neurology 67: 1849–51.

Gorno-Tempini ML, Brambati SM, Ginex V et al. (2008) The logopenic/phonological variant of primary progressive aphasia. Neurology 71: 1227–34.

Green RC, Goldstein FC, Mirra SS et al. (1995) Slowly progressive apraxia in Alzheimer's disease. Journal of Neurology, Neurosurgery and Psychiatry 59: 312–5.

Greene JD, Patterson K, Xuereb J, Hodges JR. (1996) Alzheimer disease and nonfluent progressive aphasia. Archives of Neurology 53: 1072–8.

Grossman M, Moore P. (2005) A longitudinal study of sentence comprehension difficulty in primary progressive aphasia. Journal of Neurology, Neurosurgery and Psychiatry 76: 644–9.

Grossman M, McMillan C, Moore P et al. (2004) What's in a name: voxel-based morphometric analyses of MRI and naming difficulty in Alzheimer's disease, frontotemporal dementia and corticobasal degeneration. Brain 127: 628–49.

Hachisuka K, Uchida M, Nozaki Y et al. (1999) Primary progressive aphasia presenting as conduction aphasia. Journal of the Neurological Sciences 167: 137–41.

Hillis AE, Tuffiash E, Caramazza A. (2002) Modality-specific deterioration in naming verbs in nonfluent primary progressive aphasia. Journal of Cognitive Neuroscience 14: 1099–108.

Hillis AE, Oh S, Ken L. (2004) Deterioration of naming nouns versus verbs in primary progressive aphasia. Annals of Neurology 55: 268–75.

Hodges JR, Patterson K. (2007) Semantic dementia: a unique clinicopathological syndrome. Lancet Neurology 6: 1004–14.

Hodges JR, Martinos M, Woollams AM et al. (2008) Repeat and point: differentiating semantic dementia from progressive non-fluent aphasia. Cortex 44: 1265–70.

Hof PR, Bouras C, Constantinidis J, Morrison JH. (1989) Balint's syndrome in Alzheimer's disease: specific disruption of the occipito-parietal visual pathway. Brain Research 493: 368–75.

Hof PR, Bouras C, Constantinidis J, Morrison JH. (1990) Selective disconnection of specific visual association pathways in cases of Alzheimer's disease presenting with Balint's syndrome. Journal of Neuropathology and Experimental Neurology 49: 168–84.

Hof PR, Vogt BA, Bouras C, Morrison JH. (1997) Atypical form of Alzheimer's disease with prominent posterior cortical atrophy: a review of lesion distribution and circuit disconnection in cortical visual pathways. Vision Research 37: 3609–25.

Janssen JC, Schott JM, Cipolotti L et al. (2005) Mapping the onset and progression of atrophy in familial frontotemporal lobar degeneration. Journal of Neurology, Neurosurgery and Psychiatry 76: 162–8.

Josephs KA, Duffy JR, Strand EA et al. (2006) Clinicopathological and imaging correlates of progressive aphasia and apraxia of speech. Brain 129: 1385–98.

Josephs KA, Whitwell JL, Boeve BF et al. (2006) Visual hallucinations in posterior cortical atrophy. Archives of Neurology 63: 1427–32.

Josephs KA, Whitwell JL, Duffy JR et al. (2008) Progressive aphasia secondary to Alzheimer disease vs FTLD pathology. Neurology 70: 25–34.

Joshi A, Roy EA, Black SE, Barbour K. (2003) Patterns of limb apraxia in primary progressive aphasia. Brain and Cognition 53: 403–7.

Kertesz A, Davidson W, Munoz DG. (1999) Clinical and pathological overlap between frontotemporal dementia, primary progressive aphasia and corticobasal degeneration: the Pick complex. Dementia and Geriatric Cognitive Disorders 10 (Suppl. 1): 46–9.

Kertesz A, Morlog D, Light M et al. (2008) Galantamine in frontotemporal dementia and primary progressive aphasia. *Dementia and Geriatric Cognitive Disorders* 25: 178–85.

Kim E, Lee Y, Lee J, Han SH. (2005) A case with cholinesterase inhibitor responsive asymmetric posterior cortical atrophy. *Clinical Neurology and Neurosurgery* 108: 97–101.

Knibb JA, Xuereb JH, Patterson K, Hodges JR. (2006) Clinical and pathological characterization of progressive aphasia. *Annals of Neurology* 59: 156–65.

Knopman DS, Jack Jr CR, Kramer JH et al. (2009) Brain and ventricular volumetric changes in frontotemporal lobar degeneration over 1 year. *Neurology* 72: 1843–9.

Krefft TA, Graff-Radford NR, Dickson DW et al. (2003) Familial primary progressive aphasia. *Alzheimer Disease and Associated Disorders* 17: 106–12.

Lehmann M, Crutch SJ, Ridgway GR, et al. (2009) Cortical thickness and voxel-based morphometry in posterior cortical atrophy and typical Alzheimer's disease. *Neurobiology of Aging.* Epub ahead of print.

Levine DN, Lee JM, Fisher CM. (1993) The visual variant of Alzheimer's disease: a clinicopathologic case study. *Neurology* 43: 305–13.

Li X, Rowland LP, Mitsumoto H et al. (2005) Prion protein codon 129 genotype prevalence is altered in primary progressive aphasia. *Annals of Neurology* 58: 858–64.

Lindberg O, Ostberg P, Zandbelt BB et al. (2009) Cortical morphometric subclassification of frontotemporal lobar degeneration. *American Journal of Neuroradiology* 30: 1233.

Lucchelli F, Papagno C. (2005) Is slowly progressive anarthria a 'pure' motor-speech disorder? Evidence from writing performance. *Neurocase* 11: 234–41.

Luzzi S, Viticchi G, Piccirilli M et al. (2008) Foreign accent syndrome as the initial sign of primary progressive aphasia. *Journal of Neurology, Neurosurgery and Psychiatry* 79: 79–81.

Mackenzie IR, Rademakers R. (2007) The molecular genetics and neuropathology of frontotemporal lobar degeneration: recent developments. *Neurogenetics* 8: 237–48.

McMillan C, Gee J, Moore P et al. (2004) Confrontation naming and morphometric analyses of structural MRI in frontotemporal dementia. *Dementia and Geriatric Cognitive Disorders* 17: 320–3.

McMonagle P, Blair M, Kertesz A. (2006a) Corticobasal degeneration and progressive aphasia. *Neurology* 67: 1444–51.

McMonagle P, Deering F, Berliner Y, Kertesz A. (2006b) The cognitive profile of posterior cortical atrophy. *Neurology* 66: 331–8.

Marczinski CA, Davidson W, Kertesz A. (2004) A longitudinal study of behavior in frontotemporal dementia and primary progressive aphasia. *Cognitive Behavioural Neurology* 17: 185–90.

Medina J, Weintraub S. (2007) Depression in primary progressive aphasia. *Journal of Geriatric Psychiatry and Neurology* 20: 153–60.

Mendez MF, Ghajarania M, Perryman KM. (2002) Posterior cortical atrophy: Clinical characteristics and differences compared to Alzheimer's disease. *Dementia and Geriatric Cognitive Disorders* 14: 33–40.

Mesulam M, Johnson N, Krefft TA et al. (2007) Progranulin mutations in primary progressive aphasia: the PPA1 and PPA3 families. *Archives of Neurology* 64: 43–7.

Mesulam M, Wicklund A, Johnson N et al. (2008) Alzheimer and frontotemporal pathology in subsets of primary progressive aphasia. *Annals of Neurology* 63: 709–19.

Mesulam MM. (1982) Slowly progressive aphasia without generalized dementia. *Annals of Neurology* ; 11: 592–8.

Mesulam MM. (2001) Primary progressive aphasia. *Annals of Neurology* 49: 425–32.

Mesulam MM. (2003) Primary progressive aphasia – a language-based dementia. *New England Journal of Medicine* 349: 1535–42.

Mesulam MM, Johnson N, Grujic Z, Weintraub S. (1997) Apolipoprotein E genotypes in primary progressive aphasia. *Neurology* 49: 51–5.

Mesulam MM, Grossman M, Hillis A et al. (2003) The core and halo of primary progressive aphasia and semantic dementia. *Annals of Neurology* 54 (Suppl. 5): S11–14.

Mochizuki A, Ueda Y, Komatsuzaki Y et al. (2003) Progressive supranuclear palsy presenting with primary progressive aphasia – clinicopathological report of an autopsy case. *Acta Neuropathologica* 105: 610–14.

Neary D, Snowden JS, Gustafson L et al. (1998) Frontotemporal lobar degeneration: a consensus on clinical diagnostic criteria. *Neurology* 51: 1546–54.

Nestor PJ, Caine D, Fryer TD et al. (2003) The topography of metabolic deficits in posterior cortical atrophy (the visual variant of Alzheimer's disease) with FDG-PET. *Journal of Neurology, Neurosurgery and Psychiatry* 74: 1521–9.

Nestor PJ, Graham NL, Fryer TD et al. (2003) Progressive non-fluent aphasia is associated with hypometabolism centred on the left anterior insula. *Brain* 126: 2406–18.

Nestor PJ, Balan K, Cheow HK et al. (2007) Nuclear imaging can predict pathologic diagnosis in progressive nonfluent aphasia. *Neurology* 68: 238–9.

Ogar J, Slama H, Dronkers N et al. (2005) Apraxia of speech: an overview. *Neurocase* 11: 427–32.

Ogar JM, Dronkers NF, Brambati SM et al. (2007) Progressive nonfluent aphasia and its characteristic motor speech deficits. *Alzheimer Disease and Associated Disorders* ; 21: S23–30.

Payton A, Holland F, Diggle P et al. (2003) Cathepsin D exon 2 polymorphism associated with general intelligence in a healthy older population. *Molecular Psychiatry* 8: 14–18.

Peelle JE, Cooke A, Moore P et al. (2007) Syntactic and thematic components of sentence processing in progressive nonfluent aphasia and nonaphasic frontotemporal dementia. *Journal of Neurolinguistics* 20: 482–94.

Pereira JM, Williams GB, Acosta-Cabronero J et al. (2009) Atrophy patterns in histologic vs clinical groupings of frontotemporal lobar degeneration. *Neurology* 72: 1653–60.

Pietrini P, Furey ML, Graff-Radford N et al. (1996) Preferential metabolic involvement of visual cortical areas in a subtype of Alzheimer's disease: Clinical implications. *American Journal of Psychiatry* 153: 1261–8.

Rabinovici GD, Jagust WJ, Furst AJ *et al.* (2008) Abeta amyloid and glucose metabolism in three variants of primary progressive aphasia. *Annals of Neurology* 64: 388–401.

Reed DA, Johnson NA, Thompson C *et al.* (2004) A clinical trial of bromocriptine for treatment of primary progressive aphasia. *Annals of Neurology* 56: 750.

Renner JA, Burns JM, Hou CE *et al.* (2004) Progressive posterior cortical dysfunction: a clinicopathologic series. *Neurology* 63: 1175–80.

Rogalski E, Johnson N, Weintraub S, Mesulam M. (2004) Increased frequency of learning disability in patients with primary progressive aphasia and their first-degree relatives. *Archives of Neurology* 65: 244–8.

Rogalski E, Rademaker A, Mesulam M, Weintraub S. (2004) Covert processing of words and pictures in nonsemantic variants of primary progressive aphasia. *Alzheimer Disease and Associated Disorders* 22: 343–51.

Rogers MA, King JM, Alarcon NB. (2004) Proactive management of primary progressive aphasia. In: Beukelman DR, Yorkston KM, Reichle J (eds). *Augmentative and alternative communication for adults with acquired neurologic disorders.* Baltimore: Brookes.

Rohrer JD, Mead S, Omar R *et al.* (2004) Prion protein (PRNP) genotypes in frontotemporal lobar degeneration syndromes. *Annals of Neurology* 60: 616.

Rohrer JD, Knight WD, Warren JE *et al.* (2004) Word-finding difficulty: a clinical analysis of the progressive aphasias. *Brain* 131: 8–38.

Rohrer JD, Warren JD, Barnes J *et al.* (2004) Mapping the progression of progranulin-associated frontotemporal lobar degeneration. *Nature Clinical Practice. Neurology* 4: 455–60.

Rohrer JD, Warren JD, Modat M *et al.* (2004) Patterns of cortical thinning in the language variants of frontotemporal lobar degeneration. *Neurology* 72: 1562–9.

Rohrer JD, Warren JD, Rossor MN. (2004) Abnormal laughter-like vocalisations replacing speech in primary progressive aphasia. *Journal of the Neurological Sciences* 284: 120–3.

Rosen HJ, Allison SC, Ogar JM *et al.* (2004) Behavioral features in semantic dementia vs other forms of progressive aphasias. *Neurology* 67: 1752–6.

Ross SJ, Graham N, Stuart Green L *et al.* (2004) Progressive biparietal atrophy: an atypical presentation of Alzheimer's disease. *Journal of Neurology, Neurosurgery and Psychiatry* 61: 388–95.

Schott JM, Ridha BH, Crutch SJ *et al.* (2004) Apolipoprotein E genotype modifies the phenotype of Alzheimer disease. *Archives of Neurology* 63: 155–6.

Schroeter ML, Raczka K, Neumann J, Yves von Cramon D. (2004) Towards a nosology for frontotemporal lobar degenerations – a meta-analysis involving 267 subjects. *Neuroimage* 36: 497–510.

Snowden JS, Pickering-Brown SM, Mackenzie IR *et al.* (2004) Progranulin gene mutations associated with frontotemporal dementia and progressive non-fluent aphasia. *Brain* 129: 3091–102.

Snowden JS, Pickering-Brown SM, Du Plessis D *et al.* (2004) Progressive anomia revisited: focal degeneration associated with progranulin gene mutation. *Neurocase* 13: 366–77.

Snowden JS, Stopford CL, Julien CL *et al.* (2004) Cognitive phenotypes in Alzheimer's disease and genetic risk. *Cortex* 43: 835–45.

Snowden J, Neary D, Mann D. (2004) Frontotemporal lobar degeneration: clinical and pathological relationships. *Acta Neuropathologica* 114: 31–8.

Sobrido MJ, Abu-Khalil A, Weintraub S *et al.* (2004) Possible association of the tau H1/H1 genotype with primary progressive aphasia. *Neurology* 60: 862–4.

Soliveri P, Piacentini S, Carella F *et al.* (2004) Progressive dysarthria: definition and clinical follow-up. *Neurological Sciences* 24: 211–2.

Sonty SP, Mesulam MM, Thompson CK *et al.* (2004) Primary progressive aphasia: PPA and the language network. *Annals of Neurology* 53: 35–49.

Sonty SP, Mesulam MM, Weintraub S *et al.* (2004) Altered effective connectivity within the language network in primary progressive aphasia. *Journal of Neuroscience* 27: 1334–45.

Stark ME, Grafman J, Fertig E. (2004) A restricted 'spotlight' of attention in visual object recognition. *Neuropsychologia* 35: 1233–49.

Stopford CL, Snowden JS, Thompson JC, Neary D. (2004) Distinct memory profiles in Alzheimer's disease. *Cortex* 43: 846–57.

Tang-Wai D, Mapstone M. (2004) What are we seeing? Is posterior cortical atrophy just Alzheimer disease? *Neurology* 66: 300–1.

Tang-Wai DF, Josephs KA, Boeve BF *et al.* (2004) Pathologically confirmed corticobasal degeneration presenting with visuospatial dysfunction. *Neurology* 61: 1134–5.

Tang-Wai DF, Josephs KA, Boeve BF *et al.* (2004) Coexistent Lewy body disease in a case of 'visual variant of Alzheimer's disease'. *Journal of Neurology, Neurosurgery and Psychiatry* 74: 389.

Tang-Wai DF, Graff-Radford NR, Boeve BF *et al.* (2004) Clinical, genetic, and neuropathologic characteristics of posterior cortical atrophy. *Neurology* 63: 1168–74.

Tsao JW, Dickey DH, Heilman KM. (2004) Emotional prosody in primary progressive aphasia. *Neurology* 63: 192–3.

Tsuchiya K, Ozawa E, Fukushima J *et al.* (2004) Rapidly progressive aphasia and motor neuron disease: a clinical, radiological, and pathological study of an autopsy case with circumscribed lobar atrophy. *Acta Neuropathologica* 99: 81–7.

Turner RS, Kenyon LC, Trojanowski JQ *et al.* (2004) Clinical, neuroimaging, and pathologic features of progressive nonfluent aphasia. *Annals of Neurology* 39: 166–73.

Tyrrell PJ, Kartsounis LD, Frackowiak RS *et al.* (2004) Progressive loss of speech output and orofacial dyspraxia associated with frontal lobe hypometabolism. *Journal of Neurology, Neurosurgery and Psychiatry* 54: 351–7.

Ungerleider LG, Mishkin M. (2004) Two cortical visual systems. In: Ingle DJ, Mansfield RJW, Goodale MD (eds). *The analysis of visual behaviour.* Cambridge, MA: MIT Press, 549–86.

Uttner I, Mottaghy FM, Schreiber H *et al.* (2004) Primary progressive aphasia accompanied by environmental sound agnosia: a neuropsychological, MRI and PET study. *Psychiatry Research* 146: 191–7.

Vandenbulcke M, Peeters R, Van Hecke P, Vandenberghe R. (2004) Anterior temporal laterality in primary progressive aphasia shifts to the right. *Annals of Neurology* **58**: 362–70.

van der Flier WM, Schoonenboom SNM, Pijnenburg YAL *et al.* (2004) The effect of APOE genotype on clinical phenotype in Alzheimer disease. *Neurology* **67**: 526–7.

Victoroff J, Ross GW, Benson DF *et al.* (2004) Posterior cortical atrophy – neuropathologic correlations. *Archives of Neurology* **51**: 269–74.

Warren JD, Warren JE, Fox NC, Warrington EK. (2004) Nothing to say, something to sing: primary progressive dynamic aphasia. *Neurocase* **9**: 140–55.

Weintraub S, Rubin NP, Mesulam MM. (2004) Primary progressive aphasia. Longitudinal course, neuropsychological profile, and language features. *Archives of Neurology* **47**: 1329–35.

Westbury C, Bub D. (2004) Primary progressive aphasia: a review of 112 cases. *Brain and Language* **60**: 381–406.

Wilson SM, Ogar JM, Laluz V *et al.* (2004) Automated MRI-based classification of primary progressive aphasia variants. *Neuroimage* **47**: 1558–67.

Whitwell JL, Jack CR, Kantarci K *et al.* (2004) Imaging correlates of posterior cortical atrophy. *Neurobiology of Aging* **28**: 1051–61.

Zahn R, Buechert M, Overmans J *et al.* (2004) Mapping of temporal and parietal cortex in progressive nonfluent aphasia and Alzheimer's disease using chemical shift imaging, voxel-based morphometry and positron emission tomography. *Psychiatry Research* **140**: 115–31.

The cerebellum and cognitive impairment

ELSDON STOREY

73.1 INTRODUCTION

The motor features of the cerebellar syndrome were crystallized by the great English neurologist Gordon Holmes soon after the First World War. He did not ascribe any cognitive function to the cerebellum and, until the last decade or two, this view held general sway. However, a confluence of evidence from new neuroanatomical tracing techniques, functional neuroimaging experiments and careful clinical studies now points strongly to a significant role for the cerebellum in cognition, although the exact process(es) underlying this contribution have not been fully elucidated. This chapter aims to distil some of the important studies supporting a non-motor role for the cerebellum. The reader interested in a detailed exposition is referred to *The cerebellum and cognition*, edited by Jeremy Schmahmann (1997), while several shorter reviews have also been published (Fiez, 1996; Diamond, 2000; Rapoport *et al.*, 2000; Timmann and Daum, 2007; Baillieux *et al.*, 2008).

73.2 THE NEUROANATOMICAL BASIS OF CEREBELLAR COGNITIVE FUNCTION

The cerebellum, which contains as many neurons as the entire remainder of the brain, has a regular and relatively simple modular structure. The 'corticonuclear microcomplex' is essentially a positive loop through the deep cerebellar nuclei,

modulated by a variable negative side loop through the cerebellar cortex (Ito, 1993). The degree of inhibitory influence of the cerebellar cortical Purkinje cells on the deep cerebellar nuclei is governed by the development of long-term depression (LTD) at the excitatory parallel fibre-Purkinje dentrite synapses (Ito, 1993). LTD itself develops in response to near-simultaneous Purkinje cell activation by parallel fibres, and by climbing fibres from the inferior olive. It may thus be considered to be analogous to associative long-term potentiation in the hippocampus. In the influential Marr–Albus–Ito model of cerebellar function, the climbing fibres are regarded as carrying the 'error signals' responsible for adaptive motor learning.

While there is no universally accepted model of the mechanism whereby LTD in the corticonuclear microcomplex might result in motor learning at the whole animal level (Massaquoi and Topka, 2002), it is clear from its stereotyped modular structure that the cerebellum performs the same type of basic computation on whatever inputs it receives, and informs all its various efferent targets similarly of the results of such computation. If different areas of the cerebellum differ in function, therefore, they do so by virtue of their differing inputs and outputs.

With this in mind, the evidence for cerebellar input from, and output to, non-motor areas can be considered. Such evidence is both indirect and direct. The former consists of the observation that, in primate phylogeny, and especially in hominids, the prefrontal portion of the frontal lobes and the lateral neocerebellum with its associated ventral macrogyric region of the dentate nucleus have undergone massive parallel selective enlargement, out of proportion to other brain areas (Matano, 2001; MacLeod *et al.*, 2003). More direct evidence has had to await the development of anterograde and retrograde trans-synaptic (viral) tracers (Middleton and Strick, 1997). Such tracers are necessary because cerebral cortical input to the cerebellum proceeds via cortico-pontine fibres synapsing in the pontine nuclei, which in turn project to the deep cerebellar nuclei and cerebellar cortex, while cerebellar output to the cortex proceeds via synaptic relays in the thalamus (Schmahmann and Pandya, 1997). Studies utilizing such tracers in primates have shown that a series of anatomically discrete parallel cortico-ponto-cerebello-thalamo-cortical loops exist, with pre-frontal input predominantly to the ventral, macrogyric portion of the dentate nucleus and associated lateral neocerebellar cortex, and output via the ventrolateral and medial dorsal thalamic nuclei (Middleton and Strick, 2000; Middleton and Strick, 2001). Motor and premotor cortex, in contrast, are reciprocally connected to the phylogenetically older dorsolateral, microgyric portion of the dentate nucleus (Middleton and Strick, 2001). The analogy with separate, parallel corticobasal ganglionic circuits subserving motor and non-motor functions, as conceptualized by Alexander *et al.* (1986) is readily drawn (Middleton and Strick, 2000). This circuitry has now been imaged in life in humans, using functional connectivity magnetic resonance imaging (MRI) (Allen *et al.*, 2005).

73.3 FUNCTIONAL NEUROIMAGING STUDIES

A large number of functional neuroimaging studies over the last 20 years have reported cerebellar activation during tests of various cognitive domains, utilizing positron emission tomography (PET) or fMRI (Cabeza and Nyberg, 2000). The typical design compares patterns of cerebellar activation on a cognitive task with that on what is thought to be a relevant control 'motor' and/or perceptual task. This section includes a broadly representative sample of such studies across various cognitive domains.

The cerebellum appears to play a role in language function. One of the earliest reports was that of Petersen *et al.* (1989), who used PET to study a verb association task. The control tasks were reading aloud, and silently. Broca's area and the right lateral cerebellum were both activated. Hubrich-Ungureanu *et al.* (2002) extended these findings with an fMRI study of a silent verbal fluency task in left- and right-handed subjects. Fullbright *et al.* (1999) asked subjects to read silently. Their fMRI study showed that semantic comparison and judgement of non-word rhyming activated posterolateral (and especially right posterolateral) cerebellar cortex, compared with the control conditions of line orientation judgement, upper versus lower case print judgement, or judgement of real word rhyming. Xiang *et al.* (2003) confirmed the role of the right posterolateral cerebellum in semantic discrimination divorced from articulation. Such studies have led to the concept of the 'lateralized linguistic cerebellum', reviewed by Marien *et al.* (2001).

The cerebellum also appears to be involved in executive functioning and working memory. Cognitive processing during attempted solution of a pegboard puzzle task compared with simple peg movement was studied using fMRI estimation of dentate activation by Kim *et al.* (1994). The cognitively demanding task produced increased, and bilateral, dentate activation compared with the contralateral (to the moving hand) activation seen with simple peg movement. In as much as this task tapped visuospatial working memory, it is conceptually similar to the verbal working memory fMRI study of Desmond *et al.* (1997), who found that delayed matching of letter strings, but not the control task, activated the right inferolateral cerebellar hemisphere. In more recent studies, Chen and Desmond (2005) and Tomasi *et al.* (2007) have supported this lateralization of the cerebellar contribution to verbal working memory. The Wisconsin Card Sorting Test, a complex task often used to assess aspects of executive functioning, has also been found to activate the lateral cerebellum (Nagahama *et al.*, 1996).

An aspect of episodic memory was addressed by Andreasen *et al.* (1999) in a 'pure thought' PET experiment. Subjects were asked to recall a personal memory silently. The right lateral cerebellum was activated, in addition to several relevant supratentorial areas.

A further area of recent active study has been the role(s) of the cerebellum in attention. Allen *et al.* (1997) showed an anatomical double dissociation in cerebellar regional activation; a visual attention task activated the lateral cerebellum, while the motor task activated more medial regions. Attention is, however, a multifaceted concept, placing a variety of different demands on the subject. Le *et al.* (1998) showed that shifting attention between stimulus dimensions (colour/shape) activated the right lateral cerebellum, while sustained attention did not. More recently, Bischoff-Grethe *et al.* (2002) have demonstrated that the lateral cerebellum's role in this paradigm may actually be in re-assignment of a given motor response to the new stimulus dimension, rather than in shifting attention *per se*.

It is clear that the weight of evidence from functional neuroimaging studies in favour of lateral cerebellar contributions to cognition is strong, as illustrated by the selected studies cited above. However, it is also clear that the exact role(s) of the lateral cerebellum in complex aspects of cognition, such as language and attentional shifting, still requires considerable clarification.

73.4 REPETITIVE TRANSCRANIAL MAGNETIC STIMULATION STUDIES

Low-frequency (~1 Hz) repetitive transcranial magnetic stimulation results in temporary inhibition of function of the stimulated structure. In the cerebellum, this has been shown to result in contralateral motor cortex facilitation, presumably via inhibition of Purkinje cells leading to disinhibition of deep cerebellar nuclei (Oliveri *et al.*, 2007). In this way, the dependence of observational learning on the lateral cerebellum has been demonstrated (Oliveri *et al.*, 2007).

A conceptually similar technique – transcranial direct current stimulation of the cerebellum – has been shown to impair practice-dependent proficiency acquisition in a verbal working memory task (Ferrucci *et al.*, 2008).

73.5 DIFFICULTIES IN STUDYING COGNITIVE FUNCTION IN SUBJECTS WITH CEREBELLAR DYSFUNCTION

The results of functional neuroimaging studies in normals notwithstanding, the practising clinician is primarily concerned with the potential impact of cerebellar disease or dysfunction on cognition. Unfortunately, several confounding factors must be borne in mind when interpreting such studies. The first problem is that performance on the neuropsychological tests utilized may be adversely affected by requirements for rapid verbal output, motor accuracy and speed, or by dependence on rapid visual scanning. A correlation between test results and ataxia severity will not necessarily indicate that such requirements are confounding the results, however; motor and cognitive function would be expected to decline in parallel in diffuse cerebellar degenerations, whether the observed cognitive dysfunction was secondary to the cerebellar disorder or was merely secondary to the resultant motor impairment.

Several types of neuropsychological task would be expected *a priori* to limit the potential for confounding of results. Some tests are untimed, and do not require motoric or visual speed or accuracy. In the executive domain, these include the Wisconsin Card Sorting Test (WCST), Raven's progressive matrices, and the Zoo Map subtest (of planning) from the Behavioural Assessment of the Dysexecutive Syndrome (BADS) battery. Most measures of verbal anterograde episodic memory also fall into this category, provided that dysarthria is not so severe as to compromise intelligibility. Other tests include a timed internal control condition involving similar scanning and output to the test condition. The effects of visual, verbal and motor dysfunction can therefore be subtracted out. Such tests within the executive function cognitive domain would include Trails B (versus A) and the Stroop test. However, other tests requiring verbal output are timed, but empirical observation suggests that speed of articulation is not the rate-limiting factor. The controlled oral word association test (COWAT, FAS) appears to fall into this category (Storey *et al.*, 1999).

An indirect way of exploring the possibility that motor dysfunction might secondarily affect performance on cognitive tests is to study patients with Friedreich's ataxia (FA), whose motoric deficit is partly consequent upon disruption of afferent cerebellar input rather than direct disruption of the cerebellar microcorticonuclear units, although the deep cerebellar nuclei are also affected (Koeppen, 2002). While FA patients display impairments in a number of domains (Wollmann *et al.*, 2002), they have been shown to be less impaired on verbal working memory and visuospatial reasoning tasks than patients with assorted other cerebellar degenerations (Botez-Marquard and Botez, 1997). Indeed,

White *et al.* (2000) demonstrated slowed processing speed and decreased cognitive inhibition on the Stroop test, but preserved planning, verbal fluency and Wisconsin Card Sorting Test performance.

The potential confounding factor of motor deficit has recently been explicitly addressed by Timmann *et al.* (2002), who correctly pointed out that even ataxic patients who cope well with the motor demands of a test may do so at the cost of attentional resources not required by control patients. These authors reported that subjects with pure cerebellar cortical atrophies (SCA 6, other more or less pure cerebellar dominant ataxias, such as SCA 8, or idiopathic cerebellar cortical atrophy) demonstrated impairments of visual association learning independent of the separately manipulated motor output requirements of the task.

The second problem affecting patient studies is that of choice of patient type. The ideal patient group for such a study would have widespread/diffuse involvement of cerebellar corticonuclear microcomplex units, with complete sparing of all other central nervous system (CNS) structures. Unfortunately, such patients probably do not exist, at least to the extent of satisfying those sceptical of the idea of cerebellar contributions to cognition. Even relatively 'pure' cerebellar ataxias, such as SCA 6 and SCA 8, often have mild non-cerebellar features (e.g. pyramidal signs). Other degenerative cerebellar diseases studied in this context, such as SCAs 1, 2 and 3, are even more problematic, as they are known to manifest extracerebellar involvement of structures potentially or actually contributing to cognition, such as the cerebral cortex, the striatum and the substantia nigra (Koeppen, 2002). On the other hand, focal cerebellar lesions, such as infarcts and resected tumours, may be 'pure', but there is no guarantee that cerebellar region(s) potentially important for cognition will be involved, unless a range of lesions in different locations are studied. Pooled results may then conceal regional differences in cognitive contribution unless sufficient subjects are available in each group for comparison. While this is difficult, such studies do perhaps provide the most convincing clinical evidence, as outlined below.

73.6 ALTERED COGNTION IN ADULTS WITH FOCAL CEREBELLAR LESIONS

In a seminal report, Schmahmann and Sherman (1998) described the features of an entity they named the 'cerebellar cognitive affective syndrome' in 20 adults with isolated cerebellar lesions: strokes, resected tumours not treated with radiotherapy and post-viral cerebellitis. Posterior (roughly equivalent to lateral neocerebellar) lobe lesions produced executive dysfunction, with impairments of planning, set shifting, verbal fluency by semantic category and abstract reasoning. There was also impairment of spatial cognition, including of visual organization and visual memory. Lesions of the posterior vermis tended to produce personality change with blunting or disinhibition, while anterior lobe lesions resulted only in motor deficit. Similar findings were reported by Malm *et al.* (1998), in 24 consecutive young adult patients with cerebellar infarcts who were compared with 14 age-matched controls. The patients performed less well on working memory and cognitive flexibility tasks, while intelligence (WAIS-R scores) and episodic memory were unaffected. Interestingly, while most made a good motor recovery, only half returned to work. The broad conclusions of these studies have since been confirmed by Neau et al. (2000), who reported the neuropsychological profile of 15 consecutive patients with recent, isolated cerebellar infarcts, compared with 15 demographically matched controls. A further assessment was undertaken one year after the infarcts. These authors demonstrated impairments on a range of tasks tapping aspects of executive functioning, such as verbal fluency, working memory on the Paced Serial Addition Test (PASAT), and the Stroop colour/word interference test. These abnormalities were not accompanied by a clinically apparent 'frontal' neuropsychiatric syndrome. Block design was also affected, which deficit the authors likened to a mild parietal syndrome, although problems with block design can also be a feature of executive dysfunction. Of interest is that infarcts in any of the three cerebellar arterial territories produced similar deficits, although the numbers in each group were small. This is in contrast to the findings of Schmahmam and Sherman (1998) and Exner et al. (2004), the latter reporting that posterior inferior, but not superior, cerebellar artery infarcts resulted in cognitive deficits. As might be expected with infarcts, the deficits reported by Neau et al. (2000) tended to have improved at the one year assessment. The authors plausibly suggest that this improvement may have been partly responsible for the failure of Beldarrain et al. (1997) to demonstrate consistent deficits in a patient population including subjects with old cerebellar infarcts, a finding since confirmed by Richter et al. (2007a). Hokkanen et al. (2006) reported on 26 Finnish subjects with cerebellar lesions, assessed acutely and at three months. Those with left cerebellar lesions were slow on a visuospatial task, whereas those with right-sided damage showed impairments of verbal episodic and working memory. These deficits improved over time, such that all but one eventually returned to work, and 77 per cent had done so at three months. The reasons for the discrepancy in long-term outcome from the Swedish study of Malm et al. (1998) are unclear.

The specific role of the right lateral cerebellum in language, outlined in the section on functional neuroimaging above, was studied in control subjects and subjects with left lateral or right lateral cerebellar infarcts (Gebhart et al., 2002). Those with right lateral cerebellar damage were impaired only on antonym generation, and not on semantic (category) noun fluency, or verb selection. This argues in favour of a cerebellar role in producing word associations, and not just in 'imaging' verb action to a noun cue. Helmuth et al. (1997) also failed to demonstrate impaired noun-triggered verb generation in subjects with right cerebellar lesions, opposing the findings from earlier functional neuroimaging studies. In contrast, verbal fluency was the only impaired function in subjects with chronic focal cerebellar lesions, being most evident in those with right-sided lesions (Richter et al., 2007b). The potential role of the cerebellum in more complex rather than simpler tasks has recently been extended to reading: Ben-Yehudah and Fiez (2008) showed that focal cerebellar damage impaired a visual rhyme judgement task for irregularly spelt words, but not for phonetically regular words, and impaired working memory only for non-words rather than for real words. Reading fluency and comprehension were unimpaired.

Verbal working memory – the ability to manipulate phonological data in consciousness (e.g. reversing digit strings) – is one aspect of executive function often found to be mildly affected in subjects with cerebellar lesions (Bellebaum and Daum, 2007). A parsimonious explanation would be that the cerebellum has a role in subvocal articulatory rehearsal. However, Ravizza et al. (2006) provide evidence that the cerebellum's role is actually in initial phonological encoding and/or in strengthening memory traces. Episodic memory has generally been reported as relatively preserved with focal cerebellar lesions, but a recent study of patients after removal of cerebellar tumours revealed episodic memory deficits in most, although there was no clear correlation of modality with lesion laterality (de Ribaupierre et al., 2008).

Various attentional processes have also been studied in subjects with cerebellar lesions, with varying results. Orienting of visuospatial attention has been found to be markedly delayed in such subjects, independent of motor responses (Townsend et al., 1999), while the speed of visual attention is also slowed, independent of eye movements (Schweizer et al., 2007). Gottwald et al. (2003) compared 16 subjects with cerebellar tumours or haematomas to 11 matched control subjects and to demographically adjusted results from normative studies, and detected deficits in divided attention and working memory, but not in sustained directed attention. However, Helmuth et al. (1997) did not demonstrate deficits in spatial attention shifting or in intra- or inter-dimensional non-spatial attentional shifting, again failing to confirm earlier functional neuroimaging studies in a clinical population. Moreover, Ravizza and Ivry (2001) found that, while patient groups with Parkinson's disease and with cerebellar lesions each showed impairment of attentional shifting, reducing the motor demands of the task improved the performance of only the cerebellar patients. Neglect may be regarded as a disorder of lateralized spatial attention. Conflicting results have been obtained in line bisection tasks in subjects with lateralized lesions (Daini et al., 2008; Kim et al., 2008), with the minority in whom neglect was demonstrable not always showing this ipsilateral to the lesion, as might be expected a priori (Kim et al., 2008). The question of a cerebellar contribution to various forms of attention has generated conflicting results, and remains to be settled conclusively.

Recent work has also highlighted the role of the cerebellum in sequencing (Leggio et al., 2008) – an aspect of executive functioning. Analogous with its role in sensory and motor sequence detection and production, cerebellar damage also disturbs verbal (sentence) and spatial sequencing (Leggio et al., 2008). Furthermore, there is an effect of lesion laterality, with right-sided lesions impairing verbal and left-sided lesions impairing spatial sequencing.

Studies in children with resected cerebellar tumours have produced similar results to those in adults (Levisohn et al., 2000).

73.7   EVIDENCE FOR COGNITIVE IMPAIRMENT IN DEGENERATIVE CEREBELLAR DISEASE

Evidence for cognitive impairment in degenerative cerebellar disease comes from both neurophysiological and clinical neuropsychological studies. The best known neurophysiological method of studying cognition involves measuring the latency of the P_{300} event-related cerebral potential. This occurs with conscious registration of an unusual stimulus, such as an occasional ('oddball') high-pitched tone inserted into a series of usual stimuli, such as many low-pitched tones. It may be regarded as a neurophysiological measure of selective attention and processing speed, and is delayed in various forms of dementia (Goodin, 2003) (see Chapter 14, The neurophysiology of dementia). Tachibana et al. (1999) measured the P_{300} during a visual discrimination task and found it to be delayed in 15 subjects with idiopathic late-onset cerebellar ataxia, when compared with ten controls. SPECT (single photon emission computed tomography) scanning in the ataxic subjects showed correlated cerebellar/frontal cortex hypoperfusion. Tanaka et al. (2003) did not find any differences in P_{300} timing or scalp distribution to the classical auditory 'oddball' paradigm in 13 subjects with cerebellar cortical atrophy when compared with 13 demographically matched controls. However, P_{300} latency was prolonged, and its peak attenuated frontally, in the 'No Go' condition of the 'Go/No Go' paradigm. The authors suggested that the cerebellum contributes to the frontal inhibitory system.

The neuropsychological consequences of degenerative cerebellar disease have been studied extensively. In one early study, Grafman et al. (1992) compared nine patients with 'pure cortical cerebellar atrophy' with 12 controls. There were no differences on paired associate learning, verbal fluency or procedural (skill) learning. However, the ataxic subjects performed significantly less well on the Tower of Hanoi planning task, which is conceptually similar to the Tower of London test. Botez-Marquard and Botez (1997) showed that cerebellar degenerations resulted in impaired executive functioning, visuospatial organization, working memory and spontaneous retrieval of episodic memories. Cerebellar strokes produced similar patterns of impairment, but these cognitive deficits resolved in two to five months. In both types of subjects, SPECT scanning showed reverse cerebellar/frontoparietal diaschisis. Drepper et al. (1999) studied nine subjects with 'isolated' cerebellar degeneration and ten controls. The ataxic subjects showed a significant impairment in novel associative learning (colours with numbers), that did not correlate with either simple reaction time or visual scanning time.

Kish et al. (1994) studied the performance of 43 subjects with undefined dominant cerebellar degenerations of varying ataxia severity on a number of neuropsychological measures. Impaired performance on the WCST correlated with ataxia severity; none of those with mild ataxia showed deficits, while all of those with severe ataxia were impaired. Some of the latter also showed evidence of mild generalized cognitive deficit. The authors concluded that the dominant ataxias are not homogeneous with respect to cognitive involvement, and

indeed the topography of extracerebral neuropathological involvement does vary considerably between these disorders (Koeppen, 2002). Trojano et al. (1998) also studied a mixed population of subjects with dominant ataxias of varying severity, although 15 of their 22 subjects had SCA 2. They attempted to avoid confounding effects of motor impairment on performance by restricting their investigation to tests with untimed verbal response modes. The domains examined were predominantly verbal memory, and non-verbal reasoning (Raven's progressive matrices). None of the four genetically confirmed, but asymptomatic subjects performed poorly on any of the tests, while most of the symptomatic subjects showed impairment on at least one measure, most commonly the progressive matrices. Some showed more widespread deficits, but there was no correlation with ataxia severity. This might have reflected the small sample size and the contaminating effects of inclusion of several SCA subtypes.

Several studies have assessed subjects with different SCA types singly or separately, thereby avoiding this particular confounding factor. Maruff et al. (1996) compared six patients with SCA 3 (Machado–Joseph disease) with 15 matched controls using a touch-screen testing system: the Cambridge Neuropsychological Test Automated Battery (CANTAB). Learning and visual memory were unaffected, but SCA 3 subjects displayed impaired visual information processing speed on high-demand tasks, and impaired attentional switching between visual stimulus dimensions. Executive dysfunction in SCA 3 was confirmed by Zawacki et al. (2002). Ishikawa et al. (2002) reported dementia with features of delirium including hallucinations in four young SCA 3 patients with severe disease, in the absence of MRI or pathological evidence of cortical neuronal loss.

SCA 2 may be associated with cortical atrophy and clinically obvious dementia in some pedigrees (Dürr et al., 1995; Geschwind et al., 1997). Although it is therefore not ideal for the purpose, it has been studied by several groups. Gambardella et al. (1998) and Storey et al. (1999) demonstrated impairments of executive function on the WCST and the Stroop test. Bürk et al. (1999) found that 25 per cent of their subjects were demented, while the others showed impairments of executive function and verbal memory that were independent of the severity of motor impairment. In contrast, Le Pira et al. (2002) reported that the impairments of executive function, attention and verbal memory in their SCA 2 patients were partly related to ataxia severity.

The pattern of neuropsychological impairment in SCA 1 patients compared with matched controls was reported by Bürk et al. (2001). Evidence of executive and verbal memory dysfunction was found, while visuospatial memory and attention were unaffected. The deficits did not correlate with CAG repeat length or with disease duration, which may be regarded as surrogate markers of disease severity in different dimensions.

While the studies on SCAs 1, 2 and 3 cited above paint a fairly consistent picture of executive dysfunction and verbal memory impairment, the effects of differences in the pattern and extent of extracerebral neuropathological involvement, if any, can only be addressed adequately by direct comparison. This was undertaken by Bürk et al. (2003), who found that executive dysfunction was more marked in SCA 1 than in

SCAs 2 or 3, while mild verbal memory impairment was present in all. On the basis of these findings, the authors suggested that the cognitive deficits were likely to result from disruption of cerebrocerebellar circuitry at the pontine, rather than at the cerebellar level. Given that SCA 2 causes more severe pontine atrophy than SCA 1, the reasons for this conclusion are unclear. A problem with this study is the lack of control for ataxia severity.

Perhaps the best way of clarifying the relative contributions of cerebellar and extracerebellar pathology to cognitive dysfunction in the SCAs is to study those disorders characterized by relatively pure cerebellar involvement, such as SCA 6, and to a lesser extent SCA 8. Although McMurtray et al. (2006) found that SCA 6 patients, in contrast to those with other SCA types, tended not to show memory deficits, Suenaga et al. (2008) reported significant impairments of verbal fluency and immediate visual memory in SCA 6, independent of motor dysfunction. Two groups have recently reported a dysexecutive syndrome in SCA 8 (Lilja et al., 2005; Torrens et al., 2008), with the first group also demonstrating deficits in attention and information processing.

73.8   CONCLUSION

There is converging evidence from neuroanatomical, neuroimaging and neurophysiological and neuropsychological patient studies that the lateral cerebellum is involved in network(s) subserving a range of cognitive functions, including aspects of language and executive functioning. The exact nature of the cerebellar contributions to cognition, and especially to attention, are still being debated and elucidated. Nevertheless, the broad picture is well enough established that clinicians should consider the possibility of cognitive dysfunction in patients with overt cerebellar disorders. In this context, executive dysfunction is both the most likely to be overlooked in the structured clinical setting, and potentially the most disruptive to the patients' ability to compensate for impaired motor functioning. Clinicians should also bear in mind that obvious cognitive dysfunction may result from cerebellar disease, at least from degenerative disorders and acute focal lesions, and that such dysfunction does not necessarily signify that a second, supratentorial disorder has been overlooked.

REFERENCES

Alexander GE, DeLong PL, Strick PL. (1986) Parallel organization of functionally segregated circuits linking basal ganglia and cortex. Annual Review of Neuroscience 9: 357–81.

Allen G, Buxton RB, Wong EC et al. (1997) Attentional activation of the cerebellum independent of motor involvement. Science 275: 1940–3.

Allen G, McColl R, Barnard H et al. (2005) Magnetic resonance imaging of cerebellar-prefrontal and cerebellar-parietal functional connectivity. Neuroimage 28: 39–48.

Andreasen NC, O'Leary DS, Paradiso S et al. (1999) The cerebellum plays a role in conscious episodic memory retrieval. Human Brain Mapping 8: 226–34.

Baillieux H, De Smet HJ, Paquier PF et al. (2008) Cerebellar neurocognition: insights into the bottom of the brain. Clinical Neurology and Neurosurgery 110: 763–73.

Beldarrain MG, Garcia-Monco JC, Quintana JM et al. (1997) Diaschisis and neuropsychological performance after cerebellar stroke. European Neurology 37: 82–9.

Bellebaum C, Daum I. (2007) Cerebellar involvement in executive control. The Cerebellum 6: 184–92.

Ben-Yehudah G, Fiez JA. (2008) Impact of cerebellar lesions on reading and phonological processing. Annals of the New York Academy of Sciences 1145: 260–74.

Bischoff-Grethe A, Ivry RB, Grafton ST. (2002) Cerebellar involvement in response reassignment rather than attention. Journal of Neuroscience 22: 546–53.

Botez-Marquard T, Botez MI. (1997) Olivopontocerebellar atrophy and Friedreich's ataxia: neuropsychological consequences of bilateral versus unilateral cerebellar lesions. International Review of Neurobiology 41: 387–410.

Bürk K, Globas C, Bösch S et al. (1999) Cognitive deficits in spinocerebellar ataxia 2. Brain 122: 769–77.

Bürk K, Bösch S, Globas C et al. (2001) Executive dysfunction in spinocerebellar ataxia type 1. European Neurology 46: 43–8.

Bürk K, Globas C, Bösch S et al. (2003) Cognitive deficits in spinocerebellar ataxia type 1, 2, and 3. Journal of Neurology 250: 207–11.

Cabeza R, Nyberg L. (2000) Imaging cognition II: An empirical review of 275 PET and fMRI studies. Journal of Cognitive Neuroscience 12: 1–47.

Chen SH, Desmond JE. (2005) Cerebrocerebellar networks during articulatory rehearsal and verbal working memory tasks. Neuroimage 24: 332–8.

Daini R, Arduino LS, Di Menza D et al. (2008) Line bisection and cerebellar damage. Cognitive and Behavioural Neurology 21: 214–20.

de Ribaupierre S, Ryser C, Villemure JG et al. (2008) Cerebellar lesions: is there a lateralisation effect on memory deficits? Acta Neurochirurgica 150: 545–50.

Desmond JE, Gabrieli J, Wagner A et al. (1997) Lobular patterns of cerebellar activation in verbal working-memory and finger-tapping tasks as revealed by functional MRI. Journal of Neuroscience 17: 9675–85.

Diamond A. (2000) Close interrelation of motor development and cognitive development and of the cerebellum and prefrontal cortex. Child Development 71: 44–56.

Drepper J, Timmann D, Kolb FP, Diener HC. (1999) Non-motor associative learning in patients with isolated degenerative cerebellar disease. Brain 122: 87–97.

Dürr A, Smadja D, Cancel G et al. (1995) Autosomal dominant cerebellar ataxia type I in Martinique (French West Indies): clinical and neuropathological analysis of 53 patients from three unrelated SCA 2 families. Brain 118: 1573–81.

Exner C, Weniger G, Irle E. (2004) Cerebellar lesions in the PICA but not SCA territory impair cognition. Neurology 63: 2132–5.

Ferrucci R, Marceglia S, Vergari M *et al.* (2008) Cerebellar transcranial direct current stimulation impairs the practice-dependent proficiency increase in working memory. *Journal of Cognitive Neuroscience* 20: 1687–97.

Fiez JA. (1996) Cerebellar contributions to cognition. *Neuron* 16: 13–15.

Fullbright RK, Jenner AR, Mencl WE *et al.* (1999) The cerebellum's role in reading: A functional MR imaging study. *American Journal of Neuroradiology* 20: 1925–30.

Gambardella A, Annesi G, Bono F *et al.* (1998) CAG repeat length and clinical features in three Italian families with spinocerebellar ataxia type 2 (SCA 2): early impairment of Wisconsin Card Sorting Test and saccade velocity. *Journal of Neurology* 245: 647–52.

Gebhart AL, Petersen SE, Thach WT. (2002) Role of the posterolateral cerebellum in language. *Annals of the New York Academy of Sciences* 978: 318–33.

Geschwind DH, Perlman S, Figueroa CP *et al.* (1997) The prevalence and wide clinical spectrum of the spinocerebellar ataxia type 2 trinucleotide repeat in patients with autosomal dominant cerebellar ataxia. *American Journal of Human Genetics* 60: 842–50.

Goodin DS. (2003) Long-latency event-related potentials. In: Ebersole JS, Pedley TA (eds). *Current practice of clinical electroencephalography*, 3rd edn. Philadelphia: Lippincott Williams & Wilkins, 923–35.

Gottwald B, Mihajlovic Z, Wilde B, Mehdorn HM. (2003) Does the cerebellum contribute to specific aspects of attention? *Neuropsychologia* 41: 1452–60.

Grafman J, Litvan I, Massaquoi S *et al.* (1992) Cognitive planning deficit in patients with cerebellar atrophy. *Neurology* 42: 1493–6.

Helmuth LL, Ivry RB, Shimizu N. (1997) Preserved performance by cerebellar patients on tests of word generation, discrimination learning, and attention. *Learning and Memory* 3: 456–74.

Hokkanen LS, Kauranen V, Roine RO *et al.* (2006) Subtle cognitive deficits after cerebellar infarcts. *European Journal of Neurology* 13: 161–70.

Hubrich-Ungureanu P, Kaemmerer N, Henn FA, Braus DF. (2002) Lateralized organization of the cerebellum in a silent verbal fluency task: a functional magnetic resonance imaging study in healthy volunteers. *Neuroscience Letters* 319: 91–4.

Ishikawa A, Yamada M, Makino K *et al.* (2002) Dementia and delirium in 4 patients with Machado–Joseph disease. *Archives of Neurology* 59: 1804–8.

Ito M. (1993) Movement and thought: identical control mechanisms by the cerebellum. *Trends in Neuroscience* 16: 448–50.

Kim EJ, Choi KD, Han MK *et al.* (2008) Hemispatial neglect in cerebellar stroke. *Journal of the Neurological Sciences* 275: 133–8.

Kim S, Ugurbil K, Strick P. (1994) Activation of a cerebellar output nucleus during cognitive processing. *Science* 265: 949–51.

Kish SJ, el-Awar M, Stuss D *et al.* (1994) Neuropsychological test performance in patients with dominantly inherited spinocerebellar ataxia: relationship to ataxia severity. *Neurology* 44: 1738–46.

Koeppen AH. (2002) Neuropathology of the inherited ataxias. In: Manto MU, Pandolfo M (eds). *The cerebellum and its disorders.* Cambridge: Cambridge University Press, 387–405.

Leggio MG, Tedesco AM, Chiricozzi FR *et al.* (2008) Cognitive sequencing impairment in patients with focal or atrophic cerebellar damage. *Brain* 131: 1332–43.

Le Pira F, Zappala G, Saponara R *et al.* (2002) Cognitive findings in spinocerebellar ataxia type 2: relationship to genetic and clinical variables. *Journal of the Neurological Sciences* 201: 53–7.

Le TH, Pardo JV, Hu X. (1998) 4T-fMRI study of nonspatial shifting of selective attention: cerebellar and parietal contributions. *Journal of Neurophysiology* 79: 1535–48.

Levisohn L, Cronin-Golomb A, Schmahmann JD. (2000) Neuropsychological consequences of cerebellar tumour resection in children: Cerebellar cognitive affective syndrome in a paediatric population. *Brain* 123: 1041–50.

Lilja A, Hamalainen P, Kaitaranta E *et al.* (2005) Cognitive impairment in spinocerebellar ataxia type 8. *Journal of the Neurological Sciences* 237: 31–8.

MacLeod CE, Zilles K, Schleicher A *et al.* (2003) Expansion of the neocerebellum in Hominoidea. *Journal of Human Evolution* 44: 401–29.

McMurtray AM, Clark DG, Flood MK *et al.* (2006) Depressive and memory symptoms as presenting features of spinocerebellar ataxia. *Journal of Neuropsychiatry and Clinical Neurosciences* 18: 420–2.

Malm J, Kristensen B, Karlsson T *et al.* (1998) Cognitive impairment in young adults with infratentorial infarcts. *Neurology* 51: 433–40.

Marien P, Engelborghs S, Fabbro F, De Deyn PP. (2001) The lateralized linguistic cerebellum: a review and a new hypothesis. *Brain and Language* 79: 580–600.

Maruff P, Tyler P, Burt T *et al.* (1996) Cognitive deficits in Machado–Joseph disease. *Annals of Neurology* 40: 421–7.

Massaquoi SG, Topka H. (2002) Models of cerebellar function. In: Manto MU, Pandolfo M (eds). *The cerebellum and its disorders.* Cambridge: Cambridge University Press, 69–94.

Matano S. (2001) Brief communication: Proportions of the ventral half of the cerebellar dentate nucleus in humans and great apes. *American Journal of Physical Anthropology* 114: 163–5.

Middleton FA, Strick PL. (1997) Cerebellar output channels. In: Schmahmann JD (ed.). *The cerebellum and cognition.* International Review of Neurobiology, 41. San Diego: Academic Press, 61–82.

Middleton FA, Strick PL. (2000) Basal ganglia and cerebellar loops: motor and cognitive circuits. *Brain Research Reviews* 31: 236–50.

Middleton FA, Strick PL. (2001) Cerebellar projections to the prefrontal cortex of the primate. *Journal of Neuroscience* 21: 700–12.

Nagahama Y, Fukuyama H, Yamauchi H *et al.* (1996) Cerebral activation during performance of a card sorting test. *Brain* 119: 1667–75.

Neau J-Ph, Arroyo-Anllo E, Bonnaud V *et al.* (2000) Neuropsychological disturbances in cerebellar infarcts. *Acta Neurologica Scandinavica* 102: 363–70.

Oliveri M, Torriero S, Koch G et al. (2007) The role of transcranial magnetic stimulation in the study of cerebellar cognitive function. The Cerebellum 6: 95–101.

Petersen SE, Fox PT, Posner MI et al. (1989) Positron emission tomographic studies of the processing of single words. Journal of Cognitive Neuroscience 1: 153–70.

Rapoport M, ven Reekum R, Mayberg H. (2000) The role of the cerebellum in cognition and behavior: A selective review. Journal of Neuropsychiatry and Clinical Neurosciences 12: 193–8.

Ravizza SM, Ivry RB. (2001) Comparison of the basal ganglia and cerebellum in shifting attention. Journal of Cognitive Neuroscience 13: 285–97.

Ravizza SM, McCormick CA, Schlerf JE et al. (2006) Cerebellar damage produces selective deficits in verbal working memory. Brain 129: 306–20.

Richter S, Aslan B, Gerwig M et al. (2007a) Patients with chronic focal cerebellar lesions show no cognitive abnormalities in a bedside test. Neurocase 13: 25–36.

Richter S, Gerwig M, Aslan B et al. (2007b) Cognitive functions in patients with MR-defined chronic focal cerebellar lesions. Journal of Neurology 254: 1193–203.

Schmahmann JD (ed.). (1997) The cerebellum and cognition. International Review of Neurobiology, 41. San Diego: Academic Press.

Schmahmann JD, Pandya DN. (1997) The cerebrocerebellar system. In: Schmahmann JD (ed.). The cerebellum and cognition. International Review of Neurobiology, 41. San Diego: Academic Press, 31–60.

Schmahmann JD, Sherman JC. (1998) The cerebellar affective cognitive syndrome. Brain 121: 561–79.

Schweizer TA, Alexander MP, Cusimano M et al. (2007) Fast and efficient visuotemporal attention requires the cerebellum. Neuropsychologia 45: 3068–74.

Storey E, Forrest SM, Shaw JH et al. (1999) Spinocerebellar ataxia type 2: Clinical features of a pedigree displaying prominent frontal-executive dysfunction. Archives of Neurology 56: 43–50.

Suenaga M, Kawai Y, Watanabe H et al. (2008) Cognitive impairment in spinocerebellar ataxia type 6. Journal of Neurology, Neurosurgery and Psychiatry 79: 496–9.

Tachibana H, Kawabata K, Tomino Y, Sugita M. (1999) Prolonged P_3 latency and decreased brain perfusion in cerebellar degeneration. Acta Neurologica Scandinavica 100: 310–16.

Tanaka H, Harada M, Arai M, Hirata K. (2003) Cognitive dysfunction in cortical cerebellar atrophy correlates with impairment of the inhibitory system. Neuropsychobiology 47: 206–11.

Timmann D, Daum I. (2007) Cerebellar contributions to cognitive functions: a progress report after two decades of research. The Cerebellum 6: 159–62.

Timmann D, Drepper J, Maschke M et al. (2002) Motor deficits cannot explain impaired cognitive associative learning in cerebellar patients. Neuropsychologia 40: 788–800.

Tomasi D, Chang L, Caparelli EC et al. (2007) Different activation patterns for working memory load and visual attention load. Brain Research 1132: 158–65.

Torrens L, Burns E, Stone J et al. (2008) Spinocerebellar ataxia type 8 in Scotland: frequency, neurological, neuropsychological and neuropsychiatric findings. Acta Neurologica Scandinavica 117: 41–8.

Townsend J, Courchesne E, Covington J et al. (1999) Spatial attention deficits in patients with acquired or developmental cerebellar abnormality. Journal of Neuroscience 19: 5632–43.

Trojano L, Chiacchio L, Grossi D et al. (1998) Determinants of cognitive disorders in autosomal dominant cerebellar ataxia type 1. Journal of the Neurological Sciences 157: 162–7.

White M, Lalonde R, Botez-Marquard T. (2000) Neuropsychologic and neuropsychiatric characteristics of patients with Friedreich's ataxia. Acta Neurologica Scandinavica 102: 222–6.

Wollmann T, Barroso J, Monton F, Nieto A. (2002) Neuropsychological test performance of patients with Friedreich's ataxia. Journal of Clinical and Experimental Neuropsychology 24: 677–86.

Xiang H, Lin C, Ma X et al. (2003) Involvement of the cerebellum in semantic discrimination: an fMRI study. Human Brain Mapping 18: 208–14.

Zawacki TM, Grace J, Friedman JH, Sudarsky L. (2002) Executive and emotional dysfunction in Machado–Joseph disease. Movement Disorders 17: 1004–10.

PART VIII

OTHER DEMENTIAS AND NEUROPSYCHIATRIC DISORDERS ASSOCIATED WITH COGNITIVE IMPAIRMENTS

Depression with cognitive impairment

SARAH SHIZUKO MORIMOTO, BINDU SHANMUGHAM, ROBERT E KELLY JR AND GEORGE S ALEXOPOULOS

74.1 INTRODUCTION

Major depression in the elderly is often accompanied by cognitive impairment. Although estimates vary, studies have shown that combined depression and cognitive dysfunction is present in roughly 25 per cent of subjects (Arve *et al.*, 1999). In addition, the number of community residents with both depressive symptoms and impaired cognition doubles every five years after the age of 70 years. In some cases, the syndromes of depression and cognitive impairment may be related to the same underlying disorders (e.g. vascular dementia, hypothyroidism), whereas in other cases depression and cognitive impairment may be relatively independent, and simply coexist. Differential diagnosis and treatment decisions can be complicated because depressive cognitive changes can be severe, incipient dementia often has physical and cognitive symptoms that overlap with depression, and the two can coexist (Bayles *et al.*, 1987). The relationships between the prominent cerebrovascular changes, other structural abnormalities, specific forms of cognitive dysfunction, and increased risk for developing dementias in geriatric depression have yet to be reconciled. The varied and most current findings suggest that there are likely multiple pathways to poor cognitive outcomes (Butters *et al.*, 2008).

74.2 COGNITIVE IMPAIRMENT IN NON-DEMENTED DEPRESSED PATIENTS

Neuropsychological impairments spanning many cognitive domains (Lockwood *et al.*, 2000; Lockwood *et al.*, 2002), including impairment in episodic memory (Beats *et al.*, 1996; Kramer-Ginsberg *et al.*, 1999; Story *et al.*, 2008), recognition memory, visuospatial skills (Boone *et al.*, 1994; Lesser *et al.*, 1996; Elderkin-Thompson *et al.*, 2004) verbal fluency, psychomotor speed (Hart *et al.*, 1987; Butters *et al.*, 2004b) have been reported consistently in late-life depression. These impairments, particularly memory impairments, were attributed to dysfunction in subcortical structures related to mood regulation, such as the hippocampus (Hickie *et al.*, 2005). Recent research has focused on the role of executive functions, such as impaired planning, organizing, initiating, perseverating, sequencing and attentional set shifting in geriatric depression (Lesser *et al.*, 1996; Alexopoulos *et al.*, 2000; Butters *et al.*, 2000; Murphy and Alexopoulos 2004; Potter *et al.*, 2004). These studies indicate that abnormal performance on some tests of executive function predicts both poor and unstable antidepressant response in late-life depression (Kalayam and Alexopoulos 1999; Alexopoulos *et al.*, 2000), although some disagreement exists (Butters *et al.*, 2004a). The specifics of this topic are discussed below.

Although focal deficits or even severe global impairment are observed in some depressed elderly patients, the cognitive functioning of others remains intact. Studies of cognitive response to psychopharmacological treatment of late-life depression indicate that a substantial number of patients continue to experience residual symptoms and neuropsychological deficits. Executive dysfunction, processing speed and working memory impairment may persist after remission of geriatric depression (Butters *et al.*, 2000; Nebes *et al.*, 2000; Aizenstein *et al.*, 2009).

The structural and functional abnormalities that contribute to the symptoms of this disorder remain unclear, although several abnormalities have been reported (Alexopoulos et al., 2005). Recently, structural and functional neuroimaging have documented both frontostriatal impairment and the relationship between frontostriatal impairment and executive dysfunction in geriatric depression (Murphy et al., 2007; Aizenstein et al., 2009).

Structural abnormalities have been identified in the orbitofrontal cortex (Van Otterloo et al., 2009), particularly the gyrus rectus bilaterally (Ballmaier et al., 2004; Yuan et al., 2008), the anterior cingulate (Drevets et al., 1997; Ballmaier et al., 2004), the caudate head (Krishnan et al., 1992), putamen (Husain et al., 1991), hippocampus (Sheline et al., 1996; Lai et al., 2000) and amygdala (Sheline et al., 1998).

In addition to grey matter reductions, bilateral white matter hyperintensities are prevalent in geriatric depression (Boone et al., 1992; Steffens et al., 1999; Kumar et al., 2000; Alexopoulos et al., 2008a; Gunning-Dixon et al., 2008), and mainly occur in the subcortical structures and their frontal projections (MacFall et al., 2001; Gunning-Dixon et al., 2008). There is evidence that white matter hyperintensities disrupt frontostriatal circuits (Hannestad et al., 2006) and have been associated with executive dysfunction (Boone et al., 1992; Lesser et al., 1996).

Abnormal metabolism has also been noted in limbic regions, including the amygdala (Wu et al., 1992; Drevets, 1999; Drevets et al., 2002), the pregenual and subgenual anterior cingulate (Drevets, 1998), the posterior orbital cortex (Drevets et al., 1992), the posterior cingulate and the medial cerebellum (Bench et al., 1992). Recent research has shown increased cortical glucose metabolism in both anterior and posterior cortical regions in patients with geriatric depression relative to controls, particularly in areas where there has been cerebral atrophy, which may represent a compensatory response (Smith et al., 2009). In fact, positive correlations between anxiety and depressive symptoms and cortical glucose metabolism have been observed (Smith et al., 2009).

74.3 DEPRESSION IN PATIENTS WITH DEMENTING DISORDERS

Estimates of the rates of depression in dementing disorders range from 30 to 50 per cent (Taylor et al., 2003). Major depression or clinically significant depressive symptoms can be found in between 17 and 40 per cent of Alzheimer's disease (AD) patients (Wragg and Jeste, 1989; Holtzer et al., 2005). Depression in AD is notable for increased disturbances in initiation or motivation, such as fatigue, psychomotor slowing and apathy (Chemerinski et al., 2001; Janzing et al., 2002; Teng et al., 2008). Patients with subcortical dementias, including vascular dementia (VaD) and Parkinson's disease (PD), are more likely to experience depression than patients with AD (Sobin and Sackeim, 1997). Rates of major depression in PD reach 50 per cent (Lagopoulos et al., 2005). Depression associated with this disease can produce severe negative symptoms and has been shown to contribute to an increased rate of decline of both cognitive and motor function. The symptoms of depression often overlap with the motor features of PD, which may make differential diagnosis particularly challenging (Lagopoulos et al., 2005).

A first episode of depression presenting in late life is, in some cases, a prodrome of a dementing disorder. Depressed mood has been associated with an increased risk of incident dementia in some samples (Devanand et al., 1996). For example, depressive symptoms predicted cognitive decline of elderly women during a four-year follow-up study (Yaffe et al., 1999). In addition, in patients with subthreshold cognitive symptoms, those suffering concurrent depressive symptoms are more likely to progress to dementia (Ritchie et al., 1999). However, more recent data suggest that there is a significant decline in functioning that precedes late onset depressive symptoms in AD, and that cognition declines subsequently (Holtzer et al., 2005).

The prevalence of depressive symptoms in AD decrease over time as patients exhibit fewer affective symptoms, increased agitation and psychomotor slowing. Data suggest that rates of depression in this population remain stable for roughly the first three years of follow up. Rates appear to drop in the fourth and fifth year of follow up by as much as 30 per cent (Holtzer et al., 2005).

The National Institute of Mental Health's Provisional Diagnostic Criteria for Depression of Alzheimer's Disease were developed in order to promote research on the mechanisms and treatment of this disorder (Olin et al., 2002). The criteria require presence of AD diagnosis and clinically significant depressive symptoms. The criteria specify that the patient must have three (reduced from five) or more of the following symptoms during the same 2-week period (reduced from 'most of the day, nearly every day') and represent a change from previous functioning: depressed mood, anhedonia, social isolation, appetite disturbance, sleep disturbance, psychomotor changes, irritability, fatigue or loss of energy, worthlessness, hopelessness or inappropriate or excessive guilt, and recurrent thoughts of death or suicidal ideation, plan or attempt. At least one of the symptoms must be (1) depressed mood or (2) anhedonia. Symptoms due to a medical condition other than AD, or as a direct result of non-mood-related dementia symptoms (e.g. loss of weight due to difficulties with food intake) should not be used in making the diagnosis of depression of AD. These diagnostic criteria have less stringent guidelines about the duration and number of symptoms and, therefore, are likely more sensitive than other diagnostic approaches (Teng et al., 2008).

74.4 DEPRESSION AS A RISK FACTOR FOR DEMENTIA

Individual studies attempting to link geriatric depression with subsequent dementia have shown mixed results. Although one recent meta-analysis showed an almost twofold risk for the development of AD with previous history of depression (Ownby et al., 2006), another found this association only when depressive symptoms had appeared within the 10 years prior to onset of dementia (Jorm et al., 1991).

Other individual studies have failed to find this association (Ganguli *et al.*, 2006). Recent research suggests that only the most severe cases of depression increase risk for later development of dementia (Chen *et al.*, 2008). Lifetime history of depression may also increase the risk of AD in patients with or without a family history of dementia (Van Duijn *et al.*, 1994). Depressive episodes with onset more than 10 years prior to dementia are associated with AD at any age, suggesting that depression may be a risk factor for dementia (Jorm *et al.*, 1991).

Some data suggest that the experience of multiple depressive episodes may promote the clinical expression of dementia in patients with AD. Some volumetric studies have found reductions in hippocampal volumes in patients with recurrent major depression (Sheline *et al.*, 1996; Sheline *et al.*, 2003). Lifetime duration of depression correlated with hippocampal volume reduction and with behavioural measures of hippocampal function, such as verbal memory (Sheline *et al.*, 1999). Depression leads to an acute dysregulation of the hypothalamic–pituitary–adrenal (HPA) axis, which in turn can result in hypercortisolaemia (Carroll *et al.*, 1981). Studies have shown that depression disrupts the fast feedback control of cortisol secretion (Young *et al.*, 1991) at various levels, including limbic structures such as the hippocampus (Young and Vazquez, 1996). The precise relationship between hypercortisolemia, hippocampal volume loss and hippocampal inhibitory control is unknown, although animal studies show that neurotoxic tissue damage may be one possible mechanism. Another theory postulates that excess and chronic secretion of glucocorticoid hormones can reduce neurotrophic factors, inhibit neurogenesis and render neurons vulnerable to the toxic effect of amyloid. These changes may then compound the neuropathological changes of AD and accelerate the clinical expression of dementia.

One such neurotrophic factor is the brain-derived neurotrophic factor (BDNF), which is widely distributed in the adult brain and has been implicated in structural abnormalities of the human hippocampus (Pezawas *et al.*, 2004; Bueller *et al.*, 2006). Several antidepressants elevate BDNF in the rat hippocampus. Recent research suggests that BDNF protein is rapidly elevated by antidepressant treatments through post-transcriptional mechanisms (Musazzi *et al.*, 2009). Through this action, antidepressants may prevent stress-induced inhibition of neurogenesis and increase dendritic branching (Duman *et al.*, 1997). Whether this action delays the onset or inhibits the progression of AD is unclear; systematic studies have not yet explored this question.

74.5   COGNITIVE IMPAIRMENT AND THE COURSE OF GERIATRIC DEPRESSION

Multiple pathways may lead to depression and cognitive impairment. However, clinical as well as structural and functional neuroimaging studies suggest that depressive symptoms and executive impairment originate from related brain dysfunctions (Alexopoulos *et al.*, 2001), at least in a subgroup of elderly patients. We described a 'depression-executive

dysfunction syndrome' (DED), characterized by symptoms resembling a medial frontal lobe syndrome, including psychomotor retardation, anhedonia, apathy, mild vegetative symptoms and pronounced functional disability disproportional to the severity of the depressive syndrome (Alexopoulos *et al.*, 1996; Kiosses *et al.*, 2000; Lockwood *et al.*, 2000). The neuropsychological impairments of these patients include impaired verbal fluency and visual naming, as well as poor performance on tasks of initiation and perseveration (Alexopoulos *et al.*, 2002c; Alexopoulos, 2003). Recognition of these patients is particularly important due to their tendency to have poor and unstable response to antidepressants (Alexopoulos *et al.*, 2005), as well as a higher level of functional disability (Kiosses *et al.*, 2001).

There is increasing evidence that impaired neurocognitive performance on select neuropsychological tests at baseline predicts to poor and/or slow antidepressant response (Alexopoulos *et al.*, 2002b). In younger women, abnormal executive functions were associated with poor response to fluoxetine (Dunkin *et al.*, 2000). Abnormal performance on tests of prose recall, processing speed, initiation and perseveration predict poor and unstable antidepressant response and low remission rate in non-demented elderly patients with major depression treated with 'adequate' dosages of various antidepressants (Simpson *et al.*, 1998; Kalayam and Alexopoulos, 1999; Alexopoulos *et al.*, 2000; Alexopoulos *et al.*, 2004; Potter *et al.*, 2004; Sneed *et al.*, 2007; Story *et al.*, 2008), although disagreement exists (Butters *et al.*, 2004a).

One domain that has received increasing attention is abnormal initiation/perseveration (Alexopoulos *et al.*, 2002c). Approximately 42 per cent of elders with major depression have abnormal initiation/perseveration scores as measured by the Mattis Dementia Rating Scale (MDRS) (Alexopoulos *et al.*, 2002c). The term 'executive functions' encompasses a variety of cognitive abilities, such as planning, organizing, self-monitoring, inhibiting prepotent responses and strategy generation (Lezak, 1976; Benton, 1994). Each of these functions is subserved by distinct, but also shared, neural systems. Furthermore, performance on measures of executive function can affect and be affected by performance in non-executive cognitive domains, such as processing speed, learning, and memory (Elderkin-Thompson *et al.*, 2008). Therefore, it is likely that some of these functions, and not others, may be relevant to antidepressant response.

These findings are consistent with studies suggesting that abnormalities in neural systems related to executive functions are associated with poor remission rate of late-life depression. Severe hyperintensities in subcortical grey matter regions were associated with poor response of depressed elderly patients to electroconvulsive therapy (Steffens *et al.*, 2001). An electrical tomography analysis study suggests that anterior cingulate activity is a predictor of the extent of treatment response in depression (Pizzagalli *et al.*, 2001); functional integrity of the anterior cingulate cortex is required for the performance of executive functions.

Functional imaging studies suggest that remission of younger adults suffering from depression is associated with metabolic increases in dorsal cortical regions (Mayberg *et al.*, 1999) and decreases in ventral limbic and paralimbic structures (Mayberg *et al.*, 1999; Smith *et al.*, 1999; Liotti and Mayberg, 2001). Persistently elevated metabolism of the amygdala during remission of depression was associated with high risk for relapse of depression in younger adults (Drevets, 1999). The anterior cingulate cortex may also play a role in the response of depressive symptoms to treatment. Improvement of depression is often associated with at least partial normalization of abnormal activation of the anterior cingulate (Buchsbaum *et al.*, 1997; Kennedy *et al.*, 2001; Drevets *et al.*, 2002; Saxena *et al.*, 2002; Gildengers *et al.*, 2005; Kennedy *et al.*, 2007). More recent research has shown greater activation of the rostral and dorsal cingulate at baseline predicts better subsequent antidepressant treatment response (Langenecker *et al.*, 2007), that remission of depression is often associated with at least partial normalization of anterior cingulate activation abnormalities (Mayberg *et al.*, 1999; Wu *et al.*, 1999), and that changes in anterior cingulate function are associated with symptomatic improvement (Fu *et al.*, 2004). Furthermore, a recent diffusion tension imaging (DTI) study suggest that, in addition to other cortico-striatal-limbic regions, reduced white matter integrity lateral to the dorsal and rostral anterior cingulate cortex (ACC) (Alexopoulos *et al.*, 2008) predicts failure to remit with antidepressant treatment.

74.6 'PSEUDODEMENTIA'

The concept of reversible dementia was introduced in the mid-nineteenth century (Berrios, 1985; Emery, 1988) and became the focus of clinical attention in the early 1960s when the term 'pseudodementia' was used to describe a broad range of reversible cognitive impairments associated with psychiatric syndromes (Kiloh, 1961). The current concept of 'pseudodementia' is that of an initially reversible cognitive impairment that both occurs in the context of diverse psychiatric disorders, and influences their course.

The clinical presentation of depression with cognitive impairment is heterogeneous; the signs and symptoms are principally influenced by the patients' age and underlying psychiatric disorders (Kiloh, 1961; Wells, 1979; Rabins *et al.*, 1984; Alexopoulos, 1990; Emery and Oxman, 1992). In a non-geriatric series, 'pseudodementia' was reported in patients with Ganser syndrome, personality disorders, melancholic depression, hypomania, atypical psychosis, paraphrenia, catatonia, depersonalization and malingering (Kiloh, 1961; Wells, 1971). Non-geriatric patients with 'pseudodementia' in this sample had a history of prior psychiatric disorders, a recent and abrupt onset of current illness, complained about their cognitive loss and experienced distress, and were able to both precisely identify the onset and describe in detail the course of their illness (Kiloh, 1961; Wells, 1979). On cognitive tests, these patients often said they did not know the correct answers even though the tasks were within their abilities. Performance on tasks of similar difficulty was markedly variable and accompanied by an over-dramatization of their failures.

As many younger patients with 'pseudodementia' have psychiatric syndromes other than depression, their clinical presentation is dissimilar from that of geriatric patients with 'pseudodementia' in whom depression is the most common diagnosis. Depressed elders with 'pseudodementia' usually have a severe depression syndrome, but a mild dementia. The clinical profile of major depression accompanying 'pseudodementia' of older adults is characterized by motor retardation, depressive delusions, hopelessness and helplessness (Alexopoulos and Abrams, 1991). Geriatric inpatients with major depression and 'pseudodementia' differ from those with uncomplicated major depression in that they often have a later age of onset of illness (Alexopoulos *et al.*, 1993b). When compared to Alzheimer's patients with concomitant depression, 'pseudodementia' patients have more psychic and somatic anxiety, early morning awakening and loss of libido (Reynolds *et al.*, 1986).

Neuropsychological assessment is generally considered the gold standard in differentiating between depression and the early stages of dementia. Decrements in memory, attention, visuospatial ability, processing speed and executive functioning have been reported in pseudodementia. Although these deficits are also seen in AD, cognitive impairments seen in early AD are more severe in nearly every cognitive domain. In addition, although memory may be impaired in both conditions, AD patients will often exhibit 'rapid forgetting' (Gray *et al.*, 1986) pointing to deficits in memory systems, as well as difficulty with recognition memory (Cohen *et al.*, 1982), which may indicate deficits in memory consolidation. AD patients also produce more 'false-positive' errors or 'intrusions', whereas depressed elderly patients tend to produce more false negatives (Whitehead, 1973). In addition, patients with true AD tend to present with additional specific impairments, such as impaired temporal orientation, abstraction, calculation, visual recognition, visuoconstruction and language functions (Chaves and Izquierdo, 1992; Jones *et al.*, 1992). As a rule, the symptoms of depression also precede those of cognitive dysfunction in patients with true 'pseudodementia', making it important to take a thorough history of symptoms.

74.7 THE PROGNOSIS OF DEPRESSION WITH COGNITIVE IMPAIRMENT

Cognitive impairment, when mild, does not appear to progress to dementia in most cases. Instead, it is a stable disturbance that improves only moderately when depressive symptoms are ameliorated (Alexopoulos *et al.*, 2004; Nakano *et al.*, 2008). However, follow-up studies suggest that geriatric patients with depression and more severe cognitive symptoms, such as 'pseudodementia', are at an increased risk for developing irreversible dementia (Reynolds *et al.*, 1986; Kral and Emery, 1989; Copeland *et al.*, 1992; Alexopoulos *et al.*, 1993a; Butters *et al.*, 2008). Taken together, these studies suggest that 9–25 per cent of elderly patients with depression and an initially reversible dementia develop irreversible dementia each year.

Cognitive dysfunction in depressed patients has heterogeneous aetiology and outcome (Alexopoulos *et al.*, 2002a). Some patients presenting with both cognitive dysfunction and late onset depression may already be experiencing the beginning stages of a dementia. This view is supported by recent studies suggesting that depression is often a prodrome of dementing disorders (Butters *et al.*, 2008). Patients with comorbid depression and executive dysfunction have poor and unstable response to antidepressant treatment (Simpson *et al.*, 1998; Kalayam and Alexopoulos, 1999; Alexopoulos *et al.*, 2000; Potter *et al.*, 2004; Sneed *et al.*, 2007), as well as poorer social and occupational functioning at follow up (Withall *et al.*, 2009).

74.8   DIAGNOSTIC ASSESSMENT AND TREATMENT PLANNING

Identifying and characterizing the cognitive impairment of depressed elderly patients has important clinical implications. Depressed elders often develop delirium in response to drug side effects, dehydration, infections and other factors. Therefore, cognitive examination should focus on manifestations of delirium, including inattention, fluctuating state of consciousness and sleep–wake disturbances. Of course, making a diagnosis of delirium does not exclude a diagnosis of dementia. As dementing disorders predispose to delirium, delirious patients should be re-examined for an underlying dementia after the delirium resolves. Identifying treatable causes of dementia (e.g. dementia due to drug intoxication, organ failure, endocrinopathies, B_{12} deficiency, normal pressure hydrocephalus and space-occupying lesions) is important, as treatment of these conditions may reverse or arrest the progress of dementia.

The occurrence of depression or cognitive impairment in the elderly should lead to an examination for possibly undetected cardiovascular disease and to consideration of factors that might predispose to cardiovascular disease, because both of these conditions are associated with cerebrovascular disease (Thomas *et al.*, 2004; Román, 2006; Kelly and Alexopoulos, 2009). Most brain infarcts do not manifest with neurological signs (Fried *et al.*, 1991; Longstreth *et al.*, 1998; Vermeer *et al.*, 2002), so depression and/or cognitive impairment can be the first sign of cerebrovascular disease. The relationship between depression and cardiovascular disease appears to be bidirectional (Thomas *et al.*, 2004). Therefore, care should be coordinated to ensure that both psychiatric and cardiovascular health issues are addressed (Alexopoulos *et al.*, 2002a). Since many medications, including psychotropic medications, increase cardiovascular risk factors including hyperlipidaemia, hyperglycaemia, hypertension and obesity, a careful overview of patient medications is needed (Kelly and Alexopoulos, 2009).

When dementia is identified, the clinical characterization of the dementia syndrome can guide treatment. Among the dementia syndromes, subcortical dementia is the syndrome most likely to be complicated by depression. Subcortical dementia is characterized by significant memory impairment, executive dysfunction and psychomotor retardation. Disorders causing subcortical dementias include mixed AD and VaD, VaD, PD and dementia with Lewy bodies (DLB). These disorders require specific treatments, e.g. VaD is often treated

with aspirin, statins and management of hypertension, PD with dopamine acting agents, and DLB with cholinesterase inhibitors. Unlike subcortical dementias, cortical dementias manifest broader impairment of cognitive functions, including memory impairment, apraxia, aphasia with paraphasic errors and graphomotor construction problems. The most common cause of cortical dementia is AD, a condition treated with cholinesterase inhibitors at least during the early and middle phase and with memantine during the advanced phase or earlier. Frontal lobe syndromes are characterized by rather mild memory impairment and pronounced personality changes, apathy, socially inappropriate behaviour and disinhibition, often resulting in irritability. Frontal lobe syndromes may be due to frontotemporal dementia, head trauma, or stroke; disorders for which there are no specific treatments.

Identification of executive dysfunction is important even in non-demented depressed elderly patients. Depressed patients with psychomotor retardation, reduced interest in activities, suspiciousness and disability are likely to have executive dysfunction (Alexopoulos *et al.*, 2002c). Depression with executive dysfunction may have a poor and unstable response to antidepressants (Kalayam and Alexopoulos, 1999; Alexopoulos *et al.*, 2000; Alexopoulos *et al.*, 2005). For this reason, patients with the depression-executive dysfunction syndrome of late life require carefully planned psychopharmacological treatment and vigilant follow up, since they are at high risk for relapse or recurrence (Alexopoulos *et al.*, 2000). Non-pharmacological interventions should be considered, particularly in medication non-responders. Problem-solving therapy (PST) aimed at remedying behavioural deficits (Alexopoulos *et al.*, 2003) has been effective in such patients (Gellis *et al.*, 2007; Alexopoulos *et al.*, 2008b) and high-frequency repetitive transcranial magnetic stimulation has been demonstrated effective for 'vascular depression' (Jorge *et al.*, 2008). Stimulation of the dorsolateral prefrontal cortex (DLPFC) may be a common mode of action for both treatments. Finally, depressed patients whose cognitive impairment prevents them from benefiting from problem-solving therapy or other psychotherapy treatments might benefit from a comprehensive approach aimed at helping patients to assimilate new skills within their abilities, while helping their environment (including caregivers) to be more accommodating. We have developed 'ecosystem-focused therapy', which utilizes problem-solving therapy principles, but focuses on the 'ecosystem' (patient + family member/ caregiver) of which the patient is part. Ecosystem-focused therapy imparts to the patient skills maximizing his/her remaining functions, modifies the patient's physical environment, and engages family members/caregivers in helping the patient to utilize his/her skills. Enabling the patient to assimilate new skills and changing their environment so that it accommodates to their state maximizes adaptation and may reduce depression (Alexopoulos and Bruce, 2009).

Evaluation of depressive syndromes in cognitively impaired patients is complicated by the symptom overlap with dementia, the instability of depressive manifestations over time, and the poor ability of elderly patients to report their symptoms. If criteria for one of the depressive syndromes are met, an antidepressant treatment trial should be offered. Beyond the benefits of alleviating the suffering and the complications of depression, remission of the depressive syndrome can increase the clinician's ability to evaluate the severity of the remaining cognitive impairment and plan for further treatment and follow up. The Expert Consensus Guideline recommends antidepressant drug therapy combined with a psychosocial intervention as the treatment of choice for geriatric depression (Alexopoulos et al., 2001). Variability in the course of elders with depression and cognitive impairment suggests the need for careful follow up. About 40 per cent of these patients are expected to receive the diagnosis of dementia within two years after the diagnosis of 'pseudodementia'. Prompt identification and treatment of the dementing disorder may increase the time during which the patient can function independently.

REFERENCES

Aizenstein HJ, Butters MA, Wu M et al. (2009) Altered functioning of the executive control circuit in late-life depression: episodic and persistent phenomena. *American Journal of Geriatric Psychiatry* **17**: 30–42.

Alexopoulos GS. (1990) Clinical and biological findings in late-onset depression. In: Tasman A, Goldfinger SM, Kaufmann CA (eds). *American Psychiatric Press Review of Psychiatry*. Washington DC: American Psychiatric Press, 249–62.

Alexopoulos GS, Abrams RC. (1991) Depression in Alzheimer's disease. *Psychiatric Clinics of North America* **14**: 327–40.

Alexopoulos GS, Bruce ML. (2009) A model for intervention research in late-life depression. *International Journal of Geriatric Psychiatry* **24**: 1325–34.

Alexopoulos GS, Meyers BS, Young RC et al. (1993a) The course of geriatric depression with "reversible dementia": a controlled study. *American Journal of Psychiatry* **150**: 1693–9.

Alexopoulos GS, Young RC, Meyers BS. (1993b) Geriatric depression: age of onset and dementia. *Biological Psychiatry* **34**: 141–5.

Alexopoulos GS, Vrontou C, Kakuma T et al. (1996) Disability in geriatric depression. *American Journal of Psychiatry* **153**: 877–85.

Alexopoulos GS, Meyers BS, Young RC et al. (2000) Executive dysfunction and long-term outcomes of geriatric depression. *Archives of General Psychiatry* **57**: 285–90.

Alexopoulos GS, Katz IR, Reynolds 3rd CF et al. (2001) The expert consensus guideline series. Pharmacotherapy of depressive disorders in older patients. *Postgraduate Medicine* **20** (Special issue): 1–86.

Alexopoulos GS, Buckwalter K, Olin J et al. (2002a) Comorbidity of late life depression: an opportunity for research on mechanisms and treatment. *Biological Psychiatry* **52**: 543–58.

Alexopoulos GS, Kiosses DN, Choi SJ et al. (2002b) Frontal white matter microstructure and treatment response of late-life depression: a preliminary study. *American Journal of Psychiatry* **159**: 1929–32.

Alexopoulos GS, Kiosses DN, Klimstra S et al. (2002c) Clinical presentation of the 'depression-executive dysfunction syndrome' of late life. *American Journal of Geriatric Psychiatry* **10**: 98–106.

Alexopoulos GS, Raue P, Arean P. (2003) Problem-solving therapy versus supportive therapy in geriatric major depression with executive dysfunction. *American Journal of Geriatric Psychiatry* **11**: 46–52.

Alexopoulos GS, Kiosses DN, Murphy C, Heo M. (2004) Executive dysfunction, heart disease burden, and remission of geriatric depression. *Neuropsychopharmacology* **29**: 2278–84.

Alexopoulos GS, Kiosses DN, Heo M et al. (2005) Executive dysfunction and the course of geriatric depression. *Biological Psychiatry* **58**: 204–10.

Alexopoulos GS, Murphy CF, Gunning-Dixon FM et al. (2008a) Microstructural white matter abnormalities and remission of geriatric depression. *American Journal of Psychiatry* **165**: 238–44.

Alexopoulos GS, Raue PJ, Kanellopoulos D et al. (2008b) Problem solving therapy for the depression-executive dysfunction syndrome of late life. *International Journal of Geriatric Psychiatry* **23**: 782–8.

Arve S, Tilvis RS, Lehtonen A et al. (1999) Coexistence of lowered mood and cognitive impairment of elderly people in five birth cohorts. *Aging* **11**: 90–5.

Ballmaier M, Toga AW, Blanton RE et al. (2004) Anterior cingulate, gyrus rectus, and orbitofrontal abnormalities in elderly depressed patients: an MRI-based parcellation of the prefrontal cortex. *American Journal of Psychiatry* **161**: 99–108.

Bayles KA, Kaszniak AW, Tomoeda CK. (1987) *Communication and cognition in normal aging and dementia*. San Diego: College-Hill Press.

Beats BC, Sahakian BJ, Levy R. (1996) Cognitive performance in tests sensitive to frontal lobe dysfunction in the elderly depressed. *Psychological Medicine* **26**: 591–603.

Bench CJ, Friston KJ, Brown RG et al. (1992) The anatomy of melancholia–focal abnormalities of cerebral blood flow in major depression. *Psychological Medicine* **22**: 607–15.

Benton AL. (1994) *Contributions to neuropsychological assessment: a clinical manual*, 2nd edn. New York: Oxford University Press.

Berrios GE. (1985) 'Depressive pseudodementia' or 'Melancholic dementia': a 19th century view. *Journal of Neurology, Neurosurgery, and Psychiatry* **48**: 393–400.

Boone KB, Miller BL, Lesser IM et al. (1992) Neuropsychological correlates of white-matter lesions in healthy elderly subjects: A threshold effect. *Archives of Neurology* **49**: 549–54.

Boone KB, Lesser I, Miller B et al. (1994) Cognitive functioning in a mildly to moderately depressed geriatric sample: relationship to chronological age. *Journal of Neuropsychiatry and Clinical Neurosciences* **6**: 267–72.

Buchsbaum MS, Wu J, Siegel BV et al. (1997) Effect of sertraline on regional metabolic rate in patients with affective disorder. *Biological Psychiatry* **41**: 15–22.

Bueller JA, Aftab M, Sen S et al. (2006) BDNF Val66Met allele is associated with reduced hippocampal volume in healthy subjects. *Biological Psychiatry* **59**: 812–5.

Butters MA, Becker JT, Nebes RD *et al.* (2000) Changes in cognitive functioning following treatment of late-life depression. *American Journal of Psychiatry* **157**: 1949–54.

Butters MA, Bhalla RK, Mulsant BH *et al.* (2004a) Executive functioning, illness course, and relapse/recurrence in continuation and maintenance treatment of late-life depression: is there a relationship? *American Journal of Geriatric Psychiatry* **12**: 387–94.

Butters MA, Whyte EM, Nebes RD *et al.* (2004b) The nature and determinants of neuropsychological functioning in late-life depression. *Archives of General Psychiatry* **61**: 587–95.

Butters MA, Young JB, Lopez O *et al.* (2008) Pathways linking late-life depression to persistent cognitive impairment and dementia. *Dialogues in Clinical Neuroscience* **10**: 345–57.

Carroll BJ, Feinberg M, Greden JF *et al.* (1981) A specific laboratory test for the diagnosis of melancholia. Standardization, validation, and clinical utility. *Archives of General Psychiatry* **38**: 15–22.

Chaves ML, Izquierdo I. (1992) Differential diagnosis between dementia and depression: a study of efficiency increment. *Acta Neurologica Scandinavica* **85**: 378–82.

Chemerinski E, Petracca G, Sabe L *et al.* (2001) The specificity of depressive symptoms in patients with Alzheimer's disease. *American Journal of Psychiatry* **158**: 68–72.

Chen R, Hu Z, Wei L *et al.* (2008) Severity of depression and risk for subsequent dementia: cohort studies in China and the UK. *British Journal of Psychiatry* **193**: 373–7.

Cohen RM, Weingartner H *et al.* (1982) Effort and cognition in depression. *Archives of General Psychiatry* **39**: 593–7.

Copeland JR, Davidson IA *et al.* (1992) Alzheimer's disease, other dementias, depression and pseudodementia: prevalence, incidence and three-year outcome in Liverpool. *British Journal of Psychiatry* **161**: 230–9.

Devanand DP, Sano M, Tang MX *et al.* (1996) Depressed mood and the incidence of Alzheimer's disease in the elderly living in the community. *Archives of General Psychiatry* **53**: 175–82.

Drevets WC. (1998) Functional neuroimaging studies of depression: the anatomy of melancholia. *Annual Review of Medicine* **49**: 341–61.

Drevets WC. (1999) Prefrontal cortical-amygdalar metabolism in major depression. *Annals of the New York Academy of the Sciences* **877**: 614–37.

Drevets WC, Videen TO, Price JL *et al.* (1992) A functional anatomical study of unipolar depression. *Journal of Neuroscience* **12**: 3628–41.

Drevets WC, Price JL, Simpson Jr JR *et al.* (1997) Subgenual prefrontal cortex abnormalities in mood disorders. *Nature* **386**: 824–7.

Drevets WC, Bogers W, Raichle ME. (2002) Functional anatomical correlates of antidepressant drug treatment assessed using PET measures of regional glucose metabolism. *European Neuropsychopharmacology* **12**: 527–44.

Duman RS, Heninger GR, Nestler EJ. (1997) A molecular and cellular theory of depression. *Archives of General Psychiatry* **54**: 597–606.

Dunkin JJ, Leuchter AF, Cook IA *et al.* (2000) Executive dysfunction predicts nonresponse to fluoxetine in major depression. *Journal of Affective Disorders* **60**: 13–23.

Elderkin-Thompson V, Kumar A, Mintz J *et al.* (2004) Executive dysfunction and visuospatial ability among depressed elders in a community setting. *Archives of Clinical Neuropsychology* **19**: 597–611.

Elderkin-Thompson V, Hellemann G, Pham D, Kumar A. (2008) Prefrontal brain morphology and executive function in healthy and depressed elderly. *International Journal of Geriatric Psychiatry* **16**: 633–42.

Emery OB. (1988) A theoretical and empirical discussion. Western Reserve Geriatric Education Center Interdisciplinary Monograph Series. Cleveland: Case Western Reserve University School of Medicine.

Emery VO, Oxman TE. (1992) Update on the dementia spectrum of depression. *American Journal of Psychiatry* **149**: 305–17.

Fried LP, Borhani NO, Enright P *et al.* (1991) The Cardiovascular Health Study: design and rationale. *Annals of Epidemiology* **1**: 263–76.

Fu CH, Williams SC, Cleare AJ *et al.* (2004) Attenuation of the neural response to sad faces in major depression by antidepressant treatment: a prospective, event-related functional magnetic resonance imaging study. *Archives of General Psychiatry* **61**: 877–89.

Ganguli M, Du Y, Dodge HH *et al.* (2006) Depressive symptoms and cognitive decline in late life: a prospective epidemiological study. *Archives of General Psychiatry* **63**: 153–60.

Gellis ZD, McGinty J, Horowitz A *et al.* (2007) Problem-solving therapy for late-life depression in home care: a randomized field trial. *American Journal of Geriatric Psychiatry* **15**: 968–78.

Gildengers AG, Houck PR, Mulsant BH *et al.* (2005) Trajectories of treatment response in late-life depression: psychosocial and clinical correlates. *Journal of Clinical Psychopharmacology*, **254** (Suppl 1)S8–13.

Gray JW, Rattan AI, Dean RS. (1986) Differential diagnosis of dementia and depression in the elderly using neuropsychological methods. *Archives of Clinical Neuropsychology* **1**: 341–9.

Gunning-Dixon FM, Hoptman MJ, Lim KO *et al.* (2008) Macromolecular white matter abnormalities in geriatric depression: a magnetization transfer imaging study. *American Journal of Geriatric Psychiatry* **16**: 255–62.

Hannestad J, Taylor WD, McQuoid DR *et al.* (2006) White matter lesion volumes and caudate volumes in late-life depression. *International Journal of Geriatric Psychiatry* **21**: 1193–8.

Hart RP, Kwentus JA, Taylor JR, Harkins SW. (1987) Rate of forgetting in dementia and depression. *Journal of Consulting and Clinical Psychology* **55**: 101–5.

Hickie I, Naismith S, Ward PB *et al.* (2005) Reduced hippocampal volumes and memory loss in patients with early- and late-onset depression. *British Journal of Psychiatry* **186**: 197–202.

Holtzer R, Scarmeas N, Wegesin DJ *et al.* (2005) Depressive symptoms in Alzheimer's disease: natural course and temporal relation to function and cognitive status. *Journal of the American Geriatrics Society* **53**: 2083–9.

Husain MM, McDonald WM, Doraiswamy PM et al. (1991) A magnetic resonance imaging study of putamen nuclei in major depression. Psychiatry Research 40: 95–9.

Janzing JG, Hooijer C, van't Hof MA, Zitman FG. (2002) Depression in subjects with and without dementia: a comparison using GMS-AGECAT. International Journal of Geriatric Psychiatry 17: 1–5.

Jorge RE, Moser DJ, Acion L, Robinson RG. (2008) Treatment of vascular depression using repetitive transcranial magnetic stimulation. Archives of General Psychiatry 65: 268–76.

Jorm AF, van Duijn CM, Chandra V et al. (1991) Psychiatric history and related exposures as risk factors for Alzheimer's disease: a collaborative re-analysis of case–control studies. EURODEM Risk Factors Research Group. International Journal of Epidemiology 20 (Suppl. 2): S43–7.

Kalayam B, Alexopoulos GS. (1999) Prefrontal dysfunction and treatment response in geriatric depression. Archives of General Psychiatry 56: 713–8.

Kelly RE, Alexopoulos GS. (2009) The vascular depression concept and its implications. In: Ellison JM, Kyomen HH, Verma S (eds). Mood disorders in late life, 2nd edn. New York: Informa Healthcare, 161–77.

Kennedy GJ. (2001) The dynamics of depression and disability. American Journal of Geriatric Psychiatry 9: 99–101.

Kiloh LG. (1961) Pseudo-dementia. Acta Psychiatrica Scandinavica 37: 336–51.

Kiosses DN, Alexopoulos GS, Murphy C. (2000) Symptoms of striatofrontal dysfunction contribute to disability in geriatric depression. International Journal of Geriatric Psychiatry 15: 992–9.

Kiosses DN, Klimstra S, Murphy C, Alexopoulos GS. (2001) Executive dysfunction and disability in elderly patients with major depression. American Journal of Geriatric Psychiatry 9: 269–74.

Kral VA, Emery OB. (1989) Long-term follow-up of depressive pseudodementia of the aged. Canadian Journal of Psychiatry 34: 445–6.

Kramer-Ginsberg E, Greenwald BS, Krishnan KR et al. (1999) Neuropsychological functioning and MRI signal hyperintensities in geriatric depression. American Journal of Psychiatry 156: 438–44.

Krishnan KR, McDonald WM, Escalona PR et al. (1992) Magnetic resonance imaging of the caudate nuclei in depression. Preliminary observations. Archives of General Psychiatry 49: 553–7.

Kumar A, Bilker W, Jin Z, Udupa J. (2000) Atrophy and high intensity lesions: complementary neurobiological mechanisms in late-life major depression. Neuropsychopharmacology 22: 264–74.

Lai T, Payne ME, Byrum CE et al. (2000) Reduction of orbital frontal cortex volume in geriatric depression. Biological Psychiatry 48: 971–5.

Lagopoulos J, Malhi GS, Ivanovski B et al. (2005) A matter of motion or an emotional matter? Management of depression in Parkinson's disease. Expert Review of Neurotherapeutics 5: 803–10.

Langenecker SA, Kennedy SE, Guidotti LM et al. (2007) Frontal and limbic activation during inhibitory control predicts treatment response in major depressive disorder. Biological Psychiatry 62: 1272–80.

Lesser IM, Boone KB, Mehringer CM et al. (1996) Cognition and white matter hyperintensities in older depressed patients. American Journal of Psychiatry 153: 1280–87.

Lezak MD. (1976) Neuropsychological assessment. New York: Oxford University Press.

Liotti M, Mayberg HS. (2001) The role of functional neuroimaging in the neuropsychology of depression. Journal of Clinical and Experimental Neuropsychology 23: 121–36.

Lockwood KA, Alexopoulos GS, Kakuma T, Van Gorp WG. (2000) Subtypes of cognitive impairment in depressed older adults. American Journal of Geriatric Psychiatry 8: 201–8.

Lockwood KA, Alexopoulos GS, van Gorp WG. (2002) Executive dysfunction in geriatric depression. American Journal of Psychiatry 159: 1119–26.

Longstreth Jr WT, Bernick C, Manolio TA et al. (1998) Lacunar infarcts defined by magnetic resonance imaging of 3660 elderly people: the Cardiovascular Health Study. Archives of Neurology 55: 1217–25.

MacFall JR, Payne ME, Provenzale JE, Krishnan KR. (2001) Medial orbital frontal lesions in late-onset depression. Biological Psychiatry 49: 803–6.

Mayberg HS, Liotti M, Brannan SK et al. (1999) Reciprocal limbic-cortical function and negative mood: converging PET findings in depression and normal sadness. American Journal of Psychiatry 156: 675–82.

Murphy CF, Alexopoulos GS. (2004) Longitudinal association of initiation/perseveration and severity of geriatric depression. American Journal of Geriatric Psychiatry 12: 50–56.

Murphy CF, Gunning-Dixon FM, Hoptman MJ et al. (2007) White-matter integrity predicts stroop performance in patients with geriatric depression. Biological Psychiatry 61: 1007–10.

Musazzi L, Cattaneo A, Tardito D et al. (2009) Early raise of BDNF in hippocampus suggests induction of posttranscriptional mechanisms by antidepressants. BMC Neuroscience 10: 48.

Nakano Y, Baba H, Maeshima H et al. (2008) Executive dysfunction in medicated, remitted state of major depression. Journal of Affective Disorders 111: 46–51.

Nebes RD, Butters MA, Mulsant BH et al. (2000) Decreased working memory and processing speed mediate cognitive impairment in geriatric depression. Psychological Medicine 30: 679–91.

Olin JT, Schneider LS, Katz IR et al. (2002) Provisional diagnostic criteria for depression of Alzheimer disease. American Journal of Geriatric Psychiatry 10: 125–8.

Ownby RL, Crocco E, Acevedo A et al. (2006) Depression and risk for Alzheimer disease: systematic review, meta-analysis, and metaregression analysis. Archives of General Psychiatry 63: 530–8.

Pezawas L, Verchinski BA, Mattay VS et al. (2004) The brain-derived neurotrophic factor val66met polymorphism and variation in human cortical morphology. Journal of Neuroscience 24: 10099–102.

Pizzagalli D, Pascual-Marqui RD, Nitschke JB *et al.* (2001) Anterior cingulate activity as a predictor of degree of treatment response in major depression: evidence from brain electrical tomography analysis. *American Journal of Psychiatry* **158**: 405–15.

Potter GG, Kittinger JD, Wagner HR *et al.* (2004) Prefrontal neuropsychological predictors of treatment remission in late-life depression. *Neuropsychopharmacology* **29**: 2266–71.

Rabins PV, Merchant A, Nestadt G. (1984) Criteria for diagnosing reversible dementia caused by depression: validation by 2-year follow-up. *British Journal of Psychiatry* **144**: 488–92.

Reynolds 3rd CF, Kupfer DJ, Hoch CC *et al.* (1986) Two-year follow-up of elderly patients with mixed depression and dementia. Clinical and electroencephalographic sleep findings. *Journal of the American Geriatrics Society* **34**: 793–9.

Ritchie K, Gilham C, Ledesert B *et al.* (1999) Depressive illness, depressive symptomatology and regional cerebral blood flow in elderly people with sub-clinical cognitive impairment. *Age and Ageing* **28**: 385–91.

Román GC. (2006) Vascular depression: An archetypal neuropsychiatric disorder. *Biological Psychiatry* **60**: 1306–8.

Saxena S, Brody AL, Ho ML *et al.* (2002) Differential cerebral metabolic changes with paroxetine treatment of obsessive-compulsive disorder vs major depression. *Archives of General Psychiatry* **59**: 250–61.

Sheline YI, Wang PW, Gado MH *et al.* (1996) Hippocampal atrophy in recurrent major depression. *Proceedings of the National Academy of Sciences of the United States of America* **93**: 3908–13.

Sheline YI, Gado MH, Price JL. (1998) Amygdala core nuclei volumes are decreased in recurrent major depression. *Neuroreport* **9**: 2023–8.

Sheline YI, Sanghavi M, Mintun MA, Gado MH. (1999) Depression duration but not age predicts hippocampal volume loss in medically healthy women with recurrent major depression. *Journal of Neuroscience* **19**: 5034–43.

Sheline YI, Gado MH, Kraemer HC. (2003) Untreated depression and hippocampal volume loss. *American Journal of Psychiatry* **160**: 1516–18.

Simpson S, Baldwin RC, Jackson A, Burns AS. (1998) Is subcortical disease associated with a poor response to antidepressants? Neurological, neuropsychological and neuroradiological findings in late-life depression. *Psychological Medicine* **28**: 1015–26.

Smith GE, Housen P, Yaffe K *et al.* (2009) A cognitive training program based on principles of brain plasticity: results from the Improvement in Memory with Plasticity-based Adaptive Cognitive Training (IMPACT) study. *Journal of the American Geriatric Society* **57**: 594–603.

Smith GS, Reynolds 3rd CF, Pollock B *et al.* (1999) Cerebral glucose metabolic response to combined total sleep deprivation and antidepressant treatment in geriatric depression. *American Journal of Psychiatry* **156**: 683–9.

Smith GS, Kramer E, Ma Y *et al.* (2009) The functional neuroanatomy of geriatric depression. *International Journal of Geriatric Psychiatry* **24**: 798–808.

Sneed JR, Roose SP, Keilp JG *et al.* (2007) Response inhibition predicts poor antidepressant treatment response in very old depressed patients. *American Journal of Geriatric Psychiatry* **15**: 553–63.

Sobin C, Sackeim HA. (1997) Psychomotor symptoms of depression. *American Journal of Psychiatry* **154**: 4–17.

Steffens DC, Hays JC, Krishnan KR. (1999) Disability in geriatric depression. *American Journal of Geriatric Psychiatry* **7**: 34–40.

Steffens DC, Conway CR, Dombeck CB *et al.* (2001) Severity of subcortical gray matter hyperintensity predicts ECT response in geriatric depression. *Journal of ECT* **17**: 45–9.

Story TJ, Potter GG, Attix DK *et al.* (2008) Neurocognitive correlates of response to treatment in late-life depression. *American Journal of Geriatric Psychiatry* **16**: 752–9.

Taylor WD, Steffens DC, McQuoid DR *et al.* (2003) Smaller orbital frontal cortex volumes associated with functional disability in depressed elders. *Biolical Psychiatry* **53**: 144–9.

Teng E, Ringman JM, Ross LK *et al.* (2008) Diagnosing depression in Alzheimer disease with the national institute of mental health provisional criteria. *American Journal of Geriatric Psychiatry* **16**: 469–77.

Thomas AJ, Kalaria RN, O'Brien JT. (2004) Depression and vascular disease: what is the relationship? *Journal of Affective Disorders* **79**: 81–95.

Van Duijn CM, Clayton DG, Chandra V *et al.* (1994) Interaction between genetic and environmental risk factors for Alzheimer's disease: a reanalysis of case–control studies. *Genetic Epidemiology* **11**: 539–51.

Van Otterloo E, O'Dwyer G, Stockmeier CA *et al.* (2009) Reductions in neuronal density in elderly depressed are region specific. *International Journal of Geriatric Psychiatry* **24**: 856–64.

Vermeer SE, Koudstaal PJ, Oudkerk M *et al.* (2002) Prevalence and risk factors of silent brain infarcts in the population-based Rotterdam Scan Study. *Stroke* **33**: 21–5.

Wells CE. (1971) The symptoms and behavioral manifestations of dementia. *Contemporary Neurology Series* **9**: 1–11.

Wells CE. (1979) Pseudodementia. *American Journal of Psychiatry* **136**: 895–900.

Whitehead A. (1973) Verbal learning and memory in elderly depressives. *British Journal of Psychiatry* **123**: 203–8.

Withall A, Harris LM, Cumming SR. (2009) The relationship between cognitive function and clinical and functional outcomes in major depressive disorder. *Psychological Medicine* **39**: 393–402.

Wragg RE, Jeste DV. (1989) Overview of depression and psychosis in Alzheimer's disease. *American Journal of Psychiatry* **146**: 577–87.

Wu J, Buchsbaum MS, Gillin JC *et al.* (1999) Prediction of antidepressant effects of sleep deprivation by metabolic rates in the ventral anterior cingulate and medial prefrontal cortex. *American Journal of Psychiatry* **156**: 1149–58.

Wu JC, Gillin JC, Buchsbaum MS *et al.* (1992) Effect of sleep deprivation on brain metabolism of depressed patients. *American Journal of Psychiatry* **149**: 538–43.

Yaffe K, Blackwell T, Gore R *et al.* (1999) Depressive symptoms and cognitive decline in nondemented elderly women: a prospective study. *Archives of General Psychiatry* **56**: 425–30.

Young EA, Vazquez D. (1996) Hypercortisolemia, hippocampal glucocorticoid receptors, and fast feedback. *Molecular Psychiatry* 1: 149–59.

Young EA, Haskett RF, Murphy-Weinberg V *et al.* (1991) Loss of glucocorticoid fast feedback in depression. *Archives of General Psychiatry* 48: 693–9.

Yuan Y, Zhu W, Zhang Z *et al.* (2008) Regional gray matter changes are associated with cognitive deficits in remitted geriatric depression: an optimized voxel-based morphometry study. *Biological Psychiatry* 64: 541–4.

Schizophrenia, cognitive impairment and dementia

FLAVIE WATERS AND OSVALDO P ALMEIDA

75.1 INTRODUCTION

More than a century ago, Emil Kraepelin identified a disorder that he termed 'dementia praecox'. He argued that the two key features of this disorder were a progressive and deteriorating course of cognitive and functional processes ('dementia') and an early age of onset in previously healthy individuals ('praecox'). Since Kraepelin's seminal description of the key features of the disorder that is now known as schizophrenia, researchers have attempted to clarify whether:

- schizophrenia is associated with cognitive and functional deficits;
- the cognitive deficits of schizophrenia show a progressive and deteriorating course; and
- schizophrenia ultimately leads to the development of dementia.

This chapter selectively reviews the most recent evidence covering these areas of research.

75.2 IS SCHIZOPHRENIA ASSOCIATED WITH COGNITIVE AND FUNCTIONAL DEFICITS?

Studies consistently show that people with schizophrenia demonstrate cognitive dysfunctions in many neuropsychological domains that generally fall between one to two standard deviations below the scores of age- and gender-matched healthy controls (Heinrichs and Zakzanis, 1998; Bilder et al., 2000; Keshavan et al., 2008). Deficits have been reported in areas of memory, executive functions, speed of information processing, language and attention (Cirillo and Seidman, 2003; Bozikas et al., 2006; Waters, 2007).

Memory impairments have been reported in both verbal and non-verbal domains, as well as immediate and delayed recall (Bozikas et al., 2006). In a review of the literature, Cirillo and Seidman (2003) showed that 101 of 110 studies demonstrated a pattern of pervasive memory impairment in individuals with schizophrenia that is independent of the duration of illness, use of medications and premorbid intelligence. Impairments in executive functions have also been reported consistently in schizophrenia, with evidence of moderate to severe deficits on tasks measuring inhibitory control, planning, monitoring of performance and set-shifting (Waters, 2007). The cognitive deficits of schizophrenia are pervasive and extend beyond impairments of memory and executive functions. When compared with healthy controls, people with schizophrenia also show evidence of impairments in speed of information processing, language and attention. Some of these deficits have been found to precede the onset of clinical symptoms, with several studies reporting significantly lower school performances in children who go on to develop schizophrenia in adult life than their age-matched peers (Bilder et al., 2006; Woodberry et al., 2008). The pattern of generalized cognitive impairment in people with schizophrenia is consistent with findings from imaging studies showing smaller brain volumes, larger ventricles, reduced volumes of the temporal gyri, hippocampi, frontal lobes and corpus callosum, as well as reduced frontal lobe connectivity (Delisi, 2008; Rosenberger et al., 2008).

In a subset of cases, the symptoms of schizophrenia develop for the first time in middle or old age. Studies in this older age group show a pattern of generalized cognitive impairment that is similar to the deficits displayed by patients with an early illness onset, and involves dysfunctions in memory, executive functions, attention and speed of processing (Almeida *et al.*, 1995; Sachdev and Brodaty, 1999). Available evidence suggests that these deficits are different from those seen in patients with Alzheimer's disease (AD), as the latter show much more pronounced deficits of delayed recall on memory tasks (Heaton *et al.*, 1994; Davidson *et al.*, 1996; Zakzanis *et al.*, 2003).

Consistent with findings of cognitive dysfunctions, neuro-imaging studies of people with late-onset schizophrenia show cortical and subcortical abnormalities, and cerebrovascular changes (Miller *et al.*, 1991; Howard *et al.*, 1995; Sachdev and Brodaty, 1999; Jones *et al.*, 2005). Recently, Almeida and Starkstein (2010) critically examined the possible link between cerebrovascular disease and symptoms of psychosis, and concluded that cerebrovascular disease is unlikely to play a major role in the development of schizophrenia in later life. They also commented that lesions to the right temporo-parietal-occipital cortex were the most frequently reported cortical abnormalities associated with psychosis, a finding that is consistent with the results of brain stimulation studies in healthy people that produce significant sensory changes and out-of-body experiences (Blanke *et al.*, 2005). These results suggest that psychotic symptoms may be elicited by a non-specific lesion or insult to the right temporo-parietal-occipital cortex.

In addition to cognitive impairments, pervasive functional impairments have also been demonstrated in people with schizophrenia. Evidence shows that cognitive deficits contribute significantly to the functional disability of people with schizophrenia. A review of relevant studies concluded that there is a strong direct association between cognitive impairments and community functioning, the ability to maintain employment and the quality of social relationships (Green *et al.*, 2004). Furthermore, cognitive scores have been found to reliably predict the functional capacity of patients after six months (Green *et al.*, 2004), as well as their long-term social and vocational outcome (Bowie *et al.*, 2008). These findings underline the need to consider cognitive dysfunction as a critical treatment target in schizophrenia.

In summary, young and old adults with schizophrenia display a pattern of generalized cognitive deficits which precede the onset of symptoms, but become more apparent once diagnosis is established. The degree of functional impairment and disability of patients with schizophrenia is directly related to the severity of their cognitive deficits.

75.3   DO COGNITIVE DEFICITS IN SCHIZOPHRENIA SHOW A PROGRESSIVE AND DETERIORATING COURSE?

Studies that have examined the trajectory of cognitive deficits at different stages of the course of schizophrenia show that the most substantial changes occur in the early stages of the

illness. Longitudinal studies have shown a significant drop of intellectual functioning in patients assessed before and after the onset of illness (Seidman *et al.*, 2006), and cross-sectional studies report that patients with first-episode psychosis show broad neuropsychological impairments when compared with age-matched controls (Hoff *et al.*, 2005). In addition, twin studies have demonstrated that affected twins score, on average, ten points lower on intelligence tests than their unaffected siblings, supporting the hypothesis that schizophrenia is associated with cognitive decline (Kremen *et al.*, 2006). These findings are supported by reports of brain changes in people early in the disease process. The major findings have included lateral ventricular enlargement, bilateral grey matter reductions, reduced white matter integrity and regional volume reductions in the frontal and temporal gyri, as well as in the hippocampus and limbic regions (Kuroki *et al.*, 2006; Steen *et al.*, 2006; Vita *et al.*, 2006).

Fewer studies have examined the course of cognitive deficits post-onset and during middle adulthood, but these do not show consistent evidence of intellectual or cognitive decline over time. A review of 53 studies that had conducted repeat testing of patients with schizophrenia at least one month apart found that cognitive functioning does not seem to decline significantly with time – in fact, the opposite may occur (Szoke *et al.*, 2008). Longitudinal studies with a longer follow-up period also show little or no evidence of progression of impairment in the first decades of illness onset. For instance, Barnett *et al.* (2007) examined changes in cognitive function over one year. Overall, the results showed mixed performance with both improvements and decline in cognition, but also that the magnitude of these changes was relatively small. Finally, a ten-year longitudinal study of 21 patients with first-episode psychosis concluded that the cognitive performance of participants remained relatively stable over that period, and that the pattern of deterioration was not significantly greater in patients than in healthy controls (Hoff *et al.*, 2005).

The results of longer-term investigations of older patients have been mixed and indicate that outcomes may vary on the basis of clinical differences. Some studies have reported a progressive decline later in life which follows a pattern of relatively stable cognitive performance during middle adulthood (Friedman *et al.*, 2001; Morrison *et al.*, 2006). These findings, however, have not always been replicated, and there is some evidence that a more malignant pattern of cognitive decline may be associated with an increased number of hospital admissions and a more chronic course (Kurtz, 2005; O'Donnell, 2007).

There is only sparse information available about the long-term cognitive outcome of patients with late-onset schizophrenia. Harvey and colleagues (2003) examined the rate of decline in patients aged 64 years and older who were initially either low or high functioning. The results showed that the progression of cognitive decline was almost identical for the two schizophrenia groups, suggesting that baseline cognitive abilities are not a determinant of long-term outcome. A similar pattern of results was reported by Palmer *et al.* (2003) who compared the cognitive performance of patients with early and late-onset schizophrenia, with the performance of patients with AD and age-matched healthy controls. A similar rate of change was observed in controls and in the two schizophrenia patient groups, indicating that schizophrenia was not associated with an abnormal decline in performance. By contrast, patients with AD showed a much steeper deterioration of scores over two years when compared with patients with schizophrenia, highlighting the differences in the course of illness between these two diagnostic groups.

Taken together, these results suggest that most cognitive changes occur early in the illness and represent a drop from a previous level of functioning. However, there is limited evidence that cognitive functions change substantially after the onset of symptoms in schizophrenia and the vast majority of studies argue against a progressive deteriorating course in all patients.

75.4   WHAT IS THE ASSOCIATION BETWEEN SCHIZOPHRENIA AND DEMENTIA?

Kraepelin's concept of dementia praecox has led researchers to examine the link between schizophrenia and dementia. Some investigators have suggested that people with schizophrenia are at increased risk of developing dementia in older age (Harvey, 2001; Brodaty et al., 2003; Rabins and Lavrisha, 2003), often on the basis of observational studies which have reported that psychotic symptoms at times precede a diagnosis of dementia. For example, Korner and colleagues (2009) reviewed administrative data to examine the risk of dementia in approximately 20 000 people who had symptoms of schizophrenia after the age of 40 years, and concluded that people with schizophrenia had twice the rate of developing dementia as the general population. However, the validity of the diagnosis of schizophrenia in this study is uncertain, and patients and controls were not recruited from the same population. Another study by Velakoulis and colleagues (2009) found that five of 17 patients diagnosed with early frontotemporal dementia had received a diagnosis of psychotic illness (schizophrenia-spectrum disorder or bipolar disorder) approximately five years prior to the diagnosis of dementia, which was interpreted as evidence for a causal relationship between schizophrenia and frontotemporal dementia. Notwithstanding the methodological limitation of retrospective case report methods, a difficulty with this argument is that psychotic symptoms may, instead, point to shared brain pathology, or indicate an illness prodrome for dementia. Finally, the presence of hallucinations and delusions alone is not indicative of any specific disorders, given that studies in younger adults show that they have multiple causes. Future studies should pursue the exploration of phenomenological characteristics of psychotic symptoms in individuals who develop dementia, with a view to identifying clinical symptoms with diagnostic implications.

Moreover, the results of imaging studies show that the brain changes in people with schizophrenia are localized and specific, in contrast to the widespread changes observed in patients with AD, vascular dementia, frontotemporal dementia or dementia with Lewy bodies. Results of functional imaging studies suggest that most of the changes in schizophrenia occur in subcortical or anterior brain structures, which is different from the pattern observed in AD such as temporo-parietal hypometabolism and vulnerability in the frontal, parietal, temporal and occipital association areas. Structural imaging of people with AD also show significant reductions in mean grey matter volume and grey/white matter volume ratio, and significant increases in lateral ventricular volumes which are related to dementia severity, a pattern which is not seen in people with schizophrenia.

Detailed neuropathological investigations have failed to support the suggestion that people with schizophrenia are at an increased risk of developing dementia. Post-mortem studies of patients with schizophrenia, for instance, demonstrate that they are no more likely than controls to show neurodegenerative changes during ageing, and histopathological studies of the brains of people with schizophrenia have failed to show any evidence of AD-related pathology. For example, Purohit et al. (1998) found no evidence of excessive numbers of senile plaques, neurofibrillary tangles or neuronal loss among 100 consecutive autopsy brain specimens of subjects with chronic schizophrenia aged 52–101 years. Similarly, Arnold et al. (1998) used a steriological counting method to quantify the presence of neurofibrillary tangles, amyloid plaques and Lewy bodies, and found that their 23 elderly patients with schizophrenia did not present a larger number of neurodegenerative lesions than 14 healthy comparison controls, although notably both groups differed significantly on these measures from ten subjects with AD. In addition, Religa et al. (2003) found that the concentration of antibodies against $A\beta40$ and $A\beta42$ in the brains of 26 patients with schizophrenia was the same as in 11 controls and substantially lower than in ten patients with AD. Since β-amyloid is thought to be central to the pathogenetic process that leads to the development of AD, the results are not supportive of the suggestion that schizophrenia and AD have shared pathological processes. Finally, there is no evidence that schizophrenia and AD share the same genetic risk factors (Bertram and Tanzi, 2008; Schwab and Wildenauer, 2009). Taken together, these findings indicate that the mechanisms that lead to cognitive impairment in schizophrenia are different from those observed in common neurodegenerative disorders such as AD.

75.5   CONCLUSION

Schizophrenia is a debilitating disorder that is associated with marked generalized cognitive impairment and functional deficits. People with schizophrenia experience substantial cognitive losses at the time of onset of symptoms, but these neuropsychological deficits remain relatively stable over time (although a small proportion of patients may experience further losses in later life). There is no convincing evidence that schizophrenia is a disorder that will ultimately lead to the development of dementia – in fact, all available evidence indicates that schizophrenia is not associated with any form of continuous deterioration or neurodegeneration. Overall, the bulk of research findings do not support the idea that schizophrenia is related to dementia, and the label 'dementia' should be actively avoided to prevent further confusion.

Future studies should aim to restore a research strategy which focuses on the unique characteristics of these two complex disorders as separate lines of investigations.

REFERENCES

Almeida O, Starkstein S. (2010) Cerebrovascular disease and psychosis. In: Sachdev P, Keshavan MS (eds). *Secondary schizophrenia*. Cambridge: Cambridge University Press.

Almeida O, Howard R, Levy R *et al.* (1995) Clinical and cognitive diversity of psychotic states arising in late life (late paraphrenia). *Psychological Medicine* 25: 699–714.

Arnold S, Trojanowski J, Gur R *et al.* (1998) Absence of neurodegeneration and neural injury in the cerebral cortex in a sample of elderly patients with schizophrenia. *Archives of General Psychiatry* 55: 225–32.

Barnett J, Croudace T, Jaycock S *et al.* (2007) Improvement and decline of cognitive function in schizophrenia over one year: a longitudinal investigation using latent growth modelling. *BMC Psychiatry* 7: 16–26.

Bertram L, Tanzi RE. (2008) Thirty years of Alzheimer's disease genetics: the implications of systematic meta-analyses. *Nature Review Neuroscience* 9: 768–78.

Bilder R, Reiter G, Bates J *et al.* (2006) Cognitive development in schizophrenia: Follow back from the first episode. *Journal of Clinical and Experimental Neuropsychology* 28: 270–82.

Bilder RM, Goldman RS, Robinson D *et al.* (2000) Neuropsychology of first-episode schizophrenia: initial characterization and clinical correlates. *American Journal of Psychiatry* 157: 549–59.

Blanke O, Mohr C, Michel C *et al.* (2005) Linking out-of-body experience and self-processing to mental own-body imagery at the temporoparietal junction. *Journal of Neuroscience* 25: 550–7.

Bozikas VP, Kosmidis MH, Kiosseoglou G, Karavatos A. (2006) Neuropsychological profile of cognitively impaired patients with schizophrenia. *Comprehensive Psychiatry* 47: 136–43.

Brodaty H, Sachdev P, Koschera A *et al.* (2003) Long-term outcome of late-onset schizophrenia: 5-year follow-up study. *British Journal of Psychiatry* 183: 213–19.

Bowie C, Leung W, Reichenberg A *et al.* (2008) Predicting schizophrenia patients' real world behavior with specific neuropsychological and functional capacity measures. *Biological Psychiatry* 63: 505–11.

Cirillo M, Seidman LJ. (2003) Verbal declarative memory dysfunction in schizophrenia: From clinical assessment to genetics and brain mechanisms. *Neuropsychology Review* 13: 43–77.

Davidson M, Harvey P, Welsh K *et al.* (1996) Cognitive functioning in late-life schizophrenia: a comparison of elderly schizophrenic patients and patients with Alzheimer's disease. *American Journal of Psychiatry* 153: 1274–9.

Delisi L. (2008) The concept of progressive brain change in schizophrenia: implications for understanding schizophrenia. *Schizophrenia Bulletin* 34: 312.

Friedman J, Harvey P, Coleman T *et al.* (2001) Six-year follow-up study of cognitive and functional status across the lifespan in schizophrenia: A comparison with Alzheimer's Disease and normal aging. *American Journal of Psychiatry* 158: 1441–8.

Green M, Kern R, Heaton R. (2004) Longitudinal studies of cognition and functional outcome in schizophrenia: implication for MATRICS. *Schizophrenia Research* 72: 41–51.

Harvey P. (2001) Cognitive impairment in elderly patients with schizophrenia: age-related changes. *International Journal of Geriatric Psychiatry* 16: S78–85.

Harvey P, Bertisch H, Friedman J *et al.* (2003) The course of functional decline in geriatric patients with schizophrenia. *American Journal of Geriatric Psychiatry* 11: 610–19.

Heaton R, Paulsen J, McAdams L *et al.* (1994) Neuropsychological deficits in schizophrenics: Relationship to age, chronicity and dementia. *Archives of General Psychiatry* 51: 469–76.

Heinrichs RW, Zakzanis KK. (1998) Neurocognitive deficit in schizophrenia: a quantitative review of the evidence. *Neuropsychology* 12: 426–45.

Hoff A, Svetina C, Shields G *et al.* (2005) Ten year longitudinal study of neuropsychological functioning subsequent to a first episode of schizophrenia. *Schizophrenia Research* 75: 27–34.

Howard R, Cox T, Almeida O *et al.* (1995) White-matter signal hyperintensities in the brains of patients with late paraphrenia and normal community living elderly. *Biological Psychiatry* 38: 86–91.

Jones D, Catani M, Pierpaoli C *et al.* (2005) A diffusion tensor magnetic resonance imaging study of frontal cortex connections in very-late onset schizophrenia-like psychosis. *American Journal of Geriatric Psychiatry* 13: 1092–9.

Keshavan M, Tandon R, Boutros H *et al.* (2008) Schizophrenia, 'just the facts': What we know in 2008. Part 3: Neurobiology. *Schizophrenia Research* 106: 89–107.

Korner A, Lopez A, Lauritzen L *et al.* (2009) Late and very-late first-contact schizophrenia and the risk of dementia: a nationwide register based study. *International Journal of Geriatric Psychiatry* 24: 61–7.

Kremen W, Lyons M, Boake C *et al.* (2006) A discordant twin study of premorbid cognitive ability in schizophrenia. *Journal of Clinical Experimental Neuropsychology* 28: 208–24.

Kuroki N, Kubicki M, Nestor P *et al.* (2006) Fornix integrity and hippocampal volume in male schizophrenic patients. *Biological Psychiatry* 60: 22–31.

Kurtz M. (2005) Neurocognitive impairment across the lifespan in schizophrenia: an update. *Schizophrenia Research* 74: 15–26.

Miller BL, Lesser IM, Boone K *et al.* (1991) Brain lesions and cognitive function in late-life psychosis. *British Journal of Psychiatry* 158: 76–82.

Morrison G, O'Carroll R, McCreadie R *et al.* (2006) The long-term course of cognitive impairment in schizophrenia. *British Journal of Psychiatry* 189: 556–7.

O'Donnell B. (2007) Cognitive impairment in schizophrenia: A lifespan perspective. *American Journal of Alzheimer's Disease and Other Dementias* 22: 398–405.

Palmer B, Bondi M, Twamley E *et al.* (2003) Are late-onset schizophrenia spectrum disorders neurodegenerative conditions? Annual rates of change on two dementia measures.

Journal of Neuropsychiatry and Clinical Neurosciences **15**: 45–52.

Purohit D, Perl D, Haroutunian V *et al.* (1998) Alzheimer disease and related neurodegenerative diseases in elderly patients with schizophrenia: A post-mortem neuropathologic study of 100 cases. *Archives of General Psychiatry* **55**: 205–11.

Rabins P, Lavrisha M. (2003) Long-term follow-up and phenomenological differences distinguish among late-onset schizophrenia, late-life depression, and progressive dementia. *American Journal of Geriatric Psychiatry* **11**: 589–94.

Religa D, Laudon H, Styczynska M *et al.* (2003) Amyloid β pathology in Alzheimer's disesase and schizophrenia. *American Journal of Psychiatry* **160**: 867–72.

Rosenberger G, Kubicki M, Nestor P *et al.* (2008) Age-related deficits in fronto-temporal connections in schizophrenia: A diffusion tensor imaging study. *Schizophrenia Research* **102**: 181–8.

Sachdev P, Brodaty H. (1999) Quantitative study of signal hyperintensities on T2-weighted magnetic resonance imaging in late-onset schizophrenia. *American Journal of Psychiatry* **156**: 1958–67.

Schwab SG, Wildenauer DB. (2009) Update on key previously proposed candidate genes for schizophrenia. *Current Opinion in Psychiatry* **22**: 147–53.

Seidman L, Thermenos H, Poldrack R *et al.* (2006) Altered brain activation in dorsolateral prefrontal cortex in adolescents and young adults at genetic risk for schizophrenia: An fMRI study of working memory. *Schizophrenia Research* **85**: 58–72.

Steen RG, Mull C, McClure R *et al.* (2006) Brain volume in first-episode schizophrenia: systematic review and meta-analysis of magnetic resonance imaging studies. *British Journal of Psychiatry* **188**: 510–18.

Szoke A, Trandafir A, Dupont ME *et al.* (2008) Longitudinal studies of cognition in schizophrenia: meta-analysis. *British Journal of Psychiatry* **192**: 248–57.

Velakoulis D, Walterfang M, Mocellin R *et al.* (2009) Frontotemporal dementia presenting as schizophrenia-like psychosis in young people: Clinicopathological series and review of cases. *British Journal of Psychiatry* **194**: 298–305.

Vita A, De Peri L, Silenzi C, Dieci M. (2006) Brain morphology in first-episode schizophrenia: A meta-analysis of quantitative magnetic resonance imaging studies. *Schizophrenia Research* **82**: 75–88.

Zakzanis K, Andrikopoulos J, Young DA *et al.* (2003) Neuropsychological differentiation of late-onset schizophrenia and dementia of the Alzheimer's type. *Applied Neuropsychology* **10**: 105–14.

Waters F. (2007) Cognitive impairments in schizophrenia: Review of recent developments. In: Briscoe WP (ed.). *Focus on cognitive disorders research*. Hauppauge, NY: Nova Publishing, 41–64.

Woodberry K, Giuliano A, Seidman L. (2008) Premorbid IQ in schizophrenia: A meta-analytic review. *American Journal of Psychiatry* **165**: 579–87.

76

Dementia in intellectual disabilities

JENNIFER TORR

76.1 INTRODUCTION

The life expectancy of people with intellectual disabilities (ID) has increased from 20 years in the 1930s to 60 years today. However, the life expectancy of people with mild ID, in good general health, is approaching that of the general population (Carter and Jancar, 1983; Patja et al., 2000). The dementias are not only important disorders of old age for people with ID in general, but of early and mid-adulthood for specific subgroups. Dementia in people with ID may be considered in three categories: (1) Early onset Alzheimer's disease (AD) in people with Down syndrome (DS); (2) Dementias of old age in people with non-DS ID; (3) Rare, early adult onset dementias.

76.2 AD IN PEOPLE WITH DOWN SYNDROME

Down syndrome is due to trisomy 21 in 95 per cent of cases. The remainder are due to translocations, partial trisomies and mosaicism (Stoll et al., 1998). People with DS are at high risk of developing early onset AD. Post-mortem studies have shown the typical neuropathological markers of AD, neuritic amyloid plaques and neurofibrillary tangles, are present in the brains of all people with trisomy 21 by the age of 40 years (Wisniewski et al., 1985). Triplication of the amyloid precursor protein (APP) and transcription factor ETS2 genes on chromosome 21 results in a 4–5-fold increase in amyloid production, resulting in early and excessive cerebral amyloid deposition which is postulated to be the fundamental cause of early onset AD in DS (Robakis et al., 1987; Wolvetang et al., 2003).

Serum levels of Aβ1-40 and Aβ1-42 are significantly increased in DS. Levels are 26 per cent higher in those with DS and dementia compared with those without dementia (Schupf et al., 2001). Aβ amyloid mediates inflammatory processes and the progressive accumulation of neurofibrillary tangles, profileration of dystrophic neurons, impaired synaptic connections and neuronal loss (De la Monte, 1999; Head et al., 2002; see Chapter 49, The neuropathology of Alzheimer's disease and Chapter 51, The central role of Aβ amyloid in the pathogenesis of Alzheimer's disease). Clinical dementia has been correlated with the density of neurofibrillary tangles (Margallo-Lana et al., 2007).

The early stages of clinical AD are characterized by personality and behaviour change, decline in executive functioning (Ball et al., 2008) and poor performance on a modified cued recall test (Devenny et al., 2002). The average age of clinical diagnosis of dementia in DS is 50–55 years (Prasher and Kirshnan, 1993). The reported prevalence varies greatly between studies (Holland, 1998). The largest prospective population-based study of 506 adults with DS, aged over 45 years, reports prevalence of dementia as 8.9 per cent up to age 49 years, 17.7 per cent from 50–54 years, 32.1 per cent from 55–59 years and 25.6 per cent above 60 years. The incidence of dementia did not decline in the over 60 years group and the lower prevalence is thought to be due to high mortality rates associated with onset of dementia (Coppus et al., 2006). A number of factors modulate the risk of dementia in DS. Increased risk is associated with the presence of an Apolipoprotein E ε4 allele (Coppus et al., 2008), elevated cholesterol, especially if not treated with statins (Zigman et al., 2007) and menopause (Schupf et al., 2003).

76.3 DEMENTIA IN PEOPLE WITH OTHER INTELLECTUAL DISABILITIES

Dementia in people with non-DS ID is at least as prevalent as in the general population (Evenhuis, 1997; Zigman *et al.*, 2004) and possibly more prevalent and of earlier onset (Lund, 1985; Cooper, 1997; Strydom *et al.*, 2007). Reported prevalence of dementia varies depending on study population, method of ascertaining caseness and choice of diagnostic criteria. DSM-IV-TR (American Psychiatric Association, 2000) gives higher prevalence rates of dementia than ICD-10 (World Health Organization, 1993) and DC-LD (Royal College of Psychiatrists, 2001) which both require behavioural and emotional change (Strydom *et al.*, 2007). A comprehensive population study of dementia in people with non-DS found higher prevalence of dementia compared with the general population and an increase in prevalence with age. Prevalence for dementia subtypes for subjects aged 60 years plus and 65 years plus are reported as: all dementias (13.1 and 18.3 per cent); AD (8.6 and 12 per cent); dementia with Lewy bodies (DLB) (5.9 and 7.1 per cent); frontotemporal dementia (FTD) (3.2 and 4.2 per cent); vascular dementia (VaD) (2.7 and 3.5 per cent); other dementias (1.4 and 1.4 per cent). DLB and FTD were proportionately over-represented compared with reported rates in the general population (Stevens *et al.*, 2002).

There is little research into the risk factors for dementia in people with ID. Congenital brain abnormalities, epilepsy and head injury are associated with dementia (Popovitch *et al.*, 1990; Cooper, 1997). Factors, such as educational attainment, exercise, education, social enagagement and enriched environment, which may protect against dementia in the general population have not been examined in the people with ID.

High rates of pathological lipid profiles, obesity (Rimmer *et al.*, 1994), smoking (Tracy and Hosken, 1997), hypertension, other cardiovascular disease and cerebrovascular disease (Cooper, 1999) have been reported in people with ID. However lower rates, than the general population, of smoking (Taylor *et al.*, 2004) and other vascular risk, besides obesity and lack of exercise (Wallace and Schluter, 2008), have also been reported in people with ID. A number of rare genetic syndromes are associated with hypertension, diabetes, hyperhomocysteinuria and hyperlipidaemia, potentially increasing the risk of VaD (Wallace, 2004).

In theory, people with ID make up 3 per cent of the population; however, only 1–2 per cent of the population are identified as having an ID. Hence, 1–2 per cent of the population have an ID that is not recognized. Little is known about this group, although they are likely to be in the lower socioeconomic or marginalized groups, such as the homeless, and are likely to have significant lifestyle risks for dementia.

76.4 RARE AND VERY EARLY ONSET DEMENTIAS

A number of rare autosomal recessive disorders may present with intellectual disability in childhood, and dementia in early to mid-adulthood. These disorders are multisystem neurodegenerative disorders that are often fatal in childhood. However, some people survive into adulthood, and after an apparent or actual delay in further decline progress to dementia in early to mid-adulthood. Examples include Sanfillippo syndrome type B (mucopolysaccharidosis III) (Moog *et al.*, 2007) and Cockayne syndrome (Rapin *et al.*, 2006). In addition to the genetic disorders, infectious diseases, such as congenital rubella syndrome, may progress to a progressive panencephalitis with seizures, decline in motor function and dementia in adulthood (Wolinsky, 1988).

76.5 ASSESSMENT OF DEMENTIA IN PEOPLE WITH ID

The general principles of dementia assessment (see Chapter 5, Assessment of the patient with apparent dementia) apply to the assessment of suspected dementia in people with ID. In addition, it is essential to establish an individual baseline of daily and cognitive functioning and to carefully assess for other causes of functional decline.

A comprehensive history should be obtained, when possible, from carers who have known the person over time, to establish baseline functioning, the onset, nature and progression of cognitive change. Carer history should be supplemented by documented IQ, functional, speech and other assessments, as well as examples of the person's writing and artworks. Informant rating scales, such as the informant interview schedule of the CAMDEX-DS (Ball *et al.*, 2004), the Dementia Questionnaire for Persons with Mental Retardation (DMR) (Evenhuis, 1996) and the Dementia Scale for Down's Syndrome (Gedye, 1995), can supplement history taking.

Functional decline in a person with ID must not be assumed to be due to dementia. Important differential diagnoses for functional decline include depression, delirium, psychotropic medications, sensory and mobility impairments, and general medical conditions. Older people with ID have high rates of co-morbid conditions. People with DS, in particular, have high rates of early onset age-related disorders and two-thirds have vision and hearing impairments (Haveman *et al.*, 2009). Dementia may also be associated with onset of seizures, gait disorders, feeding and swallowing impairments and recurrent chest infections.

The population of people with ID is heterogeneous in aetiology, severity of cognitive and other impairments, and profile of cognitive functioning. There are few established population norms to assist in interpretation of cross-sectional cognitive testing. Hence, individual baseline functional and cognitive performance is important for dementia assessment. When prior baseline assessments are not available, then repeat assessments may need to be conducted to establish cognitive decline over time. In addition, standard cognitive tests have floor effects and are not validated for use in people with ID. Many tests rely on language and numeracy skills and tests of non-verbal abilities may still rely on the person with learning disability being able to understand verbal instructions. Modified cognitive batteries, such as the CAMDEX-DS (Ball *et al.*, 2006), can be used in people with mild to moderate ID. It may not be possible to conduct cognitive assessments of people with severe and profound ID.

Neuroimaging can identify generalized and localized atrophy (e.g. hippocampal atrophy), cerebrovascular disease, subdural haematoma, and other pathology. In practice, pre-existing developmental abnormalities need to be differentiated from acquired changes. In comparison to normal intelligence controls, the brains of people with Down syndrome are smaller, the ventricles larger and hippocampi smaller, even when corrected for body size (Strydom et al., 2002). Serial neuroimaging can help identify neurodegenerative disorders (Prasher et al., 1996).

76.6 MANAGEMENT AND CARE OF PEOPLE WITH ID AND DEMENTIA

The evidence for the use of cholinesterase inhibitors in people with ID is limited to case studies and a small randomized control trial with open label extension in DS and AD. There are no reports of memantine use in DS or ID in general. Care must be taken to monitor for side effects, which include high rates of fatigue (44 per cent), diarrhoea (38 per cent), insomnia (25 per cent), nausea (25 per cent), dizziness (19 per cent) and anorexia (19 per cent) (Prasher, 2004). There is also a risk of seizures and bradycardia.

There is little guidance on the management of behavioural and psychological symptoms of dementia. Depression which is a common feature of dementia should be treated. Use of other psychotropic medications should be kept to a minimum and medications with anticholinergic effects should be avoided. Strategies include stability of care provision, maintenance of routines, support of functioning, reduction of high visual and auditory stimulus, and attention to non-verbal communication, such as showing in addition to telling. Rapid changes in behaviour may be to due to illness, such as chest or urinary tract infections, seizures or pain (Torr et al., 2009).

In accordance with the principles of the United Nations Convention on the Rights of Persons with Disabilities (United Nations, 2009), people with ID and dementia should be accorded the same standards of assessment, treatment and care options, including ageing in place, as the general population. This will require improved co-operation and co-ordination between disability, health and aged care sectors, as well as training of carers and clinicians.

REFERENCES

American Psychiatric Association. (2000) *Diagnostic and statistical manual of mental disorders: DSM-IV-TR.* Washington, DC: American Psychiatric Association.

Ball S, Holland T, Huppert F et al. (2006). *CAMDEX-DS: The Cambridge examination for mental disorders of older people with Down's syndrome and others with intellectual disabilities.* Cambridge: Cambridge University Press.

Ball SL, Holland AJ, Huppert FA et al. (2004) The modified CAMDEX informant interview is a valid and reliable tool for use in the diagnosis of dementia in adults with Down's syndrome. *Journal of Intellectual Disability Research* 48: 611–20.

Ball SL, Holland AJ, Treppner P et al. (2008) Executive dysfunction and its association with personality and behaviour changes in the development of Alzheimer's disease in adults with Down syndrome and mild to moderate learning disabilities. *British Journal of Clinical Psychology* 47: 1–29.

Carter G, Jancar J. (1983) Mortality in the mentally handicapped: a 50 year survey at the Stoke Park group of hospitals (1930–1980). *Journal of Mental Deficiency Research* 27: 143–56.

Cooper SA. (1997) High prevalence of dementia among people with learning disabilities not attributable to Down's syndrome. *Psychological Medicine* 27: 609–16.

Cooper SA. (1999) The relationship between psychiatric and physical health in elderly people with intellectual disability. *Journal of Intellectual Disability Research* 43: 54–60.

Coppus A, Evenhuis H, Verberne G-J et al. (2006) Dementia and mortality in persons with Down's syndrome. *Journal of Intellectual Disability Research* 50: 768–77.

Coppus AMW, Evenhuis HM, Verberne GJ et al. (2008) The impact of apolipoprotein E on dementia in persons with Down's syndrome. *Neurobiology of Aging* 29: 828–35.

De la Monte SM. (1999) Molecular abnormalities in the brain of patients with Down syndrome. In: Lubec B (ed.). *The molecular biology of Down syndrome.* New York: Spinger-Verlag, 1–20.

Devenny DA, Zimmerli EJ, Kittler P, Krinsky-McHale SJ. (2002) Cued recall in early-stage dementia in adults with Down's syndrome. *Journal of Intellectual Disability Research* 46: 472–83.

Evenhuis HM. (1996) Further evaluation of the dementia questionnaire for persons with mental retardation (DMR). *Journal of Intellectual Disability Research* 40: 369–73.

Evenhuis HM. (1997) The natural history of dementia in ageing people with intellectual disability. *Journal of Intellectual Disability Research* 41: 92–6.

Gedye A. (1995) *Dementia scale for Down's syndrome.* Manual. Vancouver: Gedye Research and Consulting.

Haveman MJ, Heller T, Lee LA et al. (2009) Report on the state of science on health risks and ageing in people with intellectual disabilities, IASSID Special Interest Research Group on Ageing and Intellectual Disabilities. Accessed September 10, 2009. Available from: www.iassid.org/pdf/ssca-health-risks.pdf.

Head E, Lott IT, Cribbs DH et al. (2002) Beta-amyloid deposition and neurofibrillary tangle association with caspase activation in Down syndrome. *Neuroscience Letters* 330: 99–103.

Holland AJ. (1998) Down's syndrome. In: Janicki MP, Dalton AJ (eds). *Dementia, aging and intellectual disabilities.* Philidephia: Bunner/Mazel, 183–93.

Lund J. (1985) The prevalence of psychiatric morbidity in mentally retarded adults. *Acta Psychiatrica Scandinavica* 72: 563–70.

Margallo-Lana ML, Moore PB, Kay DWK et al. (2007) Fifteen-year follow-up of 92 hospitalized adults with Down's syndrome: incidence of cognitive decline, its relationship to age and neuropathology. *Journal of Intellectual Disability Research* 51: 463–77.

Moog U, van Mierlo I, van Schrojenstein Lantman-de Valk HM et al. (2007) Is Sanfilippo type B in your mind when you see adults with mental retardation and behavioral problems? *American Journal of Medical Genetics Part C, Seminars in Medical Genetics* **145C**: 293–301.

Patja K, Iivanainen M, Vesala H et al. (2000) Life expectancy of people with intellectual disability: A 35-year follow-up study. *Journal of Intellectual Disability Research* **44**: 591–9.

Popovitch ER, Wisniewski HM, Barcikowska M et al. (1990) Alzheimer neuropathology in non-Down's syndrome mentally retarded adults. *Acta Neuropathologica* **80**: 362–7.

Prasher VP. (2004) Review of donepezil, rivastigmine, galantamine and memantine for the treatment of dementia in Alzheimer's disease in adults with Down syndrome: Implications for the intellectual disability population. *International Journal of General Psychiatry* **19**: 509–15.

Prasher VP, Kirshnan VH. (1993) Age of onset and duration of dementia in people with Down syndrome: Integration of 98 reported cases in the literature. *International Journal of Geriatric Psychiatry* **8**: 915–22.

Prasher VP, Barber PC, West R, Glenholmes P. (1996) The role of magnetic resonance imaging in the diagnosis of Alzheimer disease in adults with Down syndrome. *Archives of Neurology* **53**: 1310–13.

Rapin I, Weidenheim K, Lindenbaum Y et al. (2006) Cockayne syndrome in adults: review with clinical and pathologic study of a new case. *Journal of Child Neurology* **21**: 991–1006.

Rimmer JH, Braddock D, Fujiura G. (1994) Cardiovascular risk factor levels in adults with mental retardation. *American Journal on Mental Retardation* **98**: 510–18.

Robakis NK, Wisniewski HM, Jenkins EC et al. (1987) Chromosome 21q21 sublocalisation of gene encoding beta-amyloid peptide in cerebral vessels and neuritic (senile) plaques of people with Alzheimer disease and Down syndrome. *Lancet* **1**: 384–5.

Royal College of Psychiatrists. (2001) *DC-LD: Diagnostic criteria for psychiatric disorders for use with adults with learning disabilities/mental retardation.* London: Gaskell.

Schupf N, Patel B, Silverman W et al. (2001) Elevated plasma amyloid beta-peptide 1-42 and onset of dementia in adults with Down syndrome. *Neuroscience Letters* **301**: 199–203.

Schupf N, Pang D, Patel BN et al. (2003) Onset of dementia is associated with age at menopause in women with Down's syndrome. *Annals of Neurology* **54**: 433–8.

Stevens T, Livingston G, Kitchen G et al. (2002) Islington study of dementia subtypes in the community. *British Journal of Psychiatry* **180**: 270–6.

Stoll C, Alembik Y, Dott B, Roth MP. (1998) Study of Down syndrome in 238,942 consecutive births. *Annales de Genetique* **41**: 44–51.

Strydom A, Hassiosis A, Walker Z. (2002) Clinical use of structural magnetic resonance imaging in the diagnosis of dementia in adults with Down's syndrome. *Irish Journal of Psychological Medicine* **19**: 60–3.

Strydom A, Livingston G, King M, Hassiotis A. (2007) Prevalence of dementia in intellectual disability using different diagnostic criteria. *British Journal of Psychiatry* **191**: 150–7.

Taylor NS, Standen PJ, Cutajar P et al. (2004) Smoking prevalence and knowledge of associated risks in adult attenders at day centres for people with learning disabilities. *Journal of Intellectual Disability Research* **48**: 239–44.

Torr J, Iacono T, Rickards L, Winters D. (2009) *About Down syndrome and Alzheimer's disease.* Sydney: Alzheimer's Australia.

Tracy J, Hosken R. (1997) The importance of smoking education and preventative health strategies for people with intellectual disability. *Journal of Intellectual Disability Research* **41**: 416–21.

United Nations. (2009) Convention on the rights of persons with disabilities and optional protocol. Accessed September 12. Available from: www.un.org/disabilities/documents/convention/convoptprot-e.pdf.

Wallace R. (2004) Risk factors for coronary artery disease among individuals with rare syndrome intellectual disabilities. *Journal of Policy and Practice in Intellectual Disabilities* **1**: 31–41.

Wallace RA, Schluter P. (2008) Audit of cardiovascular disease risk factors among supported adults with intellectual disability attending an ageing clinic. *Journal of Intellectual and Developmental Disability* **33**: 48–58.

Wisniewski KE, Dalton AJ, McLachlan C et al. (1985) Alzheimer's disease in Down's syndrome: clinicopathologic studies. *Neurology* **35**: 957–61.

Wolinsky JS. (1988) Rubella virus and its effects on the developing nervous system. In: Johnson RT, Lancaster LG (eds). *Viral infections of the developing nervous system.* Lancaster, UK: MTP Press, 125–42.

Wolvetang EW, Bradfield OM, Tymms M et al. (2003) The chromosome 21 transcription factor ETS2 transactivates the beta-APP promoter: implications for Down syndrome. *Biochimica et Biophysica Acta* **1628**: 105–10.

World Health Organization. (1993) *The ICD-10 classification of mental and behavioural disorders: Diagnostic criteria for research.* Geneva, World Health Organization.

Zigman WB, Schupf N, Devenny DA et al. (2004) Incidence and prevalence of dementia in elderly adults with mental retardation without Down syndrome. *American Journal of Mental Retardation* **109**: 126–41.

Zigman WB, Schupf N, Jenkins EC et al. (2007) Cholesterol level, statin use and Alzheimer's disease in adults with Down syndrome. *Neuroscience Letters* **416**: 279–84.

Alcohol-related dementia and Wernicke–Korsakoff syndrome

STEPHEN C BOWDEN

77.1 INTRODUCTION

Alcohol abuse and dependence is an increasing public-health concern worldwide (Caetano and Babor, 2006; Christensen *et al.*, 2006; Gupta and Warner, 2008). Excessive alcohol intake is a risk factor for cognitive impairment. The severity of impairment across individuals may vary from subtle impairments that are difficult to detect at clinical interview, or masked by intoxication, through to a severe dementia which may persist long after drinking ceases (Bowden and Ritter, 2005; Ritchie and Villebrun, 2008). Within any one individual, cognitive impairment associated with excessive alcohol use may vary across time, perhaps associated with level of alcohol intake, general nutritional and health status, and other factors less well understood (Lishman, 1998; Bowden and Ritter, 2005; Pfefferbaum, *et al.*, 2007; Bates *et al.*, 2009). Excessive alcohol use is an under-appreciated problem in older people, in the age range at highest risk for dementia (Gupta and Warner, 2008; Perney *et al.*, 2008).

Alcohol contributes to 4 per cent of the global burden of disease expressed as disability-adjusted life years lost (WHO, 2007). The prevalence of hazardous alcohol use in western countries is estimated at 5–10 per cent of the adult population; higher in males than females (Chisholm *et al.*, 2004; Harford *et al.*, 2005). A review of the prevalence of mental disorder among homeless people in western countries identified alcohol dependence as the most common disorder with an estimated prevalence between 8.1 and 58.5 per cent with a pooled prevalence estimate of 37.9 per cent (Fazel *et al.*, 2008). Although cautions have been raised about the interpretation of symptom endorsement in epidemiological surveys of younger people, the increasing trend for young people to consume to excess raises concern about a future wave of alcohol-related health problems as populations age (Harford *et al.*, 2005; Christensen *et al.*, 2006; Fazel *et al.*, 2008).

In the context of a high prevalence of alcohol abuse and dependence, particularly in some sections of the community, the existence of significant cognitive impairment associated with alcohol use disorders provides an indication of the scale of associated disability and public health costs. It has been estimated that 10–24 per cent of people with a diagnosis of alcohol abuse display a clinically detectable dementia (Gupta and Warner, 2008; Ritchie and Villebrun, 2008). In this chapter, the pattern of cognitive impairment associated with alcohol use disorders and the diagnostic criteria for alcohol-related dementia will be reviewed. Finally, alternative explanations for the clinical diagnosis and treatment recommendations will be considered.

77.2 COGNITIVE IMPAIRMENT ASSOCIATED WITH REGULAR, EXCESSIVE ALCOHOL INTAKE

Study of the ethanol neurotoxicity hypothesis has taken many forms. Only in its most severe form is ethanol neurotoxicity assumed to result in a clinical presentation of so-called alcohol-related dementia. At the mildest end of the dose–response range is the hypothesis that 'social drinking' may lead to subtle long-term cognitive impairment. In general, despite much early interest, there is no substantial evidence that moderate alcohol consumption in the range of 20–40 mL of ethanol on a regular daily basis leads to lasting effects on cognitive function after the alcohol is eliminated from the body (Bowden, 1987; Harper, 2009). A systematic review suggests that moderate alcohol consumption may have some protective effect against the development of dementia in later life, although the heterogeneity of study methods and populations requires caution with this inference (Solfrizzi et al., 2007; Peters et al., 2008). The apparent lack of serious cognitive consequences associated with long-term moderate alcohol intake should not be confused with the multiple health and other risks associated with even occasional acute intoxication, at any age.

At the high end of the dose–response range, the concept that beverage alcohol induces a dementia has official sanction, but causation has been a matter of debate for many years (Code 291.2) (American Psychiatric Association, 2000). Despite official imprimatur, the pathophysiology of an alcohol-induced dementia remains to be established and a specific pathological gold standard is lacking (Alderazi and Brett, 2007; Gupta and Warner, 2008; Ritchie and Villebrun, 2008; Harper, 2009). The ambiguity regarding the pathological basis of an alcohol-induced dementia contrasts markedly with the many recent developments in the understanding of the pathology of other dementias (e.g. Brust, 2008; Schneider et al., 2009).

From a descriptive point of view, clinically identifiable cognitive impairment associated with higher levels of beverage alcohol consumption typically is reported in people whose alcohol dependence became established in late teenage years or early adulthood. Regular daily intake in this population is often in excess of 80–100 mL of ethanol often over many years. A substantial proportion of people seeking treatment for alcohol dependence have alcohol-induced multiple organ disease, and other complicating conditions such as poor nutrition, and in some cases multiple episodes of head trauma. In such samples, the prevalence of cognitive impairment has been estimated at a substantial minority or perhaps a majority (Parsons, 1994; Allen et al., 2006; Bates et al., 2009).

In less severe forms, this pattern of cognitive impairment associated with long-term excessive alcohol use was termed 'subclinical psychological deterioration' (Cutting, 1985), because in individual cases it may not be apparent until elicited by objective assessment of cognition. Only in the most severe forms does cognitive impairment present as a clinically obvious dementia (Victor, 1994; Oslin et al., 1998; Bowden and Ritter, 2005). Several reviews provide a comprehensive overview of the many cognitive, neuroimaging and post-mortem changes observed in alcohol-dependent patients (Lishman, 1998; Donnino et al., 2007; Brust, 2008; Bates et al., 2009; Harper, 2009; Sullivan and Pfefferbaum, 2009).

Considering the pattern of cognitive impairment associated with excessive alcohol use, there has been some discussion of specific profiles associated with alcohol dependence as opposed to other neuropsychiatric conditions (for example, see Saxton et al., 2000). However, the diagnostic specificity of this kind of profile is low; substantial variability within samples is common (Parsons, 1994; Allen et al., 2006; Bates et al., 2009). Instead, the overwhelming majority of evidence suggests that impairments in patients with alcohol use disorders will be detected in most aspects of cognition if appropriately assessed. Described in terms of a contemporary, comprehensive model of cognitive abilities (McGrew, 2009), the pattern of impairment associated with alcohol use disorders may affect (1) acquired knowledge or 'crystallized' ability, (2) fluid intelligence, particularly reasoning ability, (3) working memory, (4) processing speed and (5) long-term retrieval or anterograde memory formation (Leckliter and Matarazzo, 1989; Parsons, 1994; Allen et al., 2006; Bates et al., 2009). In this context, it is important to note fluid intelligence and working memory are often termed 'executive functions' and deficits in these abilities will be evident in most multifocal or dementia-like conditions, including in association with excessive alcohol use. Only in its most severe form has this pattern of multiple cognitive impairments been described as an alcohol-related dementia, but unlike degenerative conditions, such as Alzheimer's disease (AD), clinically observed alcohol-related dementia has a variable course, and may insidiously worsen with prolonged drinking, or may stabilize or improve with reduction or cessation of alcohol intake (Victor, 1994; Allen et al., 2006; Bates et al., 2009).

Because of the difficulty identifying a distinctive neuropathology associated with the clinical diagnosis of alcohol-related dementia, diverse aetiological processes have been considered. Potential explanations of alcohol-related cognitive impairment include pre-existing learning disabilities, family history of alcohol dependence, childhood behaviour problems and co-morbid psychopathology (Adams et al., 1998; Lishman, 1998; Allen et al., 2006; Bates et al., 2009). Medical risk factors which may predispose to cognitive impairment are diverse and include multiple organ disease, single or multiple traumatic brain injuries associated with an alcohol-dependent lifestyle, single or multiple nutritional deficiencies and other incidental dementias (Parsons, 1994; Harper et al., 2003; Brust, 2008; Bates et al., 2009). However, discussion of pathophysiology underlying alcohol-related dementia has primarily focused on two likely explanations, namely, ethanol neurotoxicity on the one hand, or 'atypical' Wernicke–Korsakoff syndrome (WKS) on the other (Victor, 1994; Lishman, 1998; Bowden and Ritter, 2005; Nixon et al., 2008). The likely role of 'atypical' WKS will be discussed further below under 77.3.1 Misconception 1: WKS is readily diagnosed and readily excluded from clinical studies of alcohol-related dementia. Many studies have examined frequency and severity of alcohol intake with a view to delineating a dose–response relationship with underlying alcohol-related dementia. This search for a clear dose–response relationship generally has been unrewarding in terms of clinical impairment and histopathological markers, including at a molecular level (Oslin et al., 1998; Nixon et al., 2008; Aho et al., 2009; Harper, 2009).

An important issue in the clinical management of patients suspected of alcohol-related dementia relates to stabilization of cognitive status and the timing of assessment of cognition after cessation of drinking. Any assessment of cognitive status in a patient who is currently consuming excessive quantities of alcohol should be interpreted with considerable caution, particularly because acute intoxication may mask even severe cognitive impairment (Thomson and Marshall, 2006a). As a consequence, many neuropsychologists recommend refraining from assessment of cognitive status until several weeks after withdrawal from alcohol, although earlier assessment may provide a reasonable guide to the course of cognitive status over the first few weeks after alcohol withdrawal (Unkenstein and Bowden, 1990; Bowden et al., 1995; Goldman, 1995; Allen et al., 1997). Nevertheless, cognitive status may slowly improve after cessation of drinking, over a period of months or years, in a proportion of patients, or conversely worsen with resumption of alcohol intake (Victor et al., 1989; Sullivan et al., 2000; Oslin and Carey, 2003; Allen et al., 2006; Bates et al., 2009). Therefore, any assessment of cognitive status in alcohol-dependent people, even in those showing a severe alcohol-related dementia, should be predicated on the assumption that cognitive status may evolve or resolve and may need to be reviewed regularly.

77.3   DIAGNOSTIC CRITERIA FOR ALCOHOL-RELATED DEMENTIA

Some years ago, Oslin and colleagues (1998) described detailed criteria for the diagnosis of alcohol-related dementia. Distinguishing 'probable' and 'definite' subcategories, they defined their probable category as applying to patients displaying a persisting dementia after ceasing alcohol intake, or in the context of continuing moderate intake, not obviously attributable to any other condition. The primary predisposing factor was identified as significant past use of beverage alcohol defined by at least 35 standard drinks per week. Oslin and colleagues outlined a variety of inclusion and exclusion criteria for the subcategories, and acknowledged that many of the diagnostic criteria were arbitrary and intended to stimulate debate and research. They also acknowledged that there were no acceptable criteria for a definite diagnosis of alcohol-related dementia, in other words, there was no known neuropathological entity corresponding to the clinical diagnosis of alcohol-related dementia. Instead, they noted that other diseases, including other dementias, but also less symptomatic variants of WKS, may confound the study of alcohol-related dementia. The anomalous state of alcohol-related dementia endures, with no tangible progress in identifying a specific form of neuropathology in the decade since Oslin and colleagues published their criteria (Alderazi and Brett, 2007; Ritchie and Villebrun, 2008; Harper, 2009). The diagnosis of alcohol-related dementia always was, and remains, a diagnosis of exclusion (Oslin et al., 1998; Gupta and Warner, 2008; Ritchie and Villebrun, 2008). As detailed below, other conditions may produce dementia-like impairment in association with alcohol abuse (Brust, 2008).

In view of the ambiguities in diagnosis, it is not surprising that precise prevalence figures are difficult to obtain. Nevertheless, clinical surveys suggest that alcohol dependence may be one of the most common apparent causes of dementia,

after AD and vascular dementia (Lishman, 1998; Oslin and Carey, 2003).

Estimates suggest that for 9–22 per cent of patients with a clinical dementia, alcohol abuse or dependence is a significant complicating or contributing factor (Gupta and Warner, 2008; Ritchie and Villebrun, 2008; Kopelman et al., 2009). Other less common conditions can give rise to cognitive deterioration in association with alcohol dependence (e.g. pellagra, Marchiafava–Bignami disease, hepatic encephalopathy and many other less common conditions) (Victor, 1994; Lishman, 1998; Donnino et al., 2007; Brust, 2008). Critically, many years ago, Torvik and colleagues (Torvik et al., 1982; Torvik, 1991) inferred from their large post-mortem surveys that most patients diagnosed clinically as suffering alcohol-related dementia will be found to have long-standing WKS neuropathology at post-mortem. There is increasing evidence that many physiological derangements, worsened by excessive alcohol intake, may interact to diminish available thiamin in the brain, even in the context of an adequate diet. The primary mode of action of alcohol on the brain may be to exacerbate the effects of thiamin deficiency and the primary neuropathology underlying 'alcohol-related' brain disease may be WKS (Chiossi et al., 2006; Thomson and Marshall, 2006b; Pfefferbaum et al., 2007; Nixon et al., 2008; Guerrini et al., 2009).

As Bowden and Ritter (2005) noted, the principal danger in giving a different name such as 'alcohol-related dementia' to unrecognized clinical variants of known conditions like WKS, is that appropriate treatment opportunities may be missed (Lishman, 1998; Victor, 1994; Thomson and Marshall, 2006b). There remain several important impediments to a better understanding of the clinical heterogeneity of WKS which encourage continuing speculation regarding an alcohol-induced dementia. Although thiamin deficiency is recognized as a common explanation for brain disease associated with hazardous alcohol use, older conceptions of the clinical manifestation of WKS still limit the understanding of this latter disease.

77.3.1   Misconception 1: WKS is readily diagnosed and readily excluded from clinical studies of alcohol-related dementia

The viability of the view that WKS is readily diagnosed and excluded from clinical studies of alcohol-related dementia was challenged many years ago (Torvik et al., 1982; Harper, 1983; Reuler et al., 1985; Bowden, 1990; Victor, 1994). The view is less common nowadays, but is still encountered with surprising frequency. The view is based on old neuropsychological formulations of the WKS which predate the recognition of the high prevalence of undiagnosed of WKS particularly in alcohol-dependent people. (e.g. Lezak et al., 2004; Sivolap, 2005; Allen et al., 2006; Kopelman et al., 2009). This view has an important consequence for clinical management of patients with chronic cognitive deficits. According to this incorrect reasoning, if WKS, particularly in the chronic Korsakoff phase, is readily identified clinically by a severe, selective anterograde memory impairment (Butters and Cermak, 1980), then any evidence of cognitive impairment in alcohol-dependent people without obvious WKS must be due to other causes.

It is true that the clinical heterogeneity of patients in the Wernicke's phase is now much more widely appreciated (Lishman, 1998; Chiossi *et al.*, 2006; Thomson and Marshall, 2006b; Sechi and Serra, 2007). However, the logical implication of a more variable Wernicke's phase being associated with a more variable Korsakoff phase does not attract sufficient recognition. If the Wernicke's phase is highly variable in severity, course and symptomatic presentation, and if Wernicke's and Korsakoff's amnesia are different phases of the same disease, then it is likely that the Korsakoff's amnesia phase will also be more variable in severity, course and symptomatic presentation (Bowden, 1990; Victor, 1994). Multiple lines of evidence suggest this is the case, key evidence being that unselected cases of WKS, other than in acute presentation, display a pattern of cognitive impairment that is much more variable than commonly assumed, being highly variable in severity and best described as a potentially reversible dementia-like impairment of multiple cognitive abilities (Bowden, 1990; Torvik, 1991; Victor, 1994; Bowden and Ritter, 2005). This observation applies to patients who develop WKS in the context of alcohol dependence and also to those whose WKS syndrome appears to be unrelated to alcohol (Chiossi *et al.*, 2006).

Regarding the identification of WKS, diagnosis is still based on clinical findings and a history of risk factors for malnutrition, including alcohol use, without a rapidly available diagnostic test (Donnino *et al.*, 2007; Thomson *et al.*, 2008). Presentation is highly variable, ranging from coma at one extreme to subtle signs of cognitive impairment at the other extreme (Donnino *et al.*, 2007; Thomson *et al.*, 2008). In addition, while magnetic resonance imaging (MRI) may be useful to identify a proportion of acute cases, sensitivity is limited and may not be indicated or available for the majority of less acute or chronic cases in whom alcohol-related dementia, or 'atypical' WKS is suspected (Thomson and Marshall, 2006b; Donnino *et al.*, 2007; Pfefferbaum *et al.*, 2007). As with the Wernicke's phase, a less symptomatic or insidious evolution into the Korsakoff's phase, in chronic form, may be difficult to diagnose with confidence even when associated with some degree of dementia, although many such cases have been documented with pathological confirmation (Torvik, 1991; Victor, 1994). There is insufficient recognition of the potential for insidious development of the chronic form of WKS where cognitive impairment of variable severity may be the primary sign (Bowden, 1990; Torvik, 1991; Victor, 1994).

77.3.2 Misconception 2: The Korsakoff phase of WKS is characterized by a severe, selective and lasting anterograde amnesia, especially when associated with alcohol

Clearly related to considerations of less symptomatic or variable course, a related source of misunderstanding concerns the prospect of recovery from the severe, amnesic phase of WKS. In his original description, Korsakoff drew attention to the potential for recovery, although this aspect is rarely discussed

(see Bowden and Ritter, 2005). However, there are numerous descriptions of recovery from the Korsakoff's amnesia in cases associated with alcohol dependence from many research groups, although these patients were often excluded from study of the amnesic phase because they did not conform to the stereotypical severe and lasting anterograde amnesia (Bowden, 1990). It is not widely appreciated that the stereotype of the severe, selective and lasting amnesia defining the Korsakoff's phase, operationalized as the Wechsler intelligence quotient (IQ) versus memory quotient (MQ) discrepancy was never based on any empirical or epidemiological criterion (Butters and Cermak, 1980). Instead, this IQ versus MQ discrepancy criterion was adopted as a clinical heuristic (Butters, personal communication, February 1991).

On the one hand, some degree of recovery from a severe Korsakoff's amnesia is common, including when associated with prior alcohol abuse. In the largest study of its kind Victor and colleagues described substantial, clinically obvious, recovery from Korsakoff's amnesia in approximately half their patients, most of whom had abused alcohol prior to admission. However, Victor and colleagues' (1989) sample was followed for up to ten years. Few clinicians are in a position to observe recovery over this kind of period, and as a consequence, it is easy to subscribe to the erroneous view that the amnesia following the acute Wernicke's phase 'usually persists indefinitely' (American Psychiatric Association, 2000). In recent systematic reviews of many published cases of WKS not obviously associated with alcohol dependence, significant anterograde amnesia or a dementia-like cognitive impairment was found to be frequent (Bowden and Ritter, 2005; Chiossi *et al.*, 2006). Recovery was observed over medium- to long-term follow up, in proportions not dissimilar to patients recovering from WKS associated with alcohol dependence (Chiossi *et al.*, 2006). Some reviewers have arrived at different conclusions based on much smaller and less representative samples of published cases (Freund, 1973; Homewood and Bond, 1999).

On the other hand, empirical evidence on the profile of cognitive impairment in the chronic phase of WKS strongly points to a dementia-like deterioration as being a more accurate description than the 'typical' severe, selective amnesia (Victor, 1994; Bowden and Ritter, 2005). Criticizing this narrow focus on the severe, selective amnesia, operationalized as the IQ versus MQ discrepancy (e.g. Butters and Cermak, 1980), Victor (1994) observed 'perhaps this notion of the Korsakoff amnesic syndrome is the conventional one, but if so, it is not consonant with the observed facts, clinical or pathologic'. In other words, when memory is affected, most other aspects of cognition are also affected (Jacobson and Lishman, 1987; Victor, 1994; Ambrose *et al.*, 2001; Bowden and Ritter, 2005; Chiossi *et al.*, 2006).

77.3.3 Misconception 3: Wernicke's encepaholopathy and Korsakoff's amnesia are different disease entities

Although recognized many years ago as the acute and chronic phases, respectively, of the same disease entity, with identical pathology, attributable to thiamin deficiency (Victor *et al.*,

1971), continuing use of the term 'Wernicke's encephalopathy' separately from 'Korsakoff's amnesia' reinforces the idea that these conditions are somehow different (Donnino et al., 2007; Sechi and Serra, 2007). An excellent animal model for WKS exists in a variety of species (Victor et al., 1989; Pfefferbaum et al., 2007; Nixon et al., 2008). However, difficulties in reproducing in non-primates, the experimental equivalent of the human anterograde amnesia, limit the scientific value of animal models of WKS. Nevertheless, the key criterion for the similarity of Wernicke's encephalopathy and Korsakoff syndrome is the pathological picture. Apart from differences in acuteness of onset, the neuropathology underlying the Wernicke and Korsakoff phases is identical (Victor et al., 1989; Alderazi and Brett, 2007; Harris et al., 2008; Harper, 2009).

Speculation regarding subtypes of pathology corresponding to arbitrary subtypes based on the IQ versus MQ discrepancy, discussed above, neglect to appreciate the variable distribution and course of pathological changes and accompanying variability in clinical manifestations of WKS (Harding et al., 2000). The variability in severity and extent of pathology was identified by Torvik (1991) and supported by recent experimental imaging studies (Pfefferbaum et al., 2007). As noted, patients who display a severe selective amnesia may be an uncommon variant of the chronic phase of WKS (Bowden, 1990; Victor, 1994; Bowden and Ritter, 2005). To base a pathological criterion on what is undoubtedly only a proportion, possibly only a small proportion of patients in the stable phase, who exhibit a particular cognitive profile is likely to be misleading regarding the variability in the underlying pathology (Torvik, 1991; Victor, 1994; Harper, 2009). By way of analogy, the study of AD is rapidly moving beyond the era when people who displayed a clinically obvious dementia were considered to be the only bona fide cases of AD (Schneider et al., 2009).

77.3.3.1   CASE DESCRIPTION

A 48-year-old male was admitted to an inpatient treatment unit for alcohol withdrawal having a recent regular daily beverage alcohol intake history in excess of 250–300 mL. He had been homeless and itinerant for most of the previous 18 months, since the last recorded episode of alcohol withdrawal and inpatient treatment. He was a long-standing patient of the treatment service with an extensive addiction-treatment history. On admission, he was examined by a medical officer and judged to be medically well apart from elevated liver function tests, and mildly elevated mood which the patient himself, and treatment staff who knew him, described as a long-standing trait. Three weeks after admission, he undertook neuropsychological assessment. He was fully oriented except to date of the month, and Wechsler Intelligence Factor and Memory Scale Index scores were all between the 50th and 55th percentiles for his age, with no significant discrepancies, in particular no significant discrepancy between general intellectual function and anterograde memory ability. No other more severe cognitive impairments were detected on additional testing. Estimated pre-morbid cognitive ability was in the superior to very superior range. This estimate was based on detailed, corroborated knowledge of occupational attainments

in his earlier life. Overall, he was judged to have a mild dementia-like impairment involving multiple cognitive abilities. The patient himself described his current cognitive abilities as 'nothing like' his former self: 'I can't be bothered thinking any more.'

Subsequent to the neuropsychological assessment, this patient was re-examined by a consultant physician who reported only one additional sign, a mild horizontal nystagmus, which was not noticed by the admitting officer. When this patient's full medical history was retrieved from the archives, at least two previous clinical episodes of WKS co-incident with admissions to treatment services were noted. One episode, approximately two years previously, included severe disorientation, clinically obvious anterograde amnesia, confabulation and peripheral neuropathy in the context of alcohol dependence. Another episode, again associated with alcohol dependence approximately ten years before, included documented nystagmus and opthalmoplegia, ataxia, and confusion and severe disorientation, which resolved over 2–3 weeks into a severe anterograde amnesia. On that admission, he was transferred from the acute ward to a long-stay facility where he was initially highly dependent, but recovered enough to be discharged into his own care approximately six months after the acute admission. Medical and nursing staff involved in these earlier admissions were re-interviewed and corroborated all details. This patient illustrates the fluctuating course of WKS associated with alcohol dependence, and illustrates that partially recovered WKS may easily be mistaken for a mild–moderate alcohol-related dementia. Instead, this patient might be best considered as an example of long-standing WKS (Victor et al., 1989). This case report was approved by the institutional Human Research and Ethics Committee, with demographic details altered for the purposes of anonymity.

77.4   THE POST–MORTEM PREVALENCE OF WKS IS SUFFICIENT TO EXPLAIN MOST OF THE CLINICAL OBSERVATIONS OF ALCOHOL-RELATED DEMENTIA

Recently, Ritchie and Villebrun (2008) suggested that the observations of clinical cases of alcohol-related dementia require explanation because the prevalence of alcohol-related dementia appears to be higher than that of WKS. However, they acknowledged that there is no clear pathological entity corresponding to the hypothesized alcohol-related dementia and that clinical descriptions of alcohol-related dementia may be confounded by WKS or other dementias (Ritchie and Villebrun, 2008). While Ritchie and Villebrun did not define their usage of WKS, one assumes that they are referring to the prevalence of the clinically obvious syndrome when suggesting that alcohol-related dementia is more common than can be accounted for by WKS. This issue is important because, as noted above, clinically diagnosed WKS is much less frequent than the prevalence of WKS estimated from pathological studies. Torvik and colleagues suggested that only 1–20 per cent of cases of WKS are diagnosed clinically (Torvik, 1991). In the era of increased vigilance, Thomson and Marshall (2006b) suggest that only 20 per cent of pathological WKS may be detected clinically and this figure undoubtedly depends on setting and careful attention.

Contrary to Ritchie and Villebrun's (2008) surmise, the high frequency of undiagnosed WKS may be sufficient to account for most clinically detected alcohol-related dementia. Four pieces of information support this conclusion:

1. As noted above, 10–23 per cent of people with a diagnosis of alcohol abuse display a clinically detectable dementia (Ritchie and Villebrun, 2008).
2. We also know that the prevalence of WKS neuropathology is approximately 0.5–2 per cent (Victor, 1994; Thomson and Marshall, 2006b; Donnino et al., 2007; Harper, 2009).
3. It is estimated that hazardous alcohol consumption occurs with a prevalence of at least 5 per cent ignoring sex differences (Harford et al., 2005; Gupta and Warner, 2008).
4. More than 90 per cent of cases of WKS neuropathology are observed in people with alcohol dependence (Thomson and Marshall, 2006b).

On the basis of the above four pieces of information, we can infer that most of the 0.5–2 per cent of cases of WKS observed at post-mortem will occur in the 5 per cent of people with hazardous drinking, which gives an order of magnitude estimate of WKS in alcohol-dependent people in the range of approximately 10–40 per cent. This estimate coincides with the observed prevalence of WKS pathology in alcohol-dependent people in the range of 12–35 per cent (Torvik, 1991; Thomson and Marshall, 2006b). In other words, the prevalence of WKS may be sufficient to account for the clinical observations of so-called 'alcohol-related dementia'. Unfortunately, as outline above, the continuing misapprehension that chronic WKS in the context of alcohol abuse has a distinctive, readily identified clinical presentation distracts from recognition of the high prevalence and variable clinical presentation of this disease.

77.5   TREATMENT RECOMMENDATIONS

Effective treatment of alcohol-related dementia should target underlying causes (Thomson and Marshall, 2006b; Brust, 2008). Behavioural management of cognitive impairment and associated alcohol dependence has been reviewed recently (McCrady, 2008; Bates et al., 2009). Excessive alcohol use may exacerbate thiamin and other nutritional deficiencies and may increase metabolic requirements for thiamin, making even 'well-nourished' alcohol-dependent people more susceptible to WKS (Thomson and Marshall, 2006b). In addition, concurrent alcohol intake impairs absorption and utilization of thiamin, requiring higher doses of thiamin for reversal of symptoms of WKS (Thomson and Marshall, 2006b; Donnino et al., 2007).

At present, identification of WKS in all its variants remains a clinical diagnosis because there is no quick, readily available laboratory test to assay thiamin levels (Thomson et al., 2002; Thomson and Marshall, 2006b; Donnino et al., 2007). Rather than waiting for some definitive diagnostic

sign, it is more important to make a presumptive diagnosis and treat the patient as soon as possible (Cook et al., 1998; Thomson and Marshall, 2006b; Donnino et al., 2007). The need for a more pro-active approach to treatment of known or suspected WKS has been argued strongly by many authors (Victor, 1994; Cook et al., 1998; Thomson and Marshall, 2006b; Sechi and Serra, 2007). Current medical management of acute WKS, in particular with aggressive B vitamin therapy, has been reviewed by Thomson and colleagues (Thomson et al., 2002; Thomson and Marshall, 2006b). Many of the same principles should apply to treatment of cognitive impairment, including apparent dementia, in association with alcohol dependence irrespective of the setting. The systematic review of treatment for alcohol-related dementia reveals few studies and suggests that high doses of parenteral thiamin may be required for effective response, but many issues remain to be investigated (Thomson and Marshall, 2006b). As Thomson and colleagues show, the risks of parenteral B vitamin therapy are low, and the potential to minimize long-term disability may be greatly enhanced by early and effective treatment. In addition, a variety of experimental treatments are under investigation (Thomson and Marshall, 2006b; Kopelman et al., 2009).

77.6   CONCLUSIONS

Although the concept of an alcohol-induced dementia enjoys wide currency as a clinical entity, a distinctive pathology remains to be identified. While many conditions may give rise to cognitive impairment in association with alcohol abuse and dependence (Thomson and Marshall, 2006a; Donnino et al., 2007; Ritchie and Villebrun, 2008), it may be that the most common underlying cause of alcohol-related dementia is unrecognized WKS (Torvik, 1991). Two primary impediments limit greater recognition of the high prevalence of WKS and its role in alcohol-related dementia: (1) the stereotype of the severe, selective amnesia in the chronic phase of WKS and (2) the idea that WKS is uncommon. Both these latter views do not accord with the evidence. The classic triad of eye signs, ataxia and mental impairment is no longer conceived as highly sensitive to the presence of WKS. Instead, the neurological definition of the disease has evolved to include a highly variable presentation (Reuler et al., 1985; Thomson and Marshall, 2006a; Donnino et al., 2007). In addition, a wide variety of evidence suggests that the neuropsychology and neuropsychiatry of WKS is better viewed as a potentially reversible dementia of highly variable severity (Victor, 1994; Bowden and Ritter, 2005). The value of rethinking the clinical presentation of WKS lies in the fact that better recognition may lead to better treatment and prevention, and less so-called alcohol-related dementia.

REFERENCES

Adams KM, Gilman S, Johnson-Green D et al. (1998) The significance of family history status in relation to neuropsychological test performance and cerebral glucose metabolism studied with positron emission tomography in older alcoholics. *Alcoholism: Clinical and Experimental Research* 22: 105–10.

Aho L, Karkola K, Juusela J, Alafuzoff I. (2009) Heavy alcohol consumption and neuropathological lesions: a post-mortem human study. *Journal of Neuroscience Research* 87: 2786–92.

Alderazi Y, Brett F. (2007) Alcohol and the nervous system. *Current Diagnostic Pathology* 13: 203–9.

Allen DN, Goldstein G, Seaton BE. (1997) Cognitive rehabilitation of chronic alcohol abusers. *Neuropsychology Review* 7: 21–39.

Allen DN, Framton LV, Forrest TJ, Strauss GP. (2006) Neuropsychology of substance use disorders. In: Snyder PJ, Nussbaum PD, Robins DL (eds). *Clinical neuropsychology: a pocket handbook for assessment*, 2nd edn. Washington, DC: American Psychological Association, 649–73.

Ambrose ML, Bowden SC, Whelan G. (2001) Thiamin treatment and working memory function of alcohol-dependent people: Preliminary findings. *Alcoholism: Clinical Experimental Research* 25: 112–6.

American Psychiatric Association. (2000) *Diagnostic and statistical manual of mental disorders* (*DSM-IV-TR*). Washington, DC: American Psychiatric Association.

Bates ME, Bowden SC, Barry D. (2009) Alcohol related dementia: the spectrum of impairment. In: Geldmacher DS (ed.). *Other dementias*. Lake Worth, FL: Carma Publishing.

Bowden SC. (1987) Brain impairment in social drinkers? No cause for concern. *Alcoholism: Clinical and Experimental Research* 11: 407–10.

Bowden SC. (1990) Separating cognitive impairment in neurologically asymptomatic alcoholism from Wernicke–Korsakoff syndrome: Is the neuropsychological distinction justified? *Psychological Bulletin* 107: 355–66.

Bowden SC, Ritter AJ. (2005) Alcohol related dementia and the clinical spectrum of Wernicke-Korsakoff syndrome. In: Burns A, O'Brien J, Ames DJ (eds). *Dementia*, 3rd edn. London: Edward Arnold, 738–44.

Bowden SC, Whelan G, Long C, Clifford C. (1995) The temporal stability of the WAIS-R and WMS-R in a heterogeneous sample of alcohol dependent clients. *The Clinical Neuropsychologist* 9: 194–7.

Brust JCM. (2008) A 74-year-old man with memory loss and neuropathy who enjoys alcoholic beverages. *Journal of the American Medical Association* 299: 1046–54.

Butters N, Cermak LS. (1980) *Alcoholic Korsakoff's syndrome: an information-processing approach to amnesia*. London: Academic Press.

Caetano R, Babor TF. (2006) Diagnosis of alcohol dependence in epidemiological surveys: an epidemic of youthful alcohol dependence or a case of measurement error? *Addiction* 101 (Suppl. 1): 111–4.

Chiossi G, Neri I, Cavazzuti M *et al.* (2006) Hyperemesis gravidarum complicated by Wernicke encephalopathy: background, case report, and review of the literature. *Obstetrical and Gynecological Survey* 61: 255–68.

Chisholm D, Rehm J, Van Ommeren M, Monteiro M. (2004) Reducing the global burden of hazardous alcohol use: a comparative cost-effectiveness analysis. *Journal of Studies on Alcohol* 65: 782–93.

Christensen H, Low L-F, Anstey KJ. (2006) Prevalence, risk factors and treatment for substance abuse in older adults. *Current Opinion on Psychiatry* 19: 587–92.

Cook CCH, Hallwood PM, Thomson AD. (1998) B vitamin deficiency and neuropsychiatric syndromes in alcohol misuse. *Alcohol and Alcoholism* 33: 317–36.

Cutting J. (1985) Korsakoff syndrome. In: Frederiks JAM (ed.). *Handbook of clinical neurology: Clinical neuropsychology*, vol. 45. revised series 1. Amsterdam: Elsevier, 193–204.

Donnino MW, Vega J, Miller J, Walsh M. (2007) Myths and misconceptions of Wernicke's encephalopathy: what every emergency physician should know. *Annals of Emergency Medicine* 50: 715–21.

Fazel S, Khosla V, Doll H, Geddes J. (2008) The prevalence of mental disorders among the homeless in Western countries: Systematic review and metaregression analysis. *PLoS Medicine* 5: e225.

Freund G. (1973) Chronic central nervous system toxicity of alcohol. *Annual Review of Pharmacology* 13: 217–27.

Goldman M. (1995) Recovery of cognitive functioning in alcoholics. *Alcohol Health Research World* 19: 148–54.

Guerrini I, Thomson AD, Gurling HM. (2009) Molecular genetics of alcohol-related brain damage. *Alcohol and Alcoholism* 44: 166–70.

Gupta S, Warner J. (2008) Alcohol-related dementia: a 21st-century silent epidemic? *British Journal of Psychiatry* 193: 351–3.

Harding A, Halliday GM, Caine D, Kril JJ. (2000) Degeneration of anterior thalamic nuclei differentiates alcoholics with amnesia. *Brain* 123: 141–54.

Harford TC, Grant BF, Yi H-Y, Chen CM. (2005) Patterns of DSM-IV alcohol abuse and dependence criteria among adolescents and adults: results from the 2001 National Household Survey on Drug Abuse. *Alcoholism, Clinical and Experimental Research* 29: 810–28.

Harper C. (1983) The incidence of Wernicke's encephalopathy in Australia – a neuropathological study of 131 cases. *Journal of Neurology, Neurosurgery, Psychiatry* 46: 593–8.

Harper C. (2009) The neuropathology of alcohol-related brain damage. *Alcohol and Alcoholism* 44: 136–40.

Harper CG, Dixon G, Sheedy D, Garrick T. (2003) Neuropathological alterations in alcoholic brains. Studies arising from the New South Wales Tissue Resource Centre. *Progress in Neuro-Pharmacology and Biological Psychiatry* 27: 951–61.

Harris J, Chimelli L, Kril JJ, Ray D. (2008) Nutritional deficiencies, metabolic disorders and toxins affecting the nervous system. In: Love S, Louis DN, Ellison DW (eds). *Greenfield's neuropathology*, 8th edn. London: Hodder Arnold, 657–731.

Homewood J, Bond NW. (1999) Thiamin deficiency and Korsakoff's syndrome: Failure to find memory impairments following non-alcoholic Wernicke's encephalopathy. *Alcohol and Alcoholism* 19: 75–84.

Jacobson RR, Lishman WA. (1987) Selective memory loss and global intellectual deficits in alcoholic Korsakoff's syndrome. *Psychological Medicine* 17: 649–55.

Kopelman MD, Thomson AD, Guerrini I, Marshall EJ. (2009) The Korsakoff syndrome: clinical aspects, psychology and treatment. *Alcohol and Alcoholism* 44: 148–54.

Leckliter IN, Matarazzo JD. (1989) The influence of age, education, IQ, gender, and alcohol abuse on Halstead-Reitan Neuropsychological Test Battery performance. *Journal of Clinical Psychology* 45: 484–512.

Lezak MD, Howieson DB, Loring DW *et al.* (2004). *Neuropsychological assessment*, 4th edn. New York, NY: Oxford University Press.

Lishman WA. (1998) *Organic psychiatry: the psychological consequences of cerebral disorder*, 3rd edn. Oxford, UK: Blackwell Scientific Publications.

McCrady BS. (2008) *Alcohol use disorders*. New York, NY: Guilford Press.

McGrew KS. (2009) CHC theory and the human cognitive abilities project: Standing on the shoulders of the giants of psychometric intelligence research. *Intelligence* 37: 1–10.

Nixon PF, Jordan L, Zimitat C *et al.* (2008) Choroid plexus dysfunction: the initial event in the pathogenesis of Wernicke's encephalopathy and ethanol intoxication. *Alcoholism, Clinical and Experimental Research* 32: 1513–23.

Oslin D, Carey MS. (2003) Alcohol related dementia: Validation of diagnostic criteria. *American Journal of Geriatric Psychiatry* 11: 441–7.

Oslin D, Atkinson RM, Smith DM, Hendrie H. (1998) Alcohol related dementia: Proposed clinical criteria. *International Journal of Geriatric Psychiatry* 13: 203–12.

Parsons OA. (1994) Determinants of cognitive deficits in alcoholics: The search continues. *The Clinical Neuropsychologist* 8: 39–58.

Perney P, Rigole H, Blanc F. (2008) [Alcohol dependence: diagnosis and treatment]. *La Revue de Médecine Interne* 29: 297–304.

Peters R, Peters J, Warner J *et al.* (2008) Alcohol, dementia, and cognitive decline in the elderly: a systematic review. *Age and Ageing* 37: 505–12.

Pfefferbaum A, Adalsteinsson E, Bell RL, Sullivan EV. (2007) Development and resolution of brain lesions caused by pyrithiamine- and dietary-induced thiamine deficiency and alcohol exposure in the alcohol-preferring rat: a longitudinal magnetic resonance imaging and spectroscopy study. *Neuropsychopharmacology* 32: 1159–77.

Reuler JB, Girard DE, Cooney TG. (1985) Wernicke's encephalopathy. *New England Journal of Medicine* 312: 1035–9.

Ritchie K, Villebrun D. (2008) Epidemiology of alcohol-related dementia. *Handbook of Clinical Neurology* 89: 845–50.

Saxton J, Munro CA, Butters MA *et al.* (2000) Alcohol, dementia, and Alzheimer's disease: Comparison of neuropsychological profiles. *Journal of Geriatric Psychiatry and Neurology* 13: 141–9.

Schneider JA, Arvanitakis Z, Leurgans SE, Bennett DA. (2009) The neuropathology of probable Alzheimer disease and mild cognitive impairment. *Annals of Neurology* 66: 200–8.

Sechi G, Serra A. (2007) Wernicke's encephalopathy: new clinical settings and recent advances in diagnosis and management. *Lancet Neurology* 6: 442–55.

Sivolap YP. (2005) The current state of SS Korsakov's concept of alcoholic polyneuritic psychosis. *Neuroscience and Behavioural Physiology* 35: 977–82.

Solfrizzi V, D'Introno A, Colacicco AM *et al.* (2007) Alcohol consumption, mild cognitive impairment, and progression to dementia. *Neurology* 68: 1790–9.

Sullivan EV, Pfefferbaum A. (2009) Neuroimaging of the Wernicke–Korsakoff syndrome. *Alcohol and Alcoholism* 44: 155–65.

Sullivan EV, Rosenbloom MJ, Lim KO, Pfefferbaum A. (2000) Longitudinal changes in cognition, gait, and balance in abstinent and relapsed alcoholic men: Relationships to changes in brain structure. *Neuropsychology* 14: 178–88.

Thomson AD, Marshall EJ. (2006a) The natural history and pathophysiology of Wernicke's encephalopathy and Korsakoff's psychosis. *Alcohol and Alcoholism* 41: 151–8.

Thomson AD, Marshall EJ. (2006b) The treatment of patients at risk of developing Wernicke's encephalopathy in the community. *Alcohol and Alcoholism* 41: 159–67.

Thomson AD, Cook CC, Touquet R, Henry JA. (2002) The Royal College of Physicians report on alcohol: guidelines for managing Wernicke's encephalopathy in the Accident and Emergency Department. *Alcohol and Alcoholism* 37: 513–21.

Thomson AD, Cook CCH, Guerrini I *et al.* (2008) Wernicke's encephalopathy: 'Plus ça change, plus c'est la même chose'. *Alcohol and Alcoholism* 43: 180–6.

Torvik A. (1991) Wernicke's encephalopathy – prevalence and clinical spectrum. *Alcohol and Alcoholism* 26 (Suppl. 1): 381–4.

Torvik A, Lindboe CF, Rogde S. (1982) Brain lesions in alcoholics: A neuropathological study with clinical correlations. *Journal of the Neurological Sciences* 56: 233–48.

Unkenstein AE, Bowden SC. (1990) The individual course of neuropsychological recovery in recently abstinent alcoholics: A pilot study. *The Clinical Neuropsychologist* 5: 24–32.

Victor M. (1994) Alcoholic dementia. *Canadian Journal of Neurological Science* 21: 88–99.

Victor M, Adams RD, Collins GH. (1971) *The Wernicke-Korsakoff syndrome*. Oxford: Basil Blackwell.

Victor M, Adams RD, Collins GH. (1989) *The Wernicke-Korsakoff syndrome and related neurological disorders due to alcoholism and malnutrition*. Philadelphia: FA Davis.

World Health Organization. (2007) WHO Expert Committee on Problems Related to Alcohol Consumption, Second Report. Geneva: World Health Organization.

Huntington's disease

PHYLLIS CHUA AND EDMOND CHIU

78.1 CLINICAL FEATURES

Huntington's disease (HD) is an autosomal-dominant progressive neurodegenerative disorder beginning classically in mid-life with the characteristic triad of clinical features (Folstein, 1989) – motor disorder, cognitive disorder and emotional disorder. Within this characteristic triad, there is variety in the clinical phenotype with respect to timing of onset, symptoms and progression. Death usually occurs 20–30 years after the onset of motor symptoms.

78.1.1 Motor disorder

Although chorea is usually the predominant feature, dystonia, athetosis, motor restlessness, myoclonus and voluntary movement abnormalities may also be present. The chorea typically consists of rapid, non-repetitive contractions involving the orofacial and truncal areas and the limbs, and worsens with anxiety. Common manifestations include lip pouting, twitching of the cheeks, irregular grimacing, alternate lifting of the eyebrows, head nodding from neck muscle involvement, irregular breathing, fingers and toes flexion and extension, crossing and uncrossing of the legs and truncal restlessness (Kremer, 2003). The choreoathetosis tends to be absent during sleep and present when awake. The movements cannot be suppressed voluntarily, although early on the patient may be able to integrate some of these movements into purposeful actions or minimize them by holding on to a chair, for example. The choreiform movements usually affect the periphery initially, i.e. piano playing fingers, twitchy toes. They may be intermittent and more obvious when the person

is distracted by being asked to perform a motor or mental task. In this early stage, there is hypotonia with hyperreflexia (Suttonbrown and Suchowersky, 2003). In advanced cases, dysarthria may result from involvement of the diaphragm and vocal apparatus (Suttonbrown and Suchowersky, 2003). Dystonia often accompanies chorea early in the illness, but can be very severe in advanced cases, juvenile onset patients or in the 'Westphal variant' of adult onset cases. The dystonia may manifest as abnormal posturing of the extremities and head, internal shoulder rotation, sustained fist clenching, excessive knee flexion and foot inversion (Kremer, 2003).

Motor impersistence – the inability to sustain a voluntary muscle contraction – can be noted during a handshake or by asking the person to hold their tongue out. Abnormalities in saccadic eye movements, poor optokinetic nystagmus and slowness with refixation may also be present in the majority of patients. Saccadic abnormalities with an inability to suppress reflexive glances to sudden novel stimuli and delayed initiation of voluntary saccades and slow saccades, particularly in the vertical movements, are seen early in the majority of patients (Lasker and Zee, 1997).

As the condition progresses, choreiform movements become less prominent and voluntary movements are increasingly impaired by the occurrence of clumsiness, bradykinesia, rigidity, inability to sustain complex voluntary movement patterns, leading to gait abnormalities and dysarthria. There is difficulty with tandem walking, turning and falls, until eventually the patients is confined to a wheelchair. The dysarthria starts off as reduced clarity, which becomes worse as the rate and rhythm of speech becomes affected. Towards the late stage of the disease, rigidity and akinesia frequently overtake other aspects of the motor disorder accompanied by dysphagia and urinary incontinence. Frontal release reflexes, such as snouting, sucking or grasping, are seen when there is significant cognitive decline.

78.1.2   Cognitive disorder

The cognitive changes in HD primarily reflect a form of subcortical dementia characterized by memory deficit, psychomotor slowing, apathy and depression. Cognitive domains affected include executive, language, perceptual and spatial skills, and memory functions. Executive function refers to a collection of higher order cognitive functions, including the ability to plan and organize, monitor one's performance and self-correct, mental flexibility, shift attention set as circumstances change, and inhibit impulsive behaviours. Psychomotor slowing is evident in timed tasks, such as digit symbol substitution and trail-making. Intact verbal recognition memory, word recognition and object naming allow the person with HD to continue communicating initially, despite mild dysarthria and dysprosody being present. In the advanced stages, language may be impaired leading to a mute state. This is due to a combination of motor disorder affecting phonation leading to severe dysarthria, impairment of comprehension of both affective and propositional prosody, leading to failure to appreciate rhythm and changes of tone in normal speech and other cognitive deficits, such as reduced verbal fluency, psychomotor slowing and apathy.

Visuospatial disorder in HD is evident early during performance in object assembly and block design tests (Craufurd and Snowden, 2003). Deficits occur in complex tasks (Lawrence et al., 2000) that also require planning and organization such as tests of pattern and spatial recognition memory, simultaneous and delayed matching-to-sample and spatial. Further studies are needed to determine whether these deficits represent 'true' deficits in visuospatial/visual processing or reflect other processes, such as deficits in context recognition/recognition (Lawrence et al., 2000).

Memory problems are a common complaint of patients with HD. This is due to an inefficient memory strategy for acquiring and retrieving memories rather than a primary disorder of retention (Craufurd and Snowden, 2003), and may reflect executive dysfunction, leading to ineffective information retrieval strategies.

These cognitive deficits appear early in the illness and may predate the motor signs. The rate of decline and cognitive domains affected in each individual are variable. Correlations between the rate of cognitive decline and CAG repeat length have been inconsistent (Craufurd and Snowden, 2003). The neural basis for the cognitive deficits is thought to be involvement of the basal ganglia and frontostriatal connections.

78.1.3   Psychiatric disorder

There is increasing awareness that the high prevalence of behavioural and psychological symptoms in HD make a large contribution to the distress and functional decline in the person with HD. An early study of 186 persons with HD in Maryland by Folstein (1989) found that 30 per cent of the sample were free from any psychiatric disorder, 33 per cent had affective disorder, 30 per cent had intermittent explosive disorder, 4.8 per cent had dysthymic disorder, 15.6 per cent alcoholism, 5.9 per cent antisocial personality and 5.9 per cent schizophrenia. In a similar population-based study, Watt and Seller (1993) reported on a higher prevalence of depression (54 per cent), schizophrenia (12 per cent) and behavioural and personality disorder (42 per cent). The latter consisted of aggressiveness, which was the most frequent reported, followed by suspiciousness and temper. A recent review by van Duijn et al. (2007) found studies reported prevalence of depressed mood, anxiety, irritability and apathy ranged from 33 to 78 per cent, obsessive–compulsive symptoms 10–52 per cent and psychosis 3–11 per cent.

Irritability is reported frequently by family members as being one of the most difficult symptoms to tolerate. The potential role of alcohol and benzodiazepines in precipitating such symptoms should be considered. Irritability as part of a depressive illness should also be considered. Other psychiatric manifestations, such as obsessive–compulsive symptoms (Anderson et al., 2001), excessive worrying and somatizations have been reported, but often do not meet criteria for a formal psychiatric diagnosis. The common obsessions reported have aggressive and contamination themes (Anderson et al., 2001). Checking rituals were the most commonly reported. A recent study found the probability of obsessive and compulsive symptoms increased with disease severity (Beglinger, 2007). Psychotic symptoms in HD tend to be isolated and atypical rather than schizophreniform, with persecutory delusions being the most common. The psychotic symptoms are more common early on in the illness and decrease with the cognitive decline. Sleep disturbances of frequent nocturnal awakenings and changes in sleep architecture and sleep–wake rhythm have been reported in HD (Gagnon et al., 2008).

Many studies have reported a high rate of suicide in HD (Di Maio et al., 1993), but in Victoria, Australia, only 1.6 per cent of deaths were attributed to suicide (Chiu and Alexander, 1982). Suicide in HD has been related to the high prevalence of major affective disorder and other symptoms, such as irritability, emotional lability and impulsiveness. The prevalence of suicidal ideas was found to vary at different stages of HD: 9 per cent in the asymptomatic at-risk individuals rising to 22 per cent in the prediagnostic group (Walker, 2007).

The aetiology of psychological symptoms in HD is likely to be multifactorial. Depression can precede the onset of motor symptoms of HD by many years and can occur in those who may not be aware of being at-risk for the disorder (Craufurd and Snowden, 2003). Subtle psychiatric symptoms in the depression, anxiety, obsessive–compulsive domain were reported more in the prediagnosed HD gene carriers compared to HD gene-negative individuals (Duff et al., 2007). Thompson et al. (2002) examined three dimensions of behavioural change reported in HD – apathy, depression and irritability using the Problem Behaviours Assessment for Huntington's Disease (PBA-HD) scale. Of the three dimensions, only apathy was highly correlated with cognitive and motor indices of disease severity. Apathy and executive dysfunction may reflect a common underlying deficit in the striatofrontal circuits. No correlation between the presence of psychiatric symptoms and CAG repeat size has been found (Vassos *et al.*, 2008). Genetic heterogeneity at the HD locus, or a gene predisposing to the psychiatric disorder and closely linked to the HD gene may explain the clustering of specific psychiatric symptoms, such as psychosis (Tsuang *et al.*, 2000) and affective disorder (Folstein *et al.*, 1983) observed in some families.

78.1.4   Onset

The age of onset usually refers to the onset of typical motor symptoms, with the mean previously being reported from the late thirties to the early forties. Kremer (2003) argues that the median age of onset, which is in the late forties or early fifties, is the more accurate measure of onset age rather than the mean, due the fact that the onset age is not normally distributed, and that the truncated intervals of observation in many studies biases the results towards the younger onset group.

Penney *et al.* (1990) introduced the term 'zone of onset', referring to the insidious onset of symptoms over many years between the asymptomatic stage and the definitive appearance of involuntary movements, such as chorea. During the period prior to formal diagnosis of HD, there may be subtle changes in the psychological, cognitive and neurological domains of which the person may be aware. Individuals may suffer from depression, increased irritability, be more disinhibited, experience increased forgetfulness and have difficulties with multi-tasking. All these problems may lead to difficulties at work. Increased fidgeting and restlessness may be noted by family and friends. This stage merges imperceptibly with the diagnostic stage when the person demonstrates unequivocal and more specific evidence of HD, such as choreiform movements.

Various studies have indicated that the length of the trinucleotide repeats in the HD gene accounts for 50–70 per cent of the statistical variance in onset age (Duyao *et al.*, 1993). In the majority of families, the age of onset tends to be similar. An analysis of Venezuelan kindreds revealed that CAG repeat size is the most important factor in determining the age of onset and 40 per cent of the variance remaining in onset age is due to other genes and 60 per cent is environmental (US-Venezuela Collaborative Research Project and Wexler, 2004). Several models to predict age of onset have been developed. Ranen *et al.* (1995) developed a prediction equation which was derived from a stepwise multiple regression analysis from 50 parent–child pairs, whereby age at onset $= [-0.81 \times \text{repeat length}] + [0.51 \times \text{parental age}] + 54.87$. A parametric survival model based on CAG repeat length and age of the patient can provide probability of onset of motor symptoms for CAG repeats between 36 and 56. This model by Langbehn *et al.* (2004) was based on data from 2913 individuals from 40 centres worldwide.

78.1.5   Advanced stage

The median duration of HD is 21.4 years with a range of 1.2–40.8 years (Foroud *et al.*, 1999). In the late stages, the person with HD is usually confined to a wheelchair and reliant on nursing care. Bradykinesia, dystonia and rigidity dominate the picture. Choreiform movements may still be evident in the orobuccal region and the extremities. Communication and swallowing are severely impaired. Nasogastric or percutaneous endoscopic gastric (PEG) feeds may be necessary to prevent aspiration and to offset the weight loss commonly seen in the advanced stage. Increased muscle tone may result in joint contractures. Pressure sores occur secondary to immobility. Cognition is impaired and slow. It may be difficult to assess for psychiatric symptoms because of limited communication. Sleep disturbance and agitation may be problems. Some patients are incontinent of faeces and urine. Cachexia despite adequate intake may be seen late in the illness. The leading causes of death are pneumonia, heart disease, choking, nutritional deficiencies and skin ulcers.

78.1.6   Clinical variants

Clinical variants of HD include the juvenile onset, adult onset Westphal variant and late-onset disease (Kremer, 2003). Juvenile onset refers to the 10 per cent of all patients with HD who have onset before 20 years of age. These cases usually have over 60 CAG repeats (Squitieri *et al.*, 2006). Children with juvenile-onset HD often present with a decline in school performance and non-specific behavioural problems, predating the motor disorder by a few years. Other features of the juvenile onset are prominent rigidity and bradykinesia early on and minimal chorea, a rapidly progressive dementia, cerebellar abnormalities, myoclonus and epilepsy. Infantile HD (5 per cent of juvenile cases), a devastating illness with onset before ten years of age, is associated with very large CAG repeats beyond 80–100 (Squitieri *et al.*, 2006). The adult-onset Westphal variant refers to the cases with prominent rigidity earlier on, rather than chorea. These patients are usually young with onset in their twenties or rarely in their thirties. Late-onset HD patients have a slower, milder form of HD with onset usually after age 50 years. Motor and cognitive symptoms are present but less severe, while psychiatric symptoms are less common. Despite a more benign course, the number of years of survival after disease onset may still be similar to earlier onset cases (James *et al.*, 1994).

78.1.7   Differential diagnosis

Other diseases which may present with similar features are dentatorubropallidoluysian atrophy, HD-like and neuroacanthocytosis. Choreiform movements are also seen in other diseases, such as chorea gravidarum, hyperthyroidism, tardive dyskinesia, Syndenham's chorea, chorea-associated with antibodies against phospholipids and vascular hemichorea (Walker, 2007).

78.2   EPIDEMIOLOGY

The prevalence of HD has been largely based on estimates of point prevalence and has shown wide variations between countries and studies due to differences in selection criteria, source population and sampling methods. In the United States, most studies gave a rate of 5–7 per 100 000 population (Folstein, 1989). The prevalence is much lower among non-European ethnic groups.

78.3   GENETICS

78.3.1   The HD gene

HD is transmitted as an autosomal dominant trait with high penetrance (Gusella *et al.*, 1993). The gene, *IT15* (interesting transcript) located at 4p16.3 (short arm of chromosome 4) was discovered in March 1993 by The Huntington's Disease Collaborative Research Group (Huntington's Disease Collaborative Research, 1993). It contains a polymorphic trinucleotide CAG repeat that is expanded and unstable. The number of CAG repeats on normal chromosomes ranges from 11 to 34 (Gusella *et al.*, 1993). The zone of reduced penetrance (ZRP) refers to the CAG size range where the majority of people will manifest the disease within their expected lifetime, but a few will remain asymptomatic. In HD, the ZRP range is 36–38 (Andrew *et al.*, 1997). In the CAG size range 29–35 (intermediate alleles), individuals do not manifest signs of HD (Goldberg *et al.*, 1993), but their offspring are at risk of inheriting an expanded CAG gene and therefore of developing HD (Andrew *et al.*, 1997). The estimate risk of an expansion to 36 or more CAG repeats in the offspring of male intermediate HD gene carriers is between 2 and 10 per cent (Goldberg *et al.*, 1993). There is a bias towards an increased number of CAG repeats, especially in paternal transmission leading to anticipation (Duyao *et al.*, 1993) – earlier onset and greater severity of disease in later generations. This is due to greater meiotic instability during spermatogenesis than oogenesis. During replication, trinucleotides CAG repeats with more than 28 are more unstable. Furthermore, most instability leads to increased size (73 per cent) of CAG repeats (Walker, 2007). Most adult-onset cases have a CAG repeat size in the 40–50 range (Imarisio *et al.*, 2008).

Mutation rate is very low, variously calculated to be between 0.07×10^{-6} to 9.6×10^{-6} (Harper, 1991). Most cases with no known family history usually have parents in the intermediate allele range. Increased number of CAG repeats is associated with an earlier age of onset (Duyao *et al.*, 1993; Illarioshkin *et al.*, 1994; Kieburtz *et al.*, 1994; Brandt *et al.*, 1996). In the CAG repeat size range of 37–52 CAG units (88 per cent of all HD repeats), the variation around the predicted age of onset is 18 years (Gusella *et al.*, 1993). Late-onset HD has less correlation with the CAG repeat size (Kremer *et al.*, 1993) and increased likelihood of an intermediate CAG range (James *et al.*, 1994). Other factors, aside from the number of CAG repeats, clearly also have a role in determining the age of onset (Andrew *et al.*, 1997); possible contenders are modifying genes, environmental factors or stochastic effects (Gusella *et al.*, 1993). Severity of brain pathology as assessed by various measures, such as striatal atrophy (Penney *et al.*, 1997) has been correlated with

the size of the CAG repeat in the majority of studies. Some studies examining for correlation with regional brain atrophy have not found any correlation with the CAG repeat size (Sieradzan *et al.*, 1997). The relationship between CAG repeat size and rate of disease progression is controversial, partly due to the different markers of disease progression used in different studies. Illarioshkin *et al.* (1994) reported on a significant positive correlation between the rate of progression of neurological and psychiatric symptoms and CAG repeat size. In a two-year longitudinal follow up, Brandt *et al.* (1996) found there was a greater decline in neurological and cognitive functioning in those with CAG repeats greater than 47. In contrast, Kieburtz *et al.* (1994) failed to find such a correlation between clinical progression of disease and CAG size.

Homozygotes have been reported to have a more aggressive course, but do not appear to have an earlier age of onset (Squitieri *et al.*, 2003). The few case reports of monozygous twins with different phenotypes suggests the potential role of environmental factors (Gomez-Esteban *et al.*, 2007), epigenetic mechanisms (Georgiou *et al.*, 1999) and mosaicism (Norremolle *et al.*, 2004).

78.3.2   Mouse genetic models

Genetic animal models (Cepeda *et al.*, 2007), which can mimic the molecular pathogenesis of HD through alteration of the mouse genome, are now used to elucidate aspects of the disease and for therapeutic research. The term 'transgenic mice' refers to mice generated by pronuclear microinjection of recombinant DNA or modification of endogenous mouse genes. The main models are:

1. Mice where transgenes expressing truncated or full length versions of the huntingtin in the form of genomic or cDNA constructs have been introduced into the mouse germline.
2. 'Knockouts' – transgenic animals where a specific gene has been deleted.
3. 'Knock-ins' – transgenic mice where the sequence in exon 1 of the *Hdh* gene (the mouse homologue for the *IT15* gene) has been replaced with a CAG repeat that is pathogenic in humans. In the knock-in mice, the *Hdh* gene in mice has been modified by inserting a pure mouse gene or a *HD/Hdh* chimera. There are several lines of transgenic mice with different phenotypes and ages of onset.
4. Conditional mouse models – one model expresses exon1 with 94 repeats in response to a tetracycline regulated switch.

78.4   NEUROPATHOLOGY AND PATHOGENESIS

Gradual atrophy of the striatum (caudate and putamen) is the pathological hallmark of HD. Macroscopically at the end stage, there is generalized cerebral atrophy and decreased brain weight (Gil and Rego, 2008). The ventricles are enlarged to a greater extent than can be explained by the striatal loss. The neuronal loss in the striatum primarily involves the medium-sized neurones which are the major cell type in the striatum and act as the inhibitory projection neurones from the striatum to the globus pallidus and substantia nigra. These neurones use the inhibitory neurotransmitter gamma aminobutyric acid (GABA) and other co-transmitters, such as substance P, enkephalin and dynorphin (Gil and Rego, 2008). It is hypothesized that the loss of the inhibitory input from the medium-sized neurones is responsible for the involuntary movements in HD. These neuropathological changes evolve with time with the major cell loss starting in the dorsomedial 'tail' of the caudate and dorsal putamen, progressing ventrally, posteriorly and laterally until there is widespread severe neuronal loss and gliosis in the caudate and putamen, and moderate loss in the nucleus accumbens. Other neurotransmitter receptor systems, such as the dopamine, glutamate, cannabinoid and adenosine, have also been implicated in the pathogenesis of HD (Cepeda et al., 2007). Vonsattel et al. (Gil and Rego, 2008) developed a system for grading the severity of striatal degeneration from grade 0 (no macroscopic changes, neuronal loss may be present) to grade 4 (severe striatal atrophy and neuronal loss). Advances in cell staining techniques now show evidence of neuronal dysfunction prior to neuronal loss. Studies indicate disruption of synaptic function, cytoskeletal integrity and axonal transport in the early symptomatic stages of HD (Walker, 2007). A recent exciting finding is evidence of increased neurogenesis in the subventricular zones of patients with HD (Grote and Hannan, 2007) and in mice and rodent models, and which may provide another potential therapeutic avenue.

In HD, the expanded CAG repeats in the *IT15* gene results in an expanded polyglutamine tract at the *N*-terminus of the huntingtin protein. The abnormal huntingtin is not limited to cerebral structures most affected by the neurodegenerative process (Sharp et al., 1995). Within the brain, huntingtin is predominantly found in the neurones and to a smaller extent in the glial cells (Sharp et al., 1995). It is present primarily in the cytoplasm and to a small extent in the nucleus (Imarisio et al., 2008). The function of the wild-type huntingtin and role of the mutant huntingtin in these pathological mechanisms of HD remain unknown. It is likely to be a gain of function of the mutant huntingtin, possibly through disturbance of specific transcriptional pathways or inhibition of mitochondrial function and proteosome activity. The significance of neuronal intranuclear and intracytoplasmic inclusions containing the mutant huntingtin, pathological hallmarks of HD – mainly whether they have a causative or protective role in the pathogenesis of HD, is equally uncertain.

The exact mechanism of HD pathogenesis postulated has included excitotoxicity, oxidative stress, impaired energy metabolism, mitochondrial dysfunction, inflammatory events, apoptosis, autophagy and abnormal protein–protein interactions causing secondary effects such as transcription dysregulation (Gil and Rego, 2008). The challenge now remains to fit the above pieces of the puzzle together to formulate a pathogenesis model of HD.

78.5 NEUROIMAGING

Structural and functional neuroimaging modalities allow investigation of the possible neural correlates of motor, cognitive and psychiatric manifestations of HD.

78.5.1 Structural imaging studies in HD

Early computed tomography (CT) imaging techniques and recent magnetic resonance imaging (MRI) have consistently revealed bicaudate atrophy. MRI studies also demonstrate atrophy of the putamen, caudate and globus pallidus in HD patients (Aylward et al., 1996). Significant cerebral cortical grey and white matter loss in patients with HD have been reported in many studies (Rosas et al., 2003; Fennema-Notestine et al., 2004). Frontal lobe atrophy involving primarily the white matter and total brain atrophy have been noted (Aylward et al., 1998). Age of onset of disease and CAG repeat length have been correlated with change in volume of caudate and total basal ganglia, even after controlling for length between scans, duration of illness and symptom severity (Aylward et al., 1997).

Early structural imaging studies were useful in demonstrating that anatomical changes predated onset of symptoms. Basal ganglia atrophy was evident as early as seven years before the onset of motor symptoms (Aylward et al., 2000). HD gene-positive subjects close to estimated age of onset had smaller basal ganglia volumes than those far from onset except for the caudate volume (Aylward et al., 1996), but putamen volume was a more sensitive marker of DNA status.

78.5.2 Magnetic resonance spectroscopy studies in HD

Proton magnetic resonance spectroscopy (MRS) (^{1}H-MRS) is a non-invasive technique that allows the detection of brain chemicals containing hydrogen such as *N*-acetyl-aspartate (NAA), choline-containing compounds (CHO), creatine/phosphocreatine (CRE), glutamine, glutamate and lactate (lactate (LAC). Studies using ^{1}H-MRS in HD have found decreased NAA/Cr in the putamen (Davie et al., 1994), lower concentration of NAA in the combined caudate head and anterior putamen (Sanchez-Pernaute et al., 1999), decreased NAA and increased choline relative to creatine in the basal ganglia (Jenkins et al., 1993), suggesting neuronal loss in these structures. Reduced creatine in the basal ganglia has also been reported (Sanchez-Pernaute et al., 1999). Elevated lactate levels in the basal ganglia and occipital region have been noted in symptomatic HD patients (Jenkins et al., 1993).

The findings in the presymptomatic gene-positive group have been more inconsistent. Gomez-Anson et al. (2007) did not observe any differences in the basal ganglia between presymptomatic and control subjects, despite their finding of decreased choline in the frontal lobe. These varied findings were corroborated by the heterogenous findings in the putamen in the presymptomatic and symptomatic group reported by Reynolds et al. (2005). The majority of these subjects showed a combination of reduced NAA, reduced creatine, increased glutamate/glutamine or the presence of lactate.

78.5.3   Functional imaging

single photon emission computed tomography (SPECT) studies of cerebral blood flow have consistently revealed reduced cerebral perfusion in the basal ganglia before evidence of atrophy on MRI (Sax et al., 1996). Hypoperfusion in the cortical areas, such as the prefrontal cortex (Sax et al., 1996), has been reported although these findings have not always been replicable. Initial positron emission tomography (PET) studies of cerebral glucose metabolism mirrored the hypoperfusion findings in SPECT studies. These findings were extended to some (Feigin et al., 2001), but not all (Young et al., 1987) considered at risk of developing HD. Cortical hypometabolism has been demonstrated in some (Kuwert et al., 1990), but not all studies (Young et al., 1986). An H2(15)O PET cerebral activation (Weeks et al., 1997) study results suggest that there is impairment of the output part of the basal ganglia-thalamo-cortical motor circuit and compensatory recruitment of additional accessory motor pathways in the cortex. Decreased benzodiazepine receptor density in the caudate, but not the putamen in early HD using ^{11}C-flumazenil PET has been reported (Holthoff et al., 1993). ^{11}C-SCH23390 PET and ^{11}C-raclopride PET were used to study dopamine D1 and D2 receptor binding, respectively. D1 and D2 (Ginovart et al., 1997) receptor binding was reduced in the striatum in symptomatic HD. Dopamine D1 receptors are reduced in the frontal (Sedvall et al., 1994) and temporal (Ginovart et al., 1997) cortices in symptomatic HD subjects. Some studies have found some asymptomatic HD subjects with reduced dopamine D1 and D2 receptor binding in the putamen and caudate (Weeks et al., 1996).

There have been few studies using functional MRI (fMRI) to examine neural activity in HD. Clark et al. (2002) reported reduced fMRI signal in the three patients relative to the three controls in occipital, parietal and somatomotor cortex and in the caudate, while increased signal was found in HD in the left post-central and right middle frontal gyri during performance of the Porteus maze task.

78.5.4   Diffusion-weighted imaging

diffusion tensor imaging (DTI) is a MRI technique that measures indices of passive water diffusion which is believed to reflect the tissue fibre density, fibre architecture and uniformity of nerve fibre direction (Mamata et al., 2004), thus allowing in vivo imaging of large white matter tracts at macroscopic resolution (millimetre scale). The studies to date indicate changes in diffusivity as measured by apparent diffusion coefficient or fractional anisotropy in the putamen, caudate, globus pallidus and different regions of white matter. Increased diffusivity in the white matter in the symptomatic group compared to controls seems to be a common finding (Mascalchi et al., 2004; Reading et al., 2005; Rosas et al., 2006; Kloppel et al., 2008). The changes in the presymptomatic group have been inconsistent across various studies.

78.6   MANAGEMENT

Given the range of problems and the changing needs with progression of the disease, care of a person with HD would ideally be provided by a multidisciplinary team consisting of a physician (a neurologist or psychiatrist with expertise in HD), genetic counsellors, psychologists, social workers, physiotherapists, speech therapists and nurses.

The main management issues in patients with HD are:

- movement disorders, causing involuntary movements, gait disorder, dystonia and rigidity;
- oral motor disorder, affecting speech and eating;
- behavioural and psychiatric disorder of depression, psychosis, anxiety, obsessive–compulsive behaviours, irritability, agitation in late stage;
- cognitive disorder, which can lead to behavioural problems due to frustration from difficulty adapting to change, inflexibility and apathy;
- medical issues of weight loss, sleep disturbance and complications in late-stage HD from infections, regurgitation, cachexia, delirium;
- social issues of work, finances, care and placement, driving ability;
- support for the caregiver and families, and education of the patient, family and other healthcare professionals (Nance and Westphal, 2002).

78.6.1   Predictive testing for HD

Guidelines of the International Huntington Association (IHA) and the World Federation of Neurology for HD (WFN) (International Huntington Association and World Federation of Neurology Research Group on Huntington's Chorea, 1994), developed soon after the HD gene testing became available, have provided the framework for pre-symptomatic, prenatal and confirmatory testing. The pre-symptomatic predictive testing programmes include:

- helping the individual and accompanying support person understand the diagnosis, probable course and current management available for HD;
- helping appreciation of the implications of the genetic results for relatives;
- pedigree analysis, which allows the risk to the individual to be assessed and provide some insight into the family dynamics;
- discussion of their personal experiences, goals, financial and social resources, coping styles and other support; reason for testing;
- psychological assessment of their coping ability; and
- possible neurological assessment for symptom onset.

The uptake of predictive testing has varied between countries – varying from less than 5 per cent in Germany, Australia and Switzerland to 24 per cent in The Netherlands (Tibben, 2007). The low figures reported may be due to errors in the commonly used formulae, such as the failure to exclude children from the at-risk group number (Tassicker et al.,

2009). Reasons for seeking the predictive test were commonly for relief of anxiety about developing HD, preparing for the future and family planning. Despite initial concerns, with the appropriate support from pretest counselling, the risk of suicide and other events, such as suicide attempts or hospitalization for psychiatric reasons, have been low, with a worldwide risk reported at 0.97 per cent (Almqvist *et al.*, 1999). High risk factors include a positive gene test, psychiatric history five years prior to testing, and unemployment. All who committed suicide were symptomatic at the time.

Prenatal testing of the fetus has had low uptake. Preimplantation genetic testing, which combines assisted reproduction and genetic testing, so that only HD-negative embryos are implanted, is now available.

78.6.2 Pharmacological treatments

Currently, pharmacological treatment is aimed at symptomatic control of the motor and psychiatric aspects of the disorder. Unfortunately, there is little evidence-based treatment strategies specific to HD and clinicians need to rely mainly on their general treatment principles. Neuroleptics, such as haloperidol (a dopamine antagonist), are used to suppress abnormal movements. In later stages of the illness, as dopamine receptors are destroyed with the neurones containing them, these medications will gradually be of lesser value and may aggravate dystonia, bradykinesia and dysphagia, gait and balance problems. Given this natural progression of the chorea to decrease with time, antichoreic agents should be given only if the involuntary movements are severe and disabling. Low doses of haloperidol (less than 10 mg/day) have been shown to be most effective. Atypical neuroleptics, such as risperidone and olanzapine, are now preferred as they have a lower incidence of side effects. Tetrabenazine, a presynaptic dopamine-depleting agent is effective, but may cause depression as a side effect (Gimenez-Roldan and Mateo, 1989). Trials of clozapine (doses up to 150 mg/day) have shown modest antichoreic effects, but the adverse side effects outweigh the potential benefits in most cases (van Vugt *et al.*, 1997). Benzodiazepines, such as clonazepam, may reduce anxiety and some of the motor symptoms (Peiris *et al.*, 1976). Rigidity and akinesia in the Westphal variant of HD have been shown to respond to antiparkinsonian medications (Bonelli and Hofmann, 2007).

Depression responds to the same treatments as it does in the general population, but people with HD may be more sensitive to side effects, such as sedation (Craufurd and Snowden, 2003) and anticholinergic-induced cognitive decline (Leroi and Michalon, 1998). Despite the high prevalence of depression in HD, there have been no systematic antidepressant trials in HD (Bonelli and Hofmann, 2007). There have been 11 reported cases in the literature of the effective use of electroconvulsive therapy in treatment of depression (Van Duijn *et al.*, 2005). HD patients appear sensitive to lithium toxicity owing to their high risk of dehydration (Leroi and Michalon, 1998).

Management of irritability or behavioural disturbance should focus initially on any possible underlying cause such as depression or psychosis. Psychotic symptoms, irritability or behavioural disturbance may respond to neuroleptics (Bonelli and Hofmann, 2007). Propranolol, serotonin reuptake inhibitors, carbamazepine and sodium valproate can be helpful in the management of irritability (Ranen *et al.*, 1996; Grove *et al.*, 2000; Craufurd and Snowden, 2003). Trials using rivastigmine and donepezil have had limited benefit for cognitive and motor deficits (Imarisio *et al.*, 2008).

78.6.3 Psychosocial and physical management

Supportive psychotherapy aims to deal with losses of health, work, independence for the individual and their implications for the other family members. Cognitive assessment can assist in clinical management and decision-making on employment, driving, self-care and other legal and safety issues. Identification of the cognitive deficits and strengths can assist in understanding any behavioural problems and determine strategies to deal with them (Bourne *et al.*, 2006). Executive dysfunction can lead to a person with HD to become more rigid in their ways and fixated on themes. The fixed thought or behaviour can be channelled to more manageable or appropriate behaviours. Difficulty with planning, organizing and sequencing may lead to difficulties completing even simple tasks at home. Having a regular and simple routine, use of prompts and eventually supervision of these tasks may be useful measures. Similarly, apathy may be interpreted as laziness or stubbornness. Slowing of thought processes, difficulty in retrieving information and poorer communication skills can be frustrating for the person and those around them. Having an explanation for this may allow the person to give themselves more time to process information and to use other memory strategies, i.e. lists and diaries.

As the disease progresses, assistance with personal care and other activities of daily living will become necessary. Day care and respite care programmes may need to be considered. Attention to nutrition is important as weight loss is an inherent feature of the disease and may be compounded by dysphagia in the late stages, poor dentition, unusual food-related behaviours, such as obsessive intake of sweet foods and food refusals, psychiatric disorders and medication side effects. The use of a percutaneous endoscopic gastrostomy (PEG) feeding tube at the end stage of the disease should be discussed early on when the patient is able to express his or her wishes on this matter. Local branches of the HD Association can provide valuable support, advice on local resources and educational material on HD. Finally, residential care may be needed for some HD patients.

78.6.4 Research into new therapies

There are currently no disease-modifying treatments for HD, but unlike most other forms of neurodegenerative diseases, the ability to identify the at-risk group through genetic testing provides the opportunity to prevent neuronal loss early in the course of the disease.

Specific treatments which theoretically target the hypothetical disease pathways are being trialled in cell and animal models (Imarisio *et al.*, 2008). The prevention of mutant gene expression has been used in mouse models, but remains a distant possibility only in humans due to safety concerns, such as the need for direct intraventricular injection of the siRNA and potential unwanted genetic effects. The clearance of the mutant huntingtin through autophagy can also be enhanced using drugs which upregulate this process, such as carbamazepine, sodium valproate and rapamycin, which are already approved for use in humans. Minocycline, an antibiotic, is been trialled in humans due to its potential ability to prevent the action of caspases which are involved in the cleavage of huntingtin to produce toxic N-terminal fragments and subsequent cell death through apoptosis. Preliminary dose-finding and tolerability trials in humans have shown promise with creatine (a transglutaminase inhibitor which also targets mitochondrial dysfunction) and cystamine (a transglutaminase inhibitor to prevent the formation of aggregates). The use of NMDA receptor antagonists to prevent excitotoxic cell death have had mixed (amantadine and riluzole) or disappointing (lamotrigine and remacemide) results in human randomized controlled trials. Memantine has shown some promise. These results have been disappointing given that some of these drugs theoretically target more than one potential pathway. New studies using dimebon and creatine are now being undertaken.

Restorative therapies that rejuvenate or replace malfunctioning neurones in order to restore functions are also being developed. Since 1989, there have been over 50 cases of cell transplantation using fetal striatal tissues (Dunnett and Rosser, 2002). Most reports have shown no major adverse effect with evidence of improved function and striatal graft viability in the short follow up of 12–33 months postoperatively (Dunnett and Rosser, 2002). There are many issues related to fetal striatal tissue transplantation in the ethical and practical domains that are likely to limit its availability. Another alternative is stem cells, which have the potential for self-renewal and are capable of forming at least one, sometimes many, specialized cell types. Currently, the task is to control the differentiation potential of these cells in the adult brain environment. The use of neurotrophic factors through direct administration into the ventricles or use of specially engineered neurotrophic factor releasing cells is another strategy being explored (Imarisio *et al.*, 2008).

Recent research on environmental enrichment and experience-dependent neural plasticity in rodent models has opened another therapeutic avenue (Nithianantharajah and Hannan, 2006). Environmental enrichment has been found to induce changes in brain structure and function, and promote neurogenesis. Relatively recent findings of evidence of increased neurogenesis in the subventricular zones of patients with HD (Grote and Hannan, 2007).

REFERENCES

Almqvist E, Bloch M, Brinkman R *et al.* (1999) A worldwide assessment of the frequency of suicide, suicide attempts, or psychiatric hospitalisation after predictive testing for Huntington disease. *American Journal of Human Genetics* **64**: 1293–304.

Anderson K, Louis E, Stern Y, Marder K. (2001) Cognitive correlates of obsessive and compulsive symptoms in Huntington's disease. *American Journal of Psychiatry* **158**: 799–801.

Andrew S, Goldberg Y, Hayden M. (1997) Rethinking genotype and phenotype correlations in polyglutamine expansion disorders. *Human Molecular Genetics* **6**: 2005–10.

Aylward E, Am C, Pe B *et al.* (1996) Basal ganglia volume and proximity to onset in presymptomatic Huntington disease. *Archives of Neurology* **53**: 1293–6.

Aylward EH, Li Q, Stine OC *et al.* (1997) Longitudinal change in basal ganglia volume in patients with Huntington's disease. *Neurology* **48**: 394–9.

Aylward EH, Anderson NB, Bylsma FW *et al.* (1998) Frontal lobe volume in patients with Huntington's disease. *Neurology* **50**: 252–8.

Aylward EH, Codori AM, Rosenblatt A *et al.* (2000) Rate of caudate atrophy in presymptomatic and symptomatic stages of Huntington's disease. *Movement Disorders* **15**: 552–60.

Beglinger LJ. (2007) Probability of obsessive and compulsive symptoms in Huntington's disease. *Biological Psychiatry* **61**: 415–18.

Bonelli RM, Hofmann P. (2007) A systematic review of the treatment studies in Huntington's disease since 1990. *Expert Opinion on Pharmacotherapy* **8**: 141–53.

Bourne C, Clayton C, Murch A, Grant J. (2006) Cognitive impairment and behavioural difficulties in patients with Huntington's disease. *Nursing Standard* **20**: 41–4.

Brandt J, Bylsma F, Stine O *et al.* (1996) Trinucleotide repeat length and clinical progression in Huntington's disease. *Neurology* **46**: 527–31.

Cepeda C, Wu N, Andre VM *et al.* (2007) The corticostriatal pathway in Huntington's disease. *Progress in Neurobiology* **81**: 253–71.

Chiu E, Alexander L. (1982) Causes of death in Huntington's disease. *Medical Journal of Australia* **1**: 153.

Clark VP, Lai S, Deckel AW *et al.* (2002) Altered functional MRI responses in Huntington's disease. *Neuroreport* **13**: 703–6.

Craufurd D, Snowden J. (2003) Neuropsychological and neuropsychiatric aspects of Huntington's disease. In: Bates G, Harper P, Jones L (eds). *Huntington's disease.* Oxford: Oxford University Press, 62–94.

Davie CA, Barker GJ, Quinn N *et al.* (1994) Proton MRS in Huntington's disease. *Lancet* **343**: 1580.

Davie CA, Hawkins CP, Barker GJ *et al.* (1994) Serial proton magnetic spectroscopy in acute multiple sclerosis lesions. *Brain* **117**: 49–58.

Di Maio L, Squitieri F, Napolitano G *et al.* (1993) Suicide risk in Huntington's disease. *Journal of Medical Genetics* **30**: 292–5.

Duff K, Paulsen JS, Beglinger LJ *et al.* (2007) and the Predict-HD Investigators of the Huntingdon Study Group. Psychiatric symptoms in Huntington's disease before diagnosis: the predict-HD study. *Biological Psychiatry* **62**: 1341–6.

Dunnett S, Rosser A. (2002) Cell and tissue transplantation. In: Bates G, Harper P, Jones LE (eds). *Huntington's Disease*, 3rd edn. Oxford: Oxford University Press, 512–46.

Duyao M, Ambrose C, Myers R *et al.* (1993) Trinucleotide repeat length instability and age of onset in Huntington's disease. *Nature Genetics* 4: 387–92.

Feigin A, Leenders KL, Moeller JR *et al.* (2001) Metabolic network abnormalities in early Huntington's disease: an [(18)F]FDG PET study. *Journal of Nuclear Medicine* 42: 1591–5.

Fennema-Notestine C, Archibald S, Jacobson M *et al.* (2004) *In vivo* evidence of cerebellar atrophy and cerebral white matter loss in Huntington disease. *Neurology* 63: 989–95.

Folstein S. (1989) *Huntington's disease: a disorder of families.* Baltimore, MD: John Hopkins University Press.

Folstein S, Abbott M, Chase G *et al.* (1983) The association of affective disorder with Huntington's disease in a case series and in families. *Psychological Medicine* 13: 537–42.

Foroud T, Gray J, Ivashina J, Conneally P. (1999) Differences in duration of Huntington's disease based on age at onset. *Journal of Neurology, Neurosurgery and Psychiatry* 66: 52–6.

Gagnon JF, Petit D, Latreille V, Montplaisir J. (2008) Neurobiology of sleep disturbances in neurodegenerative disorders. *Current Pharmaceutical Design* 14: 3430–45.

Georgiou N, Bradshaw J, Chiu E *et al.* (1999) Differential clinical and motor control function in pair of monozygotic twins with Huntington's disease. *Movement Disorders* 14: 320–5.

Gil JM, Rego AC. (2008) Mechanisms of neurodegeneration in Huntington's disease. *European Journal of Neuroscience* 27: 2803–20.

Gimenez-Roldan S, Mateo D. (1989) Huntington disease: tetrabenazine compared to haloperidol in the reduction of involuntary movements. *Neurologia* 4: 282–7.

Ginovart N, Lundin A, Farde L *et al.* (1997) PET study of the pre- and post-synaptic dopaminergic markers for the neurodegenerative process in Huntington's disease. *Brain* 120: 503–14.

Goldberg Y, Kremer B, Andrew S *et al.* (1993) Molecular analysis of new mutations causing Huntington disease: Intermediate alleles and sex of origin effects. *Nature Genetics* 5: 174–9.

Gomez-Anson B, Alegret M, Muñoz E *et al.* (2007) Decreased frontal choline and neuropsychological performance in preclinical Huntington disease. *Neurology* 68: 906–10.

Gomez-Esteban J, Lezcano EZ, Velasco F *et al.* (2007) Monozygotic twins suffering from Huntington's disease show different cognitive and behavioral symptoms. *European Neurology* 57: 26–30.

Grote HE, Hannan AJ. (2007) Regulators of adult neurogenesis in the healthy and diseased brain. *Clinical and Experimental Pharmacology and Physiology* 34: 533–45.

Grove VJ, Quintanilla J, Devaney G. (2000) Improvement of Huntington's disease with olanzapine and valproate. *New England Journal of Medicine* 343: 973–4.

Gusella J, Macdonald M, Ambrose C, Duyao M. (1993) Molecular genetics of Huntington's Disease. *Archives of Neurology* 50: 1157–63.

Harper P. (1991) *Huntington's disease.* London: WB Saunders.

Holthoff VA, Koeppe RA, Frey KA. (1993) Positron emission tomography measures of benzodiazepine receptors in Huntington's disease. *Annals of Neurology* 34: 76–81.

Huntington's Disease Collaborative Research Group. (1993) A novel gene containing a trinucleotide repeat that is expanded and unstable on Huntington's disease chromosomes. *Cell* 72: 971–83.

Illarioshkin S, Igarashi S, Onodera A *et al.* (1994) Trinucleotide repeat length and rate of progression of Huntington's disease. *Annals of Neurology* 36: 630–5.

International Huntington Association (IHA) and the World Federation of Neurology (WFN) Research Group on Huntington's Chorea. (1994) Guidelines for the molecular genetics predictive test in Huntington's disease. *Neurology* 44: 1533–6.

Imarisio S, Carmichael J, Korolchuk V *et al.* (2008) Huntington's disease: from pathology and genetics to potential therapies. *Biochemical Journal* 412: 191–209.

James C, Houlihan G, Snell R *et al.* (1994) Late-onset Huntington's disease: a clinical and molecular study. *Age and Ageing* 23: 445–8.

Jenkins BG, Koroshetz WJ, Beal MF, Rosen BR. (1993) Evidence for impairment of energy metabolism *in vivo* in Huntington's disease using localised 1H NMR spectroscopy. *Neurology* 43: 2689–95.

Kieburtz K, Macdonald M, Shih C *et al.* (1994) Trinucleotide repeat length and progression of illness in Huntington's disease. *Journal of Medical Genetics* 31: 872–4.

Kloppel SD, Golding B, Chu CV *et al.* (2008) White matter connections reflect changes in voluntary-guided saccades in pre-symptomatic Huntington's disease. *Brain* 131: 196–204.

Kremer B. (2003) Clinical neurology of Huntington's disease. In: Bates G, Harper P, Jones L (eds). *Huntington's disease.* Oxford: Oxford University Press, 28–61.

Kremer B, Squitieri F, Telenius H *et al.* (1993) Molecular analysis of late onset Huntington's disease. *Journal of Medical Genetics* 30: 991–5.

Kuwert TL, Langen HW, Herzog KJ *et al.* (1990) Cortical and subcortical glucose consumption measured by PET in patients with Huntington's disease. *Brain* 113: 1405–23.

Langbehn DB, Faulush R, Paulsen D *et al.* (2004) A new model for prediction of the age of onset and penetrance for Huntington's disease based on CAG length. *Clinical Genetics* 65: 267–7.

Lasker A, Zee D. (1997) Ocular motor abnormalities in Huntington's disease. *Vision Research* 37: 3639–45.

Lawrence A, Watkins L, Sahakian BJ *et al.* (2000) Visual object and visuospatial cognition in Huntington's disease: implications for information processing in corticostriatal circuits. *Brain* 123: 1349–64.

Leroi I, Michalon M. (1998) Treatment of the psychiatric manifestations of Huntington's disease: a review of the literature. *Canadian Journal of Psychiatry – Revue Canadienne de Psychiatrie* 43: 933–40.

Mamata H, Jolesz FA, Maier SE. (2004) Characterisation of central nervous system structures by magnetic resonance diffusion anisotrophy. *Neurochemistry International* 45: 553–60.

Mascalchi ML, Della Nave F, Tessa R *et al.* (2004) Huntington disease: volumetric, diffusion weighted and magnetization transfer MR imaging of brain. *Radiology* 232: 867–73.

Nance M, Westphal B. (2002) Comprehensive care in Huntington's disease. In: Bates G, Harper P, Jones L (eds). *Huntington's disease.* Oxford: Oxford University Press, 475–500.

Nithianantharajah J, Hannan AJ. (2006) Enriched environments, experience-dependent plasticity and disorders of the nervous system. *Nature Reviews Neuroscience* 7: 697–709.

Norremolle A, Hasholt L, Petersen C et al. (2004) Mosaicism of the CAG repeat sequence in the Huntington disease gene in a pair of monozygotic twins. *American Journal of Medical Genetics* 130A: 154–9.

Peiris J, Boralessa H, Lionel N. (1976) Clonazepam in the treatment of choreiform activity. *Medical Journal of Australia* 1: 225–7.

Penney J, Young A, Shoulson I. (1990) Huntington's disease in Venezuala: 7 years of follow-up on symptomatic and asymptomatic individuals. *Movement Disorders* 5: 93–9.

Penney JJ, Vonsattel JP, Macdonald M et al. (1997) CAG repeat number governs the development rate of pathology in Huntington's disease. *Annals of Neurology* 41: 689–92.

Ranen N, Stine O, Abbott M et al. (1995) Anticipation and instability of IT-15 (CAG)n repeats in parent-offsrping pairs with Huntington's disease. *American Journal of Human Genetics* 57: 593–602.

Ranen N, Lipsey J, Treisman G, Ross C. (1996) Sertraline in the treatment of severe aggressiveness in Huntington's disease. *Journal of Neuropsychiatry and Clinical Neurosciences* 8: 338–40.

Reading SAJ, Yassa MA, Bakker A et al. (2005) Regional white matter change in pre-symptomatic Huntington's disease: a diffusion tensor imaging study. *Psychiatry Research* 140: 55–62.

Reynolds Jr N, Prost R, Mark L. (2005) Heterogeneity in 1H-MRS profiles of presymptomatic and early manifest Huntington's disease. *Brain Research* 1031: 82–9.

Rosas H, Koroshetz W, Chen Y et al. (2003) Evidence for more widespread cerebral pathology in early HD. An MRI-based morphometric analysis. *Neurology* 60: 1615–20.

Rosas HD, Tuch DS, Hevelone ND et al. (2006) Diffusion tensor imaging in presymptomatic and early Huntington's disease: Selective white matter pathology and its relationship to clinical measures. *Movement Disorders* 21: 1317–25.

Sanchez-Pernaute R, Garcia-Segura JM, Del Barrio AA et al. (1999) Clinical correlation of striatal 1H MRS changes in Huntington's disease. *Neurology* 53: 806–12.

Sax DS, Powsner R, Kim A et al. (1996) Evidence of cortical metabolic dysfunction in early Huntington's disease by single-photon-emission computed tomography. *Movement Disorders* 11: 671–7.

Sedvall G, Karlsson P, Lundin A et al. (1994) Dopamine D1 receptor number – a sensitive PET marker for early brain degeneration in Huntington's disease. *European Archives of Psychiatry Clinical Neuroscience* 243: 249–55.

Sharp A, Loev S, Schilling G et al. (1995) Widespread expression of Huntington's disease gene (IT15) protein product. *Neuron* 14: 1065–74.

Sieradzan K, Mann D, Dodge A. (1997) Clinical presentation and patterns of regional cerebral atrophy related to the length of trinucleotide repeat expansions in patients with adult onset Huntington's disease. *Neuroscience Letters* 225: 45–8.

Squitieri F, Gellera C, Cannella M et al. (2003) Homozygosity for CAG mutation in Huntington disease is associated with a more severe clinical course. *Brain* 126: 946–55.

Squitieri F, Frati L, Ciarmiello A et al. (2006) Juvenile Huntington's disease: does a dosage–effect pathogenic mechanism differ from the classical adult disease? *Mechanisms of Ageing Development* 127: 208–12.

Suttonbrown M, Suchowersky O. (2003) Clinical and research advances in Huntington's disease. *Canadian Journal of Neurological Sciences* 30: S45–52.

Tassicker R, Teltscher B, Trembath M et al. (2009) Problems assessing uptake of Huntington's disease predictive testing and a proposed solution. *European Journal of Human Genetics* 17: 66–70.

Thompson J, Snowden J, Craufurd D, Neary D. (2002) Behaviour in Huntington's disease: dissociating cognition-based and mood-based changes. *Journal of Neuropsychiatry Clinical Neurosciences* 14: 37–43.

Tibben A. (2007) Predictive testing for Huntington's disease. *Brain Research Bulletin* 72: 165–71.

Tsuang D, Almqvist E, Lipe H et al. (2000) Familial aggregation of psychotic symptoms in Huntington's disease. *American Journal of Psychiatry* 157: 1955–9.

US-Venezuela Collaborative Research Project, Wexler NS. (2004) Venezuelan kindreds reveal that genetic and environmental factors modulate Huntington's disease age of onset. *Proceedings of the National Academy of Sciences of the United States of America* 101: 3498–503.

Van Duijn E, Roos R, Smarius L, Van Der Mast RC. (2005) Electroconvulsive therapy in patients with Huntington's disease with depression. *Nederelands Tijdschrift voor Geneeskunde* 149: 2141–4.

Van Duijn E, Kingma EM, Van Der Mast RC. (2007) Psychopathology in verified Huntington's disease gene carriers. *Journal of Neuropsychiatry Clinical Neurosciences* 19: 441–8.

Van Vugt J, Siesling S, Vergeer M et al. (1997) Clozapine versus placebo in Huntington's disease: a double blind randomised comparative study. *Journal of Neurology, Neurosurgery and Psychiatry* 63: 35–9.

Vassos E, Pana M, Kladi A, Vassilopoulos D. (2008) Effect of CAG repeat length on psychiatric disorders in Huntington's disorders. *Journal of Psychiatric Research* 42: 544–9.

Walker FO. (2007) Huntington's disease. *Lancet* 369: 218–28.

Watt D, Seller A. (1993) A clinico-genetic study of psychiatric disorder in Huntington's chorea. *Psychological Medicine* 23 (Suppl.): 1–46.

Weeks RC-B, Piccini A, Boecker P et al. (1997) Cortical control of movement in Huntington's disease. A PET activation study. *Brain* 120: 1569–78.

Weeks RP, Harding P, Brooks AE. (1996) Striatal D1 and D2 dopamine receptor loss in asymptomatic mutation carriers of Huntington's disease. *Annals of Neurology* 40: 49–54.

Young AP, Starosta-Rubinstein JB, Markel S et al. (1986) PET scan investigations of Huntington's disease: cerebral metabolic correlates of neurological features and functional decline. *Annals of Neurology* 20: 296–303.

Young AP, Penney JB, Starosta-Rubinstein S et al. (1987) Normal caudate glucose metabolism in persons at risk for Huntington's disease. *Archives of Neurology* 44: 254–7.

Creutzfeldt–Jakob disease and other prion diseases

JOHN COLLINGE

79.1 INTRODUCTION AND AETIOLOGY

Human prion diseases, also known as the transmissible spongiform encephalopathies, have been traditionally classified into Creutzfeldt–Jakob disease (CJD), Gerstmann–Sträussler syndrome (GSS) (also known as Gerstmann–Sträussler–Scheinker disease) and kuru. Remarkable attention has been focused on these rare diseases because of the unique biology of the transmissible agent or prion, and also because of the epizootic of bovine spongiform encephalopathy (BSE) and the evidence that BSE prions have infected humans, causing the new human prion disease known as variant CJD (vCJD). Human prion infection is associated with long, clinically silent, incubation periods which may span over half a century (Collinge et al., 2006), and while the numbers of recognized cases of vCJD have been relatively small, uncertainty remains as to the number of infected individuals in the United Kingdom and other BSE-affected countries, the eventual epidemic size of BSE-related human prion disease, and the risks of its secondary transmission from such asymptomatic carriers via medical and surgical procedures. Such secondary transmission of vCJD prion infection by blood transfusion is well documented and transmission by blood products may have occurred (Wroe et al., 2006; Peden et al., 2010).

The transmissibility of the human diseases was demonstrated with the transmission (by intracerebral inoculation with brain homogenates) to chimpanzees, of kuru and CJD in 1966 and 1968, respectively (Gajdusek et al., 1966; Gibbs et al., 1968). Transmission of GSS followed in 1981. Scrapie is a naturally occurring disease of sheep and goats, recognized in Europe for over 200 years (McGowan, 1922) and present in the sheep flocks of many countries. Scrapie was demonstrated

to be transmissible in 1936 (Cuillé and Chelle, 1936) and the recognition that kuru, and then CJD, resembled scrapie in its histopathological appearances led to the suggestion that these diseases may also be transmissible (Hadlow, 1959). Kuru reached epidemic proportions amongst the Fore population in the Eastern Highlands of Papua New Guinea and was transmitted by ritual cannibalism. Since the cessation of cannibalism in the late 1950s, the disease has steadily declined, but a few cases still occur as a result of the long incubation periods in this condition (Collinge et al., 2006). The term 'Creutzfeldt–Jakob disease' was introduced by Spielmeyer in 1922, bringing together the case reports published by Creutzfeldt and Jakob. Several of these cases would not meet modern diagnostic criteria for CJD and it was not until the demonstration of transmissibility allowed diagnostic criteria to be reassessed and refined that a clear diagnostic entity developed. All these diseases share common histopathological features: the classical triad of spongiform vacuolation (affecting any part of the cerebral grey matter), astrocytic proliferation and neuronal loss, may be accompanied by the deposition of amyloid plaques (Beck and Daniel, 1987).

Prion diseases are associated with the accumulation of an abnormal, partially protease-resistant, isoform of a host-encoded cellular glycoprotein, known as 'prion protein' (PrP). Such disease-related isoforms are referred to as PrP^{Sc} and are derived from the normal cellular precursor, PrP^{C}, by a post-translational process which involves conformational change and aggregation. PrP^{C} is rich in α-helical structure, while PrP^{Sc} is predominantly composed of β-sheet. According to the 'protein-only' hypothesis (Griffith, 1967), an abnormal PrP isoform is the principal, and possibly the sole, constituent of the transmissible agent or prion (Prusiner, 1982). It is hypothesized that PrP^{Sc} acts as a conformational template, promoting the conversion of PrP^{C} to further PrP^{Sc}. PrP^{C} may be poised between two radically different folding states: α- and β-forms of PrP can be inter-converted in suitable conditions (Jackson et al., 1999). Remarkably, human prion diseases have three distinct aetiologies with inherited, acquired and sporadic forms. It is thought that prion replication, with recruitment of PrP^{C} into the aggregated PrP^{Sc} isoform, may be initiated by a pathogenic mutation in the PrP gene (resulting in a PrP^{C} predisposed to form β-PrP) in inherited prion diseases, by exposure to a 'seed' of PrP^{Sc} in acquired cases, or as a result of the spontaneous conversion of PrP^{C} to β-PrP (and subsequent formation of aggregated material) as a rare stochastic event in sporadic prion disease.

The human PrP gene (designated *PRNP*) is located on chromosome 20p and was an obvious candidate for genetic linkage studies in the familial forms of CJD and GSS, which show an autosomal dominant pattern of disease segregation. A milestone in prion research was the identification of *PRNP* mutations in familial CJD and GSS in 1989. The first mutation to be identified in *PRNP* was in a family with CJD and consisted of a 144-bp insertion (Owen et al., 1989). A second mutation was reported in two families with GSS and genetic linkage was confirmed between this missense variant at codon 102 and GSS, confirming that GSS is an autosomal dominant Mendelian disorder (Hsiao et al., 1989). These diseases are therefore both inherited and transmissible, a biologically unique feature. Approximately 15 per cent of prion diseases are inherited and over 30 coding mutations in *PRNP* are now recognized (Collinge, 2001).

Most prion disease occurs as sporadic CJD where, by definition, there will not be a family history. However, *PRNP* mutations are seen in some apparently sporadic cases, since the family history may not be apparent due to late age of onset or non-paternity.

A common PrP polymorphism at residue 129, where either methionine or valine can be encoded, is however a key determinant of genetic susceptibility in acquired and sporadic forms of prion disease, the large majority of which occur in homozygotes (Collinge et al., 1991; Palmer et al., 1991). This protective effect of *PRNP* codon 129 heterozygosity is also seen in some of the inherited prion diseases (Baker et al., 1991; Hsiao et al., 1992; Poulter et al., 1992).

Sporadic CJD is thought to arise from somatic mutation of *PRNP* or spontaneous conversion of PrP^{C} to PrP^{Sc} as a rare stochastic event. The alternative hypothesis, that of exposure to an environmental source of either human or animal prions, was not supported by early epidemiological studies (Brown et al., 1987), but more recent studies have suggested a proportion of apparently sporadic CJD may be related to surgery or other iatrogenic routes (Collins et al., 1999; Mahillo-Fernandez et al., 2008) and it remains possible that a minority of patients have acquired the disease from exposure to animal prions, of which multiple strain types have been recognized in sheep, cattle and other species consumed for food (Collinge, 2005).

The existence of multiple isolates or strains of prions with distinct biological properties has provided a challenge to the 'protein-only' model of prion replication. Understanding how a protein-only infectious agent could encode phenotypic information is of considerable biological interest. However, it is now clear that prion strains can be distinguished by differences in the biochemical properties of PrP^{Sc}. Prion strain diversity appears to encoded by differences in PrP conformation and pattern of glycosylation (Collinge et al., 1996b). Molecular strain typing is now possible and has allowed the identification of four main types in CJD, sporadic and iatrogenic CJD being of PrP^{Sc} types 1–3, while all vCJD cases are associated with a type 4 PrP^{Sc} type (Collinge et al., 1996b; Wadsworth et al., 1999). That a similar PrP^{Sc} type to that seen in vCJD is seen in BSE transmitted to several other species (Collinge et al., 1996b) strongly supported the hypothesis that vCJD was human BSE. This conclusion was strengthened by transmission studies of vCJD into both transgenic and conventional mice which indicated that cattle BSE and vCJD were caused by the same prion strain (Bruce et al., 1997; Hill et al., 1997). Molecular classification of human prion diseases is now possible and it is likely that additional PrP^{Sc} types will be identified (Parchi et al., 1996; Hill et al., 2003), although an international consensus on human strain classification has not yet been achieved. Such studies, where patients are aetiologically classified by human prion strain, rather than by descriptive clinicopathological phenotype, allows re-evaluation of epidemiological risk factors and may provide new insights into causes of 'sporadic' CJD. The ability of a protein to encode a disease phenotype has important implications in biology, as it represents a non-Mendelian form of transmission. It would be surprising if this mechanism had not been used more widely during evolution and may prove to be of wider relevance in pathobiology.

Transmission of prion diseases between different mammalian species is restricted by a 'species barrier' (Pattison, 1965). Early studies of the molecular basis of this barrier argued that it resided in differences in PrP primary structure between the species from which the inoculum was derived and the inoculated host. Transgenic mice expressing hamster PrP were, unlike wild-type mice, highly susceptible to infection with hamster prions (Prusiner et al., 1990). That most sporadic and acquired CJD occurred in individuals homozygous at *PRNP* polymorphic codon 129 supported the view that prion propagation proceeded most efficiently when the interacting PrP^{Sc} and PrP^{C} were of identical primary structure (Collinge et al., 1991). However, prion strain type affects ease of transmission to another species. Interestingly, with BSE prions this strain component to the barrier seems to predominate, with BSE not only transmitting efficiently to a range of species, but maintaining its transmission characteristics even when passaged through an intermediate species with a distinct PrP gene (Bruce et al., 1994; Hill et al., 1997). The term 'species-strain barrier' or simply 'transmission barrier' may be preferable (Collinge, 1999). It is now clear that prion strains and transmission barriers are intimately related. According to the conformational selection model, the PrP amino acid sequence in a given species is compatible with only a subset of possible mammalian prion strains and the degree of overlap between such preferred conformations between two species will determine the effectiveness of the barrier and which strain or strains propagate in the recipient when exposed to a prion from another species (Collinge, 1999; Hill and Collinge, 2003). Recent advances, including the recognition of subclinical carrier states of prion infection in animal models (Hill *et al.*, 2000), suggest that prions themselves are not directly neurotoxic, but rather their propagation involves production of toxic species which may be uncoupled from infectivity (Hill and Collinge, 2003). A general model of prion propagation to encompass these phenomena, centring on the kinetics of prion propagation, has been proposed (Collinge and Clarke, 2007).

The species barrier between cattle BSE and humans cannot be directly measured, but can be modelled in transgenic mice expressing human PrP^C which produce human PrP^{Sc} when challenged with human prions (Collinge *et al.*, 1995a). While classical CJD prions transmit efficiently to such mice expressing human PrP valine 129 at around 200 days, only infrequent transmissions at over 500 days were seen with BSE (and vCJD) prions, consistent with a substantial species barrier for this human *PRNP* genotype (Hill *et al.*, 1997). In transgenic mice expressing only human PrP methionine 129, while transmission assessed by onset of clinical disease was again inefficient, remarkably a large proportion of the inoculated animals were subclinically infected (Asante *et al.*, 2002) suggesting a considerably lower barrier to infection in this genotype. To date, vCJD has only been recognized in humans of *PRNP* codon 129 methionine homozygous genotype (although see below for possible exception). Transmissions of BSE to mice expressing human PrP methionine 129 resulted in the generation of two distinct pathological and molecular phenotypes in these animals: one closely resembling vCJD (with type 4 PrP^{Sc} and the characteristic neuropathology of vCJD) and the other sporadic CJD with type 2 PrP^{Sc}. This raises the possibility that BSE infection of humans may result in phenotypes resembling classical CJD, as well as the distinctive phenotype of vCJD (Asante *et al.*, 2002).

In addition to public health concerns, prions have assumed much wider relevance in understanding neurodegenerative and other diseases involving accumulation of misfolded host proteins. These molecular processes are of far wider relevance in human disease, and the emerging and rapidly developing field of 'protein-misfolding diseases' has prion disease as a key paradigm. The most common neurodegenerative diseases can be considered in this category, notably Alzheimer's disease (AD), and these processes also appear to be a significant component of normal brain ageing. Analogous processes are described in yeast and fungi involving distinct proteins with prion-like properties. It has long been speculated that other neurodegenerative conditions might be at least experimentally transmissible (Gajdusek, 1988) and experimental transmission of aspects of Alzheimer pathology to primates has been reported (Baker *et al.*, 1994). Systemic amyloidosis has been experimentally transmitted by exposure to amyloid fibrils by transfusion or oral exposure in mice (Solomon *et al.*, 2007; Sponarova *et al.*, 2008). Brain extracts containing β-amyloid deposits taken from either AD patients or transgenic mice expressing β-amyloid precursor protein (APP) induced β-amyloidosis and related pathology when injected into the brains of presymptomatic APP transgenic mice (Meyer-Luehmann *et al.*, 2006; Walker *et al.*,

2006). The morphology of amyloid plaques depended on the source of the injected amyloid in a manner reminiscent of prion strains. It is interesting to speculate that distinct strains of β-amyloid may develop spontaneously in AD and might contribute to phenotypic variability in patients. A recent report raises the possibility that prion-like processes may be relevant in Parkinson's disease pathogenesis with host-to-graft spread of Lewy bodies (Li *et al.*, 2008).

79.2   CLINICAL FEATURES AND DIAGNOSIS

Human prion diseases can be divided aetiologically into inherited, sporadic and acquired forms with CJD, GSS and kuru now seen as clinicopathological syndromes within a wider spectrum of disease. Kindreds with inherited prion disease have been described with phenotypes of classical CJD, GSS and other syndromes, including fatal familial insomnia (FFI) (Medori *et al.*, 1992a). Some kindreds show remarkable phenotypic variability which can encompass both CJD- and GSS-like cases, as well as other cases which do not conform to either phenotype (Collinge *et al.*, 1992). Atypical cases (diagnosed by *PRNP* analysis) have been reported which entirely lack the classical histological features (Collinge *et al.*, 1990). There is significant clinical overlap with familial AD, frontotemporal dementias and amyotrophic lateral sclerosis with dementia. It now seems sensible to designate the familial illnesses as inherited prion diseases and to subclassify according to *PRNP* mutation. Acquired prion diseases include iatrogenic CJD, kuru, vCJD and secondary vCJD. Sporadic prion diseases at present consist of CJD and atypical variants of CJD. As there are at present no equivalent aetiological diagnostic markers for sporadic prion diseases to those for the inherited diseases, it cannot be excluded that more diverse phenotypic variants of sporadic prion disease exist.

79.2.1   Sporadic prion disease

79.2.1.1   CREUTZFELDT–JAKOB DISEASE

The core clinical syndrome of classical CJD is a rapidly progressive multifocal dementia, usually with myoclonus. Most have onset between the ages of 45 and 75, with peak between 60–65 and a clinical progression to akinetic mutism and death in less than six months. Around one third of cases have prodromal features including fatigue, insomnia, depression, weight loss, headaches, general malaise and ill-defined pain sensations. Frequent additional neurological features include extrapyramidal signs, cerebellar ataxia, pyramidal signs and cortical blindness.

Routine haematological and biochemical investigations are normal, although occasional cases have raised serum transaminases or alkaline phosphatase. There are no immunological markers and acute phase proteins are not elevated. Cerebrospinal fluid is normal, although neuronal specific enolase (NSE) and S-100 are usually elevated. However, they are not specific for CJD and represent markers of neuronal injury (Jimi *et al.*, 1992; Zerr *et al.*, 1995; Otto *et al.*, 1997).

Estimation of cerebrospinal fluid (CSF) 14-3-3 protein, while again not a specific disease marker, is useful in the appropriate clinical context (Hsich et al., 1996; Collinge, 1996). It is also positive in recent cerebral infarction or haemorrhage and in viral encephalitis, which are unlikely to present diagnostic confusion with CJD, but more recent studies have found 14-3-3 positive in other non-prion-related conditions (Yamada et al., 1999). While 14-3-3 is usually positive in typical CJD, its use in differential diagnosis in more challenging diagnostic contexts in less clear, as it may be negative in long duration atypical CJD and positive in patients with rapidly progressive AD with myoclonus for example.

Neuroimaging with computed tomography (CT) is useful to exclude other causes of subacute neurological illness, but there are no diagnostic features; cerebral and cerebellar atrophy may be present. However, magnetic resonance imaging (MRI) changes are increasingly recognized and may be extremely helpful diagnostically. Several recent reports have established diffusion-weighted imaging (DWI) as the most sensitive sequence for the diagnosis of sCJD (Murata et al., 2002; Tschampa et al., 2005; Young et al., 2005; Tschampa et al., 2007). Visual inspection of the diffusion-weighted trace image demonstrates typically increased signal intensity in the cerebral cortex with up to 95 per cent of cases showing hyperintensity affecting the insula, cingulate and superior frontal cortex independently of deep grey matter involvement (**Figure 79.1**) (Tschampa et al., 2007). DWI is superior to FLAIR in detecting MRI cortical signal change and this has been shown to correlate with lateralized clinical and electroencephalogram (EEG) abnormalities (Cambier et al., 2003).

It is suggested that the anatomical distribution of abnormal hyperintensity affecting the basal ganglia is influenced by *PRNP* genotype and PrP^{Sc} strain type (Fukushima et al., 2004; Hamaguchi et al., 2005). MRI studies are now included in the World Health Organization (WHO) diagnostic criteria for sCJD (Zerr, 2009) and the routine use of diffusion-weighted imaging has enabled earlier and more accurate diagnosis of sCJD, often with avoidance of brain biopsy. The EEG may show characteristic pseudoperiodic sharp wave activity which is very helpful in diagnosis, but present only in around 70 per cent of cases. This finding may be intermittent and serial EEG is appropriate to try and demonstrate this appearance.

Neuropathological confirmation is by demonstration of spongiform change, neuronal loss and astrocytosis. PrP amyloid plaques are usually not present, although PrP immunohistochemistry, using appropriate pretreatments (Budka et al., 1995), will nearly always be positive. PrP^{Sc} can be demonstrated by Western blot. *PRNP* analysis is essential to exclude pathogenic mutations as a family history may not always be apparent. *PRNP* mutations should certainly be excluded prior to brain biopsy, which may be considered in some patients where there is significant diagnostic doubt to exclude alternative, potentially treatable diagnoses. Tonsil biopsy (see below under 79.2.3 Variant CJD) is negative in sporadic CJD, but may be considered in younger patients where a diagnosis of vCJD is being considered. Most cases of classical CJD are homozygous with respect to the codon 129 *PRNP* polymorphism (see above under 79.1 Introduction and aetiology).

FLAIR   DWI

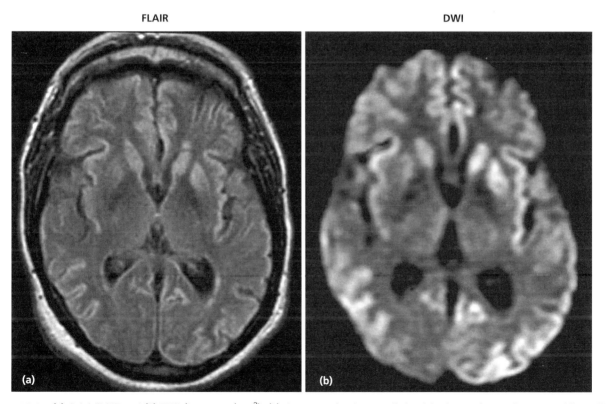

Figure 79.1 (a) Axial FLAIR and (b) DWI (b = 1000 s/mm^2); (b) demonstrating increased signal in the caudate and putamen bilaterally diffuse cortical hyperintensity.

Sporadic CJD can now be subclassified by molecular strain type using Western blot analysis of brain tissue at biopsy or autopsy, although there is no international consensus on the number or nomenclature of these molecular types. Distinctive phenotypes are associated with different PrP^{Sc} types (Parchi et al., 1999; Hill et al., 2003). For example, subacute patients of short clinical duration (several weeks) are associated with type 1 PrP^{Sc} (London classification) in the brain (Wadsworth et al., 1999; Hill et al., 2003).

79.2.1.2 ATYPICAL CREUTZFELDT–JAKOB DISEASE

Atypical forms of CJD are well recognized. Around 10 per cent of CJD has a prolonged clinical course with duration of over two years (Brown et al., 1984). Patients with a valine homozygous or methionine valine heterozygous genotype at PRNP codon 129 are more often atypical clinical forms than methionine homozygotes (Collinge and Palmer, 1994) and may lack a characteristic EEG. It is unclear yet to what extent this represents propagation of different prion strains or a direct effect of the genotype on disease expression (Collinge, 2001). Approximately 10 per cent of CJD cases present with cerebellar ataxia rather than cognitive impairment, ataxic CJD (Gomori et al., 1973). Heidenhain's variant refers to cases in which cortical blindness predominates, with severe involvement of the occipital lobes. In panencephalopathic CJD, predominately reported from Japan, there is extensive degeneration of the cerebral white matter in addition to spongiform vacuolation of the grey matter (Mizutani, 1981). Amyotrophic variants of CJD have been described with prominent early muscle wasting. However, most cases of dementia with amyotrophy are not experimentally transmissible (Salazar et al., 1983) and their relationship with CJD is unclear. Most cases are probably variants of motor neurone disease with associated dementia. Amyotrophic features in CJD are usually seen in late disease when other features are well established. There are numerous individual case reports in the literature of other unusual presentations of CJD, mimicking many other neurological and psychiatric disorders.

79.2.2 Acquired prion diseases

While human prion diseases can be transmitted to experimental animals by inoculation, they are not contagious in humans. Documented case-to-case spread has only occurred by direct exposure to infected human tissues during ritual cannibalistic practices (kuru) or following accidental inoculation with prions during medical or surgical procedures (iatrogenic CJD or secondary vCJD).

79.2.2.1 KURU

Kuru reached epidemic proportions among a relatively isolated population (the Fore linguistic group and their neighbours with whom they intermarried) in the Eastern Highlands of Papua New Guinea. It predominantly affected women and children (of both sexes), with only 2 per cent of cases in adult males (Alpers, 1987) and was the most common cause of death among women. It had been the practice in these communities to consume dead relatives, as a mark of respect and mourning. Males over the age of 6–8 years participated little if at all in such mortuary feasts, which is thought to explain the different age and sex incidence. Preparation of the cadaver was performed by the women and children, such that other routes of exposure may also have been relevant. It is thought that the epidemic related to a single sporadic CJD case occurring in the region some decades earlier and such a source is supported by prion strain typing which showed prion strains isolated from kuru cases to be indistinguishable from those seen in sporadic CJD (Wadsworth et al., 2008). Epidemiological studies provided no evidence for vertical transmission, since most of the children born after 1956 (when cannibalism had effectively ceased) and all of those born after 1959 of mothers affected with or incubating kuru were unaffected (Alpers, 1987). From the age of the youngest affected patient, the shortest incubation period is estimated as 4.5 years, although may have been shorter, since time of infection was usually unknown. Over recent years, only a few cases have occurred, all in individuals born prior to the cessation of cannibalism and indicating that incubation periods can be 50 years or more (Collinge et al., 2006).

Onset of disease has ranged from age 5 to over 60 with a mean duration of 12 months (range 3 months to 3 years). The key clinical feature is progressive cerebellar ataxia. In sharp contrast to CJD, dementia is much less of a feature, even in the latter stages (Alpers, 1987). Kuru typically begins with prodromal symptoms consisting of headache, aching of limbs and joint pains, which can last for several months. Kuru was frequently self-diagnosed by patients at the earliest onset of unsteadiness in standing or walking, or of dysarthria or diplopia. Gait ataxia worsens and patients develop a broad-based gait, truncal instability and titubation. A coarse postural tremor is usually present and accentuated by movement; patients characteristically hold their hands together in the midline to suppress this. Standing with feet together reveals clawing of toes to maintain posture. Patients often become withdrawn at this stage and occasionally develop a severe reactive depression. Prodromal symptoms tend to disappear. Astasia and gait ataxia worsen and the patient requires a stick for walking. Intention tremor, dysmetria, hypotonia and dysdiadochokinesis develop. Strabismus, usually convergent, may occur particularly in children. Photophobia is common and there may be an abnormal cold sensitivity with shivering and piloerection even in a warm environment. Tendon reflexes are reduced or normal and plantar responses are flexor. Dysarthria usually occurs. As ataxia progresses, the patient passes from the first (ambulatory) stage to the second (sedentary) stage. At this stage, patients are able to sit unsupported, but cannot walk. Attempted walking with support leads to a high steppage, wide-based gait with reeling instability and flinging arm movements in an attempt to maintain posture. Hyperreflexia is seen, although plantar responses usually remain flexor with intact abdominal reflexes. Clonus is characteristically short-lived. Athetoid and choreiform movements and parkinsonian tremors may occur. There is no paralysis, although muscle power is reduced. Obesity is common at this stage, but may be present in early disease associated with bulimia. Characteristically, there is emotional lability and uncontrollable laughter, which has led to the disease being referred to as 'laughing death'. There is no sensory impairment. In sharp contrast to CJD, myoclonic jerking is rarely seen. EEG is usually normal or may show non-specific changes. When truncal ataxia reaches the point where the patient is unable to sit unsupported, the third or tertiary stage is reached. Hypotonia and hyporeflexia develop and the terminal state is marked by flaccid muscle weakness. Plantar responses remain flexor and abdominal reflexes intact. Progressive dysphagia occurs and patients become incontinent of urine and faeces. Inanition and emaciation develop. Transient conjugate eye signs and dementia may occur. Primitive reflexes develop in occasional cases. Brainstem involvement and both bulbar and pseudobulbar signs occur. Respiratory failure and bronchopneumonia eventually lead to death. This characteristic clinical syndrome has remained with recent long incubation period cases which showed the same progressive cerebellar syndrome previously described; however, two recent patients showed marked cognitive impairment well before preterminal stages, in contrast to earlier clinical descriptions (Collinge et al., 2008).

79.2.2.2 IATROGENIC CREUTZFELDT–JAKOB DISEASE

Iatrogenic transmission of CJD has occurred by inadvertent inoculation with human prions during medical procedures. Such iatrogenic routes include the use of inadequately sterilized neurosurgical instruments, dura mater and corneal grafting, and use of human cadaveric pituitary-derived growth hormone or gonadotrophin. Cases arising from intracerebral or optic inoculation manifest typically as classic CJD, with a rapidly progressive dementia, while those resulting from peripheral inoculation (pituitary-derived growth hormone exposure) typically present with a progressive cerebellar syndrome and are, in that respect, reminiscent of kuru. Unsurprisingly, the incubation period in intracerebral cases is short (19–46 months for dura mater grafts) compared to peripheral cases (typically 15 years or more). There is evidence for genetic susceptibility to iatrogenic CJD with an excess of codon 129 homozygotes; heterozygosity appears protective with a more prolonged incubation period (Collinge et al., 1991; Brandel et al., 2003).

Epidemiological studies have not shown association of CJD with occupations that may be exposed to human or animal prions, although individual cases in two histopathology technicians, a neuropathologist, and a neurosurgeon have been documented. Similarly, extensive epidemiological analysis in the United Kingdom has found no evidence that blood transfusion is a risk factor for sporadic CJD (Esmonde et al., 1993). However, it could not be assumed that the same picture would hold for vCJD as this is caused by a distinct prion strain (Collinge et al., 1996b) from those causing classical CJD and has a distinct pathogenesis with marked prion colonization of lymphoreticular tissues (Hill et al., 1999). Indeed, four cases of vCJD or vCJD prion infection have now been documented from among a

small cohort of patients known to have received blood from donors who went on to develop vCJD (Llewelyn et al., 2004; Peden et al., 2004; Wroe et al., 2006).

79.2.3 Variant CJD

In late 1995, two cases of sporadic CJD were reported in the UK in teenagers (Bateman et al., 1995; Britton et al., 1995). Only four cases of sporadic CJD had previously been recorded in teenagers; none in the UK. In addition, both were unusual in having kuru-type plaques, seen in only around 5 per cent of CJD cases. Soon afterwards, a third very young sporadic CJD case occurred (Tabrizi et al., 1996). These cases caused considerable concern and the possibility was raised that they were BSE-related. By March 1996, further extremely young onset cases were apparent and review of the histology of these cases showed a remarkably consistent and unique pattern. These cases were named 'new variant' CJD (Will et al., 1996). Review of neuropathological archives failed to demonstrate such cases. The statistical probability of such cases occurring by chance was vanishingly small and ascertainment bias seemed unlikely as an explanation. It was clear that a new risk factor for CJD had emerged and appeared to be specific to the UK. The UK Government Spongiform Encephalopathy Advisory Committee (SEAC) concluded that, while there was no direct evidence for a link with BSE, exposure to specified bovine offal (SBO) prior to the ban on its inclusion in human foodstuffs in 1989, was the most likely explanation. A case of vCJD was soon after reported in France (Chazot et al., 1996). Direct experimental evidence that vCJD is caused by BSE was provided by molecular analysis of human prion strains and transmission studies in transgenic and wild-type mice (see 79.1 Introduction and aetiology). While it is now clear that vCJD is the human counterpart of BSE, it is unclear why this particular age group should be affected and why none of these cases had a pattern of unusual occupational or dietary exposure to BSE. However, very little is known of which foodstuffs contained high-titre bovine offal. It is possible that certain foods containing particularly high titres were eaten predominately by younger people. An alternative is that young people are more susceptible to BSE following dietary exposure or that they have shorter incubation periods. It is important to appreciate that BSE-contaminated feed was fed to sheep, pigs and poultry and that although there is no evidence of natural transmission to these species, it would be prudent to remain open-minded about other dietary exposure to novel animal prions.

There are considerable concerns that extensive human infection may have resulted from the widespread dietary exposure to BSE prions. Cattle BSE was subsequently reported, albeit at much lower levels than in the UK, in most member states of the EU, Switzerland, United States, Canada and Japan. Fortunately, the number of recognized cases of vCJD (~170) in the UK has been small and the incidence has been falling for some years. Patients have been identified in a number of other countries notably France and including Ireland, Italy, United States, Canada and Hong Kong. However, the number of infected individuals is unknown. Human prion disease incubation periods, as evidenced by kuru, are known to span decades. While estimates based on mathematical modelling and clinically recognized vCJD suggest the total epidemic will be small (Ghani *et al.*, 2003), key uncertainties, notably with respect to major genetic effects on incubation period (Lloyd *et al.*, 2001), suggest the need for caution: such models cannot estimate the number of infected individuals and it is these that are most relevant to assessing risks of secondary transmission. Also, the possibility of subclinical carrier states of prion infection in humans, as recognized in several animal models, must also be considered (Hill *et al.*, 2000; Asante *et al.*, 2002). An attempt to estimate prevalence of vCJD prion infection in the UK by anonymous screen of archival, largely appendix tissue, necessarily using a method of unknown sensitivity, found three positives in around 12 000 samples and estimated prevalence of 237 per million (95 per cent confidence interval (CI) 49–692 per million) (Hilton *et al.*, 2004). This was followed by a larger UK study screening discarded tonsil tissue, which found no positives and suggested a lower prevalence, but which was still statistically consistent with the earlier study (Clewley *et al.*, 2009). Further UK studies to attempt to better estimate prevalence of infection are planned. The risk of secondary transmission via medical and surgical procedures is unquantifiable at present, but continues to cause considerable concern. As discussed above, vCJD appears transmissible by blood transfusion, also prions are known to be resistant to conventional sterilization and indeed iatrogenic transmission from neurosurgical instruments has long been documented (Bernoulli *et al.*, 1977). The wider tissue distribution of infectivity in vCJD (Wadsworth *et al.*, 2001), unknown prevalence of clinically silent infection, together with the recent experimental demonstration of the avid adherence to, and ease of transmission from, surgical steel surfaces (Flechsig *et al.*, 2001) highlight these concerns. Studies in transgenic mouse models of human susceptibility to BSE prion infection suggest that BSE may also induce propagation of a prion strain indistinguishable from the most common type of sporadic CJD (Asante *et al.*, 2002), in addition to that causing variant CJD. Other novel human prion disease phenotypes may be anticipated in alternative *PRNP* genotypes exposed to BSE prions (Hill *et al.*, 1997; Wadsworth *et al.*, 2004; Asante *et al.*, 2006).

Presentation of vCJD is with behavioural and psychiatric disturbances and, in some cases, sensory disturbance (Will *et al.*, 1996). Initial referral is often to a psychiatrist with depression, anxiety, withdrawal and behavioural change (Zeidler *et al.*, 1997). Suicidal ideation is, however, infrequent and response to antidepressants poor. Delusions, which are complex and unsustained, are common. Other features include emotional lability, aggression, insomnia and auditory and visual hallucinations. Dysaesthesiae, or pain in the limbs or face, which was persistent rather than intermittent and unrelated to anxiety levels is a frequent early feature, sometimes prompting referral to a rheumatologist. A minority of cases have early memory loss or gait ataxia, but in most such overt neurological features are not apparent until some months later (Zeidler *et al.*, 1997). Typically, a progressive cerebellar syndrome then develops with gait and limb ataxia followed with dementia and progression to akinetic mutism. Myoclonus is frequent and may be preceded by chorea. Cortical blindness develops in a minority of patients in late disease. Upgaze paresis, an uncommon feature of classical CJD, has been noted in some patients (Zeidler *et al.*, 1997). The age at onset has widened since the initial descriptions, but remains dominated by young adults (range 12–74 years; mean 28 years) and the clinical course is relatively prolonged when compared to typical sporadic CJD (9–35 months, median 14 months). The EEG is nearly always abnormal, most frequently showing generalized slow wave activity, but without the pseudoperiodic pattern seen in most sporadic CJD cases. Neuroimaging by CT is either normal or shows only mild atrophy. However, high signal in the posterior thalamus on T_2-weighted MRI is seen in the majority, but not all recognized cases (Zeidler *et al.*, 1997; Hill *et al.*, 1999) known as the 'pulvinar sign'. In one report of a blood transfusion acquired case of vCJD, imaging at the time of initial clinical presentation was negative for the pulvinar sign and was only positive when the patient was severely affected, suggesting that the pulvinar sign may be a late feature of vCJD (Wroe *et al.*, 2006). Recently, cases of sporadic CJD mimicking vCJD both clinically and on MRI have been described, with high signal from the pulvinar on FLAIR and diffusion-weighted imaging (Martindale *et al.*, 2003; Rossetti *et al.*, 2004; Summers *et al.*, 2004).

No *PRNP* mutations are present in vCJD (Collinge *et al.*, 1996a) and gene analysis is important to exclude pathogenic mutations, as inherited prion disease presents in this age group and a family history is not always apparent. The codon 129 genotype has uniformly been homozygous for methionine at *PRNP* codon 129 to date in clinical cases with the exception of a recent case thought clinically to be vCJD in an MV heterozygote; neither tonsil biopsy (see below) nor autopsy was performed (Kaski *et al.*, 2009).

Clear ante-mortem tissue-based diagnosis of vCJD can now be made by tonsil biopsy with detection of characteristic PrP immunostaining and PrP^{Sc} type (Collinge *et al.*, 1997; Hill *et al.*, 1999). Prion replication, in experimentally infected animals, is first detectable in the lymphoreticular system, considerably earlier than the onset of neurological symptoms. Importantly, PrP^{Sc} is only detectable in tonsil in vCJD, and not other forms of human prion disease studied. The PrP^{Sc} type detected on Western blot in vCJD tonsil has a characteristic pattern designated type 4t (Hill *et al.*, 1999). A positive tonsil biopsy obviates the need for brain biopsy which may otherwise be considered in such a clinical context to exclude alternative, potentially treatable diagnoses. To date, tonsil biopsy has proved 100 per cent specific and sensitive for vCJD diagnosis and is well tolerated.

The neuropathological appearances of vCJD are striking and consistent. In addition to widespread spongiform change, gliosis and neuronal loss (most severe in the basal ganglia and thalamus), there are abundant PrP amyloid plaques in cerebral and cerebellar cortex. These consisted of kuru-like, 'florid' (surrounded by spongiform vacuoles) and multicentric plaque types. The 'florid' plaques, seen previously only in scrapie, were a particularly unusual but highly consistent feature. There is abundant pericellular

PrP deposition in the cerebral and cerebellar cortex and, unusually, extensive PrP immunoreactivity in the molecular layer of the cerebellum.

In some respects, vCJD resembles kuru, in which behavioural changes and progressive ataxia predominate. Peripheral sensory disturbances are well recognized in the kuru prodrome and kuru plaques are seen in around 70 per cent of cases (and are especially abundant in younger kuru cases). That iatrogenic prion disease related to peripheral exposure to human prions has a more kuru-like than CJD-like clinical picture may well be relevant and would be consistent with a peripheral prion exposure in vCJD also.

This relatively stereotyped clinical presentation and neuropathology of vCJD contrasts sharply with sporadic CJD. This may be because vCJD is caused by a single prion strain and/or because a relatively homogeneous, genetically susceptible, subgroup with short incubation periods to BSE has been infected to date. However, it will be important to be alert to different clinical presentations.

Secondary vCJD following blood transfusion has now been recognized (see above under 79.2.3 Variant CJD). Prion colonization of tonsils was confirmed at autopsy suggesting tonsil biopsy can also be used for early diagnosis in at-risk individuals (Wroe et al., 2006).

79.2.4   Inherited prion diseases

79.2.4.1   GERSTMANN–STRÄUSSLER–SCHEINKER DISEASE

The first case was described by Gerstmann in 1928 and was followed by a more detailed report on seven other affected members of the same family in 1936 (Gerstmann et al., 1936). The classical presentation is a chronic cerebellar ataxia accompanied by pyramidal features, with dementia occurring later. The histological hallmark is the presence of multicentric amyloid plaques. Numerous GSS kindreds from several countries have now been demonstrated to have PRNP mutations. GSS is an autosomal dominant disorder which can be classified within the spectrum of inherited prion disease.

79.3   INHERITED PRION DISEASES

The identification of a pathogenic PRNP mutation in a patient with neurodegenerative disease allows both diagnosis of inherited prion disease and its subclassification according to mutation. Around 30 pathogenic mutations in PRNP are described and consist of two groups: (1) point mutations resulting in amino acid substitutions in PrP (or production of a stop codon); (2) insertions encoding additional integral copies of an octapeptide repeat present in a tandem array of five copies in the normal protein. An aetiological notation for these diseases (Collinge and Prusiner, 1992) is 'inherited prion disease (PrP mutation)'; for instance, inherited prion disease (PrP 144bp insertion) or inherited prion disease (PrP P102L). Phenotypic descriptions of some of these mutations follow.

79.3.1   Missense mutations

79.3.1.1   PRP P102L

First reported in 1989 in a UK and US family and now demonstrated in many kindreds worldwide. Progressive ataxia is the dominant clinical feature, with dementia and pyramidal features. However, marked variability both at the clinical and neuropathological level is apparent in some families (Hainfellner et al., 1995). A family with marked amyotrophic features has also been reported (Kretzschmar et al., 1992). Cases with early psychiatric involvement and dementia in the absence of prominent ataxia are also recognized (Webb et al., 2008). Neuropathological examination reveals PrP immunoreactive plaques in the majority of cases. Transmissibility to experimental animals has been demonstrated. Phenotypic variability is a major feature: median age of onset in 52 reported cases was 50 (range 25–70) and median duration of disease was four years (range 5 months–17 years) (Adam et al., 1982; Hainfellner et al., 1995; Barbanti et al., 1996; Tanaka et al., 1997; Young et al., 1997; Piccardo et al., 1998; Webb et al., 2008). Families with amyotrophic features (Kretzschmar et al., 1992) and patients with a rapidly deteriorating course are occasionally seen. The variable involvement of wild-type PrP in the disease process may contribute to phenotypic heterogeneity (Wadsworth et al., 2006).

79.3.1.2   PRP P105L

Initially reported in three Japanese families (Kitamoto et al., 1993) with a history of spastic paraparesis and dementia, this is now known not to be a universal feature (Yamada et al., 1999). Typical onset is around 38–50 years, with a duration of around five years. There was no periodic synchronous discharge on EEG, but MRI showed atrophy of the motor cortex. Neuropathological examination showed plaques in cerebral cortex (but not cerebellum) and neuronal loss, but no spongiosis. Neurofibrillary tangles were variably present.

79.3.1.3   PRP A117V

First described in a French family (Doh ura et al., 1989) and subsequently in a US family of German origin (Hsiao et al., 1991). Clinical features are presenile dementia with pyramidal signs, parkinsonism, pseudobulbar features and cerebellar signs. Neuropathologically, PrP immunoreactive plaques are usually present. This mutation has also been identified in a large family in the UK (Mallucci et al., 1999). The mutation is linked to valine at codon 129 and is modified by the genotype at this polymorphism (Webb et al., 2009).

79.3.1.4   PRP Y145STOP

This mutation was detected in a Japanese patient with a clinical diagnosis of AD. She developed memory disturbance at age 38, with a duration of illness of 21 years. Neuropathology revealed typical Alzheimer-like pathology without spongiform change (Kitamoto et al., 1993). Many amyloid plaques were seen in the cortex along with paired helical filaments. However, plaques were PrP immunoreactive. βA4 immunocytochemistry was negative. These clinicopathological findings emphasize the importance of *PRNP* analysis in the differential diagnosis of dementia. Other rare truncation mutations have been described (Jansen *et al.*, 2010).

79.3.1.5 PRP D178N

This mutation was first reported in Finnish families with a CJD-like illness (Goldfarb *et al.*, 1991c). Subsequently, the same mutation was identified in families with a condition known as 'fatal familial insomnia' (FFI). A large family case series was reported by Medori (Medori *et al.*, 1992b), who described an untreatable insomnia, dysautonomia and myoclonus. Histopathologically, selective degeneration of the anteroventral and dorsomedial thalamus was seen with variable cortical spongiform change and weak PrP immunocytochemical staining (Lugaresi *et al.*, 1986).

Goldfarb *et al.* (1992) established a haplotypic relationship between codon 129 and 178, whereby the mutation on a 129M chromosome leads to FFI, and the mutation on a 129V chromosome leads to familial CJD. However, there are pedigrees that segregate both the FFI and CJD phenotype (McLean *et al.*, 1997), and it has become increasingly recognized that autonomic and sleep disturbances may accompany other *PRNP* mutations, sometimes overtly (Chapman *et al.*, 1996). D178N patients reported to the CJD surveillance unit in Germany were less clinically distinct than the first reported FFI families in that none were clinically diagnosed as FFI due to an absence of obvious insomnia and no positive family history was obtained in four of nine (Zerr *et al.*, 1998). Pocchiari *et al.* (1998) noted that of patients presenting with overt sleep disturbance to a CJD unit, four of nine had sporadic CJD, one of nine had a V210I mutation, but none had D178N. Of 72 case reports, the median age of onset was 50 (range 20–72 years) and median duration of disease was 11 months (range 5 months–4 years) (Mead, 2006).

CJD-like codon 178 patient material has frequently transmitted to experimental animals, while the FFI type did not transmit to laboratory primates (Brown *et al.*, 1994). However, transmission of FFI to mice has been reported (Collinge *et al.*, 1995b; Tateishi *et al.*, 1995).

79.3.1.6 PRP F198S

PrP F198S has been described in a single large Indiana kindred. Neuropathologically, there are widespread Alzheimer-like neurofibrillary tangles in cortex and subcortical nuclei in addition to PrP amyloid plaques (Dlouhy *et al.*, 1992). There is a strong codon 129 effect with this mutation, in that individuals who were heterozygous at codon 129 had a later age of onset than homozygotes.

79.3.1.7 PRP E200K

This mutation is the most common worldwide. The typical clinical presentation is a rapidly progressive dementia with myoclonus and pyramidal, cerebellar or extrapyramidal signs,

very similar to sporadic CJD. Median age of onset of 112 reported cases (including some summarized data) was 58 with a median duration of seven months (Goldfarb *et al.*, 1991b; Bertoni *et al.*, 1992; Collinge *et al.*, 1993; Inoue *et al.*, 1994; Antoine *et al.*, 1996; Chapman *et al.*, 1996; Miyakawa *et al.*, 1998; Mitrova and Belay, 2002). Although the age of onset is slightly younger than that for sporadic CJD, Kahana and Zilber (1991) found no unique clinical features that distinguish E200K patients from those with sporadic CJD. The neuropathology is also similar to sporadic CJD, often with an absence of PrP plaques. However, in E200K patients with 129M homozygosity, a peculiar perpendicular stripe-like PrP deposit has been described in the molecular layer of the cerebellum (Jarius *et al.*, 2003). Transmission to experimental animals has been demonstrated.

There are multiple occurrences of the mutation in human history (Goldfarb *et al.*, 1991b; Lee *et al.*, 1999; Seno *et al.*, 2000). These events have led to distinct geographical clusters with a high incidence of disease, most notably of Libyan Jews, which had prompted investigators to make an epidemiological link with ingestion of sheep's brain, but also in Slovakia (Kovacs *et al.*, 2005). At least four separate mutational events are responsible for the global distribution of the mutation (Lee *et al.*, 1999). Clustering has led to the occurrence of a small number of individuals homozygous for the E200K mutation. These patients have a slightly earlier age of onset at 50, but overall, the homozygous and heterozygous phenotypes are similar, confirming the true dominance of this *PRNP* mutation (Simon *et al.*, 2000).

Expressivity of E200K is highly variable, manifesting in a wide range of age of onset of disease. Examination and genetic testing of unaffected relatives detect asymptomatic mutation carriers in old age, implying that penetrance is incomplete. The codon 129 polymorphism may determine these to a limited extent (Mitrova and Belay, 2002). The E219K polymorphism (approximately $655G > A$) may also modify phenotype (Seno *et al.*, 2000). Atypical clinical presentations include those with peripheral neuropathy (Chapman *et al.*, 1993; Antoine *et al.*, 1996), supranuclear gaze palsy (Bertoni *et al.*, 1983) and with sleep disturbance (Chapman *et al.*, 1996), the pathogenesis of these atypical presentations is not well understood.

79.3.1.8 PRP V210I

This mutation is the most common cause of inherited prion disease in Italy, cases being concentrated in the Campania and Apulia regions (Ladogana *et al.*, 2005). Presentation is typical of sporadic CJD, except that the mean age of onset is slightly younger (around age 55 years). There are likely to be multiple ancestral occurrences of the mutation as cases have been reported from Africa (Mouillet-Richard *et al.*, 1999), China (Furukawa *et al.*, 1996) and Japan (Shyu *et al.*, 1996).

79.3.2 Insertional mutations

The addition of a small number of octapeptide repeats in the N-terminal region of PrP may result in a CJD-like illness. As these mutations have not been described to segregate in families and have been found coincidentally or in population screens, it is difficult to distinguish whether they are rare polymorphisms or incompletely penetrant IPD mutations.

1-OPRI was initially reported in a single French individual, the patient presented at age 73 with dizziness followed by visual agnosia, cerebellar ataxia and intellectual impairment with diffuse periodic activity on EEG. Myoclonus and cortical blindness developed and he progressed to akinetic mutism. Disease duration was four months. The patient's father had died at age 70 from an undiagnosed neurological disorder. No neuropathological information is available (Laplanche et al., 1995). Subsequently, two further patients with a CJD-like illness, which in one was confirmed at autopsy, have been associated with a 1-OPRI (Pietrini et al., 2003).

2-OPRI has been reported in a US family (Goldfarb et al., 1993), the proband had a CJD-like phenotype both clinically and pathologically with a typical EEG and an age at onset of 58 years. However, the proband's mother had onset of cognitive decline at age 75 with a slow progression to a severe dementia over 13 years. The maternal grandfather had a similar late onset (at age 80) and slow progressive cognitive decline over 15 years. A second report of a Dutch patient with a distinct 2-OPRI was diagnosed with presenile dementia and ataxia (Van Harten et al., 2000). MRI was atypical of prion disease with extensive white matter signal change.

3-OPRI has only recently been detected. It was first found in a screen of healthy Chinese (Yu et al., 2004). Subsequently, a different 3-OPRI mutation was reported in a patient with a clinical and pathological phenotype typical of CJD.

79.3.2.1   PRP 96-BP INSERTION (FOUR EXTRA REPEATS)

First reported in an individual who died of hepatic cirrhosis at the age of 63 (Goldfarb et al., 1991a) with no history of neurological illness and it is unclear if this finding indicates incomplete penetrance of this mutation. Two separate four octapeptide repeat insertional mutations have been reported in affected individuals, each differing in the DNA sequence from the original four repeat insertion, although all three of the mutations encode the same PrP. Laplanche et al. reported a 96-bp insertion in an 82-year-old French woman who developed progressive depression and behavioural changes (Laplanche et al., 1995). She progressed over three months to akinetic mutism with pyramidal signs and myoclonus. EEG showed pseudoperiodic complexes. Duration of illness was four months. There was no known family history of neurological illness. Another 96-bp insertional mutation was seen in a patient with classical clinical and pathological features of CJD with the exception of the unusual finding of pronounced PrP immunoreactivity in the molecular layer of the cerebellum (Campbell et al., 1996).

79.3.2.2   PRP 120-BP INSERTION (FIVE EXTRA REPEATS)

Several families have now been reported (Mead et al., 2007). The disease onset may vary from the fourth to the seventh decade. Disease duration is also variable with some clinical courses similar to CJD, other patients have survived decades with the disease. Clinical phenotype is dominated by apraxia and dementia, with variable additional neurological signs. Codon 129 modifies the age of onset.

79.3.2.3   PRP 144-BP INSERTION (SIX EXTRA REPEATS)

This mutation has some historical importance as it was the first described PRNP mutation, in a small UK family (Owen et al., 1989). Genealogical work demonstrated a common ancestor of this small family and a larger pedigree with over 50 affected individuals (Poulter et al., 1992). In 2006, this pedigree was updated and now comprises over 86 affected individuals and around 100 at risk of disease affording a detailed analysis of phenotype and its determinants (Mead et al., 2006).

Clinical and pathological features of the UK pedigree are highly variable. Cortical dementia, often with apraxia, is the core feature with additional neurological signs, including cerebellar ataxia, pyramidal, extrapyramidal, myoclonus, chorea and seizures in declining order of frequency. Age of onset ranges from the third to the sixth decade, and duration of disease ranges from an aggressive condition mistaken for sporadic CJD to a slowly progressive neurodegenerative disease over more than two decades. A prominent clinical sign is apraxia. The polymorphism at PRNP codon 129 accounts for a proportion of this variability. Insert mutation carriers associated with heterozygosity at codon 129 have a delayed age of onset by around a decade compared with patients homozygous at codon 129 (Poulter et al., 1992), accounting for 41 per cent of the variance in age of onset. 6-OPRI has been transmitted to laboratory mice with incubation times comparable with that expected of sporadic CJD (Mead et al., 2006). Analysis of PrP^{Sc}-type indicates a molecular heterogeneity within this single pedigree, although given a small sample no conclusion can be made about whether this has an impact on phenotypic heterogeneity.

The existence of a premorbid personality disorder in prion disease was first reported in this pedigree, characterized by criminality, aggression, delinquency and hypersexuality (Collinge et al., 1992). Other clinicians have ascribed psychiatric symptoms in IPD to the early stages of a neurodegenerative disease (Laplanche et al., 1999; Rodriguez et al., 2005), although the abnormalities described by Collinge dated from early childhood in some cases. The presence of personality disorders with such an early onset may indicate a role for the normal function of PrP in the healthy brain that is abrogated by certain mutations.

79.3.2.4   PRP 168-BP INSERTION (SEVEN EXTRA REPEATS)

PrP 168-bp insertion was reported in a US family. Clinical features were mood change, abnormal behaviour, confusion, aphasia, cerebellar signs, involuntary movements, rigidity, dementia and myoclonus. The age at onset was 23–35 years and the clinical duration between 10 and over 13 years. EEG atypical. Neuropathology showed spongiform change, neuronal loss and gliosis to varying degrees (Goldfarb et al., 1991a). Experimental transmission has been demonstrated.

Another three mutations have since been described with a similar phenotype (Lewis *et al.*, 2003).

79.3.2.5 PRP 192-BP INSERTION (EIGHT EXTRA REPEATS)

Originally reported in a French family with clinical features which include abnormal behaviour, cerebellar signs, mutism, pyramidal signs, myoclonus, tremor, intellectual slowing and seizures. The disease duration ranged from three months to 13 years. The EEG findings include diffuse slowing, slow wave burst suppression and periodic triphasic complexes. Neuropathological examination revealed spongiform change, neuronal loss, gliosis and multicentric plaques in the cerebellum (Goldfarb *et al.*, 1991a; Guiroy *et al.*, 1993). Experimental transmission has been reported. Two other families (van Gool *et al.*, 1995; Laplanche *et al.*, 1999) with prominent psychological or psychiatric changes are now known.

79.3.2.6 PRP 216-BP INSERTION (NINE EXTRA REPEATS)

PrP 216-bp insertion was first reported in a single case from the UK (Owen *et al.*, 1992). The clinical onset was around 54 years with falls, axial rigidity, myoclonic jerks and progressive dementia (Tagliavini *et al.*, 1993). Although there was no clear family history of a similar illness, the mother had died at age 53 with a cerebrovascular event. The maternal grandmother died at age 79 with senile dementia. EEG was atypical. Neuropathological examination showed no spongiform encephalopathy, but marked deposition of plaques, which in the cerebellum and the basal ganglia showed immunoreactivity with PrP antisera (Duchen *et al.*, 1993). In the hippocampus, there were neuritic plaques positive for both β-amyloid protein and tau. Some neurofibrillary tangles were also seen. In some respects, therefore, the pathology resembled Alzheimer's disease. Experimental transmission studies have not been attempted. A second, German, family with a 9-octapeptide repeat insertion of different sequence has also been reported (Krasemann *et al.*, 1995).

79.3.2.7 PRP 48-BP DELETION

While deletion of a single octapeptide repeat element is a well-recognized polymorphic variant of human PrP (with a frequency of around 1 per cent in the UK population) which does not appear to be associated with disease (Palmer *et al.*, 1993), a two repeat deletion has been described in two individuals with CJD (Beck *et al.*, 2001; Capellari *et al.*, 2002).

79.4 GENETIC COUNSELLING AND PRESYMPTOMATIC TESTING

PRNP analysis allows unequivocal diagnosis in patients with inherited prion disease. This has also allowed presymptomatic testing of unaffected, but at-risk, family members, as well as antenatal testing following appropriate genetic counselling (Collinge *et al.*, 1991). The effect of codon 129 genotype on the age of onset of disease associated with some mutations also means it is possible to determine within a family whether a carrier of a mutation will have an early or late onset of disease. Most of the well-recognized pathogenic *PRNP* mutations appear fully penetrant, but experience with some mutations is extremely limited. In families with the E200K mutation, there are examples of elderly unaffected gene carriers who appear to have escaped the disease.

79.5 SECONDARY PROPHYLAXIS AFTER ACCIDENTAL EXPOSURE

Certain occupational groups are at risk of exposure to human prions, for instance neurosurgeons and other operating theatre staff, pathologists and morticians, histology technicians, as well as an increasing number of laboratory workers. Because of the prolonged incubation periods to prions following administration to sites other than the central nervous system (CNS), which is associated with clinically silent prion replication in the lymphoreticular tissue, treatments inhibiting prion replication in lymphoid organs may represent a viable strategy for rational secondary prophylaxis after accidental exposure. A preliminary suggested regimen is a short course of immunosuppression with oral corticosteroids in individuals with significant accidental exposure to human prions (Aguzzi and Collinge, 1997). Urgent surgical excision of the inoculum might also be considered in exceptional circumstances. There is hope that progress in the understanding of the peripheral pathogenesis will identify the precise cell types and molecules involved in colonization of the organism by prions. The ultimate goal will be to target the rate-limiting steps in prion spread with much more focused pharmacological approaches, which may eventually prove useful in preventing disease even after iatrogenic and alimentary exposure (Collinge, 2005). A proof of principle of immunoprophylaxis by passive immunization using anti-PrP monoclonals has already been demonstrated in mouse models (White *et al.*, 2003).

79.6 PROGNOSIS AND POSSIBLE THERAPIES

All known forms of prion diseases are invariably fatal following a relentlessly progressive course and there is no effective therapy. The duration of illness in sporadic patients is very short with a mean duration of three to four months. However, in some of the inherited cases the duration can be 20 years or more (Collinge *et al.*, 1990). Symptomatic treatment of various neurological and psychiatric features can be provided and a range of supportive services are likely to be required in the later stages of the disease (see UK National Prion Clinic website for factsheets and specialist advice: www.nationalprionclinic.org). While no effective treatment for the human disease is known, several drugs have or are currently being studied in patients. In the UK, a clinical trial protocol for evaluation of potential CJD therapeutics has been developed and the MRC PRION-1 trial of the drug quinacrine completed (Collinge *et al.*, 2009). This did not show evidence of benefit. Some patients in the UK and elsewhere have been treated with intracerebroventricular infusion of pentosan polysulphate, although not as part of a controlled trial. Again, there has been no clear evidence of overall benefit, although some treated patients have lived longer than would have been expected (Bone *et al.*, 2008). Clearly, advances towards early diagnosis, to allow therapies to be used prior to extensive neuronal loss, will be important. While the challenge of interrupting this aggressive, non-focal and uniformly fatal neurodegenerative process is daunting, major advances are being made in understanding the basic processes of prion propagation and neurotoxicity. Considerable optimism is provided by the finding that onset of clinical disease in established neuroinvasive prion infection in a mouse model can be halted and early pathology and behavioural changes reversed (Mallucci *et al.*, 2003; Mallucci *et al.*, 2007). A number of approaches to rational therapeutics are being studied in experimental models. Anti-PrP antibodies have been shown to block progression of peripheral prion propagation in mouse models and humanized versions of these antibodies are being developed for potential use for both post-exposure prophylaxis or during established clinical disease. In the longer term, the development of drugs which bind to PrP^C to inhibit its conversion might be able to block prion propagation and allow natural clearance mechanisms to eradicate remaining PrP^{Sc} and so cure prion infection (Nicoll and Collinge, 2009).

REFERENCES

Adam J, Crow TJ, Duchen LW *et al.* (1982) Familial cerebral amyloidosis and spongiform encephalopathy. *Journal of Neurology, Neurosurgery, and Psychiatry* 45: 37–45.

Alpers MP. (1987) Epidemiology and clinical aspects of kuru, in prions. In: Prusiner SB, McKinley MP (eds). *Novel infectious pathogens causing scrapie and Creutzfeldt–Jakob disease.* San Diego: Academic Press, 451–65.

Antoine JC, Laplanche JL, Mosnier JF *et al.* (1996) Demyelinating peripheral neuropathy with Creutzfeldt–Jakob disease and mutation at codon 200 of the prion protein gene. *Neurology* 46: 1123–7.

Asante E, Linehan J, Desbruslais M *et al.* (2002) BSE prions propagate as either variant CJD-like or sporadic CJD-like prion strains in transgenic mice expressing human prion protein. *EMBO Journal* 21: 6358–66.

Asante E, Linehan J, Gowland I *et al.* (2006) Dissociation of pathological and molecular phenotype of variant Creutzfeldt-Jakob disease in transgenic human prion protein 129 heterozygous mice. *Proceedings of the National Academy of the Sciences of the United States of America* 103: 10759–64.

Baker HE, Poulter M, Crow TJ *et al.* (1991) Amino acid polymorphism in human prion protein and age at death in inherited prion disease (letter). *Lancet* 337: 1286.

Baker HF, Ridley RM, Duchen LW *et al.* (1994) Induction of β(A4)-amyloid in primates by injection of Alzheimer's disease brain homogenate: Comparison with transmission of spongiform encephalopathy. *Molecular Neurobiology* 8: 25–39.

Barbanti P, Fabbrini G, Salvatore M *et al.* (1996) Polymorphism at codon 129 or codon 219 of PRNP and clinical heterogeneity in a previously unreported family with Gerstmann–Straussler–Scheinker disease (PrP-P102L mutation). *Neurology* 47: 734–41.

Bateman D, Hilton D, Love S *et al.* (1995) Sporadic Creutzfeldt–Jakob disease in a 18-year-old in the UK. *Lancet* 346: 1155–6.

Beck E, Daniel PM. (1987) Neuropathology of transmissible spongiform encephalopathies. In: Prusiner SB, McKinley MP (eds). *Prions: Novel infectious pathogens causing scrapie and Creutzfeldt–Jakob disease.* San Diego: Academic Press, 331–85.

Beck J, Mead S, Campbell TA *et al.* (2001) Two-octapeptide repeat deletion of prion protein associated with rapidly progressive dementia. *Neurology* 57: 354–6.

Bernoulli C, Siegfried J, Baumgartner G *et al.* (1977) Danger of accidental person-to-person transmission of Creutzfeldt–Jakob disease by surgery (letter). *Lancet* 1: 478–9.

Bertoni JM, Label LS, Sackelleres JC, Hicks SP. (1983) Supranuclear gaze palsy in familial Creutzfeldt–Jakob disease. *Archives of Neurology* 40: 618–22.

Bertoni JM, Brown P, Goldfarb LG *et al.* (1992) Familial Creutzfeldt–Jakob disease (codon 200 mutation) with supranuclear palsy. *Journal of the American Medical Association* 268: 2413–5.

Bone I, Belton L, Walker AS, Darbyshire J. (2008) Intraventricular pentosan polysulphate in human prion disease: An observational study in the UK. *European Journal of Neurology* 15: 458–64.

Brandel JP, Preece M, Brown P *et al.* (2003) Distribution of codon 129 genotype in human growth hormone-treated CJD patients in France and the UK. *Lancet* 362: 128–30.

Britton TC, Al-Sarraj S, Shaw C *et al.* (1995) Sporadic Creutzfeldt–Jakob disease in a 16-year-old in the UK. *Lancet* 346: 1155.

Brown P, Rodgers-Johnson P, Cathala F *et al.* (1984) Creutzfeldt–Jakob disease of long duration: clinicopathological characteristics, transmissibility, and differential diagnosis. *Annals of Neurology* 16: 295–304.

Brown P, Cathala F, Raubertas RF *et al.* (1987) The epidemiology of Creutzfeldt–Jakob disease: conclusion of a 15-year investigation in France and review of the world literature. *Neurology* 37: 895–904.

Brown P, Gibbs Jr CJ, Rodgers Johnson P *et al.* (1994) Human spongiform encephalopathy: the National Institutes of Health series of 300 cases of experimentally transmitted disease. *Annals of Neurology* 35: 513–29.

Bruce M, Chree A, McConnell I *et al.* (1994) Transmission of bovine spongiform encephalopathy and scrapie to mice: Strain variation and the species barrier. *Philosophical Transactions of the Royal Society of London. B: Biological Sciences* 343: 405–11.

Bruce ME, Will RG, Ironside JW *et al.* (1997) Transmissions to mice indicate that 'new variant' CJD is caused by the BSE agent. *Nature* 389: 498–501.

Budka H, Aguzzi A, Brown P et al. (1995) Neuropathological diagnostic criteria for Creutzfeldt–Jakob disease (CJD) and other human spongiform encephalopathies (Prion diseases). *Brain Pathology* 5: 459–66.

Cambier DM, Kantarci K, Worrell GA et al. (2003) Lateralized and focal clinical, EEG, and FLAIR MRI abnormalities in Creutzfeldt–Jakob disease. *Clinical Neurophysiology* 114: 1724–8.

Campbell TA, Palmer MS, Will RG et al. (1996) A prion disease with a novel 96-base pair insertional mutation in the prion protein gene. *Neurology* 46: 761–6.

Capellari S, Parchi P, Wolff BD et al. (2002) Creutzfeldt–Jakob disease associated with a deletion of two repeats in the prion protein gene. *Neurology* 59: 1628–30.

Chapman J, Brown P, Goldfarb LG et al. (1993) Clinical heterogeneity and unusual presentations of Creutzfeldt–Jakob disease in Jewish patients with the PRNP codon 200 mutation. *Journal of Neurology, Neurosurgery and Psychiatry* 56: 1109–12.

Chapman J, Arlazoroff A, Goldfarb LG et al. (1996) Fatal insomnia in a case of familial Creutzfeldt–Jakob disease with the codon 200^{Lys} mutation. *Neurology* 46: 758–61.

Chazot G, Broussolle E, Lapras CI et al. (1996) New variant of Creutzfeldt–Jakob disease in a 26-year-old French man. *Lancet* 347: 1181.

Clewley JP, Kelly CM, Andrews N et al. (2009) Prevalence of disease related prion protein in anonymous tonsil specimens in Britain: cross sectional opportunistic survey. *British Medical Journal* 338: b1442.

Collinge J. (1996) New diagnostic tests for prion diseases. *New England Journal of Medicine* 335: 963–5.

Collinge J. (1999) Variant Creutzfeldt–Jakob disease. *Lancet* 354: 317–23.

Collinge J. (2001) Prion diseases of humans and animals: their causes and molecular basis. *Annual Review of Neuroscience* 24: 519–50.

Collinge J. (2005) Molecular neurology of prion disease. *Journal of Neurology, Neurosurgery and Psychiatry* 76: 906–19.

Collinge J, Clarke A. (2007) A general model of prion strains and their pathogenicity. *Science* 318: 930–6.

Collinge J, Prusiner SB. (1992) Terminology of prion disease. In: Prusiner SB, Collinge J, Powell J et al. (eds). *Prion diseases of humans and animals*, 1st edn. London: Ellis Horwood, 5–12.

Collinge J, Owen F, Poulter M et al. (1990) Prion dementia without characteristic pathology. *Lancet* 336: 7–9.

Collinge J, Palmer MS, Dryden AJ. (1991) Genetic predisposition to iatrogenic Creutzfeldt–Jakob disease. *Lancet* 337: 1441–2.

Collinge J, Poulter M, Davis MB et al. (1991) Presymptomatic detection or exclusion of prion protein gene defects in families with inherited prion diseases. *American Journal of Human Genetics* 49: 1351–4.

Collinge J, Brown J, Hardy J et al. (1992) Inherited prion disease with 144 base pair gene insertion: II. Clinical and pathological features. *Brain* 115: 687–710.

Collinge J, Palmer MS, Campbell TA et al. (1993) Inherited prion disease (PrP lysine 200) in Britain: two case reports. *British Medical Journal* 306: 301–2.

Collinge J, Palmer MS, Sidle KC et al. (1995a) Unaltered susceptibility to BSE in transgenic mice expressing human prion protein. *Nature* 378: 779–83.

Collinge J, Palmer MS, Sidle KCL et al. (1995b) Transmission of fatal familial insomnia to laboratory animals. *Lancet* 346: 569–70.

Collinge J, Beck J, Campbell T et al. (1996a) Prion protein gene analysis in new variant cases of Creutzfeldt–Jakob disease. *Lancet* 348: 56.

Collinge J, Sidle KCL, Meads J et al. (1996b) Molecular analysis of prion strain variation and the aetiology of 'new variant' CJD. *Nature* 383: 685–90.

Collinge J, Whitfield J, McKintosh E et al. (2006) Kuru in the 21st century – an acquired human prion disease with very long incubation periods. *Lancet* 367: 2068–74.

Collinge J, Hill AF, Ironside J, Zeidler M. (1997) Diagnosis of new variant Creutzfeldt–Jakob disease by tonsil biopsy – authors' reply to Arya and Evans. *Lancet* 349: 1322–3.

Collinge J, Whitfield J, McKintosh E et al. (2008) A clinical study of kuru patients with long incubation periods at the end of the epidemic in Papua New Guinea. *Philosophical Transactions of the Royal Society of London. B: Biological Sciences* 363: 3725–39.

Collinge J, Gorham M, Hudson F et al. (2009) Safety and efficacy of quinacrine in human prion disease (PRION-1 study): a patient-preference trial. *Lancet Neurology* 8: 334–44.

Collins S, Law MG, Fletcher A et al. (1999) Surgical treatment and risk of sporadic Creutzfeldt–Jakob disease: a case–control study. *Lancet* 353: 693–7.

Cuillé J, Chelle PL. (1936) La maladie dite tremblante du mouton est-elle inocuable? *Compte Rendu de l'Academie des Sciences* 203: 1552–4.

Dlouhy SR, Hsiao K, Farlow MR et al. (1992) Linkage of the Indiana kindred of Gerstmann–Sträussler–Scheinker disease to the prion protein gene. *Nature Genetics* 1: 64–7.

Doh ura K, Tateishi J, Sasaki H et al. (1989) Pro-leu change at position 102 of prion protein is the most common but not the sole mutation related to Gerstmann–Straussler syndrome. *Biochemical and Biophysical Research Communications* 163: 974–9.

Duchen LW, Poulter M, Harding AE. (1993) Dementia associated with a 216 base pair insertion in the prion protein gene. Clinical and neuropathological features. *Brain* 116: 555–67.

Esmonde TFG, Will RG, Slattery JM et al. (1993) Creutzfeldt–Jakob disease and blood transfusion. *Lancet* 341: 205–7.

Flechsig E, Hegyi I, Enari M et al. (2001) Transmission of scrapie by steel-surface-bound prions. *Molecular Medicine* 7: 679–84.

Fukushima R, Shiga Y, Nakamura M et al. (2004) MRI characteristics of sporadic CJD with valine homozygosity at codon 129 of the prion protein gene and PrP(Sc) type 2 in Japan. *Journal of Neurology, Neurosurgery and Psychiatry* 75: 485–7.

Furukawa H, Kitamoto T, Hashiguchi H, Tateishi J. (1996) A Japanese case of Creutzfeldt–Jakob disease with a point mutation in the prion protein gene at codon 210. *Journal of the Neurological Sciences* 141: 120–2.

Gajdusek DC. (1988) Transmissible and non-transmissible amyloidoses: autocatalytic post-translational conversion of host precursor proteins to beta-pleated sheet configurations. *Journal of Neuroimmunology* **20**: 95–110.

Gajdusek DC, Gibbs Jr CJ, Alpers MP. (1966) Experimental transmission of a kuru-like syndrome to chimpanzees. *Nature* **209**: 794–6.

Gerstmann J, Sträussler E, Scheinker I. (1936) Über eine eigenartige hereditär-familiäre Erkrankung des Zentralnervensystems. Zugleich ein Beitrag zur Frage des vorzeitigen lakalen Alterns. *Zeitschrift für Neurologie* **154**: 736–62.

Ghani AC, Donnelly CA, Ferguson NM, Anderson RM. (2003) Updated projections of future vCJD deaths in the UK. *BMC Infectious Diseases* **3**: 4.

Gibbs Jr CJ, Gajdusek DC, Asher DM et al. (1968) Creutzfeldt–Jakob disease (spongiform encephalopathy): transmission to the chimpanzee. *Science* **161**: 388–9.

Goldfarb LG, Brown P, McCombie WR et al. (1991a) Transmissible familial Creutzfeldt–Jakob disease associated with five, seven, and eight extra octapeptide coding repeats in the PRNP gene. *Proceedings of the National Academy of Sciences of the United States of America* **88**: 10926–30.

Goldfarb LG, Brown P, Mitrova E et al. (1991b) Creutzfeldt–Jacob disease associated with the PRNP codon 200Lys mutation: an analysis of 45 families. *European Journal of Epidemioloigy* **7**: 477–86.

Goldfarb LG, Haltia M, Brown P et al. (1991c) New mutation in scrapie amyloid precursor gene (at codon 178) in Finnish Creutzfeldt–Jakob kindred. *Lancet* **337**: 425.

Goldfarb LG, Petersen RB, Tabaton M et al. (1992) Fatal familial insomnia and familial Creutzfeldt–Jakob disease: disease phenotype determined by a DNA polymorphism. *Science* **258**: 806–8.

Goldfarb LG, Brown P, Little BW et al. (1993) A new (two-repeat) octapeptide coding insert mutation in Creutzfeldt–Jakob disease. *Neurology* **43**: 2392–4.

Gomori AJ, Partnow MJ, Horoupian DS, Hirano A. (1973) The ataxic form of Creutzfeldt–Jakob disease. *Archives of Neurology* **29**: 318–23.

Griffith JS. (1967) Self-replication and scrapie. *Nature* **215**: 1043–4.

Guiroy DC, Marsh RF, Yanagihara R, Gajdusek DC. (1993) Immunolocalization of scrapie amyloid in non-congophilic, non-birefringent deposits in golden Syrian hamsters with experimental transmissible mink encephalopathy. *Neuroscience Letters* **155**: 112–5.

Hadlow WJ. (1959) Scrapie and kuru. *Lancet* **ii**: 289–90.

Hainfellner JA, Brantner-Inthaler S, Cervenáková L et al. (1995) The original Gerstmann–Straussler–Scheinker family of Austria: Divergent clinicopathological phenotypes but constant PrP genotype. *Brain Pathology* **5**: 201–11.

Hamaguchi T, Kitamoto T, Sato T et al. (2005) Clinical diagnosis of MM2-type sporadic Creutzfeldt–Jakob disease. *Neurology* **64**: 643–8.

Hill AF, Collinge J. (2003) Subclinical prion infection. *Trends in Microbiology* **11**: 578–84.

Hill AF, Desbruslais M, Joiner S et al. (1997) The same prion strain causes vCJD and BSE. *Nature* **389**: 448–50.

Hill AF, Butterworth RJ, Joiner S et al. (1999) Investigation of variant Creutzfeldt–Jakob disease and other human prion diseases with tonsil biopsy samples. *Lancet* **353**: 183–9.

Hill AF, Joiner S, Linehan J et al. (2000) Species barrier independent prion replication in apparently resistant species. *Proceedings of the National Academy of the Sciences of the United States of America* **97**: 10248–53.

Hill AF, Joiner S, Wadsworth JD et al. (2003) Molecular classification of sporadic Creutzfeldt–Jakob disease. *Brain* **126**: 1333–46.

Hsiao K, Baker HF, Crow TJ et al. (1989) Linkage of a prion protein missense variant to Gerstmann–Straussler syndrome. *Nature* **338**: 342–5.

Hsiao K, Dlouhy SR, Farlow MR et al. (1992) Mutant prion proteins in Gerstmann–Sträussler–Sheinker disease with neurofibrillary tangles. *Nature Genetics* **1**: 68–71.

Hsiao KK, Cass C, Schellenberg GD et al. (1991) A prion protein variant in a family with the telencephalic form of Gerstmann–Straussler–Scheinker syndrome. *Neurology* **41**: 681–4.

Inoue I, Kitamoto T, Doh-ura K et al. (1994) Japanese family with Creutzfeldt–Jakob disease with codon 200 point mutation of the prion protein gene. *Neurology* **44**: 299–301.

Jackson GS, Hosszu LLP, Power A et al. (1999) Reversible conversion of monomeric human prion protein between native and fibrilogenic conformations. *Science* **283**: 1935–7.

Jansen C, Parchi P, Capellari S et al. (2010) Prion protein amyloidosis with divergent phenotype associated with two novel nonsense mutations in PRNP. *Acta Neuropathology* **119**: 189–97.

Jarius C, Kovacs GG, Belay G et al. (2003) Distinctive cerebellar immunoreactivity for the prion protein in familial (E200K) Creutzfeldt–Jakob disease. *Acta Neuropathologica* **105**: 449–54.

Jimi T, Wakayama Y, Shibuya S et al. (1992) High levels of nervous system-specific proteins in cerebrospinal fluid in patients with early stage Creutzfeldt–Jakob disease. *Clinica Chimica Acta* **211**: 37–46.

Kahana E, Zilber N. (1991) Do Creutzfeldt–Jakob disease patients of Jewish Libyan origin have unique clinical features? *Neurology* **41**: 1390–2.

Kaski D, Mead S, Hyare H et al. (2009) Variant CJD in an individual heterozygous for PRNP codon 129. *Lancet* **374**: 2128.

Kitamoto T, Ohta M, Doh-ura K et al. (1993) Novel missense variants of prion protein in Creutzfeldt–Jakob disease or Gerstmann–Straussler syndrome. *Biochemica and Biophysica Research Communications* **191**: 709–14.

Kovacs GG, Puopolo M, Ladogana A et al. (2005) Genetic prion disease: the EUROCJD experience. *Human Genetics* **118**: 166–74.

Krasemann S, Zerr I, Weber T et al. (1995) Prion disease associated with a novel nine octapeptide repeat insertion in the PRNP gene. *Molecular Brain Research* **34**: 173–6.

Kretzschmar HA, Kufer P, Riethmuller G et al. (1992) Prion protein mutation at codon 102 in an Italian family with Gerstmann–Straussler–Scheinker syndrome. *Neurology* **42**: 809–10.

Ladogana A, Puopolo M, Poleggi A et al. (2005) High incidence of genetic human transmissible spongiform encephalopathies in Italy. Neurology 64: 1592–7.

Laplanche JL, Delasnerie Laupretre N, Brandel JP et al. (1995) Two novel insertions in the prion protein gene in patients with late-onset dementia. Human Molecular Genetics 4: 1109–11.

Laplanche JL, El Hachimi KH, Durieux I et al. (1999) Prominent psychiatric features and early onset in an inherited prion disease with a new insertional mutation in the prion protein gene. Brain 122: 2375–86.

Lee HS, Sambuughin N, Cervenakova L et al. (1999) Ancestral origins and worldwide distribution of the PRNP 200K mutation causing familial Creutzfeldt–Jakob disease. American Journal of Human Genetics 64: 1063–70.

Lewis V, Collins S, Hill AF et al. (2003) Novel prion protein insert mutation associated with prolonged neurodegenerative illness. Neurology 60: 1620–4.

Li JY, Englund E, Holton JL et al. (2008) Lewy bodies in grafted neurons in subjects with Parkinson's disease suggest host-to-graft disease propagation. Nature Medicine 14: 501–3.

Llewelyn CA, Hewitt PE, Knight RS et al. (2004) Possible transmission of variant Creutzfeldt–Jakob disease by blood transfusion. Lancet 363: 417–21.

Lloyd S, Onwuazor ON, Beck J et al. (2001) Identification of multiple quantitative trait loci linked to prion disease incubation period in mice. Proceedings of the National Academy of Sciences of the United States of America 98: 6279–83.

Lugaresi E, Medori R, Baruzzi PM et al. (1986) Fatal familial insomnia and dysautonomia, with selective degeneration of thalamic nuclei. New England Journal of Medicine 315: 997–1003.

McGowan JP. (1922) Scrapie in sheep. Scottish Journal of Agriculture 5: 365–75.

McLean CA, Storey E, Gardner RJM et al. (1997) The D178N (cis-129M) 'fatal familial insomnia' mutation associated with diverse clinicopathologic phenotypes in an Australian kindred. Neurology 49: 552–8.

Mahillo-Fernandez I, Pedro-Cuesta J, Bleda MJ et al. (2008) Surgery and risk of sporadic Creutzfeldt–Jakob disease in Denmark and Sweden: Registry-based case-control studies. Neuroepidemiology 31: 229–40.

Mallucci G, Campbell TA, Dickinson A et al. (1999) Inherited prion disease with an alanine to valine mutation at codon 117 in the prion protein gene. Brain 122: 1823–37.

Mallucci G, Dickinson A, Linehan J et al. (2003) Depleting neuronal PrP in prion infection prevents disease and reverses spongiosis. Science 302: 871–4.

Mallucci G, White MD, Farmer M et al. (2007) Targeting cellular prion protein reverses early cognitive deficits and neurophysiological dysfunction in prion-infected mice. Neuron 53: 325–35.

Martindale J, Geschwind MD, De Armond S et al. (2003) Sporadic Creutzfeldt–Jakob disease mimicking variant Creutzfeldt–Jakob disease. Archives of Neurology 60: 767–70.

Mead S. (2006) Prion disease genetics. European Journal of Human Genetics 14: 273–81.

Mead S, Poulter M, Beck J et al. (2006) Inherited prion disease with six octapeptide repeat insertional mutation – molecular analysis of phenotypic heterogeneity. Brain 129: 2297–317.

Mead S, Webb TE, Campbell TA et al. (2007) Inherited prion disease with 5-OPRI: phenotype modification by repeat length and codon 129. Neurology 69: 730–8.

Medori R, Tritschler HJ, LeBlanc A et al. (1992a) Fatal familial insomnia, a prion disease with a mutation at codon 178 of the prion protein gene. New England Journal of Medicine 326: 444–9.

Medori R, Tritschler HJ, LeBlanc AC et al. (1992b) Fatal familial insomnia, a prion disease with a mutation in codon 178 of the prion protein gene: study of two kindreds. In: Prusiner SB, Collinge J, Powell J et al. (eds). Prion diseases of humans and animals. London: Ellis Horwood, 180–7.

Meyer-Luehmann M, Coomaraswamy J, Bolmont T et al. (2006) Exogenous induction of cerebral beta-amyloidogenesis is governed by agent and host. Science 313: 1781–4.

Mitrova E, Belay G. (2002) Creutzfeldt–Jakob disease with E200K mutation in Slovakia: characterization and development. Acta Virologica 46: 31–9.

Miyakawa T, Inoue K, Iseki E et al. (1998) Japanese Creutzfeldt–Jakob disease patients exhibiting high incidence of the E200K PRNP mutation and located in the basin of a river. Neurological Research 20: 684–8.

Mizutani T. (1981) Neuropathology of Creutzfeldt–Jakob disease in Japan. With special reference to the panencephalopathic type. Acta Pathologica Japonica 31: 903–22.

Mouillet-Richard S, Teil C, Lenne M et al. (1999) Mutation at codon 210 (V210I) of the prion protein gene in a North African patient with Creutzfeldt–Jakob disease. Journal of the Neurological Sciences 168: 141–4.

Murata T, Shiga Y, Higano S et al. (2002) Conspicuity and evolution of lesions in Creutzfeldt–Jakob disease at diffusion-weighted imaging. American Journal of Neuroradiology 23: 1164–72.

Nicoll AJ, Collinge J. (2009) Preventing prion pathogenicity by targeting the cellular prion protein. Infectious Disorders Drug Targets 9: 48–57.

Otto M, Stein H, Szudra A et al. (1997) S-100 protein concentration in the cerebrospinal fluid of patients with Creutzfeldt–Jakob disease. Journal of Neurology 244: 566–70.

Owen F, Poulter M, Lofthouse R et al. (1989) Insertion in prion protein gene in familial Creutzfeldt–Jakob disease. Lancet 1: 51–2.

Owen F, Poulter M, Collinge J et al. (1992) A dementing illness associated with a novel insertion in the prion protein gene. Molecular Brain Research 13: 155–7.

Palmer MS, Dryden AJ, Hughes JT, Collinge J. (1991) Homozygous prion protein genotype predisposes to sporadic Creutzfeldt–Jakob disease. Nature 352: 340–2.

Palmer MS, Mahal SP, Campbell TA et al. (1993) Deletions in the prion protein gene are not associated with CJD. Human Molecular Genetics 2: 541–4.

Parchi P, Castellani R, Capellari S et al. (1996) Molecular basis of phenotypic variability in sporadic Creutzfeldt–Jakob disease. Annals of Neurology 39: 669–80.

Parchi P, Giese A, Capellari S et al. (1999) Classification of sporadic Creutzfeldt–Jakob disease based on molecular and phenotypic analysis of 300 subjects. *Annals of Neurology* **46**: 224–33.

Pattison IH. (1965) Experiments with scrapie with special reference to the nature of the agent and the pathology of the disease. In: Gajdusek CJ, Gibbs CJ, Alpers MP (eds). *Slow, latent and temperate virus infections, NINDB Monograph 2*. Washington DC: US Government Printing, 249–57.

Peden AH, Head MW, Ritchie DL et al. (2004) Preclinical vCJD after blood transfusion in a PRNP codon 129 heterozygous patient. *Lancet* **364**: 527–9.

Peden A, McCardle L, Head MW et al. (2010) Variant CJD infection in the spleen of a neurologically asymptomatic UK adult patient with haemophilia. *Haemophilia* **16**: 296–304.

Piccardo P, Dlouhy SR, Lievens PMJ et al. (1998) Phenotypic variability of Gerstmann–Straussler–Scheinker disease is associated with prion protein heterogeneity. *Journal of Neuropathology and Experimental Neurology* **57**: 979–88.

Pietrini V, Puoti G, Limido L et al. (2003) Creutzfeldt–Jakob disease with a novel extra-repeat insertional mutation in the PRNP gene. *Neurology* **61**: 1288–91.

Pocchiari M, Ladogana A, Petraroli R et al. (1998) Recent Italian FFI cases. *Brain Pathology* **8**: 564–6.

Poulter M, Baker HF, Frith CD et al. (1992) Inherited prion disease with 144 base pair gene insertion: I: Genealogical and molecular studies. *Brain* **115**: 675–85.

Prusiner SB. (1982) Novel proteinaceous infectious particles cause scrapie. *Science* **216**: 136–44.

Prusiner SB, Scott M, Foster D et al. (1990) Transgenetic studies implicate interactions between homologous PrP isoforms in scrapie prion replication. *Cell* **63**: 673–86.

Rodriguez MM, Peoc'h K, Haik S et al. (2005) A novel mutation (G114V) in the prion protein gene in a family with inherited prion disease. *Neurology* **64**: 1455–7.

Rossetti AO, Bogousslavsky J, Glatzel M, Aguzzi A. (2004) Mimicry of variant creutzfeldt-jakob disease by sporadic Creutzfeldt–Jakob disease: importance of the pulvinar sign. *Archives of Neurology* **61**: 445–6.

Salazar AM, Masters CL, Gajdusek DC, Gibbs Jr CJ. (1983) Syndromes of amyotrophic lateral sclerosis and dementia: relation to transmissible Creutzfeldt–Jakob disease. *Annals of Neurology* **14**: 17–26.

Seno H, Tashiro H, Ishino H et al. (2000) New haplotype of familial Creutzfeldt–Jakob disease with a codon 200 mutation and a codon 219 polymorphism of the prion protein gene in a Japanese family. *Acta Neuropathologica* **99**: 125–30.

Shyu WC, Hsu YD, Kao MC, Tsao WL. (1996) Panencephalitic Creutzfeldt–Jakob disease in a Chinese family – Unusual presentation with PrP codon 210 mutation and identification by PCR SSCP. *Journal of Neurological Sciences* **143**: 176–80.

Simon ES, Kahana E, Chapman J et al. (2000) Creutzfeldt–Jakob disease profile in patients homozygous for the PRNP E200K mutation. *Annals of Neurology* **47**: 257–60.

Solomon A, Richey T, Murphy CL et al. (2007) Amyloidogenic potential of foie gras. *Proceedings of the National Academy of Sciences of the United States of America* **104**: 10998–1001.

Sponarova J, Nystrom SN, Westermark GT. (2008) AA-amyloidosis can be transferred by peripheral blood monocytes. *PLoS One* **3**: e3308.

Summers DM, Collie DA, Zeidler M, Will RG. (2004) The pulvinar sign in variant Creutzfeldt–Jakob disease. *Archives of Neurology* **61**: 446–7.

Tabrizi S, Scaravilli F, Howard RS et al. (1996) Creutzfeldt–Jakob disease in a young woman. Report of a Meeting of Physicians and Scientists, St. Thomas' Hospital, London. *Lancet* **347**: 945–8.

Tagliavini F, Giaccone G, Prelli F et al. (1993) A68 is a component of paired helical filaments of Gerstmann–Straussler–Scheinker disease, Indiana kindred. *Brain Research* **616**: 325–8.

Tanaka Y, Minematsu K, Moriyasu H et al. (1997) A Japanese family with a variant of Gerstmann–Straussler–Scheinker disease. *Journal of Neurology, Neurosurgery and Psychiatry* **62**: 454–7.

Tateishi J, Brown P, Kitamoto T et al. (1995) First experimental transmission of fatal familial insomnia. *Nature* **376**: 434–5.

Tschampa HJ, Kallenberg K, Urbach H et al. (2005) MRI in the diagnosis of sporadic Creutzfeldt–Jakob disease: a study on inter-observer agreement. *Brain* **128**: 2026–33.

Tschampa HJ, Kallenberg K, Kretzschmar HA et al. (2007) Pattern of cortical changes in sporadic Creutzfeldt–Jakob disease. *American Journal of Neuroradiology* **28**: 1114–8.

Van Gool WA, Hensels GW, Hoogerwaard EM et al. (1995) Hypokinesia and presenile dementia in a Dutch family with a novel insertion in the prion protein gene. *Brain* **118**: 1565–71.

Van Harten B, Van Gool WA, Van Langen IM et al. (2000) A new mutation in the prion protein gene: A patient with dementia and white matter changes. *Neurology* **55**: 1055–7.

Wadsworth JD, Hill AF, Joiner S et al. (1999) Strain-specific prion-protein conformation determined by metal ions. *Nature Cell Biology* **1**: 55–9.

Wadsworth JD, Joiner S, Hill AF et al. (2001) Tissue distribution of protease resistant prion protein in variant CJD using a highly sensitive immuno-blotting assay. *Lancet* **358**: 171–80.

Wadsworth JD, Asante E, Desbruslais M et al. (2004) Human prion protein with valine 129 prevents expression of variant CJD phenotype. *Science* **306**: 1793–6.

Wadsworth JD, Joiner S, Linehan J et al. (2006) Phenotypic heterogeneity in inherited prion disease (P102L) is associated with differential propagation of protease-resistant wild-type and mutant prion protein. *Brain* **129**: 1557–69.

Wadsworth JD, Joiner S, Linehan JM et al. (2008) Kuru prions and sporadic Creutzfeldt–Jakob disease prions have equivalent transmission properties in transgenic and wild-type mice. *Proceedings of the National Academy of Sciences of the United States of America* **105**: 3885–90.

Walker LC, Le Vine H III, Mattson MP, Jucker M. (2006) Inducible proteopathies. *Trends in Neurosciences* **29**: 438–43.

Webb TE, Poulter M, Beck J et al. (2008) Phenotypic heterogeneity and genetic modification of P102L inherited prion disease in an international series. *Brain* **131**: 2632–46.

Webb TE, Whittaker J, Collinge J, Mead S. (2009) Age of onset and death in inherited prion disease are heritable. *American Journal of Medical Genetics. Part B, Neuropsychiatric Genetics* **150B**: 496–501.

White AR, Enever P, Tayebi M *et al.* (2003) Monoclonal antibodies inhibit prion replication and delay the development of prion disease. *Nature* **422**: 80–3.

Will RG, Ironside JW, Zeidler M *et al.* (1996) A new variant of Creutzfeldt–Jakob disease in the UK. *Lancet* **347**: 921–5.

Wroe SJ, Pal S, Siddique D *et al.* (2006) Clinical presentation and pre-mortem diagnosis of variant Creutzfeldt–Jakob disease associated with blood transfusion: a case report. *Lancet* **368**: 2061–7.

Yamada M, Itoh Y, Inaba A *et al.* (1999) An inherited prion disease with a PrPP105L mutation – clinicopathologic and PrP heterogeneity. *Neurology* **53**: 181–8.

Young GS, Geschwind MD, Fischbein NJ *et al.* (2005) Diffusion-weighted and fluid-attenuated inversion recovery imaging in Creutzfeldt–Jakob disease: high sensitivity and specificity for diagnosis. *American Journal of Neuroradiology* **26**: 1551–62.

Young K, Clark HB, Piccardo P *et al.* (1997) Gerstmann-Straussler-Scheinker disease with the PRNP P102L

mutation and valine at codon 129. *Molecular Brain Research* **44**: 147–50.

Yu SL, Jin L, Sy MS *et al.* (2004) Polymorphisms of the PRNP gene in Chinese populations and the identification of a novel insertion mutation. *European Journal of Human Genetics* **12**: 867–70.

Zeidler M, Stewart G, Cousens SN *et al.* (1997) Codon 129 genotype and new variant CJD. *Lancet* **350**: 668.

Zerr I. (2009) Therapeutic trials in human transmissible spongiform encephalopathies: recent advances and problems to address. *Infectious Disorders Drug Targets* **9**: 92–9.

Zerr I, Bodemer M, Räcker S *et al.* (1995) Cerebrospinal fluid concentration of neuron-specific enolase in diagnosis of Creutzfeldt–Jakob disease. *Lancet* **345**: 1609–10.

Zerr I, Giese A, Windl O *et al.* (1998) Phenotypic variability in fatal familial insomnia (D178N-129M) genotype. *Neurology* **51**: 1398–405.

80

Uncommon forms of dementia

ANOOP R VARMA

80.1 INTRODUCTION

In 1–5 per cent of patients with dementia, the underlying disorders are uncommon. Many of these patients develop dementia as part of a more prominent neurological syndrome (e.g. progressive supranuclear palsy (PSP)). However, awareness of these disorders may lead to effective treatments, or to better care from the knowledge of evolution of the disease and its attendant symptoms and signs. Those conditions with an underlying genetic basis may benefit from rapid scientific advances and/or require genetic counselling. This chapter attempts to summarize the clinical, diagnostic and therapeutic aspects of these disorders.

80.2 DEMENTIAS ASSOCIATED WITH MOVEMENT DISORDERS (EXCLUDING PARKINSON'S AND HUNTINGTON'S DISEASES)

The definition of diseases always leads to controversy, debate (Hachinski, 1997; Kertesz, 1997; Neary, 1997) and attempts at development of criteria only to end up being continually appraised (Litvan et al., 2003). This process often begins with clinical descriptions, evolving into clinicoradiological correlations and then discovery of pathological and biological hallmarks of the disorder. The newly identified pathology and biology may in turn question the remit of the initial clinical phenotype; hence, nosology undergoes scrutiny (Sha et al., 2006). The movement disorders discussed below are

prototypical examples of this process. The observation of the unifying pathological accumulation of tau in many of these parkinsonian and/or cognitive disorders lump them into one pathological entity, tauopathies. In an attempt to correlate the pathology with previously defined clinical syndromes, weight is added to the rate of development and topography of tau accumulation in determining the clinical picture (Williams and Lees, 2009). Awareness of current thinking contributes to a clearer understanding, better management and informed communication with patients. The Reisensburg Working group for Tauopathies with Parkinsonism (Ludolph et al., 2009) discusses the overlap and expansion of the phenotypes of PSP and corticobasal degeneration (CBD). These new variations to the classical conceptualization of these disorders are discussed below. An attempt to diagnose syndromes, rather than loosely lump them, remains useful for management and prognostication.

80.2.1 Progressive supranuclear palsy (Steele–Richardson–Olszweski syndrome)

Progressive supranuclear palsy is characterized by supranuclear ophthalmoplegia (especially downgaze), pseudobulbar palsy, dysarthria, retrocollis, parkinsonism and dementia (Steele et al., 1964; Steele, 1972). Patients are commonly affected in the seventh decade with no significant difference between the sexes (Maher and Lees, 1986). The disorder is often misdiagnosed (Osaki et al., 2004) and initial diagnoses include Parkinson's disease, balance disorders and stroke (Burn and Lees, 2002). Presenting complaints include abrupt falls, unsteadiness of gait, slurred speech or memory impairment. As the disease progresses, marked and relatively symmetrical rigidity (pronounced in the neck) and the characteristic downgaze palsy emerge. Cerebellar and pyramidal signs and pseudobulbar palsy may be observed. This classical syndrome has been termed Richardson's syndrome, but other clinicopathological variants have been described (Williams and Lees, 2009). PSP-parkinsonism (PSP-P) does not feature an early eye movement disorder or early falls, but presents with an akinetic, predominantly axial, rigid syndrome with a jerky postural tremor which is often levo-dopa responsive. Survival is longer than classical PSP and cognitive decline is observed late in the disorder. PSP-PAGF refers to the variant with progressive gait disturbance with hesitant starts and freezing without rigidity, tremor or dementia.

Although severe dementia is unusual, a subcortical cognitive impairment and depression are common. Mentation is slowed and difficulty in switching set, perseveration, apathy and poor abstraction are prominent neuropsychological features (Albert et al., 1974). Significant depression may occur in addition to emotional lability that often accompanies the pseudobulbar syndrome. Cognitive impairment in PSP is proposed to be due to the accumulation of tau in the frontal cortices (Williams and Lees, 2009). Evidence for the overlap of cognitive syndromes in PSP, CBD/corticobasal syndrome (CBS), frontotemporal dementia (FTD) and progressive non-fluent aphasia (PNFA) is accumulating (Kertesz and McMonagle, 2010). It could thus be argued that dementia in PSP can no more be termed purely subcortical; however, as a common clinical phenomenon, subcortical dementia as the prototype of PSP remains valid.

The diagnosis rests on clinical history and examination. Midbrain atrophy on magnetic resonance imaging (MRI) and/or signal changes in the midbrain, red nucleus or globus pallidus are supportive (Asato et al., 2000; Warmuth-Metz et al., 2001). Functional imaging studies including blood flow single photon emission tomography (SPECT), dopamine transporter and dopamine (D2) receptor imaging are not diagnostically specific to PSP (Brooks, 1993; Kim et al., 2002).

Treatment with levodopa, dopamine agonists, amantadine, tricyclic antidepressants and anticholinergics has proved disappointing.

Over a period of five to seven years, severe physical decline leads to loss of ambulation and eventual death. Autopsy reveals tau-positive neurofibrillary tangles, neuronal loss and tau-positive glial inclusions in the substantia nigra, globus pallidus, subthalamic nucleus and midbrain (Jellinger and Blancher, 1992). The pathology may be more widespread and can be regionally mapped to clinical models based on the emphasis of distribution of pathology (Williams and Lees, 2009).

80.2.2 Corticobasal syndrome and degeneration

Corticobasal degeneration is a striking parkinsonian syndrome characterized by grossly asymmetrical dystonia, alien limb phenomenon, apraxia and myoclonus (Ribeiz et al., 1968; Gibb et al., 1989). Patients usually present in late middle life, often with a useless arm. The asymmetry is marked and eventually the disorder spreads contralaterally. The involved arm may initially be evidently apraxic, but rigidity and dystonia quickly supervene. Myoclonus may be reported or elicited at action. Patients may describe alien limb phenomenon and intermanual conflict. Rigidity, corticospinal signs, cortical sensory loss, supranuclear gaze palsy and dysarthria may occur (Gibb et al., 1989; Stover and Watts 2001). These clinical features constitute the clinical syndrome, termed the 'corticobasal syndromes'. The characteristically asymmetrical cortical (apraxia and myoclonus) and basal (dystonia, with akinesia and rigidity) signs are the hallmark of CBS. Even when a limb is severely rigid and postured due to dystonia, it is usually possible to elicit apraxia in the contralateral limb or orofacial musculature. The elicitation of this sign is vital, although neurologists do not routinely look for apraxia (Kertesz and McMonagle, 2010).

Pathologically defined CBD presents as CBS in only 40 per cent of patients; other clinical phenotypes include the syndromes of dementia (FTLD-like), PSP, aphasia/apraxia of speech and posterior cortical atrophy (PCA) (Wadia and Lang, 2007). Conversely, varied pathologies may underlie CBS: CBD, PSP, Pick's, FTLD, Alzheimer's disease (AD), dementia with Lewy bodies (DLB), Creutzfeldt–Jakob disease (CJD) or vascular neuropathology. In CBS too, like PSP (see above), the distribution (not type) of pathology seems to dictate the clinical syndrome. Until specific biological markers become available, prediction of pathology from the clinical picture remains at best an educated guess. The disorder is cruel and CBS poses similar management challenges, regardless of the underlying pathology.

Prior to the elucidation of distinction between CBS and CBD, subcortical deficits, apraxia and constructional and spatial impairment were described in CBD (Gibb et al., 1989; Stover and Watts, 2001). With expanding phenotype, it appears that cognitive impairment in CBS includes behavioural changes overlapping with FTD (apathy, disinhibition, perseveration, attention deficits); language disturbance, including nonfluent aphasia and apraxia of speech; spatial and constructive deficits with limb and buccofacial apraxia (Kertesz and McMonagle, 2010). However, in most cases with CBS, the motor disorder eclipses the less prominent cognitive impairment.

MRI may show severe asymmetrical posterior frontal and parietal atrophy, putaminal hypointensity and hyperintense signals in the motor cortex or subcortical white matter (Savoiardo, 2003; Seppi, 2007). These findings seem specific to CBS, regardless of the pathology (Josephs et al., 2004). Cerebral blood flow (rCBF) SPECT shows reduced uptake in the affected posterior frontal, superior, anterior, inferior and posterior parietal cortices with less prominent changes in the thalamus and basal ganglia (Markus et al., 1995) or more widespread rCBF change (Hossain et al., 2003).

Sustained benefit with levodopa, dopamine agonists or amantadine is unusual. The disorder is relentlessly progressive leading to a severe akinetic-rigid syndrome with dysarthria, dysphagia and, eventually, a wheelchair and bed-bound state. Survival from the onset of symptoms ranges from six to nine years.

Pathological features (Gibb *et al.*, 1989) of CBD include neuronal loss in the thalamus, basal ganglia, brainstem and the frontoparietal cortex. Swollen achromatic neurones in the frontoparietal region are pathologically characteristic. CBS poses a clinical challenge to both cognitive and movement disorder clinicians. Regardless of arguments between lumpers (Kertesz, 1997) and splitters (Neary, 1997), it is sensible to painstakingly document the clinical, radiological, pathological and biological markers associated with this syndrome.

80.2.3   Multiple system atrophy

The term 'multiple system atrophy' (MSA) was proposed in 1969 (Graham and Oppenheimer, 1969) and has gained wide acceptance (Gilman *et al.*, 1999). The disorder affects both sexes in the sixth decade. The main features include autonomic dysfunction, parkinsonism, cerebellar ataxia and pyramidal signs in varying combinations (Wenning *et al.*, 2004). The two main subtypes are the parkinsonian (MSA-P) and the ataxic (MSA-C) variants, depending on the major motor feature. Patients may also develop inspiratory stridor or REM sleep behaviour disorder. Dementia is usually mild and neuropsychological tests reveal deficits in frontosubcortical function. Cognitive dysfunction is heterogeneous and some patients reveal no impairment even when severely physically disabled (Robbins *et al.*, 1992). It is, though, generally believed that frank dementia and psychosis argue against MSA (Gilman *et al.*, 2008; Wenning and Brown 2009). In their cohort of 58 patients, Kitayama *et al.* (2009) reported dementia in ten patients with MSA-C; three of these patients presented with dementia, whereas the remaining developed cognitive impairment later in the course (ataxia-onset). Although detailed neuropsychological findings are not reported, the pattern of dementia in the ataxia-onset group was frontosubcortical. The dementia-onset patients had more severe dementia and marked white matter changes and atrophy on MRI. All the ten patients with dementia had significantly decreased H/M ratio of ^{123}I-MIBG cardiac scintigraphy. These patients do not have autopsy confirmation. Thus, the question remains whether at least some of these patients may have harboured coincidental Alzheimer or Lewy-body pathology. Another study (Chang *et al.*, 2009) noted frontosubcortical deficits on neuropsychological testing (more severe in the MSA-C subgroup) and frontal atrophy on MRI morphometry. These findings correlate with disease duration.

MRI may show putaminal or olivopontocerebellar atrophy ('hot-cross bun' sign), sometimes with hyperintensities in the pons and middle cerebellar peduncles (Brooks and Seppi, 2009; Kitayama *et al.*, 2009; Schrag *et al.*, 2000). Although hypointensities in the putamen with a hyperintense rim are thought to be characteristic of MSA (Kraft *et al.*, 1999), none of the imaging characteristics described could be regarded as surrogate markers for MSA (Brooks and Seppi, 2009). Denervation on sphincter electromyogram (EMG) may be diagnostically helpful if other causes of sphincter denervation have been ruled out (Vodusek, 2001).

Most patients are levodopa-unresponsive and symptomatic treatment centres around relief from dysautonomic symptoms. MSA progresses relentlessly to severe disability in five years. Argyrophilic glial cytoplasmic inclusions are the pathological hallmark of MSA. The distribution of pathology varies with the predominance of parkinsonian or cerebellar features (Wenning *et al.*, 2004).

80.3   DEMENTIAS ASSOCIATED WITH NEUROINFECTIONS, INCLUDING HIV-ASSOCIATED DEMENTIA

80.3.1   HIV-associated dementia

The last two decades have witnessed the success story of HIV medicine. However, HIV-associated dementia (HAD) continues to confound. The AIDS dementia complex (ADC) was associated with high cerebrospinal fluid (CSF) viral load and advanced disease (Brew, 2007). The post-highly active antiretroviral therapy (HAART) era is seeing an increase in lifespan and, paradoxically, the prevalence of HIV-associated neurocognitive disorders (HAND) (Kaul, 2009). The nosology (Antinori *et al.*, 2007) of HAND (including asymptomatic neurocognitive impairment (ANI); mild neurocognitive disorder (MND) and HAD) is an attempt to achieve uniformity in a diverse field. The term HIV encephalitis (HIVE) refers to the pathological features of multinucleated giant cells in HIV-identified brains and not to the clinical syndrome (Nath *et al.*, 2008).

In this HAART era, MND is more prevalent than frank dementia. However, slow development of HAD is relentless and HAART does not seem to be protective (McArthur, 2004). Consequently, the expression of neuroinflammation in HIV infection progressing into neurodegeneration, along with toxicological effects of HAART, seems to drive HAD. Whereas pre-HAART brains show inflammation in the basal ganglia, post-HAART pathology is focused around hippocampus, entorhinal and temporal cortices (Kaul, 2009). The overlap between HAD, ageing and neurodegenerative dementias has been remarked upon (Noorbakhsh *et al.*, 2009). Such models suggest a complex interplay of various pathogenetic factors, perhaps of greater significance than the initial HIV infection, in the development and expression of HAD. Ageing, effects of long-term HAART including metabolic dyslipidaemic effects and mitochondrial toxicity, substance use and co-infection with hepatitis C are associated with HAND along with host genetic factors, including apolipoprotein E ε4 (Jayadev and Garden, 2009; Nath *et al.*, 2008).

The clinical picture of HAD comprises cognitive, behavioural and motor dysfunction. Dementia is subcortical, although in the post-HAART era cortical involvement may be seen (McArthur, 2004; Brew, 2007; Nath *et al.*, 2008). Apathy, gait unsteadiness, clumsiness, tremor, myoclonus, hyperreflexia, bradykinesia, peripheral neuropathy and release reflexes are observed in varying combinations and severity. Uncommonly, mania may be seen at onset. With progression, the dementia becomes global accompanied with motor decay (Brew, 2007; Nath *et al.*, 2008).

The patient presenting with HAND/HAD to the memory clinic may elude diagnosis, unless HIV is considered as a possible differential. The presence of motor deficits should alert the clinician to enquire into possible indications of HIV-related illness in the preceding months of weight loss, diarrhoea and constitutional symptoms. Clinical and laboratory observations of thrush, seborrhoeic dermatitis, leukopenia and polyclonal increase in gamma globulins are other clues.

MRI and CSF studies are used first to exclude opportunistic infections. MRI may demonstrate atrophy and deep white matter changes in HAD (Nath *et al.*, 2008). It is not widely appreciated that unlike the pre-HAART era, HAD can manifest in patients with undetectable viral loads (VL) in plasma or CSF (Kaul, 2009). CD4 counts may also be much higher, although there appears to be a correlation between nadir CD4 and development of HAD (Nath *et al.*, 2008). CSF may thus be normal or simply reflect established background findings of HIV infection (mild rise in protein, mononuclear cells or oligoclonal bands).

The course of HAD may vary from untreated patients developing a 'subacute progressive' dementia; poorly compliant patients on HAART manifesting a 'chronic-active' dementia; effective HAART with adherence rendering the course 'chronic-inactive' and some proving 'reversible' with effective viral suppression (Nath *et al.*, 2008; Venkataramana and Sacktor, 2008).

Although HAD may continue to progress despite HAART, lower central nervous system (CNS) penetration of anti-retroviral drugs (ART) allows viral replication and worse cognitive impairments. Clinical trials investigating this are progressing (Kaul, 2009). Drugs, including disease-modifying cognitive enhancers, neuroprotectors and other viral agents, are experimental. A wider understanding of HAND, awareness of HIV as a possible cause of dementia and the possible interaction with age-related neurodegenerative dementias opens the possibility of halting or reversing the progression of dementia in these patients.

80.3.2 Syphilis

Recently, there has been an outbreak of syphilis (Simms *et al.*, 2005) emphasizing the need again to consider neurosyphilis, the great mimic, in the differential of various neurological syndromes, including dementia. Also, there is an increased prevalence of neurosyphilis in HIV co-infected patients (Lynn and Lightman, 2004). Paretic neurosyphilis (GPI, dementia paralytica) manifests usually in the 35–50 age group, after an incubation of 10–25 years. The onset is insidious with personality change, cognitive decline, mood disturbance and progression to frank dementia with neuropsychiatric features, including psychosis, mania, grandiose delusions and/or paranoia (Luo *et al.*, 2008; Nitrini, 2008; van Eijsden *et al.*, 2008; Chen-Hsiang *et al.*, 2009). Neurological signs may include lip and tongue tremor, dysarthria, pupillary abnormalities, pyramidal signs and ataxia (Luo *et al.*, 2008; Nitrini, 2008).

Meningovascular syphilis may result in vascular dementia (VaD) due to vasculitic brain infarctions including lacunae or larger territory strokes (Lynn and Lightman, 2004; Nitrini, 2008).

MRI may be misleading with varying patterns of atrophy erroneously suggesting an irreversible degenerative dementia (Nitrini, 2008). Indeed, the case of van Eijsden *et al.* (2008) shows striking mesial temporal atrophy (MTA) in a patient with memory impairment and prosopagnosia identical to that seen in AD. Another case (Chen-Hsiang *et al.*, 2009) showed progressive and marked right frontotemporal cortical atrophy on MRI in a patient presenting with personality change, mania and right frontotemporal hypoperfusion on SPECT. We have observed a similar example in our practice; these patients can be misdiagnosed as FTD because of the early personality and behavioural changes. The fronto-temporal atrophy on MRI and hypoperfusion on SPECT in similar regions offers false security to the initial clinical misdiagnosis. Most reported cases of dementia due to syphilis are of an age where screening for syphilis would not be uncommon. However, it also stands to reason that many, somewhat older, patients with clinical and radiological diagnosis of AD or FTD may have syphilis. These patients are not routinely tested for syphilis, a practice currently not recommended by the American Academy of Neurology (Knopman *et al.*, 2001).

Conclusive diagnosis requires serological tests for syphilis in the blood and CSF confirming treponemal reactivity. Penicillin remains the mainstay of therapy and response is monitored by periodic CSF studies (Nitrini, 2008). Early diagnosis and treatment are desirable to prevent irreversibility (Chen-Hsiang *et al.*, 2009). Management should occur in close consultation with genitourinary medicine and/or infectious disease specialists.

80.3.3 Lyme disease

Lyme disease is caused by *Borrelia burgdorferi*, a tick-borne spirochaete. The tick bite and early skin infection (erythema migrans) may go unnoticed or be forgotten. After a few weeks to months, multisystem involvement may cause musculoskeletal pains, myopericarditis, meningoencephalitis, radiculoneuritis and cranial (usually facial) nerve palsies. After several years, bouts of arthritis and late encephalomyelitis or chronic Lyme encephalopathy may develop (Fallon and Nields, 1994; Nitrini, 2008).

Lyme encephalopathy refers to patients with cognitive disturbances, depressive symptoms, fatigue and sleep disturbance months or years after initial infection. CSF shows intrathecal anti-*B. burgdorferi* antibody or elevated protein. Most patients improve with antibiotic therapy (ceftriaxone or penicillin) (Kaplan *et al.*, 2003; Nitrini, 2008). MRI may show white matter hyperintensities (Almeida and Lautenschlager, 2005; Nitrini, 2008). A progressive dementia syndrome is a rare manifestation of Lyme disease (Nitrini, 2008), although pronounced neuropsychiatric symptoms accompanied by some cognitive deficiency is less uncommon (Fallon and Nields, 1994).

Diagnosis of Lyme disease is based on published criteria (Halperin *et al.*, 1996). Lyme serology in the blood and CSF confirming intrathecal production of antibody to *B. Burgdorferi* is a specific widely available test. Therapy involves a 4-week course of antibiotics (e.g. ceftriaxone or penicillin).

Retreatment is reserved for patients with a chronic syndrome, objective evidence of neuropsychological deficits and abnormal CSF, despite previous antibiotic therapy (Kaplan *et al.*, 2003).

80.3.4   Whipple's disease

Whipple's disease (WhD) is a systemic infectious disorder usually presenting with weight loss, arthralgia, diarrhoea and abdominal pain. Small intestinal biopsy confirms the diagnosis by demonstrating periodic acid Schiff (PAS)-positive inclusions in the lamina propria. These inclusions represent the causative bacteria, *Tropheryma whipplei* (Marth and Raoult, 2003). Neurological symptoms occur in approximately 10–43 per cent of patients and may present without prominent gastrointestinal disorder (Louis *et al.*, 1996; Marth and Raoult, 2003; Panegyres *et al.*, 2006; Panegyres, 2008).

Eighty per cent of patients with CNS WhD have systemic signs, although a proportion of patients with WhD may have isolated CNS involvement (primary WhD of the CNS). An analysis of published cases (Panegyres *et al.*, 2006) suggests two syndromes: (1) diverse neurological symptoms and signs with multiple nodular enhancing lesions on computed tomography (CT) or MRI and (2) focal neurological syndromes secondary to solitary mass lesion. The first group is rich in its neurological spectrum including seizures, ataxia, dysarthria, nystagmus, vertical gaze pareses, amnesia, sleep disturbances, raised intracranial pressure, pyramidal signs, behavioural disturbance, dementia, VII nerve paresis, neuropathic sensory loss and suppressed ankle jerks and syndrome of inappropriate antidiuretic hormone secretion (SIADH). Primary WhD of the CNS shares the clinical features of systemic WhD with CNS involvement, i.e. supranuclear gaze paresis, memory impairment, confusion, apathy and occasionally oculomasticatory myorhythmia (Louis *et al.*, 1996; Panegyres *et al.*, 2006). Patients may develop frank dementia. Isolated case reports expand the phenotype to include clinical profiles and radiology, supportive of a degenerative process rather than that of a subacute/chronic granulomatous disorder. A 63-year-old case (Benito-Leon *et al.*, 2008) with frontotemporal features fulfilled consensus criteria for FTD (Neary *et al.*, 1998) and had no signs/symptoms of gastrointestinal involvement. Both MRI and SPECT imaging supported the diagnosis of FTD; the MRI did not show any focal lesions, but only modest anterior atrophy. A CSF examination revealed *T. whipplei*. Treatment reversed both the cognitive/behavioural symptoms and the blood flow changes on SPECT, removing doubts around any chance association between WhD and the FTD-like syndrome in this case. A further 55-year-old lady presented with bitemporal involvement (Leesch *et al.*, 2009), again raising the possibility of FTLD. Gastrointestinal symptoms were absent; however, the ring enhancing bitemporal lesions on MRI prompted cerebral biopsy which showed PAS-positive organisms of WhD.

CSF may show pleocytosis (lymphocytic or polymorphonuclear), raised or low protein and oligoclonal bands. *T. whipplei* polymerase chain reaction (PCR) in blood and CSF, and other materials (gastric fluid, small bowel, synovia or saliva) is strongly advocated, since tissue biopsy (small bowel, brain, lymph node or vitreous fluid) is not invariably positive (Louis *et al.* 1996; Delanty *et al.*, 1999; Panegyres, 2008).

Currently recommended treatment regimes include parenteral ceftriaxone or meropenem for 2 weeks followed by long-term oral trimethoprim-sulfamethoxazole administration (Marth and Raoult, 2003; Panegyres, 2008). It is recommended that all patients with WhD be regarded as having subclinical CNS involvement and that such brain infection may persist long after treatment and relapse (Panegyres, 2008).

80.4   DEMENTIAS ASSOCIATED WITH CNS INFLAMMATORY DISORDERS

80.4.1   Cerebral vasculitis

Cerebral vasculitis may occur as part of a systemic vasculitis (e.g. systemic lupus erythematosus (SLE)). However, occasionally a neurological syndrome may be the presenting feature of systemic vasculitis or, less commonly, due to an isolated primary vasculitis of the CNS, i.e. without peripheral clinical or laboratory (absence of autoantibodies, normal erythrocyte sedimentation rate (ESR) and C-reactive protein (CRP)) markers of systemic vasculitis (Hajj-Ali and Calabrese, 2009). The latter condition (primary angiitis of the CNS (PACNS)) poses diagnostic difficulties. Detection of PACNS requires a high degree of clinical suspicion and experience. Patients present in varying combinations of cognitive impairment, behavioural changes and focal symptoms or signs with a chronic headache. The onset is usually subacute, although stroke-like presentations are reported (Salvarani *et al.*, 2007; Birnbaum and Hellman, 2009). PACNS is an important and potentially reversible cause of rapidly progressive dementia (RPD) (**Box 80.1**). Headache and confusion, with focal signs, and less commonly seizures, raise suspicion of an underlying cerebral vasculitis. Although individual investigations including MRI, electroencephalogram (EEG) and CSF studies may be normal, the combination of completely normal MRI and CSF studies is a strong negative predictor for the diagnosis of PACNS (Stone *et al.*, 1994). Cerebral angiography and leptomeningeal biopsies may also be falsely negative. However, biopsy is strongly recommended for its additional value in excluding alternative diagnoses in 40 per cent of suspected cases of PACNS (Alrawi *et al.*, 1999). The diagnosis is sometimes established after repeated investigations (vascular changes on MRI, CSF pleocytosis and raised protein, multifocal narrowing of blood vessels on angiography and vasculitic lesions on leptomeningeal biopsy). MRI is abnormal in over 90 per cent of patients, including changes in subcortical white matter, deep white matter, and less frequently deep grey matter and cerebral cortex (Birnbaum and Hellman, 2009; Salvarani *et al.*, 2007). Multiple infarctions of different ages and brain haemorrhage favour PACNS against other causes of RPD (Geschwind *et al.*, 2008). Treatment is aggressive with immunosuppression (cyclophosphamide) and steroids (Joseph and Scolding, 2002; Salvarani *et al.*, 2007; Birnbaum and Hellman, 2009).

Box 80.1 Rapidly progressive dementias.

- Infectious
  - HIV
  - Syphilis
  - Lyme disease
  - Meningoencephalitides, including tuberculosis
- Inflammatory
  - Cerebral vasculitis
  - Hashimoto's encephalopathy
  - Limbic encephalitis
    - paraneoplastic
    - non-paraneoplastic, including VGKC, anti-NMDAR
  - Cognitive presentation of multiple sclerosis
- Neoplastic/space occupation
  - Lymphoma
  - Glioblastoma multiforme
  - Subdural haematoma
- Rapid degenerative
  - Creutzfeldt–Jakob disease
  - Dementia with Lewy bodies
  - Alzheimer's disease
  - Frontotemporal dementia
  - Corticobasal degeneration
- Toxic and metabolic
  - Ethanol
  - Drugs

Box 80.2 Fluctuating encephalopathies.

Metabolic encephalopathy
Dementia with Lewy bodies
Creutzfeldt–Jakob disease
Hashimoto's encephalopathy
Cerebral vasculitis
Limbic encephalitis

The disorder responds to steroids and often prolonged courses are required. HE is most likely to be confused with fluctuating encephalopathies including DLB, CJD, metabolic encephalopathy, cerebral vasculitis and limbic encephalitis (LE) (**Box 80.2**). Plasma exchange is useful in some cases (Scheiss and Pardo, 2008).

80.4.3   Limbic encephalitis and variants

Limbic encephalitis was first described in patients with severe short-term memory impairment or dementia in association with bronchial carcinoma (Corsellis *et al.*, 1968). The last decade has seen an increased recognition of LE and similar disorders with advances in neuroimaging and diagnostic immunological markers. The phenotype has thus expanded to include autoimmune LE not associated with underlying neoplasm. LE is characterized by severe anterograde amnesia, neuropsychiatric symptoms (personality changes, behavioural disturbance including irritability, depression and hallucinations), seizures or even frank dementia (Gultekin *et al.*, 2000; Tüzün and Dalmau, 2007; Anderson and Barber, 2008). Memory loss and confusion are the most common presenting symptoms. The EEG is invariably abnormal with focal or generalized epileptic discharges or slow wave activity (Tüzün and Dalmau, 2007), excluding psychiatric causes which may present similarly. LE usually presents subacutely with a fluctuating course and rapid deterioration, unless recognized and appropriately treated.

MRI shows unilateral/bilateral, often asymmetric, high signal changes in mesial temporal lobes on T_2-weighted and/or fluid-attenuated inversion recovery (FLAIR) images that may infrequently enhance with contrast (Gultekin *et al.*, 2000; Urbach *et al.*, 2006). The CSF may show pleocytosis, raised protein or oligoclonal bands. Two broad categories are now recognized: (1) associated with antibodies to intracellular neuronal antigens, including paraneoplastic antigens (Hu, Ma2, CRMP-5, amphiphysin) and (2) associated with antibodies to cell membrane antigens, including voltage-gated potassium channel (VGKC) and N-methyl-D-aspartate receptor (NMDAR). The first group is more commonly associated with an underlying cancer (lung, testis, breast) and is less responsive to immunotherapy (Tüzün and Dalmau, 2007). The VGKC and NMDAR encephalitides are less commonly associated with underlying tumours (thymoma, teratoma) and are far more responsive to immune mediation (Tüzün and Dalmau, 2007; Anderson and Barber, 2008; Dalmau *et al.*, 2008). Hyponatraemia is prominent in VGKC LE (Vernino *et al.*, 2007) and paraneoplastic LE associated with lung cancers.

Although giant cell arteritis (GCA) usually presents with headache, ischaemic optic neuropathy and/or strokes in the elderly, this condition is an uncommon, yet reversible, cause of multi-infarct dementia (MID). In MID, the presence of prominent headache, systemic symptoms, visual loss and a raised ESR draws attention to GCA. Steroids may improve cognitive symptoms (Solans-Laqué *et al.*, 2008).

80.4.2   Hashimoto's encephalopathy

Hashimoto's encephalopathy (HE) characteristically presents with a fluctuating confusional state (which may include visual hallucinations and psychosis), tremor and myoclonus (Shaw *et al.*, 1991; Scheiss and Pardo, 2008). Seizures, stroke-like episodes, pyramidal weakness, extrapyramidal rigidity and ataxia may emerge over the ensuing weeks and months. The onset may be abrupt or insidious and the evolution is typically subacute (Kothbauer-Margreiter *et al.*, 1996).

The EEG is usually slow (Chong *et al.*, 2003). MRI and SPECT may be normal or show non-specific changes. The CSF protein is usually raised, occasionally with oligoclonal bands, but with a normal cell count. The relation between high titres of antithyroid antibodies (anti-TPO, anti-TG) and pathogenesis of the syndrome is unclear. Although widely believed to occur with normal thyroid function, varying thyroid states have been reported (Scheiss and Pardo, 2008).

Immunosuppression, with removal of the underlying tumour, if detected, is the mainstay of therapy. However, infections including *Herpes simplex* encephalitis must be excluded before embarking on these therapies. Anderson and Barber (2008) provide a useful outline of diagnostic approach. Early treatment with intravenous steroids and/or intravenous immunoglobulin is advocated. Other measures include plasma exchange, cyclophosphamide and rituximab (Dalmau *et al.*, 2008). In paraneoplastic LE, neurological dysfunction may develop 0.5–33 months (median 3.5 months) before tumour detection (Gultekin *et al.*, 2000). A diligent search for an underlying tumour and prompt treatment may improve prognosis.

80.5   DEMENTIA ASSOCIATED WITH NORMAL PRESSURE HYDROCEPHALUS

Normal pressure hydrocephalus (NPH), described by Hakim and Adams (1965), is characterized by the triad of gait disturbance, dementia and urinary incontinence. The age range most affected is the sixth/seventh decade (mean age, 71) (Krauss and von Stuckrad-Barre, 2008). Secondary NPH may occur after subarachnoid haemorrhage (SAH), head injury or meningitic illnesses (Ropper and Brown, 2005).

The triad of symptoms/signs may manifest in varying combinations: gait disturbance is universal (100 per cent), dementia (98 per cent) and urinary difficulties (83 per cent) (Krauss and von Stuckrad-Barre, 2008). Gait abnormalities vary in severity and quality and have the greatest potential to improve after shunting. Even when patients cannot walk, they retain the ability to perform cycling or walking movements when supine or sitting (Ropper and Brown, 2005). Mild cognitive deficits are nearly always present. Dementia, when present, is subcortical and without frank aphasia or visuo-spatio-perceptual impairment. Mental processing is slowed and patients are apathetic (Vanneste, 2000; Devito *et al.*, 2005). Bradykinesia, postural instability and parkinsonism may be observed, necessitating differentiation from Parkinsonian syndromes.

Diagnosis is clinical. Although on occasion the differential can be wide and includes AD, FTD, DLB and VaD, NPH need not be considered in patients with progressive dementia without gait disturbance regardless of ventriculomegaly (Shprecher *et al.*, 2008). Co-nfusion can arise when general radiological reports over-call ventricular dilatation as NPH. Caution must be exercised in erroneously describing any ventriculomegaly, without signs of high pressure hydrocephalus, as NPH. Similarly hydrocephalus-*ex-vacuo* (seen in diffuse cerebral atrophy) should not be mistaken for NPH. NPH remains a clinical syndrome and imaging techniques do not exclusively confirm/exclude the diagnosis. Prominent ventricular dilatation on MRI without proportionate cortical atrophy is a useful clue in raising the possibility of NPH. Removal of 30–50 mL of CSF with marked improvement in gait, sometimes after many hours, may suggest a good prognosis after CSF diversion. However, many patients benefit with shunts even if CSF removal had not demonstrated benefit (Ropper and Brown, 2005). Small vessel cerebrovascular disease (SVD) may coexist in approximately 60 per cent of patients (Shprecher *et al.*, 2008). Shunt must not be denied before careful consideration, since selected patients with concurrent NPH and SVD may benefit from CSF diversion (Krauss and von Stuckrad-Barre, 2008; Shprecher *et al.*, 2008). Co-morbid AD pathology may occur with NPH and in these patients shunts may improve gait, but not the dementia (Shprecher *et al.*, 2008).

80.6   DEMENTIAS IN YOUNG ADULTS, INCLUDING INHERITED METABOLIC DISEASES

A wide variety of inherited metabolic diseases, usually thought to be limited to infancy or childhood, may manifest in adolescence or young adulthood (Coker, 1991). They may present with predominantly neurological disease or with associated systemic involvement (**Box 80.3**). The brunt of pathology may vary from dominant grey matter involvement (seizures, dementia) to white matter disease (motor weakness, spasticity, ataxia). The fate of these disorders, if untreated, is severe mental and physical disability, eventually leading to death. With advances in biology and genetics, many of these disorders can now be treated with enzyme replacement therapies (ERT) or stem cell and gene therapies. In some conditions, simple and established dietary measures may halt or reverse the process. Dementia in many of these neurological syndromes provides models for understanding the neuroanatomical substrates underpinning clinical dementia subtypes (Varma and Trimble, 1997; Bonelli and Cummings, 2008).

Box 80.3 Dementia associated with inherited metabolic diseases.

- Predominantly neurological disease:
  - Predominantly white matter
    * Metachromatic leukodystrophy
    * Adrenoleukodystrophy
    * Cerebrotendinous xanthomatosis
  - Predominantly grey matter
    * GM2 gangliosidosis
    * Kufs' disease
    * Lafora body disease
- Associated systemic disease:
  Gaucher disease
  - Niemann–Pick disease type C
  - Wilson's disease
- Prominent extrapyramidal signs:
  - Wilson's disease
  - Metachromatic leukodystrophy
  - Kufs' disease
  - GM2 gangliosidosis
  - Niemann–Pick disease type C
  - Gaucher disease

80.6.1   Metachromatic leukodystrophy

Metachromatic leukodystrophy (MLD) is an autosomal recessive (AR) disorder due to arylsulphatase deficiency. Sulphatide accumulation, especially in the brain and peripheral nerves is accompanied by central and peripheral demyelination. Late infantile, juvenile and adult forms are recognized. The adult form usually presents in the 20s, although late onset cases in the sixties have been described (Duyff and Weinstein, 1996). Adults usually present with personality change and intellectual deterioration (Hageman *et al.*, 1995), although mainly motor forms (pyramidal, extrapyramidal and cerebellar involvement with peripheral neuropathy) exist (Baumann *et al.*, 2002). Some of these patients have psychotic features and could be misdiagnosed as schizophrenia (Hyde *et al.*, 1992). Neurological signs may appear several years after the onset of psychosis (Letournel and Dubas, 2008).

The disease progresses over about 20 years and in the terminal stages patients become quadriparetic and mute. The diagnosis is confirmed by demonstration of reduced arylsulphatase activity in peripheral blood white cells. CSF studies reveal raised protein. T_2-weighted MRI brain scans show bilaterally symmetrical, predominantly periventricular high signal changes in the deep white matter and centrum semiovale, initially with frontal predominance, progressing to corpus callosum, internal capsules and pyramidal tracts (Faerber *et al.*, 1999; Vanderver, 2005; Sedel *et al.*, 2008). Bone marrow transplantation may prolong survival and cognition (Letournel and Dubas, 2008; Sedel *et al.*, 2008).

80.6.2   Adrenoleukodystrophy

Adrenoleukodystrophy (ALD) is an X-linked disorder (gene locus on Xq28) characterized by impaired ability to oxidize very long chain fatty acids (VLCFA), leading to their accumulation in the brain and adrenal glands (Igarashi *et al.*, 1976). Moser (1997) and colleagues (Moser *et al.*, 1984) found that isolated cerebral forms occur in 30 per cent, solitary adrenomyeloneuropathy in 20 per cent and combined childhood cerebral and myelopathic forms in the remainder. Most cases present in the first decade with decline in intellect, change in personality with inappropriate laughter and crying. Unsteadiness, incoordination and intention tremor soon develop. Vomiting, circulatory collapse, oral mucosal and skin pigmentation may occur. In the late stage blindness, deafness, pseudobulbar paralysis and bilateral hemiplegia supervene. Adult cerebral forms of ALD present with psychiatric and cognitive symptoms, progressing with motor signs, optic atrophy and seizures, to death (Kitchin *et al.*, 1987; van Geel *et al.*, 2001; Sedel *et al.*, 2008).

White matter changes on brain MRI precede clinical signs and start in the parieto-occipital regions, spreading to the splenium and corpus callosum (Vanderver, 2005). The diagnosis is confirmed by the demonstration of an excess of VLCFA in blood (plasma, red and white cells). Markers of adrenal insufficiency support the diagnosis. Dietary supplementation with monounsaturated fatty acids and bone marrow transplantation stabilize disability (van Geel *et al.*, 1997; Letournel and Dubas, 2008).

80.6.3   Cerebrotendinous xanthomatosis

Cerebrotendinous xanthomatosis (CTX) is a rare but treatable AR disorder with accumulation of cholestanol and cholesterol. Patients usually present in the second and third decades. Juvenile cataracts or diarrhoea may present from childhood. Tendon (mainly Achilles) xanthomas are noted in 30–70 per cent of cases (Sedel *et al.*, 2008). With progression, intellectual deficit and inattentiveness give way to progressive dementia, spasticity, ataxia, pseudobulbar palsy and peripheral neuropathy (Moghadasian *et al.*, 2002).

CT and MRI demonstrate diffuse brain and spinal cord atrophy, white matter changes, characteristically in dentate nuclei of cerebellum, and occasionally focal lesions (Kaye, 2001; Sedel *et al.*, 2008). Laboratory investigations reveal elevated levels of plasma and bile cholestanol (normally cholestanol is 0.1–0.2 per cent of total cholesterol; in CTX there is a 10- to 100-fold rise) and increased urinary excretion of bile alcohol glucuronides (Koopman *et al.*, 1988). Treatment with chenodeoxycholic acid may reverse neurological deficits, especially when started in young patients (Berginer *et al.*, 1984).

80.6.4   Late-onset GM2 gangliosidosis (LGG)

GM2 gangliosidosis is due to deficiency of hexosaminidase A, which leads to accumulation of gangliosides in neurones (Argov and Navon, 1984). Late-onset GM2 gangliosidosis (LGG) presents in adolescence and young adulthood. Cognitive dysfunction can be marked, progressive with a subcortical pattern of breakdown and is invariably associated with motor, cerebellar or extrapyramidal deficits (Frey *et al.*, 2005).

The diagnosis is confirmed by enzyme assays in white cells. MRI shows generalized atrophy with particularly severe cerebellar involvement (Clarke, 2002). Electromyography reveals denervation even in patients without overt clinical signs.

80.6.5   Kufs' disease (neuronal ceroid lipofuscinosis)

Kufs' disease is the juvenile/adult form of neuronal ceroid lipofuscinosis (NCL), a group of lysosomal storage disorders. Approximately 160 NCL mutations have been found in eight genes (*CLN1, CLN2, CLN3, CLN5, CLN6, CLN7, CLN8, CLN10*) (Jalanko and Braulke, 2009). Unlike the early onset forms, Kufs' disease develops later (15–25 years) and is unattended by retinal and visual changes (Berkovic *et al.*, 1988). Most cases are AR, although dominant patterns have been described (Josephson *et al.*, 2001). Type A, the epileptic form, includes generalized seizures (myoclonus, prolonged tonic phases, and photosensitivity), ataxia, pyramidal and extrapyramidal signs. Type B, the psychiatric form, is characterized by progressive dementia, neuropsychiatric symptoms including behavioural changes and psychosis, ataxia and movement disorder (Berkovic *et al.*, 1988; Hinkebein and Callahan, 1997; Sedel *et al.*, 2007).

The diagnosis may prove difficult and involves demonstration of accumulation of autofluorescent ceroid and lipofuscin in nerve-containing tissue (Goebel and Braak, 1989). Skin or rectal biopsies can be positive and are easier to obtain than brain tissue. The disease is relentlessly progressive, resulting in death after 10–15 years.

80.6.6   Lafora body disease

Lafora body disease (LD) is an AR disorder usually presenting with intractable seizures in the second decade. Myoclonus and occipital seizures are characteristic. Dysarthria, ataxia, emotional disturbances, confusion and dementia develop gradually. Patients progress to severe dementia and become bed-bound, remaining in near continuous myoclonus with seizures, mutism and quadriparesis. Death occurs within ten years of onset (Minassian, 2001). LD is caused by mutations in *EPM2A* or *EPM2B* genes encoding the proteins laforin and malin (Serratosa *et al.*, 1995; Minassian *et al.*, 1998; Ramachandran *et al.*, 2009).

The EEG shows generalized epileptiform discharges with photomyoclonus and a slow background. Skin, liver, muscle or brain biopsies may reveal the pathognomonic PAS-positive Lafora bodies. At pathology Lafora bodies, composed of polyglucosans, are present throughout the brain, especially in the cerebral and cerebellar cortices, basal ganglia, thalamus and the spinal cord. Similar accumulations are also found in skin, muscle, heart and liver.

80.6.7   Gaucher disease

Gaucher disease is an AR inherited lysosomal storage disorder due to glucocerebrosidase deficiency. Glucocerebroside accumulates in visceral organs, reticuloendothelial tissue and the nervous system.

The clinical manifestations of Gaucher disease vary enormously. Many patients remain asymptomatic lifelong; at the opposite end of the spectrum, some patients with the rare acute neuronopathic form die by the age of 18 months. Type I Gaucher disease is without neurological manifestations and visceral manifestations include hepatosplenomegaly, anemia, thrombocytopenia and skeletal abnormalities. The adult forms are stable and slowly progressive. Type II Gaucher disease is characterized by early onset neurological and visceral disease. Severe neck rigidity and arching, bulbar signs, appendicular rigidity, chorea and dystonia follow eye movement disorders and strabismus. Type III Gaucher disease is the intermediate form with onset between 0.1 and 14 years (usually one year). Eye movement disorders, ataxia, spasticity, slowly progressive dementia may be accompanied with visceral involvement (Balicki and Beutler, 1995).

Investigations show a rise in acid phosphatase, characteristic histiocytes (Gaucher cells) in marrow smears and liver or spleen biopsies. The diagnosis is confirmed by detecting reduced glucocerebrosidase activity in peripheral white cells. Type I Gaucher disease responds to ERT with recombinant glucocerebrosidase (Charrow *et al.*, 2004; Platt

and Lachmann, 2009), but its potential in neurological disease is not established (Sedel *et al.*, 2007).

80.6.8   Niemann–Pick disease type C

Niemann-Pick disease type C (NPD-C) is a lipid storage disorder with hepatosplenomegaly and a variety of neurological and psychiatric symptoms and signs (Patterson, 2003). The diagnosis should be considered in any individual with unexplained dementia or psychiatric impairment, especially when accompanied by ataxia, dystonia or vertical supranuclear gaze palsy. The absence of organomegaly, normal imaging or bone marrow biopsy does not rule out the diagnosis.

NPD-C can present at any age. Psychiatric and cognitive dysfunction predominate in later onset presentations. Dysarthria, dementia and ataxia may be accompanied by vertical supranuclear gaze palsy. Psychosis is an occasional presenting feature and rarely choreoathetosis occurs. A mixture of partial and generalized seizures may occur. Gelastic cataplexy (ranging from subtle head nodding to profound atonia, usually provoked by humorous situations) is seen in approximately 20 per cent of patients (Shulman *et al.*, 1995a; Shulman *et al.*, 1995b).

Most patients with NPD-C have mutations in the *NPC1* and *NPC2* genes on chromosome 18. The diagnosis is strongly supported by detecting polymorphous cytoplasmic bodies on electron microscopic (EM) examination of skin. Until the recent approval of miglustat, no disease-modifying treatment was available for NPD-C. Miglustat can stabilize neurological disease. The NP-C Guidelines Working Group has laid down recommendations for diagnosis and treatment (Wraith *et al.*, 2009).

80.6.9   Wilson's disease

Wilson's disease (WD) is an AR disorder of copper homeostasis. The responsible *ATP7B* gene is located on chromosome 13. Most clinical manifestations are attributable to copper accumulation, especially in the brain and liver (Jones and Weissenborn, 1997; Gitlin, 2003; Pfeiffer, 2007).

Between 40 and 60 per cent of individuals with WD may present with neurological disorder in the second or third decades of life. Incoordination, clumsiness, tremor, dysarthria, excess salivation, dysphagia and movement disorders (a variety of tremors, dystonia, bradykinesia, chorea) produce a prominent motor syndrome. Psychiatric symptoms dominate the clinical picture in a third of all patients and include behavioural and personality changes, psychosis, depression and/or cognitive impairment (Jones and Weissenborn, 1997; Gitlin, 2003; Ala *et al.*, 2007). T_2-weighted MRI may reveal the 'face of the giant panda' sign consisting of high signal in the midbrain tegmentum except the red nucleus, preservation of signal in the substantia nigra and hypointensity of the superior colliculus (Hitoshi *et al.*, 1991). Slit lamp examination reveals Kayser–Fleischer rings and peripheral blood ceruloplasmin concentration is <20 mg/dL. Urinary copper excretion is >100 µg/24 hours (normal <40). Treatment requires lifelong chelation with D-penicillamine, trientine or tetrathiomolybdate. Advanced liver failure may require transplantation (Jones and Weissenborn, 1997; Gitlin, 2003).

80.6.10   Mitochondrial disorders

Mitochondrial disorders, especially respiratory chain diseases (RCD) may present as single or multiple organ involvement. The skeletal and nervous systems are preferentially affected. RCDs may present with (1) a progressive course, (2) neuro-muscular disorders or CNS manifestations including epilepsy, stroke-like episodes, migraine, ataxia, movement disorders, demyelination, psychosis and dementia, (3) involvement of seemingly unrelated organs or tissues (Munnich and Rustin, 2001; Finsterer, 2008).

The central and/or peripheral nervous system may be involved. Patients may present with a range of manifestations, i.e. encephalopathy, brainstem involvement (ophthalmoplegia), cerebellar disorders (ataxia), myoclonus, seizures, pyramidal dysfunction, leukodystrophy, poliodystrophy or peripheral neuropathy and/or myopathy. MELAS (mitochondrial encephalomyopathy with lactic acidosis and stroke-like episodes), MERRF (myoclonic epilepsy with ragged red fibres), subacute necrotizing encephalomyopathy (Leigh syndrome), MNGIE (mitochondrial myopathy, peripheral neuropathy, encephalopathy and gastrointestinal disease), are commonly recognized syndromic RCDs, whereas progressive external ophthalmoplegia (PEO) and Kearns–Sayre syndrome (KSS) are predominantly mitochondrial myopathic syndromes (Rahman and Schapira, 1999).

Cognitive impairment and dementia are common features of mitochondrial disorders and Finsterer (2008) has proposed the term 'mitochondrial dementia'. His exhaustive review lists various syndromic and non-syndromic RCDs associated with dementia. Various cognitive functions affected in RCDs include memory, language, executive function, attention and visuospatial ability (Sartor et al., 2002; Finsterer, 2008). Turconi et al. (1999) found memory and constructional impairment in PEO, KSS and one patient with MERRF. In a similar group of syndromic RCDs, Bosbach et al. (2003) uncovered executive impairment, constructional and attentional difficulties suggesting frontosubcortical dysfunction. Occasionally, an initial focal cognitive impairment may gradually progress to dementia (Finsterer, 2008). These patients are usually younger and the onset may suggest an encephalitic illness, although longitudinal follow up clearly documents progressive decline. Such cases are confused with focal atrophies of the FTLD variety or focal presentations of AD. A complete physical and neurological examination may provide clues, aided by imaging features atypical for FTLD and AD. MRI may show marked focal white matter hyperintensities, cystic lesions more commonly in parietotemporal regions, focal intracerebral microbleeds and basal ganglia calcifications (Abe et al., 2004). None of these features are seen in degenerative dementias.

An underlying mitochondrial disorder is suspected in patients with dementia if they are younger, with a short stature, migraine-like headaches, epilepsy, deafness, diabetes mellitus and/or neurological signs of PEO, myopathy, neuropathy, myoclonus, ataxia and other multisystem

---

Box 80.4 Myoclonic dementias.

Alzheimer's disease
Dementia with Lewy bodies
Creutzfeldt–Jakob disease
Metabolic encephalopathy
Hashimoto's encephalopathy
Cerebral vasculitis
Limbic encephalitis
HIV associated dementia
Whipple's disease
Corticobasal syndrome
Mitochondrial encephalomyopathy
Lafora body disease
Kufs' disease
GM2 gangliosidosis

---

involvement. T_2-weighted MRI may show high signal changes in the deep white matter or grey–white interface, especially posteriorly, along with the abnormalities described above. Magnetic resonance spectroscopy may show elevated lactate in the stroke-like lesion (Abe et al., 2004; Finsterer, 2008). Neurophysiology may reveal neuropathy in a third of cases; electromyography may be normal, neurogenic and/or myogenic. EEG may be slow and reflect encephalopathy. CSF protein is raised in KSS; CSF lactate may be elevated, for example, in MELAS, MERRF or Leigh syndromes. Muscle biopsy may show ragged red fibres (MELAS, MERRF) on light microscopy; further immunohistochemical and electron microscopy studies may detail mitochondrial abnormalities. Negative genetic tests require cautious interpretation. Mitochondrial deletions are usually not detected in blood. Further DNA analysis from muscle tissue may be required (Rahman and Schapira, 1999; Munnich and Rustin 2001; Finsterer, 2008). Treatment remains symptomatic.

80.7   CONCLUSION

An awareness of underlying clinical syndromes (**Box 80.1**, **Box 80.2**, **Box 80.3** and **Box 80.4**) and a high index of suspicion are required, first to consider, and then to accurately diagnose uncommon forms of dementia. Some of these disorders can be conclusively diagnosed with the help of biological markers (biochemical or genetic) or radiological findings. Since effective treatments may reverse some conditions (infective, inflammatory and metabolic), knowledge of these dementias, although uncommon, is essential. Insights into disease mechanisms of some of these disorders (e.g. HIV) also provide fresh opportunities to understand neurodegenerative diseases, including the primary dementias.

REFERENCES

Abe K, Yoshimura H, Tanaka H et al. (2004) Comparison of conventional and diffusion weighted MRI and proton MR spectroscopy in patients with mitochondrial encephalomyopathy, lactic acidosis and stroke like events. *Neuroradiology* **46**: 113–17.

Ala A, Walker AP, Ashkan K *et al.* (2007) Wilson's disease. *Lancet* **369**: 397–408.

Albert ML, Feldman RG, Day J *et al.* (1974) The 'subcortical dementia' of progressive supranuclear palsy. *Journal of Neurology, Neurosurgery and Psychiatry* **37**: 121–30.

Almeida OP, Lautenschlager NT. (2005) Dementia associated with infectious diseases. *International Psychogeriatrics* **17** (Suppl.): S65–7.

Alrawi A, Trobe JD, Blaivas M, Musch DC. (1999) Brain biopsy in primary angiitis of the central nervous system. *Neurology* **53**: 858–60.

Anderson NE, Barber PA. (2008) Limbic encephalitis – a review. *Journal of Clinical Neuroscience* **15**: 961–71.

Antinori A, Arendt G, Becker JT *et al.* (2007) Updated research nosology for HIV-associated neurocognitive disorders. *Neurology* **69**: 1789–99.

Argov Z, Navon R. (1984) Clinical and genetic variations in the syndrome of adult GM2 gangliosidosis resulting from hexosaminidase A deficiency. *Annals of Neurology* **16**: 14–20.

Asato R, Akiguchi I, Masunaga S, Hashimoto N. (2000) Magnetic resonance imaging distinguishes progressive supranuclear palsy from multiple system atrophy. *Journal of Neural Transmission* **107**: 1427–36.

Balicki D, Beutler E. (1995) Gaucher disease. *Medicine (Baltimore)* **74**: 305–23.

Baumann N, Turpin J-C, Lefevre M, Colsch B. (2002) Motor and psycho-cognitive clinical types in adult metachromatic leukodystrophy: genotype/phenotype relationships? *Journal of Physiology, Paris* **96**: 301–6.

Benito-Leon J, Sedano LF, Louis ED. (2008) Isolated central nervous system Whipple's disease causing reversible frontotemporal-like dementia. *Clinical Neurology and Neurosurgery* **110**: 747–9.

Berginer VM, Salen G, Shefer S. (1984) Long term treatment of cerebrotendinous xanthomatosis with chenodeoxycholic acid. *New England Journal of Medicine* **311**: 1649–52.

Berkovic SF, Carpenter S, Andermann F *et al.* (1988) Kufs' disease: a critical appraisal. *Brain* **111**: 27–62.

Birnbaum J, Hellman DB. (2009) Primary angiitis of the central nervous system. *Archives of Neurology* **66**: 704–9.

Bonelli RM, Cummings JL. (2008) Frontal-subcortical dementias. *The Neurologist* **14**: 100–7.

Bosbach S, Kornblum C, Schroder R, Wagner M. (2003) Executive and visuospatial deficits in patients with chronic progressive external ophthalmoplegia and Kearns–Sayre syndrome. *Brain* **126**: 1231–40.

Brew BJ. (2007) AIDS dementia complex. In: Portegies P, Berger JR (eds). *Handbook of clinical neurology*, vol. 85. 3rd series, HIV/AIDS and the nervous system. Oxford: Elsevier, 79–91.

Brooks DJ. (1993) Functional imaging in relation to Parkinsonian syndromes. *Journal of the Neurological Sciences* **115**: 1–17.

Brooks DJ, Seppi K. (2009) Proposed neuroimaging criteria for the diagnosis of multiple system atrophy. *Movement Disorders* **24**: 949–64.

Burn DJ, Lees AJ. (2002) Progressive supranuclear palsy: where are we now? *Lancet Neurology* **1**: 359–69.

Chang CC, Chang YY, Chang WN *et al.* (2009) Cognitive deficits in multiple system atrophy correlate with frontal atrophy and disease duration. *European Journal of Neurology* **16**: 1144–50.

Charrow J, Andersson HC, Kaplan P *et al.* (2004) Enzyme replacement therapy and monitoring for children with Type 1 Gaucher disease: consensus recommendations. *Journal of Paediatrics* **144**: 112–20.

Chen-Hsiang L, Wei-Che L, Cheng-Hsien L, Jein-Wei L. (2009) Initially unrecognised dementia in a young man with neurosyphilis. *The Neurologist* **15**: 95–7.

Chong JY, Rowland LP, Utiger RD. (2003) Hashimoto encephalopathy: syndrome or myth? *Archives of Neurology* **60**: 164–71.

Clarke JTR. (2002) *A clinical guide to inherited metabolic diseases*, 2nd edn. Cambridge: Cambridge University Press, 18–64.

Coker SB. (1991) The diagnosis of childhood neurodegenerative disorders presenting as dementia in adults. *Neurology* **41**: 794–8.

Corsellis JA, Goldberg GJ, Norton AR. (1968) 'Limbic encephalitis' and its association with carcinoma. *Brain* **91**: 481–96.

Dalmau J, Gleichman AJ, Hughes EG *et al.* (2008) Anti-NMDA-receptor encephalitis: case series and analysis of the effects of antibodies. *Lancet Neurology* **7**: 1091–8.

Delanty N, Georgescu L, Lynch T *et al.* (1999) Synovial fluid polymerase chain reaction as an aid to the diagnosis of central nervous system Whipple's disease. *Annals of Neurology* **45**: 137–8.

Devito EE, Pickard JD, Salmond CH *et al.* (2005) The neuropsychology of normal pressure hydrocephalus. *British Journal of Neurosurgery* **19**: 217–24.

Duyff RF, Weinstein HC. (1996) Late-presenting metachromatic leukodystrophy. *Lancet* **348**: 1382–3.

Faerber EN, Melvin J, Smergel EM. (1999) MRI appearances of metachromatic leukodystrophy. *Pediatric Radiology* **29**: 669–72.

Fallon BA, Nields JA. (1994) Lyme disease: a neuropsychiatric illness. *American Journal of Psychiatry* **151**: 1571–83.

Finsterer J. (2008) Cognitive decline as a manifestation of mitochondrial disorders (mitochondrial dementia). *Journal of the Neurological Sciences* **272**: 20–33.

Frey LC, Ringel SP, Filley CM. (2005) The natural history of cognitive dysfunction in late-onset GM2 gangliosidosis. *Archives of Neurology* **62**: 989–94.

Geschwind MD, Shu H, Haman A *et al.* (2008) Rapidly progressive dementia. *Annals of Neurology* **64**: 97–108.

Gibb WRG, Luthert PJ, Marsden CD. (1989) Corticobasal degeneration. *Brain* **112**: 1171–92.

Gilman S, Low P, Quinn N *et al.* (1999) Consensus statement on the diagnosis of multiple system atrophy. *Journal of the Neurological Sciences* **163**: 94–8.

Gilman S, Wenning GK, Low PA *et al.* (2008) Second consensus statement on the diagnosis of MSA. *Neurology* **71**: 670–6.

Gitlin JA. (2003) Wilson disease. *Gastroenterology* **125**: 1868–77.

Goebel HH, Braak H. (1989) Adult neuronal ceroid-lipofuscinosis. *Clinical Neuropathology* **8**: 109–19.

Graham J, Oppenheimer DR. (1969) Orthostatic hypotension and nicotine sensitivity in a case of multiple system atrophy. *Journal of Neurology, Neurosurgery and Psychiatry* 32: 28–34.

Gultekin HS, Rosenfeld MR, Voltz R *et al.* (2000) Paraneoplastic limbic encephalitis: neurological symptoms, immunological findings and tumour association in 50 patients. *Brain* 123: 1481–94.

Hachinski V. (1997) Frontotemporal degeneration, Pick disease, and corticobasal degeneration: One entity or 3? *Archives of Neurology* 54: 1429.

Hageman ATM, Gabreel FJM, De Jong JGN *et al.* (1995) Clinical symptoms of adult metachromatic leukodystrophy and arylsulphatase A pseudodeficiency. *Archives of Neurology* 52: 408–13.

Hajj-Ali RA, Calabrese LH. (2009) Central nervous system vasculitis. *Current Opinion in Rheumatology* 21: 10–18.

Hakim S, Adams RD. (1965) The special clinical problem of symptomatic hydrocephalus with normal cerebrospinal fluid pressure. *Journal of the Neurological Sciences* 2: 307–27.

Halperin JJ, Logigian EL, Finkel MF *et al.* (1996) Practice parameters for the diagnosis of patients with nervous system Lyme borreliosis (Lyme disease). *Neurology* 46: 619–27.

Hinkebein JH, Callahan CD. (1997) The neuropsychology of Kufs' disease: a case of atypical early onset dementia. *Archives of Clinical Neuropsychology* 12: 81–9.

Hitoshi S, Iwata M, Yoshikawa K. (1991) Mid-brain pathology of Wilson's disease: MRI analysis of three cases. *Journal of Neurology, Neurosurgery and Psychiatry* 54: 624–6.

Hossain AK, Murata Y, Zhang L *et al.* (2003) Brain perfusion SPECT in patients with corticobasal degeneration: analysis using statistical parametric mapping. *Movement Disorders* 18: 697–703.

Hyde TM, Ziegler JC, Weinberger DR *et al.* (1992) Psychiatric disturbances in metachromatic leukodystrophy: insight into the neurobiology of psychosis. *Archives of Neurology* 49: 401–6.

Igarashi M, Schaumburg HH, Powers J *et al.* (1976) Fatty acid abnormality in adrenoleukodystrophy. *Journal of Neurochemistry* 26: 851–60.

Jalanko A, Braulke T. (2009) Neuronal ceroid lipofuscinosis. *Biochimica et Biophysica Acta* 1793: 697–709.

Jayadev S, Garden GA. (2009) Host and viral factors influencing the pathogenesis of HIV-associated neurocognitive disorders. *Journal of Neuroimmune Pharmacology* 4: 175–89.

Jellinger KA, Blancher C. (1992) Neuropathology. In: Litvan I, Agid Y (eds). *Progressive supranuclear palsy: clinical and research approaches.* Oxford: Oxford University Press, 44–88.

Jones EA, Weissenborn K. (1997) Neurology and the liver. *Journal of Neurology, Neurosurgery and Psychiatry* 63: 279–93.

Joseph FG, Scolding NJ. (2002) Cerebral vasculitis. *A practical approach. Practical Neurology* 2: 80–93.

Josephs KA, Tang-Wai DF, Edland SD *et al.* (2004) Correlation between antemortem magnetic resonance imaging findings and pathologically confirmed corticobasal degeneration. *Archives of Neurology* 61: 1881–4.

Josephson SA, Schmidt RE, Millsap P *et al.* (2001) Autosomal dominant Kufs' disease: a cause of early onset dementia. *Journal of the Neurological Sciences* 188: 51–60.

Kaplan RF, Trevino RP, Johnson GM *et al.* (2003) Cognitive function in post-treatment Lyme disease. Do additional antibiotics help? *Neurology* 60: 1916–22.

Kaul M. (2009) HIV-1 associated dementia: update on pathological mechanisms and therapeutic approaches. *Current Opinion in Neurology* 22: 315–20.

Kaye EM. (2001) Update on genetic disorders affecting white matter. *Pediatric Neurology* 24: 11–24.

Kertesz A. (1997) Frontotemporal degeneration, Pick disease, and corticobasal degeneration one entity or 3? 1. *Archives of Neurology* 54: 1427–9.

Kertesz A, McMonagle P. (2010) Behavior and cognition in corticobasal degeneration and progressive supranuclear palsy. *Journal of Neurological Sciences* 289: 138–43.

Kim YJ, Ichise M, Ballinger JR *et al.* (2002) Combination of dopamine transporter and D2 receptor SPECT in the diagnostic evaluation of PD, MSA and PSP. *Movement Disorders* 17: 45–53.

Kitayama M, Wada-Isoe K, Irizawa Y, Nakashima K. (2009) Assessment of dementia in patients with multiple system atrophy. *European Journal of Neurology* 16: 589–94.

Kitchin W, Cohen-Cole SA, Mickel SF. (1987) Adrenoleukodystrophy: frequency of presentation as a psychiatric disorder. *Biological Psychiatry* 22: 1375–87.

Knopman DS, DeKosky ST, Cummings JL *et al.* (2001) Practice parameter: diagnosis of dementia (an evidence-based review), Report of the quality standards subcommittee of the American academy of neurology. *Neurology* 56: 1143–53.

Koopman BJ, Wolthers BG, van der Slik W *et al.* (1988) Cerebrotendinous xanthomatosis: a review of biochemical findings of the patient population in the Netherlands. *Journal of Inherited Metabolic Diseases* 11: 56–75.

Kothbauer-Margreiter I, Sturzenegger M, Komor J *et al.* (1996) Encephalopathy associated with Hashimoto thyroiditis: diagnosis and treatment. *Journal of Neurology* 243: 585–93.

Kraft E, Schwarz J, Trenkwalder C *et al.* (1999) The combination of hypointense and hyperintense signal changes on T2 weighted magnetic resonance imaging sequences: a specific marker of multiple system atrophy? *Archives of Neurology* 56: 225–8.

Krauss JM, von Stuckrad-Barre SF. (2008) Clinical aspects and biology of normal pressure hydrocephalus. In: Duyckaerts C, Litvan I (eds). *Handbook of clinical neurology,* vol. 89. 3rd series, Dementias. Oxford: Elsevier, 887–902.

Leesch W, Fischer I, Staudinger R *et al.* (2009) Primary cerebral Whipple disease presenting as Klüver-Bucy syndrome. *Archives of Neurology* 66: 130–1.

Letournel F, Dubas F. (2008) Leukodystrophies: clinical and therapeutic aspects. In: Duyckaerts C, Litvan I (eds). *Handbook of clinical neurology,* vol. 89. 3rd series, Dementias. Oxford: Elsevier, 726–35.

Litvan I, Bhatia KP, Burn DJ *et al.* (2003) Movement disorders society scientific issues committee report, SIC Task Force Appraisal of Clinical Diagnostic Criteria for Parkinsonian Disorders. *Movement Disorders* 18: 467–86.

Louis ED, Lynch T, Kaufmann P *et al.* (1996) Diagnostic guidelines in central nervous system Whipple's disease. *Annals of Neurology* 40: 561–8.

Ludolph AC, Kassubek J, Landwehrmeyer BG *et al.* (2009) Tauopathies with parkinsonism: clinical spectrum, neuropathologic basis, biological markers, and treatment options. *European Journal of Neurology* **16**: 297–309.

Luo W, Ouyang Z, Xu H *et al.* (2008) The clinical analysis of general paresis with 5 cases. *Journal of Neuropsychiatry and Clinical Neurosciences* **20**: 490–3.

Lynn WA, Lightman S. (2004) Syphilis and HIV: a dangerous combination. *Lancet Infectious Diseases* **4**: 456–66.

Maher ER, Lees AJ. (1986) The clinical features and natural history of Steele–Richardson–Olszweski syndrome (progressive supranuclear palsy). *Neurology* **36**: 1005–8.

Markus HS, Lees AJ, Lennox G *et al.* (1995) Patterns of regional cerebral blood flow in corticobasal degeneration studied using HMPAO SPECT; comparison with Parkinson's disease and normal controls. *Movement Disorders* **10**: 179–87.

Marth T, Raoult D. (2003) Whipple's disease. *Lancet* **361**: 239–46.

McArthur JC. (2004) HIV dementia: An evolving disease. *Journal of Neuroimmunology* **157**: 3–10.

Minassian BA. (2001) Lafora's disease: towards a clinical, pathologic and molecular synthesis. *Pediatric Neurology* **25**: 21–9.

Minassian BA, Lee JR, Herbrick JA *et al.* (1998) Mutations in a gene encoding a novel protein tyrosine phosphatase cause progressive myoclonus epilepsy. *Nature Genetics* **20**: 171–4.

Moghadasian MH, Salen G, Frohlich JJ, Scudamore CH. (2002) Cerebrotendinous xanthomatosis. A rare disease with diverse manifestations. *Archives of Neurology* **59**: 527–9.

Moser HW. (1997) Adrenoleukodystrophy: Phenotype, genetics, pathogenesis and therapy. *Brain* **120**: 1485–508.

Moser HW, Moser AW, Singh I *et al.* (1984) Adrenoleukodystrophy: survey of 303 cases: biochemistry, diagnosis, therapy. *Annals of Neurology* **16**: 628–41.

Munnich A, Rustin P. (2001) Clinical spectrum and diagnosis of mitochondrial disorders. *American Journal of Medical Genetics* **106**: 4–17.

Nath A, Svhiess N, Venkatesan A *et al.* (2008) Evolution of HIV dementia with HIV infection. *International Review of Psychiatry* **20**: 25–31.

Neary D. (1997) Frontotemporal degeneration, Pick disease, and corticobasal degeneration. One entity or 3? 3. *Archives of Neurology* **54**: 1425–7.

Neary D, Snowden JS, Gustafson L *et al.* (1998) Frontotemporal lobar degeneration: a consensus on clinical diagnostic criteria. *Neurology* **51**: 1546–54.

Nitrini R. (2008) Clinical and therapeutic aspects of dementia in syphilis and Lyme disease. In: Duyckaerts C, Litvan I (eds). *Handbook of clinical neurology*, vol. 89. 3rd series. Dementias. Oxford: Elsevier, 819–23.

Noorbakhsh F, Overall CM, Power C. (2009) Deciphering complex mechanisms in neurodegenerative diseases: the advent of systems biology. *Trends in Neurosciences* **32**: 88–100.

Osaki Y, Ben-Shlomo Y, Lees AJ *et al.* (2004) Accuracy of clinical diagnosis of progressive supranuclear palsy. *Movement Disorders* **19**: 181–9.

Panegyres PK. (2008) Diagnosis and management of Whipple's disease of the brain. *Practical Neurology* **8**: 311–17.

Panegyres PK, Edis R, Beaman M, Fallon M. (2006) Primary Whipple's disease of the brain: characterisation of the clinical syndrome and molecular diagnosis. *Quarterly Journal of Medicine* **99**: 609–23.

Patterson MC. (2003) A riddle wrapped in a mystery: understanding Niemann–Pick disease, type C. *The Neurologist* **9**: 301–10.

Pfeiffer RF. (2007) Wilson's disease. *Seminars in Neurology* **27**: 123–32.

Platt FM, Lachmann RH. (2009) Treating lysosomal storage disorders: current practice and future prospects. *Biochimica et Biophysica Acta* **1793**: 737–45.

Rahman S, Schapira AHV. (1999) Mitochondrial myopathies: clinical features, molecular genetics, investigation and management. In: Schapira AHV, Griggs RC (eds). *Muscle diseases*. Blue Books of Practical Neurology, 24. Woburn, MA: Butterworth-Heinemann, 177–223.

Ramachandran N, Girard J-M, Turnbull J, Minassian BA. (2009) The autosomal recessively inherited progressive myoclonus epilepsies and their genes. *Epilepsia* **50** (Suppl. 5): 29–36.

Ribeiz JJ, Kolodny EH, Richardson EP. (1968) Corticodentatonigral degeneration with neuronal achromasia. *Archives of Neurology* **18**: 20–33.

Robbins TW, James M, Lange KW *et al.* (1992) Cognitive performances in multiple system atrophy. *Brain* **115**: 271–91.

Ropper AH, Brown RH. (eds) (2005) Disturbances of cerebrospinal fluid and its circulation including hydrocephalus, pseudotumour cerebri and low pressure syndromes. In: *Adam's and Victor's Principles of neurology*. New York, NY: McGraw-Hill, 529–45.

Salvarani C, Brown Jr RD, Calamia KT *et al.* (2007) Primary central nervous system vasculitis: analysis of 101 patients. *Annals of Neurology* **62**: 442–51.

Sartor H, Loose R, Tucha O *et al.* (2002) MELAS: a neuropsychological and radiological follow-up study. Mitochondrial encephalomyopathy, lactic acidosis and stroke. *Acta Neurologica Scandinavica* **106**: 309–13.

Savoiardo M. (2003) Differential diagnosis of Parkinson's disease and atypical parkinsonian disorders by magnetic resonance imaging. *Neurological Sciences* **24** (Suppl. 1): S35–7.

Schrag A, Good CD, Miszkiel K *et al.* (2000) Differentiation of atypical parkinsonian syndromes with routine MRI. *Neurology* **54**: 697–702.

Scheiss N, Pardo CA. (2008) Hashimoto's encephalopathy. *Annals of the New York Academy of Sciences* **1142**: 254–65.

Sedel F, Gourfinkel-An I, Lyon-Caen O *et al.* (2007) Epilepsy and inborn errors of metabolism in adults: A diagnostic approach. *Journal of Inherited Metabolic Diseases* **30**: 846–54.

Sedel F, Tourbah A, Fontaine B *et al.* (2008) Leukoencephalopathies associated with inborn errors of metabolism in adults. *Journal of Inherited Metabolic Diseases* **31**: 295–307.

Serratosa JM, Delgado-Escueta AV, Posada I *et al.* (1995) The gene for progressive myoclonus epilepsy of the Lafora type maps to chromosome 6q. *Human Molecular Genetics* **4**: 1657–63.

Seppi K. (2007) MRI for the differential diagnosis of neurodegenerative parkinsonism in clinical practice. *Parkinsonism and Related Disorders* **13**: S400–5.

Sha S, Hou C, Viscontas IV, Miller BL. (2006) Are frontotemporal lobar degeneration, progressive supranuclear palsy and corticobasal degeneration distinct diseases. *Nature Clinical Practice Neurology* 2: 658–65.

Shaw PJ, Walls TJ, Newman PK *et al.* (1991) Hashimoto's encephalopathy: a steroid responsive disorder associated with high antithyroid antibody titres – report of five cases. *Neurology* 41: 228–33.

Shprecher D, Schwalb J, Kurlan R. (2008) Normal pressure hudrocephalus: diagnosis and treatment. *Current Neurology Neuroscience Reports* 8: 371–6.

Shulman LM, David NJ, Weiner WJ. (1995a) Psychosis as the initial manifestation of adult-onset Niemann Pick disease type C. *Neurology* 45: 1739–43.

Shulman LM, Lang AE, Jankovic J *et al.* (1995b) Case 1, 1995: psychosis, dementia, chorea, ataxia, and supranuclear gaze dysfunction. *Movement Disorders* 10: 257–62.

Simms I, Fenton KA, Ashton M *et al.* (2005) The re-emergence of syphilis in the United Kingdom: the new epidemic phases. *Sexually Transmitted Diseases* 32: 220–6.

Solans-Laqué R, Bosch-Gil JA, Molina-Catenario CA *et al.* (2008) Stroke and multi-infarct dementia as presenting symptoms of giant cell arteritis. Report of 7 cases and review of literature. *Medicine* 87: 335–44.

Steele JC. (1972) Progressive supranuclear palsy. *Brain* 95: 693–704.

Steele JC, Richardson JC, Olszweski J. (1964) Progressive supranuclear palsy. *Archives of Neurology* 10: 333–59.

Stone JH, Pomper MG, Roubenoff R *et al.* (1994) Sensitivities of non-invasive tests for central nervous system vasculitis: a comparison of lumbar punctures, computed tomography, and magnetic resonance imaging. *Journal of Rheumatology* 21: 1277–82.

Stover NP, Watts RL. (2001) Corticobasal degeneration. *Seminars in Neurology* 21: 49–58.

Turconi AC, Benti R, Castelli E *et al.* (1999) Focal cognitive impairment in mitochondrial encephalomyopathies: a neuropsychological and neuroimaging study. *Journal of the Neurological Sciences* 170: 57–63.

Tüzün E, Dalmau J. (2007) Limbic encephalitis and variants: classification, diagnosis and treatment. *The Neurologist* 13: 261–71.

Urbach H, Soeder BM, Jeub M *et al.* (2006) Serial MRI of limbic encephalitis. *Neuroradiology* 48: 380–6.

Van Eijsden P, Veldink JH, Linn FH *et al.* (2008) Progressive dementia and mesiotemporal atrophy on brain MRI: Neurosyphilis mimicking presenile Alzheimer's disease? *European Journal of Neurology* 15: e14–5.

van Geel BM, Assies J, Wanders RJ, Barth PG. (1997) X linked adrenoleukodystrophy: Clinical presentation, diagnosis and therapy. *Journal of Neurology Neurosurgery and Psychiatry* 63: 4–14.

van Geel BM, Bezman L, Loes DJ *et al.* (2001) Evolution of phenotypes in adult male patients with X-linked adrenoleukodystrophy. *Annals of Neurology* 49: 186–94.

Vanderver A. (2005) Tools for diagnosis of leukodystrophies and other disorders presenting with white matter disease. *Current Neurology Neuroscience Reports* 5: 110–18.

Vanneste JAL. (2000) Diagnosis and management of normal-pressure hydrocephalus. *Journal of Neurology* 247: 5–14.

Varma AR, Trimble MR. (1997) Subcortical neurological syndromes. In: Trimble MR, Cummings JL editors. *Contemporary behavioral neurology.* Blue Books of Practical Neurology, 16. Oxford: Butterworth-Heinemann, 223–38.

Venkataramana A, Sacktor N. (2008) Human immunodeficiency virus-associated dementia: clinical aspects, biology, and treatment. In: Duyckaerts C, Litvan I editors. *Handbook of clinical neurology,* vol. 89. 3rd series, Dementias. Oxford: Elsevier, 800–6.

Vernino S, Geschwind M, Boeve B. (2007) Autoimmune encephalopathies. *The Neurologist* 13: 140–7.

Vodusek B. (2001) Sphincter EMG and differential diagnosis of multiple system atrophy. *Movement Disorders* 16: 600–7.

Wadia PM, Lang AE. (2007) The many faces of cortico basal degeneration. *Parkinsonism and Related Disorders* 13: S336–40.

Warmuth-Metz M, Naumann M, Csoti I, Solymosi I. (2001) Measurement of the midbrain diameter on routine magnetic resonance imaging: a simple and accurate method of differentiating between Parkinson disease and progressive supranuclear palsy. *Archives of Neurology* 58: 1076–9.

Wenning GK, Brown R. (2009) Dementia in multiple system atrophy: does it exist? *European Journal of Neurology* 16: 551–2.

Wenning GK, Colosimo C, Geser F, Poewe W. (2004) Multiple system atrophy. *Lancet Neurology* 3: 93–103.

Williams DR, Lees AJ. (2009) Progressive supranuclear palsy: clinicopathological concepts and diagnostic challenges. *Lancet Neurology* 8: 270–9.

Wraith JE, Baumgartner MR, Bembi B *et al.* (2009) Recommendations on the diagnosis and management of Niemann-Pick disease type C. *Molecular Genetics and Metabolism* 98: 152–65.

Index

Abbreviations used: AD, Alzheimer's disease; BPSD, behavioural and psychological psychiatric symptoms of dementia; DLB, dementia with Lewy bodies; FTD, frontotemporal dementia; FTLD, frontotemporal lobar degeneration; HD, Huntington's disease; MCI, mild cognitive impairment; PD, Parkinson's disease; PDD, Parkinson's disease dementia; PWD, people with dementia; VaD, vascular dementia; VID, vascular cognitive impairment.